Preface

Fifteen years have elapsed since the publication of the first edition of this book, and a decade has gone by since the second edition was published in 1976. The intervening years have witnessed many important changes in the field of industrial pharmacy—probably more so than at any other period of time in its history. Therefore, the editors were challenged to select the most qualified contributors to this third edition of the textbook.

As before, the major objective of this edition is to serve as a textbook for graduate and undergraduate students in the pharmaceutical sciences. In addition, it is intended to provide a comprehensive reference source on modern industrial pharmacy. As such, this book should be useful to practitioners in the pharmaceutical and allied health sciences, hospital pharmacists, drug patent attorneys, government scientists and regulatory personnel, and others seeking information concerning the design, manufacture, and control of pharmaceutical dosage forms.

Despite the fact that the preface to a book appears, as its title implies, at the beginning of a volume, it is common practice for editors and authors to delay its writing as one of their last tasks. This is done in order to reflect on the changes or modifications that have been instituted in the content and arrangement of the chapters in the new edition. In so doing, the editors are provided with an opportunity to highlight such major changes.

Writing this preface has provided us with the opportunity to note the enormous changes in pharmaceutical technology since the appearance of the first edition. This book was created to fill a need that existed during the 1960s and early 1970s, when many undergraduate and graduate programs in colleges of pharmacy included courses in industrial pharmacy to teach the unique factors involved in the production of commercially prepared drug dosage forms. It was a period during which the young disciplines of pharmacokinetics and biopharmaceutics were beginning to solve new problems associated with the burgeoning array of increasingly sophisticated new drug entities, and with the growing concerns about bioavailability of these compounds from various dosage delivery systems. At that time, graduate programs offered many opportunities for aspiring pharmaceutical scientists to deal with these exciting and innovative technologic advances. Thus, there existed an obvious need for a textbook that could bring together in one volume the emerging concepts, new theories, and their practical applications in the development and production of what were then termed "dosage forms," and what are now more appropriately referred to as "drug delivery systems."

Along with the development of new drug delivery systems and new drugs came new production processes and machines for manufacture, new control methods for accurate definition of drug delivery, and new and improved quality control procedures. All of these innovations and improvements contributed to superior quality drug dosage forms, and in many cases, to enhanced concomitant production economics. For example, the advent of microprocessors and small computers has begun to revolutionize the capabilities inherent in modern drug production to an extent not foreseeable when the second edition of this book was published.

Since the first edition of this textbook appeared in 1970, we have been most gratified to learn from comments received from all parts of the world that this book has been well-received and utilized as a basic teaching and reference text in colleges, research institutions, government agencies, and pharmaceutical and related industries. These comments have also provided us with useful suggestions and ideas for this third edition.

The multi-author approach, used in all three editions, has resulted in a uniquely prepared textbook in industrial pharmacy. This editorial

iii

method so common to the writing of modern technical books permits the use of a wide range of expertise that is necessary in dealing with the manifold aspects of modern industrial pharmacy. It also, however, poses the problem unique to all editors, namely, the necessity of gently coercing some very busy people to complete, revise, and polish their chapters. In spite of these pressures, we are grateful for the patience and forbearance of our contributors in helping us to complete this edition. Without the skillful sharing of their knowledge in the pages of this book, the enormous task of compiling this third edition of the textbook would have been impossible to consider.

We and our contributing authors will be extremely pleased if our efforts have results in an improved book to serve as a teaching and reference source in industrial pharmacy.

Westbury, New York
Livingston, New Jersey

LEON LACHMAN, PH.D.
HERBERT A. LIEBERMAN, PH.D.

Contributors

MICHAEL J. AKERS, PH.D.
Head
Dry Products Development Department
Eli Lilly & Company
Indianapolis, IN

NEIL R. ANDERSON, PH.D.
Director
Solid Dosage Form Design
Merrell Dow Pharmaceutical Company
Indianapolis, IN

KENNETH E. AVIS, D.SC.
Goodman Professor and Chairman
Department of Pharmaceutics
College of Pharmacy
University of Tennessee
Memphis, TN

JOSEPH A. BAKAN
Director
Research and Development Division
Eurand America Inc.
Vandalia, OH

GILBERT S. BANKER, PH.D.
Dean and Professor of Pharmaceutics
College of Pharmacy
University of Minnesota
Minneapolis, MN

J.V. BATTISTA
Formerly Management Consultant
Lakehurst, NJ

SANFORD BOLTON, PH.D.
Professor and Chairman
Department of Pharmacy and Administrative
    Sciences
St. John's University
Jamaica, NY

JAMES C. BOYLAN, PH.D.
Adjunct Professor
School of Pharmacy and Pharmaceutical Sciences
Purdue University
W. Lafayette, IN
Director
Scientific Services
Hospital Products Division
Abbott Laboratories
N. Chicago, IL

SUGGY CHRAI, PH.D.
E.R. Squibb & Sons, Inc.
New Brunswick, NJ

CARLO P. CROCE, M.B.A.
Manager
Package Development
Warner-Lambert Company
Morris Plains, NJ

LARRY J. COBEN, PH.D.
Director of Manufacturing
Alcon Laboratories, Inc.
Ft. Worth, TX

ANTHONY J. CUTIE, PH.D.
Associate Professor of Pharmaceutics
Arnold and Marie Schwartz College of Pharmacy
    and Health Sciences
Long Island University
Brooklyn, NY

PATRICK DeLUCA, PH.D.
Professor and Associate Dean
College of Pharmacy
University of Kentucky
Lexington, KY

M.R. DOBRINSKA, PH.D.
Research Fellow
Merck Sharp & Dohme Research Laboratories
West Point, PA

JOSEPH R. FELDKAMP
Research Engineering Specialist
Monsanto Company
St. Louis, MO

EUGENE F. FIESE, PH.D.
Pfizer Central Research
Groton, CT

ARTHUR FISCHER
DuPont Pharmaceuticals
Garden City, NY

TIMOTHY A. HAGEN, PH.D.
Pfizer Central Research
Groton, CT

SAMIR A. HANNA, PH.D.
Vice President
Quality Assurance
Industrial Division
Bristol-Myers Company
Syracuse, NY

SAMUEL HARDER, PH.D.
Laboratory Manager
Pharmaceutical Research and Development
Riker Laboratories, Inc.
St. Paul, MN

STANLEY L. HEM, PH.D.
Professor of Physical Pharmacy
School of Pharmacy and Pharmaceutical Sciences
Associate Dean
Graduate School
Purdue University
W. Lafayette, IN

VAN B. HOSTETLER
Manager
Equipment Development
Lilly Corporation Center
Eli Lilly & Company
Indianapolis, IN

BERNARD IDSON, PH.D.
American Cyanamid Company
Clifton, NJ

JOSEPH L. KANIG, PH.D.
Kanig Consulting and Research Associates, Inc.
Ridgefield, CT

LLOYD KENNON, PH.D.*
Formerly Associate Professor and Program Director
Division of Industrial Pharmacy
Arnold and Marie Schwartz College of Pharmacy
  and Health Sciences
Long Island University
Brooklyn, NY

K.C. KWAN, PH.D.
Executive Director
Drug Metabolism
Merck Sharp & Dohme Research Laboratories
West Point, PA

LEON LACHMAN, PH.D.
Lachman Consultant Services, Inc.
Garden City, NY

JACK H. LAZARUS, M.S.*
Formerly Senior Scientist
Pharmacy Research and Development
Hoffman-LaRoche, Inc.
Nutley, NJ

R. SAUL LEVINSON
Manager
Exploratory Research
Abbott Laboratories
N. Chicago, IL

HERBERT A. LIEBERMAN, PH.D.
President, Consultant Services
H. H. Lieberman Associates, Inc.
Livingston, NJ

KARL LIN, PH.D.
Vice President of Science and Technology
United Laboratories
Manila, Philippines

NICHOLAS G. LORDI, PH.D.
Professor of Pharmacy
Graduate Director of Pharmaceutical Science
College of Pharmacy
Rutgers University
Piscataway, NJ

KEITH MARSHALL, PH.D.
Adjunct Professor
School of Pharmacy
University of Rhode Island
Kingston, RI
Associate Director
Department of Pharmaceutical Research and
  Technologies
Smith Kline & French Laboratories
Philadelphia, PA

*Deceased.

RAYMOND D. MCMURRAY, J.D.*
Formerly *of McMurray and Pendergast*
Washington, DC

SHASHI P. MEHTA, PH.D.
Section Head
Tablet Products, Research and Development
Abbott Laboratories
N. Chicago, IL

EUGENE L. PARROTT, PH.D.
Professor of Industrial Pharmacy
College of Pharmacy
University of Iowa
Iowa City, IA

NAGIN K. PATEL, PH.D.
Associate Professor of Industrial Pharmacy
Arnold and Marie Schwartz College of Pharmacy
and Health Sciences
Long Island University
Brooklyn, NY

WILLIAM R. PENDERGAST, J.D.
Arent, Fox, Kintner, Plotkin, & Kahn
Washington, DC

ALBERT S. RANKELL, PH.D.
Vicks Research Center
Health Care Products Division
Richardson-Vicks Inc.
Shelton, CT

MARTIN M. RIEGER, PH.D.
M. & A. Rieger Associates
Morris Plains, NJ

EDWARD G. RIPPIE, PH.D.
Professor
Department of Pharmaceutics
College of Pharmacy
University of Minnesota
Minneapolis, MN

J.D. ROGERS, PH.D.
Research Fellow
Merck Sharp & Dohme Research Laboratories
West Point, PA

*Deceased.

ROBERT F. SCHIFFMANN, M.S.
R.F. Schiffmann Associates, Inc.
New York, NY

JOHN J. SCIARRA, PH.D.
Professor of Industrial Pharmacy
Arnold and Marie Schwartz College of Pharmacy
and Health Sciences
Long Island University
President
Retail Drug Institute
Brooklyn, NY

JAMES A. SEITZ, PH.D.
Manager
Tablet Products, Research and Development
Pharmaceutical Products Division
Abbott Laboratories
N. Chicago, IL

J.P. STANLEY, PH.D.
Formerly *Technical Director*
R.P. Scherer Corporation
Grosse Pointe Park, MI

RALPH H. THOMAS
Thomas Packaging Consultants, Inc.
Union, NJ

A.E. TILL, PH.D.
Research Fellow
Merck Sharp & Dohme Research Laboratories
West Point, PA

GLENN VAN BUSKIRK
Director of Formulations
Ortho Pharmaceutical Corporation
Raritan, NJ

JOE L. WHITE, PH.D.
Professor of Soil Mineralogy
Department of Agronomy
Purdue University
W. Lafayette, IN

JOHN H. WOOD, PH.D.
Professor
Coordinator of Research and Graduate Program
Department of Pharmacy and Pharmaceutics
School of Pharmacy
Medical College of Virginia Campus
Virginia Commonwealth University
Richmond, VA

JAMES L. YEAGER, PH.D.
Project Manager
Scientific Affairs
Abbott International, Ltd.
N. Chicago, IL

K.C. YEH, PH.D.
Senior Research Fellow
Merck Sharp & Dohme Research Laboratories
West Point, PA

Contents

*Deceased.

SECTION I

Principles of
Pharmaceutical
Processing

Mixing

EDWARD G. RIPPIE

The process of mixing is one of the most commonly employed operations in everyday life. Owing in part to the almost limitless variety of materials that can be mixed, much remains to be learned regarding the mechanisms by which mixing occurs.

For our purposes, mixing is defined as a process that tends to result in a randomization of dissimilar particles within a system. This is to be distinguished from an ordered system in which the particles are arranged according to some iterative rule and thus follow a repetitive pattern. It is possible to consider the mixing of particles differing only by some vector quantity, such as spatial orientation or translational velocity. In this chapter, however, we will deal solely with particles distinguishable by means of scalar quantities, e.g., composition, size, density, shape, or a combination of these. The following text is intended as an introduction to the fundamental concepts that lead to an understanding of the techniques employed in the chemical and pharmaceutical industries to obtain satisfactory mixing. A list of general references is included at the end of the chapter for those who desire further reading on this subject.

Fluids Mixing

Fundamentals

Flow Characteristics. Fluids may generally be classified as Newtonian or non-Newtonian, depending on the relationship between their shear rates and the applied stress. Forces of shear are generated by interactions between moving fluids and the surfaces over which they flow during mixing. The rate of shear may be defined as the derivative of velocity with respect to distance measured normal to the direction of flow (dv/dx). The viscosity (dynamic) is the ratio of shear stress to the shear rate. For Newtonian fluids, the rate of shear is proportional to the applied stress, and such fluids have a dynamic viscosity that is independent of flow rate. In contrast, non-Newtonian fluids exhibit apparent dynamic viscosities that are a function of the shear stress.

The flow characteristics and mixing behavior of fluids are governed by three primary laws or principles: conservation of mass, conservation of energy, and the classic laws of motion. The equations that result from the application of these simple laws of conservation and motion to systems used for mixing are often complex and are beyond the scope of this discussion. An understanding of the fundamental principles of fluid dynamics, however, will help the reader to visualize the overall process of fluids mixing.

Mixing Mechanisms. Mixing mechanisms for fluids fall essentially into four categories: bulk transport, turbulent flow, laminar flow, and molecular diffusion. Usually, more than one of these processes is operative in practical mixing situations.

1. Bulk transport. The movement of a relatively large portion of the material being mixed from one location in the system to another constitutes bulk transport. A simple circulation of material in a mixer, however, does not necessarily result in efficient mixing. For bulk transport to be effective it must result in a rearrangement or permutation of the various portions of the material to be mixed. This is usually accomplished by means of paddles, revolving blades, or other devices within the mixer arranged so as to move adjacent volumes of the fluid in different directions, thereby shuffling the system in three dimensions.

2. *Turbulent mixing.* The phenomenon of turbulent mixing is a direct result of turbulent fluid flow, which is characterized by a random fluctuation of the fluid velocity at any given point within the system. The fluid velocity at a given instant may be expressed as the vector sum of its components in the x, y, and z directions. With turbulence, these directional components fluctuate randomly about their individual mean values, as does the velocity itself.

In the case of turbulent flow in a pipe, the mean velocity in the direction of flow through the pipe is positive, of course, and varies somewhat depending on the distance from the pipe wall. In contrast, the mean velocity perpendicular to the wall is zero. The churning flow characteristic of turbulence results in constantly changing velocities in these directions. This is in contrast to laminar flow in which the velocity components at a given point in the flow field remain constant, at their mean value.

In general, with turbulence, the fluid has different instantaneous velocities at different locations at the same instant in time. This observation is true of both the direction and the magnitude of the velocity. If the instantaneous velocities at two points in a turbulent flow field are measured simultaneously, they show a degree of similarity provided that the points selected are not too far apart. There is no velocity correlation between the points, however, if they are separated by a sufficient distance.

Turbulent flow can be conveniently visualized as a composite of eddies of various sizes. An eddy is defined as a portion of fluid moving as a unit in a direction often contrary to that of the general flow. Large eddies tend to break up, forming eddies of smaller and smaller size until they are no longer distinguishable. The size distribution of eddies within a turbulent region is referred to as the *scale* of turbulence.

It is readily apparent that such temporal and spatial velocity differences as result from turbulence within a body of fluid produce a randomization of the fluid particles. For this reason, turbulence is a highly effective mechanism for mixing. Thus, when small eddies are predominant, the scale of turbulence is low.

An additional characteristic of turbulent flow is its *intensity,* which is related to the velocities with which the eddies move. A composite picture of eddy size versus the velocity distribution of each size eddy may be described as a complex spectrum. Such spectra are characteristic of the turbulent flow and are used in its analysis.

3. *Laminar mixing.* Streamline or laminar flow is frequently encountered when highly viscous fluids are being processed. It can also occur if stirring is relatively gentle and may exist adjacent to stationary surfaces in vessels in which the flow is predominantly turbulent. When two dissimilar liquids are mixed through laminar flow, the shear that is generated stretches the interface between them. If the mixer employed folds the layers back upon themselves, the number of layers, and hence the interfacial area between them, increase exponentially with time. This relationship is observed because the rate of increase in interfacial area with time is proportional to the instantaneous interfacial area.

Example. Consider the case wherein the mixer produces a folding effect and generates a complete fold every 10 seconds. Given an initial fluid layer thickness of 10 cm, a thickness reduction by a factor of 10^{-8} is necessary to attain layers 1 nm thick, which approximate molecular dimensions. Since a single fold results in a layer thickness reduction of one half, n folds are required where:

$$(1/2)^n = 10^{-8}$$

or in logarithmic form, $\log [(\frac{1}{2})^n] = n \log \frac{1}{2} = \log 10^{-8} = -8$. Therefore:

$$n = -8/\log \frac{1}{2} = 26.6$$

Thus, the time required for mixing is equal to n times 10 seconds (266 sec), or 4.43 min.

Mixers may also operate by simply stretching the fluid layers without any significant folding action. This mechanism does not have the stretch compounding effect produced by folding, but may be satisfactory for some purposes in which only a moderate reduction in *mixing scale* (to be defined in detail later) is required. It should be pointed out, however, that by this process alone, an exceedingly long time is required for the layers of the different fluids to reach molecular dimensions. Therefore, good mixing at the molecular level requires a significant contribution by molecular diffusion after the layers have been reduced to a reasonable thickness (several hundred molecules) by laminar flow.

4. *Molecular diffusion.* The primary mechanism responsible for mixing at the molecular level is diffusion resulting from the thermal motion of the molecules. When it occurs in conjunction with laminar flow, molecular diffusion tends to reduce the sharp discontinuities at the interfaces between the fluid layers, and if allowed to proceed for sufficient time, results in complete mixing.

The process is described quantitatively in terms of Fick's first law of diffusion:

$$\frac{dm}{dt} = -DA\frac{dc}{dx} \qquad (1)$$

where the rate of transport of mass, dm/dt, across an interface of area A is proportional to the concentration gradient, dc/dx, across the interface. The rate of intermingling is governed also by the diffusion coefficient, D, which is a function of variables including fluid viscosity and the size of the diffusing molecules. The sharp interface between dissimilar fluids, which has been generated by laminar flow, may be rather quickly obliterated by the ensuing diffusion. Considerable time may be required, however, for the entire system to become homogeneous.

The concentration gradient at the original boundary is a decreasing function of time, approaching zero as mixing approaches completion. Since the amount of material passing a boundary plane in a given time depends on the concentration gradient, the time required to attain complete uniformity may be considerable unless the fluid layers are very thin.

5. *Scale and intensity of segregation.* The quality of mixtures must ultimately be judged upon the basis of some measure of the random distribution of their components. Such an evaluation depends on the selection of a quantitative method of expressing the quality of randomness or "goodness of mixing." Danckwerts has suggested two criteria that are statistically defined and may be applied to mixtures of mutually soluble liquids, fine powders, or gases. Perhaps the greatest value of these concepts lies in the insight they give the pharmacist or chemical engineer regarding the physical nature of the mixtures produced.

Bulk transport, turbulent flow, and laminar flow all result in the intermingling of "lumps" of the liquids to be mixed. The shape and size of these lumps largely depend on the relative contribution of each of these mechanisms to the overall process and on the time over which mixing is carried out. Unless molecular diffusion occurs, however, the composition of the lumps varies discontinuously from one to the next. In other words, each lump retains a constant and uniform internal composition. This can be altered only if molecular diffusion in the case of liquids and gases, or interparticulate motion in the case of powders, tends to eliminate concentration gradients between adjacent lumps. On this basis, Danckwerts defined "two quantities to describe the degree of mixing—namely the *scale of segregation* and the *intensity of segregation.*"

The scale of segregation is defined in a manner analogous to the scale of turbulence discussed earlier, and may be expressed in two ways: as a linear scale or as a volume scale. The linear scale may be considered to represent an average value of the diameter of the lumps present, whereas the volume scale roughly corresponds to the average lump volume.

The intensity of segregation is a measure of the variation in composition among the various portions of the mixture. When mixing is complete, the intentsity of segregation is zero.

6. *Time dependence.* In any given case, the mechanisms that are active in bringing about mixing are time-dependent in their relative importance as the process of mixing proceeds. For example, consider the mixing of two miscible liquids of different densities contained in a vertical tank of cylindric form. The denser liquid is placed in the bottom of the tank, and an approximately equal volume of the less dense fluid is layered on top. Mixing is to be done with a down-draft propeller mounted on a vertical shaft midway between the tank bottom and the interface between the liquids.

If the propeller is operated at a speed sufficient to produce turbulent flow in its discharge region, mixing occurs initially, to any significant degree, only by mechanisms that reduce the scale of segregation. Until such time as both fluids are present in the region of turbulence, created by the impeller, only bulk transport is effective in the mixing process. The convection results from the flow generated by the pumping action of the propeller. When the scale of segregation has been reduced to the point at which both fluids are present in the turbulent zone, turbulent mixing becomes an important means of further reduction in scale. Convection is still of importance here, however, largely because it serves to bring the entire tank contents to the turbulent zone in a comparatively short time.

As the scale of segregation is reduced, with a

resulting increase in interfacial area, molecular diffusion becomes significant. As pointed out earlier, diffusion is necessary for the effective reduction of the intensity of segregation to zero, at which time mixing is complete.

The increase in scale observed in the latter part of the mixing process, as shown in Figure 1-1, results from molecular diffusion, which equalizes the composition of adjacent portions of fluid, resulting in large regions with an intermediate composition. At the completion of mixing, the composition becomes uniform throughout the fluid, and the linear scale of segregation increases in value to a number equal in magnitude to the dimension of the mixing tank.

Equipment

Batch Mixing. When the material to be mixed is limited in volume to that which may be conveniently contained in a suitable mixer, batch mixing is usually most feasible. A system for batch mixing commonly consists of two primary components: (1) a tank or other container suitable to hold the material being mixed, and (2) a means of supplying energy to the system so as to bring about reasonably rapid mixing. Power may be supplied to the fluid mass by means of an impeller, air stream, or liquid jet. Besides supplying power, these also serve to direct the flow of material within the vessel. Baffles, vanes, or ducts also are used to direct the bulk movement of material in such mixers, thereby increasing their efficiency.

1. Impellers. The distinction between impeller types is often made on the basis of type of flow pattern they produce, or on the basis of the

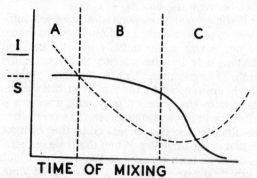

TIME OF MIXING

FIG. 1-1. *The intensity of segregation, I, and the scale of segregation, S, as a function of time. Bulk transport, turbulent mixing, and molecular diffusion are predominant over the time periods A, B, and C, respectively. The linear scale of segregation may be seen to increase at the end of the mixing operation. The final mixture will be uniform in composition and may be considered a single lump with a linear scale equal to the linear dimensions of the mixer.*

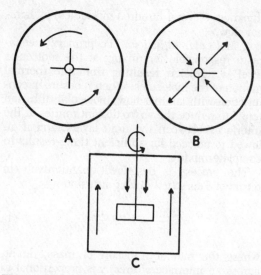

FIG. 1-2. A *and* B, *Diagrammatic representation of cylindric tanks in which tangential and radial flow occur, respectively.* C, *Side view of a similar tank in which axial flow occurs. These diagrams represent systems in which only one type of flow occurs, in contrast to the usual situation in which two or more of these flow patterns occur simultaneously.*

shape and pitch of the blades. Three basic types of flow may be produced: radial, axial, and tangential. These may occur singly or in various combinations. Figure 1-2 illustrates these patterns as they occur in vertical cylindric tanks. Propellers characteristically produce flow parallel to their axes of rotation, whereas turbines may produce either axial or tangential flow, or a combination of these.

Propellers of various types and form are used but all are essentially a segment of a multi-threaded screw, that is, a screw with as many threads as the propeller has blades. Also, in common with machine screws, propellers may be either right-or left-handed depending on the direction of slant of their blades. As with screws, propeller pitch is defined as the distance of axial movement per revolution if no slippage occurs. Although any number of blades may be used, the three-blade design is most common for use with fluids. The blades may be set at any angle or pitch, but for most applications, the pitch is approximately equal to the propeller diameter. Propellers are most efficient when they can be run at high speed in liquids of relatively low viscosity.

Although some tangential flow occurs, the primary effect of a propeller is to induce axial flow. Also, intense turbulence usually occurs in the immediate vicinity of the propeller. Consider, for example, a down-draft propeller vertically

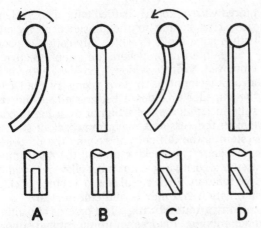

FIG. 1-3. *Impeller blade types (only one blade shown), top and side views. A and B, Radial flow design: C and D, mixed radial-axial flow design. For axial pumping, the blade must be set at an incline to the axis of the shaft.*

mounted midway to the bottom of a tank. Moderate radial and tangential flow occurring above and below the blades, acting in conjunction with the axial flow near the shaft, brings portions of fluid together from all regions of the tank and passes them through the intense turbulence near the blades.

Turbines are usually distinguished from propellers in that the blades of the latter do not have a constant pitch throughout their length. When radial-tangential flow is desired, turbines with blades set at 90-degree angle to their shaft are employed (Fig. 1-3A,B). With this type of impeller, radial flow is induced by the centrifugal action of the revolving blades. The drag of the blades on the liquid also results in tangential flow, which in many cases is undesirable.

Turbines having tilted blades produce an axial discharge quite similar to that of propellers (Fig. 1-3C,D). Because they lend themselves to a simple and rugged design, these turbines can be operated satisfactorily in fluids 1000 times more viscous than fluids in which a propeller of comparable size can be used.

Paddles also are employed as impellers and are normally operated at low speeds, 50 rpm or less. Their blades have a large surface area in relation to the tank in which they are employed, a feature that permits them to pass close to the tank walls and effectively mix viscous liquids or semisolids, which tend to cling to these surfaces. Circulation is primarily tangential, and consequently, concentration gradients in the axial and radial directions may persist in this type of mixer even after prolonged operation. Operating procedures should take these characteristics into account so as to minimize their

undesirable effects. With such mixers, for example, ingredients should not be layered when they are added to the mixing tank. Such vertical stratification can persist after very long mixing times.

2. *Air jets.* Subsurface jets of air, or less commonly of some other gas, are effective mixing devices for certain liquids. Of necessity and for obvious reasons, the liquids must be of low viscosity, nonfoaming, unreactive with the gas employed, and reasonably nonvolatile. The jets are usually arranged so that the buoyancy of the bubbles lifts liquid from the bottom to the top of the mixing vessel. This is often accomplished with the aid of draft tubes. (Fig. 1-4). These serve to confine the expanding bubbles and entrained liquid, resulting in a more efficient lifting action by the bubbles. The overall circulation in the mixing vessel brings fluid from all parts of the tank to the region of the jet itself. Here, the intense turbulence generated by the jet produces intimate mixing.

3. *Fluid jets.* When liquids are to be pumped into a tank for mixing, the power required for pumping often can be used to accomplish the mixing operation, either partially or completely. In such a case, the fluids are pumped through nozzles arranged to permit good circulation of material throughout the tank. In operation, fluid jets behave somewhat like propellers in that they generate turbulent flow in the direction of

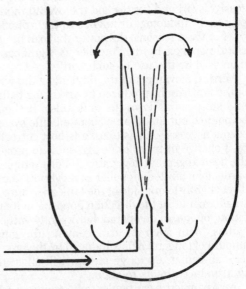

FIG. 1-4. *Vertical tank with centrally located air jet and draft tube. Bubbles confined within the draft tube rise, inducing an upward fluid flow in the tube. This flow tends to circulate fluid in the tank, bringing it into the turbulent region in the vicinity of the jet.*

their axes. They do not in themselves, however, generate tangential flow, as do propellers. Jets also may be operated simply by pumping liquid from the tank through the jet back into the tank.

4. *Baffles.* Bulk transport is important in mixing (see under previous section, "Mixing Mechanisms") and is particularly desirable in the initial stages, when segregation may be present on a large scale. For bulk fluid flow to be most effective, an intermingling must occur between material from remote regions in the mixer. To accomplish this, it is frequently necessary to install auxiliary devices for directing the flow of the fluid, usually baffle plates. Baffle placement depends largely on the type of agitator used.

Centrally mounted vertical shaft impellers tend to induce tangential flow, which is often manifested in the formation of a vortex about the impeller shaft. This is particularly characteristic of turbines with blades arranged perpendicular to the impeller shaft. The tangential motion does not in itself produce any mixing, except possibly near the tank walls where shear forces exist. Instead, swirl and the resultant vortex formation reduce the mixing intensity by reducing the velocity of the impeller relative to the surrounding fluid. In addition, severe vibration may occur, often with damaging results, if the vortex reaches the impeller, where bubbles in the fluid can result in uneven loading of the impeller blades.

Sidewall baffles, when vertically mounted in cylindric tanks, are effective in eliminating excessive swirl and further aid the overall mixing process by inducing turbulence in their proximity. For these reasons, the power that can be efficiently applied by the impeller is significantly increased by the use of such baffles.

Vertical movement of the fluid along the walls of the tank can be produced by arranging baffles in a steep spiral down the tank sides. It should be pointed out that if an elaborate baffle system seems necessary, the situation is best corrected by a change in impeller design so as to provide the desired general flow pattern. For example, a vertically mounted propeller in a cylindric tank, if set slightly to one side of the tank and canted a small amount in the direction opposite to its rotation, often can be operated efficiently without baffles. With such an arrangement, the small amount of tangential flow induced by the propeller's off-center discharge stream will offset the swirl induced by its rotation.

An asymmetric or angular tank geometry relative to the impeller may be used to produce an effect similar to that of baffles. Such a technique is useful in swirl prevention, but in many cases necessitates a longer mixing time than that required with a properly baffled tank of equivalent size. This is due to the presence of regions within such tanks in which circulation is poor.

Side-entering propellers are often effectively employed. Swirl is seldom a problem with such an arrangement, as the tank geometry relative to the impeller provides a baffling effect and results in circulation of material from top to bottom in the vessel. A major drawback of such a system is the difficulty in sealing the propeller entry port. The packing around the shaft must assure a positive seal but must allow reasonably free rotation. Such a seal is also a source of contamination and may be difficult to clean.

Continuous Mixing. The process of continuous mixing produces an uninterrupted supply of freshly mixed material and is often desirable when very large volumes of material are to be handled. It can be accomplished essentially in two ways: in a tube or pipe through which the material flows and in which there is very little back flow or recirculation, or in a chamber in which a considerable amount of holdup and recirculation occur. (Fig. 1-5).

To ensure good mixing efficiency, such devices as vanes, baffles, screws, grids, or combinations of these are placed in the mixing tube. As illustrated in Figure 1-5A, mixing takes place mainly through mass transport in directions normal to that of the primary flow. Mixing in such systems requires the careful control of the feed rate of raw materials if a mixture of uniform composition is to be obtained. The requirement of exact metering in such a device results from the lack of recirculation, which would otherwise tend to average out concentration gradients along the pipe. Where suitable metering devices are available, this method of mixing is very efficient. Little additional power input over that required for simple transfer through a pipe is necessary to accomplish mixing.

When input rate is difficult to control and fluctuations in the ratio of added ingredients are unavoidable, continuous mixing equipment of the tank type is preferred. Fluctuations in com-

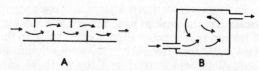

A   B

FIG. 1-5. *Continuous fluids mixing devices. A, Baffled pipe mixer; B, mixing chamber with flow induced recirculation. Both types induce turbulence in the fluid; however, recirculation is desirable when overall fluctuations occur in the material fed to the mixer, since these fluctuations will not be eliminated by simple transverse mixing in a pipe.*

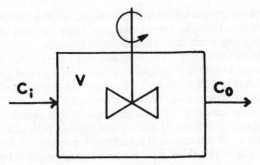

FIG. 1-6. *Diagram of a perfectly mixed tank in a flow stream with flow rate dv/dt. C_i and C_o represent the concentrations entering and leaving the tank at any given instant. Material balance requires that the total amount of fluid leaving the tank in a given time is equal to the total amount entering in the same period of time.*

position of the final mixture are greatly reduced by the dilution effect of the material contained in the tank.

For example, consider a tank of volume V, which is stirred so as to be perfectly mixed at all times, as illustrated in Figure 1-6. If each increment of added material is instantaneously distributed evenly throughout the vessel, and if the concentrations of the equal volumes entering and leaving the mixer are designated as C_i and C_o respectively, conservation of mass requires that:

$$V\frac{dC_o}{dt} = (C_i - C_o)\frac{dv}{dt} \qquad (2)$$

where dv/dt is the rate of flow of material through the tank. For a given concentration difference $(C_i - C_o)$ and flow rate, the rate of change of concentration of the effluent with time, dC_o/dt, is inversely proportional to tank volume. Two tanks in series, each having volume V/2 or half that of the single tank just discussed, would be even more effective in reducing concentration fluctuations while having the same holdup. This is true when the random fluctuations in concentration occur over small volume increments compared with the tank volumes. It is essentially a serial dilution effect.

Example. When integrated, equation (2) yields the expression:

$$C_o = C_i(1 - e^{-kt})$$

where k = dv/Vdt. When two identical tanks, each of volume V/2, are connected in series, the relationship between input and output concentrations becomes:

$$C_o = C_i(1 - e^{-2kt} - 2kte^{-2kt})$$

For comparison purposes, set k equal to 0.1 min^{-1}, and examine the ratio of C_o to C_i after 5 min of operation, with the mixing tank(s) at an initial concentration of C_o and with a constant inlet concentration of C_i. When a single tank is used, C_o/C_i equals 0.393, whereas with two tanks in series, each having one-half the volume, C_o/C_i is 0.264. This effect appears more pronounced at shorter times and less so over longer periods in relation to k, when C_o closely approaches C_i.

$$\frac{C_o}{C_i} = 1 - e^{-1/2} = 0.393$$

$$\frac{C_o}{C_i} = 1 - e^{-1} - e^{-1} = 0.264$$

An effect similar to that obtained with two tanks can be observed with a turbine agitated tank having vertical sidewall baffles. If the turbine impeller is located near the middle of the tank, two regions of mixing occur above and below the impeller as shown in Figure 1-7. Mass transport between these zones is relatively slow. This has the effect of two areas of rapid mixing, and the mixer behaves in a manner analogous to two independent tanks connected in series. Complex arrays of interconnected tanks, both in series and in parallel, can be used for special mixing situations. The differential equations that arise from such systems may be solved by a variety of methods depending on their form. The reader is referred to mathematical texts for the appropriate techniques. The great variety of agitation systems that may be used for continuous mixing in tanks has been discussed in connection with batch mixing.

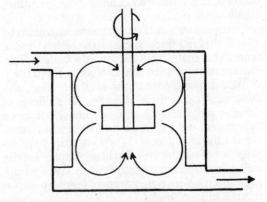

FIG. 1-7. *Diagram of a turbine agitated, continuous mixing tank with vertical side wall baffles. Two zones of mixing are shown, above and below the impeller. Net effect of such a device is similar to that obtained by the operation of two tanks, of the type shown in Figure 1-6, in series.*

Mixer Selection

Equipment Selection. One of the first and often most important considerations in any mixing problem is equipment selection. Factors that must be taken into consideration include (1) the physical properties of the materials to be mixed, such as density, viscosity, and miscibility, (2) economic considerations regarding processing, e.g., time required for mixing and the power expenditure necessary, and (3) cost of equipment and its maintenance. In any given case, a number of these factors may be taken into consideration; however, a few general guidelines can be drawn. A more extensive discussion of this subject may be found in the literature.[1-5]

1. *Monophase systems.* The viscous character and density of the fluid(s) to be mixed determine to a large extent the type of flow that can be produced and also, therefore, the nature of the mixing mechanisms involved. Fluids of relatively low viscosity are best mixed by methods that generate a high degree of turbulence and at the same time circulate the entire mass of material. These requirements are satisfied by air jets, fluid jets, and the various high-speed impellers discussed earlier. A viscosity of approximately 10 poise may be considered as a practical upper limit for the application of these devices.

Thick creams, ointments, and pastes are of such high viscosity that it is difficult if not impossible to generate turbulence within their bulk and laminar mixing, and molecular diffusion must be relied upon. Mixing of such fluids may be done with a turbine of flat blade design. A characteristic feature of such impellers is the relative insensitivity of their power consumption to density and/or viscosity. For this reason, they are particularly good choices when emulsification or added solids may change these quantities significantly during the mixing operation. This property of turbines is due to the mechanisms by which they produce their characteristic radial flow: (1) density- and viscosity-dependent fluid entrainment into the area of blades and (2) centrifugal displacement in the axial direction, also dependent upon these variables. The effects of density and viscosity tend to cancel out since they contribute in both a positive and negative way to the circulation. When compared with a propeller of similar size, flat blade turbines of the radial flow type have a significantly lower pumping capacity, which makes them less suitable for mixing in large tanks.

2. *Polyphase systems.* The mixing of systems composed of several liquid or solid phases primarily involves the subdivision or deaggregation of one or more of the phases present, with subsequent dispersal throughout the mass of material to be mixed. In a general sense, the processes of homogenization, suspension formation, and emulsification may be considered forms of mixing. Inasmuch as these topics are covered in Chapters 5, 16, and 17, they are considered from only a mechanistic standpoint here.

The mixing of two immiscible liquids requires the subdivision of one of the phases into globules, which are then distributed throughout the bulk of the fluid. The process usually occurs by stages during which the large globules are successively broken down into smaller ones. Two primary forces come into play here: the interfacial tension of the globules in the surrounding liquid, and forces of shear within the fluid mass. The former tends to resist the distortion of globule shape necessary for fragmentation into smaller globules, whereas the forces of shear act to distort and ultimately disrupt the globules. The relationship between these forces largely determines the final size distribution in the mixture.

Selection of equipment depends primarily upon the viscosity of the liquids and is made according to the mechanism by which intense shearing forces can best be generated. In the case of low-viscosity systems, high shear rates are required and are commonly produced by passing the fluid under high pressure through small orifices or by bringing it into contact with rapidly moving surfaces. Devices for accomplishing these high rates are described in Chapter 17, Emulsions.

Highly viscous fluids, such as are encountered in the production of ointments, are efficiently dispersed by the shearing action of two surfaces in close proximity and moving at different velocities with respect to each other. This is achieved in paddle mixers, in which the blades clear the container walls by a small tolerance. Such mixers are relatively efficient since they not only generate sufficient shear to reduce globule size but if properly constructed, also induce sufficient circulation of material to ensure a uniform dispersion throughout the completed mixture.

The mixing of finely divided solids with a liquid of low viscosity in the production of a suspension depends on the separation of aggregates into primary particles and the distribution of these particles throughout the fluid. These processes are often carried out in a single mixing operation, provided that shear forces of sufficient intensity to disrupt aggregates can be generated. High-speed turbines, frequently fitted with stators to produce increased shearing action, are often employed. When aggregation is not a problem, or when deaggregation is to be carried out following a general mixing step, the equipment used in mixing of suspensions is essentially the same as that previously discussed for liquids of comparable viscosity.

As the percentage of solids is increased or if highly viscous fluids are employed, the solid-liquid system takes on the consistency of a paste or dough. In these cases, the forces required to induce shear are considerable, and equipment used is of heavy design. The choice of a mixer is limited to those that either knead or mull the material. Kneaders operate by pushing masses of the material past each other and by squeezing and deforming them at the same time. Such mixers may take several forms, but usually have counter-rotating blades or heavy arms that work the plastic mass. Shear forces are generated by the high viscosity of the mass and are effective in deaggregation as well as distribution of the solids in the fluid vehicle. A diagram of a sigma-blade mixer with overlapping blades is shown in Figure 1-8.

Mulling mixers are efficient in deaggregation of solids, but are typically inefficient in distributing the particles uniformly through the entire mass. Previously mixed material of uniform composition, but containing aggregates of solid particles, is suitable for mixing in these devices. In the event of segregation during mulling, a final remixing may be necessary.

Roller mills consisting of one or more rollers are in common use. Of these, the three-roll type seems to be preferred (Fig. 1-9). In operation, rollers composed of a hard abrasion-resistant material and arranged to come into close proximity to each other are rotated at different rates of speed. Material coming between the rollers is crushed, depending on the gap, and is also sheared by the difference in rates of movement of the two surfaces. In Figure 1-9 the material passes from the hopper, A, between rolls B and C, and is reduced in size in the process. The gap between rolls C and D, which is usually less than that between B and C, further crushes and

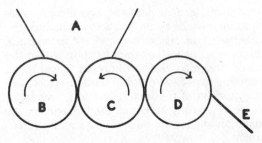

FIG. 1-9. *Cross section of a three-roll mill showing hopper (A), rolls (B,C,D), and scraper (E). Directions of roller rotation are indicated. Speed of rotation of the rollers increases from B to D. Material placed in the hopper passes between rolls B and C and then C and D in succession and is finally collected on the scraper.*

smooths the mixture, which adheres to roll C. A scraper, E, is arranged to continuously remove the mixed material from roller D. The arrangement is such that no material can reach the scraper that has not passed between both sets of rolls.

The extreme case of solid-liquid mixing is one in which a small volume of liquid is to be mixed with a large quantity of solids. This process is essentially one of coating the solid particles with liquid and of the transfer of liquid from one particle to another. In this type of mixing, the liquid is added slowly to reduce the tendency of the particles to lump; however, the process is not one of fluids mixing, but one of solids mixing. When the particles tend to stick together because of the surface tension of the coating liquid, the equipment used is the same as that for pastes. If the solids remain essentially free flowing, the equipment is the same as that used for solids mixing, which is discussed under that heading later in this chapter.

Correlation. Many of the mixing characteristics attributed to the various impellers, jets and other mixing equipment can be considerably altered, often unfavorably, by changes in the relative size, shape, or speed of their component parts. Although methods of scale-up are usually considered in relation to the problem of going from laboratory scale to pilot plant to production scale, they are also of fundamental value in understanding the proper operation of a given mixer, regardless of its size.

Exact analytic descriptions of the flow patterns, turbulent or otherwise, that occur in mixers are generally so complex as to defy solution, if indeed they may be mathematically formulated at all. For these reasons, an empiric approach, involving comparison of the system under study with systems of known performance, is employed for the prediction of the de-

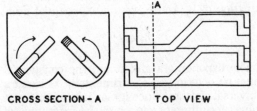

CROSS SECTION - A　　　**TOP VIEW**

FIG. 1-8. *Schematic drawing of a top-loading sigma-blade mixer with overlapping blades. The top view shows the relationship of the counter rotating blades to the overall geometry of the mixer.*

sired operational conditions. Significant variables that must be taken into account include the dimensions of the mixer and its mechanical components as well as their location within the mixer. Included also are impeller speed or jet pumping rate, fluid density, fluid viscosity, and height of fill of the mixer. In short, any factor that can possibly influence the behavior of the materials as they are mixed is potentially important.

1. *Dimensionless groups.* The method is based upon dimensionless groups that characterize the mixing systems. These groups consist of combinations of the physical and geometric quantities that affect the fluid dynamics and hence also affect the mixing performance of a given piece of equipment. The measurable quantities constituting a given dimensionless group are arranged so that their units of measurement cancel. These unitless numbers, therefore, represent ratios between pertinent variables or parameters.

Large numbers of useful dimensionless groups have been developed and employed under various circumstances for the correlation of mixer performance data as well as for the design of mixers. Three of the more important groups serve to illustrate the utility of the method. These are the Reynolds number, R_e, the Froude number, F_r, and the power number, P_n.

The Reynolds number is commonly defined by the expression:

$$R_e = \frac{vL\zeta}{\eta} \qquad (3)$$

where v is the velocity of the fluid relative to the surfaces of the equipment involved. The density and dynamic viscosity are denoted by ζ and η, respectively. The dimension of length, L, is chosen in various ways depending on the system. For example, in the case of fluid flowing through a pipe, it is taken as pipe diameter. For gas bubbles, it is taken as bubble diameter, and for impellers, as impeller diameter. The subgroup $vL\zeta$ is indicative of inertial forces in the system, and the Reynolds number indicates the ratio between these and the viscous forces. At high Reynolds numbers, the former predominate and the flow is turbulent, whereas at low values of R_e, laminar flow occurs. A transition range is known to exist since the transition from laminar to turbulent flow is not abrupt.

In systems in which gravitational effects occur, the Froude number should be taken into account. This group is defined by the equation:

$$F_r = \frac{V^2}{gL} \qquad (4)$$

where v and L are the terms previously defined and g is the acceleration of gravity. In the case of high Froude numbers, the inertial forces predominate over those due to gravity. Should such conditions prevail in an unbaffled tank agitated by a vertical, centrally located turbine, vortex formation results. This group is important whenever there is an interaction between gravitational and inertial forces.

The power that may be dissipated in a mixer by an impeller or other device is related to the power number:

$$P_n = \frac{p'}{v^2\zeta} \qquad (5)$$

where p' is the pressure increment responsible for flow. The power number is thus the ratio between the forces producing flow and the inertial forces that resist it. The power number can also be written as:

$$P_n = \frac{Pg}{\zeta\omega^3 d^5} \qquad (6)$$

where P is the power input, d is the impeller diameter, and ω is its rotational velocity.

2. *Correlation equations.* Before the dimensionless groups discussed here can be employed in useful calculations, it is necessary to find a satisfactory functional relationship between them upon which to base the desired correlations. This is accomplished by means of the methods of dimensional analysis.[1,6]

Although a complete correlation function must take into account all the variables in a given system, satisfactory results may be obtained if only the most significant variables are considered. Therefore, while the general dimensionless equation for correlating power input contains several dimensionless groups in addition to the Reynolds and Froude numbers, these latter two quantities are usually sufficient for correlations with the power number if geometrically similar systems are investigated. The power number is thus commonly written as a function of R_e and F_r in the exponential form:

$$P_n = GR_e^a F_r^b \qquad (7)$$

The exponents a and b and the constant G must be determined experimentally. G is not a universal constant since it may take on different values for different ranges in the magnitude of the associated dimensionless groups. It is reasonably constant, however, over ranges in which no gross changes in flow character occur. The exponents a and b, which should be considered as empiric quantities, also remain remarkably constant over considerable ranges of operating conditions.

Consider, for example, a propeller operating at a speed at which the flow is predominantly laminar. In such a system, the exponent, a, of the Reynolds number is found to be -1, and b is zero, since vortex formation does not occur under these conditions. The correlation equation can then be written:

$$\frac{Pg}{\zeta\omega^3 d^5} = \frac{G\eta}{\omega d^2 \zeta} \tag{8}$$

Upon rearrangement, the functional relationship of power input to the several variables is apparent:

$$P = Gg^{-1}\eta\omega^2 d^3 \tag{9}$$

Thus, power input is proportional to viscosity, and dependent on the second and third powers of the propeller velocity and diameter, respectively. The density of the fluid is not a factor under these conditions of operation.

The literature indicates that the same mixer operating under completely baffled conditions with turbulent flow can be expected to exhibit power numbers that are independent of R_e and F_r; that is, the coefficients a and b in the correlation equation will both be zero. The power number is thus equal to the experimentally determined constant G, and the power input may be expressed by the equation:

$$P = Gg^{-1}\zeta\omega^3 d^5 \tag{10}$$

Here, the power required for a given flow is independent of viscosity but linearly dependent on density, in contrast to laminar flow. Also, in this case, power input is more sensitive to changes in the rotational speed and the diameter of the propeller than with laminar flow.

Example. Consider a 500 = L, baffled mixing vat agitated by means of a centrally mounted 15-cm diameter propeller at 1750 rpm. To provide more rapid mixing, the propeller rpm is doubled, and its diameter increased to 23 cm. This design change requires a more powerful drive motor, but in order to make an estimate of the increase needed, several variables must be considered. Given that the viscosity of the fluid is 1.5 poise and the specific gravity is 1.05, the Reynolds number can be estimated. If the propeller pitch is 0.8 diameters per revolution, it will pump liquid at a velocity determined by the

product of the pitch and rpm. Thus, fluid velocity is given by the following:

$$v = \frac{(0.8)(15)(1750)}{(60)} = 350 \text{ cm sec}^{-1}$$

The Reynolds number, from equation (3), is equal to:

$$Re = \frac{(350)(15)(1.05)}{(1.5)} = 3675$$

Since this is within the turbulent range, equation (10) applies. Therefore, the power required under the new conditions, P_n, as compared with that needed previously, P_o, is given by:

$$P_n = \left(\frac{\omega_n}{\omega_o}\right)^3 \left(\frac{d_n}{d_o}\right)^5$$

$$= (2)^3 \left(\frac{23}{15}\right)^5$$

$$= 67.8$$

On the basis of these calculations, it may be decided that the increased speed of mixing resulting from this design change does not warrant the additional power required.

The foregoing conclusions are valid only if geometric similarity is maintained in the mixing systems. Also, the value of G, while reasonably constant over the ranges of laminar flow and fully developed turbulence, is not numerically the same in these two regions.

These examples illustrate the usefulness of dimensionless groups in predicting and calculating the influence of systematic variables on the mixing process. The same general technique is also useful in correlations involving more complex systems, which require additional groups for satisfactory calculations.

Solids Mixing

Fundamentals

The theory of solids mixing has not advanced much beyond the most elementary of concepts and, consequently, is far behind that which has been developed for fluids. This lag can be attributed primarily to an incomplete understanding of the ways in which particulate variables influence such systems and to the complexity of the problem itself.

When viewed superficially, such multiparticulate solids as pharmaceutical bulk powders or tablet granulations are seen to behave somewhat like fluids. That is, to the casual observer, they appear to exhibit fluid-like flow when they are poured from one container to another and seem to occupy a more or less constant bulk volume. Dissimilar powders can be intimately mixed at the particulate level much like miscible liquids, at least in principle. Contrary to these similarities with fluids, however, the mixing of solids presents problems that are quite different from those associated with miscible liquids. The latter, once mixed, do not readily separate and can be poured, pumped, and otherwise subjected to normal handling without concern for unmixing. In addition, they can be perfectly mixed in any standard equipment, with the primary concerns being power efficiency and time required. In contrast, well-mixed powders are often observed to undergo substantial segregation during routine handling following the mixing operation. Such segregation of particulate solids can occur during mixing as well and is perhaps the central problem associated with the mixing and handling of these materials.

Particulate Solids Variables. Particle size and particle size distribution are important since they largely determine the magnitude of forces, gravitational and inertial, that can cause interparticulate movement relative to surface forces, which resist such motion. As a consequence of high interparticulate forces, as compared with gravitational forces, few powders of less than 100 microns mean particle size are free-flowing. Most powders, including those encountered in pharmaceutical systems, have a wide range in particle size with the actual distribution determined to some extent by the method of preparation. An excellent discussion of the statistics of small particles is given by Herdan.[7]

Particle density, elasticity, surface roughness, and shape also exert their influence on the bulk properties of powders. Of these, particle shape is perhaps the most difficult variable to describe and is commonly expressed by scalar quantities known as shape factors. When applied to solids mixing, shape factors provide a number index to which mixing rate, flow rate, segregation rate, angle of repose, and other static or dynamic characteristics can be related. However, the limitations as well as the attributes of shape factors should be understood.

As scalar quantities, shape factors serve as proportionality constants between mean particle diameters and particle surface area and volume. They also serve to relate results of experimental particle size measurements by different methods. In spite of their utility in these ways, shape factors do not describe the shape of the particles they characterize. Thus, a single factor can in no way be considered a unique indication of shape. For example, one cannot differentiate between rods and flat discs by the use of a single shape factor. This limitation somewhat complicates correlations and interpretations of particulate shape effects on mixing.

A large number of shape factors have been defined and used in studies of multiparticulate solids systems. A typical example is that of a surface shape factor, α_s, defined by the expression:

$$\alpha_s = \frac{s}{\Sigma n_i d_i^2} \qquad (11)$$

The total surface area of the powder is s, having n_i particles of projected diameter d_i. Powders whose particles are highly irregular in shape generally exhibit large values of α_s.

Example. To calculate a value of α_s that is useful for purposes of comparison with other materials, consider a system of monodisperse spheres of diameter 2r. The surface shape factor α_s will be independent of sample size, so that for simplicity, a single particle will be taken as the sample. In this case, equation (11) takes the form.

$$\alpha_s = \frac{4\pi r^2}{(2r)^2} = \pi$$

Had the idealized particles been perfect cubes, having edges of length d, then equation (11) would become:

$$\alpha_s = \frac{6d^2}{d^2} = 6$$

The value for α_s can be seen to increase substantially as the particles become more angular and deviate from a spherical shape.

Forces Acting in Multiparticulate Solids Systems. As pointed out previously, forces that operate at a particulate level during the mixing process are essentially of two types: (1) those that tend to result in movement of two adjacent particles or groups of particles relative to each other and (2) those that tend to hold neighboring particles in a fixed relative position. This division is arbitrary, and often a clear distinction cannot be made, for reasons that will become evident.

In the first category are forces of acceleration produced by the translational and rotational movements of single particles or groups of particles. Such motion can result either from contact with the mixer surfaces or from contact with other particles. In either case, the efficiency of momentum transfer is highly dependent on the elasticity of the collisions. In general, much more rapid and efficient interchange of momentum would be expected if loss by inelasticity was minimal.

The shape and surface "roughness" of the particles involved in a collision determine, to a large measure, the distribution of the transferred momentum between translational and rotational modes. That is, all other factors being equal, particles with a high coefficient of friction are likely to exchange rotational momentum more readily. This momentum exchange can also be expected to depend more on the "available surface" area than on the density or the mass of the particle. Rotating aggregates experience centrifugal forces that tend to break them into smaller units and aid the mixing process.

Gravitational forces also operate and, of course, act on all particles at all times in proportion to their mass.

Included in the second category of forces, namely those that resist particulate movement, are interparticulate interactions associated with the size, shape, and surface characteristics of the particles themselves. Powders that have high "cohesive" forces due to interaction of their surfaces can be expected to be more resistant to intimate mixing than those whose surfaces do not interact strongly. Factors that influence this type of interaction are surface polarity, surface charge, and adsorbed substances such as moisture.

In moving from one location to another, relative to its neighbors, a particle must surmount certain potential energy barriers. These arise from forces resisting movement insofar as neighboring particles must be displaced. This effect is a function of both particle size and shape and is most pronounced when high packing densities occur. Particle shape is important because as the shape of a particle deviates more significantly from a spherical form, the free movement it experiences along its major axes also diverges.

Recent studies by several workers, on particulate beds and by means of computer simulation, have demonstrated the existence of these barriers. They are manifested by peaks and valleys in the radial location frequency distribution of particles in a bed relative to a reference particle. Figure 1-10 illustrates distributions typical of a bed of particles of relatively uniform size. This diagram shows that moderate bed expansion, short of total fluidization, facilitates interparticulate motion, and hence mixing, by reducing the magnitude of the energy barriers and shortening the distance between preferred locations.

In general, powders and divided solids possess

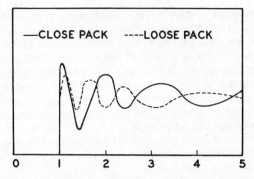

FIG. 1-10. *Relative numbers of neighboring particles per unit area as a function of distance measured in particle diameters from reference particles. Measurements are made center-to-center of relatively spherical particles under both close and loose packing arrangements.*

a wide spectrum of particulate properties, which result in an equally wide range of bulk properties. The latter may be classified as being characteristic of either a static or dynamic state of the system.

Attempts to correlate the gross properties of powders with the nature of the individual particles have been somewhat more successful in systems under static conditions than when the particles are in a state of flow. This is not unexpected since inertial forces become important when the particles are in motion, and the resulting transfer of momentum and kinetic energy is a complex function of the particulate variables.

Mixing Mechanisms. It has been generally accepted that solids mixing proceeds by a combination of one or more mechanisms.

1. Convective mixing. This mechanism may be regarded as analogous to bulk transport as discussed in connection with fluids mixing. Depending on the type of mixer employed, convective mixing can occur by an inversion of the powder bed, by means of blades or paddles, by means of a revolving screw, or by any other method of moving a relatively large mass of material from one part of the powder bed to another.

2. Shear mixing. As a result of forces within the particulate mass, slip planes are set up. Depending on the flow characteristics of the powder, these can occur singly or in such a way as to give rise to laminar flow. When shear occurs between regions of different composition and parallel to their interface, it reduces the scale of segregation by thinning the dissimilar layers. Shear occurring in a direction normal to the interface of such layers is also effective since it too reduces the scale of segregation.

3. Diffusive mixing. Mixing by "diffusion" is said to occur when random motion of particles within a powder bed causes them to change position relative to one another. Such an exchange of positions by single particles results in a reduction of the intensity of segregation. Diffusive mixing occurs at the interfaces of dissimilar regions that are undergoing shear and therefore results from shear mixing. It may also be produced by any form of agitation that results in interparticulate motion.

These mechanisms will be considered further in connection with the various types of mixer in common use.

The general flow characteristics of powders determine to a great extent the ease with which the primary particles can be mixed. That is, they determine how easily masses of powder can be transported through the powder bed, and also how easily these masses can be broken down to permit intimate mixing of individual particles. It is only through the latter process that the intensity of segregation can be reduced.

The mixing of particles whose surfaces are nonconducting (electrically) often results in the generation of surface charges, as evidenced by a tendency of the powder to clump following a period of agitation. Surface charging of particles during mixing is undesirable, for it tends to decrease the process of interparticulate "diffusion."

Unfortunately, surface charges in powder beds are not readily measurable. If the bed were electrically insulated during agitation, its net charge would be zero, whereas the intensity of charge on individual particles could be quite high. In such a system, a given particle may be singly charged positively or negatively, multiply charged with like charges, or multiply charged with either an equal or unequal number of positive and negative charges. The net charge of a powder can be determined and is often taken as a measure of the tendency of the particles to undergo charge separation.

Charging of powder beds and the undesirable effects it produces can be prevented or reduced in many cases by surface treatment, which is usually accomplished by adding small amounts of surfactants to the powder, thereby increasing the conductivity of the surface. The problem can also be solved in some cases by mixing under conditions of increased humidity (above 40%).

Segregation Mechanisms. As mentioned previously, particulate solids tend to segregate by virtue of differences in the size, density, shape, and other properties of the particles of which they are composed. The process of segregation occurs during mixing as well as during subsequent handling of the completed mix, and it is most pronounced with free-flowing powders. Powders that are not free-flowing or that exhibit high forces of cohesion or adhesion between particles of similar or dissimilar composition are often difficult to mix owing to agglomeration. The clumps of particles can be broken down in such cases by the use of mixers that generate high shear forces or that subject the powder to impact. When these powders have been mixed, however, they are less susceptible to segregation because of the relatively high interparticulate forces that resist interparticulate motion leading to unmixing.

It is sometimes possible to select pharmacologically inert excipients that have a selective affinity for an active mixture component. The particle-to-particle binding between drug and inert carrier, which results in such mixtures, can greatly improve homogeneity and stability toward separation of components. This technique is most valuable when potent drugs are to be mixed in relatively low percentages. When the drug is added as a fine powder, it can be made to coat carrier particles uniformly, and as a consequence, to be mixed uniformly throughout the batch. Usually, this is best accomplished by selecting an excipient that has a polarity similar to that of the drug. For example, a steroid would adhere well to lipid-like surfaces. In this case, however, inclusion of significant amounts of waxy or fatty materials in a tablet formulation may cause disintegration or dissolution difficulties. When stability is not a problem, it is often more practical to place the drug in relatively dilute solution and spray it on an inert excipient. After drying, this drug excipient mixture can be mixed with the remainder of the formulation.

In practice, the problem of segregation is most severe when one is working with free-flowing, cohesionless, or nearly cohesionless particulate matter. Segregation has been attributed to various types of mixers: those that generate principally convective motion have been classified as "nonsegregating," while those that produce shear or diffusive mixing are termed "segregating." The circumstances that result in segregation, however, can be generalized from a fundamental physical standpoint. Consider a bed of randomly mixed particles of two or more types in a state of agitation, with particles constantly moving around and past each other. Mixing occurs when particle motion is random and leads to a nonselective reordering of individual particles. Where particle motion is selective, however, a sorting effect occurs. The following has been suggested:[8]

[The] necessary and sufficient conditions for segregation to occur in such a system are twofold: (i) that various mixture components exhibit mobilities for interparticulate relative displacement which differ, and (ii) that the mixture experience either a field which exerts a directional motive force on the particles or a gradient in a mechanism capable of inducing or modifying interparticulate movement.

The conditions outlined here are present to a greater or lesser degree in all mixers, regardless of their type or mode of operation. They also occur during mixer emptying, during filling of capsule- or tablet-making hoppers, during flow through the hopper itself, and even in a tablet machine feed frame. In reality, the various mechanisms that lead to mixing provide the conditions but not the mechanisms that can lead to segregation.

The requirements for segregation, as previously postulated, can arise in a variety of ways. Differences in mixture component mobilities can result from differences in particle sizes, shapes, density, and surface characteristics. While other characteristics may also be important, these are recognized as significant in most cases. The second requirement for segregation can be met by the earth's gravitational field, or by a centrifugal, electrical, magnetic field generated in the course of processing. Even in the absence of such fields, this requirement can be satisfied by a gradient in shear rate within the powder bed.

According to theory, it should be possible to prevent segregation by eliminating either one of the necessary conditions for its existence. Total avoidance of undesirable environmental conditions during the course of mixing and processing is virtually impossible. If a mixture gives persistent trouble regarding homogeneity, it is usually best to try to improve the characteristics of the mixture rather than the mixer. With free-flowing materials, the goal is to make all components as alike as possible in size, shape, and density (in that order).

Equipment

Batch Mixing. A common type of mixer consists of a container of one of several geometric forms, which is mounted so that it can be rotated about an axis. The resulting tumbling motion is accentuated by means of baffles or simply by virtue of the shape of the container. The popular twin-shell blender is of this type and takes the form of a cylinder that has been cut in half, at approximately a 45-degree angle with its long axis, and then rejoined to form a "V" shape. This is rotated so that the material is alternately collected in the bottom of the V and then split into two portions when the V is inverted. This is

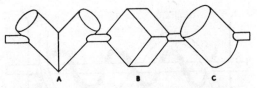

FIG. 1-11. *Three types of tumbling mixers shown mounted on a common shaft: A, twin-shell; B, cubic; C, cylindric. In operation, the asymmetric geometry results in a sideways movement of material in addition to the tumbling action of the mixers. Of the three types, the twin-shell is the most popular.*

quite effective because the bulk transport and shear, which occur i3& tumbling mixers generally, are accentuated by this design. A bar containing blades that rotate in ‚a direction opposite to that of the twin shell often is iused to improve agitation of the powder bed, and may be replaced by a hollow tube for the injection of liquids.

Other mixers of this same general type take the form of cylinders, cubes, or hexagonal cylinders (Fig. 1-11), and may be rotated about almost any axis depending on the manufacturer.

The efficiency of tumbling mixers is highly dependent on the speed of rotation. Rotation that is too slow does not produce the desired intense tumbling or cascading motion, nor does it generate rapid shear rates. On the other hand, rotation that is too rapid tends to produce centrifugal force sufficient to hold the powder to the sides of the mixer and thereby reduce efficiency. The optimum rate of rotation depends on the size and shape of the tumbler and also on the type of material being mixed, but is commonly in the range of 30 to 100 rpm.

A second class of mixer employs a stationary container to hold the material and brings about mixing by means of moving screws paddles, or blades. Since this mixer does not depend entirely on gravity as do the tumblers, it is useful in mixing solids that have been wetted and are therefore in a sticky or plastic state. The high shear forces that are set up are effective in breaking up lumps or aggregates. Well-known mixers of this type include the following. (1) The ribbon blender (Fig. 1-12), consists of a horizontal cylindric tank usually opening at the top and fitted with helical blades. The blades are mounted on a shaft through the long axis of the tank and are often of both right- and left-hand twist. (2) In the helical flight mixer, powders are lifted by a centrally located vertical screw and allowed to cascade to the bottom of the tank. Of these two types, the ribbon blender is the more popular.

When finely divided powders of a sticky consistency are to be mixed, high shear rates and

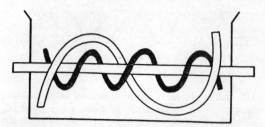

FIG. 1-12. *Side view of a top-loading ribbon blender. The blades are mounted on the horizontal axle by struts (not shown) and are rotated to circulate the material to be mixed. The spiral blades are wound (in most cases) in opposite directions to provide for movement of material in both directions along the axis of the tank. These mixers may be emptied either through ports in the bottom or by inverting them.*

forces are necessary to permit intimate mixing at the particulate level. This may be accomplished if the scale of segregation is first reduced by means of the mixers previously discussed. The roughly mixed material can then be run through a hammer mill, which effectively produces "diffusive" mixing by breaking up aggregates. The process can be repeated if necessary.

Continuous Mixing. A characteristic of solids mixing equipment is that all else being equal, mixtures produced by large mixers have greater variations in composition than those produced by small mixers. This is an important consideration when relatively small portions of the mixture are required to fall consistently within a narrow composition range. The production of tablets and capsules are examples of pharmaceutical processes in which composition uniformity is critical.

The effective volume of a solids blender may be reduced considerably by the use of continuous mixing equipment. Continuous mixing processes are somewhat analogous to those discussed under fluids mixing. Metered quantities of the powders or granules are passed through a device that reduces both the scale and intensity of segregation, usually by impact or a shearing action. The output may be transferred directly to the capsule filling or tablet machines. Control of mixing efficiency in such a system must ultimately depend on an analysis of the dosage forms as they are produced. The feasibility of such a process depends on the availability of rapid analytic procedures.

Mixer Selection

Measures of Mixing Degree. Mixer selection and evaluation depend on a quantitative measure of the degree of mixing. This is generally accomplished by the arbitrary choice of a statistical function that indicates the uniformity of composition of the powder bed.

When analytic procedures are available, the intensity and scale of segregation, as defined by Danckwerts, serve as useful criteria, but only when large-scale segregation is not present.

A large number of statistical quantities have been used by researchers in the area of solids mixing to express a "degree of mixing"; however, they all provide essentially the same type of information concerning the mixture. More important than the choice of a degree of mixing is the method of sampling employed. Unless samples that accurately represent the system are taken, the most elaborate statistical analysis is worthless.

The standard deviation or variance of the selected samples from the mean composition of the system serves as a useful measure of the overall quality of a mixture. Samples may be withdrawn periodically during discharge of the mixture or may be taken directly from the mixer by a sampling "thief."

In the evaluation of a mixture, care must be taken that the *scale of scrutiny* is appropriate. That is, the samples chosen must be large enough to contain sufficient particles to represent accurately the region from which they were taken, yet not so large as to obscure important small-scale variations in composition. The selection of a scale of scrutiny also depends on the ultimate use of the mixture. For example, samples of the same weight as the final tablet are proper for evaluating a tablet granulation. Analysis of multiple samples of this size would allow prediction of tablet-to-tablet variations due to imperfect mixing.

In terms of statistics, "perfect" mixtures are in reality random mixtures. That is, the number of particles of a given component, in samples of uniform weight from a perfect mixture, is determined by chance, and will at best vary about a mean value. The statistical considerations become more complicated as the number of components increases and their size distributions differ. In the simple case of a binary mixture of equal-sized particles of two different components, the statistics follow the binomial distribution having mean, μ, and standard deviation, σ. Thus, the following equations apply:

$$\mu = np \qquad (12)$$
$$\sigma = \sqrt{np(1 - p)} \qquad (13)$$

where n is the number of particles in the sample, and p is the number fraction of particles of the component of interest in the mixture.

Example. For purposes of illustration, consider a capsule formulation consisting of a mixture of equal-sized pellets of two different compositions, A and B. The pellets are mixed in the number ratio of 3 parts of A to 7 parts of B. The problem is to predict the variation in content of capsules containing 500 pellets each, assuming random mixing with no systematic segregation. In such a system, collecting a sample of 500 pellets at a time is equivalent to picking out 500 pellets one at a time randomly. Thus, the selection of pellets follows the binomial distribution, in which the expected composition of the sample and its expected variability in composition are given by equations (12) and (13), respectively:

$$\mu = np = (500)(0.3) = 150$$
$$\sigma = \sqrt{np(1-p)} = [(500)(0.3)(0.7)]^{1/2} = 10.2$$

One sees that on the average, a capsule will contain 150 type A pellets, the remaining 350 being type B. The number standard deviation calculated from equation (13) is 10.2. In a normal distribution, 68% of the measurements (in this case, the number of type A pellets per capsule) lie within plus or minus one standard deviation (10.2 pellets) of the mean (150 pellets per capsule). This means that even with perfect random mixing, approximately only 68% of the capsules would contain 150 ± 10.2, or approximately 140 to 160 pellets of type A among 500 pellets each.

It can be inferred from this example that as the number of particles in a sample is increased, the percentage variation in composition from sample to sample decreases, all else being equal. In evaluating the cause of problems with content uniformity related to tablets and capsules, the statistics of the sample should be considered. Calculations involving multicomponent mixtures are more complicated, as has previously been mentioned, and are covered in references listed at the end of this chapter.

Power Requirements. Unlike fluids mixing, the requirements for power of a given solids mixing operation cannot be readily predicted. This is not a problem, however, since efficiency of power utilization parallels operating conditions for optimum mixing. Consequently, minimum power is that required to operate the mixer for the time necessary to reach a satisfactory steady state.

Unlike most liquids mixers, solids mixers cannot be made to produce good mixtures, when they are operated incorrectly, simply by mixing for a long period of time. The process of solids mixing is accompanied by the process of segregation, as pointed out earlier, in which particles having different characteristics preferentially concentrate in various regions of the mixer. Because of this, the mixture reaches an equilibrium state of mix that is a function of speed of operation of the mixer.

The statement is often made that solids mixers result in unmixing if mixing is continued for an excessive length of time. Such observations are a result of improper operation of the mixer or the use of the wrong mixer or both. Such a mixer produces an equilibrium mixture having a significant degree of segregation. When the material is loaded into the mixer to cause an intermingling of the various solids as they migrate toward their steady state locations, the apparent mixing-unmixing phenomenon is seen.

A second cause of apparent unmixing after prolonged mixer operation is the milling that inadvertently occurs because of abrasion of the particles. This frequently occurs during scaling up to production from small laboratory mixers. The often substantial fill weights of production mixers can generate high shear forces between particles sliding past each other under a heavy load of material above. As a consequence, the particle size distribution after mixing may bear only slight resemblance to the original distribution. An expected and common effect is the generation of fine particulate matter (fines), which can dilute lubricants and otherwise modify formulation properties.

References

1. Johnstone, R. E., and Thring, M. W.: Pilot Plants, Models and Scale-Up Methods in Chemical Engineering. McGraw-Hill, New York, 1957.
2. Uhl, V. W., and Gray, J. B.: Mixing—Theory and Practice. Vol. I. Academic Press, New York, 1966.
3. Uhl, V. W., and Gray, J. B.: Mixing—Theory and Practice. Vol. II. Academic Press, New York, 1967.
4. Sterbacek, Z., and Tausk, P.: Mixing in the Chemical Industry. Pergamon Press, New York, 1965.
5. Bridgeman, P. W.: Dimensional Analysis. Yale University Press, New Haven, 1931.
6. Perry, R. H. Chilton, C. H., and Kirkpatrick, S. D.: Chemical Engineers' Hand-book. 4th ed. McGraw-Hill, New York, 1963.
7. Herdan, G.: Small Particle Statistics. Academic Press, New York, 1960.
8. Rippie, E. G., and Chou, D. H.: Powder Technol., 21:205, 1978.

General References

Nagata, S.: Mixing: Principles and Applications. John Wiley and Sons, New York, 1975.

Nauman, E. B.: Mixing in Continuous Flow Systems. John Wiley and Sons, New York, 1983.

Nielsen, L. E.: Predicting the Properties of Mixtures: Mixture Rules in Science and Engineering. Marcel Dekker, New York, 1978.

Oldshue, J. Y.: Fluid Mixing Technology. Chemical Engineering Magazine. American Institute of Chemical Engineering (AIChE), New York, 1983.

Randolph, J.: Mixing in the Chemical and Allied Industries. Noyes Development Corp., Park Ridge, NJ, 1967.

Weidenbaum, S. S.: Mixing of Solids. Advances in Chemical Engineering. Vol. 2. Academic Press, New York, 1958, p. 209.

2

Milling

EUGENE L. PARROTT

Few materials used in pharmaceuticals exist in the optimum size, and most materials must be comminuted at some stage during the production of a dosage form. Milling is the mechanical process of reducing the particle size of solids. Various terms (crushing, disintegration, dispersion, grinding, and pulverization) have been used synonymously with comminution depending on the product, the equipment, and the process.

Milling equipment is usually classified as coarse, intermediate, or fine according to the size of the milled product. Size is conventionally expressed in terms of mesh (number of openings per linear inch of a screen). As an arbitrary classification for the consideration of pharmaceuticals, coarse milling produces particles larger than 20-mesh, intermediate milling produces particles from 200- to 20-mesh (74 to 840 microns), and fine milling produces particles smaller than 200-mesh. A given mill may operate successfully in more than one class: a hammer mill may be used to prepare a 16-mesh granulation and to mill a crystalline material to a 120-mesh powder.

Pharmaceutical Applications

The surface area per unit weight, which is known as the *specific surface,* is increased by size reduction. This increased specific surface affects the therapeutic efficiency of medicinal compounds that possess a low solubility in body fluids by increasing the area of contact between the solid and the dissolving fluid. Thus, a given weight of a finely powdered medicinal compound dissolves in a shorter time than does the same weight of a coarser powder. The control of fineness of griseofulvin led to an oral dosage regimen half that of the originally marketed product.[1] Control of particle size and specific surface

influences the duration of adequate serum concentration, rheology, and product syringeability of a suspension of penicillin G procaine for intramuscular injection.[2] The rectal absorption of aspirin from a theobroma oil suppository is related to particle size.[3] Increased antiseptic action has been demonstrated for calomel ointment when the particle size of calomel has been reduced.[4] The size of particles used in inhalation aerosols determines the position and retention of the particles in the bronchopulmonary system.[5] Fincher has reviewed the influence of particle size of medicinal compounds and its relationship to absorption and activity.[6] Size may affect texture, taste, and rheology of oral suspensions in addition to absorption.[7]

Extraction or leaching from animal glands (liver and pancreas), and from crude vegetable drugs, is facilitated by comminution. The time required for extraction is shortened by the increased area of contact between the solvent and the solid and the reduced distance the solvent has to penetrate into the material. The control of particle size in the extraction process provides for more complete extraction and a rapid filtration rate when the solution is filtered from the marc. Similarly, the time required for dissolution of solid chemicals in the preparation of solutions is shortened by the use of smaller particles.

The drying of wet masses may be facilitated by milling, which increases the surface area and reduces the distance the moisture must travel within the particle to reach the outer surface. Solvolytic decomposition of solids initially occurs at surface irregularities and is increased by the presence of solvates or moisture. Micronization and subsequent drying increase the stability because the occluded solvent is removed.[8]

In the manufacture of compressed tablets, the granulation of the wet mass results in more rapid and uniform drying. The dried tablet granulation is then milled to a particle size and distribution that will flow freely and produce tablets of uniform weight. The flowability of powders and granules in high-speed filling equipment and in tablet presses affects product uniformity. Relationships between flow rate and particle size have been reported.[9-11] The role of size reduction in tablet manufacturing has been discussed.[12]

The mixing or blending of several solid ingredients of a pharmaceutical is easier and more uniform if the ingredients are approximately the same size.[13] This provides a greater uniformity of dose. Solid pharmaceuticals that are artificially colored are often milled to distribute the coloring agent to ensure that the mixture is not mottled and is uniform from batch to batch. Even the size of a pigment affects its color.

Lubricants used in compressed tablets and capsules function by virtue of their ability to coat the surface of the granulation or powder. A fine particle size is essential if the lubricant is to function properly.[14] The milling of ointments, creams, and pastes provides a smooth texture and better appearance in addition to improved physical stability.

Size Distribution and Measurement

In naturally occurring particulate solids and milled solids, the shape of particles is irregular, and the size of the particles varies within the range of the largest and smallest particle. There is no known method of defining an irregular particle in geometric terms; however, statistical methods have been developed to express the size of an irregular particle in terms of a single dimension referred to as its diameter. If this diameter is measured by a standardized procedure for a large number of particles, the values may be expressed by several diameters. It is only required that the surface area is proportional to the square of the diameter and the volume is proportional to the cube of the diameter.

For an irregular particle, an equivalent particle with the same surface or volume may be substituted. For convenience of mathematical treatment, an irregular particle is considered in terms of an equivalent sphere. The size of the particle can then be expressed by a single parameter, d (the diameter). The volume of a particle may be determined by displacement in a liquid and equated to the volume of a hypothetic sphere possessing an equivalent diameter. As the volume of a sphere is $\pi d^3/6$, the equivalent diameter of an irregular particle with a volume V is:

$$d = \sqrt[3]{\frac{6V}{\pi}} \qquad (1)$$

The effective diameter of particles based on their rate of sedimentation is commonly used in pharmacy. The time required for the particle to settle between two fixed points in a suitable liquid is experimentally determined and allows evaluation of the rate of sedimentation. By use of Stokes' equation (see under "Sedimentation" in this chapter), the effective diameter is calculated. This effective, or Stokes', diameter is the diameter of a sphere that requires the same time to settle between two fixed points in the liquid as does the irregular particle.

In addition to the two effective diameters described, several other diameters are defined and their values are calculated in Table 2-1 for 261 particles measured by microscopy. The arithmetic average diameter is the sum of the diameters of the separate particles divided by the number of particles. If n_1, n_2, and n_n are the number of particles having diameters d_1, d_2, and d_n, respectively, the average diameter is:

$$d_{ave} = \frac{n_1 d_1 + n_2 d_2 + \ldots n_n d_n}{n_1 + n_2 + \ldots n_n} = \frac{\Sigma(nd)}{\Sigma n} \qquad (2)$$

The average diameter of a group of 261 particles can be calculated from the data in Table 2-2. The average diameter is:

$$d_{ave} = \frac{5366}{261} = 20.6 \ \mu m \qquad (3)$$

The geometric mean diameter is the *nth* root of the product of the n particles measured:

$$d_{geo} = \sqrt[n]{d_1 d_2 \ldots d_n} \qquad (4)$$

Using the logarithmic form of this equation, the geometric mean diameter of the 261 particles is calculated by use of the following:

$$\log d_{geo} = \frac{\Sigma(n \log d)}{\Sigma n}$$
$$= \frac{336.0874}{261} \qquad (5)$$
$$= 1.2876$$

and

$$d_{geo} = \text{antilog } 1.2876 = 19.4 \ \mu m \qquad (6)$$

TABLE 2-1. *Definitions of Various Diameters and Their Values for 261 Particles Measured by Means of an Optical Micrometer*

Size-group	Mean of Size-group, d	Number in Each Size-group, n	nd	log d	n log d	nd^2	nd^3	nd^4
4 to 7.9 μm	6 μm	5	30	0.7782	3.9910	180	1080	6480
8 to 11.9	10	15	150	1.0000	15.0000	1500	15,000	150,000
12 to 15.9	14	46	644	1.1461	52.7206	9016	126,224	1,767,136
16 to 19.9	18	68	1224	1.2553	85.3604	22,032	396,476	7,138,368
20 to 23.9	22	58	1276	1.3424	77.8592	28,072	617,584	13,586,848
24 to 27.9	26	32	832	1.4150	45.2800	21,632	562,432	14,623,232
28 to 31.9	30	22	660	1.4771	32.4962	19,800	594,000	17,820,000
32 to 35.9	34	10	340	1.5315	15.3150	11,560	393,040	1,336,336
36 to 39.9	38	2	76	1.5798	3.1596	2888	109,744	2,085,136
40 to 43.9	42	2	84	1.6232	3.2464	3528	148,176	6,222,392
44 to 47.9	46	0	0	1.6628	0	0	0	0
48 to 51.9	50	1	50	1.6990	1.6990	2500	125,000	6,250,000
		261	5366		336.0874	122,708	3,088,756	70,985,928

Diameter	Definition	Diameter for 261 Particles
Mean surface	$d_s = \sqrt{\dfrac{\Sigma nd^2}{\Sigma n}}$	$d_s = \sqrt{\dfrac{122,708}{261}} = 21.7\ \mu\text{m}$
Mean volume	$d_v = \sqrt[3]{\dfrac{\Sigma nd^3}{\Sigma n}}$	$d_v = \sqrt[3]{\dfrac{3,088,756}{261}} = 22.8\ \mu\text{m}$
Mean volume-surface	$d_{vs} = \dfrac{\Sigma nd^3}{\Sigma nd^2}$	$d_{vs} = \dfrac{3,088,756}{122,708} = 25.2\mu\text{m}$
Weight mean	$d_w = \dfrac{\Sigma nd^4}{\Sigma nd^3}$	$d_w = \dfrac{70,985,928}{3,088,756} = 22.9\ \mu\text{m}$

TABLE 2-2. *Summation for the Determination of the Median Diameter of 261 Particles Measured by an Optical Micrometer*

Size-group	Number in Each Size-group, n	Number Less Than Maximum of Size-group	Percentage of Particles in Each Size-group	Percentage of Particles Less Than Maximum Size of Group
4 to 7.9 μm	5	5	1.9	1.9
8 to 11.9	15	20	5.8	7.7
12 to 15.9	46	66	17.7	25.4
16 to 19.9	68	134	26.0	51.4
20 to 23.9	58	192	22.2	73.6
24 to 27.9	32	224	12.4	85.8
28 to 31.9	22	246	8.4	94.2
32 to 35.9	10	256	3.8	98.0
36 to 39.9	2	258	0.8	98.8
40 to 43.9	2	260	0.8	99.6
44 to 47.9	0	260	0	99.6
48 to 51.9	1	261	0.4	100

The median diameter is the diameter for which 50% of the particles measured are less than the stated size. An inspection of Table 2-2 shows that 134 particles of the 261 are less than 18 microns; therefore, the median diameter is approximately 18 microns. Cumulative plots are those in which the percentage of particles less than (or greater than) a given particle size are plotted against size. As shown in Figure 2-1 for the data in Table 2-2, the cumulative percentage less than the stated size is plotted against size, and the median diameter is read from the 50% value of the curve.

The arithmetic or geometric mean and the median have no physical significance. The meaningful choice of diameter depends on its relevance to some significant physical property. The packing and flow of a powder or granulation depends on its volume; thus, if packing is a prime consideration, the size should be expressed as a mean volume diameter. Dissolution and adsorption processes are a function of the surface area of the particles, and with these processes, the particle size should be expressed as a mean surface diameter. As sedimentation is an important property of suspensions, the size of the suspended solids should be expressed as a Stokes' diameter.

Representation of Data

When a material is milled, the particles have a variety of sizes as determined by flaw structure. The purpose of particle size measurement is to determine the percentage frequency of distribution of particle sizes. The most precise method of data presentation is tabular form, as in Table 2-1. The data may be presented as a bar graph or histogram of the frequency as a function of particle size. Size-distribution data are commonly presented graphically because a graph is more concise and permits easy visualization of the mean and skewness of distribution. A size-frequency curve is a plot of the percentage frequencies of various particles against the mean of size-groups. The size-frequency curve in Figure 2-2 is drawn from the data in Table 2-1. The arithmetic and geometric mean diameters are indicated. The mode is the maximum in the size-frequency curve.

An infinite number of particle size distributions may have the same average diameter or median. For this reason, parameters other than a median or average diameter are required to define the size of a powder. A powder should be characterized with a size-frequency curve.

Size distributions that follow the probability law are referred to as normal or Gaussian distributions, as shown in Figure 2-2. This normal-probability distribution is symmetric about a vertical axis. The size-frequency distribution of ground material is usually skewed with the number of particles increasing with decreasing size. It is believed that the size distributions of

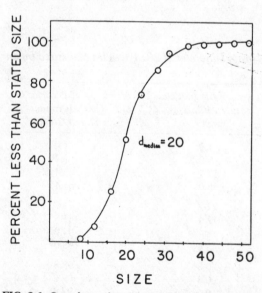

FIG. 2-1. *Cumulative distribution plot used to determine the median size.*

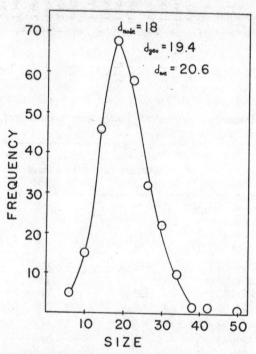

FIG. 2-2. *Size-frequency distribution of 261 particles measured by microscopy.*

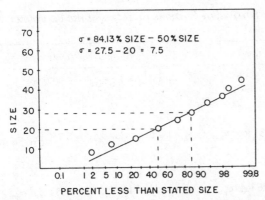

FIG. 2-3. *Arithmetic-probability plot of data in Table 2-2.*

milled material follow an exponential law. If the distribution is asymmetric or skewed, it frequently can be made symmetric and will follow the normal-probability law if the sizes are replaced by the logarithms of the sizes.

Size-frequency data are conveniently plotted on an arithmetic-probability or logarithm-probability grid. For a normal distribution, a plot of the cumulative percentage less (or greater) than the stated size against size produces a straight line. In Figure 2-3, using the data from Table 2-2, (the size is plotted against the cumulative percentage less than the stated size using an arithmetic-probability grid. For a skewed distribution, a plot of the cumulative percentage less (or greater) than the stated size against the logarithm of size generally produces a straight line, as shown in Figure 2-4.

When the plots are made on either probability grid, the distributions must be asymptotic on both extremes. In practice, there may be a largest and smallest particle in the material measured; therefore, the distribution is not asymptotic, and the plots on the probability grids often depart from linearity at the extremes. This does not detract from the usefulness of such plots, as the areas extending from the extremes to infinity are negligible compared to the area contained under the distribution curve between the largest and the smallest particles measured.

The calculations involved in computing the mean diameter and the standard deviation are reduced by the use of probability grids. The median diameter for both grids is obtained by reading from the curve the size corresponding to 50% value on the probability scale. In the arithmetic-probability plot, the mean is the arithmetic average; in the logarithm-probability plot, the 50% size is the geometric mean. The standard deviations can be obtained from the arithmetic-probability plot from the relation:

$$\sigma = 84.13\% \text{ size} - 50\% \text{ size}$$
$$\sigma = 50\% \text{ size} - 15.87\% \text{ size} \qquad (7)$$

and from the logarithm-probability plot from the relation:

$$\sigma_{\text{geo}} = \frac{84.13\% \text{ size}}{50\% \text{ size}}$$
$$= \frac{50\% \text{ size}}{15.87\% \text{ size}} \qquad (8)$$

Using these probability functions, Hatch derived equations relating various types of diameters by use of the standard deviation and mean.[15] These statistical parameters are a function of the size and numeric frequency of the particles for a given size. To calculate their values, the size-distribution data must be expressed in terms of a numbers frequency. In microscopy, this requirement is met directly; however, in sieving and sedimentation methods, the data obtained provide a weight distribution. Fortunately, as shown in Table 2-3, equations have been derived relating the weight distribution data to statistical diameters. The prime on the d'_{geo} and σ'_{geo} signify a weight distribution rather than a numbers distribution. The geometric standard deviations for a weight and numbers distribution are practically identical.

To illustrate the use of these equations, the data from a sample of magnesium hydroxide given in Table 2-6 are plotted in Figure 2-4 with the cumulative percentage less than stated size on the probability grid and the size on the logarithmic grid. The geometric mean diameter corresponding to the 50% value on the cumulative

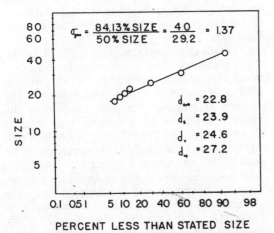

FIG. 2-4. *Logarithm-probability plot of data in Table 2-6.*

TABLE 2-3. *Definitions of Diameters of Nonuniform Particulate Systems in Terms of the Parameter of Size Distribution Curves by Number and by Weight*

Diameter	Numbers Distribution	Weight Distribution
Geometric mean, $d_{geo} = \dfrac{\Sigma(n \log d)}{\Sigma n}$		$\log d_{geo} = \log d_{geo}' - 6.9078 \log^2 \sigma_{geo}'$
Arithmetic mean, $d_{ave} = \dfrac{\Sigma nd}{\Sigma n}$	$\log d_{ave} = \log d_{geo} + 1.151 \log^2 \sigma_{geo}$	$\log d_{ave} = \log d_{geo}' - 5.756 \log^2 \sigma_{geo}'$
Mean surface, $d_s = \sqrt{\dfrac{\Sigma nd^2}{\Sigma n}}$	$\log d_s = \log d_{geo} + 2.3026 \log^2 \sigma_{geo}$	$\log d_s = \log d_{geo}' - 4.6052 \log^2 \sigma_{geo}'$
Mean volume, $d_v = \sqrt[3]{\dfrac{\Sigma nd^3}{\Sigma n}}$	$\log d_v = \log d_{geo} + 3.4539 \log^2 \sigma_{geo}$	$\log d_v = \log d_{geo}' - 3.4539 \log^2 \sigma_{geo}'$
Mean volume-surface $d_{vs} = \dfrac{\Sigma nd^3}{\Sigma nd^2}$	$\log d_{vs} = \log d_{geo} + 5.7565 \log^2 \sigma_{geo}$	$\log d_{vs} = \log d_{geo}' - 1.1513 \log^2 \sigma_{geo}'$

percentage axis is 29.2 microns. The geometric standard deviation is:

$$\sigma'_{geo} = \frac{84.13\% \text{ size}}{50\% \text{ size}}$$

$$= \frac{40}{29.2} = 1.37 \; \mu m \qquad (9)$$

Knowing the value of the geometric mean diameter and the geometric standard deviation, the Hatch and Choate equations may be used to calculate statistical diameters given in Figure 2-4. For example, the mean surface diameter of the sample of magnesium hydroxide is:

$$\log d_s = \log_{geo} - 4.606 \log^2 \sigma'_{geo}$$
$$\log d_s = \log 29.2 - (4.606 \times 0.0187)$$
$$= 1.3793 \qquad (10)$$
$$d_s = 23.9 \; \mu m$$

Microscopy

Microscopy is the most direct method for size distribution measurement. Its lower limit of application is determined by the resolving power of the lens. A particle cannot be resolved if its size is close to the wave length of the light source. For white light, an ordinary microscope is used to measure particles from 0.4 to 150 microns.

With special lenses and ultraviolet light, the lower limit may be extended to 0.1 micron. In the ultramicroscope, the resolution is improved by use of a darkfield illumination. The size range of the ultramicroscope is from 0.01 to 0.2 micron.

The diameters of the particles on the slide are measured by means of a calibrated filar micrometer eyepiece. The hairline of the eyepiece is moved by the micrometer to one edge of a particle, and the reading on the micrometer is recorded. The hairline is then moved to the opposite edge of the particle being measured, and the micrometer is read. The difference between the two readings is the diameter of the particle. All of the particles are measured along an arbitrary fixed line.

Graticules or eyepieces with grids of circles and squares are used to compare the cross-sectional area of each particle in the microscopic field with one of the numbered patterns. The number of particles that best fits one of the numbered circles is recorded. The field is changed, and the procedure is repeated with another numbered circle. This procedure is repeated until the entire size range is covered.

In both techniques, the magnification is determined by the use of a calibrated stage micrometer, as the magnification is not equal to the product of the nominal magnification of the objective and the eyepiece.

The particulate field to be counted should be

random. The total number of fields to be counted depends on the number of particles per field. In principle, the number of particles measured should be great enough so that the results do not change on measuring a larger number. The British Standard on microscopic counting recommends at least 625 particles. If the particle size distribution is wide, it may be necessary to count more particles. If the particle size distribution is narrow, as few as 200 particles may be sufficient.

There is considerable variation among operators using the microscopy technique. Photomicrographs, projections, and automatic scanners have been used to lessen operator fatigue.

The diameters measured by a microscope and defined in Table 2-1 are number parameters, since microscopy involves a counting procedure.

Sieving

Sieving is the most widely used method for measuring particle size distribution because it is inexpensive, simple, and rapid with little variation between operators. Although the lower limit of application is generally considered to be 50 microns, micromesh sieves are available for extending the lower limit to 10 microns.

A sieve consists of a pan with a bottom of wire cloth with square openings. In the United States, two standards of sieves are used. In the Tyler Standard Scale, the ratio of the width of openings in successive sieves is $\sqrt{2}$. The Tyler Standard Scale is based on the size of opening (0.0029″) in a wire cloth having 200 openings per linear inch, i.e., 200-mesh. The United States Standard Scale proposed by the National Bureau of Standards in general uses the ratio $\sqrt{2}$, but it is based on an opening of 1 mm (18-mesh). The two standard sieves are compared in Table 2-4.

The procedure involves the mechanical shaking of a sample through a series of successively smaller sieves, and the weighing of the portion of the sample retained on each sieve. The type of motion influences sieving: vibratory motion is most efficient, followed successively by side-tap motion, bottom-tap motion, rotary motion with tap, and rotary motion. Time is an important factor in sieving. The load or thickness of powder per unit area of sieve influences the time of sieving; for a given set of sieves, the time required to sieve a given material is roughly proportional to the load placed on the sieve. Therefore, in size analysis by means of sieves, the type of motion, time of sieving, and load should be standardized.

A typical size-weight distribution obtained by sieving is shown in Table 2-5. The size assigned

TABLE 2-4. *Designations and Dimensions of U.S. Standard and Tyler Standard Sieves*

U.S. Standard		Tyler Standard	
Micron	Mesh	Micron	Mesh
5660	3½	5613	3½
4760	4	4699	4
4000	5	3965	5
3360	6	3327	6
2830	7	2794	7
2380	8	2362	8
2000	10	1651	10
1680	12	1397	12
1410	14	1168	14
1190	16	991	16
1000	18	883	20
840	20	701	24
710	25	589	28
590	30	495	32
500	35	417	35
420	40	351	42
350	45	295	48
297	50	246	60
250	60	208	65
210	70	175	80
177	80	147	100
149	100	124	115
125	120	104	150
105	140	88	170
88	170	74	200
74	200		
62	230		
53	270		
44	325		
37	400		

to the sample retained is arbitrary, but by convention, the size of the particles retained is taken as the arithmetic or geometric mean of the two sieves (a powder passing a 30-mesh and retained on a 45-mesh sieve is assigned an arithmetic mean diameter of (590 + 350)/2 or 470 microns).

If the weight distribution obtained by sieving follows a logarithm-probability distribution, the Hatch-Choate equations given in Table 2-3 permit conversion of the weight to a number distribution.

Sedimentation

Sedimentation methods may be used over a size range from 1 to 200 microns to obtain a size-weight distribution curve and to permit calculation of the particle size. The sedimentation method is based on the dependence of the rate of sedimentation of the particles on their size as

TABLE 2-5. *Weight-Size Distribution of Granular Sodium Bromide as Measured by U.S. Standard Sieves*

Sieve Number (Passed/Retained)	Arithmetic Mean Size of Openings	Weight Retained on Smaller Sieve	% Retained on Smaller Sieve	Weight Size
(1)	(2)	(3)	(4)	(2) × (4)
30/45	470 μm	57.3 g	13.0	6100
45/60	300	181.0	41.2	12,380
60/80	213	110.0	25.0	5320
80/100	163	49.7	11.3	1840
100/140	127	20.0	4.5	572
140/200	90	22.0	5.0	450
		400.0	100.0	26,662

$$d_{ave} = \frac{26,662}{100} = 267 \; \mu m$$

expressed by Stokes' equation:

$$d_{Stokes} = \sqrt{\frac{18\eta}{(\rho - \rho_0)g} \frac{x}{t}} \qquad (11)$$

where d_{Stokes} is the effective or Stokes' diameter, η is the viscosity of the dispersion fluid, x/t is the rate of sedimentation or distance of fall x in time t, g is the gravitational constant, and ρ and ρ_0 are the densities of the particle and the medium, respectively. Stokes' equation is applicable to free spheres that are falling at a constant rate. If the concentration of the suspension does not exceed 2%, there is no significant interaction between the particles, and they settle independent of one another.

The pipet method (Andreasen) is the simplest means of incremental particle size analysis. A 1% suspension of the powder in a suitable liquid medium is placed in the pipet (Fig. 2-5). At given intervals of time, samples are withdrawn from a specified depth without disturbing the suspension, and they are dried so that the residue may be weighed. By means of Stokes' equation, the particle diameter corresponding to each interval of time is calculated, with x being the height of the liquid above the lower end of the pipet at time t when each sample is withdrawn. As the sizes of the particles are not uniform, the particles settle at different rates. The size-distribution and concentration of the particles vary along the length of the suspension as sedimentation occurs. The larger particles settle at a faster rate and fall below the pipet tip sooner

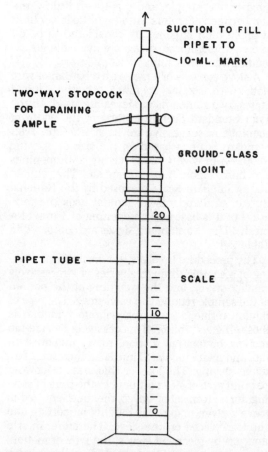

FIG. 2-5. *At measured time intervals, a 10-ml sample is withdrawn by aspiration at a depth that can be read from the scale etched on the Andreasen Pipet.*

TABLE 2-6. *Weight-Size Distribution of Magnesium Hydroxide as Determined by Andreasen Pipet Using Water as Medium*

Time (sec)	Height (cm)	Weight of Residue (g)	Percentage of Initial Suspension	Particle Diameter Calculated by Means of Stokes' Equation (μm)
120	20.0	0.0912	92.4	44.5
240	19.6	0.0591	59.9	30.5
360	19.2	0.0321	32.5	25.1
420	18.8	0.0134	13.9	22.9
480	18.4	0.0107	10.9	20.7
600	18.0	0.0089	9.0	18.5
720	17.2	0.0069	7.0	16.8

than the smaller particles; thus, each sample drawn has a lower concentration and contains particles of smaller diameters than the previous sample.

From the weight of the dried sample, the percentage by weight of the initial suspension is calculated for particles having sizes smaller than the size calculated by Stokes' equation for that time. The weight of each sample residue is called the *weight undersize*, and the sum of the successive weights is known as the *cumulative weight undersize*. Typical data obtained by use of the Andreasen pipet are given in Table 2-6. In Figure 2-4, the plot of logarithm of size against the percentage less than the stated size produces a straight line and allows the evaluation of geometric mean diameter and standard deviation. The geometric mean diameter corresponding to the graphic 50% size is 29.2 microns. The standard deviation, which is evaluated as the ratio of the 84.13% size to the 50% size (40/29.2), is 1.37. With these two values, the weight distribution obtained by sedimentation may be converted into number distribution by use of the Hatch-Choate equations. For example, if one wishes to calculate the mean surface diameter, the appropriate equation selected from Table 2-3 is:

$$\log d_s = \log d'_{geo} - 4.6052 \log^2 \sigma'_{geo}$$
$$= \log 29.2 - (4.6052 \log^2 1.37) \quad (12)$$
$$d_s = antilog\ 1.3793 = 23.9\ \mu m$$

Other Methods

The major methods for particle size distribution measurements, i.e., microscopy, sedimentation, and sieving, have been discussed to illustrate the principles involved. Other useful methods of measuring particle size involve ad-

sorption, electrical conductivity, light and x-ray scattering, permeametry, and particle trajectory. More extensive treatment of particle size measurement is given by various authors.[16-19]

Theory of Comminution

At present, there is meager basic understanding of the mechanism and quantitative aspects of milling.[20-25] The mechanical behavior of solids, which under stress are strained and deformed, is shown in the stress-strain curve in Figure 2-6. The initial linear portion of the curve is defined by Hooke's law (stress is proportional to strain), and Young's modulus (slope of linear portion) expresses the stiffness or softness in dynes per square centimeter. The stress-strain curve becomes nonlinear at the yield point, which is a measure of the resistance to permanent deformation. With still greater stress, the region of irreversible plastic deformation is

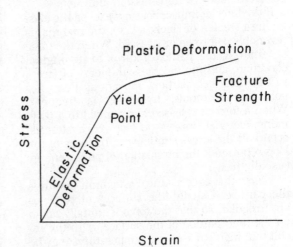

FIG. 2-6. *Stress-strain diagram for a solid.*

reached. The area under the curve represents the energy of fracture and is an approximate measure of the impact strength of the material.

In all milling processes, it is a random matter if and when a given particle will be fractured. If a single particle is subjected to a sudden impact and is fractured, it yields a few relatively large particles and a number of fine particles, with relatively few particles of intermediate size. If the energy of the impact is increased, the larger particles are of a smaller size and more numerous, and although the number of fine particles is increased appreciably, their size is not greatly changed. It seems that the size of the finer particles is related to the internal structure of the material, and the size of the larger particles is more closely related to the process by which comminution is accomplished.

Size reduction begins with the opening of any small cracks that were initially present. Thus, larger particles with numerous cracks fracture more readily than smaller particles with fewer cracks. In general, fine grinding requires more energy, not only because of the increased new surface, but also because more energy is needed to initiate cracks.

For any particle, there is a minimum energy that will fracture it; however, conditions are so haphazard that many particles receive impacts that are not sufficient to fracture them and are eventually fractured by some excessively forceful blow. As a result, the most efficient mills utilize less than 1% of the energy input to fracture particles and create new surfaces.[26] The rest of the energy is dissipated in (1) elastic deformation of unfractured particles, (2) transport of material within the milling chamber, (3) friction between particles, (4) friction between particles and mill, (5) heat, (6) vibration and noise, and (7) inefficiency of transmission and motor.

If the force of impact does not exceed the elastic limit (region of Hooke's law), the material is reversibly deformed or stressed. When the force is removed, the particle returns to its original condition, and the mechanical energy of stress in the deformed particle appears as heat. For polymeric materials, hysteresis is frequent. When a force is released and applied to a polymeric material, an elastic loop, or hysteresis, occurs in the stress-strain cycle; the area of the loop represents the dissipation of stress energy (usually heat).

A force that exceeds the elastic limit fractures the particle. Usually, the surfaces of particles are irregular, so that the force is initially taken on the high portion of the surface, with the result that high stresses and temperatures may be set up locally in the material. As fracture occurs,

the points of application of the force are shifted. The energy for the new surfaces is partially supplied by the release of stress energy. Crystalline materials fracture along crystal cleavage planes; noncrystalline materials fracture at random. If an ideal crystal were pressed with an increasing force, the force would be distributed uniformly throughout its structure until the crystal disintegrated into its individual units. A real crystal fractures under much less force into a few relatively large particles and several fine particles, with relatively few particles of intermediate size. Crystals of pure substances have internal weaknesses due to missing atoms or ions in their lattice structures and to flaws arising from mechanical or thermal stress.[20]

A flaw in a particle is any structural weakness that may develop into a crack under strain. It has been proposed that any force of milling produces a small flaw in the particle. The useful work in milling is proportional to the length of new cracks produced. A particle absorbs strain energy and is deformed under shear or compression until the energy exceeds the weakest flaw and causes fracture or cracking of the particle. The strain energy required for fracture is proportional to the length of the crack formed, since the additional energy required to extend the crack to fracture is supplied by the flow of the surrounding residual strain energy to the crack.

The Griffith theory of cracks and flaws assumes that all solids contain flaws and microscopic cracks, which increase the applied force according to the crack length and focus the stress at the atomic bond of the crack apex.[27,28] The Griffith theory may be expressed as:[29,30]

$$T = \sqrt{\frac{Y\,\epsilon}{c}} \qquad (13)$$

where T is tensile stress, Y is Young's modulus, ϵ is the surface energy of the wall of the crack, and c is the critical crack depth required for fracture. A linear relationship between the square of tensile strength of minerals and the critical height for drop weight impact suggests that the square of tensile strength is a useful criterion of impact fracture.[31]

Thermodynamic treatment of the milling process has been attempted, but there is confusion about the meaning of surface tension, surface stress, and surface energy of solids. In addition, there is some question as to whether a reversible path may be devised for a milling process. Thermodynamics have shown that the work to fracture a particle depends on surface energy,[32] and that the yield stress depends on the rate of strain and temperature of the fluid filling the particle pore.[33] Fracture is predicted to be more efficient at an elevated temperature.[34]

The weakest flaw in a particle determines its fracture strength; it controls the number of particles produced by fracture. Particles with the weakest flaws fracture most easily and produce the largest particles; however, they are not necessarily easier to mill to a given size, as they may require several more stages of fracture than particles of the same size whose weakest flaw is stronger.

The immediate objective of milling is to form cracks that spread through the deformed particles at the expense of strain energy and produce fracture. The useful work is directly proportional to the new surface area. Since the crack length is proportional to the square root of the new surface area produced, the useful work is inversely proportional to the square root of the product diameter minus the feed diameter.[35] The energy E' expended in producing new surface is:

$$E' = E\left(\frac{\sqrt{D_1}}{\sqrt{D_1} - \sqrt{D_2}}\right) \qquad (14)$$

where D_1 is the diameter of the material fed to the mill, D_2 is the diameter of the product discharged from the mill, and E is the energy input.

The efficiency of the milling process is influenced by the nature of the force as well as by its magnitude. The rate of application of force affects comminution, as there is a time lag between the attainment of maximum force and fracture. Often, materials respond as brittle materials to fast impact and as plastic materials to a slow force. The greater the rate at which the force is applied, the less effectively the energy is utilized, and the higher is the proportion of fine material produced. As the rate of milling is increased, more energy is expended. To produce a new surface in milliseconds may require three to four times as much energy as the production of the same new surface area in seconds.[36]

Energy for Comminution

The energy required to reduce the size of particles is inversely proportional to the size raised to some power. This may be expressed mathematically as:[37]

$$\frac{dE}{dD} = -\frac{C}{D^n} \qquad (15)$$

where dE is the amount of energy required to produce a change in size, dD, of unit mass of material, and where C and n are constants.

In 1885, Kick suggested that the energy requirement, E, for size reduction is directly related to the reduction ratio (D_1/D_2), where D_1 and D_2 are the diameters of the feed material and discharged product, respectively. Thus, if a certain horsepower is required to mill a given weight of material from 1000 to 500 microns, the same energy would be required to reduce the size from 500 to 250 microns. Kick's theory may be expressed as:

$$E = C \ln \frac{D_1}{D_2} \qquad (16)$$

The constant C may be regarded as a reciprocal efficiency coefficient. In the engineering literature, $C = K_k f_c$, where f_c is the crushing strength of the material and K_k is known as Kick's constant. If n = 1, the general differential equation reduces to Kick's equation. Kick's proposal was developed on a stress-strain diagram for cubes under compression and represents the energy required to effect elastic deformation before fracture occurs.[38] Kick's equation assumes that the material has flaws distributed throughout its internal structure that are independent of particle volume. Experimental and theoretic values apply best to coarse milling.[39]

In 1867, von Rittinger proposed that the energy required for size reduction is directly proportional to the increase in surface as expressed by the following relationship:[40]

$$E = k_1(S_2 - S_1) \qquad (17)$$

where k_1 includes the relationship between the particle surface and diameter, and S_1 and S_2 are the specific surface before and after milling, respectively. In terms of particle diameters:

$$E = C'\left(\frac{1}{D_2} - \frac{1}{D_1}\right) \qquad (18)$$

In the engineering literature, $C' = K_r f_c$, where K_r is known as Rittinger's constant.

Equation (18) applies precisely only under the conditions that all energy is transferred into surface energy, and that the energy of comminution required per unit of surface is independent of particle size. Rittinger's equation is less applicable if appreciable deformation occurs. It is most applicable to brittle materials undergoing fine milling, in which there is minimal deformation and a rapid production of new surfaces with concomitant surface-energy absorption.[39]

If $n = 2$ (because the surface is proportional to the square of the diameter), the solution of the general differential equation yields Rittinger's equation.[39] Rittinger's theory ignores particle deformation before fracture although work is the product of force and distance.

In 1952, Bond suggested that the energy required for size reduction is inversely proportional to the square root of the diameter of the product.[41,42] This may be expressed mathematically:

$$W_t \, \alpha \, 1/\sqrt{D_2} \qquad (19)$$

where W_t is the total work of comminution in kilowatt hours per short ton of milled material, and D_2 is the size in microns through which 80% by weight of the milled product will pass. The total work, W_t, if defined as the kilowatt hours per ton required to subdivide from an infinitely large particle size to a certain product of size D_2, is proportional to $1/\sqrt{D_2}$, since $1/\sqrt{D_1}$ is infinitely small when D is infinitely large. However, W is proportional to $(1/\sqrt{D_2}) - (1/\sqrt{D_1})$ when W is the work in kilowatt hours per ton of material to mill from D_1 microns to D_2 microns. Thus:

$$\frac{W_t}{1/\sqrt{D_2}} = \frac{W}{(1/\sqrt{D_2}) - (1/\sqrt{D_1})} \qquad (20)$$

If W_t is called a work index, W_i, and is required to be the work input to subdivide from an infinitely large size to a product size of 100 microns, then by substitution in equation (20):

$$W_i = W\left(\frac{\sqrt{D_1}}{\sqrt{D_1} - \sqrt{D_2}}\right)\sqrt{\frac{D_2}{100}} \qquad (21)$$

If the work index is known, the total input of energy necessary to mill with the same efficiency from any feed size to any product size measured in microns may be found from the following:

$$W = W_i\left(\frac{\sqrt{D_1} - \sqrt{D_2}}{\sqrt{D_1}}\right)\sqrt{\frac{100}{D_2}} \qquad (22)$$

which may be rearranged to:

$$W = W_i\left(\sqrt{\frac{100}{D_2}} - \sqrt{\frac{100}{D_1}}\right) \qquad (23)$$

If $n = 1.5$, the solution of the general differential equation yields Bond's equation:

$$\begin{aligned} E &= 2C'\left(\frac{1}{\sqrt{D_2}} - \frac{1}{\sqrt{D_1}}\right) \\ &= 2C'\sqrt{\frac{1}{D_2}}\left(1 - \frac{1}{\sqrt{D_1}/\sqrt{D_2}}\right) \end{aligned} \qquad (24)$$

Equation (22) in the form of equation (24) is:

$$W_t = 10\,W_i\left(\frac{1}{\sqrt{D_2}} - \frac{1}{\sqrt{D_1}}\right) \qquad (25)$$

where $10\,W_i$ equals $2C'$.

If fracture characteristics of a material were constant over all size ranges, and if the efficiencies of all mills were equal, then the work index would be a true constant, and the energy required to mill from any feed size to any product size could be readily calculated from one test establishing the work index. In fact, the work index is not a true constant, but a parameter that changes with shifts in particle size distribution. Best use of a work index occurs when conditions under which the work index is determined approximate those of the final application.

The work index may be determined by actual milling tests. For example, if in 6 min, ten tons of limestone with an initial size of 1600 microns were passed through an impact mill to produce a size of 400 microns, the power consumption as measured by a watt-hour meter was 30 kilowatt-hours. The work index for limestone in this mill may be calculated by use of equation (21):

$$W_i = \frac{30}{10}\left(\frac{\sqrt{1600}}{\sqrt{1600} - \sqrt{400}}\right)\sqrt{\frac{400}{100}} \qquad (26)$$

$W_i = 12$ kilowatt-hours per ton

The dry grind work index is usually 1.3 times the wet grind value. For a certain material by laboratory ball mill tests, it was determined that the work index is 12.07 kilowatt-hours per short ton. The energy expended in reducing the size of this material from 1190 to 149 microns by ball mill is calculated as:

$$E = 12.07\sqrt{\frac{100}{149}}\left[\frac{\sqrt{\frac{1190}{149}} - 1}{\sqrt{\frac{1190}{149}}}\right] \qquad (27)$$

$= 6.40$ kilowatt-hours per short ton

which is equivalent to 8.53 horsepower-hours per short ton.

Distribution and Limit of Comminution

As discussed, the variation in size is commonly expressed as a size-frequency distribution curve. As milling progresses, the particle size-frequency distribution has a narrower range and a finer mean size. As shown in Figure 2-7, a material with initially a monomodal size distribution develops a bimodal size distribution as milling occurs. The primary component gradually decreases in weight, and the secondary component increases in weight. This reduction of weight is accompanied by a decrease in modal size of the primary component and is caused by preferential fracture of larger particles. The modal size of the secondary component remains essentially constant. Continued milling tends to eliminate the primary component. The process is repeated if the material is then transferred to a second mill for finer size reduction.[43] As the particle-size distribution changes, milling characteristics (work index) change because the abundance or shortage of flaws varies at different sizes.

A minimum of two specifications is necessary to characterize a specific size distribution (85% through a 60-mesh screen and 5% through a 325-mesh screen). In the simplest case, one number establishes the limits of particle sizes involved, and another number determines the weight relationships in the various size ranges. Schuhmann[44] experimentally verified the empiric equation:

$$y = 100 \, (D/k)^a \qquad (28)$$

where y is cumulative weight percentage smaller than size D, k is a size modulus for a given distribution, and a is a distribution modulus. The size relationship of many fractured homogeneous materials is described by the Schuhmann equation. When the cumulative weight percentage less than a stated size is plotted on logarithm-logarithm paper against size, a straight line is obtained with a slope of a, and it intersects the 100% ordinate line at the theoretic maximum-sized particle equal to k.[45] For impact milling, $a \to 1$; for abrasion milling, $a \to 0$.

As an example, consider sodium chloride subdivided at three impact energies to produce the size distributions plotted in Figure 2-8 as the cumulative weight percentage finer (y) than the size D, corresponding to the sieve on which it is retained. The experimental size distributions are well described by the Schuhmann equation. The extrapolated straight line for the energy of 18.1 kg cm/cm[3] intersects the 100% ordinate line at 1.9 mm, and the slope is 1.17.

When plotted on logarithm-logarithm paper for impact fracture of sodium chloride, as shown in Figure 2-9, equation (35) yields a straight line, where a and C are constants and the slope is $(1 - n)$. If several milling experiments are conducted in which the energy inputs and the size distributions are measured, then n, the exponent in the fundamental energy-size reduc-

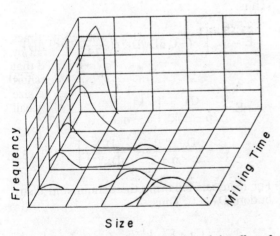

FIG. 2-7. *Diagrammatic representation of the effect of progressive milling on particle size-frequency distribution.*

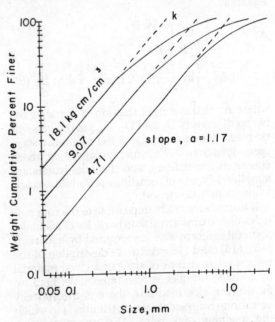

FIG. 2-8. *Particle size-frequency distributions resulting from various energies of impact on sodium chloride.*

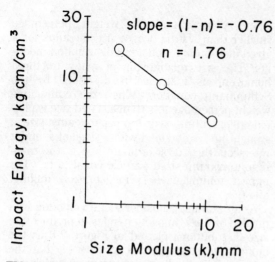

FIG. 2-9. *Energy-size reduction relationship for impact of sodium chloride.*

tion equations, may be determined. The only limitation is that for both, size distributions and shapes of the size distribution curves are the same and are displaced only laterally with a change in energy input.

As shown in Figure 2-9, if a logarithm-logarithm plot is made of the energy inputs against the size modulus, a straight line with a slope of $(1 - n)$ is produced. For sodium chloride subdivided by an impact mill, the slope is 1.76.

Frequently, milled powders have a logarithm-probability distribution as expressed by the equation:

$$\Delta y = \frac{1}{\sqrt{2\pi}\ \ln \sigma} \int_{\ln D_1}^{\ln D_2}$$
$$\exp\left\{-\left[\ln \frac{D}{D_g}\bigg/(\sqrt{2}\ \ln \sigma)\right]^2\right\} d(\ln D) \quad (29)$$

where Δy is the weight fraction of particles between diameters D_1 and D_2, D_{geo} is the geometric mean diameter, and σ is the geometric standard deviation.[46] The manipulations of these equations are tedious, and the calculations are simplified by use of logarithm-probability paper, as previously discussed.

It is experimentally impossible to fracture particles of one uniform size to particles of a smaller and still uniform size, as required by equations (15), (16), and (18). Accurate description of the weight relationships of sizes in a given material by a single number is also impossible, because for a given size modulus, there is theoretically an infinite number of size distributions to which the modulus may refer. Also, the energy required to produce each size distribution from a given size differs. For these reasons, the experimental proof of the relationship between energy and size reduction is difficult.

Verification of an energy-size reduction relationship is also difficult because of the definition of energy actually causing fracture and other forms of energy in the milling process. As fracture depends on strain energy of elastic deformation, the energy seems to be related to size reduction. Although strain energy absorbed by slow compression is easily measured, strain energy absorbed by impact is difficult to measure because of the complex milling process involving translatory motion, vibratory motion, plastic deformation, and sound.

Another difficulty in establishing energy-size reduction relationships arises from the fact that each equation implies that n is a constant independent of the mechanism and quantity of size reduction. Probably n is a variable that depends on the material and manner by which it is fractured. The following derivation shows a general method by which n and C may be calculated using a single distribution plot for any milling test.

If equations (15) and (28) are combined, the energy E required to reduce an element of weight of material dy from size D_m to size D is:

$$E = \int_{D_0}^{k} \int_{D_m}^{D} (-C\ dD_1/D_1^n) dy \quad (30)$$

As size distribution is described by the Schuhmann equation:

$$dy = \left[\frac{100a}{k^a} D^{a-1}\right] dD \quad (31)$$

Thus:

$$E = \int_{D_0}^{k} \int_{D_m}^{D} (-C\ dD_1/D_1^n) \left(\frac{100a}{k^a} D^{a-1}\ dD\right)$$
$$(32)$$

$$E = \frac{Ca}{(n-1)k^a} \left[\frac{k^{a-n-1}}{a-n+1} - \frac{k^a}{aD_m^{n-1}}\right.$$
$$\left. - \frac{D_0^{a-n+1}}{a-n+1} + \frac{D_0^a}{aD_m^{n-1}}\right] \quad (33)$$

For materials following the Schuhmann distribution, $D_0 \to 0$. Thus:

$$E = \frac{Ca}{n-1} \left[\frac{k^{1-n}}{a-n+1} - \frac{1}{aD_m^{n-1}}\right] \quad (34)$$

If D_m is large compared to k, then:

$$E = \frac{Ca}{(n-1)(a-n+1)} k^{1-n} \qquad (35)$$

Equation (35) is real only if n is greater than 1 and less than (a + 1). From experimentally determined size distributions, a has been found to be as great as 1.5, but is usually approximately 0.8. The values of n range from 1 to 2.5. This range was empirically chosen for equations (16), (18), and (20). For hard, brittle materials, (a − $\infty \alpha v$ + 1) approaches zero, and its value cannot be accurately found. Consequently, the constant C cannot be determined accurately; however, for any specific milling conditions, the following term is constant:

$$A = \frac{Ca}{(n-1)(a-n+1)} \qquad (36)$$

The general energy-size reduction equation—equation (15)—may then be expressed as:

$$E = Ak^{(1-n)} \qquad (37)$$

where A is a mill constant that can be determined easily for any size reduction test when the exponent n has been determined as discussed. In the example of sodium chloride subdivided by impact, n is 1.76, and the mill constant may be calculated by the following:

$$18.1 = A\ 1.9^{(1-1.76)}$$
$$A = 29.5 \qquad (38)$$

In pharmacy, relatively small amounts of materials are milled, and the extent of size reduction is determined by the enhancement of clinical efficacy and product characteristics, and by the facilitation of production, rather than by energy expenditure. The proposed theories of comminution are suitable for specific applications and are to be used in a qualitative manner. The only reliable means for determining the size reduction provided by a given mill is experimental testing with the actual material.

According to the general differential equation of size reduction and its special cases, a material given sufficient time may be milled to unlimited fineness; however, in these equations, the size and energy input are inadequately defined. If the ultimate size reduction by mechanical means were attributed to the unit of the crystal lattice, the limit of comminution would be approximately 10^{-3} microns (or a specific surface

of roughly 6×10^7 cm^2/cm^3. Milling limit refers to the size distribution to which a milling operation tends as a consequence of mill characteristics, material properties, and operating conditions when given sufficient time.

The milling process is affected by time. When the resident time in a mill is brief, the material is subjected to a relatively constant fracture-producing environment. Changes in milling conditions that are insignificant for short milling periods may be controlling factors in prolonged milling. In prolonged milling, the milling environment may not be constant.

As the particle becomes smaller with prolonged milling, the probability that an individual particle will be involved in a fracture diminishes. As size reduction proceeds, the mean stress required to cause fracture increases through the depletion of cracks, while the magnitude of available local stress decreases. Because of diminishing local stress and increasing aggregation, increases in energy expenditures are useless, and size reduction reaches some practical milling limit.[47]

An empiric equation was suggested by Harris[48] to express a limiting specific surface, S_m:

$$S = S_m [1 - \exp(-KE^n)] \qquad (39)$$

where E is energy input, and K is a constant that depends on milling conditions.

As shown in Figure 2-10, after 5 hours of ball milling, the size reduction of sulfadimethoxine reaches a limiting value.[49] The data fits the equation:

$$\frac{dS}{dt} = k_1 \exp(-k_2 S) \qquad (40)$$

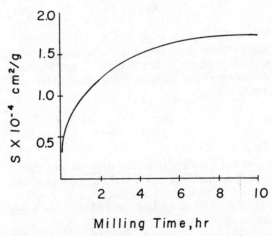

FIG. 2-10. *Increase of surface area of sulfadimethoxine with passage of ball-milling time.*

where k_1 and k_2 are parameters dependent on physical properties of the material and coherency, respectively.

The type of mill and its operation influence the milling limit. Excessive clearance between the impacting surfaces limits size reduction. In wet milling, the fineness decreases with increased viscosity, which depends on the dispersion medium, the size and concentration of particles, and the shear rate. In tumbling mills, as the particles become smaller and more numerous, friction diminishes, and the material behaves as a semisolid. Larger particles can arch and protect smaller ones from impact. Fine particles may coat the grinding medium and cushion larger particles from impact.

Milling Rate

The mass and size of particles and the time in the mill affect the milling rate. It has been reported that batch milling of brittle materials in small mills follows a first-order law.[50,51] The original particles are fractured to produce first-generation particles, which are then fractured to produce second-generation particles, which are also fractured, and so on. As this is analogous to the process of radioactive decay, milling rate is expressed in terms of a decay constant, λ, which is a function of particle size and varies with the size of the material introduced into the mill,[52] and the size of the grinding medium in a ball mill.[53]

If impact milling follows a first-order rate, the number of particles, N, that survive fracture is the product of the initial number, N_0, and the probable fraction surviving fracture at time t:

$$N = N_0 \exp(-\lambda t) \qquad (41)$$

When the average mass of a particle in a given size range is constant, then N/N_0 is equivalent to M/M_0, where M is the mass of particles yet unfractured and M_0 is the initial mass. The milling rate is:

$$\frac{dM}{dt} = -\lambda M \qquad (42)$$

For brief milling time, the survival probability is approximately $(1 - \lambda t)$, and the most probable fraction of initial material fractured is $1 - (1 - \lambda t)$, or λt. The weight of material that has been comminuted is:

$$M_o - M = M_o \lambda t \qquad (43)$$

The total mass of material in a size smaller than the largest size may increase, although the amount of original material of that size must always decrease. As particles formed from fracture of larger particles may enter the size of interest faster than the original material is fractured to a smaller size, the total mass of the size of interest is increased. A set of first-order differential equations was proposed and verified over a 30-min milling period by Sedlatschek and Bass.[54] The weight percentage of particles, M_i, having a size range between D_{i-1} and D_i has a rate change, dM_i/dt, given by:

$$-\frac{dM_i}{dt} = \lambda_{ii} M_i - \sum_{k=i+1}^{n} \lambda_{ki} M_k \qquad (44)$$

where the rate of change, dM_1/dt, is:

$$-\frac{dM_1}{dt} = -\sum_{k=1}^{n} \lambda_{k1} M_k \qquad (45)$$

In general, $\lambda_{ii} = \sum_{k=i-1}^{i} \lambda_{ik}$

where $\sum_{k=1}^{n} M_k = 100\%$.

For example, a material is milled into four arbitrary groups, $i = 1, 2, 3,$ and 4, with size limits 0.0 to 0.1, 0.1 to 0.2, 0.2 to 0.3, and 0.3 to 0.4 mm, respectively. For these limits, equations (35) and (36) have the following forms.

For Group 4, the largest size:

$$-\frac{dM_4}{dt} = \lambda_{44} M_4 \qquad (46)$$

For Group 3:

$$-\frac{dm_3}{dt} = \lambda_{33} M_3 - \lambda_{43} M_4 \qquad (47)$$

For Group 2:

$$-\frac{dM_2}{dt} = \lambda_{22} M_2 - \lambda_{32} M_3 - \lambda_{42} M_4 \qquad (48)$$

For Group 1:

$$-\frac{dM_1}{dt} = \lambda_{41} M_4 - \lambda_{31} M_3 - \lambda_{21} M_2 \qquad (49)$$

For a mass balance:

$$\lambda_{44} = \lambda_{43} + \lambda_{42} + \lambda_{41} \qquad (50)$$

$$\lambda_{33} = \lambda_{32} + \lambda_{31} \qquad (51)$$

$$\lambda_{22} = \lambda_{21} \qquad (52)$$

These equations express the rate at which the largest size, Group 4, decays; the rate at which Group 3, the next size smaller, decays as modified by the contributions from Group 4; the rate at which Group 2 decays as modified by the contributions from Groups 4 and 3; and the rate at which the smallest size of material decays as modified by the contributions of all groups.

The milling process has also been described by use of an integrodifferential equation.[55] Matrix algebra methods requiring computer solution have been proposed.[56]

Types of Mills

A mill consists of three basic parts: (1) feed chute, which delivers the material, (2) grinding mechanism, usually consisting of a rotor and stator, and (3) a discharge chute. The principle of operation depends on direct pressure, impact from a sharp blow, attrition, or cutting. In most mills, the grinding effect is a combination of these actions. The most commonly used mills in pharmaceutical manufacturing are the rotary cutter, hammer, roller, and fluid-energy mill.[50,57–59] Diagrammatic representations of these mills are shown in Figure 2-11. General characteristics of the types of mills are given in Table 2-7.

The manner in which an operator feeds a mill markedly affects the product. If the rate of feed is relatively slow, the product is discharged readily, and the amount of undersize or fines is minimized. If the mill is choke fed at a fast rate, the material is in the milling chamber for a longer

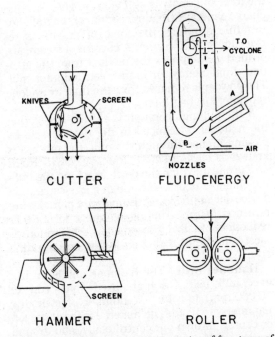

FIG. 2-11. *Diagrammatic representation of four types of mills commonly used in processing pharmaceuticals. (See text under "Fluid-Energy Mill" for explanation of labels A–D.)*

time, as its discharge is impeded by the mass of material. This provides a greater reduction of particle size, but the capacity of the mill is reduced, and power consumption is increased. Choke feed is used when a small amount of material is to be milled in one operation.

The rate of discharge should be equal to the rate of feed, which is such that the milling parts can operate most effectively. Most mills used in pharmaceutical operations are designed so that

TABLE 2-7. *General Characteristics of Various Types of Mills*

Type of Mill	Action	Product Size	Used For	Not Used For
Cutter	cutting	20- to 80-mesh	fibrous, crude animal and vegetable drugs	friable material
Revolving	attrition and impact	20- to 200-mesh	fine grinding of abrasive material	soft material
Hammer	impact	4- to 325-mesh	almost all drugs	abrasive material
Roller	pressure	20- to 200-mesh	soft material	abrasive material
Attrition	attrition	20- to 200-mesh	soft and fibrous material	abrasive material
Fluid-energy	attrition and impact	1 to 30 μm	moderately hard and friable material	soft and sticky material

the force of gravity is sufficient to give free discharge generally from the bottom of the mill. For ultrafine grinding, the force of gravity is replaced by a fluid carrier. A current of steam, air, or inert gas removes the product from the attrition, fluid-energy, or high-speed hammer mill. The powder is removed from the fluid by cyclone separators or bag filters.

If the milling operation is carried out so that the material is reduced to the desired size by passing it once through the mill, the process is known as *open-circuit milling*. A *closed-circuit mill* is one in which the discharge from the milling chamber is passed through a size-separation device or classifier, and the oversize particles are returned to the grinding chamber for further reduction of size. Closed-circuit operation is most valuable in reduction to fine and ultrafine size.

Hammer Mill. The hammer mill is an impact mill using a high-speed rotor (up to 10,000 rpm) to which a number of swinging hammers are fixed. The material is fed at the top or center, thrown out centrifugally, and ground by impact of the hammers or against the plates around the periphery of the casing. The clearance between the housing and the hammers contributes to size reduction. The material is retained until it is small enough to fall through the screen that forms the lower portion of the casing. Particles fine enough to pass through the screen are discharged almost as fast as they are formed.

The hammer mill can be used for almost any type of size reduction. Its versatility makes it popular in the pharmaceutical industry, where it is used to mill dry materials, wet filter-press cakes, ointments, and slurries. Comminution is effected by impact at peripheral hammer speeds of up to 7600 meters per minute, at which speed most materials behave as if they were brittle. Brittle material is best fractured by impact from a blunt hammer; fibrous material is best reduced in size by cutting edges. Some models of hammer mills have a rotor that may be turned 180 degrees to allow use of either the blunt edge for fine grinding or the knife edge for cutting or granulating.

In the preparation of wet granules for compressed tablets, a hammer mill is operated at 2450 rpm with knife edges, using circular or square holes of a size determined by what will pass without clogging (1.9 to 2.54 cm). In milling the dried granulation, the mill is operated at 1000 or 2450 rpm with knife edges and circular holes in the screen (0.23 to 0.27 cm). Hammer mills range in size from 5 to 500 horsepower

units; the smaller mills are especially useful for developmental and small-batch milling.

A hammer mill can be used for granulation and close control of the particle size of powders. The size of the product is controlled by selecting the speed of the hammers and the size and type of the screen. Speed is crucial. Below a critical impact speed, the rotor turns so slowly that a blending action rather than comminution is obtained. This results in overloading and a rise in temperature. Microscopic examination of the particles formed when the mill is operating below the critical speed shows them to be spheroidal, indicating not an impact action, but an attrition action, which produces irregularly shaped particles. At very high speeds, there is possibly insufficient time between hammers for the material to fall from the grinding zone. In wet milling of dispersed systems with higher speeds, the swing hammers may lay back with an increased clearance; for such systems, fixed hammers would be more effective.

Figure 2-12 shows the influence of speed on the particle size-frequency curves for boric acid milled at 1000, 2450, and 4600 rpm in a hammer mill fitted with a screen having 6.35-mm circular holes.

The screens that retain the material in the milling chamber are not woven but perforated. The particle size of the discharged material is

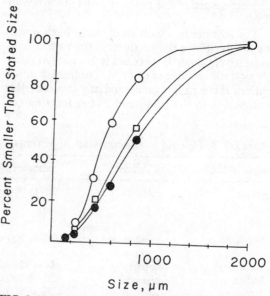

FIG. 2-12. *Influence of speed on the size-frequency distribution of boric acid flakes milled by a hammer mill operating with impact edge forward and fitted with a round hole No. 4 screen (hole diameter: 6.35 mm). Key: ●, 1000 rpm; □, 2450 rpm; and ○, 4600 rpm.*

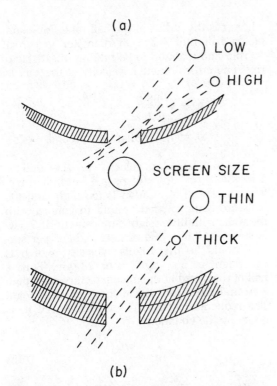

(a)

(b)

FIG. 2-13. *In a hammer mill, particle size is influenced by speed (a) and thickness of screen (b).*

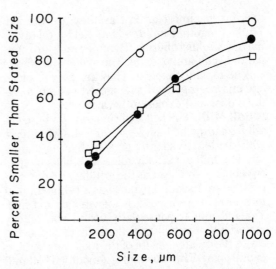

FIG. 2-14. *Influence of screen size on the size-frequency distribution of a terra alba granulation milled with a hammer mill operating at 2450 rpm, and a comparison with the granulation milled by a vertical hammer mill fitted with a no. 10 screen. Key:* ○, *hammer mill, 0.84 mm;* ●, *hammer mill, 1.65 mm; and* □, *vertical hammer mill.*

smaller than the screen hole or slot, as the particles exit through the perforation on a path approximately tangential to the rotor. For a given screen, a smaller particle size is obtained at a higher speed, as is shown in Figure 2-13. Efforts to strengthen a screen by increasing its thickness influence particle size. For a given rotor speed and screen opening, a thicker screen produces a smaller particle, which is also illustrated in Figure 2-13.

Figure 2-14 shows the influence of screen size on the size-frequency distribution of a tablet granulation that was passed through a 4-mesh screen after wet granulation with acacia, a blend of terra alba, and two active ingredients, together constituting 4.2% of the formulation. The dried granulation was milled at 2450 rpm through a Type A plate having 1.65-mm openings, and a Type B screen having 0.84-mm openings. The granulation was also milled in a hammer mill with a vertical rotor operating at medium speed and fitted with a no. 10 screen. A comparison of the particle size-frequency distributions is shown in Figure 2-14.

A circular hole design is the strongest screen and the most difficult to keep from clogging. It is recommended for the grinding of fibers. The

herringbone design consists of a series of slotted holes repeated across the surface of the screen at an angle of 45 degrees to the length of the screen. A herringbone design is preferred for grinding crystalline material and for continuous operation. A herringbone design with the width of the slot equal to the diameter of a round hole grinds more coarsely than the round hole. A herringbone design should not be used for fibrous material, as it is possible for the fibers to align themselves along the slots and pass through with inadequate size reduction.

A cross slot at right angles to the path traveled by the hammer is not used in fine grinding because it clogs readily; a cross slot is recommended for milling slurries. The jump-gap screen is a series of bars so arranged that the particle approaches a ramp, which deflects the particle into the chamber away from the opening of the screen. The jump-gap screen is for abrasive and clogging materials.

Hammer mills are compact with a high capacity. Size reduction of 20 to 40 microns may be achieved; however, a hammer mill must be operated with internal or external classification to produce ultrafine particles. Because inertial forces vary with mass as the inverse cube of the diameter, small particles with a constant velocity impact with much less kinetic energy than larger ones, and the probability that particles less than a certain size will fracture decreases rapidly. In addition, small particles pass through the screen almost as fast as they are formed. Thus, a hammer mill tends to yield a relatively narrow size distribution. Hammer mills are simple to install and operate. The speed and screen can be rapidly changed. They are easy to clean and may be operated as a closed system to reduce dust and explosion hazards.

Ball Mill. The ball mill consists of a horizontally rotating hollow vessel of cylindric shape with the length slightly greater than its diameter. The mill is partially filled with balls of steel or pebbles, which act as the grinding medium. If pebbles are used, it is known as a pebble mill; if rods or bars are used, it is known as a rod mill. The rod mill is particularly useful with sticky material that would hold the balls together, because the greater weight of the rods causes them to pull apart. The tube mill is a modified ball mill in which the length if about four times that of the diameter and in which the balls are somewhat smaller than in a ball mill. Because the material remains in the longer tube mill for a greater length of time, the tube mill grinds more finely than the ball mill. The ball mill may be modified to a conical shape and tapered at the discharge end. If balls of different size are used in a conical ball mill, they segregate according to size and provide progressively finer grinding as the material flows axially through the mill. Recently, small-scale vibration ball mills, which produce particles of a few microns, have been introduced.[60] These oscillate 1500 to 2500 cycles per minute through an amplitude of approximately 4 mm.

Most ball mills utilized in pharmacy are batch-operated; however, there are available continuous ball mills, which are fed through a hollow trunnion at one end, with the product discharged through a similar trunnion at the opposite end. The outlet is covered with a coarse screen to prevent the loss of the balls.

In a ball mill rotating at a slow speed, the balls roll and cascade over one another, providing an attrition action. As the speed is increased, the balls are carried up the sides of the mill and fall freely onto the material with an impact action, which is responsible for most size reduction. Ball milling is a combination of impact and attrition. If the speed is increased sufficiently, the balls are held against the mill casing by centrifugal force and revolve with the mill. The critical speed of a ball mill is the speed at which the balls just begin to centrifuge with the mill. Thus, at the critical speed, the centrifugal force is equal to the weight of the ball, and the critical angular velocity, ω_c, may be expressed:

$$\omega_c = \sqrt{\frac{g}{r}} \qquad (53)$$

where r is the radius of the ball mill. For example, a ball mill 1.2 m in diameter is run at 48 rpm and is found to be milling unsatisfactorily. The critical angular velocity of the mill is:

$$\omega_c = \sqrt{\frac{980}{0.6}} \qquad (54)$$

$$\omega_c = 4.04 \text{ radian per second}$$

The actual angular velocity of the mill is $2\pi(48/60)$ or 5.02 radians per second; therefore, the speed of rotation is too high, and the balls are being carried around in contact with the walls with little relative movement. If $0.6\,\omega_c$ is selected, 0.6×4.04 or 2.42 radians per second would be the angular velocity, which is equivalent to $60 \times 2.4/2\pi$ or 23 rpm. This is half of the speed of the unsatisfactory operation.

At and above the critical speed, no significant size reduction occurs. The critical speed n_c is given by the equation:

$$n_c = \frac{76.6}{\sqrt{D}} \qquad (55)$$

where D is the diameter of the mill in feet. A larger mill reaches its critical speed at a slower revolution rate than a smaller mill (a 228.6-cm ball mill and a 11.4-cm jar mill may have critical speeds of 28 and 125 rpm, respectively).

Ball mills are operated from 60 to 85% of the critical speed. Over this range, the output increases with the speed; however, the lower speeds are for finer grinding. An empiric rule for the optimum speed of a ball mill is:

$$n = 57 - 40 \log D \qquad (56)$$

where n is the speed in revolutions per minute and D is the inside diameter of the mill in feet. In actual practice, the calculated speed should be used initially in the process and modified as experience is acquired.

For a given feed, smaller balls give a slower but finer grinding. The smaller balls provide smaller voids than the larger balls; consequently, the void through which material can flow without being struck by a ball is less, and the number of impacts per unit weight of material is greater. It has been suggested that the optimum diameter of a ball is approximately proportional to the square root of the size of the feed:[59]

$$D_{ball}^2 = kD \qquad (57)$$

where D_{ball} and D are the diameters of the ball

and the feed particles, respectively. If the diameters are expressed in inches, k may be considered to be a grindability constant varying from 55 for hard to 35 for soft materials. Small balls facilitate the production of fine material, but they are ineffective in reducing large-sized feed.

The charge of balls can be expressed in terms of percentage of volume of the mill (a bulk volume of balls filling one half of a mill is a 50% ball charge). To operate effectively, a ball charge from 30 to 50% of the volume of the mill is required.

The amount of material to be milled in a ball mill may be expressed as a material-to-void ratio (ratio of the volume of material to that of the void in the ball charge). The efficiency of a ball mill is increased as the amount of material is increased until the void space in the bulk volume of ball charge is filled; then, the efficiency of milling is decreased by further addition of material.

Increasing the total weight of balls of a given size increases the fineness of the powder. The weight of the ball charge can be increased by increasing the number of balls or by using a ball composed of a material with a higher density. Since optimum milling conditions are usually obtained when the bulk volume of the balls is equal to 50% of the volume of the mill, variation in weight of the balls is normally effected by the use of materials of different densities. Thus, steel balls grind faster than porcelain balls, as they are three times more dense. Stainless steel balls are also preferred in the production of ophthalmic and parenteral products, as there is less attrition and less subsequent contamination with particulate matter.

In dry milling, the moisture should be less than 2%. With batch processing, dry ball milling produces a very fine particle size. With wet milling, a ball mill produces 200-mesh particles from slurries containing 30 to 60% solids. From the viewpoint of power consumption, wet grinding is more efficient than dry grinding. A slower speed is used in wet milling than in dry milling to prevent the mass from being carried around with the mill. A high viscosity restricts the motion of the grinding medium, and the impact is reduced. With 1.27-cm steel balls, a viscosity from 1000 to 2400 centipoises (cp) is satisfactory for wet milling.

Wetting agents may increase the efficiency of milling and the physical stability of the product by nullifying electrostatic forces produced during comminution. For those products containing wetting agents, the addition of the wetting agent at the milling stage may aid size reduction and reduce aggregation.

In addition to being used for either wet or dry milling, the ball mill has the advantage of being used for batch or continuous operation. In a batch operation, unstable or explosive materials may be sealed with an inert atmosphere and satisfactorily ground. Ball mills may be sterilized and sealed for sterile milling in the production of ophthalmic and parenteral products. The installation, operation, and labor costs involved in ball milling are low. Finally, the ball mill is unsurpassed for fine grinding of hard, abrasive materials.

Fluid-Energy Mill. In the fluid-energy mill or micronizer the material is suspended and conveyed at high velocity by air or steam, which is passed through nozzles at 100 to 150 pounds per square inch (psi). The violent turbulence of the air and steam reduces the particle size chiefly by interparticular attrition. Air is usually used because most pharmaceuticals have a low melting point or are thermolabile. As the compressed air expands at the orifice, the cooling effect counteracts the heat generated by milling.

As shown in Figure 2-11, the material is fed near the bottom of the mill through a venturi injector (A). As the compressed air passes through the nozzles (B), the material is thrown outward against the wall of the grinding chamber (C) and other particles. The air moves at high speed in an elliptical path carrying with it the fine particles that pass out of the discharge outlet (D) into a cyclone separator and a bag collector. The large particles are carried by centrifugal force to the periphery, where they are further exposed to the attrition action. The design of the fluid-energy mill provides internal classification, which permits the finer and lighter particles to be discharged and the heavier oversized particles, under the effect of centrifugal force, to be retained until reduced to a small size.

Fluid-energy mills reduce the particle to 1 to 20 microns. The feed should be premilled to approximately a 20- to 100-mesh size to facilitate milling. A 2-inch laboratory model using 20 to 25 cubic feet per minute of air at 100 psi mills 5 to 10 grams per minute. In selecting fluid-energy mills for production, the cost of a fluid-energy source and dust collection equipment must be considered in addition to the cost of the mill.

Cutting Mill. Cutting mills are used for tough, fibrous materials and provide a successive cutting or shearing action rather than attrition or impact.

The rotary knife cutter has a horizontal rotor with two to 12 knives spaced uniformly on its periphery turning from 200 to 900 rpm and a cylindric casing having several stationary knives. The bottom of the casing holds a screen that controls the size of the material discharged from the milling zone. The feed size should be less than 1 inch thick and should not exceed the length of the cutting knife. For sizes less than 20-mesh, a pneumatic product-collecting system is required. Under the best operating conditions, the size limit of a rotary cutter is 80-mesh.

A disc mill consists of two vertical discs; each may rotate in opposite directions (double-runner disc mill), or only one may rotate (single-runner disc mill), with an adjustable clearance. The disc may be provided with cutting faces, teeth, or convolutions. The material is premilled to approximately 40-mesh size and is usually suspended in a stream of air or liquid when fed to the mill.

Roller Mill. Roller mills consist of two to five smooth rollers operating at different speeds; thus, size reduction is effected by a combination of compression and shearing action.

Colloid Mill. A colloid mill consists of a high-speed rotor (3000 to 20,000 rpm) and stator with conical milling surfaces between which is an adjustable clearance ranging from 0.002 to 0.03 inches, as indicated by the schematic diagram in Figure 2-15. The rotor speed is 3000 to 20,000 rpm. The material to be ground should be premilled as finely as possible to prevent damage to the colloid mill.

In pharmacy, the colloid mill is used to process suspensions and emulsions; it is not used to process dry materials. The premilled solids are mixed with the liquid vehicle before being introduced into the colloid mill. Interfacial tension causes part of the material to adhere to, and to rotate with, the rotor. Centrifugal force throws part of the material across the rotor onto the stator. At a point between the rotor and stator, the motion imparted by the rotor ceases, and hydraulic shearing force exceeds the particle-particle attractive forces holding the individual particles in an aggregate. The particle size of milled particles may be smaller than the clearance, because the high shear is the dispersing force. In emulsification, a clearance of 75 microns may produce a dispersion with an average particle size of 3 microns. The milled liquid is discharged through an outlet in the periphery of the housing and may be recycled.

Rotors and stators may be smooth-surfaced or rough-surfaced. With a smooth-surfaced rotor and stator, there is a thin, uniform film of material between them, and it is subjected to the maximum amount of shear. Rough-surfaced mills add intense eddy currents, turbulence, and impaction of the particles to the shearing action. Rough-surfaced mills are useful with fibrous materials because fibers tend to interlock and clog smooth-faced mills.

A colloid mill tends to incorporate air into a suspension. Aeration may be minimized by use of a vertical rotor, which seals the point at which the rotor shaft enters the housing, and keeps the rotor and stator in contact with the liquid. The wasted energy of milling, which appears as heat, may raise the temperature of a liquid by as much as 40°. The passage of cooling water through the mill jacket may reduce the temperature by as much as 20°. Sanitary design mills, which may be sterilized, are available.

Factors Influencing Milling

The properties of a solid determine its ability to resist size reduction and influence the choice of equipment used for milling. The specifications of the product also influence the choice of a mill. The grindability of coal is expressed in terms of numbers of revolutions of a standardized ball mill required to yield a product of which 80% passes a 200-mesh screen. Although a similar expression could be applied to pharmaceutical materials, no quantitative scale has been adopted to express hardness. It is perhaps as useful to speak of hard, intermediate, and soft materials. Hard materials (iodine, pumice) are those that are abrasive and cause rapid wear of mill parts immediately involved in size reduction.

The physical nature of the material determines the process of comminution. Fibrous materials (glycyrrhiza, rauwolfia) cannot be crushed by pressure or impact; they must be cut. Friable materials (dried filter cake, sucrose) tend to fracture along well-defined planes and may be

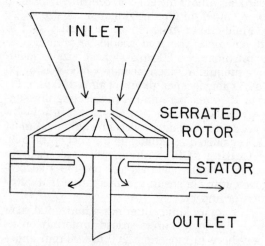

FIG. 2-15. *Colloid mill with a rotor and stator with a narrow clearance that may be adjusted.*

milled by an attrition, impact, or pressure process. The presence of more than 5% water hinders comminution and often produces a sticky mass upon milling. This effect is more pronounced with fine materials than with larger particles. At concentrations of water greater than 50%, the mass becomes a slurry, or fluid suspension. The process then is a wet milling process, which often aids in size reduction. An increase in moisture can decrease the rate of milling to a specified product size. Glauber's salt and other drugs possessing water of crystallization liberate the water at low temperatures, causing clogging of the mill. Hygroscopic materials (calcium chloride) rapidly sorb moisture to the extent that the wet mass sticks and clogs the mill.

The heat during milling softens and melts materials with a low melting point. Synthetic gums, waxes, and resins become soft and plastic. Heat-sensitive drugs may be degraded or even charred. Pigments (ocher and sienna) may change their shade of color if the milling temperature is excessive. Unstable compounds and almost any finely powdered material may ignite and explode if the temperature is high.

Other product specifications influence the choice of a mill. The shape of the milled particles may be important. An impact mill produces sharp, irregular particles, which may not flow readily. When specifications demand a milled product that will flow freely, it would be better to use an attrition mill, which produces free-flowing spheroidal particles.

Milling may alter crystalline structure and cause chemical changes in some materials. Wet milling may be useful in producing a suspension that contains a metastable form causing crystal growth and caking. For example, when cortisone acetate crystals are allowed to equilibrate with an aqueous vehicle, subsequent wet milling provides a satisfactory suspension.[61] Starch, amylose, and amylopectin may be broken down by a vibratory mill to a wide molecular weight range.[62] Powdered povidone breaks down into lower molecular weight polymers during ball milling.[63] Pure C_{12}- and C_{16}-fatty acids may be decarboxylated and converted to the hydrocarbon containing one less carbon atom by ball milling with wet sand.[64] Milling well-dried microcrystalline cellulose from 1 to 25 hours decreases its crystallinity.[65] Excessive shear of a colloid mill may damage polymeric suspending agents so that there is a loss of viscosity.[66] A decrease in particle size of crystals in a hammer mill was reported to increase the rate of crystal growth during storage, owing to alterations in crystal lattice and the formation of active sites.[67]

Specifically, crystals of phenobarbital (initial size of 310 microns) milled to 22.7 microns grew to 38.9 microns after 4 weeks at 60°C; however, crystals milled to 31.5 microns showed little growth on storage.

Selection of a Mill

In general, the materials used in pharmaceuticals may be reduced to a particle size less than 40-mesh by means of ball, roller, hammer, and fluid-energy mills. The types of mill used to reduce some typical pharmaceutical materials are shown in Table 2-8. The choice of a mill is based on (1) product specifications (size range, particle size distribution, shape, moisture content, physical and chemical properties of the material); (2) capacity of the mill and production rate requirements; (3) versatility of operation (wet and dry milling, rapid change of speed and screen, safety features); (4) dust control (loss of costly drugs, health hazards, contamination of plant); (5) sanitation (ease of cleaning, sterilization); (6) auxiliary equipment (cooling system, dust collectors, forced feeding, stage reduction); (7) batch or continuous operation; and (8) economical factors (cost, power consumption, space occupied, labor cost).

After consideration of these factors (listed in Table 2-9) for a specific milling problem, it is suggested that the equipment manufacturer be consulted and its pilot laboratory be utilized, as there exists a wide variety of mills differing in details of design and modifications. The industrial pharmacist should evaluate the pilot study personally to observe the temperature of the inlet and outlet air, the temperature of the milled material, and the size reduction performance at different mill speeds. A size-frequency analysis should be made on samples from each condition of operation. Samples should be recycled to find if there is buildup in the milling chamber. The pilot evaluation is important because laboratory procedures of size reduction do not duplicate milling conditions in production mills.

Techniques of Milling

In addition to the standard adjustments of the milling process (i.e., speed, screen size, design of rotor, load), special techniques of milling may be useful.

Special Atmosphere. Hygroscopic material can be milled in a closed system supplied with dehumidified air. Thermolabile, easily oxidizable, and combustible materials should be milled in a closed system with an inert atmosphere of carbon dioxide or nitrogen. Almost any fine dust

TABLE 2-8. *Index for Milling to Less Than 40-mesh Size*

Materials	Mill
Acetanilid	ball, roller, hammer, fluid-energy
Alum	ball, roller, hammer, fluid-energy
Antibiotics	ball, hammer, colloid, fluid-energy
Ascorbic acid	ball, roller, hammer, fluid-energy
Barium sulfate	hammer, colloid, fluid-energy
Benzoic acid	hammer, fluid-energy
Boric acid	ball, roller, hammer, fluid-energy
Caffeine	roller, hammer
Calcium stearate	hammer, colloid, fluid-energy
Carboxymethylcellulose	ball, hammer, colloid, fluid-energy
Citric acid	hammer, fluid-energy
Color, dry	ball, hammer, fluid-energy
Color, wet	hammer, colloid, fluid-energy
Filter-cake fluid energy	ball, roller, hammer, colloid
Gelatin	hammer
Iodine	hammer, fluid-energy
Methylcellulose	ball, hammer
Sodium acid phosphate	hammer, fluid-energy
Sodium benzoate	hammer, fluid-energy
Sodium metaphosphate	hammer, fluid-energy
Sodium salicylate	hammer, fluid-energy
Stearates	hammer, fluid-energy
Sugar	hammer, fluid-energy
Urea	ball, hammer, fluid-energy
Vitamins	ball, hammer, fluid-energy
Wax	hammer, colloid, fluid-energy

(dextrin, starch, sulfur) is a potential explosive mixture under certain conditions and especially if static electrical charges result from the processing. All electrical switches should be explosion-proof, and the mill should be grounded.

Temperature Control. As only a small percentage of the energy of milling is used to form new surface, the bulk of the energy is converted to heat. This heat may raise the temperature of the material many degrees, and unless the heat is removed, the solid will melt, decompose, or explode. To prevent these changes in the material and to avoid stalling of the mill, the milling chamber should be cooled by means of a cooling jacket or a heat exchanger. Stainless steel equipment (Type 304 with no. 4 finish) is routinely used in preparing pharmaceuticals because it minimizes contamination and reaction with the drugs. With the use of refrigerants, the mill must be constructed of stainless steel since cast iron becomes brittle and may shatter at low temperatures.

Waxy and low-melting-point materials are chilled before milling. If this is not sufficient to embrittle the material, it may be fed to the mill simultaneously with dry ice. Stearic acid and beeswax may be reduced in a hammer mill to 100-mesh size with the use of dry ice.

Pretreatment. For a mill to operate satisfactorily, the feed should be of the proper size and enter at a fairly uniform rate. If granules or intermediate-sized particles are desired with a minimum of fines, presizing is vital. Pretreatment of fibrous materials with high-pressure rolls or cutters facilitates comminution.

Subsequent Treatment. If extreme control of size is required, it may be necessary to recycle the larger particles, either by simply screening the discharge and returning the oversize particles for a second milling, or by using air-separation equipment in a closed circuit to return the oversized particles automatically to the milling chamber. With materials to be reduced to micron size, an integrated air-separation, conveyor, and collection element usually are required.

Dual Process. The milling process may serve simultaneously as a mixing process if the feed materials are heterogeneous. If hot gas is circulated through a mill, the mill can be used to comminute and dry moist solids simultaneously. The fluid-energy mill has been suggested as a means of simultaneous size reduction and dis-

TABLE 2-9. *Factors in Selection of a Mill*

Material

Physical property: hard, soft, fibrous, elastic, hygroscopic, solvated
Size
Moisture content
Melting point
Flammability
Thermolability
Subsequent processing

Operation

Size specification of milled material
Ease of sanitization
Ease of sterilization
Ease of adjustments during operation
Contamination of milled material
Versatility
Capacity
Batch or continuous
Wet or dry
Rate of introduction of material
Space occupied
Labor cost

Auxiliary Equipment

Dust collector
Mechanical introduction of material
Temperature control: jacket, refrigerated air, liquid nitrogen, dry ice
Inert atmosphere: carbon dioxide, nitrogen
Air sweep

Safety

Explosivity
Irritativity
Toxicity
Safety features incorporated into mill

From Parrott, E. L.: J. Pharm. Sci., 63:826, 1974. Reproduced with permission of the copyright owner, the American Pharmaceutical Association.

---

persion. It has been suggested that the particles in a fluid-energy mill can be coated with almost a monomolecular film by premixing with as little as 0.25% of the coating agent.

Wet and Dry Milling. The choice of dry or wet milling depends on the use of the product and its subsequent processing. If the product undergoes physical or chemical change in water, dry milling is recommended. In dry milling, the limit of fineness is reached in the region of 100 microns when the material cakes on the milling chamber. The addition of a small amount of grinding aid may facilitate size reduction. The use of grinding aids in pharmacy is limited by the physiologic and toxicologic restrictions on medicinal products. In certain cases, the addition of ammonium salts, aluminum stearate, arylalkyl sulfonic acid, calcium stearate, oleic acid, and triethanolamine salts have been useful. These dispersing agents are especially useful in the revolving mill if coating of the balls occurs; the addition of less than 0.1% of surface-active agent may increase the production rate of a ball mill 20 to 40%.

Wet grinding is beneficial in further reducing the size, but flocculation restricts the lower limit to approximately 10 microns. Wet grinding eliminates dust hazards and is usually done in low-speed mills, which consume less power. Some useful dispersing agents in wet grinding are the silicates and phosphates.

References

1. Kraml, M., Dubue, J., and Gaudry, R.: Antibiot. Chemother., 12:232, 1962.
2. Ober, S. S., Vincent, H. C., Simon, D. E., and Frederick, K. J.: J. Am. Pharm. Assoc., Sci. Ed., 47:667, 1958.
3. Parrott, E. L.: J. Pharm. Sci., 64:878, 1975.
4. MacDonald, L. H., and Himelick, R. E.: J. Am. Pharm. Assoc., Sci. Ed., 37:368, 1948.
5. Kanig, J.: J. Pharm. Sci., 52:513, 1963.
6. Fincher, J. H.: J. Pharm. Sci., 57:1825, 1968.
7. Tingstad, J. E.: J. Pharm. Sci., 53:955, 1964.
8. Garrett, E. R., Schumann, E. L., and Grostic, M. F.: J. Am. Pharm. Assoc., Sci. Ed., 48:684, 1959.
9. Sumner, E. D., Thompson, H. O., Poole, W. K., and Grizzle, J. E.: J. Pharm. Sci., 55:1441, 1966.
10. Gold, G., Duvall, R. N., Palermo, B. T., and Slater, J. G.: J. Pharm. Sci., 57:668, 1968.
11. Danish, F. Q., and Parrott, E. L.: J. Pharm. Sci., 60:548, 1971.
12. Cooper, J., and Rees, J. E.: J. Pharm. Sci., 61:1511, 1972.
13. Parrott, E. L.: Drug and Cosm. Ind., 115:42, 1974.
14. Danish, F. Q., and Parrott, E. L.: J. Pharm. Sci., 60:752, 1971.
15. Hatch, T.: J. Franklin Inst., 215:27, 1933.
16. Orr, C., Jr., and Dallavalle, J. M.: Fine Particle Measurement. Macmillan Company, New York, 1959.
17. Irani, R. R., and Callis, C. F.: Particle Size Measurement, Interpretation and Application. John Wiley & Sons, New York, 1963.
18. Dallavalle, J. M.: Micromeritics. 2nd Ed. Pitman Publishing Corporation, New York, 1948.
19. Edmundson, I. C.: Advances in Pharmaceutical Sciences. Vol. 2. Academic Press, New York, 1967.
20. Piret, E. L.: Chem. Eng. Prog., 49:56, 1953.
21. Heywood, H.: J. I. C. Chem Eng. Soc., 6:26, 1951.
22. Austin, L. G., and Klimpel, R. R.: Ind. Eng. Chem., 56:18, 1964.
23. Bond, F. C.: Min. Eng., 4:484, 1952.
24. Riley, R. V.: Chem. Proc. Eng., 46:189, 1965.
25. Parrott, E. L.: J. Pharm. Sci., 63:813, 1974.
26. Kwong, J. N. S., Adams, J. T., Jr., Johnson, J. F., and Piret, E. L.: Chem. Eng. Prog., 45:508, 1949.
27. Griffith, A. A.: Phil. Trans. Roy. Soc. London, Ser. A, 221:163, 1921.
28. Schoenert, K.: Trans. AIME, 251:21, 1972.
29. Orowan, E.: Dissolution in Metals. American Insti-

tute of Mineral and Petroleum Engineers, New York, 1954, Chapter 3.

30. Orowan, E.: Z. Kristallogr., *A89*:327, 1934.
31. Jomoto, E., and Majima, H.: Can. Inst. Min. Met. Bull., 65:68, 1972.
32. Zeleny, R. A., and Piret, E. L.: Ind. Eng. Chem. Process, Des. Develop., *1*:337, 1962.
33. Boozer, G. D., Miller, K. H., and Serdenqecti, S.: Proceedings of the 5th Symposium on Rock Mechanics. Pergamon, New York, 1963, p 579.
34. Dijingheuzian, L. E.: Can. Inst. Min. Met. Bull., 45:658, 1952.
35. Bond, F. C.: Chem. Eng., 59:242, 1952.
36. Gross, J.: U.S. Bur. Mines Bull., 402, 1938.
37. Coulson, J. M., and Richardson, J. F.: Chemical Engineering. Vol. II. Pergamon Press, New York, 1978.
38. Kick, F.: Das Gesetz der proportionalen Widerstande und seine Anwendung. Arthur Felix, Leipsig, Germany, 1885.
39. Walker, D. R., and Shaw, M. C.: Trans. AIME, *199*:313, 1954.
40. von Rittinger, R. P.: Lehrbuch der Aufbereitungskunde. Ernst and Korn, Berlin, Germany, 1867, p. 19.
41. Bond, F. C.: Chem. Eng., Albany, 59:169, 1952.
42. Bond, F. C.: Trans. AIME, *193*:484, 1952.
43. Mular, A. L.: Can. Met. Quart., 4:31, 1965.
44. Schuhmann, R., Jr.: Mining Technol., *4*, Tech. Publ. No. 1189, 1940.
45. Charles, R. J.: Trans. AIME, 208:80, 1957.
46. Hatch, T., and Choate, S. P.: J. Franklin Inst., 207:369, 1929.
47. Berg, T. G. O., and Avis, L. E.: Powder Technol., 4:27, 1970.
48. Harris, C. C.: Trans. AIME, 238:17, 1967.
49. Kaneniwa, N., Ikekawa, A., and Hashimoto, D.: Chem. Pharm. Bull., 21:676, 1973.
50. Kirk-Othmer: Encyclopedia of Chemical Technology. Vol. 18. 2nd Ed. John Wiley and Sons, New York, 1969, p. 336.
51. Klimpel, R. R., and Austin, L. G.: Ind. Eng. Chem. Fundam., 9:230, 1970.
52. Roberts, E. J.: Trans. AIME, *187*:1267, 1950.
53. Bowdish, F. J.: AIME, SME Preprint No. 61B2, 1961.
54. Sedlatschek, K., and Bass, L.: Powder Met. Bull., 6:148, 1953.
55. Reid, K. J.: Chem. Eng. Sci., 20:953, 1965.
56. Gaudin, A. M., and Moloy, T. P.: Trans. AIME, 223:34, 1962.
57. Berry, C. E.: Ind. Eng. Chem., 38:672, 1946.
58. Stern, A. L.: Chem. Eng., 69:130, 1962.
59. Perry, J. H.: Chemical Engineers' Handbook. 4th Ed. McGraw-Hill, New York, 1963.
60. McDonald, D. P.: Mfg. Chem. Aerosol News, 42:42, 1971.
61. Macke, T. J., U.S. Pat. 2,671,759. 1954.
62. Augustat, S.: Ernaehrungsforschung, 13:475, 1968.
63. Kaneniwa, N., and Ikekawa, A.: Chem. Pharm. Bull., 20:1536, 1972.
64. Scalan, S., U.S. Pat. 3,391,211. 1968.
65. Ogura, K., and Sobue, H.: J. Appl. Polm. Sci., 14:1390, 1970.
66. Kennon, L., and Storz, G. K.: Pharmaceutical Suspensions. *In* The Theory and Practice of Industrial Pharmacy. Edited by L. Lachman et al. 2nd Ed. Lea & Febiger, Philadelphia, 1976.
67. Weiss, H.: Pharmazie, 32:674, 1977.

3

Drying

ALBERT S. RANKELL, HERBERT A. LIEBERMAN,
and ROBERT F. SCHIFFMANN

There is hardly a pharmaceutical plant engaged in the manufacture of tablets or capsules that does not contain dryers. Unfortunately, the operation of drying is so taken for granted that efforts for achieving increased efficiency in the production of tablets do not include a study of drying. This chapter introduces the industrial pharmacist to the theory and fundamental concepts of drying.

Definition. For the purpose of this discussion, drying is defined as the removal of a liquid from a material by the application of heat, and is accomplished by the transfer of a liquid from a surface into an unsaturated vapor phase. This definition applies to the removal of a small amount of water from moisture-bearing table salt as well as to the recovery of salt from the sea by evaporation. Drying and evaporation are distinguishable merely by the relative quantities of liquid removed from the solid.

There are, however, many nonthermal methods of drying, for example, the *expression* of a solid to remove liquid (the squeezing of a wetted sponge), the *extraction* of liquid from a solid by use of a solvent, the *adsorption* of water from a solvent by the use of desiccants (such as anhydrous calcium chloride), the *absorption* of moisture from gases by passage through a sulfuric acid column, and the *desiccation* of moisture from a solid by placing it in a sealed container with a moisture-removing material (silica gel in a bottle).

Purpose. Drying is most commonly used in pharmaceutical manufacturing as a unit process in the preparation of granules, which can be dispensed in bulk or converted into tablets or capsules. Another application is found in the processing of materials, e.g., the preparation of dried aluminum hydroxide, the spray drying of lactose, and the preparation of powdered extracts. Drying also can be used to reduce bulk and

weight, thereby lowering the cost of transportation and storage. Other uses include aiding in the preservation of animal and vegetable drugs by minimizing mold and bacterial growth in moisture-laden material and facilitating comminution by making the dried substance far more friable than the original, water-containing drug.

Dried products often are more stable than moist ones, as is the case in such diverse substances as effervescent salts, aspirin, hygroscopic powders, ascorbic acid, and penicillin. The drying reduces the chemical reactivity of the remaining water, which is expressed as a reduction in the water activity of the product. Various processes for the removal of moisture are used in the production of these materials. After the moisture is removed, the product is maintained at low water levels by the use of desiccants and/or low moisture transmission packaging materials. The proper application of drying techniques and moisture-protective packaging requires a knowledge of the theory of drying, with particular reference to the concept of equilibrium moisture content.

Psychrometry

A critical factor in drying operations is the vapor-carrying capacity of the air, nitrogen, or other gas stream passing over the drying material. This carrying capacity determines not only the rate of drying but also the extent of drying, i.e., the lowest moisture content to which a given material can be dried. The determination of the vapor concentration and carrying capacity of the gas is termed *psychrometry*. The air–water vapor system is the system most commonly employed in pharmaceutical drying operations and is therefore included in this discussion.

The concentration of water vapor in a gas is

called the *humidity* of the gas. Humidity may be expressed in various ways, depending on the information required. A knowledge of humidity is necessary, therefore, to understand the basic principles of drying.

Psychrometric Chart. The humidity characteristics of air are best shown graphically in a *psychrometric* or *humidity chart*. Such charts can be found in various handbooks.[1,2] The psychrometric chart has a formidable look because of the wealth of information presented in a small area. If the different curves in the chart are separated and analyzed individually, however, their utility and ease of use becomes apparent.

The basic curves of the psychrometric chart are shown in a simplified version in Figure 3-1. These curves are graphic representations of the relationship between the temperature and humidity of the air–water vapor system at constant pressure. The temperature is shown in the hori-

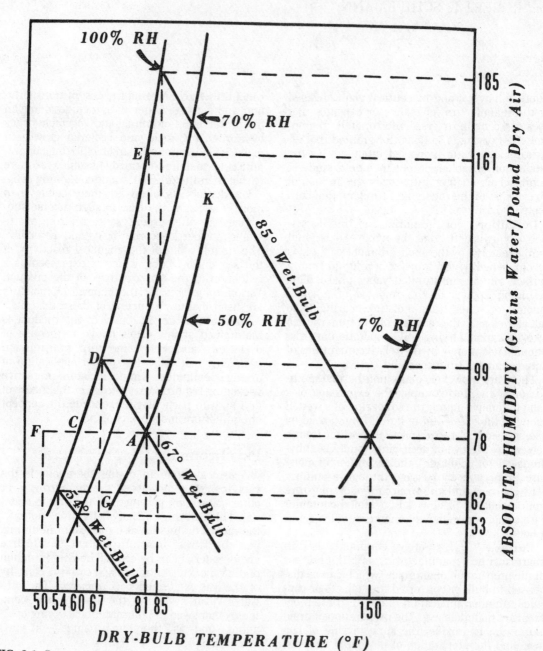

FIG. 3-1. *Diagram of psychrometric chart showing the relationship of air temperature to humidity.*

zontal axis; the vertical axis represents *absolute humidity* (weight of water vapor per unit weight of dry air). The most important curve shown is the curve for *saturation humidity,* curve CDE. Saturation humidity is the absolute humidity at which the partial pressure of water vapor in the air is equal to the vapor pressure of free water at the same temperature. Under these conditions, the air is completely saturated with moisture, and the humidity does not change when it is in contact with liquid water at the same temperature.

The saturation humidity curve is actually the boundary of a phase diagram. Any point on the curve is uniquely determined by one measurement, either the temperature or the absolute humidity. The relationship between the two variables can be shown more clearly by considering the dotted line, FCA, which corresponds to the absolute humidity, 78 grains water/pound dry air.

At point C, the air is saturated with water vapor, and its temperature, 60°F, is referred to as the *dew point.* The dew point is defined as the temperature to which a given mixture of air and water vapor must be cooled to become saturated (i.e., to hold the maximum amount of moisture without condensation taking place). When the mixture is cooled to temperatures below the dew point, such as 50°F (point F), the water vapor condenses to produce a two-phase system of saturated air (condition C) and droplets of free water.

To make the air usable for drying purposes (without changing the absolute humidity), its temperature must be raised. If the temperature is increased to 81°F (point A), the air is not completely saturated and can accept more water vapor. The relative saturation is usually measured in terms of *percent relative humidity*, the ratio of the partial pressure of water vapor in the air to the vapor pressure of free water at the same temperature. The saturation humidity curve, CDE, is thus the curve for 100% relative humidity (100% RH). Curves of temperature versus absolute humidity at a constant relative humidity are plotted on the same axes at specific intervals of relative humidity. One of these curves is shown as curve GK with 50% relative humidity. The relative saturation also can be expressed as *percent humidity* or *percent absolute humidity,* the ratio of the absolute humidity to saturation humidity at the same temperature. For air at condition A, the percent absolute humidity is represented by the ratio of the absolute humidity to the absolute humidity of saturated air at that temperature (78/161 = 48%).

If air, under the conditions represented by point A, is used to dry a wet material, the difference in vapor pressure between the surface water and the air causes some of the liquid to evaporate. The latent heat of vaporization of the water cools the evaporating surface below the air temperature. The resultant difference in temperature causes a transfer of heat from the air to the liquid at a rate that increases as the temperature difference becomes larger. Eventually, the heat transferred becomes equal to the heat of vaporization, and the temperature stabilizes. The temperature that is reached is called the *wet-bulb temperature.* It is defined as the equilibrium temperature reached by an evaporating surface when the rate of heat transferred to the surface by convection is equal to the rate of heat lost by evaporation. It is called the wet-bulb temperature because it can be measured by means of a thermometer whose bulb is covered by a wick saturated with water. The actual temperature of the air as measured by an ordinary thermometer is called the *dry-bulb temperature.*

The wet-bulb temperature is a function of the temperature and humidity of the air used for the evaporation, and thus can be employed as a means of measuring humidity. For this purpose, a second type of curve is superimposed on the temperature-humidity curves of the psychrometric chart. This is the *constant wet-bulb temperature* line. The constant wet-bulb temperature line is AD for air at condition A, and the temperature corresponding to saturation at point D is the wet-bulb temperature, 67°F.

The humidity of the air is determined by measuring two temperatures, the *wet-bulb* and the *dry-bulb* temperatures. The psychrometric chart is entered at the wet-bulb temperature, and the coordinate is followed vertically upward until it intersects the saturation or 100% relative humidity curve. Then the constant wet-bulb temperature line is followed until it intersects the dry-bulb temperature coordinate. Now the absolute humidity can be read directly, and the relative humidity can be found by interpolation between the curves for constant relative humidity. For example, let us assume a wet-bulb temperature of 54°F and a dry-bulb temperature of 60°F. The 54°F line is followed until it intersects the saturation humidity curve at an absolute humidity of 62 grains water/pound dry air. Then, the 54°F wet-bulb temperature line is followed until it intersects the 60°F dry-bulb temperature line at an absolute humidity of 53 grains water/pound dry air. The relative humidity is found to be 70%.

The constant wet-bulb temperature lines are also valuable for determining the temperature of drying surfaces. The wet-bulb temperature is approximately the same as the *adiabatic saturation temperature*, i.e., the temperature that would be attained if the air were saturated with water vapor in an adiabatic process (a process in which there is no heat gained or lost to the surroundings). This is the case when drying is carried out with the heat supplied by the drying air only. Thus, for the example given above, a wet material being dried with air having a wet-bulb temperature of 70°F would remain at that temperature as long as there is a film of free moisture at the surface. The assumption that the wet-bulb temperature is equal to the adiabatic saturation temperature does not hold true, however, for nonaqueous systems.

Humidity Measurement. The most accurate means of measuring humidity is by the *gravimetric method*. In this procedure, a known amount of air is passed over a previously weighed moisture-absorbing chemical such as phosphorus pentoxide, and the resultant increase in weight of the chemical is measured. Although accurate, the gravimetric method is cumbersome and slow. For rapid determination of humidity, temperature-measurement methods are most often used.

As indicated in the discussion of the psychrometric chart, humidity can be determined by taking two temperature measurements. The simplest instrument for this purpose is the *sling psychrometer* (Fig. 3-2). It consists of two bulb thermometers set in a frame that is attached to a swivel handle. One thermometer, the *dry-bulb thermometer*, has a bare bulb; the bulb of the other thermometer, the *wet-bulb thermometer*, is covered by a wick saturated with water. The psychrometer is whirled through the air, and the two thermometer readings are taken at successive intervals until these temperatures no longer change. In psychrometers used as permanent installations, the movement of air across the

thermometer bulbs is induced by a motor-driven fan, and a reservoir is provided to keep the wet-bulb wick saturated with water. The thermometers used in such an installation may be of almost any type—mercury bulb, bimetallic strip, vapor pressure, or electrical.

Another temperature method for determining humidity is based on the dew point instead of the wet-bulb temperature measurement. The dew point is determined directly by observing the temperature at which moisture begins to form on a polished surface in contact with the air. The surface is cooled by refrigeration until the first fog of moisture appears.

An entirely different method for measuring humidity employs the *hygrometer*. This instrument utilizes certain materials whose properties change on contact with air of different relative humidities. The *mechanical hygrometer* uses such materials as hair, wood fiber, or plastics, which expand or shrink with changes in humidity. The moisture-sensitive element is connected to a pointer in such a fashion that a change in length causes the pointer to move across a dial calibrated in humidity units. *Electric hygrometers* measure the change in electrical resistance of moisture-absorbing materials with humidity.

Theory of Drying

Drying involves both heat and mass transfer operations. Heat must be transferred to the material to be dried in order to supply the latent heat required for vaporization of the moisture. Mass transfer is involved in the diffusion of water through the material to the evaporating surface, in the subsequent evaporation of the water from the surface, and in diffusion of the resultant vapor into the passing air stream.

The drying process can be understood more easily if attention is focused on the film of liquid at the surface of the material being dried. The rate of evaporation of this film is related to the rate of heat transfer by the equation:

$$dW/d\theta = q/\lambda \qquad (1)$$

where $dW/d\theta$ is the rate of evaporation pounds of water per hour, q is the overall rate of heat transfer (BTU per hour), and λ is the latent heat of vaporization of water (BTU per pound).

The rate of diffusion of moisture into the air stream is expressed by rate equations similar to those for heat transfer. The driving force is a humidity differential, whereas for heat transfer, it is a temperature differential. The rate equation is as follows.

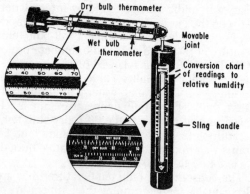

FIG. 3-2. *Sling psychrometer.*

$$dW/d\theta = k'A(H_s - H_g) \qquad (2)$$

where $dW/d\theta$ is the rate of diffusion expressed as pounds of water per hour; k' is the coefficient of mass transfer [pounds of water/(hour) (square foot) (absolute humidity difference)]; A is the area of the evaporating surface in square feet; H_s is the absolute humidity at the evaporating surface (pounds of water per pound of dry air); and H_g is the absolute humidity in the passing air stream (pounds of water per pound of dry air).

The coefficient of mass transfer, k', is not a constant, but varies with the velocity of the air stream passing over the evaporating surface. The relationship is in the form:

$$k' = cG^n \qquad (3)$$

where c is a proportionality constant, G is the rate of flow of air [pounds of dry air/(hour) (square foot)], and n is a fractional exponent, usually about 0.8.[2]

After an initial period of adjustment, the rate of evaporation is equal to the rate of diffusion of vapor, and the rate of heat transfer [equation (1)] can be equated with the rate of mass transfer [equation (2)], or:

$$dW/d\theta = q/\lambda = k'A(H_s - H_g). \qquad (4)$$

If the overall rate of heat transfer, q, is expressed as the sum of the rates of heat transfer by convection, radiation, and conduction, equation (4) is expanded to the form:

$$dW/d\theta = (q_c + q_r + q_k)/\lambda$$
$$= k'A(H_s - H_g) \qquad (5)$$

where q_c, q_r, and q_k are the rates of heat transfer by convection, radiation, and conduction, respectively.

The rate of drying may be accelerated by increasing any of the individual terms in equation (5). The rate of convection heat transfer, q_c, can be increased by increasing the air flow rate and by raising the inlet air temperature. The rate of radiation heat transfer, q_r, can be speeded up by introducing a high-temperature radiating heat source into the drying chamber. The rate of conduction heat transfer, q_k, can be stepped up by reducing the thickness of the material being dried and by allowing it to come in contact with raised-temperature surfaces. Increasing the air velocity also speeds up the rate of drying by increasing the coefficient of mass transfer, k', as

shown in equation (3). Dehumidifying the inlet air, thus increasing the humidity differential, $(H_s - H_g)$, is still another means of speeding up the rate of drying.

Rapid drying may also be accomplished through the application of a microwave or dielectric field. In this case, heat is generated internally by the interaction of the applied electromagnetic field with the solvent. Mass transfer results from an internal pressure gradient established by the internal heat generation, while the mass concentration remains relatively uniform. The drying rate, then, primarily depends on the strength of the field applied to the material.

The utility of equation (5) in actual practice can be demonstrated by the following analysis: What is the effect of heating the air in a dryer to 150°F if the outside air is 81°F with 50% relative humidity? From the psychrometric chart (Fig. 3-1), it can be seen that for ambient air at this condition (point A), the absolute humidity is 78 grains water/pound dry air. Following the wet-bulb temperature line from this point to the saturation curve (point D) yields an absolute humidity of 99 grains water/pound dry air.

For the ambient air, the humidity differential $(H_s - H_g)$ is (99 − 78), which is equal to 21 grains (0.003 pounds) water/pound dry air. When this air is heated to 150°F, the absolute humidity remains the same, but the relative humidity is now reduced to 7%, and following the new wet-bulb temperature line (85°F) to the saturation curve yields a saturation humidity of 185 grains water/pound dry air. The humidity gradient is now 185 − 78, which is equal to 107 grains (0.0153 pounds) water/pound dry air, an increase of fivefold, indicating an increase in drying rate of 500% produced by a 69°F rise in temperature. In actual practice, the increase in drying rate would be even higher because increasing the inlet air temperature would increase k' as well as the humidity gradient. It should be noted that this increase in the drying rate does not produce a serious increase in the temperature of the material being dried, because the wet-bulb temperature of the 150°F air is only 85°F.

The foregoing discussion holds true as long as there is a film of moisture on the surface of the material being dried. When the surface becomes partially or completely dry, the heat and mass transfer equations become more complex. In this case, the rate of drying is controlled by the rate of diffusion of moisture from the interior of the material. This diffusion is greatly influenced by the molecular and capillary structure of the solid. The process becomes further complicated when the drying surface causes a shrinkage of the solid. This phenomenon can cause blocking and distortion of the capillary structure and thus interfere with the transfer of internal water to the surface of the material. A striking example of this is the so-called "case hardening" phenomenon, in which the surface of the solid becomes harder than the interior and less permeable to the transmission of interior moisture.

Drying of Solids

Loss on Drying. The moisture in a solid can be expressed on a wet-weight or dry-weight basis. On a wet-weight basis, the water content of a material is calculated as a percentage of the weight of the *wet* solid, whereas on the dry-weight basis, the water is expressed as a percentage of the weight of the dry solid.

In pharmacy, the term *loss on drying*, commonly referred to as LOD, is an expression of moisture content on a wet-weight basis, which is calculated as follows:

$$\% \text{ LOD} = \frac{\text{wt. of water in sample}}{\text{total wt. of wet sample}} \times 100$$

$$(6)$$

The LOD of a wet solid is often determined by the use of a moisture balance, which has a heat source for rapid heating and a scale calibrated in percent LOD. A weighed sample is placed on the balance and allowed to dry until it is at constant weight. The water lost by evaporation is read directly from the percent LOD scale. It is assumed that there are no other volatile materials present.

Moisture Content. Another measurement of the moisture in a wet solid is that calculated on a dry-weight basis. This value is referred to as *moisture content,* or MC:

$$\% \text{ MC} = \frac{\text{wt. of water in sample}}{\text{wt. of dry sample}} \times 100$$

$$(7)$$

If exactly 5 g of moist solid is brought to a constant dry weight of 3 g:

$$\text{MC} = \frac{5 - 3}{3} \times 100 = 66.7\%$$

$$\text{whereas} \quad \text{LOD} = \frac{5 - 3}{5} \times 100 = 40\%$$

LOD values can vary in any solid-fluid mixture from slightly above 0% to slightly below 100%, but the MC values can change from slightly above 0% and approach infinity. Thus, a small change in LOD value, from 80% to 83%, represents an increase in MC of 88%, or a 22% increase in the amount of water that must be evaporated per pound of dry product. Thus, percent MC is a far more realistic value than LOD in the determination of dryer load capacity.

Behavior of Solids During Drying. How would one know if 8 or 12 hours are required to dry a batch weight of material in a certain dryer? How can one determine the size of a particular type of dryer required for drying a substance from one moisture level to the desired moisture content?

The rate of drying of a sample can be determined by suspending the wet material on a scale or balance in a drying cabinet and measuring the weight of the sample as it dries as a function of time. In determining an accurate drying rate curve for a material in a particular oven, it is important that the drying conditions approximate the conditions in a full-size dryer as closely as possible.

The information obtained from the drying rate determination may be plotted as moisture content versus time. The resultant curve is of the type shown in Figure 3-3. The changes taking place may be seen more easily if the rate of drying is calculated* and plotted against the moisture content as shown in Figure 3-3B. Comparison of the rate of drying curve with the drying time curve is clarified when the moisture content is plotted in reverse order, i.e., with the high values to the left.

When a wet solid is first placed in a drying oven, it begins to absorb heat and increases in temperature. At the same time, the moisture begins evaporating and thus tends to cool the drying solid. After a period of initial adjustment, the rates of heating and cooling become equal and the temperature of the drying material stabilizes. As long as the amount of heat transfer by radiation is relatively small, the temperature reached equals the wet-bulb temperature of the drying air. This period of initial adjustment is shown as segment AB in Figures 3-3A and 3-3B. If the wet solid is initially at a higher temperature than the wet-bulb temperature, it cools down following segment A′B.

---

*Method of determining rate of drying: The difference in moisture content between any two measurements divided by the time period between measurements represents the rate of drying for this time period. This value is plotted against the midpoint of the time period for a drying rate versus time curve, or against the midpoint of the moisture content values for a drying rate versus moisture content curve.

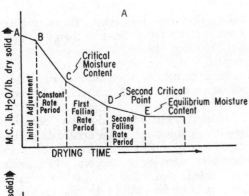

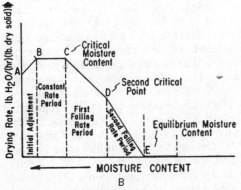

FIG. 3-3. *The periods of drying.*

At point B, the temperature is stabilized and remains constant as long as there is a film of moisture remaining at the surface of the drying solid. Between points B and C, the moisture evaporating from the surface is replaced by water diffusing from the interior of the solid at a rate equal to the rate of evaporation. The rate of drying is constant, and the time BC is the *constant rate period*.

At point C, the surface water is no longer replaced at a rate fast enough to maintain a continuous film. Dry spots begin to appear, and the rate of drying begins to fall off. The moisture content at which this occurs is referred to as the *critical moisture content*. Between points C and D, the number and area of the dry spots continue to grow, and the rate of drying falls steadily. The time CD is referred to as the *first falling rate period* or the period of *unsaturated surface drying*.

At point D, the film of surface water is completely evaporated, and the rate of drying depends on the rate of diffusion of moisture to the surface of the solid. Point D is referred to as the *second critical point*. Between points D and E the rate of drying falls even more rapidly than the first falling rate, and time DE is called the *second falling rate period*.

When the drying rate is equal to zero, starting at point E, the equilibrium moisture period begins, and the solid is in equilibrium with its surroundings, i.e., its temperature and moisture content remain constant. Continued drying after this point is a waste of time and energy.

Classification of Solids Based on Drying Behavior. Solids may be classified into two major categories on the basis of their drying behavior, namely (1) granular or crystalline type solids and (2) amorphous solids. The water in crystalline solids is held in shallow and open surface pores as well as in interstitial spaces between particles that are easily accessible to the surface. Materials with fibrous, amorphous, or gelatinous structures are in the second category. In these solids, the moisture is an integral part of the molecular structure as well as being physically entrapped in fine capillaries and small interior pores. Typical pharmaceuticals of the first category are calcium sulfate, zinc oxide, and magnesium oxide. Materials that fall into the second category are starch, casein, yeast, insulin, and gelatinous inorganic materials such as aluminum hydroxide. All of the amorphous solid materials are more difficult to dry than granular or crystalline solids.

The moisture in crystalline solids is lost with little hindrance by either gravitational or capillary forces. The constant rate period is the major portion of the drying curve, and this period continues until the material has virtually no free water. The falling rate period is much shorter. Materials in this category are usually inorganic substances and consequently are not affected by heat, unless the temperature is high enough to change any hydrate forms that the chemical may manifest. Equilibrium moisture contents for these materials are close to zero.

Moisture movement is slow in substances in the second category. The liquid diffuses through structural obstacles caused by the molecular configuration. The drying curves of these amorphous materials have short constant-rate periods, ending at high critical moisture contents. The first falling rate period, the period of water unsaturation on the surface, is relatively short. The second drying rate period is longer, as it depends on the diffusion rate of the water through the solid. The equilibrium moisture content is high, because most of the water remains intimately associated within the molecular interstitial spaces of the substance. The structure and physiologic activity of many of these substances are affected by high temperatures. The drying of these materials often requires the use of lower temperatures, reduced pressure, and increased air flow.

The condition in which a material is in equilibrium with its surroundings, neither gaining nor losing moisture, may be expressed in terms of its *equilibrium moisture content, equilibrium relative humidity,* or *water activity.* These values may differ greatly for various materials, and in addition to affecting drying, they affect physical and chemical stability, susceptibility to microbial growth, and packaging requirements.

Equilibrium Moisture Content. The moisture content of a material that is in equilibrium with an atmosphere of a given relativity is called the *equilibrium moisture content* (EMC) of the material at this humidity. It is the moisture content at which the material exerts a water vapor pressure equal to the vapor pressure of the atmosphere surrounding it; thus, it has no driving force for mass transfer. EMC values of various materials may differ greatly under the same conditions, despite the fact that they are in equilibrium with their environment. These differences are due to the manner in which the water is held by the material. The water may be held in fine capillary pores that have no easy access to the surface, dissolved solids may reduce the vapor pressure, or the water may be molecularly bound.

Equilibrium Relative Humidity. The relative humidity surrounding a material at which the material neither gains nor loses moisture is called the *equilibrium relative humidity* (ERH). At a given temperature, the ERH for a material is determined by its moisture content, just as the EMC is determined by the surrounding relative humidity.

Water Activity. The *water activity* (a_w) of a material is the ratio of the water vapor pressure exerted by the material to the vapor pressure of pure water at the same temperature. Pure water is assigned an a_w of unity, equivalent to an ERH of 100%. Thus, the water activity value for a material is the decimal fraction corresponding to the ERH divided by 100. For example, an ERH of 50% corresponds to an a_w of 0.5.

The water activity value has special significance because it is a measure of the relative chemical activity of the water in the material. It is related to the thermodynamic chemical potential by the equation:

$$U = U' + RT \cdot \ln(a_w) \qquad (8)$$

where U is the chemical potential of water in the material; U' is the chemical potential of pure water; R is the gas law constant; T is the absolute temperature; and ln is the natural logarithm.[3]

The smaller the water activity is, the smaller are the chemical potential of the water and the driving force for chemical reactions involving water. The most important effects of lowered water activity are increased chemical stability and reduced potential for micro-organism growth. Water activity can be reduced by the addition of solutes such as sucrose, glycerin, polyols, and surfactants, as well as by reduced moisture content.

Measurement Methods. The equilibrium moisture content of a material can be determined by exposing samples in a series of closed chambers, such as desiccators, which are partially filled with solutions that can maintain fixed relative humidities in the enclosed air spaces. (Lists of such solutions can be found in any handbook of chemistry.) The exposure is continued until the material comes to constant weight. This process, which can take more than a month for some materials, can be accelerated by placing a revolving fan in the chamber or by passing air currents with proper humidity and temperature over the material. Curves of the EMC versus relative humidity have been determined for many pharmaceutical substances.[4] Typical curves are illustrated in Figure 3-4.

Equilibrium relative humidity and water activity of a material can be measured by allowing the material to equilibrate in a small vapor tight chamber, such as a glass jar, with a hygrometer humidity sensor (mechanical or electric) mounted on the lid. This measurement procedure is much more rapid than the EMC technique; it yields practical near equilibrium values

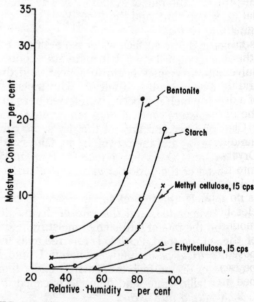

FIG. 3-4. *Equilibrium moisture content curves for tabletting materials. (Adapted from Scott, M. W., Lieberman, H. A., and Chow, F. S.: J. Pharm. Sci., 52: 994, 1963.)*

in several hours, and true end points in a day or two.[5]

Knowledge of the EMC versus relative humidity curve or ERH versus moisture content for a product allows more intelligent selection of the drying conditions to be used. The relative humidity of the air in the dryer must be lower than the ERH, corresponding to the desired moisture content of the product being dried. In general, the product should be dried to a moisture content corresponding to the EMC at the ambient conditions of processing and storage. If the moisture content differs markedly from this EMC, the product will pick up or lose moisture unless precautions are taken either to maintain the product under controlled humidity conditions or to use packaging materials with low water vapor transmission rates.

Classification of Dryers

Dryers may be classified in several different ways depending on the criteria used. Two useful classifications are based on either the method of heat transfer or the method of solids handling. Classification according to the type of heat transfer is important in demonstrating gross differences in dryer design, operation, and energy requirements. Classification by the method of solids handling is more suitable when special attention must be given to the nature of the material to be dried.

When dryers are classified according to their method of solids handling, the major criterion is the presence or absence of *agitation* of the material to be dried. A dryer that produces excessive agitation is contraindicated when the dried material is friable and subject to attrition. On the other hand, if the dried product is intended to be pulverized, then the drying time can be reduced, and the process made more efficient, by the use of a dryer that produces intense agitation during the drying cycle.

Classification based on the method of solids handling is shown schematically in Figure 3-5. Dryers in this classification scheme are divided into the following types:

1. *Static-bed dryers*—systems in which there is no relative movement among the solid particles being dried, although there may be bulk motion of the entire drying mass. Only a fraction of the total number of particles is directly exposed to heat sources. The exposed surface can be increased by decreasing the thickness of the bed and allowing drying air to flow through it.

2. *Moving-bed dryers*—systems in which the drying particles are partially separated so that they flow over each other. Motion may be induced by either gravity or mechanical agitation. The resultant separation of the particles and continuous exposure of new surfaces allow more rapid heat and mass transfer than can occur in static beds.

3. *Fluidized-bed dryers*—systems in which the solid particles are partially suspended in an upward-moving gas stream. The particles are lifted and then fall back in a random manner so that the resultant mixture of solid and gas acts like a boiling liquid. The gas-solid contact is excellent and results in better heat and mass transfer than in static and moving beds.

4. *Pneumatic dryers*—systems in which the drying particles are entrained and conveyed in a high-velocity gas stream. Pneumatic systems further improve on fluidized beds, because there is no channeling or short-circuiting of the gas flow path through a bed of particles. Each particle is completely surrounded by an envelope of drying gas. The resultant heat and mass transfer are extremely rapid; thus, drying times are short.

Because of the great variety of available drying equipment, it is impossible to describe all types of dryers. Attention is devoted to those that find ready application to the production of pharmaceuticals. These dryers are grouped according to their method of solids handling.

Static-Bed Systems

Tray and Truck Dryers. The dryers most commonly used in pharmaceutical plant operations are tray and truck dryers. An example of a tray dryer is illustrated in Figure 3-6. Tray dryers are sometimes called shelf, cabinet, or compartment dryers. This dryer consists of a cabinet in which the material to be dried is spread on tiers of trays. The number of trays varies with the size of the dryer. Dryers of laboratory size may contain as few as three trays, whereas larger dryers often hold as many as twenty trays.

A truck dryer is one in which the trays are loaded on trucks (racks equipped with wheels), which can be rolled into and out of the drying cabinet. In plant operations, the truck dryer is preferred over the tray dryer because it offers greater convenience in loading and unloading. The trucks usually contain one or two tiers of trays, with about 18 or more trays per tier. Each tray is square or rectangular and about 4 to 8 square feet in area. Trays are usually loaded from 0.5 to 4.0 inches deep with at least 1.5 inches clearance between the surface and the bottom of the tray above.

Drying in tray or truck dryers is a batch procedure, as opposed to continuous drying as per-

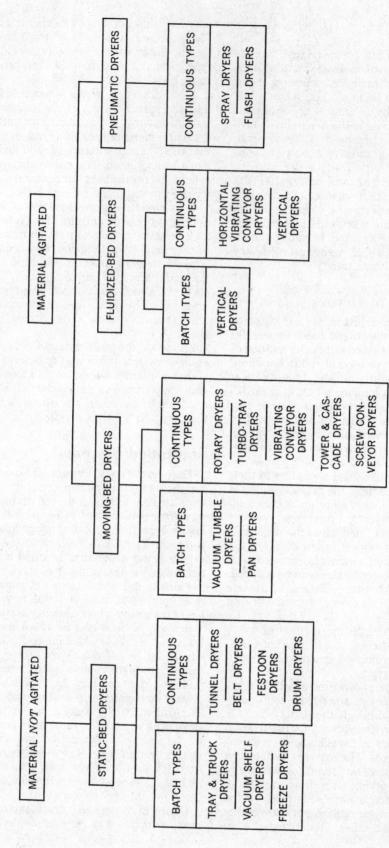

FIG. 3-5. *Classification of dryers, based on methods of solids handling.*

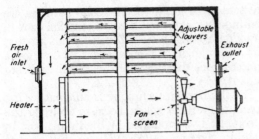

FIG. 3-6. *Tray dryer. (Courtesy of the Proctor and Schwartz Company.)*

formed in a moving belt dryer. Batch drying is used extensively in the manufacture of pharmaceuticals for several reasons: (1) Each batch of material can be handled as a separate entity. (2) The batch sizes of the pharmaceutical industry are relatively small (500 or less pounds per batch) compared with the chemical industry (2000 or more pounds per hour). (3) The same equipment is readily adjusted for use in drying a wide variety of materials.

Tray dryers may be classified as direct or indirect. Most tray dryers used in the pharmaceutical industry are of the direct type, in which heating is accomplished by the forced circulation of large volumes of heated air. Indirect tray dryers utilize heated shelves or radiant heat sources inside the drying chamber to evaporate the moisture, which is then removed by either a vacuum pump or a small amount of circulated gas. Further discussion in this section is confined to the direct (convection-type) dryer. Vacuum dryers are described separately later in the chapter.

The trays used have solid, perforated, or wire mesh bottoms. The circulation of drying air in trays with a solid base is limited to the top and bottom of the pan, whereas in trays with a perforated screen, the circulation can be controlled to pass through each tray and the solids on it. The screen trays used in most pharmaceutical drying operations are lined with paper, and the air thus circulates across rather than through the drying material. The paper is used as a disposable tray liner to reduce cleaning time and prevent product contamination.

To achieve uniform drying, there must be a constant temperature and a uniform airflow over the material being dried. This is accomplished in modern dryers by the use of a well-insulated cabinet with strategically placed fans and heating coils as integral parts of the unit. The air circulates through the dryer at 200 to 2000 feet per minute. The use of adjustable louvers helps to eliminate nonuniform airflow and stagnant pockets.

The preferred energy sources for heating the drying air used on pharmaceutical products are steam or electricity. Units fired with coal, oil, and gas produce higher temperatures at lower cost, but are avoided because of possible product contamination with fuel combustion products, and explosion hazards when flammable solvents are being evaporated. Steam is preferred over electricity, because steam energy is usually cheaper. If steam is not readily available, and drying loads are small, electric heat is used.

Tunnel and Conveyor Dryers. Tunnel dryers are adaptations of the truck dryer for continuous drying. The trucks are moved progressively through the drying tunnel by a moving chain. These trucks are loaded on one side of the dryer, allowed to reside in the heating chamber for a time sufficiently long to effect the desired drying, and then discharged at the exit. The operation may be more accurately described as *semicontinuous,* because each truck requires individual loading and unloading before and after the drying cycle. Heat is usually supplied by direct convection, but radiant energy also may be used.

Conveyor dryers are an improvement over tunnel dryers because they are truly *continuous.* The individual trucks of the tunnel are replaced with an endless belt or screen that carries the wet material through the drying tunnel. Conveyor dryers provide for uninterrupted loading and unloading and are thus more suitable for handling large volumes of materials.

The drying curve characteristic of the material in batch drying is altered considerably when continuous type dryers are used. As the mass is moved along its drying path in a continuous operation, this mass is subjected to drying air, the temperature and humidity of which are continually changing. As a consequence, the "constant rate" period is not constant, but decreases as the air temperature decreases, although the surface temperature of the wetted mass remains constant. Thus, drying rate curves for batch drying are not equally applicable to continuous drying procedures.

Moving-Bed Systems

Turbo-Tray Dryers. The turbo-tray dryer, illustrated in Figure 3-7, is a continuous shelf, moving-bed dryer. It consists of a series of rotating annular trays arranged in a vertical stack, all of which rotate slowly at 0.1 to 1.0 rpm. Heated air is circulated over the trays by turbo-type fans mounted in the center of the stack. Wet mass fed through the roof of the dryer is leveled by a stationary wiper. After about seven-eighths of a revolution, the material being dried is pushed

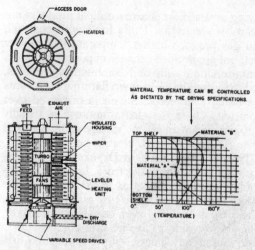

FIG. 3-7. *Turbo-tray dryer. (Courtesy of the Wyssmont Company.)*

through radial slots onto the tray below, where it is again spread and leveled. The transfer of mass from one shelf to the next is complete after one revolution. The same procedure continues throughout the height of the dryer until the dried material is discharged at the bottom. Because the turbo-tray dryer continuously exposes new surfaces to the air, drying rates are considerably faster than for tunnel dryers.

Pan Dryers. Pan dryers are moving-bed dryers of the indirect type that may operate under atmospheric pressure or vacuum, and are generally used to dry small batches of pastes or slurries. The dryer consists of a shallow, circular jacketed pan having a diameter of 3 to 6 feet and depth of 1 to 2 feet, with a flat bottom and vertical sides. Heat is supplied by steam or hot water. There is a set of rotating plows in the pan that revolve slowly, scraping the moisture-laden mass from the walls and exposing new surfaces to contact with the heated sides and bottom. Atmospheric pan drying allows moisture to escape, whereas in vacuum dryers, in which the pan is completely enclosed, solvents are recoverable if the evacuated vapors are passed through a condenser. The dried material is discharged through a door on the bottom of the pan.

Fluidized-Bed Systems

If a gas is allowed to flow upward through a bed of particulate solids at a velocity greater than the settling velocity of the particles and less than the velocity for pneumatic conveying, the solids are buoyed up and become partially suspended in the gas stream. The resultant mixture of solids and gas behaves like a liquid, and the solids

are said to be *fluidized*. The solid particles are continually caught up in eddies and fall back in a random boiling motion. The gas-solids mixture has a zero angle or repose, seeks its own level, and assumes the shape of the vessel that contains it.

The fluidization technique is efficient for the drying of granular solids, because each particle is completely surrounded by the drying gas. In addition, the intense mixing between the solids and gas results in uniform conditions of temperature, composition, and particle size distribution throughout the bed.

Fluidized bed drying has been reported to offer distinct advantages over conventional tray drying for tablet granulations.[6] In general, tablet granulations have the proper particle sizes for good fluidization. The only requirements are that the granules are not so wet that they stick together on drying, and that the dried product is not so friable as to produce excessive amounts of fine particles through attrition. It was found that the fluidized bed dryer showed a twofold to six-fold advantage in thermal efficiency* over a tray dryer. The fluidized bed dryer was also shown to be significantly faster in both drying and handling time than the tray dryer. To avoid electrostatic charge buildup and the resultant explosion hazards, fluid beds are provided with static charge grounding devices.

Types of Fluidized-Bed Dryers. The fluidized-bed dryers available for use in the pharmaceutical industry are of two types, *vertical* and *horizontal*. The design features of a vertical fluidized-bed dryer are shown in Figure 3-8. The fluidizing air stream is induced by a fan mounted in the upper part of the apparatus. The air is heated to the required temperature in an air heater and flows upward through the wet material, which is contained in a drying chamber fitted with a wire mesh support at the bottom. The air flow rate is adjusted by means of a damper, and a bag collector filter is provided at the top of the drying chamber to prevent carryover of fine particles. The unit described is a batch-type dryer, and the drying chamber is removed from the unit to permit charging and dumping. Dryer capacities range from 5 kg to 200 kg and the average drying time is about 20 to 40 min. Because of the short drying time and excellent mixing action of the dryer, no hot spots are produced, and higher drying temperatures can be employed than are used in conventional tray and truck dryers.

---

*Thermal efficiency is the ratio of the minimum energy input theoretically required to dry a material to the actual energy input used by the dryer.

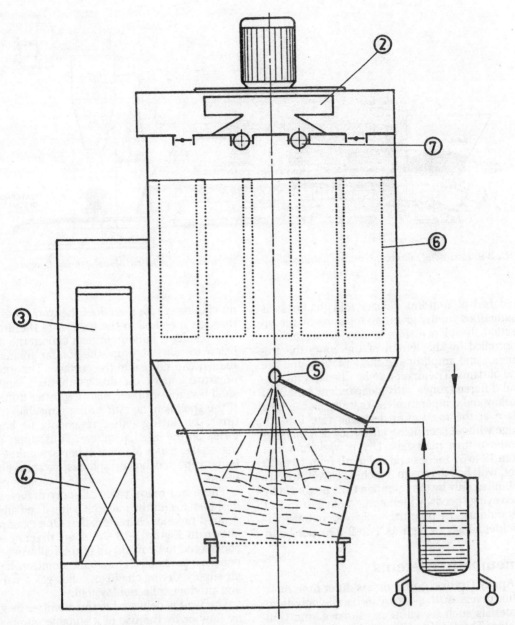

FIG. 3-8. *Fluidized-bed granulator-dryer: 1, product container; 2, blower fan; 3, air inlet pre-filter; 4, air heater (steam or electric); 5, spray nozzle for granulating liquid; 6, fabric filter bags; 7, air volume control flap. (Courtesy of Aeromatic AG.)*

The unit shown in Figure 3-8 is designed for the direct preparation of tablet granulations as well as for the drying of conventionally produced wet granulations.[7] When the unit is used as a granulator, the dry ingredients are placed in the chamber and fluidized while the granulating liquid is sprayed into the bed, causing the particles to agglomerate into granules. At the end of the granulating cycle, the granules are dried by heating the fluidizing air.

A continuous dryer is more suitable than a batch type for the drying of larger volumes of materials. A fluidized-bed dryer of this type, which is suitable for pharmaceutical use, is a horizontal vibrating conveyor dryer, shown in Figure 3-9. The heated air is introduced into a chamber below the vibrating conveying deck and passes up through the perforated or louvered conveying surface, through the fluidized bed of solids, and into an exhaust hood. A fluid-

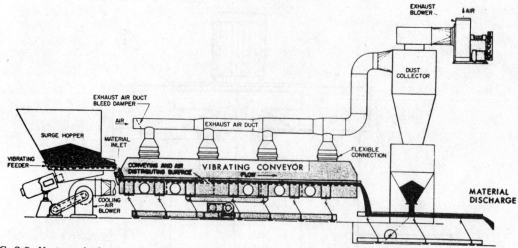

FIG. 3-9. *Horizontal vibrating conveyor fluidized bed dryer. (Courtesy of the Jeffrey Manufacturing Company.)*

ized bed of uniform density and thickness is maintained in any given drying zone by the vibration. Residence time in any drying zone is controlled by the length of the zone, the frequency and amplitude of the vibration, and the use of dams. The dryer can be divided into several different zones with independent control of airflow and temperature, so that drying can take place at the maximum desirable rate in each stage without sacrificing efficiency or damaging heat-sensitive materials. Dryers vary in width from 12 to 57 inches and in length from 10 to 50 feet, with bed depths to 3 inches. Dryer capacity is limited only by the retention time produced by conveying speeds, which range from 5 to 25 feet per minute. In pharmaceutical operations, capacities range as high as 1 to 2 tons per hour.

Pneumatic Systems

Spray Dryers. Spray dryers differ from most other dryers in that they can handle only fluid materials such as solutions, slurries, and thin pastes. The fluid is dispersed as fine droplets into a moving stream of hot gas, where they evaporate rapidly before reaching the wall of the drying chamber. The product dries into a fine powder, which is carried by the gas current and gravity flow into a collection system.

When the liquid droplets come into contact with the hot gas, they quickly reach a temperature slightly above the wet-bulb temperature of the gas. The surface liquid is quickly evaporated, and a tough shell of solids may form in its place. As drying proceeds, the liquid in the interior of the droplet must diffuse through this shell. The diffusion of the liquid occurs at a much slower rate than does the transfer of heat through the shell to the interior of the droplet. The resultant buildup of heat causes the liquid below the shell to evaporate at a far greater rate than it can diffuse to the surface. The internal pressure causes the droplet to swell, and the shell becomes thinner, allowing faster diffusion. If the shell is nonelastic or impermeable, it ruptures, producing either fragments or budlike forms on the original sphere. Thus, spray-dried material consists of intact spheres, spheres with buds, ruptured hollow spheres, or sphere fragments.

There are many types of spray dryers, each designed to suit the material being dried and the desired product characteristics. One example is shown in Figure 3-10. All spray dryers can be considered to be made up of the following components: feed delivery system, atomizer, heated air supply, drying chamber, solids-gas separator, and product collection system.

The feed is delivered to the atomizer by gravity flow or by the use of a suitable pump. The rate of feed is adjusted so that each droplet of sprayed liquid is completely dried before it comes in contact with the walls of the drying chamber, and yet the resultant dried powder is not overheated in the drying process. The proper feed rate is determined by observation of the outlet air temperature and visual inspection of the walls of the drying chamber. If the inlet air temperature is kept constant, a drop in the liquid feed rate is reflected by a rise in the outlet temperature. Excessive feed rates produce a lowering of the outlet temperature, and ultimately, a buildup of material on the walls of the chamber.

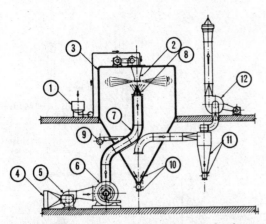

FIG. 3-10. *Spray dryer: 1, feed tank; 2, centrifugal atomizer; 3, drying chamber; 4, inlet air filter; 5, air supply fan; 6, air heater; 7, triple inlet duct; 8, adjustable air disperser; 9, cooling air fan; 10, chamber product collection; 11, cyclone product collection; 12, exhaust fan. (Courtesy of Nichols Engineering & Research Corp.)*

Spray dryer atomizers are of three basic types: pneumatic atomizers, pressure nozzles, and spinning disc atomizers. In the pneumatic atomizer (also called two-fluid or gas-atomizing nozzle), the liquid feed is broken up into droplets by a high-velocity jet of air or other gas. Pneumatic atomizers are used to produce small particles and for spraying more viscous liquids than can be handled by pressure nozzles. The pneumatic atomizer, however, requires more power than other type atomizers to achieve the same fine spray. The liquid feed is delivered by pressure nozzles under high pressure (up to 7000 pounds per square inch) and is broken up on coming into contact with the air or by impact on another jet or fixed plate. In spinning disc atomizers, the liquid is fed to the center of a rapidly rotating disc (3000 to 50,000 rpm), where centrifugal force breaks the fluid up into droplets. Spinning disc atomizers find wide utility in the spray drying of pharmaceuticals because of their ability to handle all types of liquid feeds, including high-viscosity liquids and slurries of particles that would clog other atomizers.

Hot drying air is supplied by the blowing of air over a heat exchanger. The heat may be supplied by steam, or by direct- or indirect-fired heaters. The usual heat source in laboratory units is electricity or gas. Steam or indirect-fired heaters are preferred in the spray drying of pharmaceuticals because their use avoids product contamination with combustion products.

Separation of the solid product from the effluent gas is usually accomplished by means of a cyclone separator. It is referred to as the *primary collector.* The dried product collected at this

point is referred to as *cyclone product.* Any dust remaining in the air may be removed by means of a filter bag collector or a wet scrubber to avoid air pollution. Product that reaches the walls of the drying chamber, referred to as *chamber product,* is removed at the bottom of the chamber. This chamber product is usually coarser in size and subjected to heat longer (because of increased retention time) than is the cyclone product. The final dried product is *usually* a mixture of both the chamber and cyclone products.

Spray Drying and Spray Congealing of Pharmaceuticals. Spray drying finds great utility in the pharmaceutical industry because of the rapidity of drying and the unique form of the final product. There are three major uses for the spray drying processes: (1) drying heat-sensitive materials, (2) changing the physical form of materials for use in tablet and capsule manufacture, and (3) encapsulating solid and liquid particles.

Spray drying can be used to dry materials that are sensitive to heat and/or oxidation without degrading them, even when high temperature air is employed. The liquid feed is dispersed into droplets, which are dried in seconds because of their high surface area and intimate contact with the drying gas. The product is kept cool by vaporization of the enveloping liquid, and the dried product is kept from overheating by rapid removal from the drying zone.

Spray drying is valuable in the modification of materials for use in tablet and capsule formulations, because the drying process changes the shape, size, and bulk density of the dried product.[8] The spherical particles produced usually flow better than the same product dried by conventional procedures, because the particles are more uniform in size and shape, with fewer sharp edges. The spherical shape has the least possible surface area, thus minimizing air entrapment between the particles. The improvement in flow and reduction of air entrapment make the spray dried material suitable for use in the manufacture of tablets and capsules. The spherical particle shape is obtained by spray drying either a solution of the material or a slurry of particles in a saturated solution of the same material. In the latter case, the configuration of the suspended particle is rounded out by deposition of the material in solution. An example of a spray dried material that is commonly used as a tablet excipient is spray dried lactose.

Spray drying has proved extremely useful in the coating and encapsulation of both solids and liquids. Solid particles are coated by spray drying a suspension of the material in a solution of the coating agent. As the solvent is evaporated, the coating material envelops the suspended particle. The coating provides such valuable characteristics as taste and odor masking, improvement in stability, enteric coating, and sustained release. Oily liquids may be encapsulated by emulsification in water with the aid of a gum such as acacia, or starch, and subsequent spray drying. As the water evaporates, the oil is entrapped in a shell of the gum. This process is used for the preparation of "dry" flavor oils.

An alternative to spray for the encapsulation of solid particles is *spray chilling* or *spray congealing*. This process consists of suspending the particles in a molten coating material and pumping the resultant slurry into a spray dryer in which cold air is circulated. The slurry droplets congeal on coming into contact with the air and are collected in the same manner as the spray dried product. The coating agents normally employed are low melting materials such as waxes. The congealing process requires a much higher ratio of coating agent to active material than does spray drying, because only the molten coating agent constitutes the liquid phase. Spray congealed coatings are used mainly for taste masking and for sustained-release formulations.

Flash Dryers. In flash drying, the moistened solid mass is suspended in a finely divided state in a high-velocity (3000 to 6000 feet per minute), high-temperature (300°F to 1300°F) air stream. The dispersed particles may be carried in the air stream to an impact mill, or the pneumatic flow itself may reduce the particle size of friable material. The resultant attrition exposes new surfaces for more rapid drying. The dried, fine particulate matter passes through a duct with an opening small enough to maintain desired air-carrying velocities. The dried solid is collected by a cyclone separator, which may be followed by a bag collector or wet scrubber. Thus, the flash dryer is an example of a parallel (cocurrent) airflow drying system.

The drying process is referred to as *flash drying,* because the drying time is extremely short. The drying air temperature can drop from 1300°F to 600°F in two seconds and to 350°F in only four seconds. The temperature of the drying solid can be kept at 100°F or less.

The drying cycle in many flash dryers occurs in one unit (single-stage conveyor). Multistage units are employed for drying solids that have high moisture content and contain large amounts of bound water. Figure 3-11 illustrates a two-stage unit wherein partial drying occurs in the first unit, and drying is completed in the second pneumatic conveyor dryer. In other units,

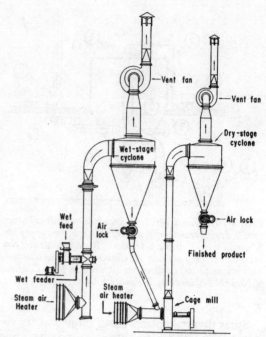

FIG. 3-11. *Two-stage flash dryer. (Courtesy of the Raymond Div., Combustion Eng., Inc.)*

some of the dried material is mixed with the wet incoming solid to make it easier to mill.

Specialized Drying Methods

Freeze Dryers. Many products of pharmaceutical interest lose their viability in the liquid state and readily deteriorate if dried in air at normal atmospheric pressures. These pharmaceutical materials may be heat-sensitive or they may react readily with oxygen, so that in order to be stabilized, they must be dehydrated to a solid state. The material to be dried is first frozen and then subjected under a high vacuum to heat (supplied by conduction or radiation, or by both) so that the frozen liquid sublimes leaving only the solid, dried components of the original liquid. Such materials as blood serum, plasma, antibiotics, hormones, bacterial cultures, vaccines, and many foodstuffs are dehydrated by *freeze drying,* also referred to as *lyophilization, gelsiccation* or *drying by sublimation.* The dried product can be readily redissolved or resuspended by the addition of water prior to use, a procedure referred to as *reconstitution.*

Freeze drying depends on the phenomenon of *sublimation,* whereby water passes directly from the solid state (ice) to the vapor state without passing through the liquid state. As shown in the schematic pressure-temperature diagram for

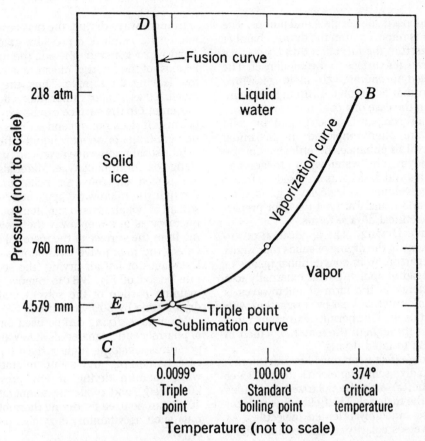

FIG. 3-12. *Schematic pressure-temperature diagram for water, showing the conditions for various phases. (This figure is not drawn to scale because of the wide range of pressures involved.) (From Daniels, F., and Alberty, R. A.: Physical Chemistry. 2nd Ed., John Wiley and Sons, Inc., New York, N.Y., 1961, p. 131.)*

water (Fig. 3-12), sublimation can take place at pressures and temperatures below the triple point, 4.579 mm Hg absolute (4579 microns) and 0.0099°C. The water in pharmaceutical products intended for freeze drying contains dissolved solids, resulting in a different pressure-temperature relationship for each solute. In such cases, the pressure and temperature at which the frozen solid vaporizes without conversion to a liquid is referred to as the *eutectic point*. Freeze drying is carried out at temperatures and pressures well below this point to prevent the frozen water from melting, which would result in frothing, as the liquid and frozen solid vaporize simultaneously. In actual practice, freeze drying of pharmaceuticals is carried out at temperatures of −10°C to −40°C, and at pressures of 2000 to 100 microns.

Freeze drying must meet the three basic requirements for all types of drying, despite this unusual approach to drying. First, the vapor pressure of the water on the surface of the mate-

rial being dried must be higher than the partial pressure of the enveloping atmosphere, i.e., there must be a positive vapor pressure driving force. Second, the latent heat of vaporization must be introduced to the drying solid at such a rate as to maintain desirable temperature levels at both the surface and interior. Third, provision must be made for removal of the evaporated moisture.

Freeze dryers are composed of four basic components: (1) a chamber for vacuum drying, (2) a vacuum source, (3) a heat source, and (4) a vapor-removal system. The chamber for vacuum drying is generally designed for batch operation and thus can be compared to the vacuum shelf dryer. Special inlet and outlet mechanisms have been designed in some drying chambers to achieve a continuous drying operation. Vacuum is achieved by pumps, steam ejectors, or a combination of the two. Heat is provided by conduction or radiation, or by both. Three different methods for the removal of water vapor are employed: condensers, desiccants, and pumps. The water vapor is removed from the drying chamber and condensed in the form of a thin layer of ice on a heat-transfer surface in the condenser. The ice is removed intermittently by melting it with a heated fluid that is circulated through the condenser, or in the case of a continuous operation, by means of scraper blades. Liquid or solid desiccants are often employed in the initial vapor removal to enhance the efficiency of the pumps removing the water vapor. In general, scraper blades and desiccants are used for freeze drying large-volume biologicals (e.g., serum, penicillin), and usually are not used for preparing pharmaceutical dosage forms.

Microwave Drying. The application of microwave energy to the drying of solids represents a radical departure from conventional means of drying. Instead of applying heat externally to a material, energy in the form of microwaves is converted into internal heat by interaction with the material itself. This permits extremely rapid heat transfer throughout the material, which in turn can lead to rapid drying.

The heating effect is produced by the interaction of a rapidly oscillating electric field (915 or 2450 megahertz) with the polarized molecules and ions in the material. The field imposes order on otherwise randomly oriented molecules. As the field reverses polarity, it relaxes and allows the molecules to return to their random orientation, giving up stored potential energy as random kinetic energy, or heat. The interaction of the alternating field with ions causes billiard-ball-like collisions with un-ionized molecules, and the impact energy is converted into heat.

A given material's molecular and ionic makeup intimately affects its ability to be dried, as is shown in the power conversion equation for microwave heating:[9]

$$P = kfE^2\epsilon' \tan \delta = kfE^2\epsilon'' \qquad (9)$$

where: P = the power developed,
   (watts/unit volume)
   k = a constant
   f = the frequency
   E = the electric field strength,
   (volts/unit distance)
   ϵ' = the relative dielectric constant
   of the material being heated
   $\tan \delta$ = the loss tangent, or dissipation
   factor of the material
   ϵ'' = the loss factor of the material,
   equal to the product $\epsilon' \tan \delta$

In microwave drying, the mass transfer is primarily the result of a pressure gradient due to rapid vapor generation inside the material, that is, most of the internal moisture is vaporized before leaving the sample. Thus, the moisture is mobilized as a vapor rather than a liquid, and its movement to the surface can be extremely rapid because it does not depend on mass concentration gradients or on slow liquid diffusion rates.

Industrial microwave dryers are usually of the static bed continuous type. Materials to be dried are placed on conveyor belts and conveyed through the microwave applicator. Generally, a stream of hot air is used simultaneously with the microwaves to sweep away the moisture evolving from the surface of the material being dried. Often, the microwave treatment is used in the last stages of hot air drying (the second falling rate period of Fig. 3-3) to remove the last remaining portion of the solvent, reducing total drying time by 50% or more.

Microwave drying can be used for the drying of pharmaceutical materials at low ambient temperatures, avoiding high surface temperatures, case hardening, and solute migration. Microwave vacuum drying at low pressure (1 to 20 mm Hg) and moderate temperature (30 to 40°C) can be used for drying thermolabile materials such as vitamins, enzymes, proteins, and flavors.

The rising cost of energy has generated a great deal of interest in microwave drying. The microwaves couple directly into the solvent, and no energy is used to heat the air, the walls of the dryer, the conveyor, or the trays. This results in extremely efficient energy utilization, and energy savings of as much as 70% have been realized in industrial installations.

References

1. Zimmerman, O. T., and Lavine, I.: Psychrometric Charts and Tables. Industrial Research Service, Dover, NH, 1945.
2. Perry, R. H., and Green, D. W.: Perry's Chemical Engineers' Handbook. 6th Ed. McGraw-Hill, New York, 1984.
3. Bone, D. P.: Food Prod. Devel., 3:81, 1969.
4. Callahan, J. C., et al.: Drug Devel. and Industrial Pharmacy, 8:355, 1982.
5. Rockland, L. B., and Nishi, S. K.: Food Technol., 34:42, 1980.
6. Scott, M. W., et al.: J. Pharm Sci., 52:284, 1963.
7. Kuelling, W., and Simon, E. J.: Pharm. Technol. Int., 3:29, 1980.
8. Nuernberg, E.: Acta Pharm. Technol., 26:39, 1980.
9. Lyons, D. W., and Hatcher, J. D.: J. Heat Mass Transfer, 15:897, 1972.

General References

Copson, D. A.: Microwave Heating. 2nd Ed. Avi Publishing, Westport, CT, 1975.

Encyclopedia of Chemical Technology. Vol 8. 3rd Ed. John Wiley and Sons, NY, 1979, p. 75.

Goldblith, S. A., et al. (eds.): Freeze Drying and Advanced Food Technology. Academic Press, NY, 1974.

Keey, R. B.: Introduction to Industrial Drying Operations. Pergamon Press, Elmsford NY, 1978.

Kunii, D., and Levenspiel, O.: Fluidization Engineering. John Wiley and Sons, NY, 1969.

Masters, K.: Spray Drying Handbook. 3rd Ed. Halsted Press, NY, 1979.

McCabe, W. L., and Smith, J. C.: Unit Operations and Chemical Engineering. 4th Ed. McGraw-Hill, NY, 1985.

Mellor, J. D.: Fundamentals of Freeze Drying. Academic Press, NY, 1979.

Perry, R. H., and Green, D. W.: Perry's Chemical Engineers' Handbook. 6th Ed. McGraw-Hill, NY, 1984, Section 20.

Treybal, R. E.: Mass Transfer Operations. 3rd Ed. McGraw-Hill, NY, 1979.

Williams-Gardner, A.: Industrial Drying. The Chemical Rubber Co., Cleveland, Ohio, 1971.

Vanecek, V., Markvart, M., and Drbohlav, R.: Fluidized Bed Drying. Leonard Hill Books, London, 1966.

4

Compression and Consolidation of Powdered Solids

KEITH MARSHALL

Unlike other physical states of matter, powdered solids are heterogeneous because they are composed of individual particles of widely differing sizes and shapes, randomly interspersed with air spaces. For this reason, it is virtually impossible to characterize these complex systems fully in terms of fundamental properties. Nevertheless, considerable advances have been made in understanding powder behavior, and many useful qualitative and semiquantitative measurements of factors important to the industrial user are now available. Properties at two levels, namely those associated with an individual particle and those typical of bulk powder, are of interest in the context under review.

Compaction of powders is the general term used to describe the situation in which these materials are subjected to some level of mechanical force. In the pharmaceutical industry, the effects of such forces are particularly important in the manufacture of tablets and granules, in the filling of hard-shell gelatin capsules, and in powder handling in general.

The physics of compaction may be simply stated as "the compression and consolidation of a two-phase (particulate solid-gas) system due to the applied force." *Compression* means a reduction in the bulk volume of the material as a result of displacement of the gaseous phase. *Consolidation* is an increase in the mechanical strength of the material resulting from particle/particle interactions.* Before each of these simultaneous processes is discussed in more detail, brief consideration is given to certain inherent properties of all powdered solids, which contribute to the characteristics of interest. In addition, some derived parameters that facilitate

*Some authors have used these terms interchangeably. The unequivocal definitions used here should avoid further confusion.

quantification of important variables are described.

The Solid-Air Interface

Atoms or ions located at the surface of any solid particle are exposed to a different distribution of intramolecular and intermolecular bonding forces than those within the particle. As indicated in Figure 4-1, they may be envisaged as unsatisfied attractive molecular forces extending out some small distance beyond the solid surface. This condition gives rise to what is called the *free surface energy* of the solid, which plays a major role in the interaction between particles, and between a particle and its environment. Many important phenomena such as adsorption, cohesion and adhesion, rate of solution, and crystallization are manifestations of this fundamental property of all solids.

Because of these unsatisfied bonding forces at the surface of particles, those that approach each other closely enough are inherently attracted and tend to stick to one another. This attraction between like particles is called *cohe-*

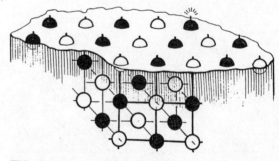

FIG. 4-1. *Diagram of distribution of attractive bonds between constituent ions or atoms in a solid, compared with those at its surface.*

sion. In addition, when they approach other types of particles or solid surfaces, they are attracted to them, leading to what is termed *adhesion.* These attractions give rise to an intrinsic property of all bulk powdered solids: they resist differential movement of their constituent particles when subjected to external forces. This phenomenon has an important influence on several operations, such as flow from hoppers or feeders, relative motion in mixers, and compression to produce granules or tablets.

The overall resistance to relative movement of particles may be markedly affected by two other factors. First, many powders of pharmaceutical interest readily develop electrostatic forces, especially when subjected to internal friction, although particle contact and separation are the only prerequisite. The charge developed depends on the particular material involved and the type of motion produced in it. Usually, electrostatic forces are relatively small, but may be significant because they act over a greater distance than the molecular forces. The second factor, namely the presence of an adsorbed layer of moisture on the particles, reduces the chance of any complicating electrostatic effect by providing a conducting path for charge dissipation. When particles approach one another closely enough, however, these films of moisture can form liquid bridges, which hold the particles together by surface tension effects and by a negative capillary pressure.

Angles of Repose

Although the contributions of each of these effects cannot always be distinguished, there are relatively simple practical techniques for measuring resistance to particle movement. For example, a quantity called *the angle of repose* of a powder can be determined. This is the angle Φ as defined by the equation:*

$$\text{Tan } \Phi = \frac{2h}{D} \qquad (1)$$

It is the maximum angle that can be obtained between the freestanding surface of a powder heap and the horizontal plane, as shown in Figure 4-2a. Such measurements give at least a qualitative assessment of the internal cohesive and frictional effects under low levels of external loading, as might apply in powder mixing, or in tablet die or capsule shell filling operations.

*See Appendix A for explanation of symbols used in formulas throughout this chapter.

Angle of repose methods, which result in a so-called *dynamic* angle, are preferred, since they most closely mimic the manufacturing situation, in which the powder is in motion.

A typical dynamic test involves a hollow cylinder half-filled with the test powder, with one end sealed by a transparent plate. The cylinder is rotated about its horizontal axis (Fig. 4-2b), until the powder surface cascades. The curved wall is lined with sandpaper to prevent preferential slip at this surface. In a second method, a sandpaper-lined rectangular box is filled with the powder and carefully tilted until the contents begin to slide, as shown in Figure 4-2c. Values of Φ are rarely less than 20°, and values of up to 40° indicate reasonable flow potential. Above 50°, however, the powder flows only with great difficulty, if at all.

With care, dynamic angle of repose measurements can be replicated with relative standard deviations of approximately 2%. They are particularly sensitive to changes in particle size distribution and to moisture content, and they provide a rapid means of monitoring significant batch-to-batch differences in these respects.

Flow Rates

Alternatively, resistance to movement of particles, especially for granular powders with little cohesiveness, may be assessed by determining their flow rate Q through a circular orifice (a tablet die, for instance) fitted in the base of a cylindric container. Flow experiments with mixtures of different size fractions of the same material can be particularly valuable, because in many instances, there exist optimum proportions that lead to a maximum flow rate, as shown in Figure 4-3. Note that for this system, when the proportion of fine particles exceeds approximately 40%, there is a dramatic fall in the flow rate.[1]

A simple indication of the ease with which a material can be induced to flow is given by application of a *compressibility index* (I) given by the equation:

$$I = \left[1 - \frac{v}{v_o} \right] \cdot 100 \qquad (2)$$

where v is the volume occupied by a sample of the powder after being subjected to a standardized tapping procedure, and v_o is the volume before tapping. Values of I below 15% usually give rise to good flow characteristics, but readings above 25% indicate poor flowability.

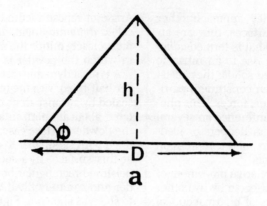

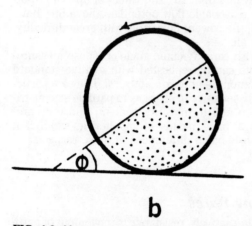

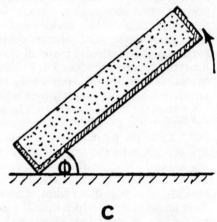

FIG. 4-2. *Measurement of dynamic angles of repose, Φ, as defined from the dimensions of a conical bed of the powder (Figure a), where tan Φ = twice the powder bed height (h)/powder bed diameter (D). Figures b and c represent the rotating cylinder and tilted box methods of measurement, respectively.*

Mass-Volume Relationships

Volume

Although the mass of a bulk powder sample can be determined with great accuracy, measurement of the volume is more complicated than it may first appear. The main problem arises in actually defining volumes of bulk powders, as may be seen from Figure 4-4, in which three types of air spaces or voids can be distinguished:

1. Open intraparticulate voids—those within a single particle but open to the external environment.

2. Closed intraparticulate voids—those within a single particle but closed to the external environment.

3. Interparticulate voids—the air spaces between individual particles.

Therefore, at least three interpretations of "powder volume" may be proposed:

1. The *true volume* (v_t)—the total volume of the solid particles, which excludes all spaces greater than molecular dimensions, and which has a characteristic value for each material.

2. The *granular volume* (particle volume) (v_g)—the cumulative volume occupied by the particles, including all intraparticulate (but not interparticulate) voids. The boundary between open intraparticulate and interparticulate air spaces may be interpreted differently, so that this interpretation of volume depends on the method of measurement.

3. The *bulk volume* (v_b)— the total volume occupied by the entire powder mass under the particular packing achieved during the meas-

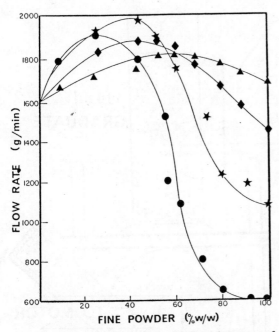

FIG. 4-3. *Effect of fines on the rate of flow of mixtures of coarse granules (0.561 mm) as a function of increasing amounts of fines:* (▲) *0.158 mm;* (◆) *0.09 mm;* (★) *0.059 mm;* (●) *0.048 mm. (From Jones.[1] Reproduced with permission of the copyright owner.)*

urement. Thus, this interpretation also depends on method.

When studying phenomena resulting in a change in volume, it may be convenient to consider the volume v of the sample under specific experimental conditions, relative to the true volume v_t. A useful dimensionless quantity *relative volume* (v_r) may be defined as:

$$v_r = \frac{v}{v_t} \qquad (3)$$

The relative volume decreases and tends toward unity as all the air is eliminated from the mass.

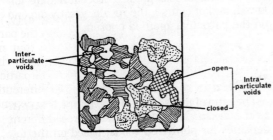

FIG. 4-4. *Diagram of various intraparticulate and interparticulate air spaces in a bed of powder.*

This phenomenon occurs in compressional processes such as tabletting.

The voids present in the powder mass may be more significant than the solid components in certain studies. For example, a fine capillary network of voids or pores has been shown to enhance the rate of liquid uptake by tablets, which in turn increases the rate of their disintegration. For this reason, a second dimensionless quantity, the ratio of the total volume of void spaces (v_v) to the bulk volume of the material, is often selected to monitor the progress of compression. This ratio $\frac{v_v}{v_b}$ is referred to as the *porosity* (E) of the material:

$$v_v = v_b - v_t \qquad (4)$$

Therefore: porosity $E = \dfrac{v_b - v_t}{v_b} = 1 - \dfrac{v_t}{v_b}$

Porosity is frequently expressed as a percentage:

$$E = 100 \cdot \left[1 - \frac{v_t}{v_b}\right] \qquad (5)$$

For example, a cylindric tablet of 10 mm diameter and 4 mm height weighed 480 mg and was made from material of true density 1.6 g cm⁻³. The bulk volume v_b is given by:

$$v_b = \pi \times \left(\frac{10}{10 \times 2}\right)^2 \times \frac{4}{10} \text{ cm}^3$$

(volume of a cylinder is $\pi r^2 h$)

$$= (0.5)^2 \cdot 0.4 = 0.3142 \text{ cm}^3$$

The true volume of the solid is the true density divided by the mass, that is:

$$v_t = \frac{480}{1000} \div 1.6 = \frac{0.48}{1.6} = 0.3 \text{ cm}^3$$

Therefore, the porosity E is:

$$E = 100 \cdot \left[1 - \frac{0.3}{0.3142}\right] = 100(1 - 0.9548)$$

$$= 4.5\% \text{ (approximately)}$$

Several practical techniques are available for measuring the volume of powder samples. Apart from x-ray diffraction methods, the nearest approach to true volume is probably provided by a helium pycnometer. This works on the principle that within a sealed system containing helium (a nonadsorbing gas), the change in pressure caused by a finite change in volume of the system is a function of its total volume. A schematic diagram for a typical apparatus is shown in Figure 4-5. During operation, the volume of the system is varied by means of the piston until a preset constant pressure is produced. This pressure is indicated by the sealed bellows pressure detector, which incorporates an integral electrical contact. The piston movement (U) necessary to achieve this pressure is read off from the scale. This value depends on the total volume of the system, which in turn is a function of the sample volume in the cell. The pycnometer is first calibrated using a sample of known volume v_c (usually a stainless steel sphere). The operating equation for the instrument then becomes:

$$v_t = \frac{v_c}{U_1 - U_2} \cdot [U_1 - U_s] \qquad (6)$$

where U_1, U_2 and U_s are the variable volume scale readings for an empty cell, with standard volume, and with test powder, respectively.

Alternatively in some instances, a large compact of the material can be prepared at high compressional force (therefore assuming zero porosity). Then, by accurately measuring its overall dimensions, true volume can be calculated. Liquid displacement by a powder pycnometer (specific gravity bottle method) can also be used, but unless special precautions are taken to ensure that no air remains in the sample, the results are prone to errors. For this reason, liquid displacement is probably best regarded as a

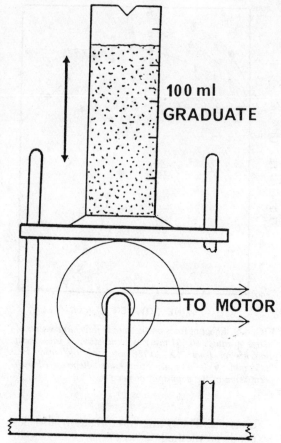

FIG. 4-6. *Diagram of apparatus for determining the bulk volume of powders.*

measurement of granule volume, especially if liquids that do not readily wet the powder are used, e.g., certain inert organic liquids, or mercury.

Bulk volumes are measured in a variety of ways, ranging from simple pouring of a known weight into a graduated vessel to sophisticated techniques involving standard tamping, tapping, or vibrating procedures, as shown in Figure 4-6. In all these techniques, reproducibility may be poor unless precise procedures are followed, and of course, the results greatly depend on the particular method chosen.

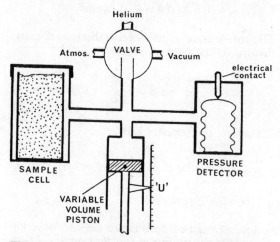

FIG. 4-5. *Diagram of a helium pycnometer for determining the true volume of powders. The variable volume piston positions (U_1, U_2, and U_s) are read off from the scale and are used in equation (6) (see text).*

Density

The ratio of mass (weight) to volume is known as the *density* of the material. Three different densities for powdered solids, based on the following ratios, may be defined.

$$\frac{M}{v_t} = \rho_t \text{ the true density}$$

$$\frac{M}{v_g} = \rho_g \text{ the granular density}$$

$$\frac{M}{v_b} = \rho_b \text{ the bulk density}$$

where M is the mass of the sample. Comparing the density ρ of a sample under specific test conditions with the *true density* (sometimes called *theoretical density*) of the material leads to the dimensionless quantity ρ_r, the *relative density*, where:

$$\rho_r = \frac{\rho}{\rho_t} \tag{7}$$

During compressional processes, relative density increases to a maximum of unity when all air spaces have been eliminated.

Effect of Applied Forces

Deformation

When any solid body is subjected to opposing forces, there is a finite change in its geometry, depending upon the nature of the applied load. The relative amount of deformation produced by such forces is a dimensionless quantity called *strain*. Three of the commonest kinds of strain are illustrated in Figure 4-7. For example, if a solid rod is compressed by forces acting at each end to cause a reduction in length of ΔH from an unloaded length of H_o (Fig. 4-7b), then the compressive strain Z is given by the equation:

$$Z = \Delta H/H_o \tag{8}$$

The ratio of the force F necessary to produce this strain to the area A over which it acts is called the stress σ, that is:

$$\sigma = F/A \tag{9}$$

Because most powder masses contain some air spaces, true analogous behavior to a solid body should not be expected. Nevertheless, under low porosity conditions (high applied forces), comparisons do provide a useful way of interpreting experimental observations, as is demonstrated in the following discussion.

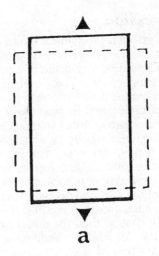

a

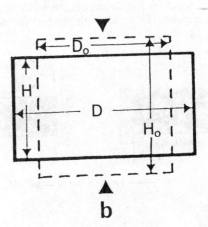

b

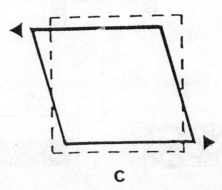

c

FIG. 4-7. *Diagram shows change in geometry (strain) of a solid body resulting from various types of applied force: tensile strain (a), compressive strain (b), and shear strain (c).*

Compression

When external mechanical forces are applied to a powder mass, there is normally a reduction in its bulk volume as a result of one or more of the following effects. The onset of loading is usually accompanied by closer repacking of the powder particles, and in most cases, this is the main mechanism of initial volume reduction, as shown diagrammatically in Figure 4-8. As the load increases, however, rearrangement becomes more difficult, and further compression involves some type of particle deformation. If on removal of the load, the deformation is to a large extent spontaneously reversible, i.e., if it behaves like rubber, then the deformation is said to be *elastic*. All solids undergo some elastic deformation when subjected to external forces. With several pharmaceutical materials, such as acetylsalicyclic acid and microcrystalline cellulose, elastic deformation becomes the dominant mechanism of compression within the range of maximum forces normally encountered in practice.

In other groups of powdered solids, an elastic limit, or *yield point*, is reached, and loads above this level result in deformation not immediately reversible on removal of the applied force. Bulk volume reduction in these cases results from plastic deformation and/or viscous flow of the particles, which are squeezed into the remaining void spaces, resembling the behavior of modeling clay. This mechanism predominates in materials in which the shear strength is less than the tensile or breaking strength (see Fig. 4-7). Conversely, when the shear strength is greater, particles may be preferentially fractured, and the smaller fragments then help to fill up any adjacent air space. This is most likely to occur with hard, brittle particles and in fact is known as *brittle fracture*; sucrose behaves in this manner. The predisposition of a material to deform in a particular manner depends on the lattice structure, in particular whether weakly bonded lattice planes are inherently present.

Irrespective of the behavior of large particles of the material, small particles may deform plastically, a process known as *microsquashing*, and the proportion of fine powder in a sample may therefore be significant. Asperities that are sheared off larger, highly irregular particles could also behave in this way, thus, particle shape is another important factor.

The above account describes all of the possible mechanisms that can contribute to a reduction in the bulk volume of a bed of powder, when subjected to external mechanical forces. The chemicophysical characteristics of the material being studied determine the contribution each effect makes as the compressional load is increased. All of the deformation effects may be accompanied by the breaking and formation of new bonds between the particles, which gives rise to consolidation as the new surfaces are pressed together.

The packaging of bulk powders and the filling of hard gelatin capsules mostly involve bulk volume reductions achievable by repacking, and possibly a minimal amount of deformation. At the other end of the scale, in the tabletting process—or in such specialized techniques as roll compacting or extruding, which involve high levels of compressive force—repacking, elastic deformation, plastic deformation, and brittle fracture may all take place.

Some deformation processes (plastic deformation, for example) are time-dependent and occur at various rates during the compaction sequence, so that the tablet mass is never in a state of stress/strain equilibrium during the ac-

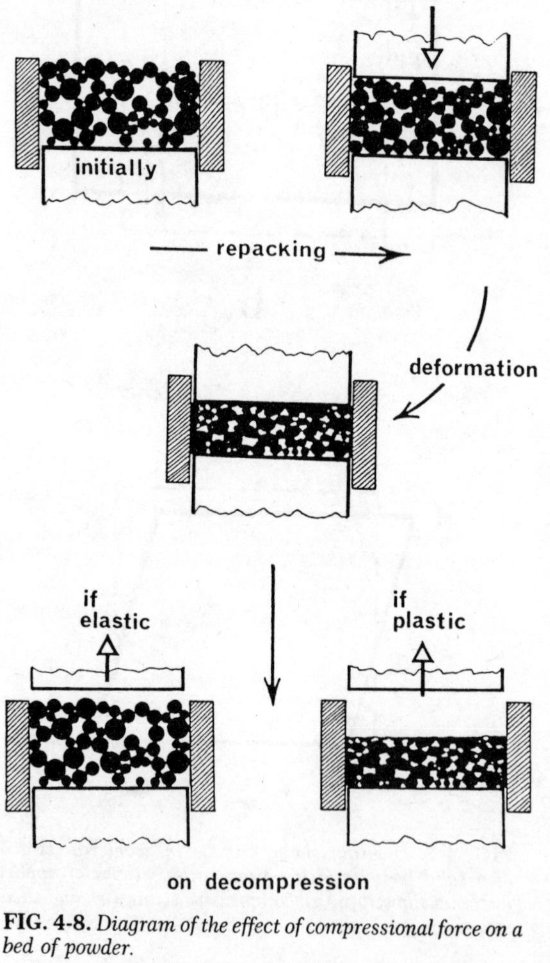

FIG. 4-8. *Diagram of the effect of compressional force on a bed of powder.*

tual tabletting event. This means that the rate at which load is applied and removed may be a critical factor in materials for which dependence on time is significant. More specifically, if a plastically deforming solid is loaded (or unloaded) too rapidly for this process to take place, the solid may exhibit brittle fracture. This is a contributing factor to the well-known problem of structurally failed tablets of some drugs as tablet machine speed is raised. Conversely, if the dwell time under the compressive load is prolonged, then plastic deformation may continue, leading to more consolidation. This phenomenon has recently been studied using a compaction simulator,[2] whereby it was shown that the expansion of acetaminophen tablets (a material with known laminating tendency) during decompression was particularly sensitive to dwell time under a maximum load. For this reason, relatively slower machine speeds and compression rolls of large diameter sometimes help with troublesome tablet formulations.

Consolidation

When the surfaces of two particles approach each other closely enough (e.g., at a separation of less than 50 nm), their free surface energies result in a strong attractive force, a process known as *cold welding*. The nature of the bonds so formed are similar to those of the molecular structure of the interior of the particles, but because of the roughness of the particle surface (on a molecular scale), the actual surface area involved may be small. This hypothesis is favored as a major reason for the increasing mechanical strength of a bed of powder when subjected to rising compressive forces.

On the macroscale, most particles encountered in practice have an irregular shape, so that there are many points of contact in a bed of powder (see Fig. 4-4). Any applied load to the bed must be transmitted through these particle contacts; under appreciable forces, this transmission may result in the generation of considerable frictional heat. If this heat is not dissipated, the local rise in temperature could be sufficient to cause melting of the contact area of the particles, which would relieve the stress in that particular region. In that case, the melt solidifies, giving rise to *fusion bonding,* which in turn results in an increase in mechanical strength of the mass.

Many pharmaceutical solids possess a low specific heat and poor thermal conductivity, so that heat transfer away from the contact points is slow. This behavior was quantified by Rankell and Higuchi,[3] who were able to estimate, from heat transfer kinetics, that temperatures high enough to fuse typical organic medicinal substances were theoretically possible. The differences between this form of bond formation and cold welding are somewhat pedantic; the end results are essentially the same.

In both "cold" and "fusion" welding, the process is influenced by several factors, including:

1. the chemical nature of the materials
2. the extent of the available surface
3. the presence of surface contaminants
4. the intersurface distances

The type and degree of crystallinity in a particular material influences its consolidative behavior under appreciable applied force. One of the earliest reports of such influence was that of Jaffe and Foss,[4] who demonstrated that substances possessing the cubic lattice arrangement were tabletted more satisfactorily than those with a rhombohedral lattice, for example. The isotropic nature of the former group might be expected to contribute to better tabletting because no alignment of particular lattice planes is required. In addition they provide three equal planes for stress relief at right angles to each other. Lattice planes with the greatest separation undergo plastic deformation more readily, since such planes are more weakly bonded. The particles of most pharmaceutical powders consist of small crystallites, or grains, aggregated in a random manner so that their crystal planes are not aligned with one another. Such an arrangement adds to the material's resistance to plastic deformation.

Of course, there are many exceptions to generalizations of this kind. For example, of the two chemically similar organic materials methacetin and phenacetin, apparently only the former can be tabletted without the tendency to laminate. More importantly, perhaps, different polymorphic forms and crystal habits of the same compound may not behave in the same way in terms of compaction properties. Detection and evaluation of these seemingly unavoidable changes in the materials from bulk chemical plants, which are responsible for many of our unanticipated tabletting problems with established products, are important. Routine testing of compaction characteristics in some type of instrumented tabletting machine constitutes a desirable and informative part of such procedures.

One interesting observation on the more successful direct compression excipients that are commercially available concerns this "material structure" aspect of tabletting. Without exception, these products may be described as microgranulations, since they consist of masses of small crystallites randomly embedded in a matrix of some glue-like (often amorphous) material. Such a combination imparts the desired overall qualities, which result in (1) strong tablets by providing a plastically deforming component (the matrix) to relieve internal stresses, and (2) strongly bonding surfaces (the faces of the crystallites) to enhance consolidation.[5]

The compressional process is affected by the extent of the available surface, the presence of surface contaminants, and the intersurface distances; if large, clean surfaces are brought into intimate contact, then bonding should occur. Brittle fracture and plastic deformation should generate clean surfaces, which the compressional force ensures are kept in close proximity. This is an important rationale when considering the tabletting process, since many of the problems that arise can be traced to interference in these mechanisms. For example, such lubricants as magnesium stearate form weak bonds, so that overlubrication, or even overmixing of lubricant into the tabletting mass, results in a continuous coating of the latter, and hence in some cases, weak tablets.

Higuchi and his co-workers were among the first to report experimental data in support of these mechanisms for a pharmaceutical material.[6] They interpreted the plot of specific surface area versus compressional force shown in Figure 4-9 in terms of an initial increase in surface area (region O to A) due to particle breakdown. At high loads (A to B), rebonding of surfaces became dominant, with a resultant decrease in specific surface areas.

Years later, Armstrong and co-workers described similar curves,[7] but at high compressional forces (see broken line in Fig. 4-9), they showed that some materials were subject to an increase in surface area. This increase was due to incipient failure or lamination of the tablet structure that resulted from considerable elastic recovery on decompression.

The actual solubility of solids also depends somewhat on the applied pressure, so that if a film of moisture is present on the solid surface, then the high pressures at points of solid contact could force more material into solution. This dissolved solid would crystallize on relief of the applied stress to form a solid bridge whose strength would partly depend on the rate of this recrystallization. In general, slow rates should produce a more perfect crystal structure with consequent higher strength.

The observation that tablets containing at

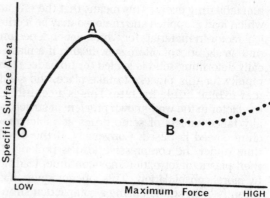

FIG. 4-9. *The effect of increasing compressional force on the specific surface area of a powder mass. When a powder mass is subjected to increasing compressional force, there is initial particle fracture, which gives rise to increased surface area (O to A on graph). At some point (A), particle rebonding becomes the dominant factor, and from then on, surface area decreases (region A to B) unless tablet lamination begins.*

least a proportion of water-soluble component are often more readily formed than those without, may indicate this mechanism. The finding that some overdried mixtures, in which moisture residues are extremely low, have inferior tabletting qualities may be further evidence. The known internal lubricant property of water, however, provides an alternative, and probably complementary, explanation of the important role of moisture.

At low levels of external force, molecular and electrostatic forces are a source of attractive tendencies between individual particles. This attraction might be encountered in the mixing of dry powders or in the filling of capsule shells. Valency type molecular forces have an extremely short range and are therefore unlikely to play a major role at this stage. Van der Waals forces, however, may exert a significant effect at distances up to 100 nm, so that once an agglomerate of particles has been formed, they may serve to prevent its breakdown. Electrostatic forces generated by friction or size reduction, though generally weaker than van der Waals forces, do have a greater range and probably produce the initial agglomerate formation in many materials. Ionic chemicals involve the additional possibility of surface polarization, which can produce marked attractive tendencies.

If the solid particles are soft, then deformation under low loads could cause more intimate contact between the particles and enhance the above bonding mechanisms. Recently, however, it has been shown that coating of a major tablet ingredient by a lower melting point component

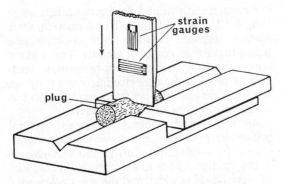

FIG. 4-10. *Plug strength tester. A device for measuring the strength of the cohesive forces holding together the soft powder plugs that are produced by some capsule machines. The force necessary to split the plug using the strain-gauged blade is measured.*

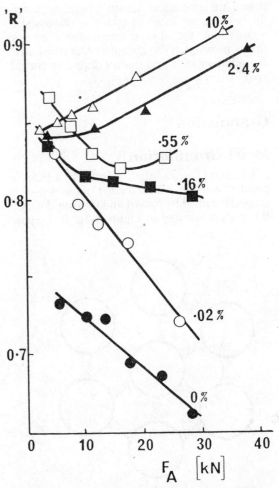

FIG. 4-11. *Effect of moisture content on the ratio of transmitted punch force to applied punch force. (After Shotton and Rees.[14])*

(such as a lubricant) can sometimes lead to reduced tensile strength of tablets, especially if produced at slightly elevated temperatures (10°C).[8] It is thought that this effect is due to masking of van der Waals forces between the particles and the formation of welded bonds by the coatings.

Some capsule filling machines operate on the "dosator principle," that is, formation of a soft plug, which is transferred to the capsule shell. In such machines, the plugs are commonly held together by one or more of the foregoing mechanisms.

A report by Augsburger and associates described a simple test to measure the comparative strength of different formulations in such powder plugs;[9] the apparatus is illustrated diagrammatically in Figure 4-10. Hiestand has reviewed in detail all the various mechanisms and their applicability to pharmaceutical powder systems,[10] concluding that in tabletting, plastic deformation is the major mechanism leading to increased areas of intimate contact, and hence bonding, by cold welding.

Role of Moisture

At least some moisture is present in virtually all capsule and tablet formulas, and concentrations well below the 1% level can dramatically affect the behavior of these feed materials and that of the finished product. This is demonstrated clearly by data such as that given in Figure 4-11, which shows that as little as 0.02% moisture can affect the proportion of the applied force transmitted to the lower punch, and at 0.55% moisture, the behavior is actually the reverse of that for the totally dry material. A more critical factor concerns the situation where the

amount of moisture present on the powder surfaces is just sufficient to fill the remaining voids in the bed. Any further reduction in porosity, e.g., as a result of increasing compressional force, results in this water being squeezed out to the surface of the tablet. This expelled moisture may act as a lubricant at the die wall, but it could also cause material to stick to the punch faces.

Recent experiments have shown the effect of thermal dehydration on the crushing strength of tablets made from certain hydrates.[11] The strength was found to depend on the temperature at which the dehydration was carried out. Scanning electron microscopy confirmed that dehydration had been accompanied by a change in texture of the crystals, which led to a more porous mass.

Moisture is also important in moist granulation processes, in which most of the fluids involved are aqueous in nature. Therefore, before the bonding produced in tablets is discussed in more detail, the special consolidative process that is involved in the granulation of powders by the addition of a granulating liquid is considered.

Granulation

Moist Granulation

Addition of a granulating liquid to a mass of powder may be characterized in a series of stages described by Newitt and Conway-Jones;[12] these are illustrated in Figure 4-12. If the pow-

der particles are wetted during the initial stage (Fig. 4-12A), liquid films will be formed on their surface and may combine to produce discrete liquid bridges at points of contact. The surface tension and negative capillary pressure in such bridges provide the cohesive force and result in a condition called the *pendular* state, which has comparatively low mechanical strength.

As the liquid content increases, several bridges may coalesce, giving rise to the *funicular* state (Fig. 4-12B), and a further modest increase in the strength of the moist granule. Eventually, as more liquid is added and the mass is kneaded to bring particles into closer proximity, the void spaces within the granule are entirely eliminated. At this point, bonding is effected by inter-

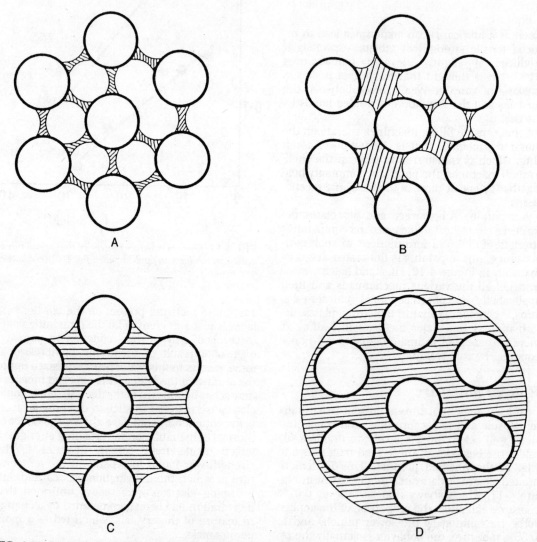

FIG. 4-12. *Stages in the development of moist granules as the proportion of liquid is increased: pendular (A), funicular (B), capillary (C), and droplet (D). (After Newitt and Conway-Jones.[12])*

facial forces at the granule surface and by a negative capillary pressure throughout the interior liquid-filled space, a condition referred to as the *capillary* state (Fig. 4-12C). Further addition of liquid results in *droplet* formation (Fig. 4-12D), in which the particles are still held together by surface tension, but without intragranular forces; such structures are weaker. The capillary state coincides with the maximum strength of the wet granules, and optimization of many granulation processes involves ensuring that this state has been achieved. For example, granulation equipment can be instrumented with torque measuring devices, which sense the change in agitator power requirements at the capillary stage, as shown in Figure 4-13.[13]

In many formulations, one or more components are to some extent soluble in the granulating liquid, which itself may contain solutes, such as binders. During drying, solid bridges form in the granule as these soluble materials crystallize or precipitate out. This process results in the often dramatic increase in granule strength observed during their drying.

A small residual moisture content sometimes optimizes strength, however, and is desirable for other reasons, notably its lubricant potential during compaction at higher applied loads. Migration of soluble components to the surface of the granule during drying may lead to a surface layer that is atypical of the bulk. This in turn can assist or hinder the consolidative performance of the granules when they are subsequently compressed. The migration rate can be reduced by increasing the viscosity of the granulating fluid and using fluidized bed drying, as opposed to the slower process of tray drying. In addition, the reports of other workers point strongly to optimum moisture levels for particular formulations.[14] Accurate moisture levels should therefore be determined routinely during formulation development.

Properties of Granules

Several characteristics of finished granules are of major significance because they can exert a pronounced influence on the progress of the subsequent tabletting process and the properties of the tablets produced. These characteristics include packing ability and flow properties of the bulk material, together with individual granule strength and porosity. Particle shape and size distribution are important factors in packing and flow. Although the former is not easy to describe quantitatively, the use of shape factors, such as those defined by Heywood,[15] and exemplified in the studies of Ridgeway and Rupp,[16] have proved useful. To be specific, particles of more regular shape (nearly spherical) led to lower angles of repose and higher bulk densities. In general, these effects should result in better granule flow properties, hence smaller tablet weight variation and a more efficient compression/consolidation tabletting sequence.

Granule size distributions are best determined by test sieving procedures, as described in ASTM 447 A for example.[17] The contribution of particle size to possible performance is difficult to generalize, but there is often an optimum proportion of fine particles necessary to achieve optimum flow properties, as shown in Figure 4-3.

The degree of packing in bulk granulation is important in its relationship to die and dosator filling. More specifically, the porosity of a tablet produced under a certain compressive load is in many cases a function of the initial porosity of the packing in the die. One of the simplest expressions of this packing tendency is the compressibility index, I, already described in equation (2). Compressibility index values up to 15% usually result in good to excellent flow properties and indicate desirable packing characteristics. Values for I above 25%, on the other hand, are obtained from materials whose compressional characteristics are often a source of poor tabletting qualities. Between these two values, less than optimum performance might be anticipated, and modification of the particle size distribution could be advisable.

Strength of Granules

Granules should possess sufficient strength to withstand normal handling and mixing processes without breaking down and producing large amounts of fine powder. On the other hand, some size reduction during compaction

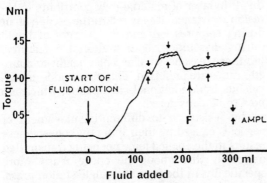

FIG. 4-13. *Plot of change in torque of mixer shaft during addition of granulating fluid. Point F represents an appropriate end point to wet massing (From Travers et al.[13])*

into tablets is desirable to expose the areas of clean surface necessary for optimum bonding (cold welding) to take place.

Definition of "strength" with respect to individual granules may be interpreted in several ways, depending on the method of applying the test load. Strength may be expressed in terms of compressive, tensile, shear, bending, impact, and abrasion tests. Only compressive and abrasion tests have been sufficiently used to provide the required data to establish general relationships between strength and other tabletting material or process characteristics.

The compressive strength, or *crushing strength,* of granules has been investigated by placing individual granules between platens and breaking them by application of a compressive load. In many formulations, there is an optimum range of average granule crushing strength for a given granule size. Granule strengths below the lower limit of this range may consolidate well, but tend to break down during mixing, handling, and precompression, to generate fines which retard uniform die filling. Conversely, hard granules retain their identity up to high compressional forces, but may consolidate poorly and give rise to weak tablets. Such tablets may disintegrate readily but sometimes have poor dissolution characteristics.

Abrasion tests, which involve standardized tumbling of granules, can also be valuable in assessing their handling properties and in readily comparing the strength of different batches. This type of test involves tumbling a known weight of granules for a specified time and then determining particle size distribution changes. More specifically, the increased proportion of fine powder, i.e., *fines* (of which the average particle size is less than 75 microns, or 200 mesh), is noted.

The quantity of granulating fluid used, and the concentration of any added binder are the major factors contributing to an increase in granule strength. One report has demonstrated that for a given material, smaller initial particle sizes led to granules of greater strength, presumably because of the increased occurrence of interparticulate contacts.[18] Smaller granules tended to be weaker, probably because they had not been subjected to as much work during their development.

Soft, porous granules tend to form tablets that are better consolidated under lower compressional forces than tablets prepared from hard and dense granules. In addition, the latter sometimes demonstrate poor dissolution characteristics as well as inferior appearance, but they are less friable and often have a more regular shape, thereby enhancing die-fill uniformity.

Compression and Consolidation under High Loads

The processes of tabletting, roll compaction, and extrusion all involve the application of massive compressive forces, which induce considerable deformation in the solid particles. With many pharmaceutical solids and perhaps most tabletting mixtures, these forces are large enough to exceed the elastic limit of the solid (or at least that of one component of the mixture). Plastic deformation and/or brittle fracture then results in the generation of new, clean surfaces, which being pressed against one another, undergo cold welding. When the compaction force reaches its maximum, a bulk solid structure of a certain overall strength will have been produced.

Irrespective of the bonding mechanism, this structure must be strong enough to withstand the new stresses induced during release of the applied load and those generated by ejection from the die (in the case of tabletting). Ideally, relief of these stresses by elastic recovery is preferred, since at this stage, plastic deformation—and even worse, brittle fracture—may result in small failure planes, if not complete lamination, since any new surfaces tend to separate rather than consolidate.

During normal tabletting operations, consolidation is accentuated in those regions adjacent to the die wall, owing to the intense shear to which material is subjected, as it is compressed axially and is pushed along the wall surface. This consolidation results in a "skin" of material that is denser over the lateral tablet surface than in the rest of the tablet mass. This skin is in some cases visible to the naked eye. Although this thin layer of material may contribute to abrasion resistance, it may retard the escape of air during compression and the ingress of liquid during dissolution, both undesirable features. For these reasons, smaller tablet height-to-diameter ratios are preferred. This situation is advantageous from additional standpoints, which are now to be considered.

The resistance to differential movement of particles caused by their inherent cohesiveness results in the applied force not being transmitted uniformly throughout the entire mass. More specifically, in the case of a single-station press, the force exerted by the upper punch diminishes exponentially at increasing depths below it.

Thus, the relationship between upper punch force F_A and lower punch force F_L* may be expressed in the form:

$$F_L = F_A \cdot e^{-KH/D} \qquad (10)$$

where K is an experimentally determined material-dependent constant that includes a term for the average die-wall frictional component. The values H and D are the height and diameter of the tablet, respectively.

The discrepancy between the two punch forces should be minimized in pharmaceutical tabletting operations, so that there is no significant difference in the amount of compression and consolidation between one region of the tablet and another. Reduction of die-wall friction effects by having smaller tablet height-to-diameter ratios and by adding a lubricant is therefore common practice. Because of their important role in the progress of the compressional sequence, frictional effects warrant further discussion.

Effects of Friction

At least two major components to the frictional forces can be distinguished.

1. Interparticulate friction. This arises at particle/particle contacts and can be expressed in terms of a coefficient of interparticulate friction μ_i; it is more significant at low applied loads. Materials that reduce this effect are referred to as *glidants*. Colloidal silica is a common example.

2. Die-wall friction. This results from material being pressed against the die wall and moved down it; it is expressed as μ_w, the coefficient of die-wall friction. This effect becomes dominant at high applied forces when particle rearrangement has ceased and is particularly important in tabletting operations. Most tablets contain a small amount of an additive designed to reduce die-wall friction; such additives are called *lubricants*. Magnesium stearate is a common choice.

*The various loads on a powder bed are sometimes expressed in terms of force, the preferred units being newtons (N). In other instances, the force acting over a unit cross-sectional area is used, i.e., a pressure. The unit in this case is the newton per square meter, which is called a pascal (Pa). To facilitate comparison, expressions originally derived in other units have been converted to this (SI) system throughout this chapter. (See Appendix B for equivalents and conversion factors.)

Force Distribution

Most investigations of the fundamentals of tabletting have been carried out on single-station presses (sometimes called *eccentric presses*), or even on isolated punch and die sets in conjunction with a hydraulic press. The system represented diagrammatically in Figure 4-14 is typical of such arrangements, with force being applied to the top of a cylindric powder mass. This simple compaction system provides a convenient way to examine the process in greater detail. More specifically, the following basic relationships apply. Since there must be an axial (vertical) balance of forces:

$$F_A = F_L + F_D \qquad (11)$$

where F_A is the force applied to the upper punch, F_L is that proportion of it transmitted to the lower punch, and F_D is a reaction at the die

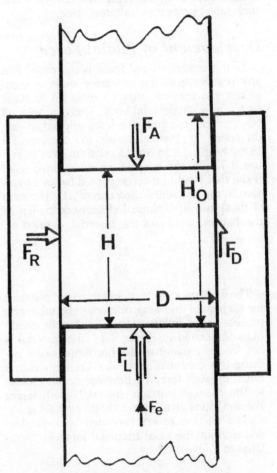

FIG. 4-14. *Diagram of a cross section of a typical simple punch and die assembly used for compaction studies.*

wall due to friction at this surface. Because of this inherent difference between the force applied at the upper punch and that affecting material close to the lower punch, a *mean compaction force,* F_M, has been proposed, where:

$$F_M = \frac{F_A + F_L}{2} \qquad (12)$$

A recent report confirms that F_M offers a practical friction-independent measure of compaction load, which is generally more relevant than F_A.[19] In single-station presses, where the applied force transmission decays exponentially as in equation (10), a more appropriate *geometric mean force,* F_G, might be:

$$F_G = (F_A \cdot F_L)^{0.5} \qquad (13)$$

Use of these force parameters are probably more appropriate than use of F_A when determining relationships between compressional force and such tablet properties as tablet strength.

Development of Radial Force

As the compressional force is increased and any repacking of the tabletting mass is completed, the material may be regarded to some extent as a single solid body. Then, as with all other solids, compressive force applied in one direction (e.g., vertical) results in a decrease ΔH in the height, i.e., a compressive stress as in Figure 4-7b. In the case of an unconfined solid body, this would be accompanied by an expansion in the horizontal direction of ΔD. The ratio of these two dimensional changes is known as the Poisson ratio λ of the material, defined as:

$$\lambda = \frac{\Delta D}{\Delta H} \qquad (14)$$

The Poisson ratio is a characteristic constant for each solid and may influence the tabletting process in the following way. Under the conditions illustrated in Figure 4-14, the material is not free to expand in the horizontal plane because it is confined in the die. Consequently, a radial die-wall force F_R develops perpendicular to the die-wall surface, materials with larger Poisson ratios giving rise to higher values of F_R. Classic friction theory can then be applied to deduce that the axial frictional force F_D is related to F_R by the expression:

$$F_D = \mu_w \cdot F_R \qquad (15)$$

where μ_w is the coefficient of die-wall friction.

Note that F_R is reduced when materials of small Poisson ratios are used, and that in such cases, axial force transmission is optimum.

The frictional effect represented by μ_w arises from the shearing of adhesions that occurs as the particles slide along the die wall. It follows that its magnitude is related to the shear strength S of the particles (or the die-wall-particle adhesions if these are weaker) and the total effective area of contact A_e between the two surfaces. Therefore, force transmission is also realized when F_D values are reduced to a minimum, which is achieved by ensuring adequate lubrication at the die wall (lower S) and maintaining a minimum tablet height (reducing A_e).

A common method of comparing degrees of lubrication has been to measure the applied and transmitted axial forces and determine the ratio F_L/F_A. This is called the *coefficient of lubricant efficiency,* or *R value.*[20] The ratio approaches unity for perfect lubrication (no wall friction), and in practice, values as high as 0.98 may be realized. Values below 0.8 probably indicate a poorly lubricated system. Values of R should be considered as relating only to the specific system from which they were obtained, because they are affected by other variables, such as compressional force and tablet H/D ratio.

Die-wall Lubrication

Most pharmaceutical tablet formulations require the addition of a lubricant to reduce friction at the die wall. Die-wall lubricants function by interposing a film of low shear strength at the interface between the tabletting mass and the die wall, as illustrated in Figure 4-15. Preferably, there is some chemical bonding between this "boundary" lubricant and the surface of the die wall as well as at the edge of the tablet. The best lubricants are those with low shear strength but strong cohesive tendencies in directions at right angles to the plane of shear. Table 4-1 gives the shear strength of some commonly used lubri-

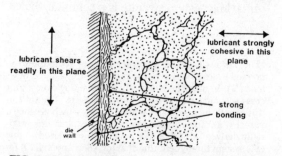

FIG. 4-15. *Diagram illustrates the preferred characteristics of die wall lubricants.*

TABLE 4-1. *The Shear Strength of Some Lubricants*

Material	Shear Strength (M Pa)	Material	Shear Strength (M Pa)
Stearic acid	1.32	Sodium stearate	3.32
Calcium stearate	1.47	Talc with grain	6.20
Hard paraffin	1.86	Talc across grain	7.85
Magnesium stearate	1.96	Boric acid	7.16
Potassium stearate	3.07	Graphite	7.35

cants as measured by a punch penetration test. By utilizing materials with low shear strength as lubricants, shear failure occurs in the lubricant layers and not at the compressed powder or resultant wall interfaces (Fig. 4-15).

Ejection Forces

Radial die-wall forces and die-wall friction also affect the ease with which the compressed tablet can be removed from the die. The force necessary to eject a finished tablet follows a distinctive pattern of three stages. The first stage involves the distinctive peak force required to initiate ejection, by breaking of tablet/die-wall adhesions. A smaller force usually follows, namely that required to push the tablet up the die wall. The final stage is marked by a declining force of ejection as the tablet emerges from the die. Variations on this pattern are sometimes found, especially when lubrication is inadequate and/or "slip-stick" conditions occur between the tablet and the die wall, owing to continuing formation and breakage of tablet/die-wall adhesions. Worn dies, which cause the bore to become barrel-shaped, give rise to a similar abnormal ejection force trace and may lead to failure of the tablet structure.

A direct connection is to be expected between die wall frictional forces and the force required to eject the tablet from the die, F_E. For example, well-lubricated systems (as indicated by a large R value) have been shown to lead to smaller F_E values.

Force-Volume Relationships

The end of the compressional process may be recognized as being the point at which all air spaces have been eliminated, i.e., $v_b = v_t$ and therefore $E = 0$. A small residual porosity is desirable, however, so there is particular interest in the relationship between applied force F_A and remaining porosity E. Originally, it was suggested that decreasing porosity resulted from a two-step process: (1) the filling of large spaces by interparticulate slippage and (2) the filling of small voids by deformation or fragmentation at higher loads.

This process can be expressed mathematically:[21]

$$\frac{E_o - E}{E_o \cdot (1 - E)} = K_1 e^{\frac{-K_2}{P}} + K_3 e^{\frac{-K_4}{P}} \quad (16)$$

where E_o is the initial porosity, E is the porosity at pressure P, and K_1, K_2, K_3 and K_4 are constants. The two terms on the right side of the equation refer to steps (1) and (2) respectively. Although equation (16) so far has only been shown to fit data from a few materials (such as alumina and magnesia), it does establish that the degree of compression achieved for a given load depends upon the initial porosity (E_o).

Therefore, the common practice of comparing different formulations by means of testing tablets of the same *weight* is undesirable. One variable is eliminated if experiments are carried out on tablet masses of the same true volume, and allowance should be made for varying initial values of bulk volume (V_b) when interpreting the results.

A more complex sequence of events during compression involves four stages, as illustrated by the data in Figure 4-16. Stage i represents the initial repacking of the particles, followed by elastic deformation (stage ii) until the elastic limit is reached. Plastic deformation and/or brittle fracture then dominates (stage iii) until all voids are virtually eliminated. At this point, the onset of stage iv, compression of the solid crystal lattice, occurs.

Attempts that have been made to derive equations for the first three stages, are of limited value, because in practice, the stages are not totally sequential. Owing to transmitted force variation, they may occur simultaneously in different regions of the same tablet.

In many tabletting processes, however, once appreciable force has been applied, the relationship between applied pressure (P) and some vol-

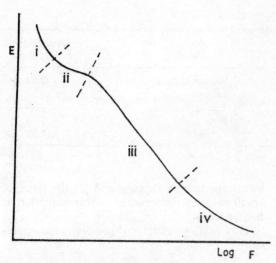

FIG. 4-16. *Decreasing porosity with increasing compressional force for single-ended pressing.*

ume parameter such as porosity (E) does become linear over the range of pressure commonly used in tabletting (region iii in Fig. 4-16). For example, an equation first suggested by Shapiro has been shown to fit data obtained from several pharmaceutical materials:[22]

$$Log\ E = Log\ E_o - K.P. \qquad (17)$$

where E_o is the porosity when the pressure is zero, and K is a constant. Another equation for which there is considerable evidence, is attributed to Walker:[23]

$$\frac{1}{1-E} = K_1 - K_2 \cdot Log\ P \qquad (18)$$

Heckel Plots

The foregoing equations have been criticized because some of the constants apparently lack physical significance. Another equation, credited to Heckel,[24] is free from this empiricism, however. The Heckel equation is based upon analogous behavior to a first-order reaction, where the pores in the mass are the reactant, that is:

$$Log\ \frac{1}{E} = K_yP + K_r \qquad (19)$$

where K_y is a material-dependent constant inversely proportional to its yield strength S ($K_y = 1/3S$), and K_r is related to the inital repacking stage, and hence E_o. The above relationships may be established by simply measuring

the applied compressional force F and the movements of the punches during a compression cycle and translating this data into values of P (applied pressure) and E (porosity). For a cylindric tablet, P is given by:

$$P = \frac{4F}{\pi \cdot D^2} \qquad (20)$$

where D is the tablet diameter. Similarly, values of E can be calculated for any stage from:

$$E = 100 \cdot \left[1 - \frac{4w}{\rho_t \cdot \pi \cdot D^2 \cdot H}\right] \qquad (21)$$

where w is the weight of the tabletting mass, ρ_t is its true density, and H is the thickness of the tablet at that point (obtained from the relative punch displacement measurements). (See previous section, "Mass-Volume Relationships.")

The particular value of Heckel plots arises from their ability to identify the predominant form of deformation in a given sample. Materials that are comparatively soft and that readily undergo plastic deformation retain different degrees of porosity, depending upon the initial packing in the die.[25] This in turn is influenced by the size distribution, shape, etc. of the original particles. Heckel plots for such materials are shown by type *a* in Figure 4-17; sodium chloride is a typical example.

Conversely, harder materials with higher yield pressure values usually undergo compression by fragmentation first, to provide a denser packing. Label *b* in Figure 4-17 shows Heckel plots for different size fractions of the same material that are typical of this behavior. Lactose is one such material.

Type *a* Heckel plots usually exhibit a higher final slope (K_y) than type *b*, which implies that the former materials have, as expected, a lower yield stress. Hard, brittle materials are, in general, more difficult to compress than soft, yielding ones because fragmentation with subsequent percolation of fragments is less efficient than void filling by plastic deformation. In fact, as the porosity approaches zero, plastic deformation may be the predominant mechanism for all materials.

The two regions of the Heckel plot are thought to represent the initial repacking stage and the subsequent deformation process, the point of intersection corresponding to the lowest force at which a coherent tablet is formed. In addition, the crushing strength of tablets can be correlated with the value of K_y of the Heckel plot; larger values of K_y usually indicate harder tab-

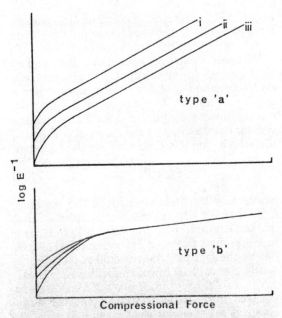

FIG. 4-17. *Examples of Heckel plots. Curves i, ii, and iii represent decreasing particle size fractions of the same material. Type a curves are typical of plastically deforming materials, while those in which fragmentation occurs initially tend to show type b behavior.*

lets. Such information can be used as a means of binder selection when designing tablet formulations. Note that Heckel plots can be influenced by the overall time of compression, the degree of lubrication, and even the size of the die, so that the effect of these variables can also be studied.

Another important factor in the use of all force-porosity relationships is that for many formulations, there is a relatively narrow optimum residual porosity range that provides adequate mechanical strength, rapid water uptake, and hence, good disintegration characteristics. It is to the formulators' advantage to identify this optimum range and be able to predict compressing conditions needed to reach it. In addition to the predictive capability, establishing behavioral patterns for a given formulation (so-called "finger-printing") may provide valuable diagnostic information in the event that a particular batch of the product causes problems.

Note also that the initial porosity can affect the course of the entire compressional sequence, and that in general, slow force application leads to a low porosity for a given applied load.

Decompression

In operations such as tabletting, the compressional process is followed by a decompression stage, as the applied force is removed. This leads to a new set of stresses within the tablet as a result of elastic recovery, which is augmented by the forces necessary to eject the tablet from the die. Irrespective of the consolidation mechanism, the tablets must be mechanically strong enough to accommodate these stresses; otherwise, structural failure will occur.

For this reason, studies in which data are collected during both parts of the cycle have proved valuable. In particular, the degree and rate of relaxation within tablets, immediately after the point of maximum compression, have been shown to be characteristic for a particular system. Recording this phase of the cycle as well can provide valuable insight into the reasons behind inferior tablet quality and may suggest a remedy. For example, if the degree and rate of relaxation are high, addition of some plastically deforming component, such as polyvinyl pyrrolidone, may be advisable to reduce the risk of pronounced recovery leading to structural failure.

If the stress relaxation process involves plastic flow, it may continue after all compressional force has been removed, and the residual radial pressure will decay with time. The plastic flow can be interpreted in terms of a viscous and elastic parameter in series.[26] This interpretation leads to a relationship of the form:

$$\text{Log } F_t = \text{Log } F_m - Kt \qquad (22)$$

where F_t is the force left in the viscoelastic region at a time t, and F_m is the total magnitude of this force at time $t = 0$ (i.e., when decompression begins). K is the *viscoelastic slope* and a measure of the degree of plastic flow. Materials with higher K values undergo more plastic flow; such materials often form strong tablets at relatively low compaction forces.

Alternatively, the changing thickness of the tabletting mass due to the compactional force, and subsequently due to elastic recovery during unloading, can be used to obtain a measure of *plastoelasticity*, γ.[27] Specifically:

$$\gamma = \frac{H_o}{H_m} \cdot \frac{H_r - H_m}{H_o - H_m} \qquad (23)$$

where H_o, H_m, and H_r are the thickness of the tablet mass at the onset of loading, at the point of maximum applied force, and on ejection from the die, respectively. A linear relationship between γ and log reciprocal of the tensile strength of the tablets has been demonstrated.[27] In general, values of γ above 9 tend to produce tablets that are laminated or capped.

Compaction Profiles

Monitoring of that proportion of the applied pressure transmitted radially to the die wall has been reported by several groups of workers. For many pharmaceutical materials, such investigations lead to characteristic hysteresis curves, which have been termed *compaction profiles.* Figure 4-18 is a typical example. Remember that the radial die-wall force arises as a result of the tabletting mass attempting to expand in the horizontal plane in response to the vertical compression. The ratio of these two dimensional changes, the *Poisson ratio,* is an important material-dependent property affecting the compressional process. The ratio is a property of solid bodies, however, and not necessarily of a porous mass of particulate solid. The anomalous results discussed in the literature may well reflect this important distinction, but certain qualitative deductions may still be possible.

For instance, when the elastic limit of the material is high, elastic deformation may make the major contribution, and on removal of the applied load, the extent of the elastic relaxation depends upon the value of the material's modulus of elasticity (Young's modulus). If this value is low, there is considerable recovery, and unless a strong structure has been formed, there is the danger of structural failure. Maximum compressional force levels are particularly important in such cases, since most of the stored energy is released on removal of the applied load. Conversely, if the modulus of elasticity is high, there is a small dimensional change on decompression and less risk of failure. The area of the hysteresis loop (0ABC′) indicates the extent of departure from ideal elastic behavior, since for a perfectly elastic body, line BC′ would coincide with AB.

In many tabletting operations, the applied force exceeds the elastic limit (point B), and brittle fracture and/or plastic deformation is then a major mechanism. For example, if the material readily undergoes plastic deformation with a constant yield stress as the material is sheared, then the region B to C should obey the equation:

$$P_R = P_A - 2S \qquad (24)$$

where S is the yield strength of the material. Note that the slope of this plot is unity, so that marked deviation from this value may indicate a more complex behavior. Deviation could also be due to the fact that the material is still significantly porous, which would invalidate the analogy to a solid body. Until this difference can be resolved, little is to be gained in proposing mathematical solutions for the region BC, which is often nonlinear anyway. This does not mean, however, that compaction profiles themselves cannot provide further useful information.

For example, since point C represents the situation at the maximum compressional force level, the region CD is therefore the initial relaxation response as the applied load is removed. In practice, many compaction profiles exhibit a marked change in the slope of this line during decompression, and a second yield point (point D) has been reported.

Perhaps the residual radial pressure (intercept EO), when all the compressional force has been removed, is more significant, since this pressure is an indication of the force being transmitted by the die wall to the tablet. As such, it provides a measure of possible ejection force level and likely lubricant requirements; if pronounced, it suggests a strong tablet capable of at least withstanding such a compressive pressure. Conversely, a low value of residual radial pressure, or more significantly, a sharp change in slope (DE) is sometimes indicative of at least incipient failure of the tablet structure. In practical terms, this may mean introducing a plastically deforming component (e.g., PVP [polyvinyl pyrrolidone] as binder, starch as diluent) to facilitate dissipation of these stresses, and hence a more gradual change in slope of the decompression plot, a preferred feature. In one recent study,[28] modified compaction profiles $(P_A - P_R)$ versus $(P_A + P_R)$ were able to distinguish between readily consolidating and nonconsolidating materials. Specifically, two characteristic parameters (a normal stress value at zero shear and a minimum shear stress value), obtained

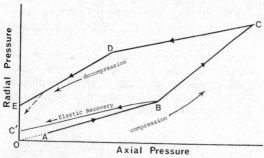

FIG. 4-18. *Examples of compaction profiles. Dotted line O to A represents a highly variable response due to repacking, while at A, elastic deformation becomes dominant and continues until the elastic limit B is reached. From B to the point of maximum compression C, deformation is predominantly plastic, or brittle fracture is taking place. The decompression process C to D is accompanied by elastic recovery, and if a second yield point (D) is reached, by plastic deformation or brittle fracture D to E. The decompression line B to C′ represents the behavior of a largely elastic material.*

from the unloading portion of the cycle, were shown to correlate with tensile strength and surface hardness of the compacted materials.

Energy Involved in Compaction

Tablet machines, roll compactors, extruders, and similar types of equipment require a high input of mechanical work. The ways in which this work is converted into other forms of energy during these processes is of interest in both research and production areas. More specifically, the work requirement is a key factor in machine design, and any proportion of the applied energy stored in a product such as a tablet retains a destructive capability.

The work involved in various phases of a tablet or granule compaction operation includes (1) that necessary to overcome friction between particles, (2) that necessary to overcome friction between particles and machine parts, (3) that required to induce elastic and/or plastic deformation of the material, (4) that required to cause brittle fracture within the material, and (5) that associated with the mechanical operation of various machine parts.

Normally, an appreciable amount of the energy supplied is converted to heat, which of course does not contribute toward the main objective of the process. On a theoretic basis, however, this heat does provide a means of monitoring the energy balance in the system. For example, one of the earliest experimental reports was that of Nelson and associates,[29] who compared the energy expenditure in lubricated and unlubricated sulfathiazole granulations as shown in Table 4-2. Lubrication reduced energy expenditure by 75%, chiefly because of a lessening of the major component, namely energy utilized during ejection of the finished tablet. Note that lubrication has no apparent effect on the actual amount of energy required to compress

the material, i.e., overcome resistance to relative interparticulate movement.

These workers' estimation of the total work involved, W_T, was obtained by monitoring punch force and the distance D through which it acted, so that:

$$W_T = \int_{D_{F=0}}^{D_{max}} F \cdot dD \qquad (25)$$

which represents the area under the entire force-displacement plot (the area ABC in Fig. 4-19).

This approach oversimplifies the true picture because, as can be seen from Figure 4-19, in which both punch forces and punch displacement data have been collected throughout an entire compression-decompression press cycle, W_T comprises at least three components.[30] The region W_F represents the work done in overcom-

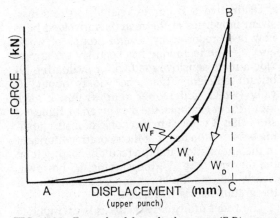

FIG. 4-19. *Example of force-displacement (F-D) curve. ($\triangle$) upper punch force; ($\blacktriangle$) lower punch force. The area W_F represents the work done in overcoming friction, while that of area W_D is the elastic deformation energy stored in the tablet during compression. Thus, W_N is the net mechanical energy actually used to form the tablet.*

TABLE 4-2 *Energy Expended in Compression of 400 mg Sulfathiazole Granulation*

Compression Process	Energy Expended (Joules)	
	Unlubricated	Lubricated
Compression	6.28	6.28
Overcoming die wall friction	3.35	negligible
Upper punch withdrawal	5.02	negligible
Tablet ejection	21.35	2.09
TOTALS	36.00	8.37

After Nelson et al.[29]

ing friction and therefore depends upon the properties of the tablet mass. W_N is the net mechanical energy actually used to form the tablet, and W_D is the elastic deformation energy stored in the tablet initially, but released during decompression. If the top punch moves too quickly during this decompression, contact with the tablet may be lost. In this eventuality, the complete work of elastic recovery of the tablet is not transferred to the punch face, and an error is introduced into the decompression curve.

Early investigators of the technique overcame the problem by compressing the tablet a second time before ejecting it from the die.[23] The second compression-decompression cycle provides a measure (W_{N2}) of the net energy required to recompress the material to the point B (in Fig. 4-19). W_{N2} is equivalent to the amount of energy involved in the elastic recovery of the tablet.

Force-Displacement (F-D) Curves

Distinctive F-D curves related to the stress/strain properties of the materials involved have now been reported by several groups of workers.[30-33] The technique has been shown to provide a more sensitive method for evaluating lubricant efficiency than the widely quoted R value (which is the lower to upper punch force ratio).[31] For example, the data given in Table 4-3 show that R values are incapable of distinguishing between the result of incorporating lubricant in the granulation and the result of coating it on the die wall. The W_N measurements, however, clearly indicate the lower energy expenditure if the granulation is lubricated.

The wider utility of F-D curves is exemplified by their application to the selection of a "best" binder (from gelatin, starch, and methylcellulose) for a sulphonamide tablet, by determining the contribution of the three components W_F, W_N, and W_D to the total work W_T.[33] A plot of W_N versus maximum compressional force produced curves such as those shown in Figure 4-20.

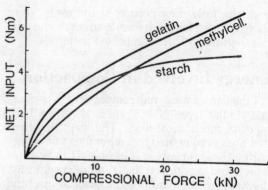

FIG. 4-20. *Binder selection using net energy input during tabletting process. Because of correlation between mechanical strength of tablets and net energy input, gelatin is the binder of choice in this example. (After deBlaey et al.[33])*

Since good correlation is usually found between W_N and the crushing strength of the tablets, gelatin in this example would be chosen as the best binder. Note too the pronounced flattening of the curve for starch, so that compression of this formulation at maximum F_A values above the point of inflection would not be helpful and might even be deleterious, owing to increased elastic recovery that could lead to structural failure of the tablet.

Because the rate of compression is known to affect the tabletting process, an extension of the use of F-D curve data has been suggested.[34] This proposition takes into account the rate of loading by monitoring the power expended, rather than the work involved. In practice, the area under the F-D curve is divided by the time over which the force is applied.

Strength of Tablets

The mechanical strength of tablets has been described in a variety of ways, including hardness, bending strength, fracture resistance, friability, and crushing strength.[35]

TABLE 4-3 *Compression of 300 mg at 440 M Pa*

	Unlubricated	Die Wall Lubricated	Granulation Lubricated
Coefficient of Lubrication, R	0.84	0.98	0.98
Net Work for Compression (Nm)	5.6	4.4	3.4
Remaining Lower Punch Pressure (MPa)	3.2	2.5	2.5

After deBlaey and Polderman.[31]

Crushing Strength

The most popular estimate of tablet strength has been crushing strength, S_c, which may be defined as "that compressional force (F_c) which, when applied diametrically to a tablet, just fractures it."[36] Most practical tests involve placing the tablet on or against a fixed anvil and transmitting the force to it by means of a moving plunger, until the tablet just fractures. Since tablets are anisotropic and test conditions rarely provide well-defined uniform stresses, full and exact interpretation of findings is difficult. With flat-faced anvil and plunger, the failure may be compressive (i.e., the tablet is crushed). If one of them is knife-edged, however, then it is more likely to be tensile (tablet splits open across a diameter). It may then be described by the equation:

$$S_T = \frac{2F_c}{D \cdot H} \qquad (26)$$

where S_T is the tensile strength, and D and H are the diameter and thickness of the tablet, respectively.

It has been suggested that the work W_f required to cause tablet failure correlates better with other mechanical strength tests and is a more sensitive parameter for comparison with other tabletting parameters. W_f is obtained from the equation:

$$W_f = \frac{2}{\pi DH} \cdot \int F dz \qquad (27)$$

where F is the force applied to the tablet and z, the deformation resulting from it, is represented by the relative displacement of the anvil and plunger.

Many crushing-strength testers are described in the literature, and several are available commercially. Comparisons of these have been made,[36] and three important sources of variability or error have been identified. Many older manually operated types had a rate of loading that was operator-controlled; this could affect the value of S_c obtained. The zero setting was indeterminate in some cases, and in a few, the scale reading did not accurately indicate the actual load being applied. For these reasons, instruments should be calibrated and checked periodically, especially if this property is being correlated with other characteristics.

Many reports relate crushing strength to other process and tablet parameters.[37] Among the most widely quoted relationships are linear proportionality with disintegration time and log F_A,

and inverse proportionality with porosity, over normal ranges of compressional force.[38]

Failure may be propagated through the tablet along individual granule boundaries or through the granules themselves, depending on whether the granular bonding is weaker or stronger than that between their composite particles. If fracture tends to occur across granules, then granule size influences tablet strength, smaller sizes leading to greatest strength for a given compressional pressure.[39] Conversely, if fracture along granule boundaries predominates, granule size may have little influence on strength.

Knudsen proposed a general equation of the form:[40]

$$S_c = K \cdot d^{-a} \qquad (28)$$

where d is the mean particle diameter, and the constant a is a material-dependent property. The results of Shotton and Ganderton supported this proposal,[41] as can be seen from the data given in Figure 4-21. The presence of lubricants, however, can nullify or even reverse the trends shown in this figure, because of the weakening of interparticle bonds.

The inherent cohesiveness of very fine particles may enhance the consolidation process and lead to even stronger tablets for a particular compressive force. On the other hand, their rela-

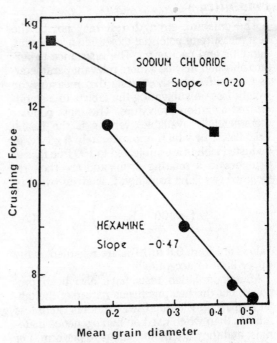

FIG. 4-21. *Effect of particle size on the crushing strength of tablets. (Applied pressure 85 MPa.) (From Shotton and Ganderton.[41])*

tively high microporosity may trap more air in the tablets, which can give rise to capping. For materials in which fracture occurs along granule boundaries, the presence of a thin film of binder at these surfaces may lead to failure across the granules, which when tabletted could result in an increase in tablet strength.

Reports describing SEM photomicrography of tablet surfaces have provided vivid pictorial evidence of tablet microstructure and of the role of various excipients.[42] More specifically, those adjuvants used widely in direct compression tabletting operations have been subjected to detailed scrutiny by Shangraw and colleagues.[43] Using this same approach, Seager and co-authors have been able to correlate method of granule manufacture with tablet structure and properties.[44] They found that spray-dried granules produced the strongest tablets, which dissolved at least as fast as those prepared by wet massing. Tablets prepared using granules from both of these methods possessed mechanical and release properties superior to those of tablets made from previously roll-compacted material. They attributed this to variation in liquid penetration rates, which are related to residual porosities, and to the tablets' degree of hydrophilicity, which is due to binder distribution.

Friability

The crushing strength test may not be the best measure of potential tablet behavior during handling and packaging. The resistance to surface abrasion may be a more relevant parameter, as exemplified by those tests that measure the weight loss on subjecting the tablets to a standardized agitation procedure. The most popular (commercially available) version is the Roche Friabilator, in which approximately 6 g (w_o) of dedusted tablets are subjected to 100 free falls of 6 inches in a rotating drum and are then reweighed (w). The friability, f, is given by:

$$f = 100 \cdot \left(1 - \frac{w_o}{w}\right) \qquad (29)$$

Values of f from 0.8 to 1.0% are regarded as the upper limit of acceptability.

Microindentation tests have also been proposed, but the heterogeneous nature of the tablet surface on the microscale renders them less reliable than when used on homogeneous materials, and they are more tedious to perform. For these reasons, they have found only limited acceptance, and then in the research rather than production areas.

One report, however, does describe the practical use of indentation hardness and tensile strength data to define three dimensionless indices (strain index, bonding index, and brittle fracture index) that were used to quantify the relative tabletting performance (especially lamination tendency) of both single components and mixtures.[45]

Lamination (Capping) of Tablets

One of the more common problems encountered in compaction is that the tablet structure fails on ejection from the die or during subsequent operations such as coating. Often, the failure has the characteristic appearance shown diagrammatically in Figure 4-22—hence, the term *capping*. The phenomenon was first thought to be due entirely to entrapment of air within the tablet. This air would be under a pressure approximating that of the applied compressional load, and so on ejection would possess considerable disruptive capability. Air entrapment is more likely to occur with fine particle sizes of materials, which tend to pack poorly. Slow compressional rates and use of multistage compression presses often reduce capping tendencies and have provided support for this postulate. This concept, however, is known to represent only one factor in what may be an extremely complex process. For example, a recent report demonstrated that when certain granulations were compressed at high speed under partial vacuum, classical capping was minimized, but was replaced by a tendency to laminate.[46]

Massive elastic recovery to relieve the inherent variation in compressional stress distribution already described, when associated with

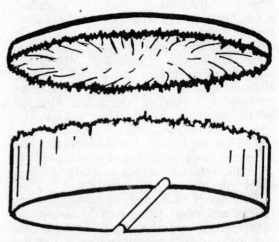

FIG. 4-22. *Diagram of a "capped" tablet.*

weakly bonded material, must be another major contributing factor in many instances. Any technique that can reduce this effect is helpful, such as inclusion of components in the formula to enhance bonding and provide a matrix of plastically deforming material for stress relief. In addition, more gradual loading and unloading of the tablet mass by utilization of large compression rolls, precompression, and slow press speeds also reduce the tendency, as does reduction in maximum compressional force. Lubricant and moisture levels, tooling geometry and condition, and compression mechanism (the type of press) all contribute to the properties of the tablets produced and demand constant consideration. For this reason, attention has been directed to the advantages of instrumentation that can accomplish at least some of these monitoring tasks.

The Instrumentation of Tablet Machines

Several distinct forms of instrumentation are discussed within this section. Increasing evidence shows the value of instrumenting tablet presses to provide information on the inherent compaction characteristics of the major components in a formulation, and on the effect of additives upon them. The emphasis, therefore, is on properties of the materials in a research and development environment, which perhaps could utilize single-station machines for some of the work. On the other hand, increasing use of high-speed multi-station tablet presses, coupled with a desire to improve quality specifications for tablets, leads to forms of instrumentation intended primarily for production machines, but of interest to the quality assurance department as well.

The technology described in the first part of the chapter suggests that the mechanisms involved in the tabletting process center on utilization of the unsatisfied bonds at the solid surface. This process is enhanced by the generation of large areas of clean surface, which are then pressed together, as might occur if appreciable brittle fracture and plastic deformation were introduced into the system. It was also noted that the behavior on decompression can markedly affect the characteristics of the finished tablets, because the structure must be strong enough to accommodate the recovery- and ejection-induced stresses. Furthermore, ability to monitor ejection forces leads to valuable information on lubricant efficiency. Measurement of punch and die forces plus the relative displacement of the punches can provide raw data, which when suitably processed and interpreted, facilitate evaluation of many of these tabletting parameters.

The value of using a single-station press for developmental work on formulations that are to be manufactured on multi-station presses is strictly limited. This is less the case when material rather than process factors are most important, unless the rate of loading is critical. The sensitivity of the formulation being tested to the loading rate, however, should be determined by compression at different speeds and by monitoring of any changes in tablet properties.

Because of this rate factor, several workers have elected to instrument isolated punch and die sets and to carry out compression experiments using these sets in conjunction with a compression/tension testing machine. For example, the assembly shown in Figure 4-23 is capable of monitoring all of the various forces acting on the system as well as the punch displacements. Recently, a sophisticated system has been described that is capable of mimicking (in real time) the precise compression cycle of any press; thus, it has all the advantages of using a single station of tooling and still follows rotary press action.[47] The system stores a representation of the precise compression cycle of the

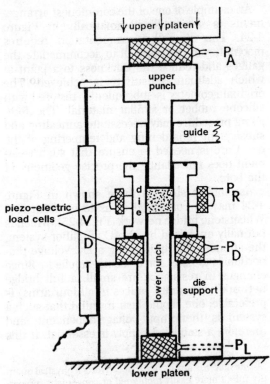

FIG. 4-23. *Diagram of instrumented, isolated punch and die assembly.*

press in a microprocessor, which in turn controls the movements of the isolated punches, so that it reproduces the exact loading profile of the press. Such assemblies facilitate compressional studies at various compressional rates and provide a convenient means of acquiring the maximum amount of information while using the minimum amount of time and materials. They are now often referred to as "compaction simulators."

Single-Station Presses

Almost all reports in the literature describe strain gauge networks as a transducer* for measuring the magnitude of the forces operating during the compression cycle. Resistive (metal foil) gauges are usually preferred, and ideally, they should be bonded as near to the active site as practicable, namely at the punch faces, so as to eliminate lack of correlation between signals obtained from remote regions of the machine frame and the actual forces present in the tooling. The bonding must be over the entire area of the correctly aligned gauge as described in strain gauge manuals,[48] at a site where the elastic change in linear dimension of the stress-bearing member (due to the applied forces) can be measured.

An example of one of the commonest arrangements is shown diagrammatically in Figure 4-24. The die-wall instrumentation requires machining of the die wall to accommodate the gauges and reduce the thickness to a point at which adequate sensitivity is achieved. The original geometry is subsequently restored with silicone rubber or similar material. The foregoing procedure may necessitate annealing and subsequent rehardening and tempering of the die. Care is needed to ensure that such treatment does not change the precise geometry of the bore.

Assemblies such as those shown in Figure 4-24 may be connected so as to conform to a Wheatstone bridge network (Fig. 4-25), which is normally energized by an AC amplifier system, the attenuated output giving a DC voltage proportional to the force being applied. Since changes in resistance are small, a full bridge network (with strain gauges in all four arms) is preferable; one should bear in mind that such a system is then input-voltage-dependent, and therefore a stabilized supply is essential. If this

*A *transducer* is any device that converts a physical quantity into a more easily monitored or convenient (proportional) signal, e.g., mechanical force into a directly proportional DC voltage.

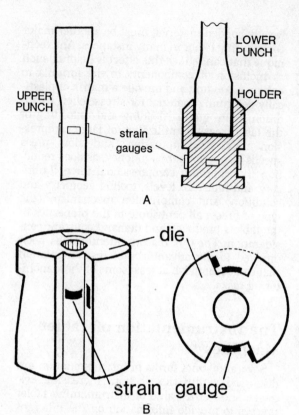

FIG. 4-24. *Strain-gauged punches (A) and instrumented die (B). Favored locations for mounting small linear foil strain gauges are the upper punch, lower punch holder, and modified die of a single-station tablet press.*

arrangement is mounted as shown in Figure 4-26 ("Poisson" configuration), compensation is provided for both temperature change and any bending of the piece.

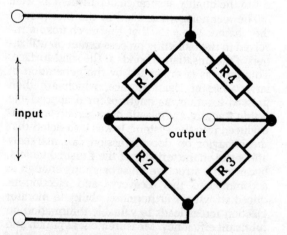

FIG. 4-25. *Simple full-bridge Wheatstone bridge circuit, in which R1, R2, R3, and R4 represent strain gauges.*

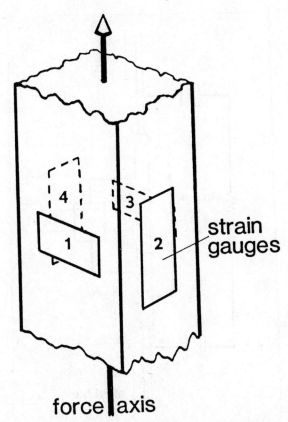

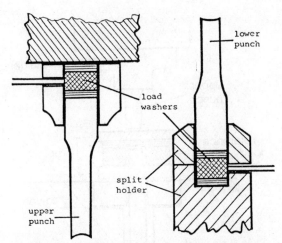

FIG. 4-27. *Piezo-electric punch instrumentation. Preferred locations for mounting small piezo-electric force transducers are the punch holders of a single-station press.*

strain gauges

force axis

FIG. 4-26. *Poisson arrangement. In this full-bridge strain gauge network, gauges 2 and 4 are active, while gauges 1 and 3 are temperature-compensating.*

The advantages of piezo-electric devices include high sensitivity, robust construction, and no bonding to machine fabric, which therefore allows easy changing of tooling. Furthermore, since the signal originates as an electrical charge, the transducer may be zeroed, simply by grounding it, regardless of initial load.

Although calibration data are supplied by the manufacturer of the above equipment, in situ calibration of the particular instrumentation against known loads is highly desirable. With punch assemblies, this may be achieved by use of a calibrated load cell, which can be placed on the die table (Fig. 4-29); its signal can be compared with those from the instrumented punches as they are simultaneously loaded. Alternatively, entire punch assemblies can be removed from the press and mounted in an accurate compression/tension test press. The normal

Alternatively, transducers based upon the piezo-electric effect in certain crystals, notably quartz, may be used. When subjected to external forces, these materials develop an electrical charge proportional to the effect of the force. Such a transducer is connected by a high impedance cable to a charge amplifier, which converts the charge into a directly proportional DC voltage. One disadvantage of such transducers is that the charge inevitably dissipates with time, and since a difference is being measured, they are unsuitable for static force measurements.

Small piezo-electric load washers can easily be mounted on, or in, the upper and lower punch holders of single-station presses, as shown in Figure 4-27. Radial die wall measurement is more difficult, but has been achieved by means of a special holder for the transducer, as illustrated in Figure 4-28. Such systems, like their strain gauge equivalents, only monitor the radial force over a localized region of the die wall. They may give rise to misleading data, unless they are sited at the same level on the die wall as the region at which the tablet is being compressed.

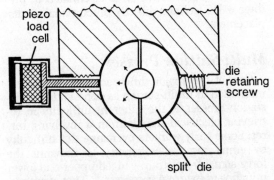

FIG. 4-28. *Piezo-electric die wall instrumentation. An example of the use of a piezo-electric force transducer (in a special holder) in conjunction with a vertically split die to measure radial die wall forces.*

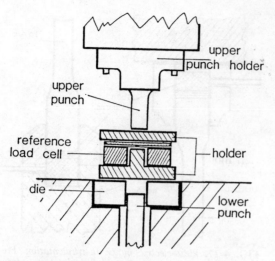

FIG. 4-29. *Calibration using load cell. Diagram illustrates the use of a piezo-electric transducer and special holder to calibrate the upper and lower punch instrumentation on a single-station press.*

procedure with die-wall instrumentation is less straightforward. Ideally, the necessary measurements are made by sealing the open ends of the die cavity, then pumping in oil at known pressures and noting the response. A close-fitting rubber plug or rubber powder in the die cavity, however, may be regarded as a perfectly elastic material (thus radial die-wall reaction will be equal to any applied force) and can therefore be substituted for oil.

The preferred form of transducer for measuring punch displacements is based on the differential inductor principle, and is commonly a *linear variable differential transformer* (LVDT) as shown diagrammatically in Figure 4-30. The movable ferrous core of the transducer is rigidly connected to the punch by a mechanical link, so that movement unbalances the "secondary" circuit, the output of which is attenuated to produce a DC voltage directly proportional to displacement.

Multi-Station Presses

One of the major differences in the instrumentation of multi-station as opposed to single-station presses is the inherent difficulty in retrieving electrical signals from a revolving turret. Some early workers overcame this difficulty by employing radiotelemetry to transmit the force signal from strain-gauged upper and lower punches to external recorders.[49] They were unsuitable for normal production conditions, since only a few stations were operative, and only low machine speeds were possible. In a system de-

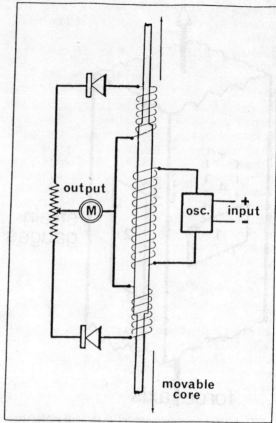

FIG. 4-30. *Typical LVDT circuit. Diagram shows the primary winding and two equally but oppositely wound secondaries surrounding the movable soft iron core.*

scribed by Ho and co-workers,[50] however, these disadvantages have been overcome, and a significant proportion of the stations remain active, as shown in Figure 4-31.

Other workers have been less reluctant to utilize remote stationary sites on the machine

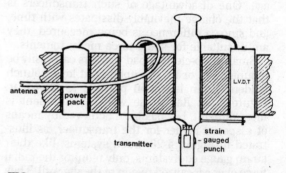

FIG. 4-31. *Telemetry system. Diagram shows a possible arrangement for a force and displacement measuring system, using radiotelemetry to retrieve the signals from a multi-station tablet press.*

frame, in particular the upper and lower compression roll carrier systems. For a given machine, the best location probably depends upon its actual design, but certain general points are worth noting. The response of a strain gauge is entirely a function of the change in linear dimension of the machine part to which it is bonded. Therefore, such changes must be sufficient to induce an adequate change in gauge resistance while not exceeding its elastic limit. In practice, this usually means that some part of the press has to be weakened by machining, an operation in which great care must be exercised. Cast iron components are unsuitable because of variability in their modulus of elasticity and Poisson ratio; therefore, only parts constructed of steel should be selected. Sensitivity to temperature changes may also influence site choice so as to avoid susceptible regions, e.g., near electric motors.

One of the more popular arrangements on modern high-speed presses is to attach strain gauges or to incorporate a piezo-electric load cell into one of the tie rods, as illustrated in Figure 4-32, although strain gauges may require machining of the rod. Other sites have included the compression columns, specially modified pressure rolls, and a modified eyebolt of the lower compression roll assembly.

Instrumenting the normal ejection cam on a rotary tablet machine by attaching strain gauges to its bolts is of limited value, because the resulting signal is a summation of the effects of the several lower punches on it at any instant. The solution adopted by Wray employed a two-part cam so that the region responsible for tablet ejection is separate and in the form of a beam fixed at one end.[51] This method necessitated minor modifications to other parts of the machine but did not affect normal operation. Flexure of the beam caused by the lower punches during ejection was monitored by strain gauges and was found to mimic the ejection response of an instrumented lower punch.

Alternatively, the normal cam can be cut into three sections, each clamped to the frame by a bolt, two of which are fitted with a piezo-electric load washer, for instance. The division should be such that there is only one punch on each section at a time (Fig. 4-33). The first transducer then monitors the force to initiate ejection (to break tablet die-wall adhesions), and the second monitors the force necessary to push the tablet clear of the die. This arrangement minimizes the fulcrum effect, as the punches move over the cam surface toward and then away from the actual transducer location. Certain aspects of the state of the tooling, such as sticking of the lower punches due to frictional effects, can also be detected by sensitive instrumentation of this type.

Mitrevej and Augsburger have recently described a system to measure the adhesion of tablets to the lower punch face by attaching strain gauges to a small cantilever blade mounted on the feed frame in front of the sweep-off attachment (Fig. 4-34).[52] They found that the force of adhesion did not necessarily reflect the ejection force or the lubricant activity of the formulation; however, the system did appear to be sensitive to batch variations in the antiadherent quality of magnesium stearate.

Regardless of which remote site is selected for instrumentation, the response should always be checked—and indeed, rechecked periodically—against signals obtained from directly instrumented tooling over the whole working range of the machine, to ensure constancy in the response relationships.

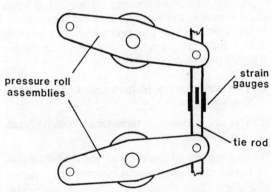

FIG. 4-32. *Instrumented tie rod. Diagram shows the location of strain gauges on the tie rod linking the upper and lower pressure roll carriers of a multi-station tablet press.*

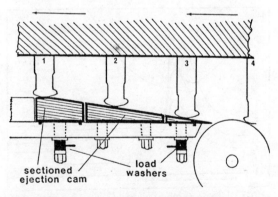

FIG. 4-33. *Instrumented ejection cam. Diagram shows the preferred method of sectioning an ejection cam and the transducer locations for monitoring ejection forces on a multi-station tablet press.*

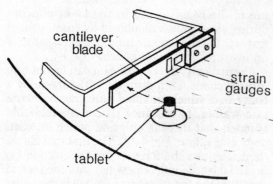

FIG. 4-34. *Instrumentation to measure "sweep-off" force. Diagram illustrates measurement of the force of adhesion between a tablet and the lower punch of a tablet press by means of a strain-gauged cantilever blade attached to the feed frame.*

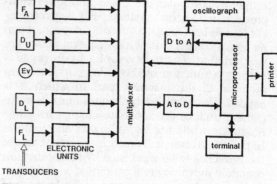

FIG. 4-36. *I.T.M.-microprocessor linkage. Diagram shows the major components of a typical instrumented tablet machine interfaced to a dedicated computer system.*

Signal Processing

The signals from the instrumentation described in this section are usually DC voltages and can therefore be retrieved, stored, and processed by a common means. Popular practice is to display the signals on a cathode ray oscillograph (CRO) since this enables instant visualization of the instrumentation output. In the past, such displays were often photographed to provide a permanent record, but ultraviolet recording oscillographs provide better definition of traces and can facilitate a larger number of simultaneous recording channels, as illustrated in Figure 4-35.

Inexpensive microcomputers that are currently available can remove much of the tedium in reducing raw data from the recorders previously described; they are therefore the method of choice. The analog signals (DC voltages) can be fed by an A-to-D (analog-to-digital) convertor

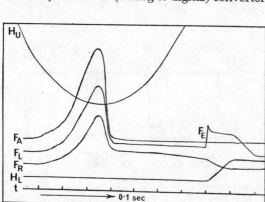

FIG. 4-35. *Typical traces from I.T.M. Reproduction of typical traces obtained from a multichannel U/V recording oscillograph connected to an instrumented single-station tablet press.*

into memory locations in the computer. This digital data can then be recalled, manipulated, and outputted in a wide range of graphic or tabular formats. By such means, active compounds and excipients can be "fingerprinted" for their compactional characteristics.[53] The general layout of a typical configuration is shown in Figure 4-36.

Role of Instrumentation in Production

The modern tablet production department seeks innovation because of the trend toward direct compression methods, the availability of machines with increased output, and the desire to lessen tablet-to-tablet variations. In addition the design of instrumentation that monitors, or perhaps exercises some degree of control over, the tabletting process is an attractive goal because of the possibility of reducing labor involvement.

To date, the most popular approach has been the attempt to limit weight and hardness deviations, based upon the premise that compressional force is directly proportional to tablet weight, providing the following:

1. The formulation is homogeneous (i.e., has uniform density).

2. The compressional force/tablet weight function is constant.

3. The volume of the die cavities at the point of maximum compression is constant.

The third supposition is valid only when the overall length of the punches and tip geometry are constant, the die bores are uniform, and the pressure rolls are perfectly cylindric and mounted centrally.

The output from the electronic unit of most force (and displacement) measuring systems is a DC voltage. Therefore, in this context, the system produces a series of voltage pulses of short duration, each proportional to the weight of an individual tablet. These signals can be conditioned to provide a wide range of monitoring and control facilities of increased complexity. The addition of a simple event marker facilitates the identification of a particular station and of any tooling faults, which produce repetitive atypical signals. The individual compression pulses can also be used to drive counting mechanisms and to provide a reliable figure for the number of tablets made.

The foregoing devices are uncomplicated and relatively inexpensive, but usually, there is a desire to extend the signal conditioning system to monitor the process to some degree. For example, one can set upper and lower limits for acceptable tablet weight and then distinguish pulses from tablets lying outside these thresholds. When the frequency of these out-of-specification tablets exceeds some preset value, a relay can be tripped to activate an alarm and/or the machine can be automatically stopped.

In general, for a larger investment, machines can be fitted with mechanical accept/reject gates at the machine outlet, so that individual out-of-specification tablets can be diverted to a separate container. This function requires a high level of sophistication, because the defective tablets must be "memorized" until they reach the outlet.

A second approach is to take the amplified output signals and feed them into an averaging network. This average DC voltage is compared with a reference voltage, and any difference is converted into an AC signal, which is amplified and used to drive a two-phase servomotor. The motor can be connected to the weight or pressure adjustment control of the press, so that any change in the average compressional force is reflected in an adjustment of either the weight or force control.

Regardless of which transducer systems, sites, or forces are selected, it is essential to ascertain that the response of the instrumentation is a direct function of the property needing to be monitored. Therefore, the work of Wray and his colleagues is important in that it establishes that stresses generated in certain parts of the machine frame are directly proportional to the punch forces, which in turn are related to compressional weights.[51]

One final important aspect of instrumenting high-speed multi-station presses is the frequency response of the various components of the system. Machine outputs are now exceeding 12,000 tablets per minute, which means that the frequency of the force pulses is approximately 0.1 kHz. Since the detection of small differences in individual pulses may be necessary, all units should have flat responses well beyond this level, up to approximately 1.0 kHz.

Instrumented tablet machine technology is advancing rapidly, and its ultimate role is not yet realized. It will undoubtedly lead, however, to an even better understanding of the tabletting process, which in turn will assist in formulation development and batch quality control. In addition, the ever-increasing demand for more fully automated production will be facilitated by such machines.

Instrumenting Hard-Shell Capsule Filling Machines

One group of machines for filling hard-shell gelatin capsules employs dosators, which form a soft plug of the powder mix and then transfer it to the empty shell body (see Chap. 13, Part I, "Hard Capsules"). This type of action requires that the material be somewhat cohesive, and that low levels of applied mechanical force are used to form and eject the plugs. Some similarity exists between these operations and tabletting, and attempts to instrument the machines in a manner that is analogous to those just described have been made. In the first report of such instrumentation, Cole and May described a modified dosator piston, to which strain gauges had been bonded as shown in Figure 4-37.[54] The machine was further altered so that the twin dosator head had a reciprocating rather than rotational movement. This facilitated using the instrumented machine through many filling cycles without entangling the transducer leads. Later workers used a mercury contact swivel to achieve the same end without changing the machine cycle.[55]

Such instrumentation permits continuous monitoring of the force necessary to form the plug during dosator filling, plus any residual force present during carry-over to the capsule shell position and that force necessary to eject it into the empty shell. Such forces were found to range from 5N to 350N, depending on the material, presence of lubricant, and time for which the machine had been running. Some typical recorder traces are shown in Figure 4-38.

Among the more important findings to emerge from such investigations is the role of even low

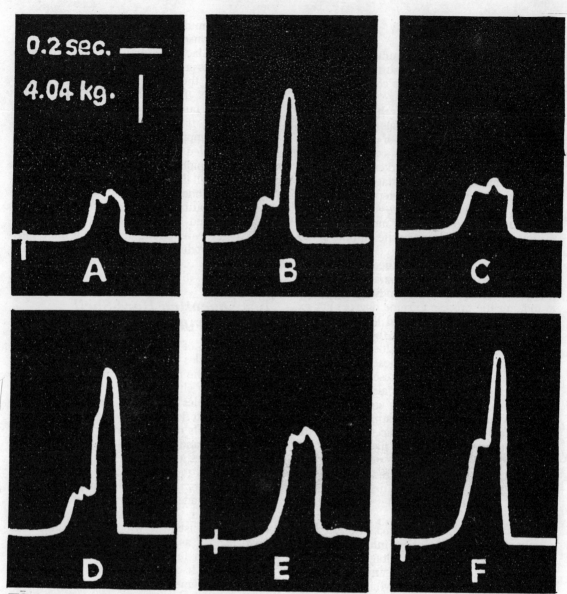

FIG. 4-38. *Typical traces from instrumented capsule machine dosator. Force-time traces are of three materials (A, B, lactose; C, D, compressible starch; E, F, dibasic calcium phosphate) at different levels. (From Small and Augsburger.[55] Reproduced with permission of the copyright owner.)*

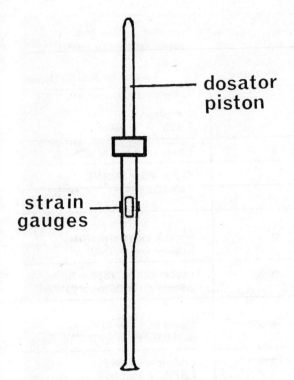

dosator piston

strain gauges

FIG. 4-37. *Diagram of instrumented dosator piston.*

or capsule at an early stage in development. Consequently, any technique that can assist in this process is particularly attractive. Because the measurements described here are sensitive to changes in the composition and performance of the tabletting or capsule mass, and because optimum values for the various parameters can usually be postulated, they provide a useful formulation and developmental tool and aid in solution of problems arising from batch-to-batch variations.

During the next decade, an increasing awareness of these possibilities is anticipated, and consequently, more profound studies of this particular form of powder compression and consolidation are to be expected. Paralleling these essential research and development activities are trends toward fuller automation of the facilities in which tablets and capsules are manufactured. Such trends place greater emphasis on the need for a fuller appreciation of the processes involved. Because complete elucidation of the tabletting operation, and indeed encapsulation, has not yet been realized, it must therefore continue to challenge contemporary investigators.

levels of lubricant (0.5%) in eliminating carry-over forces and reducing ejection forces, particularly during long runs. The adherence of material between the wall of the filling head and the piston can also be detected as a negative force after ejection and indicates a sensitive means of detecting this potential problem. Some materials such as lactose and basic dicalcium phosphate, if unlubricated, give rise to high ejection forces (300N) after only a few capsules have been filled and show the importance of determining precise lubrication needs.

Later studies have incorporated measurements of force and dosator piston displacement not unlike those described earlier for tablet machines: signals are retrieved from the rotating head by a mercury pool-slip ring assembly.[56] With this arrangement, the work involved in the various stages can be estimated, and the need for formulation modification established. This approach will undoubtedly be extended to other types of hard-shell capsule filling equipment, and perhaps to production filling operations, to achieve the same goals as enumerated for tablet manufacture.

For several reasons, including regulatory requirements and proliferation of generic products, researchers are increasingly pressured to define the optimum formulation for a new tablet

Appendix A

Symbols Used in Formulas

A. Area
D. Diameter or displacement
d. Particle diameter
E. Porosity
F. Force
f. Friability
H. Height/thickness
h. Height/thickness
K. A constant
L. Length
M. Mass
P. Pressure
R. Lubricant efficiency
S. Strength
t. Time
U. Piston movement
v. Volume
W. Work
w. Weight
Z. Strain
λ Poisson ratio
μ Frictional coefficient
ρ Density
σ Stress
Φ Angle of repose
γ Plastoelasticity

Appendix B *SI Units*

Unit	Name of Unit	Symbol	Definition	Approximate Equivalents
BASIC UNITS Length	meter	m		1 angstrom $\equiv 10^{-10}$ m 1 inch $\equiv 0.0254$ m
Mass	kilogram	kg		1 pound $\equiv 0.453592$ kg
Temperature	degree kelvin	°K		32°F $= 0$°C $\equiv 273.15$°K
Time	second	s		
DERIVED UNITS Area	square meter	m^2		1 square inch $\equiv 645.16$ mm^2 1 square foot $\equiv 0.0929$ m^2
Volume	cubic meter	m^3		1 cubic inch $\equiv 1.6387 \times 10^{-5}$ m^3 gallon $\equiv 3.7854 \times 10^{-3}$ m^3
Density	kilogram per cubic meter	kg m^{-3}		1 g per cc $\equiv 10^{-3}$kg m^{-3} pound/cu inch $\equiv 2.768 \times 10^{-3}$kg m^{-3}
Energy	joule	J	kg m^2 s^{-2}	1 calorie $\equiv 4.1868$ J 1 BTU $\equiv 1055.06$ J
Force	newton	N	kg m s^{-2} (J m^{-1})	1 kilogram force $\equiv 9.80665$ N 1 pound force $\equiv 4.44822$ N
Pressure	pascal	Pa	kg m^{-1} s^{-2} (N m^{-2})	atmosphere $\equiv 101.325$ kPa pound/sq inch $\equiv 6894.76$ Pa

Fractions and Multiples

10^{-3}	milli	m	10^{-1}	deci	d	10^{3}	kilo	k
10^{-6}	micro	μ	10^{-2}	centi	c	10^{6}	mega	M
10^{-9}	nano	n				10^{9}	giga	G
10^{-12}	pico	p				10^{12}	tera	T

REFERENCES

1. Jones, T.M.: J. Pharm. Sci., 57:2015, 1968.
2. Travers, D.N., Celik, M., and Buttery, T.C.: Drug Devel. Ind. Pharm., 9:139, 1983.
3. Rankell, A.S., and Higuchi, T.: J. Pharm. Sci., 57:574, 1968.
4. Jaffe, J., and Foss, N.E.: J. Am. Pharm. Ass., Sci. Ed., 48:26, 1959.
5. Shangraw, R.S.: Drug & Cosmet. Ind., 122:68, 123:34, 1978.
6. Higuchi, T., Rao, A.N., Busse, L.W., and Swintosky, J.V.: J. Am. Pharm. Ass., Sci. Ed., 42:194, 1953.
7. Armstrong, N.A., and Haines Nutt, R.F.: J. Pharm. Pharmacol. (Suppl.), 22:8S, 1970.
8. Malamataris, S. and Pilpel, N.: J. Pharm. Pharmacol., 35:1, 1983.
9. Mehta, A.M., and Augsburger, L.L.: Int. J. Pharm., 7:327, 1981.
10. Hiestand, E.: Proc. Int. Conf. Powder Tech. and Pharmacy, Basel, 1978. The Powder Advisory Centre, London, 1978.
11. Lerk, C.F., Zuurman, K. and Kussendrayer, K.: J. Pharm. Pharmacol., 36:399, 1984.
12. Newitt, D.M., and Conway-Jones, J.H.: Transactions of the Institution of Chemical Engineers, 36:422, 1958.
13. Travers, D.N., Rogerson, A.G., and Jones, T.M.: J. Pharm. Pharmacol., 27:3P, 1975.
14. Shotton, E., and Rees, J.E.: J. Pharm. Pharmacol. (suppl.), 18:160, 1966.
15. Heywood, H.: J. Pharm. Pharmacol., 15:56T, 1963.
16. Ridgeway, K., and Rupp, R., J. Pharm. Pharmacol., (suppl.), 21:30, 1969.
17. A.S.T.M. Standard STP 447A, ASTM Philadelphia, 1972.
18. Hunter, B.M., and Ganderton, D.: J. Pharm. Pharmacol., 24:17P, 1972.
19. Ragnarsson, G., and Sjögren, J.: Int. J. Pharm., 16:349, 1983.
20. Nelson, E., Naqvi, S.M., Busse, L.W., and Higuchi, T.: J. Am. Pharm. Ass., Sci. Ed., 43:596, 1954.
21. Cooper, A.R., and Eaton, L.E.: J. Am. Ceramic Soc., 45:97, 1962.

22. Shapiro, I.: Ph.D. Thesis, Univ. Minnesota, 1944.
23. Walker, E.E.: Trans. Farad. Soc., *19*:60, 1923.
24. Heckel, R. W.: Trans. Metallurgy Soc., Am. Inst. Mech. Eng., *221*:671, 1961.
25. Hersey, J.A., and Rees, J.E.: Nature, *230*:96, 1971.
26. David, S.T., and Augsburger, L.L.: J. Pharm. Sci., *66*:155, 1977.
27. Malamataris, S., Bin Baie, S., and Pilpel, N.: J. Pharm. Pharmacol., *36*:616, 1984.
28. Stanley-Wood, N.G., and Abdel Karim, A.M.: Powd. Technol., *35*:185, 1983.
29. Nelson, E., Busse, L.W., and Higuchi, T.: J. Am. Pharm. Ass., Sci. Ed., *44*:223, 1955.
30. Juslin, M.J., and Jaervinen, M.J.: Farm. Notisbl., *79*:1, 1970.
31. deBlaey, C.J., and Polderman, J.: Pharm. Weekblad, *105*:241, 1970.
32. Gillard, J., Touré, P., and Roland, M.: Pharm. Acta Helv., *51*:226, 1976.
33. deBlaey, C.J., van Oudtshoorn, M.C.B., and Polderman, J.: Pharm. Weekblad, *106*:589, 1971.
34. Armstrong, N.A., Abourida, N.M.A.H., and Gough, A.M.: J. Pharm. Pharmacol. *35*:320, 1983.
35. Seitz, J.A., and Flessland, G.M.: J. Pharm. Sci., *54*:9, 1965.
36. Brook, D.B., and Marshall, K.: J. Pharm. Sci., *57*:481, 1968.
37. Rees, J.E., and Hersey, J.A.: Pharm. Acta Helv., *47*:235, 1972.
38. Shotton, E., and Ganderton, D.: J. Pharm. Pharmacol., *12*:87T, 1960.
39. Shotton, E., and Ganderton, D.: J. Pharm. Pharmacol., *12*:93T, 1960.
40. Knudsen, F.P.: J. Amer. Ceram. Soc., *42*:376, 1959.
41. Shotton, E., and Ganderton, D.: J. Pharm. Pharmacol., *13*:144T, 1961.
42. Hess, H.: Pharm. Tech., *2*:36, 1978.
43. Shangraw, R.F., Wallace, J.W., and Bowers, E.M.: Pharm. Tech., *5*:69, 1981.
44. Seager, H., Rue, R.J., Burt, I., et al.: Int. J. Pharm. and Prod. Mfg., *2*:41, 1981.
45. Hiestand, H.E.N., and Smith, D.P.: Powd. Technol., *38*:145, 1984.
46. Mann, S.C., Roberts, R.J., Rowe, R.C., et al.: J. Pharm. Pharmacol. *35*:44P, 1983.
47. Ho, A.Y.K., Spence, J., and Jones, T.M.: Proc. 39th Int. Cong. Pharm. Sci., Federation Internationale Pharmaceutique, Amsterdam, 1979, p. 158.
48. SR-4 Strain Gauge Handbook. B.L.H. Electronics, Waltham, MA, 1971.
49. Shotton, E., Deer, J.J., and Ganderton, D.: J. Pharm. Pharmacol., *15*:106T, 1963.
50. Ho, A., Greer, H., and Clare, D.: J. Pharm. Pharmacol., *30*:95P, 1978.
51. Wray, P.E.: Drug Cosmet. Ind., *105*:58, 1969.
52. Mitrevej, A., and Augsburger, L.L.: Drug Dev. Ind. Pharm., *6*:331, 1980.
53. Chilamkurti, R.N., Rhodes, C.T., and Schwartz, J.B., Drug Devel. Ind. Pharm., *8*:63, 1982.
54. Cole, G.C., and May, G.: J. Pharm. Pharmacol., *27*:353, 1974.
55. Small, L.E., and Augsburger, L.L.: J. Pharm. Sci., *66*:504, 1977.
56. Mehta, A.M., and Augsburger, L.L.: Int. J. Pharm., *4*:347, 1980.

5

Basic Chemical Principles Related to Emulsion and Suspension Dosage Forms

STANLEY L. HEM, JOSEPH R. FELDKAMP, *and* JOE L. WHITE

Emulsions and suspensions are unique dosage forms because many of their properties are due to the presence of a boundary region between two phases. Figure 5-1 illustrates the types of boundary regions that are discussed in this chapter. In the case of emulsions, two immiscible liquids, usually oil and water, meet to form an interface. In suspensions, a solid and a liquid form an interface. An interface between the liquid and air is also present. Although the terms *interface* and *surface* are often used interchangeably, the latter term usually indicates boundaries in which one phase is a gas.

The boundary regions are often complex. *Surface active agents,* which are molecules with special properties, may be contained within a system in various forms: they may be present as single molecules in solution (Fig. 5-1A); they may also be adsorbed at the air-liquid surface (Fig. 5-1B); they may form a layer at the oil-water interface (Fig. 5-1C); or they may form oriented clusters in the aqueous phase, which are called *micelles* (Fig. 5-1D). Attractive and repulsive forces exist between particles, and the outlined region surrounding the particles in Figure 5-1 indicates a region of potential interaction. Thus, the objective of this chapter is to examine the phenomena that occur at the boundary regions of emulsions and suspensions.

When a beaker containing 50 ml of oil layered on 50 ml of water is examined visually, the interface appears as a sharp discontinuity between the two phases, as shown in Figure 5-2A. An interface is actually a region of finite dimension that has composition and properties different from either two phases. Figure 5-2B more correctly describes an interface as a region that is a few molecules thick in which a gradation of composition and properties exist. The density does not jump abruptly from 1.0 to 0.9 in moving from the water phase to the oil phase, but rather a gradual transition occurs. The terms *interfacial region* and *interphase* are often used to describe the region labeled *d* in Figure 5-2B. Although the physical properties of interfacial regions vary smoothly upon going from one phase to the other, the notion of a mathematical surface that has no thickness, as in Figure 5-2A, is still useful for modeling interfacial regions and has been used successfully to describe interfacial phenomena.

In addition, the molecules in the interfacial region are not locked into position but are in constant motion. The average interfacial residence time for a molecule of a liquid is believed to be approximately 10^{-6} sec. Thus, the interfacial region of emulsions and suspensions is a dynamic, clearly identifiable region between the phases of the system.

When the interfacial region constitutes a large portion of the system—as when the globule size of the dispersed phase of an emulsion is small, or when the particle size of the solid phase of a suspension is small—the overall properties of the system are profoundly influenced by the presence of the interfacial region.

A fundamental thermodynamic equation that describes emulsions and suspensions is as follows:

$$\Delta G = \gamma \Delta A \qquad (1)$$

where ΔG is the change in the free energy of the system accompanying a change in interfacial area ΔA, γ is the interfacial tension (liquid-liquid for an emulsion or solid-liquid for a suspension), and temperature, pressure, and composition are constant. The term ΔG represents the work required to increase the area of the interface by an amount equal to ΔA. Since this work is always positive, a system always tends toward that state having the lowest possible interfacial

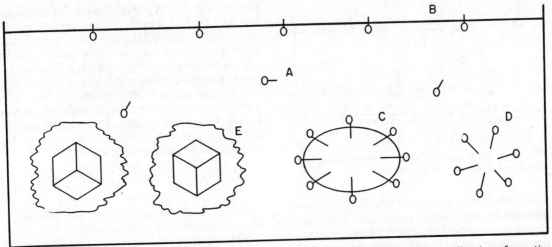

FIG. 5-1. *Schematic representation of boundary regions encountered in emulsions and suspensions. Key: A, surface active agent molecules; B, surface active agent oriented at the air-water interface; C, surface active agent oriented at the oil-water interface; D, micelle; E, suspended particles surrounded by a region of potential interaction.*

area. This state is thermodynamically stable. Thus, for an emulsion, the thermodynamically stable state is a layer of oil on water, whereas a single large particle is the thermodynamically stable state for a suspension. Although all systems tend toward the thermodynamically stable state of minimal interfacial area (which results in dramatic changes in properties), systems may vary considerably in their rates of conversion. If a system undergoes only minor changes during the period of interest, e.g., shelf-life, such a system is viewed as kinetically stable to some longer time period. As a consequence, the industrial pharmacist faces the challenging task of preparing a kinetically stable dosage form, i.e., a dosage form whose properties remain satisfactory for an acceptable shelf-life, even though emul-

sions and suspensions are thermodynamically unstable.

Molecular Basis for Surface Tension

The nature of the interfacial region can be further illustrated by examining the forces responsible for surface or interfacial tension. In a system of oil and water, the water molecules that are in the center of the volume of water are surrounded in all directions by other water molecules. Attractive intermolecular forces, hydrogen bonds in the case of water, exist between adjacent water molecules and cause the water to exist as a liquid. Similarly, van der Waals attractive forces exist between adjacent oil molecules. As depicted in Figure 5-3, however, the water

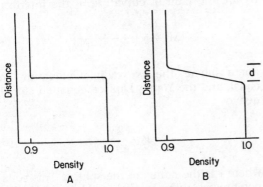

FIG. 5-2. *Change in density at the oil (density 0.9)/water (density 1.0) interface. Key: A, mathematical surface; B, interfacial region, d.*

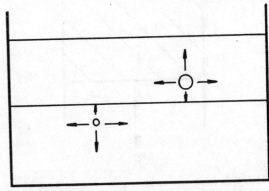

FIG. 5-3. *Molecular basis for interfacial tension between oil and water. Key: ◯, oil molecule; ○, water molecule.*

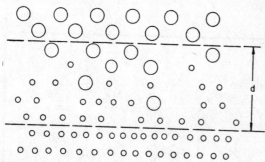

FIG. 5-4. *The interfacial region, d, between oil and water. Key:* ○, *oil molecule;* ○, *water molecule.*

molecules in the interfacial region are not surrounded by other water molecules. Thus, they experience unequal attractive forces because of the weak attractive forces between water molecules and oil molecules. If strong attractive forces existed between the oil molecules and the water molecules, the two liquids would be miscible, and no interface would exist. The imbalance of forces results in a net attractive force into the bulk water that is normal to the interface. This net attractive force leads to a reduced number of water molecules in the interfacial region (Fig. 5-4), and is responsible for the gradual change in density in the interfacial region, which was shown in Fig 5-2B. Oil molecules at this interface are also exposed to an imbalance of forces, and a similar analysis can be made for the oil.

Surface or interfacial tension is a real force whose effects are apparent at the macroscopic level as well as at the molecular level. This can be illustrated by placing a wire frame with a movable slide (Fig. 5-5) in a soap solution. When the frame is removed from the soap solution, a film is formed. This film contracts, and

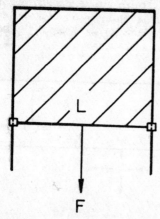

FIG. 5-5. *Device for measuring the surface tension of a soap film. A force of F is applied to the movable bar of length, L, until the film ruptures.*

the movable bar is pulled toward the stationary bar. The surface tension of the soap film can be measured if the weight needed to counterbalance the force of contraction is determined by adding weights to the movable bar. The applied force (weight × acceleration due to gravity, 980 cm/sec^2) is equal to the interfacial tension γ multiplied by the length of the movable barrier L. The total force is twice this value since the soap film forms an interface with both the top and bottom of the movable bar:

$$F = 2\gamma L \qquad (2)$$

The interfacial tension is a force per unit length when considered in this manner.

Interfacial tension may also be expressed as energy per unit area if the work needed to displace the movable bar in Fig. 5-5 by a small distance, dx, is considered:

$$dWork = Fdx \qquad (3)$$

Since:

$$dA = 2Ldx \qquad (4)$$

Thus:

$$dx = \frac{dA}{2L} \qquad (5)$$

Substituting equations (2) and (5) into equation (3) gives:

$$dWork = \gamma dA \qquad (6)$$

Most interfaces encountered in pharmaceutical systems are curved. The Young Laplace equation relates the pressure across a curved interface, ΔP, to the interfacial tension γ. R_1 and R_2 are the radii of curvature of the interface.

$$\Delta P = \gamma \left(\frac{1}{R_1} + \frac{1}{R_2} \right) \qquad (7)$$

For a sphere, the two radii of curvature are equal, and the Young Laplace equation simplifies to:

$$P = \frac{2\gamma}{r} \qquad (8)$$

where r is the radius of the sphere. This equation predicts that a smaller bubble or droplet has a greater internal pressure. Since the pressure within a small drop of liquid is greater than that for a liquid having a flat surface, i.e., a very large drop, a higher vapor pressure would be expected for the droplet.

The Kelvin equation, which relates the vapor pressure over a curved interface to the radius of curvature is given by:

$$\ln \left(\frac{P}{P^0} \right) = \frac{2 \, \gamma V}{rRT} \qquad (9)$$

where P^0 is the normal vapor pressure of the liquid, i.e., when the surface is flat, P is the vapor pressure over a spherical surface of radius r, and V is the molar volume of the liquid. For water, P/P^0 is about 1.001 for drops with a radius of 1 micron, 1.011 if the radius is 0.1 micron, and 1.114 if r is 0.01 micron. An important consequence of the Kelvin equation is that a collection of water drops of different radii is unstable, so that the large drops grow at the expense of the smaller drops. This effect is an agreement with equation (1), which states that the thermodynamically stable state of emulsions and suspensions occurs when the interfacial area is minimal.

The interfacial tension can serve as a measure of the degree of interaction between two liquids. As shown in Table 5-1, the interfacial tension between water and octane is 52 dynes/cm, but the interfacial tension between water and octanol, which contains an hydroxyl that can form a hydrogen bond with water, is 9 dynes/cm. Also, the interfacial tension decreases as the number of carbons decreases in the series hexadecane ($C_{16}H_{34}$), dodecane ($C_{12}H_{26}$), octane (C_8H_{18}) and heptane (C_7H_{16}).

The liquid molecules at the air-liquid interface also experience an imbalance of forces because the attractive forces between the liquid molecules and the air molecules are weaker than the attractive forces between the liquid molecules. In addition, the molecules of a gas are more widely separated than the liquid molecules, so there are fewer air molecules at the interface to participate in interactions with the molecules of the liquid phase. Thus, the surface tension of a liquid is usually higher than the interfacial tension of the liquid with another liquid.

The surface tension of liquids provides insight into the attractive forces between molecules of the liquid (Table 5-2). Thus, the surface tension of water decreases as the temperature increases. Liquids with strong intermolecular attractive forces, such as water and glycerin, have higher surface tensions than nonpolar liquids with relatively weak intermolecular forces, such as liquid petrolatum and heptane. Also, important differences exist in the surface tension of oils. Castor oil has a higher surface tension than liquid petrolatum, which indicates that attractive forces between castor oil molecules (triglycerides of fatty acids) are stronger than those between liquid petrolatum molecules (hydrocarbons).

Surface Active Agents

Solutes can alter the surface tension of water, as shown in Figure 5-6. Since the effect is at the surface, it is reasonable to assume that the composition of the interfacial region has changed because of the presence of either sodium stearate or sodium chloride. The Gibbs equation, one of the fundamental equations of surface chemistry, was derived to describe the effect of a solute on surface tension.[1,2] The concept of surface excess is introduced by the Gibbs equation.

TABLE 5-1. *Interfacial Tension with Water at 25°*

Liquid	Interfacial Tension, dynes/cm
Mercury	131
Hexadecane	54
Dodecane	53
Octane	52
Heptane	50
Carbon tetrachloride	45
Benzene	35
Nitrobenzene	25
Benzaldehyde	16
Diethyl ether	11
Octanol	9
Ethyl acetate	7
Heptanoic acid	7
Aminobenzene	6
Butanol	2

TABLE 5-2. *Surface Tension at 25°*

Liquid	Surface Tension, dynes/cm
Water, 5°	75
Water, 25°	72
Water, 50°	68
Glycerin	62
Dimethyl sulfoxide	44
Castor oil	39
Cottonseed oil	35
Liquid petrolatum	33
Benzene	29
Chloroform	27
Carbon tetrachloride	26
Methanol	23
Ethanol	22
Heptane	20

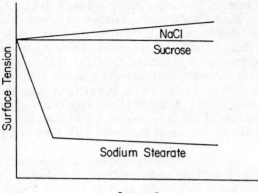

FIG. 5-6. *Effect of solutes on the surface tension of water.*

The term *surface excess*, Γ_2^{1}, is an algebraic quantity which when positive indicates that a greater concentration of the solute is present in a unit cross-section of the surface region than in a bulk region containing the same number of moles of solvent as the section of the surface region. Likewise, a negative surface excess indicates that a lower concentration of the solute is present in a unit cross-section of the surface region than in a bulk region containing the same number of moles of solvent as the surface region. The superscript indicates that the surface excess is measured relative to a constant amount of solvent. The Gibbs equation in its general form is as follows:

$$\Gamma_2^{1} = -RT\frac{d\gamma}{d\ln a_2} \quad (10)$$

where T is temperature, γ is surface tension, and a_2 is the activity of the solute.

In many cases, the system of interest is a relatively dilute solution, so that the activity of the solute may be considered to be equal to its concentration. The Gibbs equation for dilute solutions is:

$$\Gamma_2^{1} = -RT\frac{d\gamma}{d\ln C_2} \quad (11)$$

The Gibbs equation states that a solute that concentrates in the interfacial region causes a decrease in surface tension as the concentration of the solute is increased. Thus, the behavior of sodium stearate solutions shown in Figure 5-6 indicates that the concentration of sodium stearate is greater in the interfacial region than in the bulk solution. A solute such as sodium chloride, which causes an increase in surface tension, is present in greater concentration in the bulk than in the interfacial region. The surface excess of sucrose is zero, indicating a constant sucrose concentration relative to solvent throughout the entire solution.

The conclusions about the surface excess of solutes, which are based on Figure 5-6 and equation (10) (the Gibbs equation), have been verified experimentally. The most direct measurement of surface excess of a solute was made by rapidly passing a microtome across the surface of a solution, which removed the top layer of the solution for analysis. The surface concentration of solutes that caused a decrease in surface tension was greater than the bulk concentration and showed good agreement with the surface excess calculated from the Gibbs equation.[3]

The use of radioactive tracers has also provided experimental verification of the surface excess predicted by the Gibbs equation. Figure 5-7 shows that the experimentally determined concentration of tritium-labeled sodium dodecyl sulfate in this interfacial region is virtually identical to the concentration predicted by applying the Gibbs equation to the surface tension of the solutions.

Thus, experimental evidence and theoretic analysis indicate that such solutes as sodium stearate and sodium dodecyl sulfate concentrate at the interface (adsorption) while solutes composed of simple ions like sodium chloride undergo negative adsorption, i.e., concentrate in the bulk. The behavior of sodium chloride is easily understood, as both sodium and chloride ions form strong attractive forces with water by ion-dipole interactions. Because of these strong attractive forces, the ions concentrate in the re-

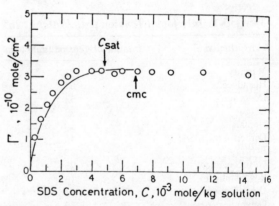

FIG. 5-7. *Surface excess of tritium-labeled sodium dodecyl sulfate (SDS) determined by radiotracer method ($\bigcirc$) and calculated by the Gibbs equation from surface tension data (———). (From Muramatsu, M., Tajima, K. M., Iwahashi, M., and Nukina, K.: J. Colloid Interface Sci., 43: 499, 1973.)*

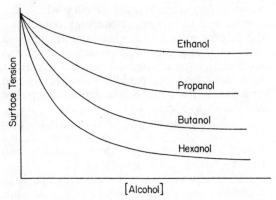

FIG. 5-8. *Effect of a series of alcohols on the surface tension of water.*

gion containing the greatest concentration of water molecules.

Structural Requirements. Surface active agents are molecules that are adsorbed at interfaces. For this to occur, a molecule must fulfill specific structural requirements. Figure 5-8 illustrates one of the requirements. The effect of alcohol in reducing the surface tension of water increased as the hydrocarbon chain of the alcohol increased in length. Thus, the surface excess of the alcohol is directly related to the length of the hydrocarbon chain of the alcohol. The hydrocarbon chain is the lipophilic part of the alcohol, and therefore, one requirement is that a surface active agent contains a lipophilic region.

A second requirement is that surface active agents also contain a hydrophilic region. The interfacial tension between paraffin oil and water is 41 dynes/cm. Upon the addition of 0.001 M oleic acid, the interfacial tension dropped to 31 dynes/cm. When 0.001 M NaOH was then added, the interfacial tension dropped to 7 dynes/cm.[4] The addition of the sodium hydroxide caused the carboxylic acid group of oleic acid to form the more hydrophilic oleate anion. Thus, a hydrophilic region is also essential for a surface active agent.

A balance of the hydrophilic and lipophilic regions of a surface active agent is usually desired. The lipophilic region is expelled from the bulk of the water phase, but the hydrophilic region prevents the surface active agent from being completely expelled from the water phase. Thus, a molecule containing both a hydrophilic and a lipophilic region is concentrated at an interface and therefore lowers surface or interfacial tension.

Surface active agents are frequently classified by the charge of the hydrophilic region. Surface active agents such as sodium lauryl sulfate, so-

dium dodecyl sulfate, or sodium stearate are termed *anionic* because the hydrophilic group is negatively charged. *Cationic* surface active agents include cetyl trimethyl ammonium bromide and benzalkonium chloride. Surface active agents whose hydrophilic region is composed of an ester or ether groups are not charged and thus are termed *nonionic.*[2]

Furthermore, the surface active agent is oriented in a special way at the interface. The hydrophilic region is in the aqueous phase while the lipophilic region is in the oil phase (for an oil-water interface) or in the air (for an air-water interface).

A further confirmation that surface active agents orient at interfaces is the gradual reduction of surface tension with the passage of time following the addition of a surface active agent, until a constant value is reached (Fig. 5-9). This behavior suggests that the surface active molecules diffuse through the water until they reach the interface, where they are adsorbed to form a stable system.

Effect on Properties. The presence of a surface active agent can change many properties of a system.[1] As shown in Figure 5-10, the surface tension decreases sharply as the concentration of surface active agent is increased, until a constant value is reached. The osmotic pressure increases as expected, but at higher concentrations, a constant osmotic pressure is observed. The detergency, i.e., the ability of the solution to dissolve oil, increases sharply once a threshold concentration of surface active agent is reached. In addition, light scattering becomes significant at the same threshold concentration. All of the properties shown in Figure 5-10 undergo a sharp change at approximately the same

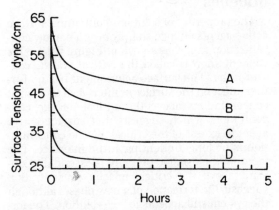

FIG. 5-9. *Change in surface tension with time following the addition of sodium dodecyl sulfate to water. Key: A, 4×10^{-4} M; B, 8×10^{-4} M; C, 1.6×10^{-3} M; D, 4×10^{-3} M. (From Neumann, A. W., and Tanner, W.: Tenside, 4:220, 1967.)*

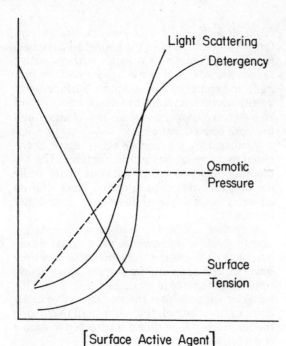

FIG. 5-10. *Effect of surface active agent on properties of water.*

[Surface Active Agent]

Light Scattering
Detergency
Osmotic Pressure
Surface Tension

concentration of surface active agent. Such other physical properties as the boiling point, freezing point, solubility, partial molar volume, electrical conductance, and color change of dyes also undergo a sharp change at the same concentration of surface active agent. This observation led to the discovery that surface active agents can form aggregates called micelles, which are discussed in the next section.

Micelles

The properties of solutions containing surface active agents change sharply over a narrow concentration range, as shown in Figure 5-10. This concentration is called the *critical micelle concentration*. The surface active agent has no further effect on the surface or interfacial tension at concentrations above the critical micelle concentration, which suggests that surface active agent in excess of the critical micelle concentration is no longer orienting at the interface. The fact that the osmotic pressure is essentially constant above the critical micelle concentration suggests the formation of a new phase, although the system still appears to be a solution. The formation of a new phase of small particle size is suggested by the initiation of light scattering at the critical micelle concentration.

Surface active agents associate to form colloi-

dal-sized aggregates termed micelles, which predominate in the system at concentrations above the critical micelle concentration. In aqueous solution, the aggregates of surface active agents form, so that the hydrophilic region is in contact with water, and the lipophilic region is shielded from water. Two possible orientations of micelles are shown in Figure 5-11.

Micellization is an alternative mechanism to interfacial adsorption by which surface active agents can satisfy their dual solubility and thereby form a stable system.

Micellization is favored because the lipophilic region is removed from contact with water, but the process is opposed by the surface active molecule's loss of freedom as a consequence of being held in a fixed position in the micelle, and in the case of ionic surface active agents, by the electrostatic repulsion of the charged polar groups. The concentration at which micellization becomes significant is determined by the balance of these factors. A low critical micelle concentration indicates that removal of the lipophilic region of the surface active agent from contact with water is the dominant factor, while a high critical micelle concentration indicates that the forces opposing aggregation are significant.

The shape and size of micelles remain somewhat uncertain, and it is likely that shape varies with the concentration of the surface active agent. A consensus is gradually being reached that spherical micelles (Fig. 5-11A) occur at concentrations in the region of the critical micelle concentration. The diameter of the spheres is approximately twice the length of the surface active agent. When the concentration of surface active agent substantially exceeds the critical micelle concentration, the spherical micelles are believed to transform into lamellar micelles (Fig. 5-11B).

The number of surface active agent molecules constituting a micelle is believed to range from

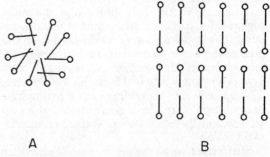

A   B

FIG. 5-11. *Orientation of surface active agents to form a spherical micelle (A) and a lamellar micelle (B).*

50 to 100 molecules and is characterized by the aggregation number. In general, the aggregation number in aqueous solution increases with an increase in the hydrophobic region of the surface active agent. The addition of an electrolyte causes the aggregation number of ionic surface active agents to increase by diminishing the repulsive charge effect. Frequently, the aggregation number has been observed to increase in the presence of a hydrocarbon that is adsorbed or solubilized in the lipophilic region of the micelle.

The critical micelle concentration is also affected by the structure of the surface active agent. In general, the critical micelle concentration in aqueous media decreases as the lipophilic nature of the surface active agent increases. This process may be thought of as enhancing the expulsion of the lipophilic region from water. Branching in the lipophilic region interferes with the close packing of surface active agents needed for van der Waals attraction of the hydrocarbon chains; thus, the critical micelle concentration increases. Ionic surface active agents have a much higher critical micelle concentration than nonionic surface active agents, as repulsive forces between the similarly charged polar groups resist the close packing necessary for micelle formation.

Another important fact is that micelles are in equilibrium with monomeric surface active agents in the system. Thus, both monomers and micelles are always present in solutions of surface active agents. The monomeric form will predominate, however, when the concentration is below the critical micelle concentration so that micelles predominate above the critical micelle concentration.

Micelles may be desirable when detergency or solubilization of a lipid-like material is desired in a system. Micelles are of great interest because of their unusual catalytic effects and because they are a good model of biologic membranes. On the other hand, micelles do not contribute to the properties of emulsions, and the concentration of surface active agent used in emulsions is usually chosen to minimize micellization.

Interfacial Films

The nature of the interfacial film is important in emulsions. Experimentally, direct examination of the film at the oil-water interface is difficult; however, techniques for studying insoluble surface films are available, providing insight into the interfacial films in emulsions.

The principle technique employed in the study of insoluble films is the *film balance* (Fig.

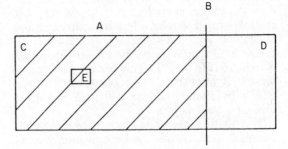

FIG. 5-12. *Diagram of essential components of a film balance. Key:* A, *trough;* B, *movable barrier;* C, *film-covered surface;* D, *film-free surface;* E, *surface tension monitor.*

5-12), which is used to produce a graph of the area of the film, A, versus the film pressure, π[5] This graph is called a π-A curve. The *film pressure* is the difference between the surface tension of the pure liquid and the surface tension of the film-covered surface.

Two typical π-A curves are shown in Figure 5-13. Usually, three characteristics of the π-A curves are examined. The *slope* gives information about the nature of the packing in the surface film. The smallest area the molecules occupy before the film collapses is termed the *limiting area* and indicates the dimension of the molecule in the film. This information indicates the orientation of the molecules in the film compared with the actual dimensions of the molecule. The film pressure that causes the film to collapse is termed the *collapse pressure* and indicates the strength of the film.

Arachidic acid, $CH_3(CH_2)_{18}COOH$, shows the increase in film pressure that is characteristic of a condensed or noncompressible film (Fig.

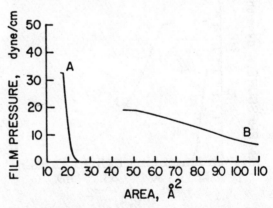

FIG. 5-13. *Film-pressure/area curves for insoluble films of arachidic acid (A) and ethyl elaidate (B). (Reprinted with permission from Rosano, H. L., and LaMer, V. K.: J. Phys. Chem., 60:348, 1956. Copyright 1956 American Chemical Society.)*

5-13A). This type of film is quite rigid and behaves in a manner analogous to a solid. Thus, it is also termed a *solid film*. In contrast, ethyl elaidate, $C_{17}H_{33}COOC_2H_5$, shows a gradual increase in film pressure as the area per molecule is reduced (Fig. 5-13B). This behavior is characteristic of an expanded or compressible film, which by analogy to the states of matter is termed a *gaseous film*.

The limiting area of arachidic acid is approximately 0.18 nm² while the limiting area of ethyl elaidate is 0.53 nm². The collapse pressure of arachidic acid is 33 dynes/cm, while the collapse pressure of ethyl elaidate is 19 dynes/cm.

The π-A curves in Figure 5-13 indicate that arachidic acid forms a rigid film with the molecules in close contact. The limiting area is similar to the area of the hydrocarbon chain, 0.184 nm², which suggests a vertical orientation of arachidic acid molecules in the film. The relatively high collapse pressure in comparison with ethyl elaidate suggests a greater degree of interaction between the closely packed hydrocarbon chains of arachidic acid. The structure of ethyl elaidate does not allow close packing of the molecules, and the π-A curve indicates a film with weaker intermolecular association.

Film balance experiments provide valuable information on how steric factors affect the film. For example, the introduction of cis-double bonds into the hydrocarbon chain produces considerable film expansion, as shown in Figure 5-14.

The presence of a charged polar group produces repulsion within the film, which results in an expanded film; however, an increase in ionic strength shields the charge and allows greater

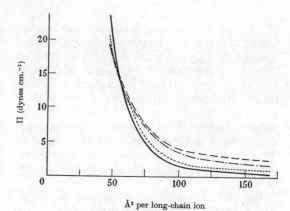

FIG. 5-15. *Film-pressure/area curves of octadecyltrimethyl ammonium cation in sodium chloride solutions of various concentration. Key:* — —, *0.033 M sodium chloride;* —ᐧ—, *0.1 M sodium chloride; C,* ----, *0.5 M sodium chloride;* ———, *2 M sodium chloride. (From Davies, J. T.: Proc. R. Soc. Lond., A208:224, 1951.)*

interaction within the film. In the π-A curve of octadecyltrimethyl ammonium ions, this phenomenon can be seen as a shift in shape toward a condensed type of film as the ionic strength is increased (Fig. 5-15).

The film balance can also be used to study mixed films. Changes in the limiting area indicate interactions between the components of the film.

Since the objective of emulsification is to produce a tough, resilient film at the oil-water interface, the information obtained from film balance experiments has provided valuable insights into the behavior of films. The principles illustrated by the π-A curves—such as the formation of a monomolecular film in which the molecules assume a specific orientation, and the demonstration that the strength of the film is related to intermolecular attraction between components of the film—can be directly applied to the formulation of emulsions.

Measurement of Surface and Interfacial Tension

Numerous methods have been used to measure surface and interfacial tension. The existence of numerous methods often indicates that the measure is complex, and that a simple, universally applicable method is not available. An excellent detailed discussion of methods for measuring surface or interfacial tension is given by Padday.[6]

The *capillary-rise method* is based on equation (7), the Young Laplace equation. If a liquid wets the walls of a capillary, the liquid surface is

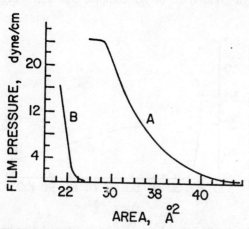

FIG. 5-14. *Film-pressure/area curves for insoluble films of cis-docosenoic acid (A) and trans-docosenoic acid (B). (From Marsden, J., and Rideal, E. K.: J. Chem. Soc., 1163, 1938.)*

concave in shape and a pressure differential exists across the interface. The pressure differential causes the liquid to rise in the capillary until the pressure differential described by the Young Laplace equation is equal to the hydrostatic pressure of the column of liquid:

$$\Delta P = (\rho_1 - \rho_g)gh = \frac{2\gamma}{r} \quad (12)$$

where ρ_1 and ρ_g are the densities of the liquid and gas phases, respectively, g is the acceleration due to gravity, h is the height to which the liquid rises in the capillary, and r is the radius of the capillary. Thus, the height to which a liquid rises in a capillary is directly related to the surface tension of the liquid and inversely related to the bore of the capillary tube. This simple treatment fails to account for the weight of the meniscus, and it assumes a hemispherical meniscus. The major difficulty with the capillary-rise method occurs if the liquid does not completely wet the walls of the capillary. Under ideal experimental conditions, however, this method is excellent for determining surface tension but unsuitable for measuring interfacial tension.

The Young Laplace equation can also be used to determine surface or interfacial tension based on the radius of curvature, i.e., the shape of pendant (hanging) or sessile (sitting) drops. The use of these methods is illustrated in Figure 5-16, in which the shape of a pendant drop of a solution of sodium stearate changed with time, reflecting the time required for the sodium stearate to equilibrate at the surface. Similar changes would also occur in a sessile drop of sodium stearate solution. Photographs of the drops are used to determine the changes in shape as a function of time from which the surface tension is determined. The pendant or sessile drop methods are good for studying the aging of surfaces and are convenient for determining interfacial tension if the pendant or sessile drop is immersed in a second immiscible liquid.

The *drop-weight method* is based on the fact that the weight of a drop that falls from a tube of radius r depends on the surface tension of the liquid. This method requires a correction factor, as only a portion of the drop that has reached the size of instability falls, the balance remaining attached to the tip. Correction tables are available, however, and satisfactory results can be obtained for surface tension when the drop forms in air, or for interfacial tension when the tip is immersed in a second liquid. Some accuracy is lost in the study of solutions because of

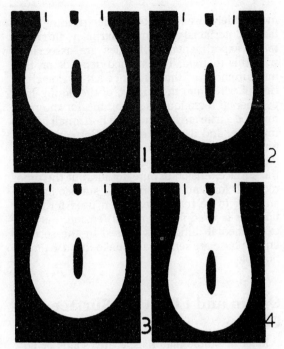

FIG. 5-16. *Change in shape of a pendant drop of a sodium stearate solution as a function of time, and the surface tension calculated using the Young Laplace equation.*
Key: 1, age = 10 sec.; γ = 71.9 dynes/cm
2, age = 50 sec.; γ = 58.2 dynes/cm
3, age = 120 sec.; γ = 54.4 dynes/cm
4, age = 1800 sec.; γ = 39.2 dynes/cm.
(Reprinted from Andreas, J. M., Hauser, E. A., and Tucker, W. B.: J. Phys. Chem., 42:1001, 1938. Published 1938 American Chemical Society.)

the time required for a new surface to reach its equilibrium surface tension.

Another approach, known as the *Wilhelmy plate method*, is the direct measurement of the force exerted on a piece of platinum foil that is in the interface. The measured or apparent weight of the foil while in the interface, W, is equal to the weight of the foil, W_0, plus the force due to the surface tension. This force is equal to the surface tension multiplied by the perimeter of the foil, which forms the interface with the liquid. The perimeter is frequently approximated by twice the length of the foil, L.

$$W = W_0 + 2L \quad (13)$$

The Wilhelmy plate method is relatively simple and gives accurate results. It is good for studying the aging of the surfaces and is usually the method used to measure surface tension during film balance experiments. It cannot be used to measure interfacial tension.

The *ring-detachment method* has been the

most widely used method for determining surface or interfacial tension in pharmacy, although many experimental difficulties are associated with this method. The method depends on the measurement of the force needed to detach a ring of wire from the surface of the liquid. Experimental technique is important, for the ring must be a true circle, it must be horizontal in the interface, and it must be clean. Correction factors have been developed for this method. Under ideal conditions, it is satisfactory for measuring the surface tension of pure liquids, but the time required for equilibration of the surface causes an error to be introduced when used for solutions. It is used for interfacial tension, but the experimental difficulties caused by the second liquid phase are serious and make this use questionable.

Origin and Effects of Surface Charge

Most insoluble materials, either solids or liquids, develop a surface charge when dispersed in an aqueous medium. The surface charge may arise by several mechanisms. The ionization of surface groups may produce a surface charge. Proteins usually contain carboxylic acid groups, which may ionize to form carboxylate anions, as well as amine groups, which become cationic when pH conditions favor protonation. The surface charge of proteins depends on the summation of negative and positive sites and therefore depends on the pH of the aqueous medium. At low pH conditions, the carboxylic acid groups are undissociated, and the amine groups are protonated to give a net positive charge. At higher pH conditions the carboxylic acid groups ionize and the amine groups are neutral; thus, the protein is negatively charged. In addition to protein, a variety of colloidal systems (e.g., polymers, metal oxides, etc.) develop surface charge due to the adsorption or desorption of protons, so that surfaces can become positively or negatively charged. An important property of such systems is the point of zero charge (PZC), which represents the pH at which the net surface charge is zero. For aluminum hydroxide gel, the surface hydroxyls may adsorb protons and become positively charged or may donate protons to become negatively charged (Fig. 5-17). The pH at which the surface hydroxyls exist in their uncharged form is the point of zero charge.

Another property of colloidal systems that exhibit a pH-dependent charge, although not as fundamental as the PZC, is the isoelectric point (i.e.p.). This property represents the pH at

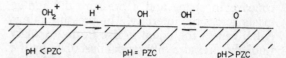

FIG. 5-17. *pH-Dependent ionization of surface hydroxyls of aluminum hydroxide gel. The point of zero charge (PZC) is the pH at which the surface is neutral.*

which a particle no longer migrates in the presence of an electric field. The PZC and i.e.p. are not necessarily identical since a surface charge may be present even when a colloidal system is at its i.e.p.

In addition to protons and hydroxyls, surface charge may also be created because of the preferential adsorption of specific ions onto the surface. This type of adsorption is termed *specific adsorption* because the ion becomes an integral part of the solid phase through a chemical bond, which is usually covalent.

Ions that are specifically adsorbed are also known as *potential determining ions*. In many cases, an electrolyte is present in the aqueous solution, which provides the anions or cations for specific adsorption. Examples of such ions are phosphate, silicate, and carbonate. If a surface has both a pH-dependent charge and a charge due to specific adsorption, then the PZC for such a surface is different from its value in the absence of any specific ion adsorption. An example is provided by aluminum hydroxide, which has a PZC of 9.6 when only H^+ or OH^- bind to its surface. In the presence of specifically adsorbed carbonate, the PZC is displaced downward within the range of 6.0 to 8.0, depending on how much carbonate is preferentially adsorbed.[7] In this case, the potential determining ions are hydroxyl, protons, and carbonate.

In some cases, charge arises owing to the adsorption of ions that are identical with those constituting the insoluble phase. For example, when silver iodide particles are in equilibrium with a solution containing both silver cations and iodide anions, the adsorption of these ions depends on their affinity for water as well as their concentration in the bulk solution phase. Thus, the surface is positively charged when the surface excess of silver cations exceeds the surface excess of iodide anions, and negatively charged when the surface excess of iodide anions exceeds the surface excess of silver cations. Because the charge on the silver iodide particle is determined by the concentration of silver or iodide ions, these ions are also regarded as potential determining ions.

Imperfections in the crystal structure may cause a surface charge. Many clays exhibit a negative surface charge because of isomorphous substitution, e.g., an aluminum occupies a site that is usually occupied by silicon.[8] Similarly, the antacid magaldrate exhibits a positive surface charge because of the substitution of aluminum in crystal lattice sites normally occupied by magnesium.[9]

The oil globules of an oil in water emulsion exhibit a surface charge if anionic or cationic surface active agents are used as the emulsifying agent. The surface active agents are oriented at the oil-water interface, so that the charged, hydrophilic groups form the outside surface.

The presence of charge at an interface has profound effects on the nature of the interfacial region. Thus, the concept of a diffuse double layer was developed by Gouy and Chapman to describe the transition from points near the charged surface to the electrically neutral bulk solution.[10] Stern made an important refinement in the double-layer theory by pointing out that the ions in the double layer are not point charges but rather real ions with finite dimensions.[10]

Figure 5-18 presents a model of the interfacial region of a charged surface and provides a good basis for understanding the behavior of pharmaceutical suspensions and emulsions. A layer of ions of opposite charge is sufficiently held to-gether by the charged surface so that the ions move with the surface (Stern layer). The surface potential is reduced from ψ_0 to ψ_δ by the Stern layer. The surface charge is not completely balanced by the Stern layer, and a second region, the *diffuse layer*, is necessary for complete balance of the surface charge. The diffuse layer contains both anions and cations, but ions that are of opposite charge to the surface predominate, so that in the neighboring area of any charged particle, there exists an ion atmosphere having a net charge that is opposite to that of the surface. This mobile layer of ions has a definite thickness, which is approximated by the so-called Debye length (1/k):

$$1/k = \left(\frac{DkT}{2ne^2Z^2} \right)^{1/2} \qquad (14)$$

where D is the dielectric constant of the medium, n is the concentration of ions in the bulk solution phase, e is the electronic charge, Z is valence, k is Boltzman's constant, and T is temperature. Beyond this distance (1/κ), the net charge density of the ion atmosphere approaches zero, and the electrical potential is reduced considerably below its value at the surface. The major factors affecting the thickness of the double layer are the electrolyte concentration of the solution, n, and the valence, z, of the counter ions. Table 5-3 shows the manner by which the thickness of the double layer decreases as the concentration or the valence of the counter ions increase.

Interparticle Forces

An area of surface chemistry in which significant advances in understanding are occurring is the nature of forces between surfaces.[11,12] The following forces have been identified.

1. *Electrostatic repulsive forces* arise from overlapping of the diffuse double layers of approaching surfaces. These forces depend greatly on the concentration and valence of electrolyte in solution. Their range may exceed 100 nm.

2. *Van der Waals attractive forces* arise from the electromagnetic fluctuations in the molecules that make up the surface. These forces largely independent of the electrolyte and may have a range of the same order of magnitude as electrostatic repulsive forces.

3. *Repulsive hydration forces* arise from the structuring of water in the interfacial region. These forces are independent of electrolyte concentration. At low electrolyte concentration, the contribution of this force may not be observed, owing to the strong electrostatic repulsive

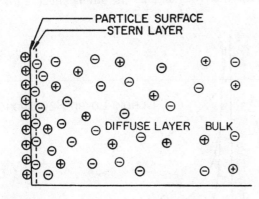

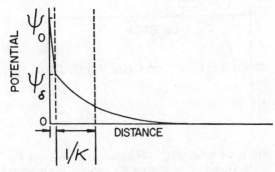

FIG. 5-18. *Diffuse double-layer model of a positively charged surface in an aqueous medium.*

TABLE 5-3. *Approximate "Thickness" of the Electric Double Layer as a Function of Electrolyte Concentration at a Constant Surface Potential*

Concentration of Ions of Opposite Charge to that of the Particle, mmole/L	Thickness of the Double Layer, nm	
	Monovalent Ions	Divalent Ions
0.01	100	50
1.0	10	5
100.0	1	0.5

From van Olphen, H: An Introduction to Clay Colloid Chemistry. 2nd Ed. John Wiley and Sons, New York, 1977, p. 35

forces. At high electrolyte concentration, however, the diffuse double-layer interactions are weak, and the repulsive hydration forces may determine the interaction of the surfaces. Typically, these forces have a range of only a few diameters (~1 nm).

4. *Born repulsive forces* are of short range and operate over distances of atomic dimensions. They are due to the repulsive effects of atomic orbital overlap.

5. *Adhesive forces* arise when surfaces are in contact. The adhesive forces depend on pH, specific cations, and the crystallographic orientation of the surfaces.

6. *Steric repulsive forces* depend on the size, geometry, and conformation of molecules that are adsorbed on the surface. Their effective range depends on the nature of the adsorbed molecules.

Many observed properties of a disperse system reflect the net force of interaction between the particles or globules that the system comprises. Deryaguin and Landau, working in Russia, and Verwey and Overbeek, working independently in Holland, were the first researchers to recognize the concept of the net force between particles.[10] Thus, the concept has become known as the *DLVO theory*. The original statement of the DLVO theory considered only the balance between electrostatic repulsive and van der Waals attractive forces, which were the only interparticle forces understood at that time.

Figure 5-19 illustrates the repulsive double layer and attractive van der Waals forces at three electrolyte concentrations. The repulsive forces predominate at low electrolyte concentration, so that the particles experience only a repulsive force upon approach. The particles remain independent, and the system is considered dispersed. At high electrolyte concentration, however, the double layer forces are greatly reduced, so that the attractive van der Waals forces predominate. These net attractive forces that the particles encounter cause the formation of an aggregate of particles, a process known as

coagulation. Thus, the DLVO theory explains the fact that the addition of electrolyte to a colloidal system causes coagulation.

The concentration of electrolyte necessary to collapse the repulsive field and permit coagulation has been found to depend primarily on the valence of the ion of opposite charge. The concentrations of various monovalent salts needed to coagulate negative silver iodide are approximately the same (Table 5-4). Electrolytes containing divalent cations all require a similar concentration to induce coagulation but the concentration is substantially lower than that required by electrolytes containing monovalent cations. Likewise, electrolytes containing trivalent cations require the lowest concentration to induce coagulation. The strong effect of the va-

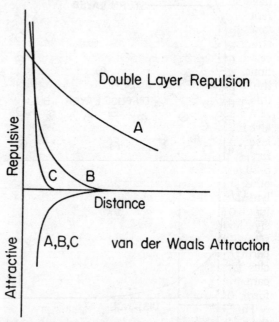

FIG. 5-19. *Effect of electrolyte concentration on repulsive double-layer forces and attractive van der Waals forces. Key: A, low electrolyte concentration; B, intermediate electrolyte concentration; C, high electrolyte concentration.*

TABLE 5-4. *Electrolyte Concentration to Floccu-late a Negative Silver Iodide Colloid*

Electrolyte	Coagulation Concentration, mmole/L
$LiNO_3$	165
$NaNO_3$	140
KNO_3	136
$Ca(NO_3)_2$	2.6
$Mg(NO_3)_2$	2.4
$Al(NO_3)_3$	0.07

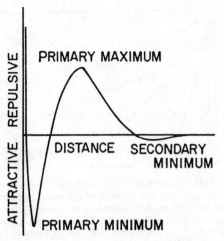

FIG. 5-20. *Net potential energy curve for a particle in an electrolyte vehicle.*

lence of the electrolyte on the double-layer repulsive force is known as the *Schulze-Hardy rule.*

As can be noticed in Table 5-4, the coagulation values for negative silver iodide are slightly different depending on the particular monovalent cation. The order of effectiveness of ions of a given valence is directly related to the hydrated radius of the ion. The order of effectiveness is known as the *Hofmeister series* and is given as:

$$Cs > Rb > NH_4 > K > Na > Li$$
$$Mg > Ca > Ba$$
$$F > Cl > Br > NO_3 > I > CNS$$

The DLVO theory at first provided an excellent framework for understanding the interactions between surfaces. Recent experiments have shown, however, that unexpectedly large repulsive forces exist at small interparticle distances, whereas the DLVO theory predicts strong attraction at small distances.[13] This observation has stimulated the search for additional forces and has led to the identification of the additional forces listed at the beginning of this section.

When the repulsive hydration and Born repulsive forces are considered along with the double-layer repulsive and van der Waals attractive forces, the net force diagram shown in Figure 5-20 is obtained. As two particles approach each other in an aqueous medium of proper electrolyte concentration, a weak attractive force exists just beyond the range of the double-layer repulsive forces. This attractive region is called the *secondary minimum* and is responsible for the particle interaction termed *flocculation.* Particles therefore experience attraction at significant interparticle distances (10 to 20 nm) and form the fluffy aggregates known as *floccules.*

The secondary minimum is not observed if the repulsive forces extend further from the surface than attractive forces. Thus, the adjustment of valence and concentration of the background electrolyte can alter the Debye length given in

equation (14) and is frequently necessary to induce flocculation.

A repulsive barrier termed the *primary maximum* separates the secondary minimum from the primary minimum. The magnitude of the repulsive force at the primary maximum determines whether a flocculated system will remain flocculated. If the thermal energy in the system is similar to, or greater than, the repulsive barrier, then the particles in the system are able to move closer together (0.5 to 2.0 nm) and encounter strong attraction due to the primary minimum. The strong attraction in the primary minimum gives rise to the particle interaction of coagulation. Other sources of energy, such as centrifugation or compression of the particles due to freezing may force particles into the primary minimum by overcoming the primary maximum and may lead to coagulation. At low electrolyte concentration, the interaction curve contains a much larger primary maximum than at higher ionic strength conditions, and particle interactions are minimized. Such a suspension is called *dispersed,* or *peptized.* If either the concentration or the valence of the background salt is increased, the primary maximum is reduced, so that such particle interactions as flocculation or coagulation occur.

Recent experimental techniques allow the direct measurement of forces between surfaces. Israelachvili and Adams measured the forces between two mica surfaces in electrolyte solutions.[14] Their results indicate the presence of a long-range repulsive force that collapses as the electrolyte concentration increases (Fig. 5-21), as predicted by the DLVO theory. They also observed an attractive region at distances predicted for the secondary minimum (Fig. 5-22).

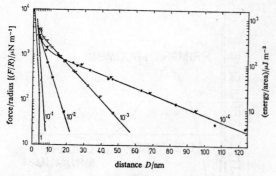

FIG. 5-21. *Experimental results of direct measurements of repulsive forces as a function of separation distance between two crossed mica cylinders in aqueous potassium nitrate solutions of various concentration, m/l. (From Israelachvili, J. N., and Adams, G. E.: J. C. S. Faraday Trans. I, 74:975, 1978.)*

State of Aggregation

Many of the physical properties of disperse systems depend on the state of aggregation. For example, the apparent viscosity of aluminum hydroxycarbonate gel is directly related to particle-particle association. When coulombic repulsion is sufficiently reduced by adjustment of the bulk pH to the point of zero charge, van der Waals attractive forces cause the particles to aggregate. Consequently, the apparent viscosity increases. The magnitude of the viscosity increase depends, however, on the structure of the aggregates. Figure 5-23 illustrates the effect of pH on the apparent viscosity of two aluminum hydroxycarbonate gels. The viscosity of both aluminum hydroxycarbonate gels was at a maximum when the bulk pH was at the point of zero charge. The fact that a different maximum viscosity occurred for each aluminum hydroxycarbonate gel suggests that gel 1 formed a more

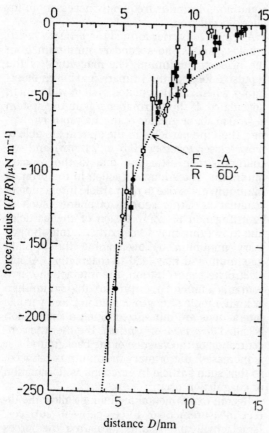

FIG. 5-22. *Attractive van der Waals dispersion forces between mica surfaces measured in the region of secondary minima in various aqueous solutions. The dotted line represents the attractive force predicted by van der Waals forces. The measured forces agree well with theory except at larger separation distances, where they decay more rapidly than predicted by theory. (From Israelachvili, J. N., and Adams, G. E.: J. C. S. Faraday Trans. I, 74:975, 1978.)*

$$\frac{F}{R} = \frac{-A}{6D^2}$$

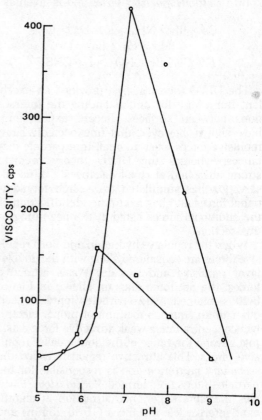

FIG. 5-23. *Effect of bulk pH on apparent viscosity of aluminum hydroxycarbonate. The point of zero charge of gel 1 (○) is 6.95, and the point of zero charge of gel 2 (□) is 6.30. (From Feldkamp, J. R., Shah, D. N., Meyer, S. L., et al.: J. Pharm. Sci., 70:638, 1981. Reproduced with permission of the copyright owner, the American Pharmaceutical Association.)*

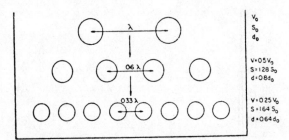

FIG. 5-24. *Effect of particle density on interparticle distance. Key: λ, interparticle distance; V, volume of each particle; S, total surface area; d, diameter of each particle. The volume of each particle is reduced by 50% in each step while the total volume of the particles is constant. (From Feldkamp, J. R., White, J. L., and Hem, S. L.: J. Pharm. Sci., 71:43, 1982. Reproduced with permission of the copyright owner, the American Pharmaceutical Association.)*

highly extended and cross-linked network of particles.

In addition to surface charge, the particle size of the dispersed phase has a great effect on interparticle interactions. Reducing the particle size while maintaining a constant solids content causes a colloidal system to have a higher particle density. The effect of particle density on particle interactions is illustrated in Figure 5-24, in which the individual particle volume is sequentially halved in a one-dimensional arrangement of particles. Such a system is relevant especially because linear chains of particles are frequently formed under the influence of van der Waals forces. Although the surface area does not increase substantially upon two divisions, the average interparticle distance decreases significantly, as can be readily observed. Since the magnitude of interparticle forces depends inversely upon separation distance, the force exerted on a given particle by all other particles is greater if the average interparticle distance is small. Conversely, at low particle density, the average interparticle distance is comparatively large, so that the particles are less influenced by each other.

The effects of decreased particle size in a colloidal system are readily examined by measurement of the coefficient of bulk compressibility, α:

$$\alpha = -\frac{1}{V}\frac{dV}{d\tau} \qquad (15)$$

where V is the entire volume occupied by the system, including both solids and solution phases, τ represents the stress applied to the system, and the mass of solids is constant. A useful apparatus for measurement of α is de-

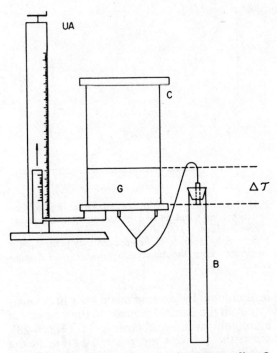

FIG. 5-25. *Schematic of tension cell apparatus. Key: C, tension cell; UA, movable plate assembly; B, collection buret; and G, sample suspension. (From Lipka, E. A., Feldkamp, J. R., White, J. L., and Hem, S. L.: J. Pharm. Sci., 70:936, 1981. Reproduced with permission of the copyright owner, the American Pharmaceutical Association.)*

picted in Figure 5-25. The dispersed phase is confined to a chamber that is fitted with a membrane at the bottom. The membrane is impermeable to particles but passes both water and solutes, so that applying a stress in the form of a tension τ causes the solution phase to leave the system. The solution phase continues to flow out of the system until interparticle forces have increased sufficiently to prevent further collapse of the colloidal matrix. By measurement of the extent of collapse as a function of applied increments of tension, α may be measured. Measured values for the coefficient of bulk compressibility are represented in Figure 5-26 for two different colloidal aluminum hydroxycarbonate systems. Although each has the same volume fraction of solids initially, gel 1 has a smaller particle size than gel 2, so that gel 1 has a greater particle density. This implies that interparticle forces ought to be greater within gel 1, according to the preceding arguments, and that therefore gel 1 should exhibit a more rigid, incompressible behavior. This conclusion is confirmed in Figure 5-26, where α is shown to be considerably smaller for gel 1.

Likewise, the tenfold increase in the viscosity

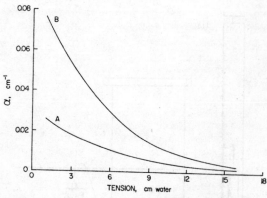

FIG. 5-26. *Compressibility of aluminum hydroxycarbonate gel 1 (A), and gel 2 (B) at various applied tensions. (From Feldkamp, J. R., White, J. L., and Hem, S. L.: J. Pharm. Sci., 71:43, 1982. Reproduced with permission of copyright owner, the American Pharmaceutical Association.)*

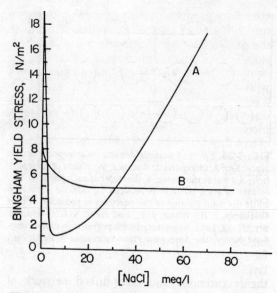

FIG. 5-28. *Effect of sodium chloride concentration on the viscosity of 3.22% sodium montomorillonite (A) and 12% sodium kaolin (B) suspensions. (From van Olphen, H.: An Introduction to Clay Colloid Chemistry. 2nd Ed. John Wiley and Sons, New York, 1977, p. 101.)*

of aluminum hydroxycarbonate gel 1 in comparison with the fourfold increase in the viscosity of aluminum hydroxycarbonate gel 2 (Fig. 5-23), when the particles are neutral, is due to the smaller particle size of aluminum hydroxycarbonate gel 1.

The shape of the particle also influences the particle interactions. Plate-like particles can undergo three different modes of particle association: face-to-face, edge-to-face, or edge-to-edge (Fig. 5-27). The physical effects of these three types of association are quite different. Face-to-face association leads to a compact arrangement while edge-to-face or edge-to-edge associations lead to the formation of an extensive network of particles.

The importance of the different types of association of plate-like particles can be seen in the rheology of kaolin or montmorillonite suspensions (Fig. 5-28). Kaolin favors the formation of face-to-face association. Thus, upon the collapse of the double layer by the addition of salt, large aggregates of clay particles form. The overall effect of the face-to-face association is a reduction of particle density, and a lower apparent viscosity is observed following coagulation. Montmorillonite favors the formation of edge-to-face or edge-to-edge associations, which produce a different effect on the rheology. The addition of salt collapses the repulsive double layer and permits interparticle association. The edge-to-face and edge-to-edge interactions lead to a three-dimensional network of particles throughout the clay suspension, which is manifested by a sharply increased apparent viscosity following coagulation.

Mechanisms of Crystal Growth

The size distribution of dispersed systems may increase during aging, owing to three principal mechanisms: Ostwald ripening; polymorphic transformation; and temperature cycling.

The basis for Ostwald ripening is found in an equation analogous to equation (9) (the Kelvin equation) and it applies to the equilibrium solubility of small particles:[15]

$$\ln \frac{S}{S^0} = \frac{2\gamma V}{rRT} \quad (16)$$

where S^0 is the solubility of infinitely large particles, S is the solubility of a small particle of radius r, γ is the surface tension, and V is the molar volume of the solid.

It is important to distinguish between equilibrium solubility and the rate at which a substance dissolves. Dissolution rate is affected by particle size since the surface area of the solid available to the solvent increases with decreasing particle

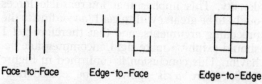

Face-to-Face   Edge-to-Face   Edge-to-Edge

FIG. 5-27. *Possible modes of particle association for plate-like particles.*

size. Equilibrium solubility at a given temperature, however, is affected by particle size only in the particle size range near the colloidal dimension, i.e., less than 5 microns. For example, the equilibrium solubility at 25° of calcium sulfate with an average particle size of 2 microns is 2.085 g/L. When the average particle size is reduced to 0.3 microns, the equilibrium solubility increases to 2.476 g/L.

In a practical sense, these values mean that a solution that is saturated with respect to small particles is supersaturated with respect to large particles of the same substance. This condition causes crystal growth in a suspension, as solute diffuses from the saturated layer surrounding small particles to the saturated layer surrounding the larger particles. Precipitation on the surface of the larger particle occurs as the saturated layer becomes supersaturated with respect to the equilibrium solubility of the larger particles. The overall effect is an increase in particle size and a decrease in the number of particles in suspension. The ultimate conclusion of this process is the formation of one large particle that represents the thermodynamically stable state of a suspension as described by equation (1).

Polymorphs exhibit different equilibrium solubilities. For example, four polymorphs of phenylbutazone were identified by x-ray diffraction, thermal analysis, and infrared spectroscopy and were found to have substantially different equilibrium solubilities (Table 5-5). The difference in the solubility of polymorphs therefore provides a driving force for crystal growth in suspension as the particles of the more soluble polymorph go into solution and reprecipitate as the less soluble, i.e., more stable, form. This process is accelerated if the drug powder used to prepare the suspension contains a mixture of polymorphs, or if a seed of the more stable form is introduced.

Temperature cycling may lead to crystal growth, as solubility depends on temperature. In most cases, solubility is directly related to temperature, so that a slight rise in temperature leads to an increased equilibrium solubility. A drop in temperature, however slight, results in a supersaturated solution surrounding each particle. Precipitation occurs to relieve the supersaturation, and crystal growth occurs.

Wetting

Wetting is the displacement of either a liquid or gas from a surface by a second liquid. The wetting of a solid during the manufacture of a suspension, or the dissolution of a tablet in the gastrointestinal tract, involves the displacement of air from the solid surface and is the type of wetting considered in this section.[2,5]

When a drop of liquid is brought into contact with a flat solid surface, the equilibrium shape of the drop depends on the balance of cohesive forces between the molecules of the liquid and the adhesive forces between the molecules of the liquid and the solid surface. As can be seen in Figure 5-29, the angle that includes the liquid at the point where the drop and solid meet can vary from 0 to 180° and is termed the *contact angle*, θ. The contact angle is a useful indication of wetting. A low contact angle indicates that adhesive forces between the liquid and the solid predominate and wetting occurs, while a high contact angle indicates that the cohesive forces of the liquid predominate.

The basic equation that applies to wetting is the Young equation, which is based on the change in free energy caused by an increase in the area of a solid that is wetted by a liquid (Fig. 5-30). For a small, reversible change in the position of the liquid on the surface, there is an increase in the liquid-solid interfacial area, ΔA, and a corresponding decrease in the solid-air interface of $\Delta A \cos \theta$. The corresponding free

TABLE 5-5. *Equilibrium Solubility of Polymorphs of Phenylbutazone*

Form	Equilibrium Solubility, mg/100 ml
1	288.7
2	279.7
3	233.6
4	213.0

Adapted from Ibrahim, H. G., Pisano, F., and Bruno, A.: J. Pharm. Sci., 66:669, 1977. Adapted with permission of the copyright owner.

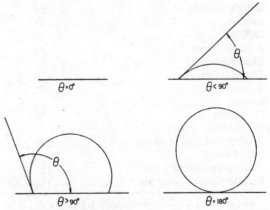

FIG. 5-29. *The use of the contact angle, θ, to characterize the wetting of a solid by a liquid.*

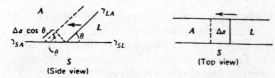

FIG. 5-30. *Schematic of derivation of Young equation based on the change in free energy caused by an increase in the area of a solid, Δa, which is wetted by a liquid. (From Rosen, M. J.: Surfactants and Interfacial Phenomena. John Wiley and Sons, New York, 1978, p. 178.)*

energy change is given by:

$$\Delta G = \gamma_{S/L}\Delta A - \gamma_{S/A}\Delta A + \gamma_{L/A}(\cos\theta)\Delta A \tag{17}$$

As ΔA approaches zero, the ratio $\Delta G/\Delta A$ approaches zero at equilibrium, so that equation (17) reduces to the Young equation:

$$\gamma_{S/A} = \gamma_{S/L} + \gamma_{L/A}\cos\theta \tag{18}$$

The Young equation states that the contact angle will be <90° if the interaction between the solid and liquid is greater than the interaction between the solid and air, i.e., $\gamma_{S/L} > \gamma_{S/A}$. Under these conditions, wetting occurs. A general guideline is that solids are readily wetted if their contact angle with the liquid phase is less than 90°. Table 5-6 confirms this rule of thumb, as solids that are known to be easily wetted, such as potassium chloride, sodium chloride, and lactose, have the lowest contact angles. Interest-

TABLE 5-6. *Contact Angle of Solids of Pharmaceutical Interest Against a Saturated Aqueous Solution of the Material*

Material	Contact Angle (°)
Potassium chloride	21
Sodium chloride	28
Lactose	30
Caffeine	43
Acetaminophen	59
Chloramphenicol	59
Phenobarbitol	70
Sulfadiazine	71
Aspirin	75
Phenacetin	78
Hexobarbitol	88
Polyethylene (high-density)	100
Salicylic acid	103
Magnesium stearate	121
Chloramphenicol palmitate	125

Adapted from Lerk, C. F., Schoonen, A. J. M., and Fell, J. T.: J. Pharm. Sci., 65: 843, 1976. Adapted with permission of the copyright owner.

ingly, the contact angle of chloramphenicol increases from 59 to 125°, indicating a change to a nonwetting surface when the palmitate ester is formed. Other materials that are known to be difficult to wet, such as high-density polyethylene and magnesium stearate, have contact angles greater than 90°.

The wetting of a powder involves several types of wetting processes. Three types of wetting have been identified: adhesional wetting, immersional wetting, and spreading wetting.

The first step in the wetting of a powder is adhesional wetting, in which the surface of the solid is brought into contact with the liquid surface. This step is the equivalent of going from stage *a* to stage *b* in Figure 5-31. The particle is then forced below the surface of the liquid as immersional wetting occurs (*b* to *c* in Fig. 5-31). During this step, solid-liquid interface is formed, and solid-air interface is lost. Finally, the liquid spreads over the entire surface of the solid as spreading wetting occurs. The work of spreading wetting is equal to the work to form new solid-liquid and liquid-air interfaces minus the loss of the solid-air interface. For the total wetting process, the work required is the sum of the three types of wetting:

$$W_{total} = -6\gamma_{L/A}\cos\theta \tag{19}$$

Therefore, the analysis supports the generalization drawn from the Young equation, as wetting occurs spontaneously, i.e., without any input of work into the system, if the contact angle is <90°.

Measurement of the contact angle is complicated because hysteresis is frequently encountered. Contact angle hysteresis means that one value for the contact angle is obtained when the liquid is advancing on the surface, and that a different, usually lower, value is obtained when the liquid is receding. Surface roughness or surface chemical heterogeneity are causes of con-

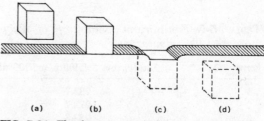

FIG. 5-31. *The three stages involved in the wetting of a solid cube: a → b, adhesional wetting; b → c, immersional wetting; c → d, spreading wetting. (From Jaycock, M. J., and Parfitt, G. D.: Chemistry of Interfaces, John Wiley and Sons, New York, 1981, p. 237.)*

tact angle hysteresis. Consider the situation arising when a syringe is used to inject more liquid into a drop that is on a "rough" surface. The advancing liquid encounters solid surface and air-filled pores. When liquid is withdrawn from the drop, the receding liquid encounters solid surface and liquid-filled pores, and a lower contact angle is measured.

Adsorbed impurities may also affect measurement of the contact angle. The first contact of the liquid with the solid surface may dissolve the impurities. The dissolved impurities may affect both $\gamma_{S/L}$ and $\gamma_{L/A}$ and thereby cause a variation in θ as described by the Young equation. In addition, the dissolution of impurities causes the surface to have a different composition when the receding contact angle is measured. Therefore, great care must be taken when measuring the contact angle, especially in the preparation and pretreatment of the solid surface.

Contact angles of finely divided solids are even more difficult to measure than the contact angle of a liquid on a flat surface. The Washburn equation states that the distance that a liquid penetrates into a bed of powder in time t is proportional to the square root of cos θ.[16] This relationship is used experimentally to evaluate the wetting ability of a powder by different vehicles; the powder is packed into a glass tube, or filled into an inclined trough, and the distance that a vehicle penetrates in time t gives a measure of the relative wetting ability of the system.[17]

Adsorption at Solid-Liquid Interfaces

The adsorption of a solute by a solid surface can occur during the preparation of suspension dosage forms as well as in a patient's gastrointestinal tract following the coadministration of a soluble drug and an insoluble solid. Most adsorption mechanisms can be classed as either physical adsorption or chemisorption. The attractive forces in physical adsorption are due to van der Waals forces, and possibly hydrogen bonding. The attractive forces in chemisorption are much stronger and include coordination complexes and ion exchange.

The extent of adsorption depends on the properties of the solute, the surface, and the solvent.[1] Taub's rule may be used to predict adsorption behavior qualitatively. The rule is that a polar adsorbent preferentially adsorbs the more polar component of a nonpolar solution. Conversely, a nonpolar adsorbent preferentially adsorbs the more nonpolar component of a polar solution. Figure 5-32 shows that silica gel, a polar adsorb-

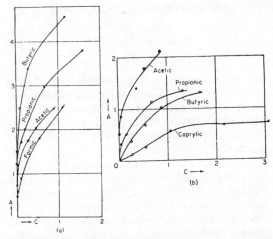

FIG. 5-32. *Illustration of Taube's rule:* a, *adsorption of fatty acids on carbon from aqueous solution, and b, adsorption of fatty acids on silica gel from toluene. (From Adamson, A. W.: Physical Chemistry of Surfaces, 3rd Ed. John Wiley and Sons, New York, 1976, p. 390.)*

ent, most strongly adsorbs the more polar members of a series of related fatty acids, and that charcoal, a nonpolar surface, most strongly adsorbs the more nonpolar members of the series of fatty acids.

Another useful generalization is that an inverse relationship usually exists between the extent of adsorption of a solute and its solubility in the solvent. Thus, adsorption of a solute can be either enhanced or minimized by the selection of the solvent. It is frequently helpful, therefore, to consider adsorption as a type of partition process.

Steric considerations are important for both the substrate and the solute. Linde molecular sieve 5A preferentially adsorbs hexane rather than benzene because of its small pore size. In addition, bulky substituent groups on the solute often reduce the degree of adsorption, probably by preventing close approach of the solute to the surface.

The basic equations used to describe adsorption from solutions are the Langmuir and Freundlich equations. These were derived for the adsorption of a gas by a solid, but have been extended to adsorption from solution.

The Langmuir equation is based on the assumptions that (1) the molecules are adsorbed onto specific points of attachment on the surface, (2) that each point of attachment can accommodate only one adsorbed molecule, and (3) that the energy state of any adsorbed molecule is independent of the presence of other adsorbed molecules on neighboring sites.

The Langmuir equation is expressed as:

$$\frac{c}{x/m} = \frac{1}{ab} + \frac{c}{b} \qquad (20)$$

where c is the equilibrium concentration of the solute in solution; x/m is the mass of solute, x, per gram of adsorbate at equilibrium, m; b is the adsorptive capacity of the solid, gram of solute per gram of adsorbate; and a is the adsorption coefficient.

Adsorption that follows the assumptions of the Langmuir equation is characterized by an adsorption isotherm, i.e., a plot of c versus x/m, which shows a sharp initial increase in the amount adsorbed, which subsequently decreases with increasing concentration until a saturation level is reached. The saturation value of x/m corresponds to b, the adsorptive capacity of the solid. The adsorption of propoxyphene by montmorillonite fits the Langmuir equation, as can be seen in Figure 5-33. The left ordinate of Figure 5-33 describes the adsorption isotherm.

When the adsorption data are plotted as $\frac{c}{x/m}$ versus c (right ordinate of Fig. 5-33), a straight line is obtained. The adsorptive capacity of the solid, b, is the reciprocal of the slope and the adsorption coefficient a is obtained by dividing the slope, 1/b, by the intercept, 1/ab. Figure 5-33 indicates an adsorptive capacity of 480 mg propoxyphene hydrochloride per gram of montmorillonite from the plateau of the adsorption isotherm, or 490 mg propoxyphene hydrochloride per gram of montmorillonite from a plot of the Langmuir equation.

In the Freundlich equation, a variation of the Langmuir model, the heat of adsorption diminishes exponentially with the number of adsorption sites that are occupied. This observation implies that the surface is heterogeneous, i.e., there are several types of adsorption sites. The Freundlich equation is as follows:

$$\frac{x}{m} = kc^{1/n} \qquad (21)$$

where x is the amount of solute adsorbed by a mass of adsorbent, m; c is the equilibrium concentration of the solute in solution; and k and n are constants for the system. When adsorption follows the Freundlich equation, the adsorption isotherm (graph of x/m versus c) is not linear at low concentrations, nor does it have a saturation value.

In many cases, information can be obtained about the mechanism of interaction, including the functional groups involved by the use of infrared spectroscopy.[18,19] The infrared bands of a functional group that is involved in an interaction with a surface are perturbed. Thus, a comparison of the infrared spectrum of the solute with the infrared spectrum of the solute-adsorbent mixture is useful in investigating the mechanism of interaction.

The orientation of a solute adsorbed by a swelling clay can be determined by x-ray diffraction. Adsorption by such swelling clays as montmorillonite occurs mainly in the interlayer space of the clay. X-ray diffraction can accurately measure the distance between the clay layers. Thus, a comparison of the dimension of the interlayer space before and after adsorption indicates whether adsorption has occurred in the interlayer space, as well as the amount of space occupied by the adsorbate. Comparison of the molecular dimensions of the adsorbate with the increase in interlayer spacing provides information about the orientation of the solute (e.g., a single layer in parallel orientation).[20]

Once adsorption occurs, several other types of reactions are of interest. *Desorption* refers to the release of the adsorbate and may be important if an adsorbed drug is exposed to different environments during either its manufacture or use. An understanding of the adsorption mechanism is essential for the prediction of desorption. For

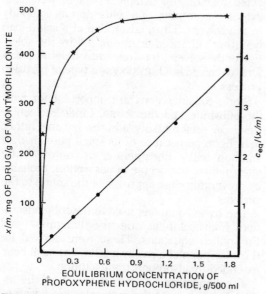

FIG. 5-33. *Adsorption isotherm for propoxyphene hydrochloride by montmorillonite. Key: ★, x/m versus equilibrium concentration; and ●, c/(x/m) versus equilibrium concentration. (From McGinity, J. W., and Lach, J. L.: J. Pharm. Sci., 65:896, 1976. Reproduced with permission of the copyright owner, the American Pharmaceutical Association.)*

example, if adsorption is due to physical adsorption, dilution may cause desorption. This phenomenon was observed in the adsorption of digoxin by montmorillonite.[21] Digoxin is a neutral molecule that is adsorbed by physical adsorption. Digoxin is readily desorbed, however, by washing the drug-clay complex with water.

Desorption is more difficult to achieve if adsorption occurs by chemisorption. Drugs that are adsorbed by cation exchange can be desorbed, however, by washing with an electrolyte solution or by changes in the pH of the medium, which cause the adsorbate to change its ionic form. McGinity and Lach were able to produce a sustained systemic effect of amphetamine by adsorbing protonated amphetamine (i.e., cationic form of amphetamine base) by montmorillonite through cation exchange.[22] The protonated amphetamine-montmorillonite complex was stable in the low pH of the stomach, but as the drug-clay complex passed through the intestine, the protonated amphetamine was exposed to an increasing pH. At higher pH conditions, the protonated amphetamine was deprotonated, and neutral amphetamine base was formed. The neutral drug was not strongly adsorbed and was desorbed in the intestine. The electrolyte concentration of the intestinal fluid may also have contributed to desorption. Thus, amphetamine was desorbed slowly as the drug-clay complex passed through the intestine, and a prolonged amphetamine blood level was obtained.

An adsorbed molecule may undergo degradation reactions at a faster rate, owing to the effects of the surface. Many clays are negatively charged and therefore strongly adsorb cations from solution, including protons. Thus, a higher concentration of protons exists at the clay surface in an aqueous suspension than is present in the bulk solution. Digoxin, which degrades by acid-catalyzed hydrolysis, degraded much more rapidly in a montmorillonite suspension than in a solution at the same pH.[21] The catalytic effect was found to be due to the ability of the clay surface to serve as a site where digoxin molecules and protons are concentrated by physical adsorption and cation exchange, respectively. Therefore, the probability of acid-catalyzed hydrolysis was enhanced, and an increased hydrolysis rate was observed. This effect may reduce the bioavailability of digoxin, as 82% of the digoxin was intact and available for absorption after a digoxin solution was aged for 1 hour at pH 2, 37°C (which corresponds to the estimated gastric residence time). Only 2% of the digoxin was intact, however, when a digoxin-montmorillonite suspension was aged for 1 hour at pH 2, 37°.

Oxidative degradation reactions may also be catalyzed by solids if the drug is adsorbed by a surface composed of inorganic ions that may be reduced. Certain clays contain structural ferric iron, as well as adsorbed iron oxides or hydroxides, at the clay surface. Attapulgite is such a clay, and the rate of oxidative degradation of hydrocortisone was accelerated significantly in an attapulgite suspension.[23] Sepiolite, another clay belonging to the same structural class of clays as attapulgite, is relatively free of surface ferric iron and did not accelerate the oxidative degradation of hydrocortisone even though adsorption occurred.[24] Thus, surfaces must not simply be considered sites for adsorption; the potential of the surface to accelerate chemical reactions should be taken into account as well.

References

1. Adamson, A. W.: Physical Chemistry of Surfaces. 3rd Ed. John Wiley and Sons, New York, 1976.
2. Rosen, M. J.: Surfactants and Interfacial Phenomena. John Wiley and Sons, New York, 1978.
3. McBain, J. W., and Humphreys, C. W.: J. Phys. Chem., 36:300, 1932.
4. Becher, P.: Emulsions: Theory and Practice. Reinhold, New York, 1957, p. 25.
5. Jaycock, M. J.; and Parfitt, G. D.: Chemistry of Interfaces. John Wiley and Sons, New York, 1981.
6. Padday, J. F.: Surface and Colloid Science. Vol. 1. Edited by E. Matijevic. John Wiley and Sons, New York, 1969, p. 101.
7. Feldkamp, J. R., Shah, D. N., Meyer, S. L. et al.: J. Pharm. Sci., 70:638, 1981.
8. Grim, R. E.: Clay Mineralogy. 2nd Ed. McGraw-Hill, St. Louis, 1968.
9. Serna, C. J., White, J. L., and Hem, S. L.: J. Pharm. Sci., 67:324, 1978.
10. Hiemenz, P. C.: Principles of Colloid and Surface Chemistry. Marcel Dekker, New York, 1977.
11. Israelachvili, J. N., and Ninham, B. W.: Colloid and Interface Science. Vol. 1. Edited by M. Kerker et al. Academic Press, New York, 1978, p.15.
12. Overbeek, J. Th. G.: Colloid and Interface Science. Vol. 1. Edited by M. Kerker et al. Academic Press, New York, 1978, p. 431.
13. Adams, G. E., and Israelachvili, J. N.: Modification of Soil Structure. Edited by W. W. Emerson et al. John Wiley and Sons, New York, 1978, p. 27.
14. Israelachvili, J. N., and Adams, G. E.: Faraday Trans. I, 74:975, 1978.
15. Kahlweit, M.: Adv. Colloid Interface Sci., 5:1, 1975.
16. Washburn, E. D.: Physiol. Rev., 17:374, 1921.
17. Szekely, J., Neumann, A. W., and Chuang, Y. K.: J. Colloid Interface Sci., 35:273, 1971.
18. Little, L. H.: Infrared Spectra of Adsorbed Species. Academic Press, New York, 1966.
19. Ledoux, R. L., and White, J. L.: J. Colloid Interface Sci., 21:127, 1966.
20. Porubcan, L. S., Serna, C. J., White, J. L., and Hem, S. L.: J. Pharm. Sci., 67:1081, 1978.
21. Porubcan, L. S., Born, G. S., White, J. L., and Hem, S. L.: J. Pharm. Sci., 68:358, 1979.

22. McGinity, J. W., and Lach, J. L.: J. Pharm. Sci., 66:63, 1977.
23. Cornejo, J., Hermosin, M. C., White, J. L., et al.: J. Pharm. Sci., 69:945, 1980.
24. Hermosin, M.C ., Cornejo, J., White, J. L., and Hem, S. L.: J. Pharm Sci., 70:189, 1981.

General References

Adamson, A. W.: Physical Chemistry of Surfaces. 3rd Ed. John Wiley and Sons, New York, 1976.
Betcher, P.: Emulsions: Theory and Practice. Reinhold, New York, 1957.

Davies, J. T., and Rideal, E. K.: Interfacial Phenomena. Academic Press, New York, 1961.
Jaycock, M. J., and Parfitt, G. D.: Chemistry of Interfaces. John Wiley and Sons, New York, 1981.
Kruyt, H. R.: Colloid Science. Vol. 1. Elsevier, New York, 1952.
van Olphen, H.: An Introduction to Clay Colloid Chemistry. 2nd Ed. John Wiley and Sons, New York, 1977.
Osipow, L. I.: Surface Chemistry: Theory and Industrial Applications. Reinhold, New York, 1962.
Rosen, M. J.: Surfactants and Interfacial Phenomena, John Wiley and Sons, New York, 1978.
Ross, S.: Chemistry and Physics of Interfaces. American Chemical Society, Washington, D.C., 1965.
Shaw, D. J.: Introduction to Colloid and Surface Chemistry. 2nd Ed. Butterworths, London, 1970.

6

Pharmaceutical Rheology

JOHN H. WOOD

Pharmaceutical fluid preparations are recognized as materials that pour and flow, having no ability to retain their original shape when not confined. The semisolids are a more nebulous grouping. They essentially retain their shape when unconfined but flow or deform when an external force is applied. Those materials that readily pour from bottles and form a puddle are clearly fluids. Ointments or pastes that clearly retain their shape after extrusion from a tube characteristically are associated with pharmaceutical semisolids. Obviously a continuum of properties exists between these limits.

Rheology (from the Greek *rheos* meaning flow and *logos* meaning science) is the study of the flow or deformation under stress. In pharmaceutical and allied research and technology, rheologic measurements are utilized to characterize the ease of pouring from a bottle, squeezing from a tube or other deformable container, maintaining product shape in a jar or after extrusion, rubbing the product onto and into the skin, and even pumping the product from mixing and storage to filling equipment. Of extreme importance in both product development and quality assurance is the determination that the desired attributes of body and flow are retained for the required shelf-life of the product.

Definitions and Fundamental Concepts

The tangential application of a force to a body and the resultant deformation of that body are the essential components for a rheologic observation. If this force is applied for only a short time and then withdrawn, the deformation is defined as *elastic* if the shape is restored, but as *flow* if the deformation remains. A *fluid* or *liquid* then becomes a body that flows under the action of an infinitesimal force. In practice, gravity is generally regarded as the criterion of such a minimal force.

To best understand the fundamental components of viscous flow, consider Figure 6-1. Two parallel planes are a distance x apart; between the planes, the viscous body is confined. The top, plane A, moves horizontally with velocity v because of the action of force F. The lower plane B is motionless. As a consequence, there exists a velocity gradient v/x between the planes. This gradient is given the definition of *rate of shear*, D. The *shear stress*, S, is the force per unit area creating the deformation.

Example 1. If some oil is rubbed into the skin with a relative rate of motion between the two surfaces of 15 cm/sec, and the film thickness is 0.01 cm, then the shear rate is as follows:

$$D = \frac{15}{0.01} \frac{cm/sec}{cm}$$
$$= 1500 \ sec^{-1}$$

This shear stress may be applied either momentarily or continuously. Elastic deformation occurs if, as the force is applied, the upper plate moves in the direction of the force only momentarily and then stops but returns to its original position when the deforming force is removed. On the other hand, pure viscous flow occurs if there is continuous movement during the applied force, and no restorative motion follows removal of the deforming force.

Between the limits of elastic deformation and pure viscous flow, there exists a continuum of combinations of these limits. Such behavior is called *viscoelastic flow*. The elastic component of viscosity is considered in a later section.

Newtonian fluid is a fluid in which a direct

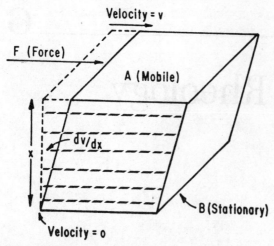

Velocity = v

F (Force)

A (Mobile)

$\frac{dv}{dx}$

x

B (Stationary)

Velocity = o

FIG. 6-1. *Model to demonstrate components of classic viscous flow.*

proportionality exists, for all values of shear, between shear stress and shear rate.

Viscosity or *coefficient of viscosity* is the proportionality constant between shear rate and shear stress. Conventionally, viscosity is represented by η. Then:

$$\eta = S/D \qquad (1)$$

The centimeter-gram-second (C.G.S.) system uses grams per centimeter per second ($g\ cm^{-1}\ sec^{-1}$) as the dimensional units of viscosity. In these units, viscosity is expressed in *poises*, a term used in recognition of the pioneering work in the 1840s of the French scientist J. L. M. Poiseuille. For dilute aqueous solutions, the common unit becomes the centipoise (10^{-2} poise), cp. The viscosity of water is about 1 cp.

In the newly adopted International System of Units (SI), the unit corresponding to the centipoise is the millipascal-second (mPas).

A perspective of these units may be obtained by considering the case of Figure 6-1 when a force of 1 dyne acts to produce a velocity of 1 cm/sec for plate A when the distance between plates is 1 cm, and both plates are 1 cm^2 in cross-sectional area. Under these terms, viscosity is calculated as:

$$\eta = \frac{S}{D}$$

$$= \frac{force/area}{velocity\ difference/distance}$$

$$= \frac{dyne/cm^2}{(cm/sec)/cm}$$

$$= dyne\ sec\ cm^{-2}$$

However, the dyne is the force acting for 1 sec to produce a velocity in a 1-g mass of 1 cm/sec. Hence, this dimensional analysis for viscosity reduces to:

$$\eta = g \cdot cm^{-1}\ sec^{-1}$$
$$= poise$$

In the International System of Units, which is not yet used routinely in viscosity references, the pascal (Pa) is the unit of stress and has the dimensions of newton/meter^2, where the newton is a kilogram meter/second^2. Hence, equivalence occurs for the centipoise with millipascal-seconds.

Example 2. If in example 1, the oil had the same viscosity as water, then the force used to create the shear can be determined as follows:

$$\eta = \frac{S}{D}$$

$$1 \times 10^{-2}\ poise = \frac{S}{1500}\ sec^{-1}$$

Then $S = (1500)(1 \times 10^{-2})(sec^{-1})(poise)$
$= 15\ (sec^{1})(dyne\ sec\ cm^{-2})$
$= 15\ dyne\ cm^{-2}$

Example 3. In S.I. units, the above terms would become:

$$\eta = 1\ mPas$$
$$D = 1500\ sec^{-1}$$
$$S = 1.5\ Pa$$

Fluidity is the reciprocal of the viscosity, usually designated by the symbol ϕ. This is an occasional unit of convenience but not an essential one.

Kinematic viscosity (ν) is the Newtonian viscosity divided by density (η/d). The unit is now the *stoke*, in honor of the English scientist who studied problems of gravitational settlement in fluids. As discussed later in this chapter, certain fluid flow viscometers give values in this kinematic scale.

Example 4. If the oil from examples 1 and 2 had a density of 0.82, then the kinematic viscosity would be:

$$\nu = \frac{\eta}{d}$$

$$= \frac{1 \times 10^{-2}}{0.82}$$

$$= 1.22 \times 10^{-2}\ stokes$$
$$= 1.22\ centistokes$$

Non-newtonian fluids are those in which there is no direct linear relationship between shear stress and shear rate. Most systems of pharmaceutical interest fall into this category. The shear stress necessary to achieve a given shear rate may increase more rapidly or less rapidly than is required by the linear direct proportionality (Fig. 6-2).

A *pseudoplastic* material is one in which the stress increases at less than a linear rate with increasing shear rate, while a *dilatant* material is one in which the increase is more rapid. Thus, if viscosity is calculated at each of a series of shear rate points by use of equation (1), then the resultant values *decrease* with increasing shear rate for pseudoplastic materials and *increase* for dilatant ones. Measurements at such single points are frequently referred to as *apparent viscosity* to recognize clearly that the number quoted refers only to the condition of measure-

ment. Although frequently, reference is carelessly made to a lotion having a viscosity of 300 cp or to a paste or ointment having a viscosity of 1200 poises, these are meaningless terms unless the shear rate at which the measurement was made becomes a clear part of the statement. The fact that one number cannot characterize the viscous behavior, however, requires the use of some equation of state. One such empiric one is the Power Law Equation:

$$S = A D^n \qquad (2)$$

where S and D are the shear stress and shear rate respectively, A is an appropriate proportionality constant, and n is the Power Index. In this form, n is less than 1 for pseudoplastic materials and greater than 1 for dilatant materials. The Power Law Equation is also used with the index n associated with stress rather than shear rate. Obviously, the magnitude of the values of n are then interchanged. Unfortunately, there is no clear convention for such equations.

When the logarithm of both sides of equation (2) is taken, the result is:

$$\log S = \log A + n \log D \qquad (3)$$

Compared with the equation of a straight line, $y = b + mx$, a plot of log S against log D results in a straight line of slope n and intercept log A. Figure 6-3 shows such plots on logarithmic scale for one gum system as a function of gum concentration.

Example 5. Calculate the parameters of the Power Law Equation for 0.01%, 0.02%, 0.04%, and 0.10% gum solutions. The following data apply to this case.

Composition	Stress at $D = 1$	Stress at $D = 10$
.01%	0.35 dyne cm^2	2.1 dyne cm^2
.02	6.2	20
.04	61	132
.10	205	440

The slope of each line is obtained from:

$$n = \frac{\log S_{(D=10)} - \log S_{(D=1)}}{\log 10 - \log 1}$$

$$= \frac{\log (S_{10}/S_1)}{1 - 0}$$

$$= \log \frac{S_{10}}{S_1}$$

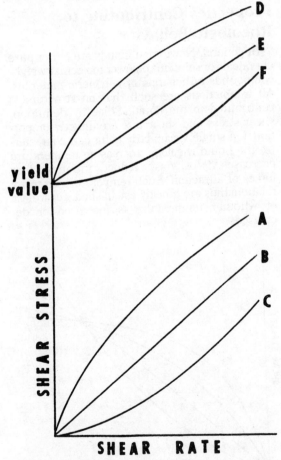

FIG. 6-2. *Examples of basic types of rheograms. A, Pseudoplastic or power law; B, Newtonian; C, dilatant; D, pseudoplastic with yield value; E, Bingham or Newtonian with yield value; F, dilatant with yield value.*

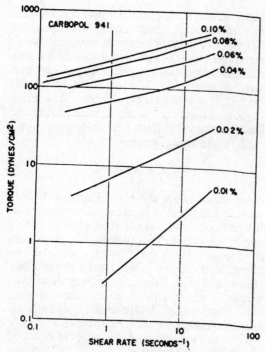

FIG. 6-3. *Logarithmic plots of the rheograms of Carbopol 941. (From Catacalos, G., and Wood, J. H.: J. Pharm. Sci., 53:1089, 1964. Reproduced with permission of the copyright owner, the American Pharmaceutical Association.)*

The slopes are then $\log \frac{2.1}{0.35}$, $\log \frac{20}{6.2}$, $\log \frac{132}{61}$, and $\log \frac{440}{205}$ for the four successive concentrations. These reduce to 0.78, 0.51, 0.34, and 0.33 respectively.

The intercept of a line is the value of y for x = 0, or here the value of log S for (log D) = 0, but the logarithm is zero when the number is unity, log 1 = 0. Therefore, the intercepts of the four concentrations are log 0.35, log 6.2, log 61, and log 205. Numerically then, these values of log S are the values log A. Hence, the values of A are 0.35, 6.2, 61, and 205 respectively. The Power Law Equations are then:

0.01%	$S = 0.35D^{0.78}$
0.02	$S = 6.2D^{0.51}$
0.04	$S = 61D^{0.34}$
0.10	$S = 205D^{0.33}$

When an initial finite force is necessary before any rheologic flow can start, this initial stress is called *yield value*. A *Bingham plastic* is represented by a straight line or curve on the stress-shear rate plot being displaced from the origin by a finite stress value, the yield value. Thus, for

Newtonian behavior at stresses (S) greater than the yield value (f) we have:

$$S - f = UD \qquad (4)$$

where U is the plastic viscosity and D is the shear rate. Similarly (see Fig. 6-2), both pseudoplastic and dilatant curves may appear to exhibit yield value. The dimensional units of the yield value must be those of the shear stress.

Because of the variety of parameters involved, no single measurement can characterize a non-Newtonian system. This can be seen in Figure 6-4. A wide variety of curves can pass through any specific value of shear stress and shear rate, exemplified here by the common focus of pseudoplastic, dilatant, and Newtonian lines. At the focal point, all have the same apparent viscosity, but at no other point do they have related values.

Properties Contributing to Rheologic Behavior

In general, Newtonian liquids are either pure chemicals or solutions of lower molecular weight compounds rather than of polymeric materials. All interactions are such that no structure is contributed to the liquid. Since by definition, shear stress and shear rate are directly proportional, a single viscometric point can characterize the liquid rheology. Increasing temperature decreases viscosity as it reduces intramolecular forces of attraction. Such temperature viscosity relationships are quickly established, regardless of whether temperature is increased or decreased.

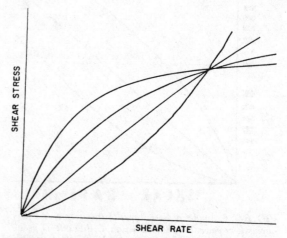

FIG. 6-4. *Different rheograms all have the same apparent viscosity at the common foci but not at any other point.*

Pseudoplastic behavior is exhibited by polymer solutions and by most semisolid systems containing some polymer components. In such systems, there is a buildup of interlacing molecular interactions. Long straight-chain polymers tend to have some coiling in their condition of minimum energy. These coils can develop a degree of interlocking. With branched polymers, the opportunity for frictional interlock is obviously even greater. In addition or alternatively, intramolecular bridging may occur by simple hydrogen bonding. This bonding may create innumerable bridges between individual adjacent molecules to create a complete cross-linking. As an example, water added to a liquid nonionic in the correct ratio can create a solid gel. In the case of silica or alumina gel, water may serve alone or with other agents from cross-linking to create a three-dimensional polymer structure. Classically, most suspending agents exhibit similar capability for development of structure. Depending on the nature of the suspending and cross-linking materials used, these adjuvants may or may not be in complete homogenous solution. Instead, these agents may have a strong affinity for the solvent and yet be partially insoluble. In systems with dispersed solids, these colloid solutions can serve as the interweaving material to hold the whole system together.

When shear is slowly imparted to such a system, deformation may initially occur with some difficulty, but once initiated, it becomes progressively easier as successive increments of force are applied. The nature of the interlocking or interwoven structure dictates whether initial flow occurs with difficulty until sufficient structure is lost or whether a sufficient initial force is required to initiate motion, that is, whether a *yield value* has to be exceeded. In any case, continued shearing breaks further linkages, so that the apparent viscosity drops with increasing shear. As shear stress is then decreased, the structure may or may not recover immediately. If recovery occurs rapidly, the ascending and descending shear-stress/shear-rate rheograms will be essentially superimposable. If the structure does not immediately recover, the descending rheogram will have lower stress values at each shear rate than the ascending (Figure 6-5). Such a body is said to be *thixotropic* and the loop, a *hysteresis* loop, is in area a measure of the thixotropy.

Occasionally, semisolid systems in shear, particularly those containing an appreciable solid content or those in which structure is developed through a three-dimensional polymer (silicate system), develop shear planes across which virtually no interactions exist, and hence, flow is

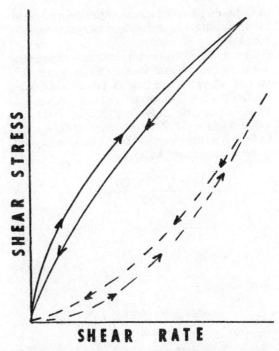

FIG. 6-5. *The solid lines represent ascending and descending rheograms for a pseudoplastic system exhibiting thixotropy. The dashed lines represent a dilatant system with a loop of rheopexy.*

easy. These planes of slippage result in what is called *plug flow*. In such a system, one portion moves with the shear stress, while the residue remains at rest. As is discussed later, this results in confusing rheologic implications for product performance. In general, such measurements are less reproducible.

Classic rheology cannot handle time-dependent phenomena except to display changes in stress under continuing shear. Thixotropy is therefore a phenomenon resulting from the time dependency of the breakdown or the rebuilding of structure. It is an empiric observation of good reliability that structure breakdown or buildup is an exponential function of time. Thus, if the observed shear stress for a given shear rate is followed with time, a plot of stress against time, both on the logarithmic scale, results in a straight line. Green and Weltmann used a variant of this observation to derive a coefficient of thixotropic breakdown (B) by the equation:[1]

$$B = \frac{S_1 - S_2}{\ln(t_2/t_1)} \qquad (5)$$

where S_1 and S_2 are the stress values at times t_1 and t_2 of continuous shear at any arbitrary shear rate chosen for comparison. Other pharmaceutical applications for pastes and lotions were later developed by Weltmann.[2]

Example 6. Consider an ointment undergoing shear in a rotational viscometer at a constant rate of shear. A reading is taken 5 sec after starting. The observed shear stress is 14,000 dyne cm^{-2}. After continuous shear, the value drops to 11,500 dyne cm^{-2} at 50 sec and to 900 dyne cm^{-2} at 500 sec. Then, the coefficient of thixotropic breakdown is:

$$B = \frac{14,000 - 11,500}{\ln(50/5)} \text{ dyne cm}^{-2}$$

$$= \frac{2500}{2.303}$$

$$= 1085 \text{ dyne cm}^{-2}$$

Similarly:

$$B = \frac{11,500 - 900}{\ln(500/50)} \text{ dyne cm}^{-2}$$

$$= 1085 \text{ dyne cm}^{-2}$$

Obviously, the coefficient is a function of the time interval chosen, in this case a decade.

Dilatant systems are essentially the opposite of pseudoplastic thixotropic ones. In dilatancy as shear continued, the fluid components contributing to lubricity between particles are excluded from between the shear planes so that the resulting structure develops increasing friction. Thus, stress increases with time in a logarithmic manner similar to that with thixotropy. A similar hysteresis loop of *rheopexy* is developed in dilatant systems. Magnesia magma is the classic pharmaceutical example of this behavioral type. Usually, some yield value is also recognized in rheopectic systems.

Equation (5) may be used with dilatant systems in the same way as with thixotropic ones to yield a coefficient of dilatant buildup.

Graphic Presentation of Rheologic Data

Stress-Shear Rate Curves

As was mentioned with the Power Law relationship, there is no uniformity of presentation of shear-stress/shear-rate data as to which should be the dependent variable (ordinate) and the independent variable (abscissa). The confusion in representing the Power Law by equation (2) is a consequence of this ambiguity. This is a historical problem originating in the equipment used in early measurements. Specific equipment is discussed in a later section of this chapter. It suffices to say that in the early work with rotational viscometers, the drive force was applied by hanging weights, and shear rate was then calculated from the observed rotational speed. In this context, stress was the controllable independent variable. Today, the drive speed is set by the use of synchronous motors whose speed is controlled by the applied electric frequency, by gear ratios, or by both. Under these conditions of a fixed set of rotational speeds, the shear rate should become the independent variable. The majority of rheologic data are obtained in this manner. With data obtained by capillary rheometers using externally applied pressure, the stress is the independent predetermined parameter, and shear rate is the consequential dependent variable. The conclusions and the essential data are the same, however, regardless of how the plots are made. Typical plots for two gum systems are given in Figure 6-6.

The logarithmic plots of the shear-stress/shear-rate relationships of these two gums are found in Figures 6-3 and 6-7. Figure 6-3 was used to illustrate the Power Law, and the calculation of its parameters.

In addition, the logarithmic plot of stress and shear rate is convenient for providing an overall summary of data taken in various shear rate ranges. In the conventional arithmetic scale, low shear rate data are excessively compacted in the presence of high shear rate observations. There is no other practical way to observe both low and high shear rate observations within one graph.

Yield Value Determination

Examining Figure 6-6 for indications of yield value as defined earlier from Figure 6-2, one

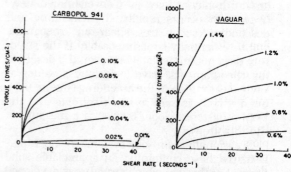

FIG. 6-6. *Rheograms for Carbopol 941 and Jaguar. (From Catacalos, G., and Wood, J. H.: J. Pharm. Sci. 53:1089, 1964. Reproduced with permission of the copyright owner, the American Pharmaceutical Association.)*

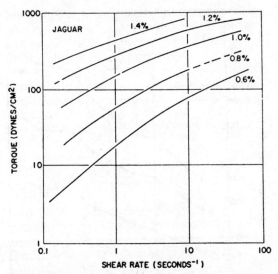

FIG. 6-7. *Logarithmic plot of the rheograms of Jaguar. (From Catacalos, G., and Wood, J. H.: J. Pharm. Sci., 53:1089, 1964. Reproduced with permission of the copyright owner, the American Pharmaceutical Association.)*

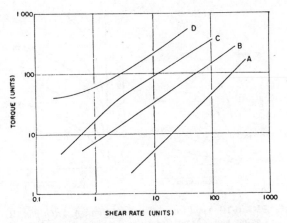

FIG. 6-8. *Logarithmic representations of rheograms. Newtonian with slope unity A; power law with slope less than unity B; power law with slope approaching unity at low shear rates C; power law with slope approaching zero at low shears indicating yield value D. (From Catacalos, G., and Wood, J. H.: J. Pharm. Sci., 53:1089, 1964. Reproduced with permission of the copyright owner, the American Pharmaceutical Association.)*

sees that discrepancies between the real and the ideal case appear to exist. The data for Carbopol 941 all behave at higher shear rates as if they belonged to a family of curves exhibiting yield value at low shears. At the lower shear rates, however, the shear stresses drop off dramatically, implying that a yield value does not occur for Carbopol 941. With the Jaguar gum, similar break-off points occur, but the high concentrations of 1.4% and 1.2% do imply a yield value.

In both cases, if no measurements had been made at shear rates below 5 sec^{-1}, the existence of a yield value would be unquestioned. When a gum system is assumed to have a yield value based on rheologic measurements, but cannot maintain a quality suspension, it is usually because the low shear-rate values were ignored. Often, this error is not deliberate but is governed by the characteristics of the measuring apparatus available.

If the logarithmic plot is essentially a straight line into the low shear rates, then obviously a true yield value does not exist, even though by the conventional plot there appears to be a yield value. However, if the power equation logarithmic plot tends to break upward toward a constant stress for lower shear rates (Fig. 6-8), a true yield value exists. When the logarithmic plots Figure 6-3 and 6-7 are examined, it is apparent that for the Carbopol 941 curves, the Power Law straight line tends to break upward toward the horizontal at low shear rates, implying the existence of a true yield value. The Jaguar® tends to break downward toward a slope of

unity, implying classic Newtonian behavior at low shear rates.

Although the logarithmic plots permit an unambiguous determination of the reality of the yield value, they permit only a qualitative assessment of its numerical magnitude.

Two plots for better visualization of yield value have become common. These are the Casson and the Fitch plots, (Figures 6-9 and 6-10);[3,4] the Casson is the most widely accepted. In the Casson plot, the square root of stress is plotted against the square root of the shear rate, while in the Fitch plot, the stress is directly plotted against the square root of the shear rate. The

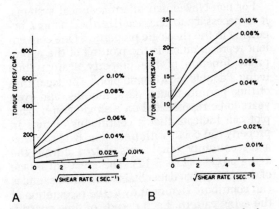

FIG. 6-9. *Yield value plots for Carbopol 941. A, Fitch plot. B, Casson plot. (From Catacalos, G., and Wood, J. H.: J. Pharm. Sci., 53:1089, 1964. Reproduced with permission of the copyright owner, the American Pharmaceutical Association.)*

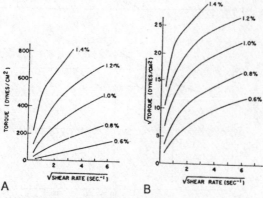

A

B

FIG. 6-10. *Yield value plots for Jaguar. A, Fitch plot. B, Casson plot. (From Catacalos, G., and Wood, J. H.: J. Pharm. Sci., 53:1089, 1964. Reproduced with permission of the copyright owner, the American Pharmaceutical Association.)*

intercept on the stress axis is then defined more clearly than is possible from other representations. In Figures 6-9 and 6-10, it is apparent both from the Casson and the Fitch plots that these implications are indeed borne out. The Carbopol 941 values generate unambiguous intercept plots by both methods, while the Jaguar values all focus on the graphic origin.[5]

If only higher shear rate measurements were available, the logarithmic plot, by the changing slopes observed, would produce uncertainty regarding a yield value; however, the conventional, the Casson, and the Fitch plots would all have clearly exhibited yield values. Unfortunately, the logarithmic plot is used rarely as insurance for the low shear rate behavior.

Aging of Rheologic Properties

For non-Newtonian pharmaceutical systems, it is necessary to characterize the changes occurring in the rheologic properties. One convenient representation is the plotting of the appropriate function of the property against time using a double logarithmic plot.[6] The logarithm of time permits hours, days, months, and even years to be represented on a single graph. This plot can indicate that a continuous change in property can occur with time (Fig. 6-11), or that a discontinuity can be recognized during the aging process (Fig. 6-12). The great advantage of this plot is that data obtained on fresh samples can contribute significantly to the recognition of the aging pattern. Each decade of time contributes equally to the continuum of the time pattern. Diffusion-controlled phenomena usually display a logarithmic time dependency.

Consider the data represented by Figure 6-11.

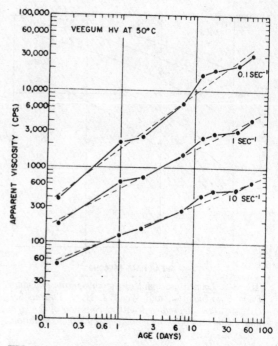

FIG. 6-11. *Aging change in apparent viscosity at different shear rates. (From Wood, J. H., Catacalos, G., and Lieberman, S. V.: J. Pharm. Sci. 52:354, 1963. Reproduced with permission of the copyright owner, the American Pharmaceutical Association.)*

Initial rheograms were run about 3 hours after manufacture of the suspension and again at 24 and 48 hours. The values at 48 hours are clearly in line with those anticipated from the first two times. The data through 60 days continue to increase linearly by the logarithmic relation. The results during the first day can predict the first week, while those of the first week predict the next month, and the month implies the year by a linear projection.

In the development of a lotion formulation

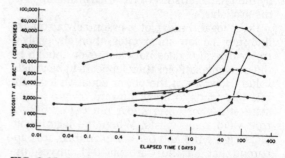

FIG. 6-12. *Aging curves for various process and formulation variants of lotion subject to age hardening. (From Wood, J. H., and Catacalos, G.: J. Soc. Cosm. Chem., 14:147, 1963. Reproduced by permission of the copyright owner.)*

and a processing study, the data of Figure 6-12 were obtained. The formulation tended to harden with age. The departures from the flat initial rheologic observations clearly indicated when this undesirable process became significant. Although the onset time of this hardening remained empiric, these logarithmic time plots did provide a level of confidence as aging of improved formulations proceeded.

Types of Rheologic Instruments

Capillary or Tube Viscometers

When a fluid flows through a round-bore capillary or tube, there is a viscous drag restraining the flow. The fluid in immediate contact with the wall is motionless while that at the center is at maximum velocity. Between these two limits is then a velocity gradient. It may be shown that D, the shear rate at the wall, for a Newtonian liquid is given by:

$$D = \frac{4Q}{\pi r^3} \qquad (6)$$

where Q is volume flowing through the capillary per unit time, and r is the radius of the capillary.

The shear stress, S, at the wall is:

$$S = \frac{\Delta Pr}{2L} \qquad (7)$$

where L is the length of the capillary and ΔP is the pressure difference across the capillary, which provides the appropriate force to overcome the viscous drag.

Example 7. What shear stress and shear rate develop when 2 ml/sec of a fluid are forced through a 10-cm length of capillary diameter 1 mm by a force equivalent to a 100 mm of mercury?

$$D = \frac{4Q}{\pi r^3}$$

$$= \frac{(4)(2 \text{ ml/sec})}{(\pi)(0.05 \text{ cm})^3}$$

$$= 20{,}400 \text{ sec}^{-1}$$

The unit of pressure must be multiplied by the mercury density and the acceleration of gravity to convert to force units.

$$S = \frac{\Delta P}{2} \frac{r}{L}$$

$$= \left(\frac{(100 \text{ mm Hg})(13.595 \text{ g/cm}^3)}{2} \right)$$

$$\times (980.7 \text{ cm sec}^2)\left(\frac{0.05 \text{ cm}}{10} \right)$$

$$= \left(\frac{1.333 \times 10^5}{2} \text{ dynes/cm}^2 \right)\left(\frac{.05}{10} \right)$$

$$= 33300 \text{ dyne cm}^{-2}$$

Example 8. What is the apparent viscosity of the fluid in example 7?

$$\eta = \frac{S}{D}$$

$$= \frac{33300}{20400} \frac{\text{dyne cm}^{-2}}{\text{sec}^{-1}}$$

$$= 1.63 \text{ poise}$$
$$= 163 \text{ cp}$$

Substituting equations (6) and (7) into equation (1) gives the net result:

$$\eta = \frac{\Delta P\pi^4}{8LQ} \qquad (8)$$

This equation is generally referred to as *Poiseuille's equation*. For this form, the results of example 8 would be obtained without a calculation of the shear rate and stress involved. As with many such relationships, this is an ideal equation. It assumes that the length is much greater than the radius, and that there are no entry and exit effects at the ends of the tubing. A series of corrections to the expressions for D and S have been derived to provide corrections for these effects and for various stress-strain relationships within the fluid; however, these basic equations are remarkably adequate in providing useful characterization on non-Newtonian systems.

The form of capillary most frequently used is the glass system typified by the Ostwald viscometer (Fig. 6-13). Here the ΔP term is the difference in height between the upper and lower meniscuses of the fluid. There is a change in head resulting from the flow of the liquid from the bulb as measured by the movement between the two markings of the upper meniscus. Simultaneously, the lower meniscus rises as the flow enters the lower reservoir. Therefore, measurements are at a varying shear stress and shear rate. This is not a problem when relative viscosity measurements are made by comparing a standard reference η_R and the unknown η_u. In each case, the volume V flowing is the same, but

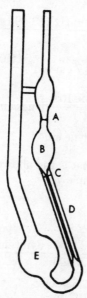

FIG. 6-13. *Ostwald viscometer. Liquid is drawn up from bulb E into the bulb above the mark A, and the time of fall of the upper meniscus from line A to line C of the fluid contained in B is measured. The diameter and length of the capillary D control the flow time.*

the time for flow is t_R and t_u respectively. The ΔP term effectively becomes a height term h divided by the density of the fluid. It then follows, on substitution into equation (8) that:

$$\eta_u = \left(\frac{(hd_u)(\pi r^4)}{8L(V/t_u)}\right)\left(\frac{(hd_R)(\pi r^4)}{8L(V/t_u)}\right)$$

$$= \frac{t_u d_u}{t_R d_R}$$

This equation can be rearranged as:

$$\left(\eta_u \Big/ d_u\right)\Big/\left(\eta_R \Big/ d_R\right) = \frac{t_u}{t_R} \qquad (9)$$

The term η/d was defined as the kinematic viscosity ν, and so:

$$\frac{\nu_u}{\nu_R} = \frac{t_u}{t_R} \qquad (10)$$

It is primarily in this type of situation that kinematic viscosity has its greatest use.

Example 9. The flow time for water in an Ostwald Viscometer was measured at 20°C as 224 sec for the average of 5 trials. Similar measurements for an oil of density 0.748 g/cm³ were 426 sec. What is the viscosity of the oil? The density of water at 20° is 0.998, and the viscosity is 1.005 cp. The kinematic viscosity of water is

given by:

$$\nu = \frac{\eta}{d} = \frac{1.005}{.998}$$

$$= 1.007 \text{ centistokes}$$

Then, by equation (10):

$$\frac{\nu_{oil}}{\nu_{water}} = \frac{t_{oil}}{t_{water}}$$

$$\frac{\nu_{oil}}{1.007} = \frac{426}{224}$$

$$\nu_{oil} = 1.92 \text{ centistokes}$$

Then

$$\eta_{oil} = d_{oil}\nu_{oil}$$
$$= (.748)(1.92)$$
$$= 1.43 \text{ cp}$$

A wide range of capillary lengths and diameters permits a full range of fluids to be studied. Such instruments should, of necessity, be restricted to materials that can readily flow into and out of the apparatus without rheologic damage. Hence, these liquids should be essentially Newtonian in behavior.

Commercially, Ostwald viscometers are purchased by the choice of the centistokes per second constant desired. The normal expected flow time is 200 to 800 sec for a given instrument. Faster times generally utilize some form of external timing. Cannon Instrument Co. (State College, PA) sells a range of Ostwald Viscometers with constants ranging from approximately 0.002 to 20 centistokes per second.

Example 10. Quality control personnel wish to purchase an Ostwald Viscometer for routine monitoring of the viscosity of an oil whose density is 0.821 and whose viscosity is about 125 cp. They wish the observed flow time to be between 200 and 400 sec. What specification instrument should they buy?

$$\nu = \frac{\eta}{d}$$

$$= \frac{125 \text{ cp}}{0.821 \text{ g/cm}^3}$$

$$= 152 \text{ centistokes}$$

To have a flow time of 300 sec, the constant of the instrument should be approximately:

$$= \frac{150}{300} \frac{\text{centistokes}}{\text{sec}}$$

$$= 0.5 \text{ centistokes/sec}$$

The Cannon Instrument Co. has size number 350, which has this instrument constant value.

Because many research and quality control measurements utilize some variant of the Ostwald Viscometer, there are commercial instruments that measure the time for flow between the two indices with high precision by using photoelectric timing. Schott America (New York, NY) markets a system capable of automatic loading of up to 30 samples for sequential measurement by such a timer.

Alternate versions of the classic Ostwald Viscometer have been developed to minimize inherent problems of the individual practical instruments. Thus, some instruments depend less on the varying pressure differential, some use either pressure or vacuum as a driving force, some require minimal volume, and some permit successive dilutions to take place in the instrument to follow concentration behavior.

In general, use of Ostwald Viscometers is restricted to a "one-shear-range" measurement only, and the instrument must be selected for the individual sample under investigation.

The alternative is a general instrument containing replaceable capillary tubes and a variable driving force. Such an instrument provides maximum flexibility of use. This system is shown schematically in Figure 6-14. A sample storage chamber is loaded with the sample to be investigated. The sample is extruded through a capillary tube attached to one end. The chamber contents are forced through this exit capillary by the force of the piston. Two versions are practical. In one, the piston is driven at a constant linear rate. Then, by equation (6), the volume extruded per unit time is a geometrically defined constant depending only on the volume displaced by the

piston per unit time. Hence, the shear rate observed is that prechosen by the capillary radius and the volume terms. In this case, the force transmitted to the piston is measured by a suitable device, either a strain gauge on the pressure shaft or a hydraulic gauge in the pressured system. Thus, by equation (7), the shear stress is a direct function of this force measurement. Instron testers, because of their constant velocity of movement, are typical components for such a system. The Instron Engineering Corp. (Canton, MA) can create suitable custom instruments.

The alternative version of Figure 6-14 requires that a constant force be applied to the piston, and the resultant displacement of piston or sample extruded is measured. Typically, the constant force is applied from gas cylinders with a good pressure regulation system. One commercially available example is the Cannon-Manning Pressure Viscometer (Cannon Instrument Co., State College, PA) shown in Figure 6-15.

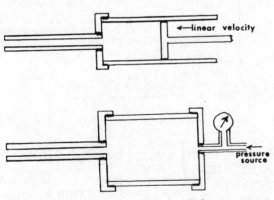

FIG. 6-14. *The extrusion rheometer. Either a constant linear velocity is imparted to the piston to give a preset volume delivery and the piston force is measured, or a preset force (air pressure) is applied and the rate of volume delivery is determined.*

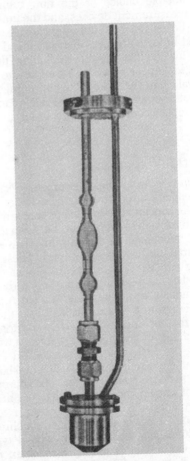

FIG. 6-15. *Cannon-Manning pressure viscometer. (By permission from Cannon Instrument Co.)*

The capillary is the metallic fixture between the two Swage Nuts. Pressure is applied through the side arm to the sample (18 ml) contained in the holding vessel. The volume displaced is measured by either or both of the two glass bulbs. The pressure drop occurs completely within the capillary so that the glass portion of the system is not under any pressure. This instrument is capable of performing rheologic studies of most pharmaceutical semisolid formulations: pastes, ointments, and creams.

These types of systems can be developed or modified "in house" to meet specific criteria. The shop work involved in creating an excellent instrument does not impose excessive demands on an adequate facility.

Many of the manufactured instruments of this type have tended to have a limited sales life because of minimal replacement needs once the market was saturated. One of these, the Severs Extrusion Rheometer,[7] is discussed later in this chapter under "Specialized Pharmaceutical Applications of Rheology."

By suitable choice of the flow tubing, the stress measurement devices, and the timing systems, the extrusion systems are capable of being utilized in virtually any pharmaceutical or cosmetic formulation system, including those in which low shear rates are necessary to define yield value. In these, as in any other measuring device, it is essential that no rheologic damage to the sample occurs in loading it for measurement.

Couette Viscometers

Couette, or *rotational*, viscometers comprise two members, a central bob or cylinder and a coaxial or concentric cup. One or both are free to rotate in relation to each other. Between these is the test substance, in the annulus. Three basic configurations have been utilized. These are a rotating cup with strain measurement on the central bob, a rotating central bob with strain measurement on the cup, and a fixed cup with both rotation and strain measured on the bob.

The first of these configurations originally provided the cup rotation by the force of weights hanging on a pan that was suspended from a cord wound around the cup. The central bob displacement was restrained by an appropriate spring of known modulus so that the angular displacement could be equated to angular torque on the bob. Later versions provided synchronous speed drives for the cup. The second type of couette viscometer is merely a mechanical inversion of the first. The third classification represents the majority of modern mass-produced

instruments. The rotation, usually of the inner member, is provided by a synchronous electric motor, usually with variable ratio drives that provide a series of discrete speeds, with the other member rigid. An alternative is a motor that provides a continuous variation in speed by an appropriate transmission control or by a variable speed motor drive. A mechanical linkage in the shaft measures angular displacement of the bob from the driving armature. Figure 6-16 exhibits the Brookfield manner of achieving this dual function. More advanced instruments have replaced the measurements of angular displacement with strain gauge linkages of some form to permit direct electronic recording or digital readout.

In the mathematical derivation of the usual expressions for shear stress S and shear rate D for the cup and bob situation, the existence of a Newtonian fluid is assumed. In this situation, two alternatives may be considered for the average shear stress and shear rate in the gap between the cup and bob. These are the arithmetic (A) and geometric (G) means of the values at the walls of the bob and the cup. The more customary arithmetic values are:

$$S_A = \frac{T(R_I^2 + R_O^2)}{4\pi h R_I^2 R_O^2} \tag{11}$$

$$D_A = \frac{(R_I^2 + R_O^2)}{(R_O^2 - R_I^2)} \Omega \tag{12}$$

where T is the measured torque (dyne cm) usually obtained as the product of a scale reading

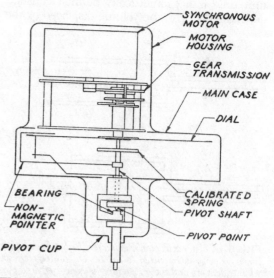

FIG. 6-16. *Brookfield Synchro-Lectric viscometer. (By permission from Brookfield Engineering Lab.)*

and the instrumental restoring torque per scale unit of deflection; R_I and R_O are radii of the inner member, bob, and the outer member, cup, respectively; h is the effective height or length of the bob; and Ω is the angular velocity of rotation in radians per second.

The values for the geometric mean replace the $(R_I^2 + R_O^2)$ term in the numerators of both equation (11) and equation (12) by $2\,R_I R_O$, yielding:

$$S_G = \frac{T}{2\pi R_I R_O h} \tag{13}$$

$$D_G = \frac{2 R_I R_O}{R_O^2 - R_I^2}\,\Omega \tag{14}$$

Obviously, if R_I and R_O are virtually identical in magnitude, that is, the annulus between the cup and bob is very thin, these two means are identical. Both sets of equations yield the same value for viscosity:

$$\eta = \frac{S}{D}$$

$$= \left(\frac{T}{4\pi h \Omega}\right)\left(\frac{R_O^2 - R_i^2}{R_i^2 R_O^2}\right) \tag{15}$$

Commercial instruments supply the values of R_I, R_O, h, and the instrument constant that converts the observed angular deflection to the restoring torque value T generated by that deflection.

Example 11. A rheometer has a cup with a radius of 2.40 cm and a bob with a radius of 2.28 cm. The effective height of the bob is 6.0 cm. The restoring torque on the rotating bob is 388 dyne cm per instrument scale division. When a sample is measured at a rotational speed of 30 rpm, the scale reading is 42.1 scale divisions. What are the shear stress, the shear rate, and the viscosity?

$$S = \frac{T(R_i^2 + R_O^2)}{4\pi h R_I^2 R_O^2}$$

$$= \frac{(388)(42.1)(2.28^2 + 2.40^2)}{(4)(3.1416)(6.0)(2.28)^2(2.40)^2}$$

$$= 79.3 \text{ dyne cm}^{-2}$$

and

$$D = \frac{(R_I^2 + R_O^2)}{(R_O^2 - R_I^2)}\,\Omega$$

$$= \left[\frac{[(2.28)^2 + (2.40)^2]}{[(2.40)^2 - (2.28)^2]}\right]\left[\frac{30 \text{ rpm}}{60 \text{ sec min}^{-1}}\right]$$

$$= \times [2\,\pi \text{ radians}]$$

$$= 61.3 \text{ sec}^{-1}$$

Note that the revolutions per minute were converted to radians per second, there being 2π radians per revolution.

$$\eta = \frac{S}{D}$$

$$= \frac{79.3 \text{ dyne cm}}{61.3 \text{ sec}^{-1}}$$

$$= 1.29 \text{ cp}$$

Note that the same value would have been obtained for the viscosity using equation (15).

Example 12. A rheometer with a spring constant and cup and bob radii as given in the previous example is used with a known standard viscosity oil to determine the effective height of the bob. If an oil of viscosity 1.98 cp gave a scale deflection of 65.1, what is the effective height of the bob?

$$\eta = \frac{T}{4\pi h \Omega}\quad\frac{R_O^2 - R_I^2}{R_I^2 R_O^2}$$

$$h = \frac{T}{4\pi \eta \Omega}\quad\frac{R_O^2 - R_I^2}{R_I^2 R_O^2}$$

$$= \left(\frac{(65.1)(388)}{(4)(3.1416)(1.98)\left(\dfrac{30}{60}\right)(2)(3.1416)}\right)$$

$$\times \left(\frac{(2.40)^2 - (2.28)^2}{(2.28)^2(2.40)^2}\right)$$

$$= 6.06 \text{ cm}$$

Often, the end effects cannot be readily calculated for the precision geometry. An effective height can then be obtained by calibration in this manner and used with all further work with that cup and bob.

When the ratio of R_O/R_I exceeds 1.1, there are reasons to feel that the use of the geometric mean with equations (13) and (14) is better than use of the arithmetic mean of equations (11) and (12) in representing the average condition of the material under shear in the annulus.

Occasionally in equipment literature and in publications, yet another pair of equations for calculating S and D are used. These result from the assumption that the gap is so wide that R_O^2 is much greater than R_I^2 and that only the larger term is retained in the summation. The equations are:

$$S = \frac{T}{2\pi h R_I^2} \tag{16}$$

$$D = \frac{2 R_O^2}{(R_O^2 - R_I^2)}\,\Omega \tag{17}$$

These equations are presented so that they may be recognized when seen in other readings. Surprisingly, the value for the viscosity is still given by equation (15) when these are used. There are some rheologic empiricists who believe that equations (16) and (17) are more suitable for non-Newtonian systems than are equations (13) and (14) or (11) and (12). The fundamental practitioners of rheology use a simple equation to establish a power law relationship and then use equations developed with that relationship to calculate more proper values of shear stress and shear rate. Such equations are not considered in this discussion.

Conventional pharmaceutical use of rheologic instrumentation consists of obtaining a comparison between samples and establishing whether changes occur in samples as a result of processing or aging. For such use, slight systematic biases or errors in calculation of exact data resulting from the method of measurement do not constitute a problem, since comparisons are made within one measurement. Examples are the already discussed Figures 6-11 and 6-12. When it is necessary to examine the rheologic behavior over a shear rate range greater than can be covered with one instrument, slight discontinuities may occur between measurement systems, as can be seen in Figure 6-17. All calculations in this example use the basic equations without any attempt at empiric or theoretic correction for differing gap sizes, end effects, or the nonlinear behavior.

In addition, it should be recognized that Figure 6-17 is another example of the lowest shear measurements inflecting to exhibit a very low but real yield value. Thus, the use of the double

logarithmic plot permits not only the recognition of apparent changes in rheologic parameters, which are artifactual to the simplified equations utilized, but also a clear recognition of the entire rheologic picture for all conditions of shear.

If it should become essential to bring values from different cup/bob combinations into absolute coherence, one approach is to use a series of sleeves that fit into a rheometer cup. By conducting measurements with one bob at a series of clearances to the sleeves (cup), one can obtain an estimate of a limiting zero gap by extrapolation to the zero gap condition. This usually permits a smooth transition from one measuring combination to the next as the product changes with age in storage trials. The Contraves Viscometer has such a set of sleeves available for use in its cups. This versatile instrument, available from the Tekman Company (Cincinnati, OH), is sometimes called the Epprecht Viscometer after its designer. Another frequently used instrument for pharmaceutical studies is the Rotovisko (Haake Inc., Saddle River, NJ). In addition, Brookfield Engineering Inc. (Stoughton, MA) has sets of cup and bob combinations available for its basic instruments.

Cone and Plate Viscometers

In this type, the cone is a slightly beveled plate such that ideally the angle ψ between cone and plate is only a few degrees; even in the cruder forms, it is less than 10° (Fig. 6-18). The linear velocity at any point on the cone r from the apex is $r\Omega$, where Ω is the angular velocity while the separation is $r\psi$; hence, the shear rate is given by:

$$D = \frac{r\Omega}{r\psi}$$
$$= \frac{\Omega}{\psi} \tag{18}$$

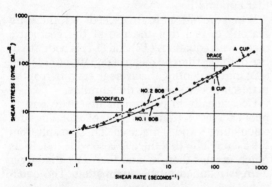

FIG. 6-17. *Type of overlapping rheograms obtained with different cup and bob combinations, using equations without correction. (From Wood, J. H., Catacalos, G., and Lieberman, S. V. (J. Pharm. Sci. 52:296, 1963. Reproduced with permission of the copyright owner, the American Pharmaceutical Association.)*

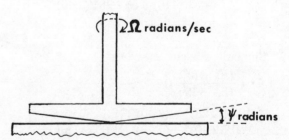

FIG. 6-18. *Basic configuration of the cone and plate viscometer.*

In this case, the dimensional analysis gives:

$$D = \frac{\Omega \text{ radians/sec}}{\psi \text{ radians}}$$

$$= \sec^{-1}$$

This is dimensionally correct. Of greatest significance in equation (18) is that the shear rate at any point is the same, uniform, throughout the gap when the cone angle is small.

If the cone radius is R, then the shear stress S is given by:

$$S \doteq \frac{3T}{2\pi R^3} \qquad (19)$$

where T is the restoring torque measured by the instrument.

Example 13. What is the shear stress and shear rate for a cone-plate viscometer measurement using a 5.00-cm radius cone and plate, with the cone rotational speed being 50 rpm, the cone angle 1.8°, and the scale reading 37.6 units? The torque conversion is 1105 dyne cm per scale division.

First, both the rotation and the cone angle must be brought to similar units, in this case, radians:

$$D = \frac{\Omega}{\psi}$$

$$= \frac{(50\,\text{rpm})\left(\dfrac{1\,\text{min}}{60\,\text{sec}}\right)(2\pi \text{ radians/revolutions})}{(1.8)\left(\dfrac{2\pi}{360}\right)(\text{degrees})(\text{radians/degree})}$$

$$= 166.7 \sec^{-1}$$

Alternately, the conversion could be to degrees:

$$D = \frac{(50 \text{ rpm})(360°/\text{rev})\left(\dfrac{1}{60} \text{ min/sec}\right)}{1.8 \text{ (degrees)}}$$

$$= 166.7 \sec^{-1}$$

Similarly, the stress is given by:

$$S = \frac{3T}{2\pi R^3}$$

$$= \frac{(3)(37.6 \text{ units})(1105 \text{ dyne cm/unit})}{(2)(\pi)(5.00)^3}$$

$$= 158.7 \text{ dyne cm}^{-2}$$

Geometrically, either the cone or the plate can be the rotating member. The torque may be measured either on the other member or through the coupling drive system exactly as in the couette viscometers.

The classic instrument of this category has been the Ferranti-Shirley Viscometer (Ferranti Electric, Corrmack, NY), whose use in a wide range of pharmaceutical and cosmetic literature testifies to its general versatility. In addition, cone-plate systems attachments are available for the Brookfield, Contraves, and Rotovisko systems.

Density-Dependent Viscometers

Physically, the falling ball viscometer requires the determination of the time t for a ball of density ρ_B to fall through a fixed distance of liquid of density ρ_L and of viscosity η. The equation governing this determination may be developed from first principles if the ball falls freely in an "ocean" of liquid, that is, there is no effect from the container walls. However, a general equation of the following form may be used regardless of whether a free fall or a slide and/or roll down an inclined tube is used:

$$\eta = K(\rho_B - \rho_L)t \qquad (20)$$

The constant K includes wall interaction factors. A liquid of known viscosity is then used to calibrate the instruments for general use, in a manner analogous to that with Ostwald and similar capillary viscometers.

Example 14. A ball of density 3.12 takes 109 sec to fall the fixed distance of an inclined tube viscometer when a calibrating liquid of density 0.94 and viscosity 8.12 poises is used. A) What is the instrumental constant? B) What would be the viscosity of a sample oil of density 0.88 if the fall time under similar conditions was 125 sec?

A) $\eta = K(\rho_B - \rho_L)t$

$$K = \frac{\eta}{(\rho_B - \rho_L)t}$$

$$= \frac{8.12}{(3.12 - 0.94)(109)} \frac{\text{poises}}{(\text{grams/ml})(\text{sec})}$$

$$= 0.0342 \text{ poises gram}^{-1} \text{ ml sec.}^{-1}$$

B) $\quad \eta_? = 0.034\,(\rho_B - P_?)t$
$\quad\quad = (0.034)(3.12 - 0.88)(125)$
$\quad\quad = 9.571 \text{ poises}$

It also is apparent that:

$$\frac{\eta}{\eta_?} = \frac{K(\rho_B - \rho_L)t_L}{K(\rho_B - \rho_?)t_?}$$

$$\eta_? = \frac{(\rho_B - \rho_?(t_?)}{(\rho_B - \rho_L)(t_L)}\,\eta_L$$

$$= \frac{(3.12 - 0.88)(125)}{(3.12 - 0.94)(109)} \quad (8.12)$$

$$= 9.57 \text{ poise}$$

One commercial example is the Hoeppler Viscometer, a 200-mm tube with an 8-mm radius and a normal 10° tilt from the vertical. Utilizing the appropriate ball, it has a workable range of 0.01 cp to 10,000 poises. This is a one-point measurement involving uncertain shear rate and shear stress, however.

Similar in principle is the Bubble Viscometer. A series of sealed standard tubes have calibrated oils covering a range of viscosities. Each has a small air bubble of exact geometry. The unknown sample is placed in an empty tube and stoppered so that it is identical in bubble content to the standards. The unknown and standard tubes are inverted, and the bubble rise times are compared to determine the standard most resembling the unknown. This is still a procedure that is utilized with some heavy oils.

Certainly, these two gravity procedures have little to offer when compared with modern rotation viscometers.

Penetrometers

These were instruments developed to measure the consistency or hardness of relatively rigid semisolids. The cone and the needle forms are the most commonly used in pharmacy. These are shown schematically in Figure 6-19. The usual cone is that specified by the ASTM, which has a 30° cone point protruding from a 90° cone; however, other solid angled cones have been used. In use, the cone is mounted on an instrument that measures its movement with time. The tip is set at the surface, and a spring tension is attached to the top of the cone. At time zero, the cone is released. Usually, the penetration occurring in a fixed time is determined. The travel distance is usually reported in decimillimeters, 10^{-4} meters.

It has been shown that these measurements can provide a self-consistent measure of a yield value (YV) through the following equation:

$$YV = \frac{KW}{P^n} \quad (21)$$

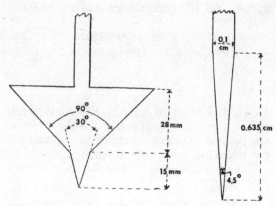

FIG. 6-19. *The basic configuration of the double cone and the needle penetrometers.*

where K is an appropriate proportionality constant, W is the load in grams on the penetrometer, P is the penetration in mm (multiples of 0.1 mm), and n is an index. The value of K depends on the cone angle, 9670 for 30°, 2815 for 60°, and 1040 for 90°.[8,9] The index n must be determined from a plot of the classically measured yield value against penetration for a variety of samples. The value of n = 1.6 applies to margarine and fat. No equivalent numbers have been reported for products of pharmaceutical interest. However, the highest possible value of n is 2, the theoretic value utilized automatically by some workers. For relative values, either number, or an average would not lead to a serious error. Pharmaceutical studies seem to be confined to empiric reporting of penetration values for comparison purposes or for following graphically the penetration with time as a function of penetrometer load. This is not surprising since rarely is the necessary time taken to calibrate full rheogram yield values against penetration parameters. This does not detract from the utility of the penetrometer as an effective tool in evaluating changes in yield value for ointments and semisolid creams. Its particular value is the relative rapidity and ease with which such penetrometer measurements may be made.

Miscellaneous Measuring Systems

A wide variety of geometries are conceivable in which a test medium either moderates motion of a driven object or serves to transmit force across a gradient. Thus, rising spheres, plates, rods, etc. have found utility in various forms of rheometers. Some have practical elements for utilization but often need empiric rather than theoretic calibration. Typical devices are the various plates, rods, and T-bars characteristic of the normal Brookfield viscometer. These measuring systems have provided most of the practical quality control of emulsions and semisolids for the cosmetic and pharmaceutical industries.

Usually, some systems meet a need of special convenience. They are usually calibrated against a Newtonian oil and hence readings obtained are apparent viscosities rather than actual values. For routine evaluation and comparison, these empiric instruments are invaluable even though the results cannot be readily translated to absolute rheologic parameters.

Viscoelastic Properties and Measurements

Earlier in this chapter, it was emphasized that there are time-dependent shear changes occurring in samples with the creation of thixotropic or rheopectic loops. The classic rheologic treatments cannot adequately handle such changes except to quantitate those that occur by fixed processes. These cannot lead to other than empiric relationships.

The time-dependent changes in properties of a substance undergoing shear are properly classified as *viscoelastic* changes. Viscoelastic properties are often represented by two mechanical analogies: a spring, and a dashpot or closed piston. The spring symbolizes the classic elastic property that is normally associated with it. When a force is applied, it stretches a fixed distance proportional to the force and stops. When the displacing force is withdrawn, the spring immediately returns to its original condition, and no permanent deformation occurs. The dashpot or piston represents the condition considered in classic rheology. As in Figure 6-1, a displacement occurs, with the application of an applied force, and continues as long as the force is applied. When the force is removed, the material merely remains in the position it has reached by that time. No recovery occurs.

In the representation of viscoelastic properties, there are two primary elements, usually called *Kelvin* and *Maxwell* elements. In the Kelvin element, the spring and the dashpot are placed in parallel position, while in the Maxwell, they are in series (Fig. 6-20). When a displacing force is applied to a Kelvin element and held constant, there occurs a viscous flow that decreases with time. In the analog, the viscous flow occurs because of the displacing force, and the net magnitude of that force decreases as the spring stretches to balance the force. When the

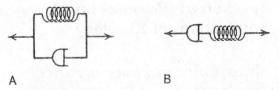

FIG. 6-20. *Spring and dashpot representation of viscoelastic elements. The Kelvin element* (A) *has the components in parallel position, whereas the Maxwell element* (B) *has them in series.*

displacing force is removed, there is a slow return to the original position as the internal force of the spring drives the dashpot back to its original position. In summary, the elastic element has a time component for its attainment of steady state. With the Maxwell element, when a displacing force is applied, there is an immediate elastic displacement followed by a continuous tinuous viscous flow. The spring stretches immediately, and the dashpot slowly moves independently. When the force is removed, there is an immediate rebound of the elastic displacement, but no viscous flow occurs after that elastic recovery. The spring has returned to its original conformation, but the dashpot remains in its new location because there is no force for a restoration.

Schematically, many of these elements may be combined in various permutations. The resulting arrays can be treated mathematically to develop the appropriate characterizing parameters. Experimental instrumentation to provide data for these mathematical treatments is available. They are of many types depending on the physical nature of the substance to be examined. In some cases, the instrument is a modification of one already described in this chapter; however, most are product-specific or extremely expensive. Unfortunately, data treatment development is beyond the scope of this chapter. An excellent review is provided by Barry,[10] one of the major contributors to pharmaceutical viscoelastic studies.

Although there have been published many excellent studies on the viscoelastic properties of pharmaceutical gums, mucilages, and gelling and suspending agents, their applicability in generalized characterizations of perceived desired product attributes is still needed.[11-13]

Unfortunately, although it is apparent that the parameters of classic rheology—thixotropy, pseudoplasticity, and dilatancy—can be readily visualized from the fundamental Kelvin and Maxwell elements, measurements from within one approach cannot be utilized to project or calculate parameters in the other.

Specialized Pharmaceutical Applications of Rheology

Shear Rates in Pharmaceutical Applications and Resultant Desired Viscosities

Henderson et al. made the first major attempt to establish shear rates corresponding to pharmaceutical use.[14] They set "topical application up to 120 sec.$^{-1}$; rubbing on ointment tile, 150 sec.$^{-1}$; roller mill, 1000–12000 sec.$^{-1}$; colloid mill, several hundred thousand sec.$^{-1}$; nasal spray (plastic squeeze bottle), 1000 sec.$^{-1}$; and pouring from bottle, below 100 sec.$^{-1}$." To this can be added rubbing into skin, 100 to 10,000 sec^{-1}, depending on the degree of rubbing; squeezing from a tube or plastic bottle, 10 to 1000 sec^{-1}, depending on orifice size and delivery rate; pumping of products, 1000 to 100,000 sec^{-1}; high-speed filling, from 5000 to 100,000 sec^{-1}; and yield value parameters, below 0.1 sec^{-1}. An example of this extrusion range is that 1 cm^3/sec delivery of a liquid cream through an orifice 10 mm in diameter imparts a shear rate of 10 sec^{-1}, while for the same volume through a 5-mm orifice, such as might occur for a toothpaste, it is 100 sec^{-1}.[12] Only 0.1 ml/sec through a 1-mm orifice imparts a shear rate of 1000 sec^{-1}.

This pharmaceutical characterization, depending upon the application, must bridge an extremely wide range of values of shear rate. The shear rate for individual use by a process may vary. The acceptability of the force necessary to extrude a product from a collapsible container is obviously dependent on the squeezing force that the subject can exert easily. Similarly, the force to permit rub-in of a topical product depends on the user.

An interesting example of how to proceed to determine suitable product characterizations is a study by Langenbucher and Lange.[15] They wished to determine suitable product characteristics for squeezing from a tube and then for ease of application of a cosmetic cream or ointment. They used a series of Newtonian oils of varying viscosity to assess acceptance with a panel. In their study, the tubes were of standard aluminum with a diameter of 18 mm, a length of 100 mm, and a 5.3-mm orifice. Using a perception scale of 1 to 5 with 1 too thin and 5 too thick, this perception scale was found to be proportionate to the logarithm of the test medium's Newtonian viscosity. These workers determined that a viscosity of 50 to 1000 poises, optimally

200 poises, was acceptable for extrusion in this tube. Similarly, for topical use, a range of 0.2 to 5 poises, optimally 1 poise, was preferred. Several products for rheologic properties were then evaluated as a function of shear rate. One cream with an apparent viscosity of 280 poises at a shear rate of 10 sec^{-1} and of 1.8 poises at 10,000 sec^{-1} had a panel preference score for extrusion of 3.4 separately for both extrusion and ease of application. (A score of 3 was defined as agreeable.) From the study of scores as a function of the logarithm of viscosity, these values of 3.4 should have corresponded to 350 and 1.8 poises respectively, an excellent confirmation of the suitability of the screening evaluation. Similar procedures can be used to evaluate any potential product dispenser or use condition with any desired segments of the user population.

In practical use, shear rate is determined entirely by setting the desired rate of motion through a filler or orifice, application mode, and so forth without regard to the force (stress) required to achieve that process. Shear stress is the force required for the process to occur. If it involves a human interaction, then there is a perception of whether that force is less than desired, optimal, or excessive. Viscosity, or apparent viscosity for a non-Newtonian oil, is then that proportionality constant relating it, which was shown by equation (1). A perceived suitable viscosity is therefore a judgment on the stress required to achieve the needed shear rate.

Alternately, visual perception of a suitable viscosity for a cream to hold its shape in a jar, a lotion to pour, or a toothpaste to maintain its ribbon shape on a brush is an identical process. Here, the shear rate is determined by the subjective evaluation of an acceptable rate of deformation or flow under the constant stress of gravity.

The rheologic measurement must permit a clear assessment of the characteristic desired. Thus, the rheogram for a toothpaste needs to have a shear rate comparable to that for container delivery in order to assess practicality of extrusion. It also must have sufficient viscosity recovery from low shear rates to maintain its ribbon shape on the brush after suitable initial flow into the bristles for stability in handling, and it must thin readily with shear for ease in brushing. This type of history need emphasizes why statements defining a suitable viscosity for a product are meaningless unless they are framed within a specific judgment of use. The wide texture range of commercial products, presently acceptable as judged by commercial sales, clearly establishes that distinct segments of the population perceive different virtues.

A classic example in pharmaceutical rheology of the need for both structural breakdown under flow and recovery of body (viscosity) is the study of depot procaine penicillin G products by Ober and associates.[16] These workers set the two parameters for the evaluation or comparison of products as the ease of extrusion from a hyperdermic syringe with needle attached, and the degree to which the extrudate would retain itself in a compact volume. An arbitrary force from a 5-g weight on one pan of a two-pan balance was used to press a pad against the tip of the hypodermic needle. If this force was sufficient to plug the needle for a fixed air pressure of 200 psi on the syringe barrel, the formulation was judged too thick. This was found to correlate with the yield value found by rheologic measurements. Unfortunately, their values were reported in torque units of dyne centimeters, which require the instrumental parameters to develop shear stress, which was given by equation (11). The suitability of the depot geometry was judged by the relative shape of the product when injected into a gelatin gel, used as a substitute for muscle. The symmetry of the depot was related to the degree of thixotropic recovery of the mass. Using these criteria, these workers then determined how such formulation factors as the particle size and size distribution affected the resulting product.

Regained structure due to recovery of cross-linking attributes of the system cannot be presumed. In any system in which the degree of breakdown is time-dependent, as it is in virtually all thixotropic systems, the recovery of structure is also time-dependent. Recovery of structure does appear to occur much more slowly than the original structural buildup with aging. Rheologic measurements can be influenced by prior shear treatment if the test material shows any thixotropy. Therefore, no shear that is comparable to the range of shear rate intended to be measured can be given to the sample in removing it from its container and loading it into the measuring instrument; otherwise, the observations depend on the loading procedure used.

An extreme of the treatment breakdown of structure was used to evaluate the effective shear rate imparted by a filling machine.[7] A cosmetic lotion subject to thixotropic breakdown was put through a filler at two different delivery rates. At the same time, bulk sample was sheared through an extrusion rheometer at eight different shear rates. The shear rate used in each case was calculated from the delivery rate resulting from preset extrusion pressures; this calculation was given by equation (6). These sheared samples, pseudo-filled, were stored along with the product from the commercial filler and with an unfilled sample until thixotropic recovery had occurred. After 7 days, low shear rate rheograms were obtained. In Figure 6-21, the apparent viscosity for each sample is shown plotted for four arbitrary values of the low shear rate evaluation: 0.5, 1.0, 2.5, and 10 sec^{-1}. For each of these shear rates, a smooth curve was plotted through the observations for the unfilled and eight pseudo-filled samples for the logarithm of apparent viscosity as a function of pseudo-filling shear rate. The observations of viscosity of the values from the real filler were then placed on the smooth curve as shown in the figure. In this way, it was concluded that the two operating conditions produced shear rates of approximately 10,000 and 25,000 sec^{-1}. It should be recognized that the shear rate of a filler is set by the internal action of its operation, including the piston size and stroke or alternate mode of fluid propulsion, the diameter of intake and output tubes, and not just the fill volume

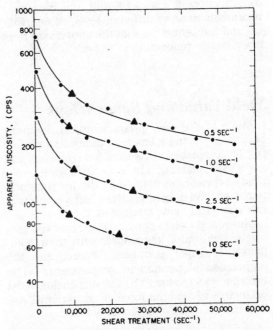

FIG. 6-21. *Low shear rate apparent viscosities measured 7 days after treatment of a thixotropic lotion. The lotion was pseudofilled at eight apparent shear rates 2 days after manufacture (solid dots) or put through two commercial fillers (solid triangles). The triangles are placed on the smoothed pseudofilled line to determine the apparent filler shear rate, approximately 10,000 sec^{-1} and 25,000 sec^{-1}. (From Wood, J. H., Catacalos, G., and Lieberman, S. V.: J. Pharm. Sci., 52:375, 1963. Reproduced with permission of the copyright owner, the American Pharmaceutical Association.)*

delivered over an allotted time. In this manner, it is possible to evaluate the shear rate from any production operation after sampling the mixing tank.

It is vitally important in any product development that all trial formulations be tested against assumed stresses and shear rates of manufacturing, product movement, filling, and use. These values must be calibrated in the manner described, preferably with products characteristically used and under the normal range of operating parameters of that facility. Excessive shear after some storage is more deleterious to product body than the same shear before aging. Thus, a product commercially filled after holding over a long weekend rarely resembles rheologically the product filled soon after manufacture. Depending on the nature of the formulation, these differences may be subtle or dramatic, even to the point of liquifying a paste by excessively shearing it after aging.

Often, the "art" of the formulation is being able to build into a product the ability to be mixed and handled in a different way from the laboratory samples. Obviously, this ability is the consequence of compensating for the shear treatments used by different levels of emulsifiers and thickeners, so that the conversion from laboratory to production is smooth.

Yield Value and Suspensions

Much of the early pharmaceutical literature bears a confusing mixture of publications relating to acceptable viscosities for emulsion and suspension stability. The viscosities were measured at shear rates defined by the instrumentation used, and only rarely were extrapolations to any true yield value attempted.

Meyer and Cohen demonstrated how the rheologic yield value obtainable with their company's Carbopol permitted theoretically the preparation of permanent suspensions.[17] The theoretic yield value (YV) for suspension must balance or exceed the force of gravitational settlement. Hence, for spherical objects:

$$YV = \frac{gV(\rho_p - \rho_m)}{A} \quad (22)$$

where g is the acceleration due to gravity, V is the particle volume, ρ_p is the particle density, ρ_m is the suspending medium density, and A is the cross-sectional area of the particle (πR^2 for round particles of radius R).

Example 15. What yield value is required to

suspend a golf ball of radius 2.13 cm and density 1.11 in a medium of density 1.00?

$$YV = \frac{gV(\rho_p - \rho_m)}{A}$$

$$= \frac{(980)(cm\ sec^{-2})(\frac{4}{3}\pi(2.13)^3\ cm^3)}{\pi(2.13)^2\ cm^2}$$

$$\times\ (7.11 - 1.00\ g\ cm^{-3})$$

$$= 310\ dynes\ cm^{-2}$$

In a similar fashion, Meyer and Cohen found theoretic yield values of 65 and 1620 dyne cm^{-2} to suspend sand of density 2.60 and radius 0.030 cm and marbles of density 2.55 and radius 0.8 cm respectively.[17] It was found that sand suspension for several years was possible in this manner when they used Carbopol 934 for the suspending agent. The required concentrations for sand, golf balls, and marbles, are 0.18%, 0.20%, and 0.40% of this agent.

Chong extended this concept by presenting a graphic nomogram.[18] (See Fig. 6-22 for the nec-

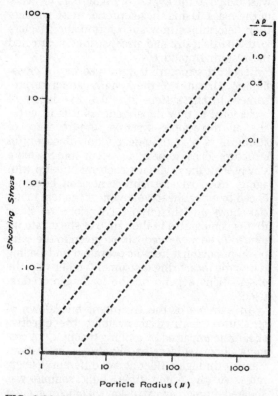

FIG. 6-22. *Necessary shearing stress to be balanced by yield value for various density differences between particle and medium as a function of particle radius. (From Chong, C. W.: J. Soc. Cosm. Chem. 14:123, 1963. Reproduced by permission of the copyright owner.)*

essary yield value to suspend particles of varying density and radius.) This graph relates to the difference in density between particle and medium and is equally valid for particles lighter than the medium, particularly in considering the aeration of a product that has yield value characteristics.

Any attempt to use this yield value approach obviously requires that real yield values exist at low shear rates as discussed earlier. If the very low shear rate measurements break from the Power Law toward Newtonian behavior, no permanent formulation can result. Unfortunately, no published literature other than the sand study with Carbopol 934 appears to exist relating to stability with aging for this yield value concept.

Artifactual Observations Due to Plug Flow or Slippage Planes

Breakdown of structure under shear may be general, or may occur locally, creating planes of slippage. Frequently, a body of material may remain motionless against the motionless wall of a viscosity measuring device, while the rest of the material moves as a unit down a tube or with a rotating bob. This behavior is characteristic of *plug flow*. Such behavior negates meaningful rheologic measurements, except that the stress at which structural rupture occurs may be characterized for that material. Typical rheograms resulting in this behavior are shown in Figure 6-23. The Haake Rotovisko has special star-shaped bobs and ribbed bobs available to minimize this effect. It is practical to machine grooves into regular viscometer bobs.[19] These

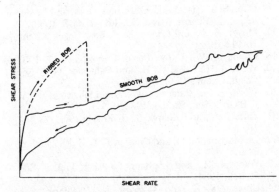

FIG. 6-23. *Rheogram for a dentrifice obtained with a Hercules Hi-Shear rheometer with smooth and ribbed bobs. (From Wood, J. H., Giles, W. H., and Catacalos, G.: J. Soc. Cosm. Chem., 15:565, 1964. Reproduced by permission of the copyright owner.)*

grooves tend to minimize the squeezing out of fluid by syneresis and thus do appreciably raise the shear rate range attainable before plug flow is initiated. This ribbing technique may also be applied in the cone-plate configuration.

Many workers have mistakenly interpreted the point at which plug flow begins as the yield value. Obviously, it represents a significant characterizing parameter, but the shear at which plug flow begins does appear to depend on geometry rather than being an intrinsic term.

In the case of the procaine penicillin study discussed in a previous section,[16] this plug parameter is probably critical to the syringe delivery. Indeed, the study evaluated this material fracture point rather than a true rheologic yield value.

This loss of cross-linked structure is clearly evident in many low shear rate measurements in solutions of suspending agents, whether montmorillonite clays or xanthan gums.[20,21] Sometimes, structure may be broken merely by pouring rapidly from a storage container into the rheometer. If the structure is retained in the viscometer, initial torque readings can be quite high before cross-linking structure is lost, which results in reduced torques as the shear rate increases. Similar loss in structure is possible when suspending agents exhibit a loss in suspending power after shaking.

Measurements of Stickiness or Tackiness

Two types of any tendency to self-adhesion have practical pharmaceutical application. The first is in dermal application, where any sticking of fingers together to a hand or any two skin surfaces can be quite objectionable. The application of rheologic principles to this problem was made by De Martine and Cussler.[22] They found a clear relationship between perceived stickiness and a complex computable function dependent on definable parameters.

An alternative approach, the force to pull two surfaces apart, has been used for measuring stickiness as dermal preparations evaporate.[23] Recently, this type of measure has been developed in detail to evaluate tackiness of coating solutions for tablets as a function of coating composition.[24,25] Using an Instron Tester, the full time-course of the adhesive force was followed during extension between the adhesive surfaces. It is of interest to note that tack appeared to parallel orientation effects attributable to elastic parameters of the coating agent.

Rheologic Use of Mixing Equipment

A major engineering use of rheologic measurements are power requirements in mixers and blenders. In the past, laboratory-sized equipment has been instrumented with strain gauges to permit torque measurements to be continuously monitored. This technology is now becoming available in manufacturing equipment.

An interesting example of such a research study was the use of a Brabender Plasti-Corder rotational torque mixer to follow the changes occurring during a wet granulation process.[26] Application of such studies permits stopping further mixing of a granulation at a specific desired point in the granule agglomeration. This can be particularly important when further mixing may create an intractable solid mass or an undesirable fluidizing. Because of the proprietary nature of such studies these are not likely to attain high visibility in the literature.

Tabletting and Compression Granulation

Although the nature of anisotropic forces during compression and the resultant difference in force vertically and laterally have been studied in theoretic tabletting, the rheologic implications have generally not been recognized. Thus, dwell time differences during compression, whether slugging or roller compression, can create flow structure differences in granulations. The full viscoelastic implications of the compression loading and unloading have recently been developed by Rippie and associates.[27,28] In particular, they have demonstrated how the fundamental parameters clearly depend on the composition of the tablet.[28]

Instrumented production tablet presses are now available and widely used in the industry for the study of optimum processing conditions. Unfortunately, few of these studies have been released for publication, so that we must rely on such studies as those described in this chapter to realize the potential of such tablet investigations. In particular, the development of formulations to minimize the delay in strain release that contributes to capping is an area in which trade secrets prevent free publication.

Summary

In stability measurements, rheologic parameters can provide a method of documenting the time-dependent changes.

Equipment suitable for most practical pharmaceutical and cosmetic rheology is commercially available from a variety of sources.

Rheologic measurements can provide criteria of product acceptability because they can be correlated to relevant "in use" factors of shear.

Recent developments in viscoelastic rheologic methodology are now moving from the academic to the industrial applications in pharmaceutical technology. These will lead to further applications in product monitoring and evaluation.

References

1. Green, H., and Weltmann, R. N.: Thixotropy. In Colloid Chemistry. Vol. VI. Edited by J. Alexander. Reinhold, New York, 1946, p. 328.
2. Weltmann, R. N.: J. Soc. Cos. Chem., 7:599, 1956.
3. Casson, N.: A flow equation for pigment-oil suspensions of the printing ink type. In Rheology in Disperse Systems. Edited by C. C. Mill. Pergamon Press, London, 1959, p. 84.
4. Fitch, E. B.: Ind. Eng. Chem., 51:889, 1959.
5. Catacalos, G., and Wood, J. H.: J. Pharm. Sci., 53:1089, 1964.
6. Wood, J. H., and Catacalos, G.: J. Soc. Cos. Chem., 14:147, 1963.
7. Wood, J. H., Catacalos, G., and Lieberman, S. V.: J. Pharm. Sci., 52:375, 1963.
8. Haighton, A. J.: J. Am. Oil Chem. Soc., 36:345, 1959.
9. Pendleton, W. W.: J. Appl. Phys., 14:170, 1943.
10. Barry, B. W.: Adv. Pharmaceut. Sci., 4:1, 1974.
11. Thurston, G. B., and Martin, A.: J. Pharm. Sci., 67:1499, 1978.
12. Radebaugh, G. W., and Simonelli, A. P.: J. Pharm. Sci., 72:415, 1983.
13. Radebaugh, G. W., and Simonelli, A. P.: J. Pharm. Sci., 73:590, 1984.
14. Hendersen, N. L., Meer, P. M., and Kostenbauder, H. B.: J. Pharm. Sci., 50:788, 1961.
15. Langenbucher, F., and Lange, B.: Pharm. Acta. Helv., 45:572, 1969.
16. Ober, S. S., Viscent, H. C., Simon, D. E., and Frederick, K. J.: Pharm. Assoc. Sci. Ed., 47:667, 1958.
17. Meyer, R. J., and Cohen, L.: J. Soc. Cosm. Chem., 10:143, 1959.
18. Chong, C. W.: J. Soc. Cosm. Chem., 14:123, 1963.
19. Wood, J. H., Giles, W. H., and Catacalos, G.: J. Soc. Cosm. Chem., 15:565, 1964.
20. Wood, J. H., Catacalos, G., and Lieberman, S. V.: J. Pharm. Sci., 52:354, 1963.
21. Zatz, J. L., and Knapp, S.: J. Pharm. Sci., 73:468, 1984.
22. De Martine, M. L., and Cussler, E. L.: J. Pharm. Sci., 64:976, 1975.
23. Wood, J. H., and Lapham, E. A.: J. Pharm. Sci., 53:835, 1964.
24. Chopra, S. K., and Tawashi, R.: J. Pharm. Sci., 71:907, 1982.
25. Chopra, S. K., and Tawashi, R.: J. Pharm. Sci., 73:477, 1984.
26. Schildcrout, S. A.: J. Pharm. Pharmacol., 36:502, 1984.

27. Rippie, E. G., and Danielson, D. W.: J. Pharm. Sci., 70:476, 1981.
28. Danielson, D. W., Morehead, W. T., and Rippie, E. G.: J. Pharm. Sci., 72:342, 1983.

General References

Dinsdale, A., and Moore, F.: Viscosity and Its Measurements. Chapman and Hall, London, 1962.

Gabelnick, H. L., and Lett, M.: Rheology of Biological Systems. Charles C Thomas, Springfield, IL, 1973.

Honwink, R.: Elasticity, Plasticity and Structure of Matter. 3rd Ed. Cambridge University Press, New York, 1971.

Reiner, M.: Selected Papers on Rheology. Elsevier, New York, 1975.

Severs, E. T.: Rheology of Polymers. Reinhold, New York, 1962.

Sherman, P.: Rheology of Emulsions. Macmillan, New York, 1963.

Stephan, K., and Lucas, K.: Viscosity of Dense Fluids. Plenum Press, New York, 1979.

Stokes, R. H.: Viscosity of Electrolytes and Related Properties. Pergamon Press, Elmsford, NY, 1965.

Van Wazer, J. R., Lyons, J. W., Kim, K. Y., and Colwell, R. E.: Viscosity and Flow Measurement. Interscience, New York, 1963.

Vinogradov, C. V.: Rheology of Polymers: Viscoelasticity and Flow of Polymers. Springer-Verlag, New York, 1980.

Walters, K.: Rheometry. Chapman and Hall, London, 1975.

Wilkinson, W. L.: Non-Newtonian Fluids, Fluid Mechanics, and Heat Transfer. Pergamon Press, Elmsford, NY, 1960.

7

Clarification and Filtration

S. CHRAI

The preparation of pharmaceutical dosage forms frequently requires the separation of particles from a fluid. The usual objective is a sparkling liquid that is free of amorphous or crystalline precipitates, colloidal hazes, or insoluble liquid drops. Sterility specifications may expand the objective to include removal of microorganisms.

Filtration is defined as the process in which particles are separated from a liquid by passing the liquid through a permeable material. The porous filter medium is the permeable material that separates particles from the liquid passing through it and is known as a *filter*. Thus, filtration is a unit operation in which a mixture of solids and liquid, the *feed, suspension, dispersion, influent* or *slurry,* is forced through a porous medium, in which the solids are deposited or entrapped. The solids retained on a filter are known as the *residue.* The solids form a *cake* on the surface of the medium, and the clarified liquid known as *effluent* or *filtrate* is discharged from the filter. If recovery of solids is desired, the process is called *cake filtration.* The term *clarification* is applied when the solids do not exceed 1.0% and filtrate is the primary product. *Ultrafiltration* may be defined as the separation of intermicellar liquid from solids by the use of pressure on a semipermeable membrane.

Filtration is frequently the method of choice for sterilization of solutions that are chemically or physically unstable under heating conditions. In many applications, *sterile filtration* is an ideal technique. Sterile filtration of liquids and gases is commonly used in the pharmaceutical industry. Final product solutions or vehicles for suspensions are sterile-filtered prior to an aseptic filling process. Sterile filtration of bulk drug solution prior to an aseptic crystallization process eliminates the possibility of organisms being occluded within crystals.

Much of the material in this chapter is based on Chapter 18 of the previous edition, which was written by Richard A. Hill, Ph.D.

The broad span of pharmaceutical requirements cannot be met by a single type of filter. The industrial pharmacist must achieve a balance between filter media and equipment capabilities, slurry characteristics, and quality specifications for the final product. The choice is usually a batch pressure filter, which uses either surface or depth principles.

Surface filtration is a screening action by which pores or holes in the medium prevent the passage of solids. The *depth filter* permits slurry to penetrate to a point where the diameter of a solid particle is greater than the diameter of a tortuous void or channel. The solids are retained within a gradient density structure by physical restriction or by absorption properties of the medium.

Theory

Even today, filtration is more an art than a science. The filtration theory, with all its mathematical models, has a deficiency. The deficiency is its preoccupation with resistance to flow, almost to the exclusion of considerations of filtrate quality. It is possible to estimate the resistance to flow of a clean filter medium but impossible to estimate with comparable accuracy what the resistance will be as the filter begins to trap solids. The mathematical models do provide a means of showing apparent relationships between variables in a process and may be valuable decision-making tools in the selection of apparatus and techniques for a particular filtration application.[1]

The mathematical models for flow through a porous medium, cake filtration, and granular bed filtration may differ, but all follow this basic rule: The energy lost in filtration is proportional to the rate of flow per unit area.

The flow of liquid through a filter follows the basic rules that govern flow of any liquid through a medium offering resistance. The rate of flow may be expressed as:

$$\text{rate} = \frac{\text{driving force}}{\text{resistance}} \qquad (1)$$

The rate may be expressed as volume per unit time and the driving force as a pressure differential. The apparent complexity of the filtration equations arises from the expansion of the resistance term. Resistance is not constant since it increases as solids are deposited on the filter medium. An expression of this changing resistance involves a material balance as well as factors expressing permeability or coefficient of resistance of the continuously expanding cake.

The rate concept as expressed in modifications of Poiseuille's equation is prevalent in engineering literature:

$$\frac{dV}{dT} = \frac{AP}{\mu\,(\alpha W/A + R)} \qquad (2)$$

where:

V = volume of filtrate
T = time
A = filter area
P = total pressure drop through cake and filter medium
μ = filtrate viscosity
α = average specific cake resistance
W = weight of dry cake solids
R = resistance of filter medium and filter

Any convenient units may be used in this equation, since inconsistencies are absorbed in the cake and filter resistances.

The practical limitation of this equation is that the constants must be determined on the actual slurry being handled. There is no crossover application of data, and the majority of filters are selected on the basis of empiric laboratory or pilot plant tests. Equation (2) has been integrated under various assumptions, and these integrated forms may be used to predict effects of process changes and to evaluate test work. The techniques for data evaluation set forth in the section "Filter Selection" in this chapter may be confirmed by reference to broader theoretic discussions.[2–4]

Interpretation of the basic equation, however, leads to a general set of rules:

1. Pressure increases usually cause a proportionate increase in flow unless the cake is highly compressible. Pressure increases on highly compressible, flocculent, or slimy precipitates may decrease or terminate flow.

2. An increase in area increases flow and life proportional to the square of the area since cake thickness, and thus resistance, are also reduced.

3. The filtrate flow rate at any instant is inversely proportional to viscosity.

4. Cake resistance is a function of cake thickness; therefore, the average flow rate is inversely proportional to the amount of cake deposited.

5. Particle size of the cake solids affects flow through effect on the specific cake resistance, α. A decreased particle size results in higher values of α and proportionally lower filtration rates.

6. The filter medium resistance, R, usually negligible or about 0.1 α in cake filtration, is the primary resistance in clarification filtration. In the latter case, flow rate is inversely proportional to R.

It is convenient to summarize the theoretic relationship as:

Rate of filtration

$$= \frac{(\text{area of filter}) \times (\text{pressure difference})}{(\text{viscosity}) \times (\text{resistance of cake and filter})} \qquad (3)$$

Most clarification problems can be resolved empirically by varying one or more of these factors. A broader understanding of filtration theory is required only if cake filtration applications are under consideration.

The membrane filters are highly porous. A number of methods are used for establishing the pore size and pore size distribution. Most methods are derived from the interfacial tension phenomenon of liquids in contact with the filter structure. Each pore in the filter acts as a capillary. For a nonwetting fluid, the following equation was established by Poiseuille:[5]

$$p = \frac{-2\gamma \cos\,\theta}{r} \qquad (4)$$

where:

p = applied pressure
γ = liquid surface tension
θ = contact angle between liquid and solid
r = radius of the pore

Filter Media

The surface upon which solids are deposited in a filter is called the *filter medium*.[6,7] For the pharmacist selecting this important element, the wide range of available materials may be bewildering. The selection is frequently based on past experience, and reliance on technical services of commercial suppliers is often advisable.

A medium for cake filtration must retain the solids without plugging and without excessive bleeding of particles at the start of the filtration. In clarification applications, in which no appreciable cake is developed, the medium is the primary factor in achieving clarity, and the choice is limited to materials that will remove all particles above a desired size. Sterile filtration imposes a special requirement, since the pore size must not exceed the dimension of microorganisms unless the filter is adsorptive, and since the medium should be sterilizable.

Filter media are available in different materials and forms. The filter fabrics are commonly woven from natural fibers such as cotton and from synthetic fibers and glass. The properties of these fibers and glass applicable for media selection are tabulated in Table 7-1.

Filter cloth, a surface type medium, is woven from either natural or synthetic fiber or metal. Cotton fabric is most common and is widely used as a primary medium, as backing for paper or felts in plate and frame filters, and as fabricated bags for coarse straining. Nylon is often superior for pharmaceutical use, since it is unaffected by mold, fungus, or bacteria, provides an extremely smooth surface for good cake discharge, and has negligible absorption properties. Both cotton and nylon are suitable for coarse straining in aseptic filtrations, since they can be sterilized by autoclaving. Monofilament nylon cloth is extremely strong and is available for openings as small as 10 microns. Teflon is superior for most liquid filtration, as it is almost chemically inert, provides sufficient strength, and can withstand elevated temperatures.

Woven wire cloth, particularly stainless steel, is durable, resistant to plugging, and easily cleaned. Metallic filter media provide good surfaces for cake filtrations and usually are used with filter aids. As support elements for disposable media, wire screens are particularly suitable, since they may be cleaned rapidly and returned to service. Wire mesh filters also are installed in filling lines of packaging equipment. Their function at this point is not clarification, but security against the presence of large foreign particles.

Nonwoven filter media include felts, bonded fabrics, and kraft papers. A *felt* is a fibrous mass that is free from bonding agents and mechanically interlocked to yield specific pore diameters that have controlled particle retention. High flow rate with low pressure drop is a primary characteristic. Felts of natural or synthetic material function as depth media and are recommended where gelatinous solutions or fine particulate matter are involved. *Bonded fabrics* are made by binding textile fibers with resins, solvents, and plasticizers. These materials have not

TABLE 7-1. *Fiber Properties For Filter Media Selection*

Fiber	Temperature Recommended Safe Limit (°F)	Wet Breaking Tenacity (g/denier)		Acid Resistance	Alkali Resistance	Price Ratio to Cotton
Cotton	210	3.3	6.4	Poor	Fair	1
Polyester (Dacron)	300	6.0	8.2	Very good	Good	2.7
Dynel modacrylic	200	3.0		Excellent	Excellent	3.2
Glass (spun)	750	3.0	4.6	Excellent	Fair	6.0
Glass (continuous filament)	550	3.9	4.7	Excellent	Fair	2.2
Nylon	250	2.1	8.0	Fair	Excellent	2.5
Acrylic (Orlon)	300	1.8	2.1	Excellent	Fair	2.7
Polyethylene	165	1.0	3.0	Excellent	Excellent	2
Polypropylene	175	3.5	8.0	Excellent	Excellent	1.75
Saran	160	1.2	2.3	Excellent	Excellent	2.5
Teflon	475	1.9		Excellent	Excellent	25.0
Polyvinylchloride	165	1.0	3.0	Good	Excellent	2.7
Wool	210	0.76	1.6	Very good	Fair	3.7
Rayon and acetate	210	1.9	3.9	Poor	Fair	1

Excerpted by special permission from Chemical Engineering, 70:177, 1963. Copyright © 1963 by McGraw-Hill, Inc., New York, NY 10020.

found wide acceptance in dosage form production because of interactions with the additives. *Kraft* paper is a pharmaceutical standard. Although limited to use in plate and frame filters and horizontal-plate filters, it offers controlled porosity, limited absorption characteristic, and a low cost. The latter is important since concern over cross-contamination makes a disposable medium attractive to pharmacy. White papers are preferred, and they may be crinkled to produce greater filtration area. A support of cloth or wire mesh is necessary in large filter presses to prevent rupture of the paper with pressure.

Porous stainless steel filters are widely used for removal of small amounts of unwanted solids from liquids (clarification) such as milk, syrup, sulfuric acid, and hot caustic soda. Porous metallic filters can be easily cleaned and repeatedly sterilized.

Membrane filter media are the basic tools for microfiltration and ultrafiltration. They are used commonly in the preparation of sterile solutions. Membrane filters classified as surface or screen filters are made of various esters of cellulose or from nylon, Teflon, polyvinyl chloride, polyamide, polysulfone, or silver. The filter is a thin membrane, about 150 microns thick, with 400 to 500 million pores per square centimeter of filter surface. The pores are extremely uniform in size and occupy about 80% of filter volume. This high porosity permits flow rates at least 40 times faster than those obtained through other media of comparable particle retention capability.

Because of surface screening characteristics, prefiltration is often required to avoid rapid clogging of a membrane. The selection of a membrane filter for a particular application is a function of the size of the particle or particles to be removed. An approximate pore size reference guide can be set down as follows:

Pore Size (micron)	Particle Removed
0.2 (0.22)	All bacteria
0.45	All coliform group bacteria
0.8	All airborne particles
1.2	All nonliving particles considered dangerous in i.v. fluids
5	All significant cells from body fluids

The fragility of membrane filters is partially overcome by the use of monofilament nylon as a supporting web within the membrane structure.

The distinction between ultrafiltration and microfiltration lies in the nature of the filter medium. Ultrafiltration membranes contain pores of relatively narrow size distribution 10^{-3} to 10^{-2} microns (10 to 100 Å) and are formed by etching cylindric pores into a solid matrix. Ultrafiltration membranes are fragile and require supporting substrates because of the high-pressured differences required during filtration.

Most types of filter media are also available as *cartridge units*. These cartridges are economical and convenient when used to remove low percentages of solids ranging in particle size from 100 microns to less than 0.2 micron. The cartridge may be a surface or depth filter and consists of a porous medium integral with plastic or metal structural hardware. Synthetic and natural fibers, cellulose esters and fiberglass, fluorinated hydrocarbon polymers, nylon, and ceramics are employed for the manufacture of disposable cartridges. Porous materials for cleanable and reusable cartridges use stainless steel, Monel, ceramics, fluorinated hydrocarbon polymers, and exotic metals.

Surface-type cartridges of corrugated, resin-treated paper are common in hydraulic lines of processing equipment, but are rarely applied to finished products. Ceramic cartridges have the advantage of being cleanable for reuse by back-flushing, and porcelain filter candles are acceptable for some sterile filtrations along with membrane filters in cartridge form. Sintered metal or woven-wire elements are also useful, but fine-wire mesh lacks strength. The metallic-edge filters overcome this problem by allowing liquid to pass between rugged metal strips, which are separated by spacers of predetermined thickness. *Depth-type cartridges* consist of fibrous media, usually cotton, asbestos, or cellulose. The cartridge may be formed by felting or by resin-bonding fibers about a mandrel. Effective units are also manufactured by winding yarn around a central supporting screen. The depth cartridge is always a disposable item since cleaning is not feasible.

Filter Aids

Justification for use of filter aids may be found in equation (2), which shows the rate of filtration to be inversely proportional to the resistance of the solids cake. Therefore, the pressure drop across the system is directly proportional to the filtration rate, the thickness of the cake, and the liquid viscosity for flow through porous media, when laminar flow conditions exist in the filter media or cake. It is also inversely proportional to the density of the liquid and square of the particle diameter. Poorly flocculated solids offer higher resistance than do flocculated solids or solids providing high porosity to the cake. In the case of cake filtration, the rate varies with the square of the volume of liquid. When the volume of the filter cake solids per unit volume of filtrate is low, the solids formed on the filter medium may penetrate the voidspace, thus making the filter medium more resistant to flow. At a higher concentration of solids in a suspension, the bridging over of openings over the voidspace, rather than blinding of the openings, seems to predominate. Slimy or gelatinous materials, or highly compressible substances, form impermeable cakes with high resistance to liquid flow. The filter medium becomes plugged or slimy with accumulation of solids, and the flow of filtrate stops. A filter aid acts by reducing this resistance.[8,9]

Filter aids are a special type of filter medium. Ideally, the filter aid forms a fine surface deposit that screens out all solids, preventing them from contacting and plugging the supporting filter medium. Usually, the filter aid acts by forming a highly porous and noncompressible cake that retains solids, as does any depth filter. The duration of a filtration cycle and the clarity attained can be controlled as density, type, particle size, and quantity of the filter aid are varied. The quantity of the filter aid greatly influences the filtration rate. If too little filter aid is used, the resistance offered by the filter cake is greater than if no filter aid is used, because of added thickness to the cake. On the other hand, if high amounts of filter aid are added, the filter aid merely adds to the thickness of the cake without providing additional cake porosity. Figure 7-1 is a typical plot of filter aid concentration versus permeability. In the figure, flow rate and permeability are directly proportional to each other. At low concentrations of filter aid, the flow rate is slow because of low permeability. As the filter aid concentration increases, the flow rate increases and peaks off. Beyond this point, the flow rate decreases as the filter aid concentration is increased.

The ideal filter aid performs its functions physically or mechanically; no absorption or chemical action is involved in most cases. The important characteristics for filter aids are the following:[10]

1. It should have a structure that permits formation of pervious cake.

2. It should have a particle size distribution suitable for the retention of solids, as required.

3. It should be able to remain suspended in the liquid.

4. It should be free of impurities.

5. It should be inert to the liquid being filtered.

6. It should be free from moisture in cases where the addition of moisture to the fluid would be undesirable.

The particles must be inert, insoluble, incompressible, and irregularly shaped. Filter aids are classified from low flow rate (fine: mean size in the range of 3 to 6 microns) to fast flow rate (coarse: mean size in the range of 20 to 40 microns). Clarity of the filtrate is inversely proportional to the flow rate, and selection requires a balance between these factors. Filter aids are considered to be equivalent in performance when they produce the same flow rate and filtered solution clarity under the same operating conditions when filtering a standard sugar solution.[1] Table 7-2 lists the advantages and disadvantages of filter aid material.

Diatomite (diatomaceous earth) is the most important filter aid. Processed from fossilized diatoms, it has an irregularly shaped porous particle that forms a rigid incompressible cake. Since diatomite is primarily silica, it is relatively inert and insoluble. *Perlite*, an aluminum silicate, forms filter cakes that are 20 to 30% less dense than diatomic cakes. Perlite is not a porous incompressible particle, but it has an economic advantage over diatomite.

Cellulose, *asbestos*, and *carbon* filter aids are also commercially available. Cellulose is highly compressible and costs two to four times more than diatomite or perlite. It is reserved for applications where the liquids may be incompatible with silica compounds. Cellulose is used as a

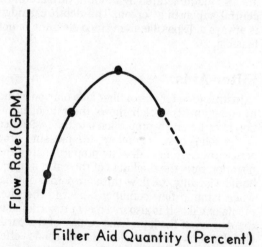

FIG. 7-1. *Experimental determination of flow rate as a function of filter aid quantity discloses correct operating level.*

TABLE 7-2. *The Advantages and Disadvantages of Filter Aid Materials*

Material	Chemical Composition	Advantages	Disadvantages
Diatomaceous earth	Silica	Wide size range available; fines reduced by calcination; can be used for very fine filtration.	Slightly soluble in dilute acids and alkalies.
Expanded perlite	Silica and aluminosilicates	Wide size range available; not capable of finest retention of diatomites.	More soluble than diatomites in acids and alkalies; may give highly compressible cakes.
Asbestos	Aluminosilicate	Usually used in conjunction with diatomites; very good retention on coarse screens.	Chemical properties similar to perlite.
Cellulose	Cellulose	Used mainly as a coarse precoat; high purity; excellent chemical resistance—slightly soluble in dilute and strong alkalies, none in dilute acids.	Expensive
Carbon	Carbon	May be used for filtering strong alkaline solutions	Available in coarser grades only; expensive

Reprinted from Akers, R., and Ward, A.: Liquid filtration theory and filtration treatment. *In* Filtration Principles and Practices, Part I. Edited by C. Orr. Marcel Dekker, Inc., New York, 1977, p. 237, by courtesy of Marcel Dekker, Inc.

coarse precoat. It is available in high-purity material and has excellent chemical resistance. Asbestos has good retention on coarse screens, but has limited application because of high cost, and because of concern over its toxicity should the fibers carry over into the filtrate. Asbestos filters may be used in pharmaceutical industry if their application is followed by a membrane filter. Nonactivated carbons that are not suitable for decolorization or absorption are rarely used in pharmaceutical applications because of cleanliness problems. They may be used for filtering strong alkaline solutions. Commercial blends of various filter aids are common, and these specialities, particularly those intended as water scavengers in oil filtrations, must be considered in selection of a filter aid.

Filter aids may be applied by *precoating* or *body-mix* techniques.[8,9] Precoating requires suspending the filter aid in a liquid and recirculating the slurry until the filter aid is uniformly deposited on the filter septum. The quantity varies from 5 to 15 pounds per 100 square feet of filter area, or that sufficient to deposit a cake $\frac{1}{16}$ to $\frac{1}{8}$ inches thick. The liquid is preferably a portion of the feed or retained filtrate from a prior cycle, since the physical properties of the precoat liquid must approximate those of the material to be filtered. Precoating should proceed at the same flow rates and pressures to be used in final filtration, and the transition from precoat liquid to regular feed must be rapid to

prevent disruption of the cake. Body mix (direct addition of filter aid to the filter feed) is more common in batch pharmaceutical operations. The filter aid, 1 to 2 pounds per pound of contaminant, or 0.1 to 0.5% of total batch weight, is mixed into the feed tank. This slurry is recirculated through the filter until a clear filtrate is obtained; filtration then proceeds to completion. The body-mix method minimizes equipment requirements and cross-contamination potentials.

Often, a filter aid may be used that performs its function not physically or mechanically, but chemically, by reacting with the solids. These chemicals may cause the solids depositing in a filter bed to adhere more strongly to the filter medium. Water-soluble polymers such as flocculating agents are often used as filter aids. The polymers may be derived from vegetable or animal sources, or they may be produced synthetically. Compounds produced by modification of the chemical structure, such as starch, may be filter aids to more costly synthetic materials. Water-soluble polymers may be classified as nonionic, anionic, or cationic, depending on their property to ionize in water. There are a few commercially available water-soluble cationic polymers. These include acrylamide copolymers, polyethyleneimine, and derivatives of casein, starch, and guar gum.[1]

Filter aids are chosen by trial and error in either laboratory or plant. Within ranges previously indicated, the filter aid is usually selected to give acceptable filtrate at the highest flow rate; however, in pharmaceutical operations in which quality is a primary consideration, the selection usually favors the fine grades, which yield low flow rates. The most important pharmaceutical factor is inertness. A filter aid may have such extensive absorption properties that desired colored substances and active principles are frequently removed. The total quantity of any ingredient absorbed may be small, but it may be a considerable portion of the original concentration.

Filtration efficiency also may be affected by changes in temperature, since there is an inverse relationship of flow rate to viscosity. The viscosities of most liquids decrease with increase in temperature. According to the "hole theory," there are vacancies in a liquid, and there is a continuous movement of the molecules into these vacancies, thus causing vacancies to move around. This movement of vacancies permits flow, but requires energy. This energy is the activation energy with which a molecule has to move into a vacancy. The activation energy is more readily available at higher temperatures than at lower temperatures. Thus, the liquid can flow more easily at higher temperatures than at lower temperatures.[11] Table 7-3 lists the viscosities of some common liquids at different temperatures. Equation (5) represents the relationship of the coefficient of viscosity to temperature.

$$\eta = Ae^{E/RT} \tag{5}$$

where:

η = coefficient of viscosity of the liquid
E = activation energy
R = ideal gas constant
T = absolute temperature
A = pre-exponential factor

According to the "hole theory," the viscosity of

a liquid increases as the pressure is increased. Since the number of holes is reduced, it is more difficult for molecules to move around. Increasing the temperature of heavy pharmaceutical syrups lowers the viscosity and increases filtration rates. Most liquids must be maintained at a high temperature during filtration to prevent the formation of crystals. The filtration of cosmetic products at low temperatures, approximately 5°C, is also common. The consequent reduction in flow rate is tolerated, since the goal is reduced solubility of contaminants or perfume oils, resulting in their more effective removal. Filtration at room temperature would yield a liquid that might cloud at the lower temperatures encountered by the product under field conditions.

Filter Selection

In designing or selecting a system for filtration, the specific requirements of the filtration problem must be defined. The following questions should be answered before any assistance is requested from the manufacturers of filtration equipment.[12,13]

1. What is to be filtered—liquid or gas?
2. What liquid or gas is to be filtered?
3. What is the pore size required to remove the smallest particle?
4. What is the desired flow rate?
5. What will the operating pressure be?
6. What are the inlet and outlet plumbing connections?
7. What is the operating temperature?
8. Can the liquid to be filtered withstand the special temperature required?
9. What is the intended process—clarification or filtration?
10. Will the process be a sterilizing filtration?
11. Will the process be a continuous or batch filtration?
12. What is the volume to be filtered?
13. What time constraints will be imposed, if any?

Once the purpose of the process has been determined, the selection of the filter medium can be made. For example, for a sterilizing filtration, a 0.2-micron pore size is used; for clarification, a plate and frame filter or woven-fiber filter may be used. In general, a pore size smaller than the

TABLE 7-3. *Viscosity of Liquids in Centipoise*

Liquid	Temperature (°C)			
	0	25	50	75
Water	1.793	0.895	0.549	0.380
Ethanol	1.79	1.09	0.698	—
Benzene	0.9	0.61	0.44	—

From Daniels, F., and Alberty, R. A.: Irreversible processes in solution. *In* Physical Chemistry. 3rd Ed. Edited by F. Daniels and R.A. Alberty. John Wiley and Sons, New York, 1966.

smallest particle to be removed is selected. The filter medium should be compatible with the liquid or gas to be filtered. It is advisable to check the chemical compatibility charts provided by the vendors for selection of filter type. Filter type, cellulose, polytetrafluoroethylene (PTFE), fiber, metal, polyvinylidene difluoride, nylon, or polysulfones may be selected based on the chemical resistance to the most aggressive ingredient in the liquid. For vent filters or gaseous filtration, a hydrophobic filter medium should be chosen.

Filtration surface area is calculated after the filter media, pore size, required flow rate, and pressure differentials are established. For a liquid having a viscosity significantly different from that of water (1 cp), the clean water flow rate is divided by the viscosity of the liquid in centipoises to obtain the approximate initial flow rate for the liquid in question. For gaseous filtration at elevated temperature and exit pressures, the standard flow rate (20°C, 1 atmosphere) must be corrected by equation (6), the *gaseous filtration flow rate formula:*

$$F = F_0 \left(\frac{293}{273 + t} \right) \left(\frac{P + \Delta P/2}{14.7 + \Delta P/2} \right) \quad (6)$$

where:

F = corrected flow rate
F_0 = standard flow rate from chart (20°C, 1 atmosphere)
t = temperature of air or gas (°C)
P = exit pressure (psia)
ΔP = pressure drop through the system (psi)

If the pressures are expressed in kg/cm², the term 14.7 in equation (6) becomes 1.03.

The optimum system often requires use of a series of filters in a single multilayered filter containing layers of various pore sizes or a prefilter followed by a final filter. Optimum performance is obtained when the filters in a series exhaust their dirt-holding capacities at the same time. When the flow resistance across each filter in the series approaches the limiting pressure drop, the dirt-holding capacity of the system is considered expended. Figures 7-2 through 7-5 illustrate the prefilters with adequate and inadequate dirt holding capacity. In Figure 7-3, the coarse prefilter does not provide sufficient retention efficiency, thus causing the poorly protected final filter to clog prematurely. Too fine a filter, on the other hand, has enough retention efficiency but insufficient dirt-holding capacity, and it plugs very quickly, as illustrated in Figure 7-4. As shown in Figure 7-5, both filters—the

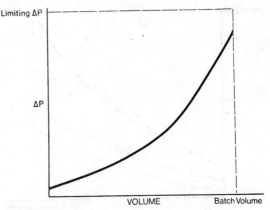

FIG. 7-2. *Ideal filtration system. (From Cole, J. C., and Shumsky, R.: Pharm. Tech., 1:39, 1977.)*

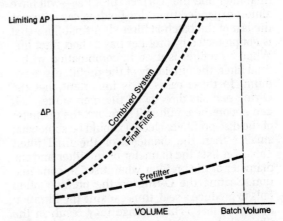

FIG. 7-3. *Filtration system with inadequate prefilter— too coarse. (From Cole, J. C., and Shumsky, R.: Pharm. Tech., 1:39, 1977.)*

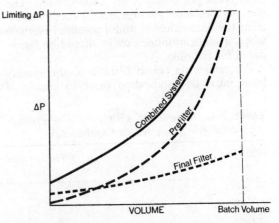

FIG. 7-4. *Filtration system with adequate retentive prefilter but inadequate dirt-holding capacity. (From Cole, J. C., and Shumsky, R.: Pharm. Tech., 1:39, 1977.)*

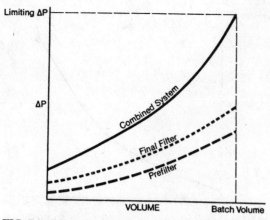

FIG. 7-5. *Filtration system with adequate prefilter. (From Cole, J. C., and Shumsky, R.: Pharm. Tech., 1:39, 1977.)*

final filter and the "correct" prefilter—will have almost expended their dirt-holding capacities as the last of the batch is filtered. A final filter that is not protected by prefilter has a short filter life. When a prefilter is used in combination with a final filter, the efficiency of the prefilter is maximum. In these cases, it is important that the O-ring seal sits directly on the membrane itself and not on the prefilter. Therefore, the diameter of the disc prefilter selected should be somewhat smaller than the diameter of the final filter. Table 7-4 lists the diameter of the filter and the diameter of the prefilter when used in combination. Seating the O-ring on the prefilter often fails to produce a seal, thus causing the filtration system to leak. This leakage may result in the filtrate being exposed to contamination.

Nonsterile Operations

Although filtration analysis can be sophisticated, pilot plant studies are usually basic. The common problems are to select the media, determine the time required, and if possible, estimate when a semicontinuous cycle should be terminated for cleaning.

For nonsterile polish filtrations, the quality level must be established prior to choice of

TABLE 7-4. *Diameter of Filter and Corresponding Prefilter When Used in Combination*

Filter Size (mm)	Prefilter Size (mm)
25	22
47	35
90	75
142	124
293	257

media. Particulate matter above 30- to 40-micron particles may be noticeable. Most pharmaceutical filtrations therefore aim for removal of particles of 3 to 5 microns or less. A nephelometer, an instrument that measures the degree of light scattering (Tyndall effect) in dilute suspensions, is an excellent tool for assessing effectiveness in this range.

The nephelometer gives a quantitative value to the formulator's quality specification of "sparkling clear." This value may be used to compare results using different filtration media. Figure 7-6 shows a typical curve obtained from filtration of an elixir through disposable cartridges and standard kraft paper. If an existing process is to be shifted from paper on a filter press to cartridges, this curve permits selection of an element that gives comparable performance. The technique also may be applied to assessment of filter aid effectiveness by determining transmittance as a function of filter-aid type, quantity, or method of use.

In addition to improving clarity, filter aids are used to increase flow rates. Figure 7-1 indicates a typical flow rate pattern as the amount of filter aid is increased. Exceeding an optimum quantity can frequently lead to decreased flow rate without improving clarity. The filter aid quantity can be expressed as a percentage of cake solids, a percentage of filter aid in body mix, or the weight applied as a precoat per unit of filter area.

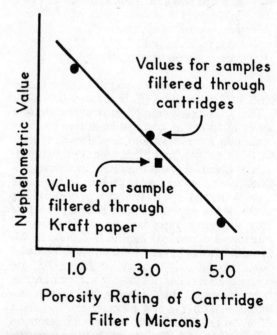

FIG. 7-6. *A nephelometer reading of a filtrate provides data that may be used to compare performance of different media.*

Flow rate should be determined for each case at constant pressure and after a uniform time interval. The maximum filter aid level used in laboratory tests must be within the cake capacity of projected or existing plant equipment.

The question of time for a filtration cycle is resolved by determining total volume versus time during a test run at pressures approximating normal operating conditions. Flow rate decreases with time as the media plugs or as the cake builds up. Plotting log total volume per unit area versus log time usually gives a straight line suitable for limited extrapolation (Fig. 7-7). If the filter area of production equipment is fixed, the time to filter a given batch size may be estimated. Alternately, the filter area required to complete the process within an allotted time period may be established. Similar flow decay studies can also be performed during sizing of a filtration system for sterile operations.

In semicontinuous operations, decisions must be made on length of the cycle prior to shutdown for replacement of media. If the goal is maximum output from the filter per unit of overall time, the graphic approach of Figure 7-8 is applicable. During productive time T, the filter discharges a clear filtrate at a steadily decreasing rate. Nonproductive time T′ is required to clean the filter and replace media. For graphic analysis, nonproductive time T′ is plotted to the left of the origin of a volume V versus time curve. When a line is drawn from T′ tangent to the curve, the value of V and T at the point of tangency indicates where the filtration should be

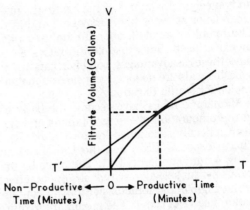

FIG. 7-8. *The optimal filtration cycle prior to cleaning can be determined by a graphic technique.*

stopped. The time lost in cleaning is offset by a return to high filtration rates associated with the new media. This point also can be calculated from theoretic relationships for constant pressure or constant volume filtration.[14] Data from laboratory equipment can be applied to production units since the analysis is independent of filter area.

The evaluation of coarse straining operations is limited to sizing a filter that will not have excessive pressure drop. The amount of impurity is usually small, and continued operation does not significantly decrease filter capacity. The metal cartridge filters, either woven-mesh or edge-type, and porous sintered stainless steel, have replaced cheesecloth in most pharmaceutical applications. Straining suspensions containing gums or other viscous ingredients can be accomplished with self-cleaning edge filters. These suspensions frequently bridge the media, and cleaning devices are needed to maintain adequate flow.

Sterile Operations

Filtration may be used to clarify and sterilize pharmaceutical solutions that are heat-labile. Until the introduction of membrane media, unglazed porcelain candles and the asbestos pad were the accepted standards. The candle requires extensive cleaning and is a fragile medium. High flow rates are attained only through use of multiple-element manifolds. The asbestos pad has significant absorption and adsorption properties, and chemical prewash and pH adjustment are required to prevent interaction with products. Failure to achieve sterility may occur with asbestos pads owing to blow-through and channeling of medium of organisms when critical pressures are exceeded. Both asbestos

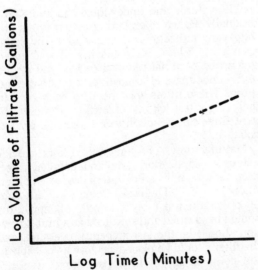

FIG. 7-7. *Extrapolation of filtrate volume produced in a given time can be made from log-log plots of experimental data.*

and porcelain are migratory media; fragments of a candle or asbestos fibers may be found in the filtrate unless serial filtration through secondary media is used. Since membrane filters do not have these disadvantages, porcelain candles and asbestos pads are no longer considered media of choice for sterile filtration.

Membrane filters have become the basic tool in the preparation of sterile solutions and have been officially sanctioned by the United States Pharmacopoeia (USP) and the U.S. Food and Drug Administration (FDA). The available materials permit selection so that absorption effects are negligible and ionic or particulate contamination need not occur. The membrane requires no pretreatment and may be autoclaved or gas-sterilized after assembly in its holder.

A sterility requirement imposes a severe restraint on filter selection. All sterility tests are presumptive, and one must rely upon total confidence in the basic process; economics becomes a secondary factor. Membranes with porosity ratings of 0.2 or 0.45 microns are usually specified for sterile filtrations. In this porosity range, membrane filters may clog rapidly, and a prefilter is used to remove some colloidal matter to extend the filtration cycle. The FDA allows the use of 0.45-micron filters only in cases of colloidal solutions in which 0.2-micron filters have been shown to clog very rapidly.

Most pharmaceutical liquids are compatible with one or more of the membrane filters now available. High viscosity or abnormal contaminant levels are the primary restraints to the use of membranes, since an extremely large filtration area is needed for practical flow rates. Oil and viscous aqueous menstruums are therefore heat-sterilized whenever possible. These solutions are usually clarified through coarser, nonsterilizing membranes, preferably prior to heat sterilization. Paraffin oils, however, may be successfully filtered through 0.2-micron membranes after heating to reduce viscosity.[15]

Simple formulations such as intravenous solutions, ophthalmics, and other aqueous products may be filtered directly through membranes in an economical manner. Heat-labile oils and liquids containing proteins require pretreatment, e.g., centrifugation or conventional filtration, prior to sterilizing filtration. The objective is removal of gross contamination that would rapidly plug the finer membranes. Difficult materials, such as blood fractions, demand serial filtration through successively finer membranes. The cost of multiple filtration may seem excessive, but it is often the only way to achieve sterility.

In selecting a filtration system for sterilization of any growth-supporting medium, the following precautions must be kept in mind:

1. Identify the potential sources of adverse biochemical and chemical contamination at each point of the system.

2. Identify the control points necessary to eliminate possible contamination and decrease cost.

3. Identify the hazards associated with each control point, i.e., airborne contamination and protein denaturation.

4. Establish a protocol for monitoring the hazards at control points of the system.

Figure 7-9 illustrates the basic filtration system for nonsterile filtration of serum, water, and salts to reduce the microbiologic and particulate matter, followed by final filtration through the sterile membrane.[13]

The use of filtration to remove bacteria, particulate matter from air, and other gases such as nitrogen and carbon dioxide is widespread in the pharmaceutical industry.[16] The following are some common applications employing initial gas filtration:

Vent filtration

Compressed air used in sterilizers

Air or nitrogen used for product and in-process solution transfers and at filling lines

Air or nitrogen used in fermentation

When sterile and under ideal conditions, traditionally packed fiberglass or cotton filters provide vent protection. The use of hydrophobic membrane filters is increasing. These filters guarantee bacterial removal in wet and dry air and do not channel, unload, or migrate the medium. These filters may need to be heated by jacketing. Restrictions of airflow through the vent filter can result in pump damage or tank collapse.[17]

Manufacturers of membrane filters provide extensive application data and detailed directions for assembly, sterilization, and use of their filters.[12,13,18–31] The basic elements of any sterile operation must be followed. All apparatus should be cleaned and sterilized as a unit. Filtration should be the last step in processing, and the filter should be placed as close as possible to the point of use of final packaging. In serial filtrations, only the final unit need be sterile, but minimal contamination in prior steps increases the reliability of the total process. Sterile filtra-

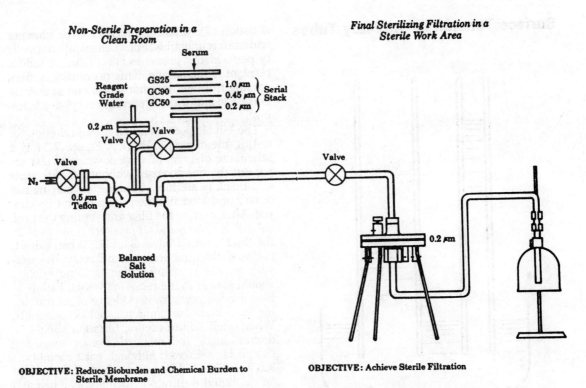

Non-Sterile Preparation in a Clean Room

Final Sterilizing Filtration in a Sterile Work Area

OBJECTIVE: Reduce Bioburden and Chemical Burden to Sterile Membrane

OBJECTIVE: Achieve Sterile Filtration

FIG. 7-9. *Schematic representation of operational sequence.*

tions should always be a pressure operation; a vacuum is undesirable since bacteria may be drawn in at leaky joints and contaminate the product.

After the successful introduction of a new filtration process, manufacturing tolerances allow reasonable changes in flow rate so long as quality is met. Therefore, the most common production problem is complete plugging of filter media resulting in no productivity. Subtle changes in raw material quality are often at fault. The level of an impurity need change only slightly to create problems with the fine porosity media used in polishing operations. For example, iron contamination in an alkaline product can lead to colloidal precipitates, which blind the media. Raw material problems should always be suspected when synthesis procedures have been altered or when the vendor of a purchased commodity has changed.

Integrity Testing

An important feature of a filtration system is its ability to be tested for integrity before and after each filtration. This is especially true in sterilization filtration, where even a few microorganisms passing through a crack in the filter could be disastrous. An integrity test is a nonde-

structive test used to predict the functional performance of a filter. Each membrane has a characteristic *bubble point, diffusion rate,* or *diffusion rate of air through water in a wetted filter,* which is a function of the porosity rating and predicts the performance of the filter. The common integrity tests used to predict the performance of the filter are the *bubble point test,* the *diffusion test,* and the *forward flow test.* Prior to filtration, the integrity test detects a damaged membrane, ineffective seals, or a system leak. The test performed after filtration confirms that the filter is still intact and that the system is remaining leak-free throughout the run.[12]

Bubble Point Test

Membrane filters, which have discrete uniform passages that penetrate from one side of the media to the other, can be regarded as fine, uniform capillaries. The bubble point test is based on the fact that when these capillaries are full of liquid, the liquid is held by surface tension. The minimum pressure required to force the liquid out of the capillary must be sufficient to overcome surface tension. Figure 7-10 illustrates the principle in the bubble point test. As can be seen in this figure, the capillary pressure is higher in the case of a small pore than in that

Surface Tension in Capillary Tubes

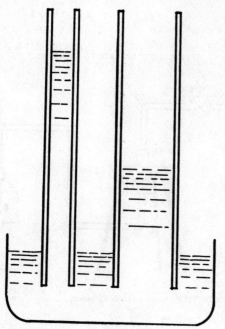

FIG. 7-10. *Surface tension in capillary tubes.*

of a large pore. The same is true for pores in a membrane. The bubble point pressure is governed by the following equation:

$$P = K \frac{4\gamma \cos \theta}{D} \qquad (7)$$

where:

P = bubble point pressure
K = shape correction factor (experimental constant)
D = pore diameter
γ = surface tension of the liquid
θ = liquid-to-membrane contact angle (angle of wetting)

In performing a bubble point experiment, the membrane is wetted and usually has a liquid above and a gas below. Since the pores are full of liquid, there is no passage of gas at zero pressure. There is still no passage of gas if the pressure is increased slightly. When the bubble point pressure is reached, a small bubble forms at the largest opening. As the pressure is further increased, rapid bubbling begins to occur. Bubble point pressure for a given membrane is different for different liquids. This can be seen in

equation (7), where the contact angle changes with different liquids. Filtration should normally be performed at pressures lower than the bubble point of a membrane. This prevents gas from passing through the filter at the end of a filtration cycle and thereby prevents excessive foaming.

The bubble point is also a useful criterion for testing membrane efficiency. Figure 7-11 is a schematic diagram of a nondestructive test apparatus that may be used without loss of product or a break in sterility. A *bubble test* may be run during and after filtration as an in-process control. After wetting the filter and venting the unit, valve A is closed, and air pressure is imposed on the filter through valves B and C. When valve C is closed, the filter holder should retain the pressure on the pressure gauge, and no bubbles should appear in the receiving vessel. Failure to hold a rated pressure is evidence of an unreliable membrane or improper holder assembly. When such failure occurs, filtration should be discontinued, and material already processed should be refiltered. Although each membrane has a specific bubble point, which is dependent on the liquid wetting the membrane, a test at a pressure of 20 pounds per square inch (psi) is usually sufficient to detect leaks.

Figure 7-12 illustrates the apparatus for performing a bubble point test on cartridge filters.

Diffusion Testing

A diffusion test must be performed in high-volume systems, e.g., cartridges or multistack discs, where a large volume of downstream liquid must be displaced before bubbles can be detected. A diffusion test measures volume of air that flows through a wet membrane from the pressurized side to the atmospheric side. The test is based on the theory that in a wet mem-

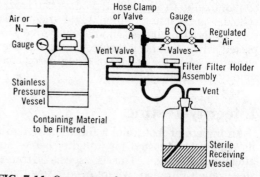

FIG. 7-11. *Connections for nondestructive bubble test to assure that membrane filter is intact. The test does not affect sterility. (Courtesy of Millipore Corporation)*

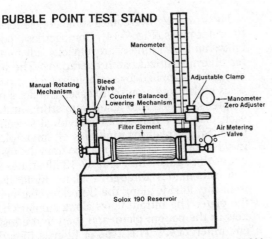

BUBBLE POINT TEST STAND

Manometer

Adjustable Clamp

Bleed Valve

Manual Rotating Mechanism

Counter Balanced Lowering Mechanism

Manometer Zero Adjuster

Filter Element

Air Metering Valve

Solox 190 Reservoir

FIG. 7-12. *Apparatus for performing the visible bubble test for cartridge filters.*[26] *(From Field Experience in Testing Membrane Filter Integrity by the Forward Flow Test Methods, Bulletin AB710-1-75. Pall Corporation, NY.)*

brane filter, under pressure, air flows through the water-filled pores at differential pressures below the bubble point pressure of the filter by a diffusion process. The process follows Fick's law of diffusion. In performing the diffusion test, the filter is thoroughly wetted in place with water, or the membrane is tested after filtration. Pressure is applied using air at 80% of the established bubble point pressure for the particular membrane. Pressure is held for 2 min, and the volume of the air displaced is recorded. The volume of air is determined by measuring the rate of flow of the displaced water. The pressure is increased until the bubble point is reached at an increment of 2 psi. Applying pressure at 80% of the bubble point pressure validates filter integrity since there would be a significant increase in airflow (water flow) at lower pressures, indicating damaged membranes, wrong pore size filter, ineffective seals, system leaks, or a broad pore size distribution.

Forward Flow Test

Forward flow testing is based upon measurement of the diffusion rate of air through water in a wetted filter at a pressure well below the bubble point pressure. The following three kinds of tests can be performed, but often, only one or two are deemed sufficient.[23,24]

1. Measurement of forward flow of individual elements prior to assembly to their housing to verify the integrity of each element prior to use.

2. Measurement of forward flow of the assembly

with elements in place in the system, before or after autoclaving, by in situ steaming or by ethylene oxide to verify tightness of any valves in parallel with elements.

3. Measurement of forward flow of assembly after completion of the filtration procedure to verify the integrity of the element during filtration.

The test is performed by placing a given element in its holder and wetting the filter. A preselected air pressure is applied to the upstream side of the filter system. Measurement of the total rate of airflow through the filter system is then made. The quality acceptance level for a given filter is based on a maximum total airflow at which the filter appears, empirically, to retain all bacteria.[23]

Filtration Equipment and Systems

Commercial Equipment

Commercial filtration equipment is classified by type of driving force (gravity, pressure, centrifugal, or vacuum), by method of operating (batch or continuous), and by end product desired (filtrate of cake solids).[2,4,26] The clarification demands of pharmaceutical processes are usually met by batch pressure units. Compatibility with a wide range of products restricts materials of construction to stainless steel, glass, and inert polymers.

Gravity filters are common in water treatment, where a *sand filter* may be used to clarify water prior to deionization or distillation. The filtering medium may consist of sand or cake beds, or for special purposes, a composition containing asbestos, cellulose fibers, activated charcoal, diatomaceous earth, or other filter aids. Small-scale purification of water may use porous ceramics as a filter medium in the form of hollow "candles." The fluid passes from the outside through the porous ceramics into the interior of the hollow candles. *Tray and frame* filters are best adapted for slow, difficult filtrations and for exceptionally soft- or fine-grained precipitates, which clog under the slightest pressure or pass through the openings of a cloth. *Gravity bag filters* also are applied to concentration of magmas, such as milk of magnesia. More efficient methods, however, particularly with respect to space requirements, are available. The *gravity nutzch* is a false-bottom tank or vessel with a support plate for filter media. Porcelain nutzches may be used for collecting sterile crystals or in operations where slurries are incompatible with metals. Since they are frequently operated under pressure or vacuum, they are not truly gravity filters.

Vacuum filters are employed on a large scale, but are rarely used for the collection of crystalline precipitates or sterile filtration. Continuous vacuum filters can handle high dirt loads, and on a volume basis, are cheap in terms of cost per gallon of filtered fluid. In the operation of the continuous drum filter system, vacuum is applied to the drum, and the fluid flows through the continuous belt. Solids are collected at the end of the belt.

Pressure filtration is desired in handling large quantities of material in order to accelerate the filtration process. Liquids with high viscosity can hardly be filtered at all by gravity.

The *plate and frame filter press* is the simplest of all pressure filters and is the most widely used (Fig. 7-13). Filter presses are used for a high degree of clarification of the fluid and for the harvesting of the cake. When clarity is the main objective, a "batch" mode operation is applied. The filter media are supported by structures in a pressure vessel. When an unacceptable pressure drop across the filter is reached during the filtration process, the filter media are changed. Methods of supporting the filter media include horizontal plates, horizontal or vertical pressure leaf, and plate and frame.

As the name implies, the plate and frame filter press is an assembly of hollow frames and solid plates that support filter media. When assembled alternately into a horizontal or a vertical unit, conduits permit flow of the slurry into the frames and through the media. One side of the plate is designed for the flow of the feed. After passing the filter media, the filtrate is accommodated on the other side. The solids collect in the frames, and filtrate is removed through place conduits. In cake filtration, the size of the frame space is critical, and wide sludge frames are used.

The filter press is the most versatile of filters since the number and type of filter sheets can be varied to suit a particular requirement. It can be used for coarse to fine filtrations, and by special conduit arrangements, for multistage filtration within a single press. The filter press is the most economical filter per unit of filtering surface, and material of construction can be chosen to suit any process conditions. Labor costs in assembly and cleaning are a primary disadvantage, and leakage between plates may occur through faulty assembly. The normal range of flow is three gallons per minute per square foot of filter surface at pressures of up to 25 psi.

The *disc filter* overcomes some deficiencies of the filter press (Fig. 7-14). Compactness, portability, and cleanliness are obvious advantages for pharmaceutical batch operations. The term disc filter is applied to assemblies of felt or paper discs sealed into a pressure case. The discs may be preassembled into a self-supporting unit, or each disc may rest on an individual screen or plate. Single plate or multiples of single plates may be applied. The flow may be from the inside out or the outside in. Figure 7-15 illustrates the flow schematics through a plate. Fluid flows from the outside along the thin flow channel in the plate. The filtrate flows along similar channels in the bottom plate, and then to the inside circumference.[22] This type of filter is intended only for clarification operations. Flow rates are similar to plate and frame presses at operating pressures of up to 50 psi. Pulp packs or *filtermasse* may be used instead of disc sheets for high-polish filtrations, but flow rates are then appreciably lower. Maximum filtrate recovery by air displacement of liquid is usually possible with a disc filter. Pressure leaf filters utilize the rotation of a pressure leaf to partially remove the cakes and extend the life of the filter media.

When filter aids are required, a plate and frame press with sludge frames is generally acceptable, but disposal of cake and cleaning becomes time-consuming. The *precoat pressure filter* (Fig. 7-15) is designed to overcome this objection. It consists of one or more leaves, plates, or tubes upon which a coat of filter aid is deposited to form the filtering surface. The filter area is usually enclosed within a horizontal or vertical tank, and special arrangements permit discharge of spent cake by backflush, air displacement, vibration, or centrifugal action. This type of filter is desirable for high-volume processes. Two or more units can be used alternatively, or surge tanks for clear filtrate may permit intermittent operation of a single unit.

Cartridge Filters and Systems

Cartridge filters have an integral cylindric configuration made with disposable or cleanable filter media and utilize either plastic or metal structural hardware.[26] With the discovery of strong pleatable membranes such as cellulose nitrate, polyamide, polyvinylidene chloride, PTFE, and nylon, cartridge filters have revolutionized the filtration industry. Cartridge filters provide maximum filtration area in the smallest possible package, allow quick changeout of the media, and save time and money. Cartridge filters of different shapes, structures, forms, and sizes for different applications in the pharma-

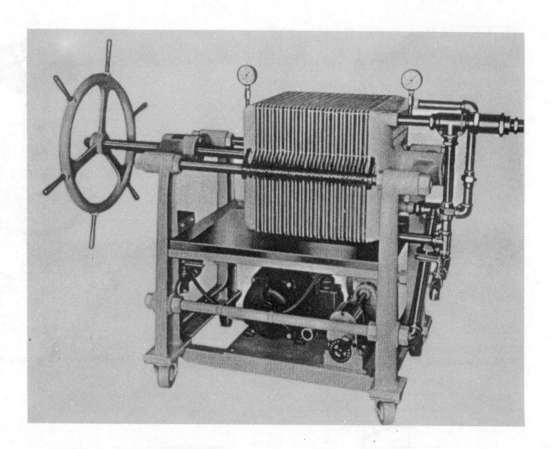

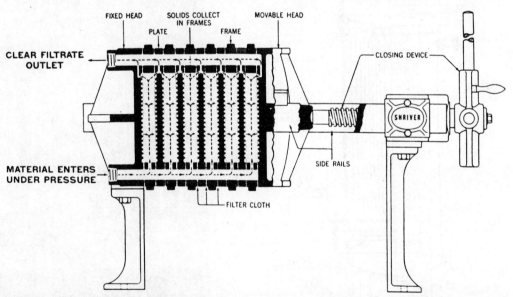

FIG. 7-13. *The plate and frame filter press may have 10 to 100 filtering surfaces and may be filled with pumps, sanitary fittings, sludge frames, or dividing plates for serial filtration. (Courtesy of Ertel Engineering and T. Shriver & Co. Inc.)*

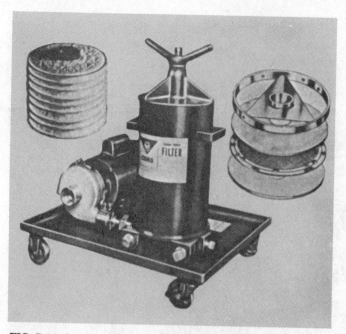
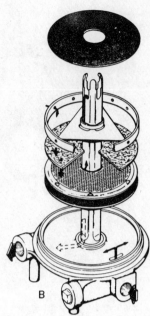

FIG. 7-14. *Disc filter casing (A) accommodates precompressed cartridges or disc media. Exploded view (B) shows liquid flow through assembled disc. (Courtesy of the Cuno Engineering Corporation.)*

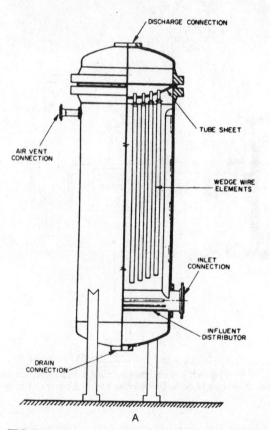

DISCHARGE CONNECTION

TUBE SHEET

AIR VENT
CONNECTION

WEDGE WIRE
ELEMENTS

INLET
CONNECTION

INFLUENT
DISTRIBUTOR

DRAIN
CONNECTION

A

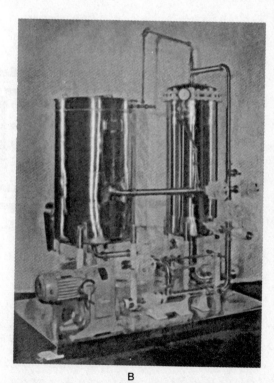

B

FIG. 7-15. *A precoat pressure filter with wedge wire elements (A) is part of all stainless steel filter systems (B). Special pump and fittings allow cleaning and sterilization in minutes. (Courtesy of Croll-Reynolds Engineering Co., Inc.)*

ceutical industry are now available in disposable and nondisposable forms.[12,19,27–30] The housings for cartridge filters come in a wide variety of configurations for both micron and submicron filtration. The major differences in various housings are in the design, materials of construction, seals that are used to install the cartridge in the housing, and the application for which they are used in the pharmaceutical industry. The housing for cartridge filters are described in terms of the height of the cartridge and in the number of cartridge receptacles in the base end of the housing. When a user purchases a housing from one manufacturer, he is usually not "locked in" to that manufacturer's cartridges. Adaptors are available that allow the cartridge filter of one manufacturer to fit into virtually any other manufacturer's housing.

Filter media can be formed into cartridge form by either tubular-wound, string-wound, or pleated formation. Alternate layers of filter media and separator material are rolled into a spiral configuration, and by potting the ends of the cartridge, form the "dead-ended" or "crossflow" type of flow channels. String-wound cartridges are the most commonly used and inexpensive filters available. Pleated cartridges are modified tubular configurations with a large filtration area. A single knife-edge flat gasket may be a satisfactory seal for cartridge filters with 1.0-micron or larger pore size. For submicron filtration, the most satisfactory seal is an O-ring.

Disposable or permanent *cartridge filters* are used for fluid clarification or sterilization. Standard elements for nonsterile filtration may be interchanged between cartridge holders offered by several companies (Fig. 7-16). Increases in capacity result from multi-element holders, and 12 element units are usually adequate for batches of 500 to 1000 gallons. The cost of disposable elements is offset by labor savings inherent in the simplicity of assembly and cleaning of cartridge clarifiers.

The metallic *edge filters,* particularly those with self-cleaning devices (Fig. 7-17), are excellent security filters for suspensions that may plug or blind conventional wire mesh. A cleaning blade combs away accumulated solids, which fall into a sump in the filter casing. A quick-coupling *metal cartridge filter* with construction that prevents short-circuiting of the filter element is also available (Fig. 7-18). The special design permits rapid disassembly as well as interchange of reusable filter media. Metal elements permit particle retention as low as 1.5 microns. Duo filters, two units connected in parallel, are recommended where uninterrupted service is required. A high-frequency vibrator,

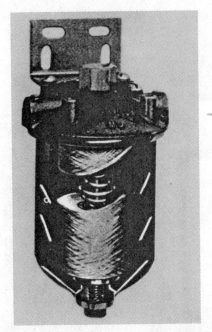

FIG. 7-16. *A disposable wound cartridge is installed in holder. Liquid flows through the element and is discharged through the core. (Courtesy of the Filterite Corporation.)*

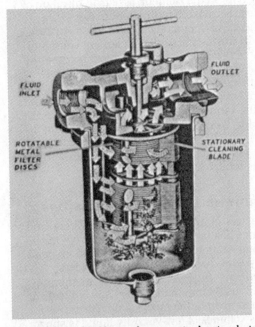

FIG. 7-17. *An edge filter with automatic cleaning device may be automated by replacing handle with motor. (Courtesy of the Cuno Engineering Corporation.)*

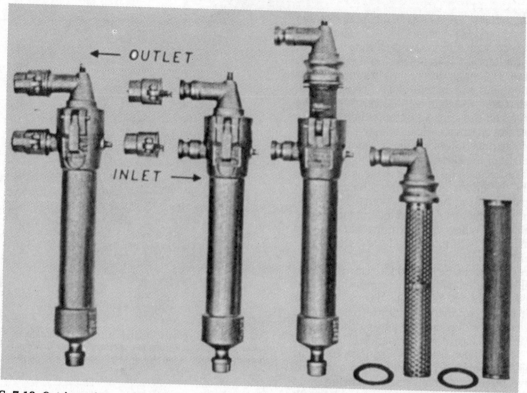

FIG. 7-18. *Quick-coupling cartridge filter for metallic media is readily cleaned. (Courtesy of the Ronnigen-Petter Company.)*

acting only on the element, assists in filtration of slurries that have blinding tendencies.

Vendors of membrane filters offer cartridge units in single- and multiple-element configurations.[21,27–32] These cartridges have become the unit of choice for high-volume, sterile filtrations and are ideal for in-line, final polish prior to bottling of bulk parenterals. Cartridge filters having absolute ratings of 0.04 microns are also available (Fig. 7-19). The latter units have 5 to 10 square feet of effective filtering area per cartridge of 10-inch height, and some can also be steam-sterilized.[27–32]

Membrane Filters and Housings

The use of membrane cartridge filters and housings has been discussed extensively in the previous section. The following section deals mainly with disc membranes and holders.

Membrane filter holders accept membranes from 13 to 293 mm in diameter. A useful rule of thumb for membrane media and holder sizes for various volumes of low-viscosity liquid is shown in Table 7-5. Although 90- or 142-mm units are suitable for moderate volumes, the 293-mm

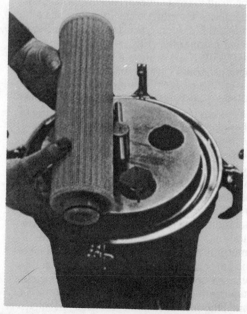

FIG. 7-19. *Multiple-cartridge holders permit high-volume processing. (Courtesy of the Pall Corporation.)*

TABLE 7-5. *Membrane Disc Filter Sizes for Various Volumes*

Volumes	Filter
10–100 ml	13- or 25-mm discs
100–300 ml	47-mm discs
300–5,000 ml	90-mm discs
5,000–10,000 ml	142-mm discs
20–1,000 L	293-mm discs
1,000 L and up	cartridges

membrane holder is the usual production choice for small-batch sizes. Stainless steel holders for the sterilizing filter have sanitary connections, and the support screens are faced with Teflon to permit autoclaving with the membrane in place. Special compatibility problems may require polyvinylchloride holders with stainless steel supports, or units that have only Teflon and polypropylene contact parts.[20]

Serial filtration is often desired to fractionate the particulates in a fluid. A membrane of large pore size may often be used as a prefilter for a final downstream membrane filter of a smaller pore size.

Pressure drop across the filter media is often observed. This pressure drop may be contributed by either the filter media, the holder, or the housing. In a properly designed system, the pressure drop due to housing should usually be insignificant except for high-flow liquids or gases.

Laboratory Filtration Equipment

Laboratory equipment catalogs offer a wide choice of funnels and flasks adaptable to pharmaceutical filtration studies. Although a Buchner funnel test permits analysis of the major difficulties in a filtration problem, development laboratories should have additional procedures and apparatus that produce the qualitative conditions expected in large-scale production. This requirement can be met with a nominal capital investment.

For gravity filtration, conventional glass percolators are applicable, in which case the bottom tube is covered with fibrous material. The filtering funnel is the most common of all laboratory filter devices. Filter paper is used with funnels. Sometimes, a plug of fibrous material may be used instead. Filter bags for laboratory use are made of fabric and are mounted for gravity filtration. The uncertainty of adequate clarification with *glass beads* or *sand* has restricted their use as gravity filters for certain operations in the laboratory.

Suction filters are greatly utilized in the laboratory. Usually, a conical funnel and the Buchner funnel are used for suction filtration, as are immersion and suction-leaf filters.[33] Immersion filter tubes, also known as filter sticks, are generally used for small-scale laboratory operations.

Small-laboratory pressure filters have been used substantially in recent years for both sterile and nonsterile filtration operations. Gravity and suction filters are used mostly for nonsterile filtration. For the pressure filtration of small amounts of material, the filter medium may be mounted in a filter tube, with the liquid poured in and pressure applied to the upper surface of the liquid.[34]

Filter paper in circular form is the most common medium for laboratory filtrations. Filter papers are available in a wide variety of textures, purities, and sizes and are available for different uses. They may be circular (1 to 50 cm in diameter), folded, or arranged in sheets or rolls. Among the special types of laboratory filter paper for pharmaceutical industry are:

1. Filter papers impregnated with activated carbon for adsorption of colors and odors in pharmaceutical liquids.

2. Filter paper impregnated with diatomaceous earth for removal of colloidal haze from liquids with low turbidity.

Minimum laboratory equipment includes a plate and frame press, a membrane filter holder, and a single-element housing for disposable cartridges. A 6- or 8-inch, stainless steel filter press with four to eight filter surfaces and sludge frames is adequate. This covers the flow range from 8 to 200 gallons per hour with minimum filtrate holdup in the press. Stainless steel construction permits autoclaving for sterile operations. Auxiliary equipment for mixing filter aid and feeding the press (10- to 20-gallon tanks, agitators, and centrifugal pump) should also be available. A 90-mm, stainless steel membrane filter holder processes 1 to 15 gallons of sterile solutions per hour. The support plate should be Teflon-lined to permit autoclave sterilization with membranes in place; the gaskets should also be Teflon. Integrity testing apparatus and a stainless steel pressure vessel of 1- to 5-gallon capacity are essential auxiliaries. The same pressure assembly may be used in cartridge filter tests. A broad selection of media should be on hand for each unit.

More flexibility is obtained by adding a metal cartridge filter and a small, manually operated, self-cleaning, edge filter. If processing of high-volume cosmetic products is expected, a single-leaf, precoat pressure filter should be available. Units can be obtained with capacities as low as 1½ gallons.

Cake Filtration

Cake filtration in which solids recovery is the goal is an important pharmaceutical process. Personnel involved in synthesis or fermentation to produce bulk active ingredients consider cake filtration to be the primary aim of the unit operation. Engineering textbooks and current literature stress the theory, laboratory test methods, and equipment required for solids separation.[2,4,26]

The plate and frame press and precoat pressure filters used for clarification also are applied to solids recovery. The basic design is often modified to reduce the high labor factor. In general, these pressure filters are restricted to batch operation and recovery of moderate weights of expensive materials.

For large-scale operations, continuous vacuum filters are most widely used. The *rotary-drum vacuum filter* is divided into sections, each connected to a discharge head. The slurry is fed to a tank in which solids are held in suspension by an agitator. As the drum rotates, each section passes through the slurry, and vacuum draws filtrate through a filter medium at the drum surface. The suspended solids deposit on the filter drum as a cake, and as rotation continues, vacuum holds the cake at the drum surface. The cake is washed and dried as it moves toward the discharge point. It may be scraped from the drum or it may be supported by strings until it breaks free under gravitational forces. Many variants of the basic design are needed to accommodate differences in cake formation, drying rates, and discharge properties.

Filtering centrifuges are another general class of solids recovery devices. In this method of filtration, centrifugal force is used to affect the passage of the liquid through the filter medium.[33] This type of filtration is particularly advantageous when very fine particles are involved. This device is fitted with a perforated basket, which supports the filter media. The basket revolves inside the casing. Slurry is sprayed into the basket, in which centrifugal action forces the filtrate through the media on which the cake deposits. Continuous discharge of solids is possible, but batch units that require shutdown for removal of solids are also common. Whenever solids recovery is the primary goal, centrifuges must be considered as an alternative to filtration.

Membrane Ultrafiltration

Membrane ultrafiltration has become a commercially feasible unit operation in the past decade.[10,12,13,19,22,30,35-38] Unlike conventional filtration, ultrafiltration is a process of selective molecular separation. It is defined as a process of removing dissolved molecules on the basis of membrane size and configuration by passing a solution under pressure through a very fine filter. Ultrafiltration membrane retains most macromolecules while allowing smaller molecules and the solvent to pass through the membrane, even though the membrane is not rated as absolute. The difference between microfiltration and ultrafiltration is significant. The former removes particulates and bacteria; the latter separates molecules. Application of hydraulic pressure reverses the normal process of osmosis, so that the membrane acts as a molecular screen through which only those molecules below a certain size are allowed to pass.

Separation of a solvent and a solute of different molecular size may be achieved by selecting a membrane that allows the solvent, but not the solute, to pass through. Alternatively, two solutes of different molecular size may be separated by choosing a membrane that passes the smaller molecule, but holds back the larger one (Fig. 7-20). Ultrafiltration is similar in process to reverse osmosis; both filter on the basis of molecular size. Ultrafiltration is different from reverse osmosis in the sense that it does not separate on the basis of ionic rejection. Dialysis and ultrafiltration are similar in the sense that both processes separate molecules, but ultrafiltration is different in that it does involve the application of pressure.

The selectivity and retentivity of a membrane are characterized by its molecular weight cutoff. It is difficult to characterize the porosity of an ultrafiltration membrane by means of precise molecular weight cutoff. The configuration of the molecule and its electrical charge may also affect the separation properties of the membrane.[30] Ultrafiltration membranes are therefore rated on the basis of nominal molecular weight cutoff. The shape of the molecule to be retained plays a major role in retentivity. Many of the same techniques that are used in microfiltration to increase flow rate and throughput are also used for ultrafiltration. Ultrafiltration membranes are available as flat sheets, pleated cartridges, or hollow fibers. The hollow fibers have the selective skin on the inside of the fiber.

Industrial use of this procedure has followed the development of anisotropic polymer membranes in a variety of biologically inert, noncel-

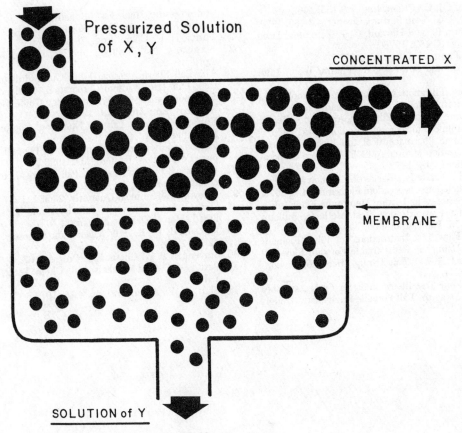

FIG. 7-20. *Schematic diagram of membrane ultrafiltration process.*

lulosic materials. These membranes are fragile structures, however, and usually require a backing plate of porous material to withstand operational pressure. During the processing of a solution, a region of high solute concentration also develops at the surface of the membrane, resisting further passage of solvent. Providing essential support for the membrane and overcoming concentration polarization through shear effects have resulted in a wide variety of commercial apparatus, including tangential-flow cassette systems, process ultrafiltration cartridges, hollow fiber beakers, and collodion bags. Since the technology continues to change rapidly, reliance on technical expertise of the manufacturer is advisable.

Applications in the pharmaceutical industry are predominantly in the concentration of heat-labile products, such as vaccines, virus preparations, and immunoglobulins. Ultrafiltration also has been used to recover antibiotics, hormones, or vitamins from fermentation broths, to separate cells from fermentation broth, to clarify solutions, and to remove low-molecular-weight contaminants prior to using conventional recovery techniques. The most important application of ultrafiltration is the removal of pyrogens.

References

1. Oulman, C., and Baumann, E.: Filtration as a laboratory tool. *In* Separation and Purification. 3rd Ed. Edited by R. Perry and A. Weissberger. John Wiley and Sons, New York, 1978, p. 364.
2. Perry, R., and Chilton, C.: Chemical Engineers Handbook. 5th Ed. McGraw-Hill, New York, 1973.
3. Tiller, F.M.: Chem. Eng., 73:151, 1966.
4. Encyclopedia of Chemical Technology, Vol. 9. 2nd Ed. Interscience, New York, 1966, p. 264.
5. Orr, C. (ed.): Filtration—Principles and Practices, Part II. Marcel Dekker, New York, 1979.
6. Mais, L. G.: Chem. Eng., 78:49, 1971.
7. London, A.: Engineering, 207:443, 1969.
8. Purcas, D. B.: Chem. and Proc. Eng., 48:95, 1967.
9. Smith, G. R. S.: Chem. Eng., 74:154, 1967.
10. Weissberger, A. (ed.): Techniques of Organic Chemistry. Vol. III. Interscience, New York, 1950.
11. Daniels, F., and Alberty, R. A. (eds.): Physical Chemistry. 3rd Ed. John Wiley and Sons, New York, 1966.
12. Industrial Process Catalog. Millipore Corporation, Bedford, MA, 1982.
13. Micro Filtration Systems Catalog 1982. Micro Filtration Systems, Dublin, CA, 1981.

14. Sharbaugh, J. C.: Chem. Eng., 69:153, 1962.
15. Mulvany, J. G.: Soap Perfum. Cosmet., 43:486, 1970.
16. Duberstein, R., and Howard, G. J., Parenteral Drug Association 32:192, 1978.
17. Cole, J.: Pharm. Tech., 1:49, 1977.
18. Cole, J. C., and Shumsky, R.: Pharm. Tech., 1:39, 1977.
19. Laboratory Filtration Microbiology Electrophoresia 1929. Sartorius GmbH, West Germany, 1979.
20. Low Volume Sterilizing Filtration, Application Report AR-11. Millipore Corporation, Bedford, MA, 1973.
21. High Volume Pharmaceutical and Biological Filtration, Application Manual AM202. Millipore Corporation, Bedford, MA, 1972.
22. Ballew, H., et al. (eds.): Basics of Filtration and Separation. Nuclepore Corporation, Pleasanton, CA, 1978.
23. Field Experience in Testing Membrane Filter Integrity by the Forward Flow Test Methods, Bulletin AB710-1-75. Pall Corporation, New York.
24. Forward Flow Test Instructions for Filter Element Integrity Using the Pall Portable Forward Flow Kit, Bulletin #PCF 700. Pall Trinity Micro Corporation, Cortland, NY.
25. Forward Flow Test Instructions for Filter Assembly Integrity Using the Pall Portable Pneusmatic Trough and Pressure Hold Test, Bulletin #PCF 701. Pall Trinity Micro Corporation, Cortland, NY.
26. Porter, H. F.: Chem. Eng., 78:39, 1971.
27. Nickolaus, N.: Filtration and Separation, March-April, 1975.
28. The Pall Pharmaceutical Filter Guide Bulletin AB-200. Pall Trinity Micro Corporation, Cortland, NY.
29. Filtration Catalog and System Design Guide. Gelman Sciences, Ann Arbor, MI, 1980.
30. Filtration, Catalog Lab 50. Nuclepore Corporation, Pleasanton, CA, 1980.
31. Cartridge Filters and Housing, Catalog PD-180. Millipore Corporation, Bedford, MA, 1980.
32. Ultipor AB Bulletin AB-100A. Pall Trinity Micro Corporation, Cortland, NY, 1972.
33. Drown, C.: Technical Quarterly, 20:552, 1981.
34. Orr, C. (ed.): Filtration Principles and Practices, Part I. Marcel Dekker, New York, 1977.
35. McDonald, D. P.: Mfg. Chem. and Aerosol News, 42:73, 1971.
36. Stavenger, P. L.: Chem. Eng. Progress, 67:30, 1971.
37. Porter, M. C., and Michaels, A. S.: Chem. Tech., 3:56, 1971.
38. Blatt, W. F.: American Lab., 4:78, 1972.

SECTION II

Pharmaceutical Dosage Form Design

8

Preformulation

EUGENE F. FIESE *and* TIMOTHY A. HAGEN

Preformulation commences when a newly synthesized drug shows sufficient pharmacologic promise in animal models to warrant evaluation in man. These studies should focus on those physicochemical properties of the new compound that could affect drug performance and development of an efficacious dosage form. A thorough understanding of these properties may ultimately provide a rationale for formulation design, or support the need for molecular modification. In the simplest case, these preformulation investigations may merely confirm that there are no significant barriers to the compound's development.

Prior to starting preformulation studies, the physical pharmacist should meet with the principal investigators involved in the drug's development to obtain information on the known properties of the compound and the proposed development schedule as listed in Figure 8-1. Since drug research is usually targeted for a specific therapeutic area, potency relative to competitive products as well as the probable human dosage form(s) may be known. Similarly, the medicinal chemists may have insight regarding the molecule's weaknesses as a result of their efforts to synthesize the compound. In addition, a literature search should be conducted to provide an understanding of the probable decay mechanism(s) and conditions that promote drug decomposition. This information may suggest a means of stabilization, a key stability test, or a stability reference compound (such as aspirin for a compound undergoing ester hydrolysis). Information on the proposed mode of drug administration as well as a literature review on the formulation, bioavailability, and pharmacokinetics of similar drugs often proves useful when deciding how to optimize the bioavailability of a new drug candidate.

Preliminary Evaluation and Molecular Optimization

Once a pharmacologically active compound has been identified, a project team consisting of representatives from the disciplines indicated in Figure 8-2 has responsibility for assuring that the compound enters the development process in its optimum molecular form. While each discipline may have its own criteria for an "optimized" molecule, the physical pharmacist must focus on how the product will be formulated and administered to patients. Commonly, stability and/or solubility shortcomings can adversely affect these aspects of drug performance.

When the first quality sample of the new drug becomes available, probing experiments should be conducted to determine the magnitude of each suspected problem area. If a deficiency is detected, then the project team should decide on the molecular modification(s) that would most likely improve the drug's properties. Salts, prodrugs, solvates, polymorphs, or even new analogs may emerge from this modification effort.

Although each of these modification approaches has proven beneficial, the salt and prodrug approaches are the most common. Most salts of organic compounds are formed by the addition or removal of a proton to form an ionized drug molecule, which is then neutralized with a counter ion. Ephedrine hydrochloride, for example, is prepared by addition of a proton to the basic secondary nitrogen atom on ephedrine, resulting in a protonated drug molecule (ephedrine-$H^{(+)}$), which is neutralized with a chloride anion (ephedrine-HCl). In general, organic salts are more water-soluble than the corresponding un-ionized molecule, and hence, offer a simple means of increasing dissolution

I.   Compound Identity:

II. Structure:

III. Formula and Molecular Weight:

IV. Therapeutic Indication:

  Probable Human Dose:
  Desired Dosage Form(s):
  Bioavailability Model(s):
  Competitive Products:

V.   Potential Hazards:

VI. Initial Bulk Lots:

  Lot Number:
  Crystallization Solvent(s):
  Particle Size Range:
  Melting Point:
  % Volatiles:
  Observations:

VII. Analytical Methods:

  HPLC Assay:
  TLC Assay:
  UV/VIS Spectroscopy:
  Synthetic Route:
  Probable Decay Products:

VIII. Key Dates:

  Bulk Scale-Up:
  Toxicology Start Date:
  Clinical Supplies Preparation:
  IND Filing:
  Phase I Testing:

IX. Critical Development Issue(s):

FIG. 8-1. *Essential information helpful in designing the preformulation evaluation of a new drug.*

rates, and possibly improving bioavailability. During synthesis, salts are usually formed in organic media to improve yield as well as purity. Some of the problems commonly encountered in evaluating salt forms include poor crystallinity, various degrees of solvation or hydration, hygroscopicity, and instability due to an unfavorable pH in the crystalline microenvironment. Table 8-1 lists a spectrum of pharmaceutical alterations resulting from salt formation, while Table 8-2 lists salts used in commercial pharmaceutical products through 1974.[1]

While salt formation is limited to molecules with ionizable groups, prodrugs may be formed with any organic molecule having a chemically reactive functional group. Prodrugs are synthetic derivatives (e.g., esters and amides) of drug molecules that may have intrinsic pharmacologic activity but usually must undergo some transformation in vivo to liberate the active drug molecule. Through the formation of a prodrug, a variety of side chains or functional groups may be added to improve the biologic and/or pharmaceutical properties of a compound.[2] Some of the biologic response parameters that may be altered by prodrug formation are absorption due to increased lipophilicity or increased water solubility, duration of action via blockade of a key metabolic site, and distribution to organs due to changes in lipophilicity. Examples of biologic improvements are abundant in the steriod and prostaglandin prodrug literature.[3] Pharmaceutical improvements resulting from prodrug formation include stabilization, an increase or decrease in solubility, crystallinity, taste, odor, and reduced pain on injection.

Erythromycin estolate is an example of a prodrug with improved pharmaceutical properties (Fig. 8-3). In aqueous solutions, protonated erythromycin is water-soluble, has a bitter taste, and is rapidly hydrolyzed in gastric acid ($t_{10\%} = 9$ sec) to yield inactive decay products. To overcome this problem, the water-insoluble lauryl sulfate salt of the propionate ester prodrug (estolate) was formed for use in both suspension and capsule dosage forms. Erythromycin propionate is inactive as an antimicrobial and must undergo ester hydrolysis to yield bioactive erythromycin. In an oral q.i.d. bioavailability comparison between Upjohn's enteric coated tablet formulation of erythromycin base E-Mycin and Dista's nonenteric Ilosone capsule formulation of erythromycin estolate (Fig. 8-4), the lipophilic ester prodrug was absorbed four times more efficiently than the formulated free base, but hydrolyzed only 24% in serum to produce equivalent plasma levels of bioactive erythromycin base.[4,5] Thus, a prodrug was used to overcome a pharmaceutical formulation problem without compromising bioavailability.

To date, most prodrugs have been esters or amides designed to increase lipophilicity. Unfortunately, this type of modification often decreases water solubility and thus decreases the concentration gradient across the cell membrane, which controls the rate of drug absorption. This trade-off between lipophilicity and concentration gradient is generally assumed to result in a net improvement in absorption. In 1980, Amidon suggested the making of water-

DISCIPLINES

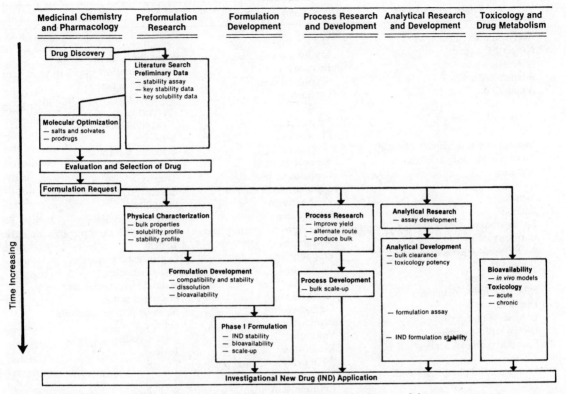

FIG. 8-2. *Flow diagram illustrating the multidisciplinary development of a drug candidate.*

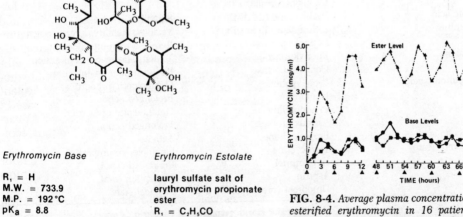

Erythromycin Base

R₁ = H
M.W. = 733.9
M.P. = 192 °C
pKₐ = 8.8

Erythromycin Estolate

**lauryl sulfate salt of
erythromycin propionate
ester**
R₁ = C₂H₅CO
R₂ = C₁₂H₂₅SO₄H
M.W. = 1056.4
M.P. = 137 °C
Drug pKₐ = 6.9

FIG. 8-3. *Structures of erythromycin and its estolate pro-drug.*

FIG. 8-4. *Average plasma concentrations of free base and esterified erythromycin in 16 patients following q.i.d. doses of 250 mg of erythromycin base (●) E-Mycin or erythromycin estolate (▲, ■) Ilosone. These products were judged equivalent with respect to production of bioactive erythromycin base plasma levels. (From DiSanto, A. R., et al.: J. Clin. Pharmacol., 20:437, 1980. Reproduced with permission of the copyright owner.)*

TABLE 8-1. *Examples of Modification of Pharmaceutical Agents Through Salt Formation*

Salt-Forming Agent	Compound Modified	Modification
Acetylaminoacetic acid	Doxycycline	Solubility
N-Acetyl-1,-asparagine	Erythromycin	Solubility, activity, stability
N-Acetylcystine	Doxycycline	Combined effect useful in pneumonia
Adamantoic acid	Alkylbiguanides	Prolonged action
Adipic acid	Piperazine	Stability, toxicity, organoleptic properties
N-Alkylsulfamates	Ampicillin	Absorption (oral)
	Lincomycin	Solubility
Anthraquinone-1,5-disulfonic acid	Cephalexin	Stability, absorption
Arabogalactan sulfate (arabino)	Various alkaloids	Prolonged action
Arginine	Cephalosporins	Toxicity
	α-Sulfobenzylpenicillin	Stability, hygroscopicity, toxicity
Aspartate	Erythromycin	Solubility
Betaine	Tetracycline	Gastric absorption
Bis(2-carboxychromon-5-yloxy)alkanes	7-(Aminoalkyl)theophyllines	Activity, prolonged prophylactic effect
Carnitine	Metformin	Toxicity
4-Chloro-*m*-toluenesulfonic acid	Propoxyphene	Organoleptic properties
Decanoate	Heptaminol	Prolonged action
Diacetyl sulfate	Thiamine	Stability, hygroscopicity
Dibenzylethylenediamine	Ampicillin	Prolonged action ·
Diethylamine	Cephalosporins	Reduced pain on injection
Diguaiacyl phosphate	Tetracycline	Activity
Dioctyl sulfosuccinate	Vincamine	Organoleptic properties
Embonic (pamoic) acid	Kanamycin	Toxicity
	2-Phenyl-3-methylmorpholine	Toxicity
Fructose 1,6-diphosphoric acid	Tetracycline	Solubility
	Erythromycin	Solubility
Glucose 1-phosphoric acid, glucose 6-phosphoric acid	Tetracycline	Solubility
1-Glutamine	Erythromycin	Solubility
Hydroxynaphthoate	Erythromycin	Solubility, activity, stability
2-(4-Imidazolyl)ethylamine	Bephenium	Toxicity
Isobutanolamine	Prostaglandin	Prolonged action
Lauryl sulfate	Theophylline	Stability
Lysine	Vincamine	Organoleptic properties
	α-Sulfobenzylpenicillin	Toxicity, stability, hygroscopicity
	Cephalosporins	
Methanesulfonic acid	Pralidoxime (2-PAM)	Solubility
N-Methylglucamine	α-Sulfobenzylpenicillin	Toxicity, stability, hygroscopicity
	Cephalosporins	Reduced pain on injection
N-Methylpiperazine	Phenylbutazone	Toxicity, faster onset of action
Morpholine	Cephalosporins	Reduced pain on injection
2-Naphthalenesulfonic acid	Propoxyphene	Organoleptic properties
Octanoate	Heptaminol	Prolonged action
Probenecid	Pivampicillin	Organoleptic properties
Tannic acid	Various amines	Prolonged action
Theobromine acetic acid	Propoxyphene	Activity
3,4,5-Trimethoxybenzoate	Tetracycline	Organoleptic properties
	Heptaminol	Prolonged action
Tromethamine	Aspirin	Absorption (oral)
	Dinoprost (prostaglandin $F_{2\alpha}$)	Physical state

From Berge, S.M., et al.: J. Pharm. Sci., 66:1, 1977. Reproduced with permission of the copyright owner.

TABLE 8-2. *Salts Used in Pharmaceutical Products Marketed in the United States Through 1974.*

Anion	Percent[a]	Anion	Percent[a]
Acetate	1.26	Iodide	2.02
Benzenesulfonate	0.25	Isethionate[i]	0.88
Benzoate	0.51	Lactate	0.76
Bicarbonate	0.13	Lactobionate	0.13
Bitartrate	0.63	Malate	0.13
Bromide	4.68	Maleate	3.03
Calcium edetate	0.25	Mandelate	0.38
Camsylate[b]	0.25	Mesylate	2.02
Carbonate	0.38	Methylbromide	0.76
Chloride	4.17	Methylnitrate	0.38
Citrate	3.03	Methylsulfate	0.88
Dihydrochloride	0.51	Mucate	0.13
Edetate	0.25	Napsylate	0.25
Edisylate[c]	0.38	Nitrate	0.64
Estolate[d]	0.13	Pamoate (Embonate)	1.01
Esylate[e]	0.13	Pantothenate	0.25
Fumarate	0.25	Phosphate/diphosphate	3.16
Gluceptate[f]	0.18	Polygalacturonate	0.13
Gluconate	0.51	Salicylate	0.88
Glutamate	0.25	Stearate	0.25
Glycollylarsanilate[g]	0.13	Subacetate	0.38
Hexylresorcinate	0.13	Succinate	0.38
Hydrabamine[h]	0.25	Sulfate	7.46
Hydrobromide	1.90	Tannate	0.88
Hydrochloride	42.98	Tartrate	3.54
Hydroxynaphthoate	0.25	Teoclate[j]	0.13
		Triethiodide	0.13

Cation	Percent[a]	Cation	Percent[a]
Organic		Metallic:	
Benzathine[k]	0.66	Aluminum	0.66
Chloroprocaine	0.33	Calcium	10.49
Choline	0.33	Lithium	1.64
Diethanolamine	0.98	Magnesium	1.31
Ethylenediamine	0.66	Potassium	10.82
Meglumine[l]	2.29	Sodium	61.97
Procaine	0.66	Zinc	2.95

[a]Percent is based on total number of anionic or cationic salts in use through 1974. [b]Camphorsulfonate. [c]1,2-Ethanedisulfonate. [d]Lauryl sulfate. [e]Ethanesulfonate. [f]Glucoheptonate. [g]p-Glycollamidophenylarsonate. [h]N,N'-Di(dehydroabietyl)ethylenediamine. [i]2-Hydroxyethanesulfonate. [j]8-Chlorotheophyllinate. [k]N,N'-Dibenzylethylenediamine. [l]N-Methylglucamine.

From Berge, S.M., et al.: J. Pharm. Sci., 66:1, 1977. Reproduced with permission of the copyright owner.

soluble prodrugs by adding selected amino acids that are substrates for enzymes located in the intestinal brush border.[6] Assuming that enzyme cleavage was not rate-limiting, and that the liberated drug molecule would remain in the lipophilic membrane, then the resulting membrane transport of the parent compound should be very rapid, owing to the large concentration gradient of liberated drug across the membrane, as illustrated in Figure 8-5. Using the lysine ester prodrug of estrone, a potential increase of five orders of magnitude in adsorption rate was found in vivo using perfused rat intestines.

Although any of the modifications discussed may provide an increase in bioavailability, chemical instability or a lack of synthetic feasibility may prohibit the commercial development of a modified drug molecule. Whatever the case, the molecular form of the drug advancing from this preliminary evaluation should have a sub-

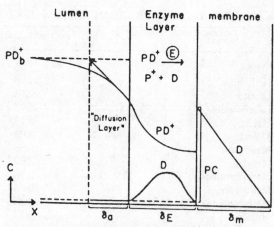

FIG. 8-5 *Concentration (C) versus distance (X) profile for the absorption of water-soluble prodrugs (PD⁺), which are enzymatically (E) hydrolyzed in the intestinal brush border to liberate the lipophilic parent compound (D). Key: δ_a, thickness of aqueous diffusion layer; δ_E, enzyme layer thickness; δ_m, membrane thickness; and PC membrane-enzyme layer partition coefficient. (From Amidon, G. L., et al.: J. Pharm. Sci., 69:1363, 1980. Reproduced with permission of the copyright owner.)*

I. Bulk Characterization

Crystallinity and Polymorphism
Hygroscopicity
Fine Particle Characterization
Bulk Density
Powder Flow Properties

II. Solubility Analysis

Ionization Constant – pKa
pH Solubility Profile
Common Ion Effect – K_{sp}
Thermal Effects
Solubilization
Partition Coefficient
Dissolution

III. Stability Analysis

Stability in Toxicology Formulations
Solution Stability
    pH Rate Profile
Solid State Stability
    Bulk Stability
    Compatibility

FIG. 8-6. *Outline of the principal areas of preformulation research.*

stantial chance of successfully progressing through the drug development process.

Once the optimum molecular form of a drug has been selected, formulation development commences, which prompts other disciplines to begin their task in the drug development process as depicted in Figure 8-2. The objective of this phase is the quantitation of those physical chemical properties that will assist in developing a stable, safe, and effective formulation with maximum bioavailability. Figure 8-6 lists the major areas of preformulation research in the order in which they are discussed in the following text. Keep in mind that these topics vary in importance according to the type of formulation sought for each individual drug candidate.

Bulk Characterization

In most instances, the synthetic process is developed in parallel with preformulation investigations. A drug candidate at this stage often has not had all of its solid forms identified, and there is a great potential for new polymorphs to emerge. Bulk properties for the solid form, such as particle size, bulk density and surface morphology, are also likely to change during process development. Therefore, comprehensive characterization of all preformulation bulk lots is necessary to avoid misleading predictions of stability or solubility, which depend on a particular crystalline form.

Crystallinity and Polymorphism

Crystal habit and the internal structure of a drug can affect bulk and physicochemical properties, which range from flowability to chemical stability. *Habit* is the description of the outer appearance of a crystal whereas the *internal structure* is the molecular arrangement within the solid. Several examples of different habits of crystals are shown in Figure 8-7. A single internal structure for a compound can have several different habits, depending on the environment for growing crystals. Changes with internal structure usually alter the crystal habit while such chemical changes as conversion of a sodium salt to its free acid form produce both a change in internal structure and crystal habit. Characterization of a solid form involves (1) verifying that the solid is the expected chemical compound, (2) characterizing the internal structure, and then (3) describing the habit of the crystal.

The internal structure of a compound can be classified in a variety of ways, as shown in Figure 8-8. The first major distinction is whether the solid is crystalline or amorphous. Crystals are characterized by repetitious spacing of con-

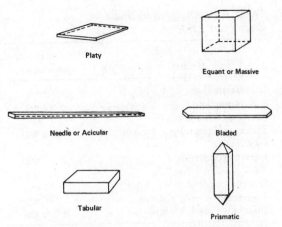

Platy

Equant or Massive

Needle or Acicular

Bladed

Tabular

Prismatic

FIG. 8-7. *Different habits of crystals. (Reprinted by permission of the publisher from Hartshorne, N. H., and Stuart, A.: Practical Optical Crystallography. American Elsevier, New York, 1964, p. 1, and courtesy of McCrone Research Institute, American Pharmaceutical Association Academy of Pharmaceutical Sciences 33rd National Meeting, November 14, 1982, San Diego, CA.*

stituent atoms or molecules in a three-dimensional array, whereas amorphous forms have atoms or molecules randomly placed as in a liquid. Amorphous forms are typically prepared by rapid precipitation, lyophilization, or rapid cooling of liquid melts. Since amorphous forms are usually of higher thermodynamic energy than corresponding crystalline forms, solubilities as well as dissolution rates are generally greater. Upon storage, amorphous solids tend to revert to more stable forms. This thermodynamic instability, which can occur during bulk processing

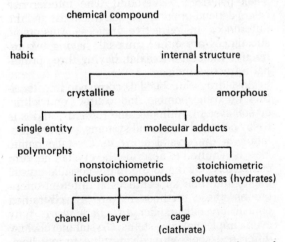

FIG. 8-8. *Outline of differentiating habit and crystal chemistry of a compound. (From Haleblian, J. K.: J. Pharm. Sci., 64:1269, 1975. Reproduced with permission of the copyright owner.)*

or within dosage forms, is a major disadvantage for developing an amorphous form.

A crystalline compound may contain either a stoichiometric or nonstoichiometric amount of crystallization solvent.[7] Nonstoichiometric adducts, such as inclusions or clathrates, involve entrapped solvent molecules within the crystal lattice. Usually this adduct is undesirable, owing to its lack of reproducibility, and should be avoided for development. A stoichiometric adduct, commonly referred to as a solvate, is a molecular complex that has incorporated the crystallizing solvent molecules into specific sites within the crystal lattice. When the incorporated solvent is water, the complex is called a hydrate, and the terms hemihydrate, monohydrate, and dihydrate describe hydrated forms with molar equivalents of water corresponding to half, one, and two. A compound not containing any water within its crystal structure is termed anhydrous.

Identification of possible hydrate compounds is important since their aqueous solubilities can be significantly less than their anhydrous forms. Conversion of an anhydrous compound to a hydrate within the dosage form may reduce the dissolution rate and extent of drug absorption.

An example of the in vivo importance of solvate forms is shown in Figure 8-9, where the

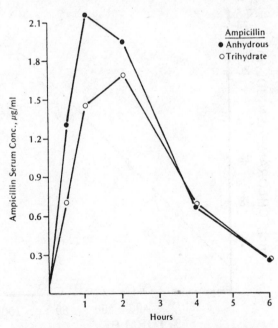

FIG. 8-9. *Mean serum concentrations of ampicillin in human subjects after oral administration of 250-mg doses of two solvate forms of the drug in suspension. Key: •, anhydrous; and ○, trihydrate. (From Poole, J., et al.: Current Therapeutic Research, 10:292, 1968. Reproduced with permission of the copyright owner.)*

anhydrous and trihydrate forms of ampicillin were administered orally as a suspension to human subjects.[8] The more soluble anhydrous form (10 mg/ml) produced higher and earlier peaks in the blood serum levels than the less soluble trihydrate form.

Polymorphism is the ability of a compound (or element) to crystallize as more than one distinct crystalline species with different internal lattices. Chemical stability and solubility changes due to polymorphism can have an impact on a drug's bioavailability and its development program. Chloramphenicol palmitate exists in three crystalline polymorphic forms (A, B, and C) and an amorphous form.[9] Aguiar and co-workers investigated the relative absorption of polymorphic forms A and B from oral suspensions administered to human subjects.[10] As summarized in Figure 8-10, "peak" serum levels increased substantially as a function of the percentage of form B polymorph, the more soluble polymorph.

Many physicochemical properties vary with the internal structure of the solid drug, including melting point, density, hardness, crystal shape, optical properties, and vapor pressure.[11] Characterization of polymorphic and solvated forms involves quantitative analysis of these differing physicochemical properties. Several

TABLE 8-3. *Analytic Methods for Characterization of Solid Forms*

Method	Material Required per Sample
Microscopy	1 mg
Fusion methods (hot stage microscopy)	1 mg
Differential scanning calorimetry (DSC/DTA)	2–5 mg
Infrared spectroscopy	2–20 mg
X-ray powder diffraction	500 mg
Scanning electron microscopy	2 mg
Thermogravimetric analysis	10 mg
Dissolution/solubility analysis	mg to gm

methods for studying solid forms are listed in Table 8-3 along with the sample requirements for each test. In the following sections, three of these techniques are discussed in detail, with particular emphasis on polymorphism.

Microscopy. All substances that are transparent when examined under a microscope that has crossed polarizing filters are either isotropic or anisotropic. Amorphous substances, such as supercooled glasses and noncrystalline solid organic compounds, or substances with cubic crystal lattices, such as sodium chloride, are isotropic materials, which have a single refractive index. With crossed polarizing filters, these isotropic substances do not transmit light, and they appear black. Materials with more than one refractive index are anisotropic and appear bright with brilliant colors (birefringence) against the black polarized background. The interference colors depend upon the crystal thickness and the differences in refractive indices. Anisotropic substances are either uniaxial, having two refractive indices, or biaxial, having three principal refractive indices.

Most drugs are biaxial, corresponding to either an orthorhombic, monoclinic, or triclinic crystal system. Although one refractive index is easily obtained for biaxial systems, proper orientation of the crystal along its crystallographic axes is required to describe the crystalline form completely. Owing to the many possible crystal habits and their appearances at different orientations, these methods require a well-trained optical crystallographer to characterize fully even simple biaxial systems. Crystal morphology differences between polymorphic forms, however, are often sufficiently distinct that the microscope can be used routinely by the less experienced microscopist to describe polymorphic

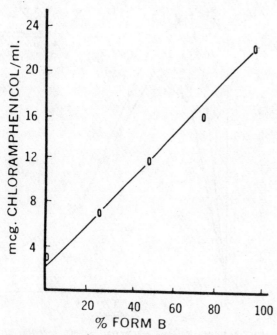

FIG. 8-10. *Correlation of "peak" blood serum levels (2 hr) of chloramphenicol vs. percentage of concentration of polymorph B. (From Aguiar, A. J., et al.: J. Pharm. Sci., 56:847, 1967. Reproduced with permission of the copyright owner.)*

crystal habits and observe transitions induced by heat or solvents.

The polarizing microscope fitted with a hot stage is a useful instrument for investigating polymorphism, melting points, transition temperatures, and rates of transition at controlled heating rates. In addition, the hot-stage microscope facilitates differentiation of DSC endotherms (explained in the next section) for polymorphic transitions from desolvation processes (when the sample is heated in degassed immersion oil). A problem often encountered during thermal microscopy is that organic molecules can degrade during the melting process, and recrystallization of the melt may not occur, because of the presence of contaminant degradation products.

Thermal Analysis. Differential scanning calorimetry (DSC) and differential thermal analysis (DTA) measure the heat loss or gain resulting from physical or chemical changes within a sample as a function of temperature. Examples of endothermic (heat-absorbing) processes are fusion, boiling, sublimation, vaporization, desolvation, solid-solid transitions, and chemical degradation. Crystallization and degradation are usually exothermic processes. Quantitative measurements of these processes have many applications in preformulation studies including purity,[12] polymorphism,[13] solvation,[14] degradation, and excipient compatibility.[15,16]

For characterizing crystal forms, the heat of fusion, ΔH_f, can be obtained from the area-under-the-DSC-curve for the melting endotherm. Similarly, the heat of transition from one polymorph to another may be calculated as shown by Guillory for several sulfonamides.[13] A sharp symmetric melting endotherm can indicate relative purity, whereas broad, asymmetric curves suggest impurities or more than one thermal process. Heating rate affects the kinetics and hence the apparent temperature of solid-solid transitions.

A variable with DSC experiments is the atmosphere in contact with the sample. Usually, a continual nitrogen purge is maintained within the heating chamber; however, the loss of a volatile counter ion such as ethanolamine or acetic acid during a polymorphic transition may produce misleading data unless the transition occurs within a closed system. In contrast, desolvation of a dihydrate species, as shown in Figure 8-11, releases water vapor, which if unvented can generate degradation prior to the melting point of the anhydrous form. During initial testing, a variety of atmospheres should be tried until the observed thermal process becomes fully understood.

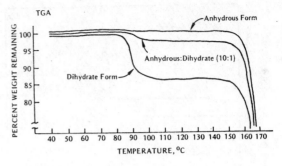

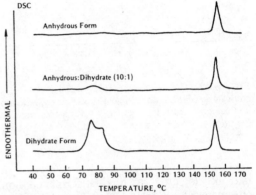

FIG. 8-11. *Thermogravimetric (TGA) and differential scanning calorimetric (DSC) analysis for an acetate salt of an organic amine that has two crystalline forms, anhydrous and dihydrate. Anhydrous/dihydrate mixture was prepared by dry blending. Heating rate was 5°/min.*

Thermogravimetric analysis (TGA) measures changes in sample weight as a function of time (isothermal) or temperature. Desolvation and decomposition processes are frequently monitored by TGA. Comparing TGA and DSC data recorded under identical conditions can greatly aid in the interpretation of thermal processes. In Figure 8-11, the dihydrate form of an acetate salt loses two moles of water via an endothermic transition between 70° and 90°C. The second endotherm at 155°C corresponds to the melting process, with the accompanying weight loss due to vaporization of acetic acid as well as to decomposition.

TGA and DSC analysis can also be used to quantitate the presence of a solvated species within a bulk drug sample. For the above example, 10% of the dihydrate form was easily detected by both methods (Fig. 8-11).

Both DSC and TGA are microtechniques and depend on thermal equilibration within the sample. Significant variables in these methods include sample homogeneity, sample size, particle size, heating rate, sample atmosphere, and sample preparation. Degradation during thermal analysis may provide misleading results, but

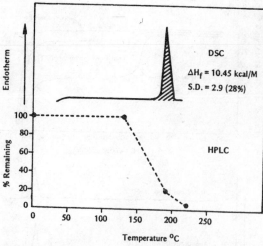

FIG. 8-12. *Differential scanning calorimetric (DSC) analysis and HPLC stability analysis of an organic amine hydrochloride salt that undergoes decomposition upon melting.*

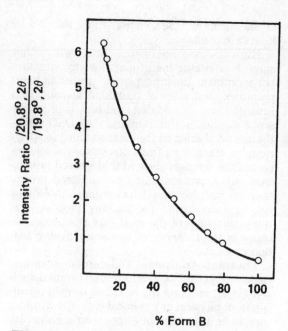

FIG. 8-13. *X-ray intensity ratio as a function of composition of forms A and B of chloramphenicol palmitate. (From Aguiar, A. J., et al.: J. Pharm. Sci., 56:847, 1967. Reproduced with permission of the copyright owner.)*

may be detected by high-performance liquid chromatography (HPLC) analysis of samples heated under representative conditions for retention of drug or appearance of decay products (Fig. 8-12).

X-Ray. An important technique for establishing the batch-to-batch reproducibility of a crystalline form is x-ray powder diffraction. Random orientation of a crystal lattice in a powder sample causes the x-rays to scatter in a reproducible pattern of peak intensities at distinct angles (θ) relative to the incident beam. Each diffraction pattern is characteristic of a specific crystalline lattice for a given compound.[17] An amorphous form does not produce a pattern. Mixtures of different crystalline forms can be analyzed using normalized intensities at specific angles, which are unique for each crystalline form. A typical standard curve is shown in Figure 8-13 for polymorphic forms A and B of chloramphenicol palmitate.

Single-crystal x-ray analysis provides a precise identification and description of a crystalline substance. Unit cell dimensions and angles conclusively establish the crystalline lattice system and provide specific differences between crystalline forms of a given compound. Other methods such as infrared spectroscopy, dilatometry, proton magnetic resonance (PMR), nuclear magnetic resonance spectroscopy (NMR), and scanning electron microscopy (SEM) have additional applications for studying polymorphism and solvation.[11]

Polymorphism

Polymorphs can be classified as one of two types: *enatiotropic* (one polymorph can be reversibly changed into another by varying temperature or pressure, e.g., sulfur) or *monotropic* (one polymorphic form is unstable at all temperatures and pressures, e.g., glyceryl stearates). There is no general way of relating enatiotrophy and monotrophy to the properties of the polymorphs, except by locating the transition temperature or the lack of one. At a specified pressure, usually 1 atmosphere, the temperature at which two polymorphs have identical free energies is the transition temperature, and at that temperature, both forms can coexist and have identical solubilities in any solvent as well as identical vapor pressures. Below the solid melting temperatures, the polymorph with the lower free energy, corresponding to the lower solubility or vapor pressure, is the thermodynamically stable form.

During preformulation, it is important to identify the polymorph that is stable at room temperature and to determine whether polymorphic transitions are possible within the temperature range used for stability studies and during processing (drying, milling, etc.). As discussed by Haleblian and McCrone, a polymorphic compound is best characterized by a complete pressure-temperature phase diagram showing melt-vapor, solid-vapor, and solid-melt curves.[11] A free energy-temperature curve at 1 atmosphere should be constructed since temperature is usually a more critical variable than pressure in pharmaceutics. As previously discussed, chloramphenicol palmitate has three known polymorphic forms, which are thermodynamically described by a van't Hoff plot of free energy (as determined from solubility measurements) versus temperature (Fig. 8-14). Transition temperatures are shown by intersection of the extrapolated lines; 50°C for forms A and C, and 88°C for forms A and B. Form A is the stable form at temperatures less than 50°C.[10]

Transition temperatures obtained by extrapolation of van't Hoff plots are susceptible to large errors. Direct measurements of transitions are preferred to support the extrapolated intersection points in the solubility-temperature diagrams. The most direct means for determining transition temperatures is microscopic observation of samples held at constant temperatures. Unfortunately, these solid-solid or solid-vapor-solid transitions usually occur slowly, owing to large activation energies and slow nucleation. To facilitate the conversion rate, a single polymorph or a mixture of forms can be granulated in a "bridging" solvent at various temperatures. The drug should be only sparingly soluble in the bridging solvent, and solvate formation should not occur. These experiments can be conducted quickly with a polarizing microscope, or samples can be stored in sealed containers at controlled temperatures and periodically examined by other suitable analytic methods.

A more difficult task in the study of poly-

morphism is determination of the relative stability of metastable polymorph and prediction of its rate of conversion within a dosage form. For suspension dosage forms, the rate of conversion can depend on several variables, including drug solubility within the vehicle, presence of nucleation seed for the stable form, temperature, agitation, and particle size. Solid dosage forms such as capsules and tablets have similar complications due to the influence of particle size, moisture, and excipients. In short, the most effective means for evaluating the stability of a metastable polymorph in the dosage form is to initiate prototype formulation work by screening a wide range of factors, including the presence and absence of seed crystals of the stable polymorphic form. Essential to this approach is development of an analytic method that is sensitive to small amounts of the stable polymorph in the presence of the metastable polymorphs and excipients. In most cases, the lower limit of detection for polymorph mixtures is in the range of 2 to 5%.

To screen for additional polymorphic forms of a particular drug, bridging solvents, supersaturated solutions, supercooled melts and sublimination have proven useful.[11] Observation of the drug particles by light microscopy during or after processing by these techniques should provide substantial insight into the preferred crystalline forms of the compound without consuming inordinate quantities of material.

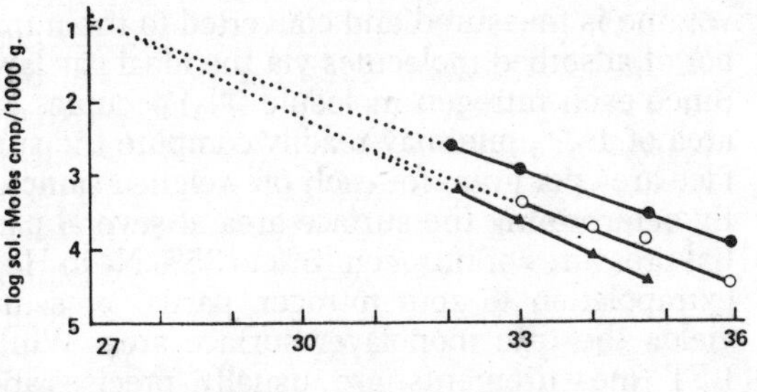

Hygroscopicity

Many drug substances, particularly water-soluble salt forms, have a tendency to adsorb atmospheric moisture. Adsorption and equilibrium moisture content can depend upon the atmospheric humidity, temperature, surface area, exposure, and the mechanism for moisture uptake, as described by Van Campen and co-workers.[18] Deliquescent materials adsorb sufficient water to dissolve completely, as is observed with sodium chloride on a humid day. Other hygroscopic substances adsorb water because of hydrate formation or specific site adsorption. With most hygroscopic materials, changes in moisture level can greatly influence many important parameters, such as chemical stability, flowability, and compactibility.

To test for hygroscopicity, samples of bulk drug are placed in *open* containers with a thin powder bed to assure maximum atmospheric exposure. These samples are then exposed to a range of controlled relative humidity environments prepared with saturated aqueous salt solutions.[19] Moisture uptake should be monitored

FIG. 8-14. *The van't Hoff plot of solubility vs. reciprocal absolute temperature for polymorphs A, B, and C of chloramphenicol palmitate. Key: Polymorphs A (▶—▶); B (●—●); and C (○—○). (From Aguiar, A. J., et al.: J. Pharm. Sci., 58:983, 1969. Reproduced with permission of the copyright owner.)*

at time points representative of handling (0 to 24 hours) and storage (0 to 12 weeks). Analytic methods for monitoring the moisture level (i.e., gravimetry, TGA, Karl Fischer titration, or gas chromatography) depend upon the desired precision and the amount of moisture adsorbed onto the drug sample.

Normalized (mg H_2O/g sample) or percentage-of-weight-gain data from these hygroscopic studies are plotted against time to justify special handling procedures kinetically. A plot of normalized equilibrium versus relative humidity data may support the need for storage in a low-humidity environment or for special packaging with a desiccant. As these studies proceed, additional testing of powder flow, dissolution, or stability of "wet" bulk may be warranted to lend further support to the need for humidity controls.

Fine Particle Characterization

Bulk flow, formulation homogeneity, and surface-area controlled processes such as dissolution and chemical reactivity are directly affected by size, shape, and surface morphology of the drug particles. In general, each new drug candidate should be tested during preformulation with the smallest particle size as is practical to facilitate preparation of homogeneous samples and maximize the drug's surface area for interactions.

A light microscope with a calibrated grid usually provides adequate size and shape characterization for drug particles.[20] Sampling and preparation of the microscopic slide must be preformed carefully to obtain a representative dispersion. Several hundred particles should be sized, and the resulting mean and range of sizes reported as a histogram. The use of photomicrographs and a hemacytometer slide, as well as other sizing techniques, may make this task slightly less strenuous. Although it is time-consuming, light microscopy has few restrictions on particle shape.

In conjunction with light microscopy, stream counting devices, such as the Coulter counter and HIAC counter, often provide a convenient method for characterizing the size distribution of a compound. Samples are prepared for analysis by the Coulter counter by dispersing the material in a conducting medium such as isotonic saline with the aid of ultrasound and a few drops of surfactant. A known volume (0.5 to 2 ml) of this suspension is then drawn into a tube through a small aperture (0.4 to 800 microns in diameter), across which a voltage is applied. As each particle passes through the hole, it is counted and sized according to the resistance generated by displacing that particle's volume of conducting medium. Given that the instrument has been calibrated with standard spheres, the counter provides a histogram output (frequency versus size) within the limits of that particular aperture tube. Several different sizes of aperture tubes should be used to assure accurate counting of single particles. Other stream counters are based on the principles of light blockage or laser light scattering for sizing each particle.[20]

Although the Coulter method is quick and statistically meaningful, it assumes that each resistance arises from a spherical particle; thus, nonspheres are sized inaccurately. Other limitations with the Coulter counter are the tendency of needle-shaped crystals to block the aperture hole, the dissolution of compound in the aqueous conducting medium, and stratification of particles within the suspension. Additional methods of particle size analysis are image analysis and sieve analysis. Sieve methods are used primarily for large samples of relatively large particles (~100 microns). Computer interfacing of image analysis techniques offers the greatest promise for particle size analysis in the '80s.[21]

Kinetic processes involving drug in the solid state, such as dissolution and degradation, may be more directly related to available surface area than to particle size. If drug particles have a shape that can be defined mathematically, then light microscopy size analysis or Coulter counter analysis with appropriate geometric equations may provide a reasonable estimation of surface area.

A more precise measurement of surface area is made by Brunauer, Emmett, and Teller (BET) nitrogen adsorption, in which a layer of nitrogen molecules is adsorbed to the sample surface at $-196°C$. Once surface adsorption has reached equilibrium, the sample is heated to room temperature, the nitrogen gas is desorbed, and its volume is measured and converted to the number of adsorbed molecules via the ideal gas law. Since each nitrogen molecule (N_2) occupies an area of $16A^2$, one may readily compute the surface area per gram for each preweighed sample. By determining the surface area at several partial pressures of nitrogen (5% to 35% N_2 in He), extrapolation to zero nitrogen partial pressure yields the true monolayer surface area. While BET measurements are usually precise and quickly obtained with current commercial equipment, errors may arise from the use of impure gases and volatile surface impurities (e.g., hydrates).

Surface morphology may be observed by scanning electron microscopy (SEM), which serves to confirm qualitatively a physical observation related to surface area. For example, bulk lots of drug recovered by different crystallization processes that have been used in an attempt to improve yield may result in surface morphologies that provide greater area for surface reactions such as degradation, dissolution, or hygroscopicity.

During preparation for SEM analysis, the sample is exposed to high vacuum during the gold coating process, which is needed to make the samples conductive, and concomitant removal of water or other solvents may result in a false picture of the surface morphology. Variable vacuum treatment of an identical sample prior to the gold coating step may confirm the effects of sample preparation on surface morphology. Most modern SEM instruments also provide energy dispersive x-ray spectroscopy analysis of surface metal ions, which may prove beneficial in deciphering an instability or incompatibility problem.

Bulk Density

Bulk density of a compound varies substantially with the method of crystallization, milling, or formulation. Once a density problem is identified, it is often easily corrected by milling, slugging, or formulation. Usually, bulk density is of great importance when one considers the size of a high-dose capsule product or the homogeneity of a low-dose formulation in which there are large differences in drug and excipient densities.

Apparent bulk density (g/ml) is determined by pouring presieved (40-mesh) bulk drug into a graduated cylinder via a large funnel and measuring the volume and weight "as is." Tapped density is determined by placing a graduated cylinder containing a known mass of drug or formulation on a mechanical tapper apparatus, which is operated for a fixed number of taps (~1000) until the powder bed volume has reached a minimum. Using the weight of drug in the cylinder and this minimum volume, the tapped density may be computed. Knowing the anticipated dose and tapped formulation density, one may use Figure 8-15 to determine the appropriate size for a capsule formulation.

In addition to bulk density, it is frequently desirable to know the true density of a powder for computation of void volume or porosity of packed powder beds. Experimentally, the true density is determined by suspending drug particles in solvents of various densities and in which the compound is insoluble. Wetting and pore penetration may be enhanced by the addition of a small quantity of surfactant to the solvent mix-

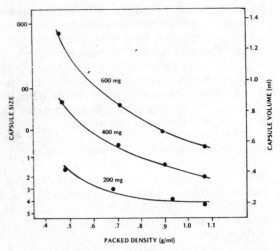

FIG. 8-15. *Correlation between capsule size and packed density for different fill weights (200–600 mg).*

tures. After vigorous agitation, the samples are centrifuged briefly and then left to stand undisturbed until floatation or settling has reached equilibrium. The sample that remains suspended corresponds to the true density of the material. Density of the test solution corresponding to the drug's true density should be checked with a calibrated pycnometer preferably after the test to include any density changes due to dissolved material.

Powder Flow Properties

Pharmaceutical powders may be broadly classified as free-flowing or cohesive (non-free-flowing). Most flow properties are significantly affected by changes in particle size, density, shape, electrostatic charge, and adsorbed moisture, which may arise from processing or formulation.[22] As a result, a free-flowing drug candidate may become cohesive during development, thus necessitating an entirely new formulation strategy. Preformulation powder flow investigations should quantitatively assess the pharmaceutical consequences of each process improvement and provide direction for the formulation development project team. This direction may consist of a formulation recommendation such as granulation or densification via slugging, the need for special auger feed equipment, or a test system for evaluating the improvements in flow brought about by formulation. This subject becomes paramount when attempting to develop a commercial solid dosage form containing a large percentage of cohesive material.

Free-flowing powders may be characterized by a simple flow rate apparatus consisting of a grounded metal tube from which drug flows through an orifice onto an electronic balance, which is connected to a strip chart recorder. Several flow rate (g/sec) determinations at each of a variety of orifice sizes ($\frac{1}{8}$ to $\frac{1}{2}$ inches) should be made. In general, the greater the standard deviation between multiple flow rate measurements, the greater is the weight variation in products produced from that powder.

When several lots of a drug candidate are tested under dissimilar conditions, equation (1), proposed by Jones and Pilpel, may be used to show the dependence of flow rate (W) on true particle density (ρ), gravity (g), and orifice diameter (D_o).[23] Both (A) and (n) are constants that are dependent upon the material and its particle size.

$$D_o = A \left(\frac{4\,W}{60\,\pi\rho\,\sqrt{g}} \right)^{1/n} \tag{1}$$

Another measurement of a free-flowing powder is compressibility, as computed from powder density, equation (2):

$$\% \text{ Compressibility} = \left(\frac{\rho_t - \rho_o}{\rho_t} \right) \times 100 \tag{2}$$

where ρ_t is the tapped bulk density and ρ_o is the initial bulk density. Table 8-4 lists compressibility data and flowability characterization for several pharmaceutical excipients.

While angle of repose determinations are usually useless because of their lack of precision, observation of powder flow from a glass funnel and then a grounded metal funnel provides insight into the drug's flow properties, electrostatic properties, and tendency to brige in a cone-shaped hopper.[24]

Cohesive powders may be characterized by tensile testing or evaluated in a shear cell. Since both methods require large samples of material (>20 g) for testing, these methods are not discussed in this section; rather, the reader is referred to the works of York, Sutton, and Hiestand for experimental details and application of cohesive powder test results to hopper design.[22,25-28]

Solubility Analysis

Preformulation solubility studies focus on drug-solvent systems that could occur during the delivery of a drug candidate. For example, a drug for oral administration should be examined for solubility in media having isotonic chloride ion concentration and acidic pH. Even though the routes of administration may not be explic-

TABLE 8-4. *Compressibility and Flowability of Pharmaceutical Excipients.*

% Compressibility	Flowability
5–15	Excellent
12–16	Good
18–21	Fair–passable
23–35	Poor
33–38	Very poor
<40	Very, very poor

Material	% Compressibility	Flowability
Celutab	11	Excellent
Emcompress	15	Excellent
Star X-1500	19	Fair–passable
Lactose monohydrate	19	Fair–passable
Maize starch	26–27	Poor
Dicalcium phosphate, dihydrate (coarse)	27	Poor
Magnesium stearate	31	Poor
Titanium dioxide	34	Very poor
Dicalcium phosphate, dihydrate (fine)	41	Very, very poor
Talc	49	Very, very poor

From Jones, T.M.: Pharmazeutische Industrie, 39:469, 1977. Reproduced with permission of the copyright owner.

itly defined at this time, understanding the drug's solubility profile and possible solubilization mechanisms provides a basis for later formulation work. Preformulation solubility studies usually include determinations of pKa, temperature dependence, pH solubility profile, solubility products, solubilization mechanisms, and rate of dissolution.[29]

Analytic methods that are particularly useful for solubility measurements include HPLC, UV spectroscopy, fluorescence spectroscopy, and gas chromatography. For most drugs, reverse phase HPLC offers an efficient and accurate means of collecting solubility data. Its major advantages are direct analysis of aqueous samples, high sensitivity, and specific determination of drug concentration due to chromatographic separation of drug from impurities or degradation products.

Solubility and dissolution experiments should have all factors defined, including pH, temperature, ionic strength, and buffer concentrations. For an equilibrium solubility determination, excess drug dispersed in solvent is agitated at a constant temperature. Samples of the slurry are withdrawn as a function of time, clarified by centrifugation, and assayed to establish a plateau concentration. The solid precipitate is also characterized to establish the equilibrium solid form of the drug.

Problems encountered with sample workup can involve adsorption or incomplete removal of the excess drug during filtration or centrifugation steps. In addition, if excess drug is not a solid but an oil, sample preparation may be even more difficult. In particular, drugs capable of ionization may require different methods of removing excess drug, owing to altered adsorption properties. Filtered saturated solutions should be carefully examined using a high-intensity light beam to detect the presence of a finely dispersed oil or solid. Solutions can also be examined conveniently with a light microscope, with which particles or droplets of 1 μ or greater can be distinguished if present in sufficient concentration.

Solubility values that are useful in a candidate's early development are those in distilled water, 0.9% NaCl, 0.01M HCl, 0.1M HCl, and 0.1M NaOH, all at room temperature as well as at pH 7.4 buffer at 37°C. These early results are useful in developing suspensions or solutions for toxicologic and pharmacologic studies. Furthermore, these studies identify those candidates with a potential for bioavailability problems. Drugs having limited solubility (<1%) in the fluids of the gastrointestinal tract often exhibit poor or erratic absorption unless dosage forms are specifically tailored for the drug.[30] Solubility profiles are not predictors of biologic performance, but do provide rationale for more extensive in vivo studies and formulation development prior to drug evaluation in humans.

pKa Determinations

Determination of the dissociation constant for a drug capable of ionization within a pH range of 1 to 10 is important since solubility, and consequently absorption, can be altered by orders of magnitude with changing pH. The Henderson-Hasselbalch equation provides an estimate of the ionized and un-ionized drug concentration at a particular pH.

For acidic compounds:

$$pH = pKa + \log \frac{[\text{ionized drug}]}{[\text{un-ionized drug}]}$$

For basic compounds:

$$pH = pKa + \log \frac{[\text{un-ionized drug}]}{[\text{ionized drug}]} \quad (3)$$

For a weakly acidic drug with pKa value greater than 3, the un-ionized form is present within the acidic contents of the stomach, but the drug is ionized predominantly in the neutral

media of the intestine. For basic drugs such as erythromycin and papaverine, (pKa ~ 8 to 9), the ionized form is predominant in both the stomach and intestine. In general, the un-ionized drug molecule is the species absorbed from the gastrointestinal tract; however, rate of dissolution, lipid solubility, common ion effects, and metabolism in the GI tract can shift or reverse predictions of the extent and site of absorption based on pH alone.

A pKa value can be determined by a variety of analytic methods. Buffer, temperature, ionic strength, and cosolvent affect the pKa value and should be controlled for these determinations. The preferred method is the detection of spectral shifts by ultraviolet (UV) or visible spectroscopy since dilute aqueous solutions can be analyzed directly. A second method, potentiometric titration, offers maximum sensitivity for compounds with pKa values in the range of 3 to 10 but is often hindered by precipitation of the un-ionized form during the titration since a high drug concentration is usually required to obtain a significant titration curve. To prevent precipitation, a cosolvent such as methanol or dimethylsulfoxide can be incorporated to maintain sufficient solubility for the un-ionized species, and the pKa value is extrapolated from titration data collected for various cosolvent concentrations. As shown in Figure 8-16, dependence of the dissociation constant on cosolvent can be highly sig-

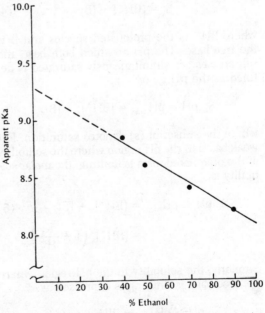

FIG. 8-16. *The pKa determination for an organic amine drug candidate whose un-ionized form is exceedingly insoluble in water.*

nificant, and extrapolations provide only an estimate of the pKa value. In general, the use of cosolvent yields higher pKa values for acids and lower values for bases than does pure water.

With insoluble drugs, the dependence of solubility on pH can also be used to obtain pKa values. For this third method, the pKa corresponds to the pH of the solution where the equilibrium solubility is twice the value for the intrinsic solubility of the un-ionized form. If other solubility determining factors such as solute-solute association or solubility products become significant owing to the titrant used to adjust the pH, then pKa values may be incorrectly determined by this procedure. Many references are available containing composite lists of pKa values for various functional groups and organic molecules, which facilitate initial estimates for dissociation constants.[31] In addition, Albert and Serjeant have provided detailed descriptions of several experimental methods for determining pKa values.[32]

pH Solubility Profile and Common Ion Effects

The solubility of an acidic or basic drug depends on the pKa of the ionizing functional group and the intrinsic solubilities for both the ionized and un-ionized forms. For a basic drug, the total molar solubility, S_t, is equal to the following summation:

$$S_t = [BH^+] + [B] \qquad (4)$$

where BH^+ is the protonated species and B is the free base. The pH at which both base and salt species are simultaneously saturated is defined as the pH_{max} or:

$$S_t, pH = pH_{max} = [BH^+]_s + [B]_s \qquad (5)$$

where the subscript (s) denotes saturation. For weak bases in the pH region where the solubility of the protonated form is limiting, the molar solubility is:

$$S_t, pH < pH_{max} = [BH^+]_s + [B] \qquad (6)$$

$$= [BH^+]_s \left(1 + \frac{K_a}{H^+}\right)$$

Similarly, the solubility in the pH region where the free base is limiting is expressed as:

$$S_t, pH > pH_{max} = [BH^+] + [B]_s \qquad (7)$$

$$= [B]_s \left(1 + \frac{H^+}{K_a}\right)$$

It therefore follows that the pH_{max} is defined as:

$$pH_{max} = pKa + \log \frac{[B]_s}{[BH^+]_s} \qquad (8)$$

At a solution pH equivalent to pH_{max}, both the free base and salt form can exist simultaneously in equilibrium with a saturated solution. The pH_{max} is verified by sampling precipitated drug from the equilibrated solution and confirming the presence of both drug forms. Solubility expressions for acidic drugs are derived in a similar fashion.[33]

When the ionized or salt form of a drug is the solubility-limiting species in solution, the concentration of the paired counter ion is usually the solubility determining factor. For a hydrochloride salt of a basic amine, the equilibrium between the solid and ionized species in solution is approximated by the following expression:

$$[BH^+ Cl^-]_{solid} \overset{K_{sp}}{\rightleftharpoons} [BH^+] + [Cl^-] \qquad (9)$$

where K_{sp} is the solubility product for the protonated species and chloride counter ion, or:

$$K_{sp} = [BH^+][Cl^-] \qquad (10)$$

If the contribution of the un-ionized species is negligible as compared with the protonated form, the total drug solubility decreases as the chloride ion concentration increases. In this case, the apparent solubility product is defined as:

$$K_{sp} = S_t [Cl^-] \qquad (11)$$

Experimental determination of a solubility product should include measurement of pH as well as assays of both drug and counter ion concentrations. To compute the thermodynamic solubility product, concentrations should be converted to activities with appropriate corrections for activity coefficient dependence on ionic strength.[34,35]

In summary, aqueous solubility profiles for ionizable compounds over large pH ranges with varying counter ion concentrations are functions of many variables, as given by the following expression for an organic amine drug:

$$S_t = f (pH, pK_a, [B]_s, K_{sp}, anions) \qquad (12)$$

These parameters also depend on ionic strength, temperature, and the aqueous media composition. Consequently, pH solubility profiles can appear dramatically different for compounds with similar functional groups. A particularly useful reference by Kramer and Flynn for organic hydrochlorides highlights pH solubility profile dependence on solvent composition.[36] While most of this discussion has focused on solubility product limitations of basic compounds, similar analyses may be made for acidic drugs.

The pH solubility profile for doxycycline (pKa 3.4) reported by Bogardus and Backwood illustrates a common ion effect for an amine hydrochloride salt.[37] As shown in Figure 8-17, the solubility in aqueous medium with pH 2 or less logarithmically decreased as a function of pH (which was adjusted with hydrochloric acid) because of corresponding increases in the chloride ion concentration. In gastric juice, where the pH can range from 1 to 2 and the chloride ion concentration is between $0.1M$ and $0.15M$, doxycycline hydrochloride dihydrate has a solubility of ~4 mg/ml, which is a factor of 7 less than its solubility in distilled water. For the hydrochloride salts of chlortetracycline, demeclocycline, and methacycline, the apparent dissolu-

tion rates and solubilities were even less than their respective free base forms in media containing chloride ion.[38] Consequently, the solubility product for each ionizable compound with either sodium or chloride ions should be evaluated to detect potential in vivo problems with dissolution and/or absorption.

Another point illustrated with doxycycline is that nonideal behavior of a solution species can dramatically affect the solubility at certain pH values. Doxycycline was shown to form dimeric species involving self-association of the protonated form. This mechanism accounted for the large positive deviation from ideal behavior, in which actual solubility values are a factor of 10 higher at pH 2.0. Therefore, actual solubility profiles should be experimentally determined within the pH region of interest.

Effect of Temperature

The heat of solution, ΔH_s, represents the heat released or absorbed when a mole of solute is dissolved in a large quantity of solvent. Most commonly, the solution process is endothermic, or ΔH_s is positive, and thus increasing the solution temperature increases the drug solubility. For such solutes as lithium chloride and other hydrochloride salts that are ionized when dissolved, the process is exothermic (negative ΔH_s) such that higher temperatures suppress the solubility.

Heats of solution are determined from solubility values for saturated solutions equilibrated at controlled temperatures over the range of interest. Typically, the temperature range should include 5°C, 25°C, 37°C, and 50°C. The working equation for determining ΔH_s is:

$$\ln S = \frac{-\Delta H_s}{R}\left(\frac{1}{T}\right) + C \qquad (13)$$

where S is the molar solubility at temperature T (°kelvin) and R is the gas constant. Over limited temperature ranges, a semilogarithmic plot of solubility against reciprocal temperature is linear, and ΔH_s is obtained from the slope. For nonelectrolytes and un-ionized forms of weak acids and bases dissolved in water, heats of solution are usually in the range of 4 to 8 kcal/mole. Salt forms of drugs are often less sensitive to temperature and may have heats of solution between −2 and 2 kcal/mole.

In Figure 8-18, examples of ΔH_s determinations are shown for the free base and hydrochloride salt of an organic amine as reported by Kramer and Flynn.[36] Although the ΔH_s for the free

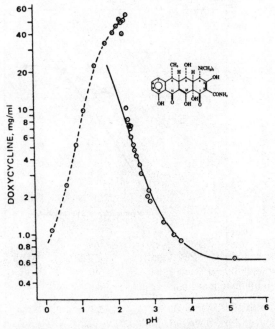

FIG. 8-17. *The pH-solubility profile for doxycycline in aqueous hydrochloric acid at 25°C. At pH = 2.16, both doxycycline monohydrate and doxycycline hydrochloride dihydrate were in equilibrium with solution. Theoretic curves are detailed by authors. (From Bogardus, J. B., and Blackwood, R. K.: J. Pharm. Sci., 68:188, 1979. Reproduced with permission of the copyright owner, the American Pharmaceutical Association.)*

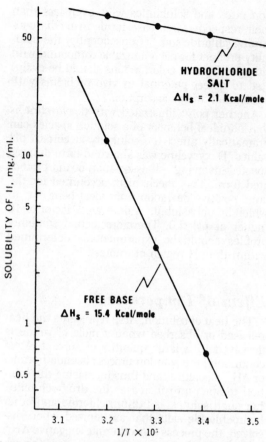

FIG. 8-18. *Plot of hydrochloride and free base solubilities for etoxadrol, an organic amine, against reciprocal temperature. (From Kramer, S. F., and Flynn, G. L.: J. Pharm. Sci., 61:1896, 1972. Reproduced with permission of the copyright owner.)*

base is somewhat large, a 10° change in temperature produces a fivefold change in solubility. This finding would certainly affect solution dosage form design and storage conditions. In addition, solvent systems involving cosolvents, micelles, and complexation have very different heats of solution in comparison to water.

Solubilization

For drug candidates with either poor water solubility or insufficient solubility for projected solution dosage forms, preformulation studies should include limited experiments to identify possible mechanisms for solubilization. A general means of increasing solubility is the addition of a cosolvent to the aqueous system. The solubility of poorly soluble nonelectrolytes can often be improved by orders of magnitude with suitable cosolvents such as ethanol, propylene glycol, and glycerin.[39] These cosolvents solubi-

lize drug molecules by disrupting the hydrophobic interactions of water at the nonpolar solute/water interfaces. The extent of solubilization due to the addition of cosolvent depends on the chemical structure of the drug, that is, the more nonpolar the solute, the greater is the solubilization achieved by cosolvent addition. This relationship is illustrated in Figure 8-19 for hydrocortisone and hydrocortisone 21-heptanoate.[40] The lipophilic ester is solubilized to a greater extent by additions of propylene glycol than by the more polar parent compound.

Cosolvent effects for dissociated drug molecules are usually much less, as shown by Kramer and Flynn.[36] Some poorly soluble drugs can be solubilized in micellar solutions such as 0.01M Tween 20, or via molecular complexes as with caffeine.[41,42] These specific formulations are usually not developed during the preformulation phase, however.

Partition Coefficient

A measurement of a drug's lipophilicity and an indication of its ability to cross cell membranes is the oil/water partition coefficient in

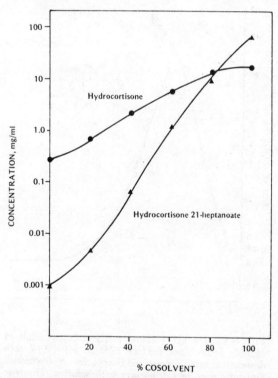

FIG. 8-19. *Solubility of hydrocortisone and hydrocortisone 21-heptanoate in propylene glycol-water mixtures. (From Hagen, T. A.: Ph.D. dissertation, University of Michigan, Ann Arbor, Michigan, 1979.)*

systems such as octanol/water and chloroform/water. The partition coefficient is defined as the ratio of un-ionized drug distributed between the organic and aqueous phases at equilibrium.

$$P_{o/w} = \left(\frac{C_{oil}}{C_{water}}\right)_{equilibrium} \qquad (14)$$

For series of compounds, the partition coefficient can provide an empiric handle in screening for some biologic properties.[43] For drug delivery, the lipophilic/hydrophilic balance has been shown to be a contributing factor for the rate and extent of drug absorption.[44,45] Although partition coefficient data alone does not provide understanding of in vivo absorption, it does provide a means of characterizing the lipophilic/hydrophilic nature of the drug.

Dissolution

Dissolution of a drug particle is controlled by several physicochemical properties, including chemical form, crystal habit, particle size, solubility, surface area, and wetting properties. When coupled with equilibrium solubility data, dissolution experiments can help to identify potential bioavailability problem areas. For example, dissolution of solvate and polymorphic forms of a drug can have a significant impact on bioavailability and drug delivery.

The dissolution rate of a drug substance in which surface area is constant during dissolution is described by the modified Noyes-Whitney equation:

$$\frac{dC}{dt} = \frac{DA}{hV}(C_s - C) \qquad (15)$$

where D is the diffusion coefficient, h is the thickness of the diffusion layer at the solid-liquid interface, A is the surface area of drug exposed to dissolution media, V is the volume of media, C_s is the concentration of a saturated solution of the solute in the dissolution medium at the experimental temperature, and C is the concentration of drug in solution at time t. The dissolution rate is given by dC/dt. If the surface area of the drug is held constant and $C_s >> C$, then equation (15) can be rearranged and integrated to give the working equation:

$$\frac{W}{A} = k\,t \qquad (16)$$

where the constant k is defined as:

$$k = \frac{D}{h}C_s \qquad (17)$$

and W is the weight (mg) of drug dissolved in time t.

A plot of W versus t gives a straight line with the slope equal to the intrinsic dissolution rate constant k,[46,47] usually expressed in units of $mg/cm^2/min$.

Experimentally, a constant surface area is obtained by compressing powder into a disc of known area with a die and punch apparatus. Either of the two systems shown in Figure 8-20 can be used to maintain uniform hydrodynamic conditions (k constant). The rotating disc method or Wood's apparatus permits the hydrodynamics of the system to be varied in a mathematically well-defined manner.[48] The static disc method is used because it is conveniently available, but it contains an element of undefined turbulence, which necessitates calibration with standards. Potential problems with this method are transformations of the crystal form, such as polymorphic transformations or desolvation, during its compression into a pellet or during the dissolution experiment. Since many drug candidates are weak acids and bases, pH and common ion gradients at the solid-liquid interface can lead to erroneous conclusions, as discussed by Mooney and co-workers.[49,50]

Dissolution experiments with drug suspensions are further complicated by changing surface area, changing surface crystal morphology, and interstitial wetting.[51] However, dissolution profiles with excess drug can be used to characterize metastable polymorphs or solvates. In Figure 8-21, the conversion of the metastable form II to form I is shown to occur in an organic solvent medium, which clearly depicts form I as the thermodynamically stable form at room temperature. Static pellet dissolution rates also substantiated that form II was the higher energy form since its dissolution rate was significantly greater (Table 8-5).

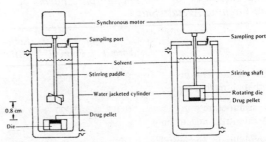

FIG. 8-20. *Constant surface area dissolution apparatus. Left: static disc dissolution apparatus. Right: rotating disc apparatus.*

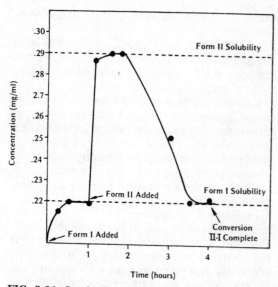

FIG. 8-21. *Powder dissolution profiles for two polymorphic forms of an organic acetate salt in acetonitrile at 25°C.*

Stability Analysis

Preformulation stability studies are usually the first quantitative assessment of chemical stability of a new drug. These studies include both solution and solid state experiments under conditions typical for the handling, formulation, storage, and administration of a drug candidate. This section focuses on the evaluation of chemical stability during preformulation research. Test protocols and experimental methods are emphasized in lieu of kinetic theory, which is presented later in this chapter. In addition, the reader is referred to the literature for comprehensive reviews of drug stability.[52-55]

TABLE 8-5. *Comparison of Dissolution Rates* and Solubility for Two Polymorphic Forms of an Organic Acetate Salt.*

	Form I	Form II	Ratio I/II
Dissolution rate in ethanol, mg/cm²/min	0.57	0.69	.83
Dissolution rate in Acetonitrile, mg/cm²/min	0.017	0.027	.62
Solubility in Acetonitrile, mg/ml	.22	.29	.75

*Dissolution rates measured with a static-disc apparatus.

Essential to a meaningful chemical stability study are multiple samples and development of a specific assay that quantitates intact drug as well as decay products (thus assuring mass balance accountability). Over the past decade, high-performance liquid chromatography has emerged as the analytic method of choice for specificity and quantitation even in complex systems. Development of a valid stability assay requires authentic pure samples of each decay product, which may be supplied by the synthetic chemists or may be isolated from samples that have been intentionally degraded by excessive acid, base, or heat.

During drug development, several bulk lots are produced, reflecting scale-up and process improvements in yield, purity, and possibly crystallinity. The first lot used for preformulation stability studies may not be representative of the commercial bulk product, but it does provide baseline data. In subsequent evaluations, parallel testing of the initial bulk lot of drug with the new bulk or formulation aids in forming conclusions about progress of the project.

Upon completion of the initial stability tests, one or more challenge models indicating stability may emerge that may be useful for limited testing on future bulk lots or formulations. Should a particularly difficult instability problem arise during drug development, then an in-depth elucidation of the decay mechanism may suggest a stabilization approach or underscore the futility of the stabilization effort.

Stability In Toxicology Formulations

Since toxicology studies typically commence early in drug development, it is often advisable to evaluate samples of the toxicology preparations for stability and potential homogeneity problems. Usually, a drug is administered to the animals in their feed, or by oral gavage of a solution or suspension of the drug in an aqueous vehicle.

Water, vitamins, minerals (metal ions), enzymes and a multitude of functional groups are present in feed, which can severely reduce the shelf-life of a drug. Enzyme activity and moisture levels typically decrease with time while feed composition varies with the "consumer"; thus, a fresh sample of feed to be used in the toxicology test provides the most relevant stability data. Since enzyme activity and mobility of adsorbed water vary substantially with temperature, it is recommended that storage temperature typical of the toxicology laboratory be used for this stability study.

Solution and suspension toxicologic preparations should be checked for ease of manufacture and then stored in flame-sealed ampules at various temperatures. In addition to chemical stability, the suspensions should be subjected to an occasional shaking to check dispersability. When analyzing the suspension data, drug solubility at the same temperature and pH may suggest that only drug in solution is undergoing decomposition.

Solution Stability

The primary objective of this phase of preformulation research is identification of conditions necessary to form a stable solution. These studies should include the effects of pH, ionic strength, cosolvent, light, temperature, and oxygen.

Solution stability investigations usually commence with probing experiments to confirm decay at the extremes of pH and temperature (e.g., 0.1N HCl, water, and 0.1N NaOH all at 90°C). These intentionally degraded samples may be used to confirm assay specificity as well as to provide estimates for maximum rates of degradation. This initial experiment should be followed by the generation of a complete pH-rate profile to identify the pH of maximum stability. Aqueous buffers are used to produce solutions over a wide range of pH values with constant levels of drug, cosolvent, and ionic strength.

Since most solution pharmaceuticals are intended for parenteral routes of administration, this initial pH-rate study should be conducted at a constant ionic strength that is compatible with physiologic media. The ionic strength (μ) of an isotonic 0.9% sodium chloride solution is 0.15, and several compendia contain recipes for isotonic buffer solutions. Ionic strength for any new buffer solution may be calculated from the following equation:

$$\mu = \tfrac{1}{2} \Sigma m_i Z_i^2 \qquad (18)$$

where m_i is the molar concentration of the ion, which has valence Z_i. Note that all ionic species (even the drug molecules) in the buffer solution must be considered in computing ionic strength. Table 8-6 illustrates a comprehensive account-

TABLE 8-6. *Comprehensive Accounting of Buffer Species[a] in Constant Ionic Strength ($\mu = 0.5$) Solutions Used to Generate a pH-Rate Profile for Ampicillin*

Obs.	pH Required	Total Citrate[b] $\times 10^2$	$H_3A \times 10^2$	$H_2A^- \times 10^2$	$HA^= \times 10^2$	$A^= \times 10^2$	Total Phosphate[c] $\times 10^2$	$H_3PO_4 \times 10^2$	$H_2PO_4^- \times 10^2$	$HPO_4^= \times 10^2$	$k_{obs} \times 10^3\ hr^{-1}$
2.05	2.0[d]	9.90	9.19	0.72	—	—	0.20	0.09	0.10	—	58.85
2.34	2.4	9.40	7.87	1.53	—	—	1.20	0.32	0.88	—	56.02
2.55	2.6	8.90	6.79	2.10	0.01	—	2.18	0.41	1.77	—	52.97
2.96	3.0	7.94	4.42	3.45	0.06	—	4.11	0.34	3.76	—	42.77
3.56	3.6	6.78	1.65	5.09	0.12	—	6.44	0.14	6.29	—	24.73
3.91	4.0	6.14	0.70	4.62	0.82	—	7.71	0.06	7.64	0.01	15.34
4.48	4.6	5.32	0.35	2.92	2.05	—	9.35	0.02	9.25	0.07	7.65
4.67	4.8	5.07	0.05	2.39	2.61	0.06	9.86	0.01	9.72	0.12	6.43
4.91	5.0	4.85	0.02	1.69	3.01	0.11	10.30	—	10.10	0.10	5.37
5.31	5.4	4.42	0.01	0.75	3.34	0.32	11.15	—	10.62	0.53	5.53
5.71	5.8	3.95	0.01	0.26	2.97	0.71	12.09	—	10.74	1.35	6.80
5.86	6.0	3.68	—	0.19	2.52	0.96	12.63	—	10.53	2.10	11.23
6.25	6.4	3.07	—	0.07	2.68	0.32	13.85	—	9.25	4.62	13.61
6.44	6.6	2.72	—	0.05	1.07	1.63	14.55	—	8.11	6.44	17.79
6.85	7.0	1.76	—	0.01	0.37	1.39	16.47	—	5.50	10.97	26.81
7.19	7.2	1.30	—	—	0.18	1.11	17.39	—	4.18	13.20	31.32
7.55	7.6	0.63	—	—	0.04	0.59	18.73	—	2.10	16.63	32.79
7.94	8.0	0.27	—	—	0.01	0.26	19.45	—	0.93	18.52	53.78

[a]The buffers were made from McIlvaine, T.C.: J. Biochem., 49:183, 1921, and all citrate and phosphate ions are concentrations in moles/L. [b]The ionization constants of citric acid and citrate ions at 35° are $pK_1 = 3.11$, $pK_2 = 4.75$; $pK_3 = 6.42$, from Bates, R.G., and Pinching, G.D.: J. Am. Chem. Soc., 71:2374, 1949. [c]The ionization constants of phosphoric acid and phosphate at 35° ($\mu = 0.5$) are $pK_1 = 1.96$; $pK_2 = 6.70$, from Schwartz, M.A., Granatek, A.P., and Buckwalter, F.H., J. Pharm. Sci., 51:523, 1962. [d]The buffer was made by mixing 990 ml of 0.1 M citric acid with 10 ml of 0.2 M Na$_2$HPO$_4$ to make a liter.

From Hou, J.P., and Poole, J.W.: J. Pharm. Sci., 58:447, 1969. Reproduced with permission of the copyright owner, the American Pharmaceutical Association.

ing of buffer molecules in constant ionic strength solutions, which were used by Hou and Poole in generating a pH-rate profile for ampicillin.[56]

Cosolvents may be needed to achieve drug concentrations that are necessary for analytic sensitivity, or to produce a defined initial condition. Cosolvents selected from the alcohol family could prove beneficial, as most pharmaceutical solvents contain hydroxy groups. If several cosolvent levels are used to prepare these initial samples, then the apparent decay rates may vary linearly with the reciprocal of the resulting solution dielectric constant.[57] The apparent pH of a buffer solution also varies, owing to the presence of cosolvent.

Once the stability solutions are prepared, aliquots are placed in flint glass ampules, flame-sealed to prevent evaporation, and stored at constant temperatures not exceeding the boiling point of the most volatile cosolvent or its azeotrope. Some of the ampules may be stored at a variety of temperatures to provide data for calculating activation energies.

Some of these solution samples should be subjected to a light stability test, which includes protective packaging in amber and yellow-green glass containers.[58] Control samples for this light test may be stored in cardboard packages or wrapped in aluminum foil.

Given that the potential for oxidation is initially unknown, some of the solution samples should also be subjected to further testing (1) with an excessive headspace of oxygen, (2) with a headspace of an inert gas such as helium or nitrogen, (3) with an inorganic antioxidant such as sodium metabisulfite, and (4) with an organic antioxidant such as butylated hydroxytoluene-BHT. Headspace composition can be controlled if the samples are stored in vials for injection that are capped with Teflon-coated rubber stoppers. After penetrating the stoppers with needles, the headspace is flooded with the desired atmosphere, and the resulting needle holes are sealed with wax to prevent degassing.

To generate a pH-rate profile, stability data generated at each pH and temperature condition are analyzed kinetically to yield the apparent decay rate constants. All of the rate constants at a single temperature are then plotted as a function of pH as shown in Figure 8-22. The minimum in this curve is the pH of maximum stability. Often, this plot, as it approaches its limits, provides insight into the molecular involvement of hydrogen or hydroxide ions in the decay mechanism.[59]

An Arrhenius plot is constructed by plotting the logarithm of the apparent decay rate con-

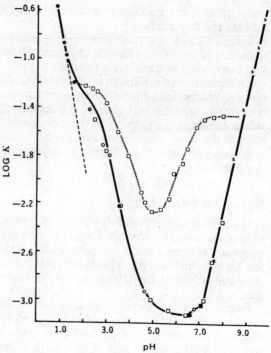

FIG. 8-22. *The pH-rate profiles for ampicillin degradation in solution at 35°C and constant ionic strength ($\mu = 0.5$). Dotted line is the apparent rate profile in the presence of buffer, while the solid line is the theoretic rate profile at zero buffer concentration. (From Hou, J. P., and Poole, J. W.: J. Pharm. Sci., 58:447, 1969. Reproduced with permission of the copyright owner.).*

stant versus the reciprocal of the absolute temperature at which each particular buffer solution was stored during the stability test. To justify extrapolation to "use" conditions, stability storage temperatures should be selected that incrementally ($\Delta t \sim 10°C$) approach the anticipated "use" temperature. If this relationship is linear, one may assume a constant decay mechanism over this temperature range and calculate an activation energy (Ea) from the slope ($-Ea/R$) of the line described by:

$$\ln k = \frac{-E_a}{R}\left(\frac{1}{T}\right) + C \qquad (19)$$

where C is a constant of integration and R is the gas constant.

A broken or nonlinear Arrhenius plot suggests a change in the rate-limiting step of the reaction or a change in decay mechanism, thus making extrapolation unreliable. In a solution-state oxidation reaction, for example, the apparent decay rate constant decreases with elevation of temperature because the solubility of oxygen in water decreases. At elevated temperatures, excipients or buffers may also degrade to give products that are incompatible with the drug under study. Often, inspection of the HPLC chromatograms for decay products confirms a change in the decay mechanism.

Shelf-life ($t_{10\%}$) for a drug at "use" conditions may be calculated from the appropriate kinetic equation, and the decay rate constant obtained from the Arrhenius plot. For a first-order decay process, shelf-life is computed from:

$$t_{10\%} = \frac{-\ln 0.90}{k_1} = \frac{0.105}{k_1} \qquad (20)$$

where $t_{10\%}$ is the time for 10% decay to occur with apparent first-order decay constant k_1. Frequently, it is useful to present the pH-rate profile as a plot of pH versus $t_{10\%}$ shelf-life data.

Results of these initial solution stability studies dictate the subsequent course of action. If the compound is sufficiently stable, liquid formulation development may commence at once. If the compound is unstable, then further investigations may be necessary.

Solid State Stability

The primary objectives of this investigation are identification of stable storage conditions for drug in the solid state and identification of compatible excipients for a formulation. Contrary to the earlier solution stability profile, these solid state studies may be severely affected by changes in purity and crystallinity, which often result from process improvements.[60] Repetitive testing of the initial bulk lot in parallel with newer bulk lots should be expected, and adequate material should be set aside for these studies.

In general, solid state reactions are much slower and more difficult to interpret than solution state reactions, owing to a reduced number of molecular contacts between drug and excipient molecules and to the occurrence of multiple-phase reactions.[61,62] A kinetic analysis of slow solid state degradation based on retention of intact drug may fail to quantitate clearly the compound's shelf-life, as assay variation may equal or exceed the limited apparent degradation, particularly at the low temperatures that are critical to establishing a room-temperature shelf-life. Usually, this situation may be corrected on analysis of the appearance of decay product(s), which may total only 1 to 5% of the sample. Additional analytic data from such studies as TLC, fluorescence, or UV/VIS spectroscopy may be required to determine precisely the kinetics of

decay product(s) appearance, and to establish a room-temperature shelf-life for the drug candidate.

To study the many possible solid state reactions, one may need more than a specific assay for the intact compound. Polymorphic changes, for example, are usually detected by differential scanning calorimetry or quantitative infrared analysis (IR). In the case of surface discoloration due to oxidation or reaction with excipients, surface reflectance measurements on tristimulus or diffuse reflectance equipment may be more sensitive than HPLC assay. In any event, additional samples are required in the solid state stability study to accommodate these additional tests.

To determine the solid state stability profile of a new compound, weighed samples are placed in open screw cap vials and are exposed directly to a variety of temperatures, humidities, and light intensities for up to 12 weeks (Fig. 8-23). Samples usually consist of three 5- to 10-mg weighed samples at each data point for HPLC analysis and approximately 10 to 50 mg of sample for polymorph evaluation by DSC and IR (~2 mg in KBr and ~20 mg in Nujol). To test for surface oxidation, samples are stored in large (25-ml) vials for injection capped with a Teflon-lined rubber stopper and the headspace flooded with dry oxygen. To confirm that the decay observed is due solely to oxygen rather than to reduced humidity, a second set of vials should be tested in which the atmosphere is flooded with dry nitrogen. After a fixed exposure time, these samples are removed and analyzed by multiple

Storage Condition	4 Weeks	8 Weeks	12 Weeks
5°C—Refrigerator			
22°C—Room Temperature			
37°C—Ambient Humidity			
37°C/75% R.H.			
Light Box			
Clear Glass			
Amber Glass			
Yellow-Green Glass			
No Exposure (Control)			
50°C—Ambient Humidity			
$-O_2$ Headspace			
$-N_2$ Headspace			
70°C—Ambient Humidity			
90°C—Ambient Humidity			

FIG. 8-23. *Sample scheme for determining the bulk stability profile for a new drug candidate. At each point, bulk drug samples should consist of 3 × 10 mg for HPLC analysis and a 50-mg sample for polymorph analysis by DSC or IR.*

methods to check for chemical stability, polymorphic changes, and discoloration.

Once the results of this initial screen are tabulated, the decay process may be analyzed by either zero-order or first-order kinetics, particularly if the amount of decay is less than 15 to 20%. The same kinetic order should be used to analyze the data at each temperature if possible. Samples exposed to oxygen, light, and humidity may suggest the need for a followup stability test at three or more levels of a given parameter for full quantitation of its involvement.

In the event that humidity is not a factor in drug stability, an Arrhenius plot may be constructed; if linear, it may be extrapolated to "use" conditions for predicting a shelf-life. If humidity directly affects drug stability, the concentration of water in the atmosphere may be determined from the relative humidity and temperature by using psychrometric charts.[63] Stability data obtained at various humidities may be linearized with respect to moisture using the following apparent decay rate constant:

$$k_H = \left[gpl \right] \cdot k_0 \qquad (21)$$

where [gpl] is the concentration of water in the atmosphere in units of grams of water per liter of dry air, and k_0 is the decay rate constant at zero relative humidity. For example, a 75% relative humidity atmosphere at 37°C is equivalent to 0.0405 grams of water per liter (gpl) of dry air. When the effect of moisture on chemical stability is examined in detail, a comparison to solution state stability and hygroscopicity data may suggest an aqueous reaction occurring in the drug-saturated water layer on the crystal surface.

Another useful relationship for analyzing solid state stability data assumes that a compound must partially liquefy prior to decomposition. Given that the mole fraction of the solid that has liquefied (F_m) is directly proportional to its decay rate, then:

$$\ln k_{app} \; \alpha \; \ln F_m = \frac{-\Delta H_{fus}}{R} \left[\frac{1}{T} - \frac{1}{T_m} \right] \qquad (22)$$

where ΔH_{fus} is the molar heat of fusion, Tm is the absolute melting point (°kelvin), T is the absolute temperature of the stability study, and R is the gas constant.

Once bulk drug stability has been determined, compatibility with excipients commonly used to produce solid dosage forms must be established. The number of excipients may be reduced by considering the results of the solid state and solution stability profiles. For example, a compound with bulk instability at high humidity should be formulated with anhydrous excipients. Similarly, the pH of maximum drug stability should match the pH of an aqueous suspension or solution of the drug and excipient.

A list of the most common excipients is created along with the hypothetic formulations utilizing these excipients. Usually, the approximate dose of the drug is known; thus, each excipient can be blended with the drug at levels that are realistic with respect to a final dosage form (e.g., 10:1 drug to disintegrant and 1:1 drug to filler such as lactose). Each blend is then divided into weighed aliquots, which are tested for stability at some elevated temperature (50°C) that is lower than the melting point of the ingredients. Early inspection ($\Delta T \sim 2$ days) of these stability samples may allow culling of those samples with a phase change and allow for retesting at a lower temperature. If possible, pellets should be formed from the drug excipient blends to increase drug-excipient contact and accelerate testing.

In addition to excipient compatibility testing, small batches of hypothetic capsule or tablet formulations (2 or more) should be prepared and tested in the same stability protocol to check for possible incompatibilities arising from a multicomponent formulation.

Solid formulations often require granulation of the drug excipient blend to improve flow, density, or homogeneity. Stability during the granulation process may be checked by excessive wet down and drying (in a 50°C forced air oven for 48 hours) of samples of the unformulated bulk, excipient-drug blends and the hypothetic formulations. These wet downs should utilize only pharmaceutically acceptable solvents with and without such approved binders as methylcellulose and polyvinylpyrrolidone. Often, the list of granulating solvents may be reduced after the drug's solubility profile is considered. Besides chemical stability, the unformulated bulk samples exposed to each granulation solvent should be checked for crystallinity, polymorph conversion, and solvate formation, all of which could severely alter dissolution or bioavailability.

Formulation Recommendation

Upon completion of the preformulation evaluation of a new drug candidate, it is recommended that a comprehensive report be prepared highlighting the pharmaceutical problems associated with this molecule. This report should conclude with recommendations for developing phase I formulations. These reports are extremely important in preparing regulatory documents and aid in developing subsequent drug candidates.

Acknowledgments

The authors wish to thank Ms. D.M. Johnson, Ms. G. Mazzella, Mr. C.J. Kenney, Ms. N.M. Ursitti, and Ms. L.E. Whitaker of Pfizer Central Research for their assistance in preparing this chapter. Also, the editorial comments of the following individuals were greatly appreciated: Dr. A.J. Aguiar (Pfizer, Inc.), Dr. D.L. Casey (Baxter Travenol), Dr. D.S. Dresback (Pfizer, Inc.), Dr. R.A. Lipper (Bristol Laboratories), and Dr. J.S. Turi (Boehringer Ingelheim Ltd.).

References

1. Berge, S.M., Bighley, L.D., and Monkhouse, D.C.: J. Pharm. Sci., 66:1, 1977.
2. Higuchi, T., and Stella, V.: Prodrugs as Novel Drug Delivery Systems. American Chemical Society, Washington, DC, 1975.
3. Roche, E.B.: Design of Biopharmaceutical Properties Through Prodrugs and Analogs. American Pharmaceutical Association, Washington, DC, 1977.
4. DiSanto, A.R., et al.: J. Clin. Pharmacol., 20:437, 1980.
5. Yakatan, G.J., et al.: J. Clin. Pharmacol., 20:625, 1980.
6. Amidon, G.L., Leesman, G.D., and Elliott, R.L.: J. Pharm. Sci., 69:1363, 1980.
7. Haleblian, J.K.: J. Pharm. Sci., 64:1269, 1975.
8. Poole, J., et al.: Curr. Ther. Res., 10:292, 1968.
9. Aguiar, A.J., et al.: J. Pharm. Sci., 56:847, 1967.
10. Aguiar, A.J., and Zelmer, J.E.: J. Pharm. Sci., 58:983, 1969.
11. Haleblian, J., and McCrone, W.: J. Pharm. Sci., 58:911, 1969.
12. Brennan, W.P., et al.: Purity Determinations by Thermal Methods. ASTM STP 838. Edited by R.L. Blaine and C.K. Schoff. American Society for Testing and Materials, Philadelphia, 1984, p. 5.
13. Guillory, J.K.: J. Pharm. Sci., 61:26, 1972.
14. Allen, P.V., et al.: J. Pharm. Sci., 67:1087, 1978.
15. Jacobson, H., and Reier, G.: J. Pharm. Sci., 58:631, 1969.
16. El-Shattawy, H.H.: Drug Dev. Ind. Pharm., 7:605, 1981.
17. Shibata, M., et al.: J. Pharm. Sci., 72:1436, 1983.
18. Van Campen, L., Amidon, G.L., and Zografi, G.: J. Pharm. Sci., 72:1381, 1983.
19. Weast, R.C.: CRC Handbook of Chemistry and Physics. 55th Ed. CRC Press, Cleveland, 1974, p. E-46.
20. Kaye, B.H.: Chemical Analysis: Direct Characterization of Fine Particles. Vol. 61. John Wiley and Sons, New York, 1981.
21. Kaye, B.H.: Private communication.
22. York, P.: Intern. J. Pharm., 6:89, 1980.
23. Jones, T.M., and Pilpel, N.: J. Pharm. Pharmacol., 18:429, 1966.
24. Gold, G., et al.: J. Pharm. Sci., 55:1291, 1966.
25. Sutton, H.M.: Characterization of Powder Surfaces. Academic Press, London, 1976, p. 1, 7, 158.
26. Hiestand, E.N., et al.: J. Pharm. Sci., 62:1513, 1973.
27. Hiestand, E.N., and Peot, C.B.: J. Pharm. Sci., 63:605, 1974.
28. Hiestand, E.N., and Wells, J.E.: Proc. Intern. Powder and Bulk Solids Handling and Processing Conf., Rosemont, IL, 1977. Industrial and Scientific Conference Management, Inc., Chicago, 1977.
29. Streng, W.H., et al.: J. Pharm. Sci., 73:1679, 1984.
30. Kaplan, S.A.: Drug. Metab. Rev., 1:15, 1972.
31. Christensen, J.J., Hansen, L.D., and Izatt, R.M.: Handbook of Proton Ionization Heats and Related Thermodynamic Quantities. John Wiley and Sons, New York, 1976.
32. Albert, A., and Serjeant, E.P.: Ionization Constants of Acids and Bases. Methuen, London, 1962.
33. Osol, A. (Ed.): Remington's Pharmaceutical Science. 16th Ed. Mack Publishing, Easton, PA, 1980, Chap. 16.
34. Martin, A., Swarbrick, J., and Cammarata, A.: Physical Pharmacy: Physical Chemical Principles in the Pharmaceutical Sciences. 3rd ed. Lea and Febiger, Philadelphia, 1983.
35. Kielland, J.: J. Amer. Chem. Soc., 59:1675, 1937.
36. Kramer, S.F., and Flynn, G.L.: J. Pharm. Sci., 61:1897, 1972.
37. Bogardus, J.B., and Backwood, R.K.: J. Pharm. Sci., 68:188, 1979.
38. Miyazaki, M., et al.: Chem. Pharm. Bull., 23:1197, 1975.
39. Williams, N.A., and Amidon, G.L.: J. Pharm. Sci., 73:18, 1984.
40. Hagen, T.A.: Ph.D. Thesis. University of Michigan, Ann Arbor, MI, 1979.
41. Mulley, B.A.: Solubility in systems containing surface-active agents. In Advances in Pharmaceutical Sciences. Vol. 1. Edited by H.S. Bean, A.H. Beckett, and J.E. Carless. Academic Press, London, 1964, p. 87.
42. Higuchi, T., et al.: J. Am. Pharm. Assoc., Sci. Ed., 43:349, 1954.
43. Hansch, C., and Dunn, W.J.: J. Pharm. Sci., 61:1, 1972.
44. Dressman, J.B., Fleisher, D., and Amidon, G.L.: J. Pharm. Sci., 73:1274, 1984.
45. Suzuki, A., Higuchi, W.I., and Ho, N.F.: J. Pharm. Sci., 59:644, 1970.
46. Wurster, D.E., and Taylor, P.W.; J. Pharm. Sci., 54:169, 1965.
47. Hamlin, W.E., et al.: J. Pharm. Sci., 54:1651, 1965.
48. Wood, J.H., et al.: J. Pharm. Sci., 54:1068, 1965.
49. Mooney, K.G., et al.: J. Pharm. Sci., 70:13, 1981.
50. Mooney, K.G., et al.: J. Pharm. Sci., 70:22, 1981.
51. Hixson, A., and Crowell, J.: Ind. Eng. Chem., 23:923, 1931.
52. Carstensen, J.T.: J. Pharm. Sci., 63:1, 1974.
53. Byrn, S.R.: Solid-State Chemistry of Drugs. Academic Press, New York, 1982.
54. Mollica, J.A., Ahuja, S., and Cohen, J.: J. Pharm. Sci., 67:443, 1978.
55. Connors, K.A., Amidon, G.L., and Kennon, L.: Chemical Stability of Pharmaceuticals. John Wiley and Sons, New York, 1979.
56. Hou, J.P., and Poole, J.W.: J. Pharm. Sci., 58:447, 1969.
57. Graham, R.E., Biehl, E.R., and Kenner, C.T.: J. Pharm. Sci., 65:1048, 1976.

58. Lachman, L., Swartz, C.J., and Cooper, J.: J. Am. Pharm. Assoc., Sci. Ed., 49:213, 1960.
59. March, J.: Advanced Organic Chemistry: Reactions, Mechanisms, and Structure. McGraw-Hill, New York, 1968, p. 199.
60. Pikal, M.J., et al.: J. Pharm. Sci., 67:767, 1978.
61. Carstensen, J.T., Osadca, M., and Rubin, S.H.: J. Pharm. Sci., 58:549, 1969.
62. Byrn, S.R.: J. Pharm. Sci., 65:1, 1976.
63. Perry, R.H., and Chilton, C.H.: Chemical Engineers' Handbook. 5th Ed. McGraw-Hill, New York, 1973, p. 20.

9

Biopharmaceutics

K. C. KWAN, M. R. DOBRINSKA, J. D. ROGERS, A. E. TILL, *and* K. C. YEH

Biopharmaceutics is the study of physiologic and pharmaceutical factors influencing drug release and absorption from dosage forms.[1] Whereas physicochemical properties of the drug (and excipients) dictate the rate of drug release from the dosage form and the subsequent transport across biologic membranes, physiologic and biochemical realities determine its fate in the body. The optimal delivery of the active moiety to the site of action depends on an understanding of specific interactions between the formulation variables and the biologic variables. In drug product development, it is invariably an iterative process whereby the pharmaceutical or the biologic system is systematically perturbed to yield specific information concerning the effect of one on the other.

Whereas physicochemical parameters of the drug and the dosage form can be accurately and precisely measured in vitro, meaningful quantitative estimates of drug absorption can be obtained only through appropriate experiments in vivo. Pharmacokinetic techniques provide the means by which the processes of drug absorption, distribution, biotransformation, and excretion are quantified in the intact organism (animal or man). Equally important, pharmacokinetic inferences can aid in the formation of test hypotheses and in the design of experiments. Alternative hypotheses can be examined in abstraction or through simulation to focus on experiments that are necessary rather than those that are simply data-gathering exercises. In this way, experiments with marginal informational content can be deferred or eliminated.

In this chapter, the basic pharmacokinetic concepts and techniques are reviewed; the physicochemical and biologic factors that influence drug absorption, elimination, and accumulation are discussed; and finally, the specific application of these general principles to the design and evaluation of drug dosage forms is illustrated. Other texts and monographs should be consulted for historical perspective and more extensive treatments of these topics.[2–32]

Pharmacokinetics

The primary goals of pharmacokinetics are to quantify drug absorption, distribution, biotransformation, and excretion in the intact, living animal or man; and to use this information to predict the effect of alterations in the dose, dosage regimen, route of administration, and physiologic state on drug accumulation and disposition. The pharmacokinetics of a drug can be deduced by studying the time courses of changes in drug or metabolite concentrations in body fluids. The drug concentration in plasma or urine at any time after the administration of a known dose or dosage regimen is the net result of its absorption, distribution, biotransformation (metabolism) and excretion. The task, therefore, is to resolve the observed kinetic profiles into their component parts. The contribution of absorption, distribution, biotransformation, and excretion can be individually isolated by appropriate experimental design and kinetic analysis of the data, often with the aid of models. Quantitation is then achieved by maintaining material balance at all times.

Drug disposition refers to events that occur subsequent to absorption, whereas *elimination* refers to the irreversible loss of a drug from the body by metabolism and excretion.

Disposition

Following an intravenous dose, plasma concentrations of a drug often decline exponentially with time. Such behavior suggests that the ki-

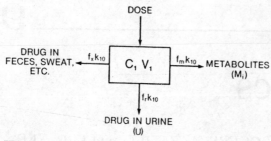

FIG. 9-1. *One-compartment, open model. (See text for definition of symbols.)*

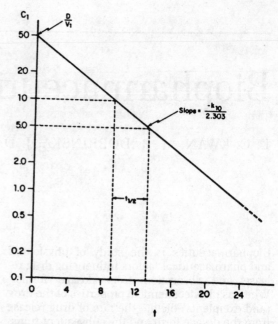

FIG. 9-2. *A semilogarithmic plot of plasma concentration (C_1) vs. time (t) for a one-compartment model.*

netics of drug disposition may be described by one or more first-order processes.

Elimination

A model consistent with monoexponential decay in plasma levels is depicted in Figure 9-1. This is the so-called one-compartment, open model, in which C_1 is plasma concentration, V_1 is the apparent volume of distribution, k_{10} is the overall elimination rate constant, f_r is the fraction of the dose that is excreted in the urine unchanged, f_m is the fraction metabolized, and f_x is the fraction eliminated by all other routes, e.g., bile. The rate of change in C_1 is therefore:

$$-\frac{dC_1}{dt} = k_{10}C_1 \tag{1}$$

which upon integration yields:

$$C_1 = C_1(0)e^{-k_{10}t}$$
$$= \frac{D}{V_1}e^{-k_{10}t} \tag{2}$$

At time zero, i.e., $t = 0$, the plasma concentration $C_1(0)$ is equal to the dose D divided by the volume of distribution V_1.

Experimentally, a semilogarithmic plot of C_1 versus t is a straight line, as shown in Figure 9-2. Model parameters k_{10} and V_1 can be calculated from its slope and intercept, respectively. Thus:

$$\log C_1 = \log\left(\frac{D}{V_1}\right) - \left(\frac{k_{10}}{2.303}\right)t \tag{3}$$

The volume of distribution is useful in relating plasma concentration to the amount of drug in the body at a given time; it is expressed in units of volume. Thus, the product of V_1 and $C_1(t)$ is the amount of drug in the body at time t. The elimination rate constant has units of recip-

rocal time. As such, its numerical value denotes the fractional (or percentage) loss from the body per unit time. For example, $k_{10} = 0.25$ hr^{-1} signifies that the instantaneous rate of elimination is 25% per hour.

The plasma half-life, $t_{\frac{1}{2}}$, is the time required for a given plasma concentration to be halved. For systems undergoing monoexponential decay, $t_{\frac{1}{2}}$ is a constant, independent of plasma concentration. Figure 9-2 shows a graphic solution for $t_{\frac{1}{2}}$. Alternatively, it can be evaluated by substituting $D/2V_1$ for C_1 in equation (3), whereby:

$$t_{\frac{1}{2}} = \frac{2.303 \log 2}{k_{10}} = \frac{0.693}{k_{10}} \tag{4}$$

The plasma half-life of a drug is inversely proportional to its elimination rate constant.

Urinary Excretion. The rate expression for urinary excretion of unchanged drug according to the model in Figure 9-1 is given by:

$$\frac{dU}{dt} = f_r k_{10} V_1 C_1 \tag{5}$$

where U is the cumulative amount of drug excreted in urine to time t. The time course of urinary excretion is obtained by integrating equation (5) and substituting C_1 from equation (2), that is:

$$U(t) = f_r k_{10} V_1 \int_0^t C_1 dt$$

$$= f_r D(1 - e^{-k_{10}t}) \qquad (6)$$

The amount of drug ultimately recovered in the urine unchanged is obtained by evaluating equation (6) at $t = \infty$:

$$\dot{U}(\infty) = f_r D \qquad (7)$$

The time course of urinary excretion is a mono-exponential that approaches $U(\infty)$ asymptotically. Its shape is, in fact, a mirror image of the plasma concentration profile. Equation (6) can be rearranged to show that:

$$\log \frac{U(\infty) - U(t)}{U(\infty)} = -\left(\frac{k_{10}}{2.303}\right)t \qquad (8)$$

Thus, a semilogarithmic plot of the fractional amount remaining to be excreted as a function of time should be a straight line with a slope identical to that shown in Figure 9-2 for plasma decay. Figure 9-3 is sometimes referred to as the *deficit plot*, or *sigma-minus plot*; it or equation (8) can be used to estimate the *overall* elimination rate constant, k_{10}, from urine data. The rate constant for urinary excretion is $f_r k_{10}$. Experi-

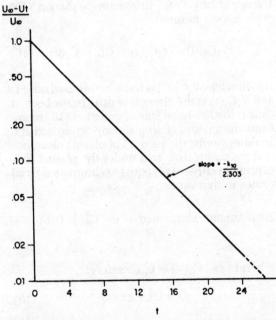

FIG. 9-3. *Deficit plot, or sigma-minus plot, of the fraction of drug remaining to be excreted in the urine vs. time.*

mentally, f_r can be obtained by the ratio of $U(\infty)$ to D.

Clearance. According to equation (6), the cumulative amount excreted in the urine to time t is proportional to the area under the plasma concentration curve from 0 to t. This relationship holds for all times such that the amount excreted over any interval between t_1 and t_2 is also proportional to the corresponding area over the same interval. In other words:

$$U(t_1) = f_r k_{10} V_1 \int_0^{t_1} C_1 dt \qquad (9)$$

$$U(t_2) = f_r k_{10} V_1 \int_0^{t_2} C_1 dt \qquad (10)$$

$$U(t_2) - U(t_1) = f_r k_{10} V_1 \int_{t_1}^{t_2} C_1 dt \qquad (11)$$

The proportionality constant relating plasma concentration and urinary excretion of a drug is known as its *plasma renal clearance rate*, CL_r, or simply *renal clearance*.

$$CL_r = f_r k_{10} V_1 = \frac{U(t_2) - U(t_1)}{\int_{t_1}^{t_2} C_1 dt} \qquad (12)$$

Similarly, blood or serum renal clearance rates would apply to situations in which drug concentrations are measured in blood or serum. Explicit reference to blood, plasma, or serum is usually unnecessary, except for emphasis or for contrasting results from different experiments.

The renal clearance of a substance is the product of its urinary excretion rate constant, $f_r k_{10}$, and its volume of distribution, V_1. Dimensionally, CL_r has units of volume per unit time, e.g., ml/min. Physiologically, the renal clearance rate represents that volume of plasma from which drug is completely eliminated per unit time as a result of passage through the kidneys. A schematic illustration of this phenomenon is shown in Figure 9-4, in which the density of shaded areas denotes plasma concentrations before and

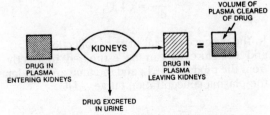

FIG. 9-4. *Schematic illustration of renal clearance.*

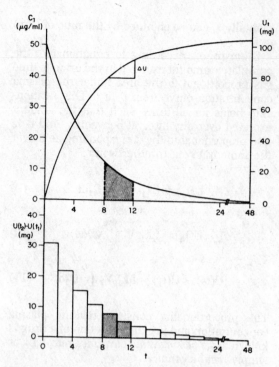

FIG. 9-5. *Graphic representation of renal clearance calculation. The shaded areas represent a typical area under the plasma concentration curve and the corresponding amount of drug excreted in the urine.*

after passage through the kidneys (or any other clearing organ). The clear zone represents a volume that is completely devoid of drug. Experimentally, the renal clearance of a substance can be determined by dividing the amount of drug present in a timed urine sample by the corresponding area under the plasma concentration curve, as shown in equation (12). This is depicted graphically in Figure 9-5.

The numerical value of renal clearance can be applied in various ways. For example, a combination of equations (5) and (12), indicates that the rate of urinary excretion at any instance is equal to the product of renal clearance and the plasma concentration at that time:

$$\frac{dU}{dt} = CL_r C_1 \qquad (13)$$

In the absence of total urinary collection, $U(\infty)$, and therefore f_r, can be estimated indirectly from the product of CL_r and the total area under the plasma concentration curve, AUC_∞:

$$U(\infty) = f_r k_{10} V_1 \int_0^\infty C_1 dt = CL_r AUC_\infty \quad (14)$$

AUC_∞ may be obtained as the integral of equation (2) evaluated from time zero to infinity, i.e., $\dfrac{D}{k_{10}V_1}$, or by suitable interpolation and extrapolation techniques.[32,33]

The clearance concept applies to any body organ or tissue capable of eliminating a drug. For example, hepatic clearance refers to the rate of elimination resulting from passage through the liver, while biliary clearance refers to that part of hepatic clearance that is due to excretion in bile. Unlike measurement of renal clearance, however, their direct experimental determination in the intact animal or person is difficult, and in some cases, impossible. Nevertheless, insights concerning their contribution are often obtained through pharmacokinetic inferences.

The overall elimination of a drug from the body is composed of fractions that are excreted in urine, metabolized, and eliminated by all other means such that $f_r + f_m + f_x = 1.0$. Since renal clearance can be represented by $f_r k_{10} V_1$, the total clearance rate from plasma is $k_{10} V_1$. Multiplying both sides of equation (1) by V_1 yields:

$$-V_1 \frac{dC_1}{dt} = k_{10} V_1 C_1 = CLC_1 \qquad (15)$$

where CL is the total plasma clearance rate, or simply plasma clearance. Equation (15) states that CL is the proportionality constant relating the overall elimination rate and plasma concentration at any time. Integrating equation (15) with respect to time:

$$V_1 C_1(0) - V_1 C_1(t) = CL \int_0^t C_1 dt \quad (16)$$

Inasmuch as $V_1 C_1(0)$ is the administered dose D and $V_1 C_1(t)$ is the amount of drug in the body at time t, the left-hand side of equation (16) represents the amount of drug already eliminated at t. In other words, the product of plasma clearance and the cumulative area under the plasma concentration curve at t is equal to elimination by all routes to that time:

$$\text{Total amount eliminated at t} = CL \int_0^t C_1 dt$$
$$(17)$$

When $t = \infty$, $C_1(\infty) = 0$; therefore:

$$D = CL \cdot AUC_\infty \qquad (18)$$

Ultimately, elimination by all routes accounts for the amount administered.

The experimental determination of plasma clearance can be accomplished in various ways following an intravenous dose. Given a reasonably complete set of plasma concentration data, CL can be estimated by the ratio of D to AUC_∞ or by the product of k_{10} and V_1 obtained from the slope and intercept in Figure 9-2. Given complete urine collection and an estimate of renal clearance, CL can also be calculated by:

$$CL = \frac{CL_r}{f_r} = \frac{CL_r D}{U(\infty)} \qquad (19)$$

In summary, clearance is a proportionality constant that relates plasma concentration of a substance to its elimination rate. It serves the same purpose in relating area under the plasma concentration curve to the amount eliminated. Plasma clearance can be readily determined from plasma concentration and urinary excretion data following an intravenous dose. Renal clearance can be estimated directly from any conveniently timed plasma and urine sample irrespective of the mode of administration.

The difference between plasma and renal clearance is clearance by other routes:

$$CL_{nr} = CL - CL_r \qquad (20)$$

The dominant component of extrarenal clearance, CL_{nr}, is usually biotransformation, although biliary excretion, expiration, or perspiration may also contribute.

Metabolism. The metabolic clearance of a drug, CL_m, is the sum of all processes that result in the formation of primary metabolites, m_i. If extrarenal clearance is due solely to biotransformation, CL_m can be estimated directly from equation (20). Otherwise, the contribution of each primary metabolic path must be examined independently. The procedure outlined below assumes a single metabolite but may be applied repeatedly for any specific precursor/successor pairs. Note, however, that secondary or tertiary metabolite formation has no impact on the metabolic clearance rate of the parent drug.

Figure 9-6 depicts a situation where drug and metabolite disposition can each be described by a one-compartment open model. Thus, following an intravenous dose M of the metabolite, its plasma concentrations decline monoexponentially with time:

$$C_1^m = \frac{M}{V_1^m} e - k_{10}^m t \qquad (21)$$

where the superscript m on C_1, V_1, and k_{10} de-

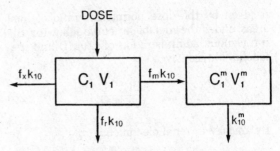

FIG. 9-6. *Disposition of drug and metabolite according to a one-compartment model for each.*

notes plasma concentration, volume of distribution, and elimination rate constant of the metabolite. The total area under the metabolite concentration curve is therefore:

$$\int_0^\infty C_1^m dt = \frac{M}{k_{10}^m V_1^m} \qquad (22)$$

The rate expression for metabolite concentrations in plasma following an intravenous dose D of drug is:

$$\frac{dC_1^{m*}}{dt} = f_m k_{10} C_1 - k_{10}^m C_1^{m*} \qquad (23)$$

The asterisk (*) distinguishes metabolite concentrations following drug administration from those after metabolite administration. The plasma time course of the metabolite following drug administration is obtained by substituting C_1 from equation (2) into equation (23) and integrating, namely:

$$C_1^{m*} = \frac{f_m k_{10} D}{V_1^m (k_{10}^m - k_{10})} [e^{-k_{10}t} - e - k_{10}^m t] \qquad (24)$$

Equation (24) can be further integrated and rearranged to yield:

$$f_m D = k_{10}^m V_1^m \int_0^\infty C_1^{m*} dt \qquad (25)$$

The left-hand side of equation (25) is the amount of metabolite formed, whereas the right-hand side is the amount of metabolite ultimately eliminated from the body. The plasma clearance of metabolite, $k_{10}^m V_1^m$, can be obtained from equation (22) following an intravenous dose M of the metabolite.

An alternative view of the same situation is obtained by combining equations (22) and (25). The fractional contribution of a specific metabolic pathway to the plasma clearance of a drug is given by the dose normalized ratio of total areas under the metabolite curve following the intravenous administration of drug D and metabolite M, namely:

$$f_m = \frac{AUC_\infty^{m^*}/D}{AUC_\infty^m/M} \qquad (26)$$

By analogy to renal clearance:

$$CL_m = f_m CL \qquad (27)$$

A potential source of error occurs when the metabolite formed undergoes further biotransformation before reaching the general circulation. This phenomenon, known as *sequential metabolism*,[34] causes an underestimation of the area term in equation (25), and hence the amount formed.

Distribution

Drug distribution is a reversible process. The rates of exchange between plasma and tissues vary widely depending on the types of tissue and the drug's partition characteristics. With few exceptions—notably plasma proteins and red blood cells—experimental determination of drug distribution in humans is not feasible. Its manifestations can be deduced, however, from the plasma concentration profiles. When distribution is rapid, the body behaves kinetically as a single homogeneous pool, and the plasma concentration time course may be adequately described by a single exponential (Fig. 9-2). On the other hand, the kinetics of drug disposition often exhibit multiexponential characteristics. Each additional exponential has been interpreted to represent a group of tissues requiring progressively more time in which to achieve a steady state in drug distribution.

Figure 9-7 is a typical semilogarithmic plot of biexponential decay corresponding to equation (28).

$$C_1 = Ae^{-\alpha t} + Be^{-\beta t} \qquad (28)$$

The profile shows an initial curvature that eventually becomes log-linear with a terminal slope $-\beta/2.303$. The intercept B is obtained by extrapolation back to time zero. Taking the logarithm of the difference between plasma concentration C_1 and the value of $Be^{-\beta t}$ yields another straight line from which A and α can be evaluated; that is:

$$\log[C_1 - Be^{-\beta t}] = \log A - \frac{\alpha t}{2.303} \qquad (29)$$

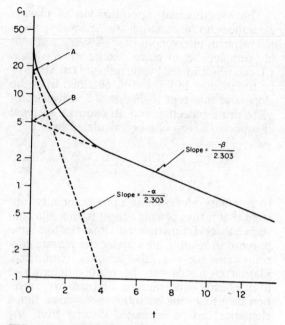

FIG. 9-7. *Semilogarithmic plot of plasma concentration* (C_1) *vs. time for a two-compartment model.*

This technique, known as *curve stripping*, can be repeated as often as necessary and is generally useful in obtaining the eigenvalues (slopes) and eigenvectors (intercepts) of a polyexponential function.

A pharmacokinetic model consistent with biexponential decay is shown in Figure 9-8. The body is perceived to be divided into two kinetically distinct compartments. A central compartment 1, which includes plasma and from which elimination occurs, is linked to a peripheral compartment 2 by first-order processes having rate constants k_{12} and k_{21}. Rate expressions apropos to this model are:

$$\frac{dC_1}{dt} = -k_{12}C_1 + k_{21}C_2 - k_{10}C_1 \qquad (30)$$

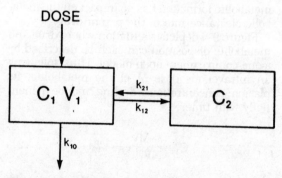

FIG. 9-8. *Two-compartment, open model.*

$$\frac{dC_2}{dt} = k_{12}C_1 - k_{21}C_2 \qquad (31)$$

$$\frac{dU}{dt} = f_r k_{10} V_1 C_1 \qquad (32)$$

where C_2 is a hypothetic concentration whose product with V_1 equals the amount of drug present in the peripheral compartment. The relationship between the model parameters and the experimentally determined slopes (α and β) and intercepts (A and B) is obtained by simultaneous solution of equations (30) and (31), whereby:

$$C_1 = \frac{D(k_{21} - \alpha)}{V_1(\beta - \alpha)}e^{-\alpha t} + \frac{D(k_{21} - \beta)}{V_1(\alpha - \beta)}e^{-\beta t} \qquad (33)$$

such that:

$$A = \frac{D(k_{21} - \alpha)}{V_1(\beta - \alpha)} \qquad (34)$$

$$B = \frac{D(k_{21} - \beta)}{V_1(\alpha - \beta)} \qquad (35)$$

$$\alpha = \frac{(k_{10} + k_{21} + k_{12})}{2} + \frac{\sqrt{(k_{10} + k_{21} + k_{12})^2 - 4k_{21}k_{10}}}{2} \qquad (36)$$

$$\beta = \frac{(k_{10} + k_{21} + k_{12})}{2} - \frac{\sqrt{(k_{10} + k_{21} + k_{12})^2 - 4k_{21}k_{10}}}{2} \qquad (37)$$

The corresponding time courses of change in the amount of drug in the peripheral compartment and in urine are respectively:

$$V_1 C_2 = \frac{k_{12}D}{(\beta - \alpha)}e^{-\alpha t} + \frac{k_{12}D}{(\alpha - \beta)}e^{-\beta t} \qquad (38)$$

and:

$$U = f_r k_{10} V_1 \int_0^t C_1 dt$$
$$= f_r D\left[1 - \frac{(\beta - k_{10})}{(\beta - \alpha)}e^{-\alpha t} - \frac{(\alpha - k_{10})}{(\alpha - \beta)}e^{-\beta t}\right] \qquad (39)$$

The model parameters can be evaluated by com-

bining and rearranging equations (34) through (37).

$$V_1 = \frac{D}{A + B} \qquad (40)$$

$$k_{10} = \frac{A + B}{A/\alpha + B/\beta} \qquad (41)$$

$$k_{21} = \frac{\alpha\beta}{k_{10}} \qquad (42)$$

$$k_{12} = \alpha + \beta - k_{10} - k_{21} \qquad (43)$$

Obviously, the distributive process alters not only the plasma concentration and urinary excretion profiles but also the interpretation of many of the pharmacokinetic parameters. Notably, the terminal slope β, or the corresponding $t_{\frac{1}{2},\beta}$ does not reflect the rate of drug elimination from the body; it merely represents the slowest rate of drug disappearance from plasma. Also, the volume of distribution V_1 must be qualified by reference to the central compartment. The product of V_1 and C_1 is not sufficient to account for the quantity of drug in the body. The contribution from the peripheral compartment, i.e., $V_1 C_2$, must be included.

The meaning of clearance remains unchanged, however. Equation (33) can be integrated and rearranged to yield an expression for plasma clearance, namely:

$$CL = k_{10}V_1 = \frac{D}{AUC_\infty} \qquad (44)$$

which is identical to that obtained for the one-compartment open model. AUC_∞ may be obtained as the integral of equation (28) evaluated from time zero to infinity, i.e., $\frac{A}{\alpha} + \frac{B}{\beta}$, or by interpolation and extrapolation techniques. According to equations (32) and (39), the product of renal clearance and plasma concentration is the instantaneous rate of urinary excretion, while the product of CI_r and AUC_∞ is the amount excreted in urine. Multiplying both sides of equation (30) by V_1, the rate of drug disappearance from plasma is:

$$-V_1\frac{dC_1}{dt} = k_{10}V_1C_1 + k_{12}V_1C_1 - k_{21}V_1C_2 \qquad (45)$$

The first term on the right-hand side of equation (45) represents rate of drug loss from the body; the second and third terms indicate drug distri-

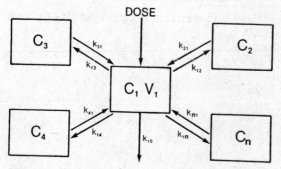

FIG. 9-9. *Mammillary model representing polyexponential decay.*

bution. Again, this emphasizes the difference between drug elimination rate and plasma disappearance rate except for monoexponential decay. The differences in interpretation cited previously apply to all mammillary models (Fig. 9-9) and polyexponential functions.

Absorption

When a drug is not administered directly into the vasculature, it must be transported to the general circulation before it can be counted. In pharmacokinetics, *absorption* is defined as the amount of drug that reaches the general circulation unchanged. Hence, that which is metabolized or chemically transformed at the site of application or in transit is by definition not absorbed. This definition arises mainly out of necessity because of experimental and physiologic limitations in quantitating the manifestations of absorption in the intact animal or human. In this context, the rate and extent of drug absorption is synonymous with its bioavailability. More generally, the term bioavailability may be used to indicate the delivery of the active moiety from the site of administration to the target tissue or organ, whereas absorption often refers to the overall transport of a drug and related substances into the body or parts thereof, e.g., the eyes or the skin. The more restrictive definitions of absorption and bioavailability are used throughout this chapter.

Material balance dictates that total elimination must equal the amount absorbed, that is:

Amount absorbed = Amount eliminated

If F is the fraction absorbed following a nonintravascular dose D^x, then:

$$FD^x = CL \cdot AUC^x_\infty \qquad (46)$$

where AUC^x_∞ is the total area under the plasma concentration curve following treatment x. The estimation of bioavailability requires knowledge of plasma clearance, which is obtained independently following an intravenous dose. See equation (18) for determination of plasma clearance.

At any time t following the administration of a dose, the amount absorbed, A(t), is equal to the sum of that which is present in the body, $A_b(t)$, and that which is already eliminated from the body. In other words:

$$A(t) = A_b(t) + CL \int_0^t C_1 dt \qquad (47)$$

Estimates of $A_b(t)$ depend on how the drug is distributed in the body. When drug disposition can be adequately described by a one-compartment open model, $A_b(t) = V_1 C_1(t)$ and the time course of absorption is estimated by:

$$A(t) = V_1 C_1(t) + k_{10} V_1 \int_0^t C_1 dt \qquad (48)$$

This is known as the Wagner-Nelson method of estimating absorption.[35] V_1 and k_{10} can be obtained following an i.v. dose (see Fig. 9-2).

When a two-compartment open model applies, the absorption profile can be constructed from equation (49):

$$A(t) = V_1 C_1(t) + V_1 C_2(t) + k_{10} V_1 \int_0^t C_1 dt \qquad (49)$$

The amount of drug present in the body at any time is the sum of the amounts in the central and the peripheral compartment. To evaluate equation (49), some method of estimating C_2 is needed. As a first approximation, Loo and Riegelman proposed that C_1 varies linearly with time between any two adjacent data points,[36] such that:

$$C_1(t_j) = C_1(t_{j-1}) + bT \qquad (50)$$

where b is the slope and T is the time between t_j and t_{j-1} as shown in Figure 9-10. Integrating equation (50) into equation (31) yields:

$$\frac{dC_2}{dT} + k_{21} C_2 = k_{12} C_1(t_{j-1}) + bk_{12}T \qquad (51)$$

Integrating equation (51) with respect to T and

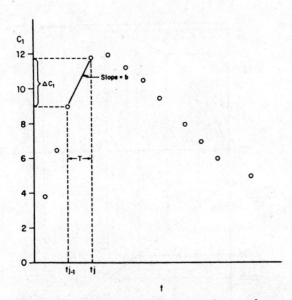

FIG. 9-10. *Relationship between two adjacent plasma concentration data points proposed by Loo and Riegelman.*[36]

noting that at $T = 0$, $C_2 = C_2(t_{j-1})$, one obtains:

$$C_2 = C_2(t_{j-1})e^{-k_{21}T} + \frac{k_{12}}{k_{21}}C_1(t_{j-1})[1 - e^{-k_{21}T}]$$

$$+ \frac{bk_{12}}{(k_{21})^2}[e^{-k_{21}T} + k_{21}T - 1] \quad (52)$$

Now define the relationships:

$$\Delta C_1 = C_1(t_j) - C_1(t_{j-1}) \quad (53)$$

and

$$\Delta t = t_j - t_{j-1} \quad (54)$$

At $T = \Delta t$,

$$C_2 = C_2(t_j) \quad \text{and} \quad b = \frac{\Delta C_1}{\Delta t} \quad (55)$$

The substitution of equations (53), (54), and (55) into equation (52) results in:

$$C_2(t_j) = C_2(t_{j-1})e^{-k_{21}\Delta t}$$

$$+ \frac{k_{12}}{k_{21}}C_1(t_{j-1})[1 - e^{-k_{21}\Delta t}]$$

$$+ \frac{k_{12}\Delta C_1}{(k_{21})^2\Delta t}[e^{-k_{21}\Delta t} + k_{21}\Delta t - 1]$$

$$\quad (56)$$

Starting at $t = 0$ when $C_2(t_{j-1}) = C_1(t_{j-1}) = 0$, the value of $C_2(t_j)$ can be estimated sequentially by the repeated application of equation (56). At $t = \infty$, no more drug remains in the body, equation (49) collapses to equation (46), and $A(\infty) =$ FD as expected. Figure 9-11 is a typical absorption profile constructed according to equation (49) using the Loo-Riegelman approximation of C_2 given in equation (56).

In summary, to estimate the bioavailability of a drug administered by a nonintravascular route, knowledge of its plasma clearance is required. The plasma clearance in an animal or a person can be calculated following an intravenous dose. In essence:

$$F = \frac{AUC_\infty^x/D^x}{AUC_\infty/D} \quad (57)$$

Since AUC_∞^x and AUC_∞ can both be determined directly by interpolation and extrapolation of the terminal slope of the plasma concentration curve to infinity, the estimation of F is model-independent. In contrast, determinations of the absorption time course based on compartmental analysis depend not only on plasma clearance but also on estimates of the volume of distribution and the rate constants for drug distribution. These values are obtained by interpreting the kinetics of drug disposition following an intravenous dose in reference to specific models.

Accumulation

Suppose a drug is administered intravenously by infusion at a constant rate R_0 (amount/time). Plasma concentration (and the amount of drug

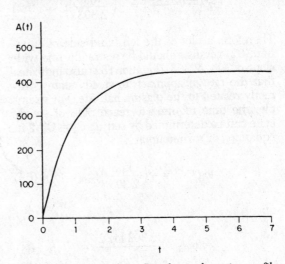

FIG. 9-11. *A typical Loo-Riegelman absorption profile.*

in the body) would increase with time and approach a plateau, which is called a steady state. At steady state, the rate of input to the body, R_0, equals the rate of drug elimination from the body, that is:

$$R_0 = CL \cdot C_1^{ss} \qquad (58)$$

where C_1^{ss} is the plasma concentration at steady state. The value of C_1^{ss} to be attained is proportional to the infusion rate. Equation (58) is applicable to all linear mammillary models of drug disposition. The rate of approach to steady state depends on the manifestations of drug distribution.

Where the one-compartment, open model (see Fig. 9-1) applies, the rate of change in drug levels is given by:

$$V_1 \frac{dC_1}{dt} = R_0 - k_{10} V_1 C_1 \qquad (59)$$

which, upon integration, yields:

$$C_1 = \frac{R_0}{k_{10} V_1}(1 - e^{-k_{10}t}) \qquad (60)$$

At $t = \infty$, $C_1 = C_1^{ss}$. Thus, equation (60) reduces to equation (58). Subtracting equation (60) from equation (58), one obtains:

$$\frac{C_1^{ss} - C_1}{C_1^{ss}} = e^{-k_{10}t} \qquad (61)$$

or:

$$\log\left(\frac{C_1^{ss} - C_1}{C_1^{ss}}\right) = -\left(\frac{k_{10}}{2.303}\right)t \qquad (62)$$

Therefore, a plot of the left-hand side of equation (62) versus t should be a straight line with slope of $-k_{10}/2.303$. Equation (62) also indicates that the rate of approach to steady state is directly related to the plasma half-life. For example, the time required to reach 50% of steady state can be determined by setting $C_1 = C_1^{ss}/2$ in equation (62) whereupon:

$$\log(\tfrac{1}{2}) = -\left(\frac{k_{10}}{2.303}\right)t_{50\%} \qquad (63)$$

or:

$$t_{50\%} = \frac{2.303 \log 2}{k_{10}} \qquad (64)$$

which is identical to the definition of plasma

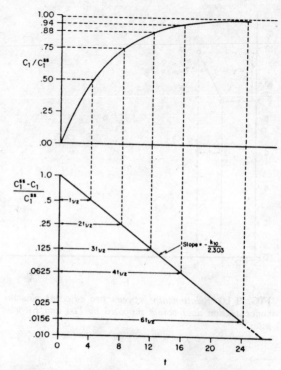

FIG. 9-12. *Relationship between plasma half-life and approach to steady state for a one-compartment model drug.*

half-life given in equation (4). Similarly, it can be shown that two half-lives would be required to achieve 75% of steady state, 3.3 half-lives for 90%, 6.6 half-lives for 99%, and so on. This relationship between plasma half-life and approach to steady state is shown in Figure 9-12. Note that the approach to steady state follows exactly the same time course as that for drug disappearance from plasma following an intravenous injection. For drugs that exhibit polyexponential decay, the approach to steady state would also be polyexponential.

Consider, for example, the situation whereby drug disposition can best be described by a two-compartment, open model (see Fig. 9-8). Temporal changes in plasma concentration attendant to a constant infusion of a drug are given by:

$$C_1 = \frac{R_0}{k_{10} V_1}\left\{1 - \frac{(\beta - k_{10})}{(\beta - \alpha)} e^{-\alpha t} - \frac{(\alpha - k_{10})}{(\alpha - \beta)} e^{-\beta t}\right\} \qquad (65)$$

At steady state, $t = \infty$, equation (65) also collapses to equation (58), as it should. Subtracting equation (65) from equation (58) one obtains:

$$\frac{C_1^{ss} - C_1}{C_1^{ss}} = \frac{(\beta - k_{10})}{(\beta - \alpha)} e^{-\alpha t} + \frac{(\alpha - k_{10})}{(\alpha - \beta)} e^{-\beta t} \tag{66}$$

In this case, the approach to steady state results from two independent exponential processes, α and β, each governed by its own half-life, $t_{\frac{1}{2},\alpha}$ and $t_{\frac{1}{2},\beta}$. The fractional contribution to the observed sum is given by the eigenvectors of equation (66), because of the following relationship:

$$\frac{(\beta - k_{10})}{(\beta - \alpha)} + \frac{(\alpha - k_{10})}{(\alpha - \beta)} = 1 \tag{67}$$

For each component, times required to reach 50%, 90%, and 99% of steady state are still 1.0, 3.3, and 6.6 half-lives, respectively. According to equations (36) and (37), however, $t_{\frac{1}{2},\beta}$ is longer than $t_{\frac{1}{2},\alpha}$; thus, steady state for the α process would be attained sooner. Figure 9-13 shows a biexponential approach to steady state. At all times, the observed plasma concentration represents the sum of two processes.

A steady state in drug accumulation can also be achieved by dosing at regular intervals. In the simplest case, consider the events following the repeated intravenous administration at intervals τ of a drug that undergoes monoexponential decay. According to equation (2), plasma concentration after the first dose is represented by:

$$C_1^{(1)} = \frac{D}{V_1} e^{-k_{10}t} \tag{68}$$

At $t = \tau$, a second dose is administered. Plasma concentrations thereafter are then represented

by:

$$C_1^{(2)} = \frac{D}{V_1}(1 + e^{-k_{10}\tau})e^{-k_{10}t'} \tag{69}$$

where t' is time from the most recent dose. Similarly, after the third and subsequent doses, one can calculate:

$$C_1^{(3)} = \frac{D}{V_1}(1 + e^{-k_{10}\tau} + e^{-2k_{10}\tau})e^{-k_{10}t'} \tag{70}$$

and:

$$C_1^{(n)} = \frac{D}{V_1}(1 + e^{-k_{10}\tau} + e^{-2k_{10}\tau} + \cdots$$
$$+ e^{-(n-1)k_{10}\tau})e^{-k_{10}t'}$$
$$= \frac{D}{V_1}\frac{(1 - e^{-nk_{10}\tau})}{(1 - e^{-k_{10}\tau})}e^{-k_{10}t'} \tag{71}$$

As n becomes large, the plasma concentration profiles from one interval to the next become indistinguishable. At steady state, $n = \infty$, the plasma time course is represented by:

$$C_1^{(ss)} = \frac{D}{V_1}\frac{e^{-k_{10}t'}}{(1 - e^{-k_{10}\tau})} \tag{72}$$

The mean plasma concentration over a dosage interval at steady state, $\bar{C}_1^{(ss)}$, can be determined by dividing the integral of equation (72) by τ such that:

$$\bar{C}_1^{(ss)} = \frac{\int_0^\tau C_1^{(ss)} dt'}{\tau}$$
$$= \frac{D}{\tau k_{10} V_1} \tag{73}$$

Mean plasma concentration at steady state, $\bar{C}_1^{(ss)}$, after intermittent dosage serves the same purpose as C_1^{ss} after a constant infusion. They would in fact be numerically identical if the rate of dosage, D/τ, given discretely were the same as the infusion rate, R_0, given continuously. A graphic representation of drug accumulation after a constant infusion and intermittent oral dosage is shown in Figure 9-14.

Equation (73) would also apply to the repeated intravenous administration of drugs that undergo polyexponential decay, although the time courses of change in plasma concentration would differ. For example, with biexponential decay, plasma concentrations during the nth

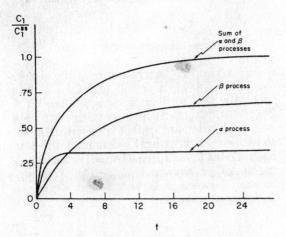

FIG. 9-13. *Biexponential approach to steady state.*

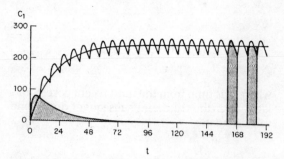

FIG. 9-14. *Drug accumulation after a constant infusion and intermittent oral doses taken at equal intervals; shaded areas illustrate the equality between* $AUC_\infty^{(1)}$ *and* $AUC_\tau^{(SS)}$

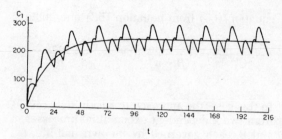

FIG. 9-15. *Drug accumulation after intermittent oral doses taken at unequal intervals.*

dosing interval are represented by:

$$C_1^{(n)} = \frac{D}{V_1}\left\{ \frac{(k_{21} - \alpha)(1 - e^{-n\alpha\tau})}{(\beta - \alpha)(1 - e^{-\alpha\tau})} e^{-\alpha t'} \right.$$
$$\left. + \frac{(k_{21} - \beta)(1 - e^{-n\beta\tau})}{(\alpha - \beta)(1 - e^{-\beta\tau})} e^{-\beta t'} \right\} \quad (74)$$

The rate of approach to steady state would on average emulate a constant infusion.

Two additional properties of repeated intermittent dosage should be considered. First, the area under the plasma concentration curve over one dosage interval at steady state, AUC_τ^{ss}, is equal to the total area under the plasma concentration curve after a single dose, that is:

$$AUC_\tau^{(ss)} = AUC_\infty^{(1)} \quad (75)$$

This identity is given by the shaded areas of Figure 9-14. At steady state, drug input to the body (FD) is equal to drug elimination from the body.[37] Mathematically, these relationships can be summarized by rearrangements of equations (44), (46) and (75) such that:

$$FD = CL \cdot AUC_\infty^{(1)} = CL \cdot AUC_\tau^{(ss)} \quad (76)$$

Second, a steady state can also be attained by intermittent drug administration at unequal intervals provided that the dosage sequence recurs regularly. For example, daily intervals of dosage may be τ_1, τ_2, and τ_3 such that $\tau_1 + \tau_2 + \tau_3 = 24$ hr. If the same dosage schedule were maintained from day to day, the plasma concentration profiles would in time become indistinguishable from one day to the next. In general, the concept of a steady state applies whenever the dosage regimen consists of recurring cycles. Within each cycle, the dose and the dosage interval need not be uniform,[38] as is shown in Figure 9-15.

Factors Affecting Drug Elimination

Binding to Plasma Proteins

Binding is usually a reversible interaction between a small molecule such as drug or metabolite and a protein or other macromolecule.[39-42] Only unbound drug can be transported across capillaries, be distributed to tissues, gain access to metabolizing enzymes, and interact with receptors to elicit a pharmacologic effect. Binding is a distributive process, which delays drug elimination. Tissue binding cannot be measured directly in the intact, living animal or human although its influence on drug distribution and elimination has been deduced and discussed.[43-45]

Binding is a function of the affinity of the protein for drug as well as the concentration of drug and protein. By far, the most important binding proteins in plasma are albumin for acidic drugs and α_1-acid glycoprotein for basic drugs. The interaction between drug and protein can be represented by the law of mass action such that:

$$C_{u,1} + C_{1,p} \leftrightarrows C_{b,1}$$

$$\text{drug} + \text{protein} \leftrightarrows \text{drug-protein}$$

where $C_{u,1}$ and $C_{b,1}$ are, respectively, the plasma concentrations of unbound and bound drug such that the total drug concentration $C_1 = C_{u,1} + C_{b,1}$. $C_{u,p}$ is the plasma concentration of free protein binding sites expressed in molar equivalents of the drug. By definition, the concentration of total (free and bound) protein binding sites, C_p, is the sum of $C_{u,p} + C_{b,1}$. The equilibrium between free and bound drug can therefore be expressed as:

$$K = \frac{C_{b,1}}{(C_{u,1})(C_{u,p})} \quad (77)$$

where the equilibrium constant K is a measure of the affinity of the protein for drug.

Define f_u as the fraction of the total drug concentration that is unbound so that $f_u C_1 = C_{u,1}$ and $(1 - f_u)C_1 = C_{b,1}$. Substituting these relationships into equation (77), one obtains, after rearrangement:

$$f_u = \frac{1}{1 + KC_{u,p}}$$
$$= \frac{1}{1 + K(C_p - C_{b,1})} \quad (78)$$

When the fractional occupancy is small compared to total available binding sites, that is, $C_{b,1} \ll C_p$, the free fraction of drug is essentially independent of changes in drug concentration. These circumstances often prevail within the therapeutic dosage range.

Renal Physiology

The mammalian kidney is composed of many units called *nephrons*. A nephron consists of an individual renal tubule and its glomerulus. The glomerulus is formed by the invagination of a tuft of capillaries into the dilated blind end of the nephron (Bowman's capsule). The capillaries are supplied by an afferent arteriole and drained by an efferent arteriole. The renal tubule consists of the proximal convoluted tubule (pars convoluta), which drains into the straight portion of the proximal tubule (pars recta), which forms the first part of the loop of Henle. The thick ascending limb of the loop of Henle reaches the glomerulus of the nephron from which the tubule arose and passes close to its afferent arteriole. The final portion of the tubule is the distal convoluted tubule. Distal tubules coalesce to form collecting ducts that pass through the renal cortex and medulla and empty into the pelvis of the kidney. The vascular supply of the tubules is essentially a portal one in that the blood that perfuses the peritubular capillaries has initially traversed the glomerular capillaries.[46-51]

Renal Excretion Mechanisms

The nephrons carry out the vital functions of the kidney through three major processes: glomerular filtration, tubular reabsorption of water and filtered substances from the lumen of the tubule into the plasma, and tubular secretion of substances from the plasma across the tubular membrane into the tubular lumen. The processes of tubular reabsorption and secretion may be governed by either passive mechanisms (simple diffusion) or carrier-mediated mechanisms (facilitated diffusion and active transport). While the renal processes serve primarily to maintain extracellular fluid volume and osmolality, to conserve important solutes, and to help regulate acid-base balance, they are also important in controlling the excretion of exogenous compounds such as drugs.

Glomerular Filtration. Approximately 25% of the cardiac output goes to the kidneys, and 10% of this output to kidneys is filtered by the glomerulus. A fluid conforming closely to that of an ideal ultrafiltrate of plasma moves across the glomerular membrane. It has nearly the same composition as plasma with respect to water and low molecular weight solutes. Glomerular filtration separates gross particulate matter and such colloidal materials as proteins from the ultrafiltrate. The availability of a drug for glomerular filtration depends on its concentration in plasma water; only free drug (drug not bound to macromolecules or red blood cells) can be filtered. The filtrate contains the drug at a concentration equal to that in plasma water, i.e., $f_u C_1$.

The rate at which plasma water is filtered is called the *glomerular filtration rate* (GFR); the rate at which a drug is filtered is equal to the concentration of unbound drug in plasma multiplied by GFR.[48,49,52] The GFR can be measured in intact animals and humans by measurement of the excretion and plasma concentration of a substance that is freely filtered through the glomeruli and is neither secreted nor reabsorbed by the tubules. In addition, the substance should be physiologically inert and nontoxic; neither destroyed, synthesized nor stored within the kidney; and preferably, easily measured in plasma and urine. Inulin, a fructose polymer of molecular weight 5200, appears to meet all criteria, and its renal clearance provides an index of GFR.

Passive Transport Across the Renal Tubule. Passive transport of exogenous compounds, such as drugs, in the renal tubule involves simple diffusion along a concentration gradient.[53-57] The concentration gradient between urine and plasma is the driving force for diffusion. The rate of movement is also governed by the diffusivity of the molecule through the tubular membrane, the membrane/aqueous phase partition coefficient for the molecule, the thickness of the membrane at the site of diffusion, and the area of the membrane through which the molecule passes. Biologic membranes, being lipid in nature, are more permeable to lipid soluble substances, and transmembrane diffusion depends in part on the lipid solubility of the diffusing compound. In the case of acids and bases, the un-ionized species exhibits greater lipid solubility than the ionized species and is either the sole diffusing species or the more rapidly diffusing species. The diffusing species of an acid or base is governed by the concentration gradient across the membrane and the pKa of the compound. In the specific case of passive diffusion across the renal tubular membrane, the concentration gradient depends on urinary pH since intracellular and blood pH are essentially constant.

Diffusion across the tubular membrane is also affected by flow-related changes in urinary concentration. The observation that excretion of N^1-methylnicotinamide (a quaternary ammonium compound) is enhanced by increases in urinary flow suggests that ionized substances diffuse passively across renal tubular membranes.

Although diffusion across the tubular membrane may occur in either direction for some organic bases, diffusion from blood to tubular lumen is highly improbable for organic acids.[55] Passive reabsorption from filtrate to blood occurs for many drugs. The urinary excretion rate of amphetamine (pKa 9.77) fluctuates with changes in urinary pH; the total amount excreted under alkaline urine conditions is lower than under acidic urine conditions. The renal clearance of phenobarbital (pKa 7.2) increases with increasing urinary flow. At any given rate of flow, the clearance is higher when the urine is alkaline than when it is acidic. In general, a weak base whose pKa is 6 or below is expected to be extensively reabsorbed at all urinary pH values; little or no reabsorption is expected for a strong base whose pKa is close to 12 throughout the range of urinary pH; reabsorption is expected to vary with changes in pH for bases with pKa values of 6 through 12. Reabsorption of acidic drugs with pKa values between 3 and 7.5 varies with urinary pH; acids with pKa ≤ 2 are not reabsorbed, and those with pKa > 8 are extensively reabsorbed throughout the range of urinary pH. Urinary flow rate often affects the excretion of compounds whose tubular reabsorption is pH-sensitive.[51,52]

Carrier-Mediated Transport Across the Renal Tubule. *Carrier-mediated transport* is a term used to describe transfer across a biologic membrane that is at a higher rate than could be attributed to diffusion alone.[58] Such transport may involve facilitated diffusion or active transport. The term *active transport* is usually applied only to those systems in which a substance is transported across a biologic membrane against a concentration gradient at the expense of energy derived from cell metabolism. Active transport processes figure prominently in the renal excretion of many drugs and their metabolites. These processes are characterized by (1) susceptibility to interference by metabolic or competitive inhibitors and (2) a maximal capacity of the transporting mechanism (T_m). Although some organic ions undergo simultaneous active bidirectional transport, i.e., reabsorption and secretion, the predominant transport of most organic ions in the renal tubule is secretory.[59] Thus, active secretion usually adds substances to the filtrate. Substances added to the filtrate in this manner may be subsequently reabsorbed. Active secretion occurs in the proximal portion of the renal tubule; reabsorption can occur all along the tubule.

The existence of renal tubule transport systems for the secretion of organic acids and bases is well documented. These systems involve separate and independent mechanisms and are not subject to inhibition by the same competitive inhibitors. There is not a high degree of specificity within either system. Substances transported by the same system compete with each other. Probenecid was synthesized in the early 1950s as an inhibitor of renal transport mechanisms. It has since been shown that probenecid itself is actively secreted by the organic acid mechanism. Probenecid has been used as the classic inhibitor of the organic anion transport system, and its ability to inhibit secretion of a compound is taken as evidence for secretion of that compound through the acid transport system.

N^1-methylnicotinamide is the classic example of an organic base that is actively transported by the renal tubule. It was one of the earliest bases for which secretion was demonstrated, and it has been used throughout the years to define the characteristics of the organic cation transport system. For drugs cleared by tubular secretion, it makes no difference what fraction is bound to plasma protein, provided that the binding is reversible. Secretion can be so extensive that all of the drug, whether in red blood cells or bound to plasma proteins, can be removed. Only the unbound drug is capable of crossing the cells lining the tubule; transport of all drug out of the blood requires rapid dissociation of the drug-protein complex and movement of drug out of the blood cells.

A compound may be subject to all of the renal excretion processes. Most organic acids and bases, however, are thought to be excreted by a three-component mechanism: glomerular filtration, active secretion, and passive reabsorption. The amount of a substance excreted by the kidney is equal to the amount filtered by the glomerulus plus the net amount transferred by tubules. Observed renal clearance, therefore, essentially consists of two components: glomerular filtration and net tubular transport. If a drug is not bound to macromolecules in the plasma, then its renal clearance either equals glomerular filtration (GFR) if there is no net tubular secretion or reabsorption, exceeds GFR if there is net tubular secretion, or is less than GFR if there is net tubular reabsorption.

While a renal clearance equal to GFR indicates the absence of a *net* tubular involvement, it does not preclude the involvement of compensating tubular processes. When a compound is bound to macromolecules, the degree of binding must be determined at relevant concentrations before meaningful statements can be made about its renal clearance. When a compound is excreted by glomerular filtration with possible passive tubular reabsorption, renal clearance should be calculated from the non-protein-bound fraction in plasma. For a compound with renal clearance higher than GFR, e.g., one involving tubular secretion, the total plasma concentration of the compound is used in the calculation of clearance. In those experimental situations whereby the contributions of glomerular filtration and tubular secretion to the renal clearance of a compound are separable, the filtration contribution should be corrected for protein binding in all cases.

Changes in renal clearance may result in changes in plasma half-life ($t_{\frac{1}{2}}$), in the overall elimination rate constant k_{10}, in the fraction of renal elimination of a compound (f_r), and in the fraction metabolized (f_m). A decrease in renal clearance (e.g., increased reabsorption, inhibition of secretion, decreased glomerular filtration) may result in an increase in $t_{\frac{1}{2}}$ and a decrease in k_{10}. For a drug that is metabolized, as well as excreted, unchanged in the urine, decreased renal clearance may also result in a larger fraction of drug metabolized ($\uparrow f_m$) and a smaller fraction recovered in the urine unchanged ($\downarrow f_r$). Opposite changes in the respective parameters would occur for an increase in renal clearance.

Experimental Techniques

A number of techniques have been employed for studying renal processes both in vitro and in vivo. In vitro techniques used to examine renal tubular transport mechanisms include renal slices, suspensions of renal tubules, perfused isolated renal tubules, and perfused isolated kidneys. In vivo methods for studying renal excretion processes include clearance techniques, the stop-flow technique, micropuncture, and microperfusion. Clearance techniques have the advantages of being technically easy, of enabling quantification of kidney function as a whole, and of being applicable to humans. Limitations include the inability to separate reabsorption from secretion for substances undergoing both processes and the inability to define transport mechanisms or to localize function to specific nephron segments.

In the clearance techniques used to study the renal excretion of a compound, an appropriate marker for GFR (e.g., inulin) is infused simultaneously with the compound. Blood and urine samples are collected and analyzed for the reference material and compound being studied; renal clearances of each are then calculated. When the ratio of the clearance of the compound being studied to that of the reference is greater than 1.0, net secretion is indicated; when the ratio is less than 1.0 (after correcting for plasma protein binding), net reabsorption is indicated. A change in the ratio with a change in urinary pH implies some passive transport, as does a change in ratio with changing urinary flow rates. A change in the ratio with increasing plasma concentration of the study compound, or in the presence of a competitive or metabolic inhibitor of transport, indicates the presence of a carrier-mediated transport process. Urinary excretion of the study compound due to glomerular filtration is equal to the unbound plasma concentration of the compound multiplied by the renal clearance of the marker (GFR); net tubular transport is equal to the total urinary excretion minus excretion due to glomerular filtration.

In the absence of active reabsorption processes, appropriate adjustment of urinary pH to preclude significant passive reabsorption of a compound enables quantitation of the secretory component (i.e., "net tubular transport" equals secretion). If there is no passive diffusion of compound from plasma to tubular lumen, the secretory component can be further evaluated in terms of saturation (Michaelis-Menten) kinetics.

Biotransformation

Most drugs are cleared from the body, at least partially, through biotransformation (metabolism). The maximum fraction of the dose that may be metabolized is given by the relative difference between the plasma and renal clearances of the drug, $(CL - Cl_r)/CL$. Biotransformations may be catabolic (e.g., hydrolysis, reduction, and oxidation) or anabolic (e.g., conjugations with glucuronic acid, glycine, or sulfate). Metabolism, unlike excretion, does not result in the removal of drug mass from the body. Rather, new chemical entities are formed, and the distribution, metabolism, and excretion of each metabolite are unique and usually independent of the parent compound. When a metabolite possesses intrinsic pharmacologic activity, as with the N-demethylated metabolite of a number of antiepileptic drugs,[60,61] characterization of its pharmacokinetic profile as well as its formation kinetics is essential to a complete understanding of pharmacokinetic/pharmacodynamic relationships.

Intrinsic Clearance and Effect of Blood Flow

Although the liver is the major metabolic organ in the body, significant metabolic activity may also exist in the lungs, kidneys, blood, or gut mucosa. A drug may be metabolized by competing pathways in the liver. The overall hepatic clearance of a drug is then given by the summation of clearances by each pathway. The ability of the liver to metabolize a drug depends in part on the intrinsic activity of the enzymatic system associated with each metabolic pathway. The overall intrinsic reaction velocity, v_{int}, may be expressed in terms of the familiar Michaelis-Menton equation applied to each of the N enzymatic systems involved in hepatic drug removal:

$$v_{int} = \sum_{i=1}^{N} \frac{V_{m,i} C_{u,1}}{K_{m,i} + C_{u,1}} \qquad (79)$$

where $C_{u,1}$ is the unbound concentration of drug available to the liver enzymes, V_m is the maximum reaction velocity, and K_m is the Michaelis constant, which is equivalent to the $C_{u,1}$ at which $v_{int} = V_m/2$. Since the instantaneous rate of drug elimination is equal to the product of its clearance and concentration, as shown in equation (15), the intrinsic hepatic clearance, CL_{int}, is given by:

$$CL_{int} = \frac{v_{int}}{C_{u,1}} = \sum_{i=1}^{N} \frac{V_{m,i}}{K_{m,i} + C_{u,1}} \qquad (80)$$

According to equation (80), if $C_{u,1}$ is significant relative to the value of K_m, then CL_{int} is not constant but varies with the dose of drug administered. The CL_{int} of either enantiomer of propranolol, for instance, is reduced more than 50% when the dosage of the racemate is increased from 160 to 320 mg/day in humans.[62] For most drugs, however, $C_{u,1}$ is small relative to K_m over the therapeutic dosage range and equation (80) reduces to equation (81):

$$CL_{int} = \sum_{i=1}^{N} \frac{V_{m,i}}{K_{m,i}} \qquad (C_{u,1} \ll K_{m,i}) \quad (81)$$

where CL_{int} is constant and independent of the dose of drug administered.

In addition to the intrinsic metabolic activity of the liver, delivery of drug to the liver (i.e., perfusion) may be an important determinant of the liver's ability to metabolize the drug: hepatic drug clearance cannot exceed the rate at which the drug is delivered to the liver. Flow rate to the liver may limit full expression of the intrinsic metabolic enzyme activity of the liver, and hepatic drug clearance is then lower than CL_{int}. A commonly used model that relates blood flow and CL_{int} to hepatic drug clearance (CL_h) is the perfusion-limited, or well-stirred, compartment model of hepatic clearance.[63-66]

$$CL_h = Q_h \left(\frac{f_u CL_{int}}{Q_h + f_u CL_{int}} \right) \qquad (82)$$

where f_u is the fraction of unbound drug in blood, Q_h is the hepatic blood flow rate (normally ~1.5 L/min in man), and CL_h is the hepatic drug clearance from blood. Equation (82) is defined in terms of blood since this is the fluid that carries drug to the eliminating organ. If measurement of drug in blood is not experimentally feasible, the blood-to-plasma concentration ratio can be determined and used to convert plasma concentration to blood concentration.

The quantity in equation (82) equivalent to CL_h/Q_h is referred to as the *hepatic extraction ratio*, E, of the drug. The effects of changes in Q_h and in $f_u CL_{int}$ on CL_h are readily evident if compounds are classified on the basis of their extraction ratio. If a drug is highly extracted ($E \to 1$), then $f_u CL_{int} \gg Q_h$, and equation (82) reduces to:

$$\lim_{E \to 1} CL_h = Q_h \qquad (83)$$

Hepatic drug clearance is then insensitive to intrinsic enzymatic activity or binding and is approximated by hepatic blood flow rate, i.e., it is perfusion-limited. On the other hand, if the drug is poorly extracted ($E \to 0$), then $Q_h \gg f_u CL_{int}$ and equation (82) reduces to

$$\lim_{E \to 0} CL_h = f_u CL_{int} \qquad (84)$$

and hepatic drug clearance is insensitive to changes in Q_h but sensitive to changes in both drug binding to blood components and metabolic enzyme activity in the liver. Thus, induction of hepatic enzyme activity, for instance, would increase the hepatic clearance of a low extraction compound but have little effect on a high extraction compound. Finally, the hepatic clearance of a drug with an intermediate extraction ratio (i.e., $E \sim 0.2$ to 0.8) is affected by changes in Q_h, f_u, or CL_{int}.

The above relationships are exemplified by the block diagram in Figure 9-16. Shown is the effect on extraction ratio (block height) and hepatic drug clearance of a ± 0.5 L/min change from normal hepatic blood flow for a compound with CL_{int} equal to 0.1, 1, or 10 times normal hepatic blood flow. In all cases, the drug is not bound in blood, i.e., $f_u = 1$. When CL_{int} is high (15 L/min) relative to blood flow, drug is highly extracted by the liver, and $E = 0.94$ when $Q_h = 1$ L/min. Substantial increases in Q_h result in only slight decreases in E. Hepatic clearance, on the other hand, increases almost proportionately with Q_h and approaches Q_h as E approaches unity, as shown in equation (83). In contrast, when CL_{int} is low (0.15 L/min) relative to blood flow, the drug is poorly extracted by the liver, that is, $E = 0.13$ when $Q_h = 1$ L/min. In this case, as blood flow increases, there is a proportionate decrease in extraction ratio. Hepatic clearance is approximately equal to CL_{int} and is independent of blood flow, as shown in equation (84). For the intermediate case where $CL_{int} \cong Q_h$ (1.5 L/min), there is a modest decrease in E and increase in hepatic clearance as blood flow increases.

Calculation of Intrinsic Clearance

The intrinsic clearance is obtained from blood concentration data following oral administration of the drug. Before it reaches the general circulation, an orally administered drug is absorbed into the portal circulation and must pass through the liver. During this "first pass," a fraction of the portally available dose, equivalent to the extraction ratio E, is lost by extraction in the liver; the remaining fraction, F, reaches the general circulation, i.e., it is *bioavailable*. If P is the fraction of the dose absorbed unchanged into the portal circulation, then $F = P(1 - E)$. If drug is totally absorbéd in unchanged form from the gastrointestinal lumen and not metabolized in the gut wall, then $P = 1$ and the bioavailable fraction is:

$$F = 1 - E \qquad (85)$$

and according to equation (46), the amount of bioavailable drug is:

$$FD^{po} = (1 - E)D^{po} = CL \cdot AUC^{po}_{\infty} \qquad (86)$$

If all of the drug eliminated from the body is cleared by the liver, CL in equation (86) can be replaced by CL_h. Expressing E and CL_h in terms of the perfusion-limited model in equation (82) gives:

$$\left(1 - \frac{f_u CL_{int}}{Q_h + f_u CL_{int}}\right) D^{po} = \left(\frac{Q_h f_u CL_{int}}{Q_h + f_u CL_{int}}\right) AUC^{po}_{\infty} \qquad (87)$$

which simplifies to:

$$CL_{int} = \frac{D^{po}}{f_u AUC^{po}_{\infty}} \qquad (88)$$

Thus, the intrinsic hepatic clearance of a drug may be determined by the ratio of the dose and the AUC_{∞} for unbound drug after oral administration. The application of equation (88), however, requires that the entire administered dose D^{po} reaches the liver unchanged and that the liver is the sole organ for drug elimination. Appropriate use of equation (88) can be ensured by infusing the drug directly into the hepatic portal vein and by adjusting for extrahepatic elimination. For example, if in addition to hepatic clearance, the drug is cleared renally, then $CL_h = (1 - f_r)CL$, which upon substitution into equation (86) would result in:

$$CL_{int} = \frac{(1 - f_r)D^{po}}{f_u AUC^{po}_{\infty}} \qquad (89)$$

The evaluation of equation (89) requires an estimate of f_r, which can be obtained following an intravenous dose of the drug.

Whereas changes in hepatic blood flow affect the hepatic clearance of most drugs (except when $E \to 0$), the determination of intrinsic

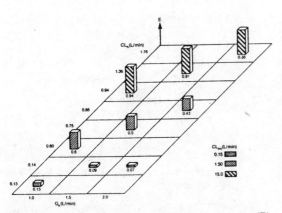

FIG. 9-16. *Relationship between extraction ratio (E), blood flow (Q_h), and hepatic drug clearance (CL_h) for a compound with an intrinsic clearance (CL_{int}) equal to 0.1, 1, or 10 times normal hepatic blood flow.*

hepatic clearance is insensitive to changes in flow rate. The intrinsic hepatic clearance of total drug is given by $f_u CL_{int}$. Hence, the effect of binding to plasma or blood proteins is to reduce the overall elimination rate of drug from the body.

Enterohepatic Circulation

Biliary Excretion

Drug elimination from the liver can occur by two distinct mechanisms: hepatic metabolism and biliary excretion. Hepatic clearance is the quantitative measure of the overall ability of the liver to eliminate the drug and is the sum of the hepatic metabolic clearance and the biliary clearance.

While all compounds may be excreted in bile, the importance of biliary clearance to the elimination of a compound depends on the degree to which it concentrates in bile relative to plasma. Biliary clearance is given by equation (90):

$$\text{Biliary Clearance} = \text{Bile Flow} \times \frac{\text{Concentration in Bile}}{\text{Concentration in Plasma}} \quad (90)$$

Since bile flow in man is relatively constant—between 0.5 and 1.0 ml/min—biliary clearance is proportional to the ratio of bile to plasma drug concentration. Compounds are classified according to the degree to which they concentrate in bile. Biliary clearance cannot exceed bile flow for such compounds as electrolytes and proteins, whose concentration ratios of bile to plasma are usually equal to or less than unity. On the other hand, a biliary clearance of 500 ml/min is not uncommon for drugs.

For the biliary clearance of a compound to be significant, the compound must be actively secreted into bile and achieve a concentration gradient relative to the blood. Separate secretory mechanisms appear to exist for acids, bases, and neutral compounds. Several physicochemical features of a molecule are important in determining the extent to which it is secreted in bile. First, compounds secreted in bile usually have molecular weights exceeding 300 to 400 daltons. Moreover, the molecular weight threshold appears to depend on species: about 325 in the rat, 400 in the guinea pig, 475 in the rabbit, and 500 in man. Second, compounds excreted in bile are usually polar in nature. Molecular structure may also be important, but the nature of the dependence is not well understood.

Knowledge of the metabolic profile of a drug is essential in assessing whether a given compound may be excreted in bile. Conjugation reactions increase the polarity as well as the molecular weight of the drug. Glucuronide conjugates, for instance, are strong acids with pKa values of 3 to 4, are nearly completely ionized at physiologic pH, and have molecular weights 176 daltons greater than the parent compound. Not surprisingly, therefore, many compounds are excreted in bile in their conjugated forms.

Many of these generalizations are illustrated by the data from two nonsteroidal anti-inflammatory agents, indomethacin and sulindac. Indomethacin is pharmacologically active whereas sulindac is a prodrug that is metabolized reversibly to the active moiety, the sulfide metabolite. Sulindac is also irreversibly biotransformed to the inactive sulfone metabolite. Structures and molecular weights are given in Figure 9-17. Both are arylacetic acids with molecular weights of about 350 daltons. In addition, these compounds undergo glucuronidation so that the effective molecular weight is about 525. Biliary and renal clearances of each in various animal species, including man, were determined from the total (free plus conjugate) amount of drug present in bile and urine. The data, summarized in Table 9-1, are expressed in terms of the renal to biliary clearance ratios as an index of the relative importance of the two routes of elimination.

A substantial species difference is evident for both indomethacin and sulindac. Biliary clearance is by far the dominant route in the dog and rat, while renal clearance is slightly favored in the rabbit. Based on molecular weight alone, a species difference is expected; the conjugated

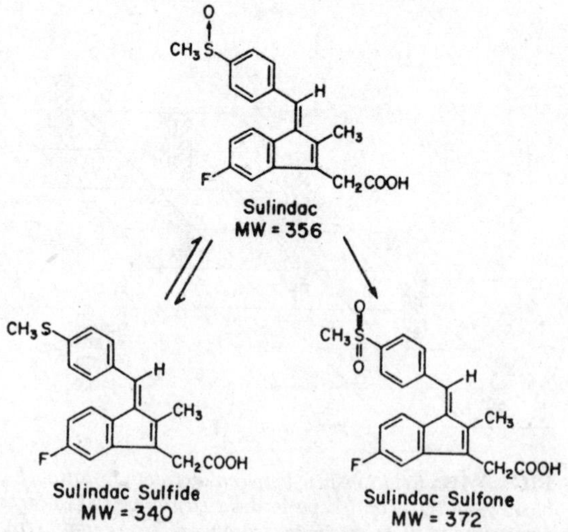

FIG. 9-17. *Sulindac and metabolites.*

TABLE 9-1. *Renal to Biliary Clearance Ratios in Various Species*[67-70]

| | Renal to Biliary Clearance Ratio | | | |
Species	Indomethacin	Sulindac	Sulindac Sulfone	Sulindac Sulfide
Dog	<0.008	<0.004	—	—
Rat	0.03	<0.03	—	—
Rhesus monkey	1.36	0.11	0.11	~0
Man	0.73	0.12	0.10	<0.03
Rabbit	2.73	1.65	2.5	2.1

— Not available.

compounds exceed the "threshold" molecular weight by approximately 200 daltons in the rat but by approximately only 50 daltons in the rabbit.

The renal-to-biliary clearance ratios are of similar magnitude in the rhesus monkey and man, especially for sulindac and metabolites, and are intermediate between those of the rat and rabbit. Only minimal amounts of the sulfide metabolite are excreted in urine.

Also, sulindac sulfide is an interesting example of structural dependence: while it differs from the parent drug and the sulfone metabolite only in the oxidation state of the sulfur atom, its clearance into bile (or urine) of man is marginal compared to either sulindac or the sulfone metabolite.

Biliary Recycling

Following its secretion into bile, the drug is stored in the gallbladder. When the gallbladder contracts, the drug is released into the duodenum and may then be metabolized, reabsorbed, or excreted in feces. If reabsorbed back into the portal circulation, it once again is subject to biliary secretion in the liver and thus completes an "enterohepatic cycle." Biliary clearance is a route of drug elimination from the body only to the extent that drug is excreted in feces, biotransformed, or otherwise degraded in the intestinal lumen (i.e., it undergoes irreversible clearance). If drug is reabsorbed, the hepatoportal system is simply an organ of drug distribution (i.e., reversible clearance). As indicated previously, compounds are often cleared in bile as their conjugates. Commonly, these are hydrolyzed within the lumen by the gut flora liberating the original drug, which is then free to be reabsorbed.

With the notable exception of the rat, all common laboratory animals and humans have a gallbladder. Contraction of the gallbladder occurs only intermittently, usually in response to food stimuli, so that considerable amounts of drug may accumulate in the gallbladder. Since gallbladder emptying is sporadic, different amounts of drug are released into the gut at uneven time intervals. If the drug is reabsorbed, gallbladder emptying serves as an additional source of drug input into the body. The overall input function is complex in that neither the amount nor the time course of reabsorption is known, and reabsorption may overlap with part of the dose being absorbed for the first time. Therefore, drugs that are recycled tend to exhibit unusual pharmacokinetic properties. The overall effect of enterohepatic recycling of drug is to delay its elimination from the body and to prolong its pharmacologic effect.

The effect of recycling on drug elimination may be described quantitatively; again, sulindac is used to illustrate this point. The biliary clearance, CL_b, of sulindac and its sulfone and sulfide metabolites was studied in man by use of a duodenal intubation technique[70] and by direct collection of bile through a surgically implanted T-tube.[71] Results of both techniques were similar, with CL_b averaging about 200 ml/min for both sulindac and the sulfone and about 14 ml/min for the sulfide. The total amount of drug secreted in bile, $CL_b \cdot AUC_\infty$, as a percentage of the administered dose averaged 135% for sulindac, 186% for the sulfone metabolite, and 16.2% for the sulfide metabolite; the total biliary drug flux was 336% of the administered dose. Thus, on the average, a given dose of sulindac is recycled approximately 3.4 times.

Drug recycling may appear as secondary reentry peaks in the plasma concentration profiles. In patients who have fasted, these peaks are typically seen 8 to 12 hours after administration of the dose coincident with gallbladder emptying following resumption of eating with the evening meal (Fig. 9-18). Figure 9-18 demonstrates that a plasma half-life ($t_{\frac{1}{2}}$) cannot be obtained in the usual manner in that the terminal plasma concentrations do not decline logarithmically. The degree of drug accumulation in plasma upon administration of multiple doses, however, is

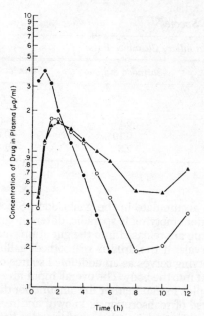

FIG. 9-18. *Plasma concentration profile of sulindac (●) and its sulfone (▲) and sulfide (○) metabolites demonstrates secondary re-entry peaks due to biliary recycling in humans.*

remarkably consistent among studies.[72] Thus, a mean effective $t_{\frac{1}{2}}$ that is consistent with the observed drug accumulation may be obtained from:

$$\frac{\bar{C}_\tau^{(n)}}{\bar{C}_\tau^{(1)}} = \frac{1 - EXP(-.693n\tau/t_{\frac{1}{2}})}{1 - EXP(-.693\tau/t_{\frac{1}{2}})} \quad (91)$$

where $\bar{C}_\tau^{(1)}$ and $\bar{C}_\tau^{(n)}$ are the average drug concentration over the first and the nth dosage interval of τ hours. The mean effective $t_{\frac{1}{2}}$ for sulindac is 7.8 hours while that of its active sulfide metabolite is 16.4 hours.[73] Thus, after three days of therapy, effective mean steady-state conditions should prevail.

Capacity Limitations

Drug removal from the body may be excretory or metabolic. Either route may be further composed of multiple parallel pathways, each with its own inherent capacity to remove the drug. The overall elimination rate of the drug from the body is the sum of these individual contributions. The Michaelis constants, K_m, for most elimination processes are large relative to the concentrations of drug following therapeutic doses, as was shown by equation (81). Hence, the rate of drug elimination is usually proportional to concentration; the proportionality constant is the plasma clearance CL. Drugs that

behave in this way are said to obey linear elimination kinetics. Occasionally encountered, however, are drug concentrations that may not be insignificant relative to the K_m for one or more processes, whereby the elimination rate becomes disproportionate in relation to concentration, and increasingly so with increasing dose or concentration. Drugs that behave nonlinearly within the therapeutic range include salicylic acid, phenytoin, theophylline, diflunisal, acetaminophen, and 5-fluorouracil.

The disposition of salicylic acid (SA) in humans is schematically depicted in Figure 9-19. Levy and co-workers have shown that capacity limitations exist in the formation of salicylurate (SU).[74] Deviations from linear kinetics become evident even after the administration of a single aspirin tablet. With increasing dosage, the metabolic pathway leading to the formation of salicyl phenolic glucuronide (SPG) also becomes nonlinear. On the other hand, the renal excretion of SA and biotransformation to salicyl acyl glucuronide (SAG) and gentisic acid (GA) appear linear throughout the therapeutic range. Therefore, the overall rate of salicylate elimination from the body can be represented by equation (92), which is based on the one-compartment, open model:

$$-V_1\frac{dC_1}{dt} = \left(CL_m^{SAG} + CL_m^{GA} + CL_r\right.$$

$$\left. + \frac{V_m^{SU}}{K_m^{SU} + C_1} + \frac{V_m^{SPG}}{K_m^{SPG} + C_1}\right)C_1 \quad (92)$$

where C_1, V_1, and CL_r refer to the plasma concentration, the volume of distribution, and the renal clearance of SA while CL_m^{SAG}, CL_m^{GA},

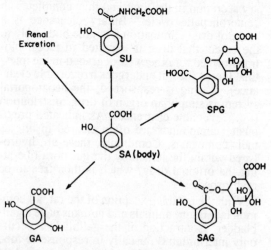

FIG. 9-19. *Disposition of salicylic acid.*

$V_m^{SU}/(K_m^{SU} + C_1)$, and $V_m^{SPG}/(K_m^{SPG} + C_1)$ are the metabolic clearances of SA leading to the formation of SAG, GA, SU, and SPG, respectively. The plasma clearance, CL, of SA is the sum of the individual clearances, that is:

$$CL = CL_m^{SAG} + CL_m^{GA} + CL_r$$
$$+ \frac{V_m^{SU}}{K_m^{SU} + C_1} + \frac{V_m^{SPG}}{K_m^{SPG} + C_1} \quad (93)$$

Thus, the plasma clearance of SA depends on concentration because of capacity limitations in the formation of SU and SPG. Representative model parameters are shown in Table 9-2. Plasma clearance decreases with increasing concentrations of SA. Consequently, the overall elimination rate of SA increases more slowly in proportion to changes in concentration. On the other hand, as elimination proceeds, C_1 decreases with time and eventually becomes insignificant relative to K_m^{SU} and K_m^{SPG}. Thereafter, plasma clearance is independent of concentration; in other words:

$$CL = CL_m^{SAG} + CL_m^{GA} + CL_r + \frac{V_m^{SU}}{K_m^{SU}} + \frac{V_m^{SPG}}{K_m^{SPG}}$$
$$(94)$$

when:

$$(C_1 \ll K_m^{SU} \text{ and } C_1 \ll K_m^{SPG})$$

such that the elimination rate is proportional to C_1 and behaves linearly.

The effect of capacity-limited elimination on salicylate plasma levels can be illustrated as a function of dose and of the dosage regimen. The time course of change in C_1 following a dose of salicylate can be described by dividing both sides of equation (92) by V_1 and providing a drug input rate (INPUT) to the body, namely:

$$\frac{dC_1}{dt} = \text{INPUT} - (k_{SAG} + k_{GA} + k_{SA})C_1$$
$$- \frac{C_1}{V_1}\left[\frac{V_m^{SU}}{K_m^{SU} + C_1} + \frac{V_m^{SAG}}{K_m^{SAG} + C_1} \right] \quad (95)$$

where k_{SAG}, k_{GA}, and k_{SA} are the first-order rate constants for the formation of SAG, the formation of GA, and the renal excretion of SA, respectively. In the ensuing discussion, the total drug input equals D/V_1, although the rate of introduction may be fast or slow.

Figure 9-20 shows the simulated plasma concentrations of SA as a function of dose. Because plasma clearance decreases with increasing concentration, total area under the plasma concentration curve, AUC_∞, increases more rapidly in proportion to dose (Fig. 9-21). Regardless of dose, the terminal phases of plasma concentration profiles are log-linear with identical half-lives. The onset of the log-linear phase occurs at the same plasma concentration but is disproportionately delayed with increasing doses (Fig. 9-22). Analogously, at identical doses, the faster input rate produces a greater AUC_∞. Because higher concentrations are achieved sooner, the intensity and the duration of the nonlinear effects of elimination are both magnified.

TABLE 9-2. *Representative Model Constants for Salicylic Acid*[74,75]

Model Parameter	Numerical Value
CL_r	41.3 ml/h
CL_m^{SAG}	39.1 ml/h
CL_m^{GA}	12.7 ml/h
V_m^{SU}	60.3 mg/h
K_m^{SU}	61.5 mg/L
V_m^{SPG}	32.3 mg/h
K_m^{SPG}	114.4 mg/L
V_1	5.5 L

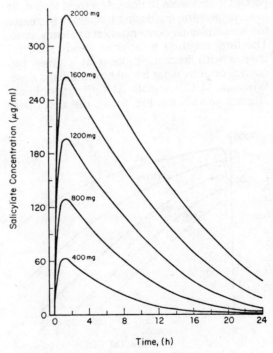

FIG. 9-20. *Simulated plasma concentrations of salicylic acid as a function of dosage.*

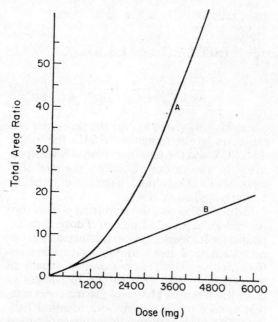

FIG. 9-21. *Disproportionate increase in AUC$_\infty$ following increasing doses of salicylic acid (A). Curve B represents the result if linear kinetics prevail.*

The effects of capacity limitations in elimination on salicylate accumulation are shown in Figure 9-23. At a given dosing frequency, higher steady-state concentrations are achieved in proportion to increases in dose. At a fixed total daily dose, decreasing the dosing frequency increases the mean plasma concentration at steady state. The time required to achieve steady state increases with increasing doses at a given frequency or increasing frequency at a fixed dose. Whereas AUC$_\infty^{(1)}$ equals AUC$_\tau^{(ss)}$ when linear kinetics prevail (see Fig. 9-14), the area under

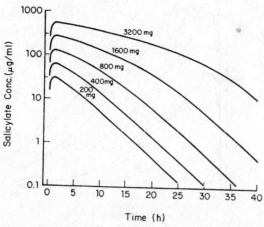

FIG. 9-22. *The effect of dose on the onset of the log-linear phase of the salicylate plasma profile.*

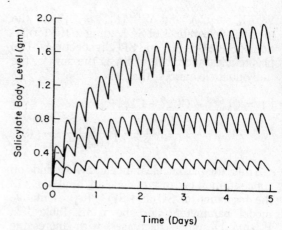

FIG. 9-23. *Disproportionate increases in salicylate accumulation with increasing doses. Key: lower curve = 1 tablet; middle curve = 2 tablets; upper curve = 3 tablets.*

the salicylate plasma concentration curve over a dosage interval at steady state always exceeds the total area after a single dose, except in the trivial case where there is no accumulation.

Finally, fractional contribution of individual elimination pathways depends on dose. As each pathway approaches saturation, its contribution to total urinary excretion diminishes while those of the remaining routes become relatively more prominent. This effect is illustrated in Figure 9-24.

The nonlinearities exemplified by salicylate kinetics apply to any drug whose elimination is subject to capacity limitations.

Effects of Disease

The pharmacokinetics of a drug may be markedly altered in the presence of disease.[76] As discussed earlier, the kidneys and the liver are the major drug-eliminating organs in the body. Any disease process that affects the functional integrity of an eliminating organ or delivery of drug thereto (e.g., blood perfusion) may decrease the rate at which the drug is cleared from the body. In addition, a decline in organ function occurs with advancing age. Cardiac output declines with age and results in a reduced renal and splanchnic blood flow. The effects of these and other age-related physiologic changes on drug pharmacokinetics have been reviewed.[77] A reduction in the usual recommended dose or a change in dosage regimen may be required in the diseased or elderly patient to avoid side effects due to excessive drug accumulation and yet achieve the desired therapeutic response. Immature renal and metabolic function must be

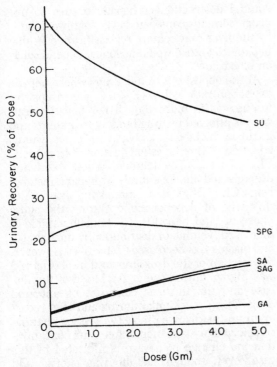

FIG. 9-24. *Effect of dosage on urinary excretion of salicylic acid and its metabolites.*

where k_{nr} is the first-order rate constant of extrarenal elimination, i.e., $(1 - f_r)k_{10}$.

For these drugs, a plot of k_{10} versus CL_{cr} should be a straight line with slope a and intercept k_{nr}. As an example, Table 9-3 presents data relating CL_{cr} to plasma $t_{\frac{1}{2}}$ of amiloride in renally impaired patients.[80] For a one-compartment model drug, $k_{10} = 0.693/t_{\frac{1}{2}}$. The plot of k_{10} versus CL_{cr} is linear (Fig. 9-25). Since amiloride is not metabolized and is cleared from the body exclusively by the kidneys, the intercept k_{nr} is zero. The predicted $t_{\frac{1}{2}}$ in subjects with normal renal function, where CL_{cr} is nominally 120 ml/min, is 6.3 hours, which is in excellent agreement with the value of 6 hours reported for healthy subjects.[80] All three observations support the application of equation (97) in the individualized dosage adjustment for the renally impaired patient. Thus, on the basis of a measured CL_{cr}, the patient's predicted k_{10} can be read from Figure 9-25 and substituted into equation (73) to determine how the dose or dosage frequency should be changed from the normal regimen to maintain the same mean plasma concentration at steady state.

For drugs with a narrow therapeutic margin,

considered as well when devising dosage regimens for neonates.[78]

The effect of renal impairment on drug elimination depends on the fractional contribution of the kidneys to the total drug clearance. In general, if f_r exceeds 0.3, a reduction in dosage is warranted in the renally impaired patient. For some compounds, the first-order rate constant for renal excretion, k_r $(= f_r k_{10})$, is directly proportional to the creatinine clearance, CL_{cr}, a measure of renal function:

$$k_r = aCL_{cr} \qquad (96)$$

The effect on the overall drug elimination rate constant k_{10} $(= k_r + k_{nr})$ is then given by:

$$k_{10} = aCL_{cr} + k_{nr} \qquad (97)$$

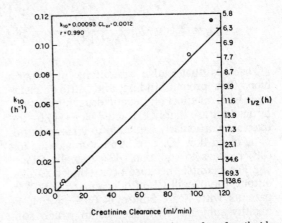

FIG. 9-25. *Relationship between k_{10} and $t_{\frac{1}{2}}$ of amiloride and creatinine clearance in patients with varying degrees of renal insufficiency (○). The mean in healthy subjects is also represented (●). (Data from George[79] and Weiss et al.[80])*

TABLE 9-3. *Plasma Half-Life of Amiloride in Renally Impaired Patients[79]*

Patient	Plasma Half-Life (h)	Creatinine Clearance (ml/min)
3	7.5	97
2	21.4	46
5	43.8	17
1	102.5	6
4	143.5	5

or when k_{10} at low CL_{cr} cannot otherwise be measured, a first approximation of the relationship between k_{10} and CL_{cr} can be obtained by linear interpolation between the extremes ($CL_{cr} = 0$ or 120 ml/min), with f_r and k_{10} in healthy subjects being the only known values ($k_{nr} = (1 - f_r)k_{10}$). This method has been successful in predicting the elimination rate constants for a number of antibiotics in severely uremic patients.[81]

Implicit in equation (97), or its equivalent expressed in terms of clearances, is that volume of distribution and nonrenal elimination are constant and independent of renal function. Biotransformation and tissue or plasma protein binding of a drug, however, may be altered in the uremic state, and dosage adjustment is thus more complex.

In contrast to renal impairment, the effect of hepatic dysfunction on drug elimination is not well defined. This lack of definition is not surprising, considering the host of diseases that affect blood flow, drug-metabolizing enzymes, and biliary secretion, all of which may be involved in drug clearance by the liver.[76] Generalizations, however, can be made based on equation (82), that is:

$$CL_h = Q_h E = Q_h \left[\frac{f_u CL_{int}}{Q_h + f_u CL_{int}} \right] \quad (98)$$

Diseases that cause alterations in hepatic blood flow, protein binding, and intrinsic clearance have an effect on hepatic drug elimination. Drugs that are highly extracted ($E \rightarrow 1$) by the liver are particularly sensitive to change in hepatic blood flow (Q_h). In other words, equation (98) reduces to equation (83), namely, $CL_h \sim Q_h$. For example, because of a reduced cardiac output, the overall CL of lidocaine ($E = 0.7$) in patients with heart failure is 60% of that in healthy subjects.[82] In diseases in which sub-stantial destruction of hepatic tissues occurs, drugs normally considered to be highly extracted by the liver may require reclassification in that hepatic clearance would no longer depend solely on blood flow.

At the opposite extreme, drugs whose hepatic extraction ratio is low ($E < 0.2$) are insensitive to changes in blood flow. Their hepatic clearance is affected by drug binding to proteins and intrinsic metabolic activity. In other words, equation (98) reduces to equation (84), namely, $CL_h \sim f_u CL_{int}$. Tolbutamide, a low extraction drug cleared almost entirely by hepatic metabolism ($CL \sim CL_h$), is an interesting example of this type of dependence.[83] During the acute phase of viral hepatitis, CL for tolbutamide is increased, volume of distribution is unchanged, and plasma $t_{\frac{1}{2}}$ is decreased (Table 9-4). However, the fraction of the drug unbound in plasma (f_u) was higher during the active phase of the disease and the intrinsic clearance of unbound drug (CL_{int}) was similar during and after recovery from the disease (Table 9-4). Since pharmacologic activity is related to free drug concentration, no change in dosage is indicated in this case, even though half-life was shorter and plasma concentrations were lower for total drug.

Binding may be altered because of changes in protein composition, concentration, and conformation. For example, changes in binding affinity have been shown to occur with changes in pH in patients with uremia and cirrhosis of the liver. Dehydration and hypoproteinemia would have opposing effects on protein concentration, and therefore on the free fraction, f_u. Concentrations of α_1-acid glycoprotein rise dramatically under stress, which is likely to affect the binding of basic drugs. The effect of binding is especially critical for drugs that are highly bound, because a small change in the fraction bound represents a major change in the fraction unbound. Thus, a change from 99% to 98% bound represents a two-fold increase in f_u.

TABLE 9-4. *Mean Pharmacokinetic Parameters for Tolbutamide in Five Subjects During and After Recovery from Acute Viral Hepatitis*

	During	After	Change
Volume of distribution (L/kg)	0.15	0.15	none
Plasma drug clearance (ml/h/kg)	26	18	increased
Half-life (h)	4.0	5.9	decreased
Free fraction in plasma (%)	8.7	6.8	increased
Clearance of unbound drug (ml/h/kg)	300	260	none

Adapted from Williams et al.[83]

Factors Affecting Drug Absorption

In general, drug absorption from dermal, vaginal, rectal, parenteral, or gastrointestinal absorption sites into the systemic circulation occurs by a passive diffusion across biologic membranes. These membranes form lipoidal barriers that separate the body's interior from its exterior environment. The rate of diffusive movement, dA/dt, across a homogeneous membrane is governed by Fick's law, that is:

$$\frac{dA}{dt} = D_c P_c S \frac{dC}{dX} \qquad (99)$$

where D_c is the diffusion coefficient of the drug through the membrane, P_c is the partition coefficient between the membrane and the donor medium containing the drug, S is the membrane surface area, dC is the concentration differential across the membrane, and dX is the membrane thickness. In actual practice, concentrations on the receptor side of the membrane are low because of continuous blood flow. Thus, when the concentration on the donor side is relatively high, equation (99) reduces to:

$$\frac{dA}{dt} = P_m SC \qquad (100)$$

where C is the drug concentration at the absorption site, and P_m is the permeability constant defined by:

$$P_m = \frac{D_c P_c}{dX} \qquad (101)$$

For solid dosage forms, drug concentration at the absorption site is a function of the dissolution rate of the drug in the medium at that site. The dissolution is given by the Noyes-Whitney equation:

$$\frac{dC}{dt} = \frac{D_c' S}{h}(C_s - C) \qquad (102)$$

where C is the concentration at time t, D_c' is the diffusion coefficient of drug in the medium, S is the surface area of drug particles, h is the thickness of the diffusion layer surrounding the particles, and C_s is the solubility of the drug in the diffusion layer.

Physical Factors

Solubility

Drug absorption requires that molecules be in solution at the absorption site. Dissolution of solid dosage forms in gastrointestinal fluids is a prerequisite to the delivery of a drug to the systemic circulation following oral administration. Dissolution depends in part on the solubility of the drug substance in the surrounding medium. Polar solutes are more soluble in water than in organic phases, while the reverse is true for nonpolar solutes. Ionized species have a greater aqueous solubility than their un-ionized counterparts. The total solubility of acids or bases in aqueous medium is therefore pH-dependent. For drugs absorbed by passive diffusion, those exhibiting low aqueous solubility tend to have a slower oral absorption rate than those exhibiting high aqueous solubility.

For drugs intended for topical application (e.g., vaginal, rectal, dermal), the solubility of the drug in the vehicle is important. For a given vehicle, the highest driving force for absorption is obtained when the drug concentration in the vehicle equals its solubility. Concentrations below saturation decrease the absorption efficiency, while concentrations exceeding drug solubility serve as reservoirs to maintain a saturated solution.

Particle Size

Surface area of drug particles is another parameter that influences drug dissolution, and in turn, drug absorption. Particle size is a determinant of surface area. Small particles with greater surface area dissolve more rapidly than larger particles, even though both have the same intrinsic solubility. Particle size appears to have little influence on the absorption of drugs with high aqueous solubility, but it may have a pronounced effect on the absorption of drugs with low aqueous solubility. The absorption of griseofulvin, a neutral compound with low aqueous solubility (15 μg/ml), is poor and erratic. Increasing particle surface area through micronization markedly improves absorption, as illustrated in Figure 9-26.[84] Further reduction of particle size by formation of fine solid dispersions in polyethylene glycols results in an approximate doubling of absorption efficiency, compared with conventionally micronized formulations.

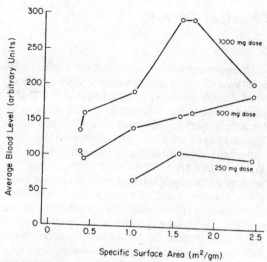

FIG. 9-26. *Effect of specific surface area on the absorption of griseofulvin in humans.*

Crystal Form

Polymorphs are crystal forms caused by differences in the packing and orientation of molecules under different crystallizing conditions. The physicochemical properties of these crystal forms (e.g., density, solubility, melting point) are influenced by the intermolecular forces present. For example, polymorphs with weak attractive forces (thus, in a high energy state) exhibit greater solubility than those with strong attractive forces. Hence, differences in dissolution and absorption rates between polymorphs of a given compound may also be observed. The rate of absorption of chloramphenicol appears to be directly related to the solubility of the different crystal forms of its palmitate ester.[85] When differences in crystal energy are small, effects of polymorphism on absorption may not be observed. Three polymorphs of chlorpropamide have been shown to yield comparable serum drug concentrations.[86]

Dissociation Constant

The un-ionized species of acidic or basic compounds in solution penetrates lipoidal membranes of the gastrointestinal tract more efficiently than the ionized species. The rate of gastrointestinal absorption of a drug, therefore, is directly related to the concentration of its un-ionized species at the absorption site, which is a function of the pKa of the compound and pH of the environment. The pH of the gastrointestinal tract ranges from approximately 1.2 to 3.5 in the stomach, to 5.0 to 6.0 in the duodenum, to 6.5 to 8.0 in the jejunum and large intestine. Over the pH range 1 to 8, the un-ionized fraction changes dramatically for acids with pKa values between 2.5 and 7.5 (decreasing with increasing pH) and for bases with pKa values between 5 and 11. For these compounds, pH-dependent absorption is expected. Weak acids with pKa values greater than 7.5 and bases with pKa values less than 5 have pH-independent absorption.[87] In general, drugs with pKa values from 5 to 7 are more readily absorbed than acidic drugs with high pKa values. Amphoteric compounds manifest the least absorption difficulties when they are presented as zwitterions, while neutral compounds do not exhibit pH-dependent absorption.

Chemical Factors

Lipophilicity

Biologic membranes, being lipoidal in nature, are usually more permeable to lipid soluble substances. Transport across these membranes therefore depends, in part, on the lipid solubility of the diffusing species. Lipid solubility of a drug is determined by the presence of nonpolar groups in the structure of the drug molecule as well as by ionizable groups that are affected by local pH. The un-ionized drug species exhibits a greater lipid solubility than the ionized species. The relative lipophilic to hydrophilic properties of the entire molecule, described by the partition coefficient, determine whether the molecule readily undergoes passive diffusion across the gastrointestinal or other biologic membranes. In general, the lipid/water partition coefficient of a molecule is a useful index of its propensity to be absorbed by passive diffusion. A high lipid solubility, however, does not necessarily favor absorption unless the water solubility is relatively low so that the drug is not "trapped" in the aqueous phase. On the other hand, when the water solubility is too low, a significant concentration cannot be achieved at the membrane surface, and absorption may be inefficient despite a favorable partition coefficient.

The absorption of a drug may often be enhanced through appropriate structural modifications that serve to alter the relative lipophilicity/hydrophilicity of the compound, e.g., esterification of a water-soluble acid. Another approach to enhanced absorption of compounds with poor lipid solubility is that of inclusion of adjuvants in the dosage form, which rather than altering the lipid solubility of the drug in question, possibly enhance absorption by altering the permeability of the absorbing membrane. For example, salicylate may interact with calcium or magnesium ions in the rectal membrane and thus facilitate rectal absorption of theophylline.[88]

Stability

Chemical integrity must be maintained until the compound is delivered to its intended site of absorption or application. Obviously, chemical instability in the dosage form, or instability prior to transport across the initial biologic barrier, invariably affects bioavailability.

Salt formation is a chemical modification that usually enhances aqueous solubility; however, aqueous solubility per se may not be the sole determinant of bioavailability. For example, salts of weak acids may precipitate on initial contact with the gastric environment following oral administration. Hence, dissolution of the precipitate is a prerequisite to absorption. In a static situation, the concentration and the partition characteristics of the drug at the pH of the mucosal surface where absorption occurs can be independently studied. The dynamics of transport along the gastrointestinal tract and across the gastrointestinal membranes, however, are such that the effect of salt formation on the bioavailability of the sample drug is usually unpredictable. The observed effect is a function of the dissolution rate of the salt or its precipitate, gastric pH, gastric emptying time, intestinal motility, pKa of the drug, and so on.

Chemical instability is often a function of pH. Compounds that are highly labile in the neutral range are seldom useful as drugs. Whereas instability in the alkaline range is seldom encountered under physiologic conditions, stability in acid is a concern, particularly for drugs intended for oral administration. For example, gastric instability of penicillin G is a major factor in its poor and erratic bioavailability following oral administration. This problem led to the synthesis of the acid-resistant phenoxyalkylpenicillins, of which penicillin V is a member.

Prodrug formation is commonly used to enhance absorption of a drug by chemical modification. An ideal prodrug is one that is quantitatively absorbed and biotransformed to the parent drug during its transport to the site of action (e.g., systemic circulation, brain, epidermis). Prior chemical degradation, including the formation of the active moiety, adversely affects bioavailability.

Metabolic Factors

In addition to the physical and chemical factors that may affect drug absorption are metabolic factors. Drugs may be exposed to presystemic biotransformation when administered by a nonintravascular route.

Gastrointestinal Tract

Presystemic elimination of drugs occurs most often following oral administration. Biotransformation can occur in the gut lumen, the gut wall, or the liver. Drug metabolizing enzymes that are found in the upper intestine probably originate in secretions of Paneth's cells, or from cells shed into the lumen from the mucosal lining. Such enzymes have been implicated in the hydrolysis of phthalate esters and pivampicillin. These enzymes are inactivated by gut flora in the lower bowel.[89]

The intestinal flora represent a highly diverse and relatively potent source of drug metabolic activity. At least 400 different species of bacteria are present in the human intestinal tract. These bacteria are mostly anaerobes involved in reductive reactions. Drugs containing nitro-groups may be reduced to amines, which can be toxic. Sulfa drugs, lactulose, and some cathartics may be activated by these bacteria. These reactions may be complementary to metabolism occurring subsequently in the gut wall or liver, but they may also be regenerative (e.g., hydrolysis of glucuronide, sulfate or acylamide metabolites excreted in the bile).[90] Diet, disease, and drugs contribute to differences in the number, type, and location of these bacteria. Since most are restricted to the lower bowel, the potential for bacterial degradation is greatest for drugs administered rectally. Drugs that are rapidly absorbed following oral ingestion may not be exposed to bacteria in the lower intestine. On the other hand, bio-inactivation by gut flora may further decrease the bioavailability of compounds that are not efficiently absorbed in the upper tract.[89]

The metabolism of a drug during transit through the gut wall also influences bioavailability. Drug-metabolizing enzymes are known to be located in the endoplasmic reticulum, mitochondria (monoamine oxidase), and cytosol (N-acetyltransferase). Some enzymes such as phenol and estrone sulfokinases exist throughout the gastrointestinal tract, while others may be more localized in the jejunal mucosa (steroid alcohol sulfokinase). These enzyme systems fall into two categories: (1) those that catalyze such preconjugation reactions as C-oxidation, hydroxylation, dealkylation, N- and S-oxidation, reduction, and hydrolysis and (2) conjugative or synthetic reactions. Since many of these reactions may also occur in the liver, it is usually difficult to quantify the relative contribution of either site to the overall metabolic scheme of a drug. It can be said, however, that preconjugative reactions that depend upon cytochromes P450 or P448 are quantitatively unimportant in the gut wall, where synthetic reactions such as O-sulfation are more highly developed. Although the pylorus, duodenum, and jejunum have the greatest metabolic activity, biotransformation can occur throughout the alimentary tract from the buccal mucosa to the rectum. Metabolism is a major source of variation in bioavailability and therapeutic response.[91,92]

Physiologic changes in the gastrointestinal tract, other drugs, diet, or disease may alter drug-metabolizing enzyme activity in the gut wall. Monoamine oxidase activity is affected by thyroid activity, systemic progesterone levels, and iron deficiency.[91] At the mucosal level, induction of preconjugative reactions are usually unimportant, but drug competition for conjugation or enzyme inhibition is clinically relevant. Sulfation depends on the systemic supply of inorganic sulfate that can be depleted by such drugs as salicylamide. Interactions between sympathomimetics, which are sulfated, and other drugs similarly metabolized are potentially dangerous. A classic example of enzyme inhibition involves tyramine, which is normally deaminated in the gut wall by monoamine oxidase. Antidepressant monoamine oxidase inhibitors (e.g., iproniazid, isocarboxazid, nialamide, phenelzine) block this metabolic pathway and thus expose patients to severe hypertensive crisis following ingestion of tyramine-rich foods.[93]

Foodstuffs are known to contain several compounds that may induce microsomal drug oxidation in the gut wall. Some plant indoles and polycyclic aromatic hydrocarbons produced in meat cooked over charcoal have been implicated in the enhanced metabolism of ethoxycoumarin and phenacetin by O-deethylation.[92]

Although little is known about the effect of disease on the metabolic activity of the gut wall, celiac disease has been shown to reduce the conjugation of ethinyl estradiol but to increase the sulfation of methyldopa.[91]

Liver

The most important site of presystemic drug metabolism is the liver. The liver receives its blood supply from the hepatic artery and the hepatic portal vein. Approximately 75% of the hepatic blood flow stems from the portal vein, which drains all but the lowest 10 cm and the uppermost 55 cm of the gastrointestinal tract. Hence, drugs absorbed from the intestinal tract and the upper portions of the rectum must pass

through the liver before reaching the systemic circulation. Drugs absorbed from the intestinal tract into the lymphatic system may bypass the liver.

The types of metabolic reactions encountered in the liver are similar to those occurring in the gut wall. Unlike the gut wall, mixed function oxidases have a major role in preconjugative reactions in the liver, where glucuronidation is the most prevalent conjugative or synthetic reaction. A drug or its metabolites may undergo one or more of these reactions to form products having different pharmacologic activity. The net effect of first-pass hepatic metabolism of a drug is to reduce its bioavailability. Examples of drugs that undergo significant first-pass hepatic metabolism include antiarrhythmics (e.g., lidocaine and verapamil), β-blockers (e.g., propranolol and metoprolol), centrally acting analgesics (e.g., propoxyphene and pentazocine), and antidepressants (e.g., imipramine and amitriptyline).[94] More comprehensive review of this subject may be found in the literature.[95–97]

Lungs

Since drug absorption following most routes of administration (oral, rectal, inhalation, intramuscular, buccal, transdermal, subcutaneous) places a drug in the venous side of the systemic circulation, the agent must pass through the lungs before reaching the arterial portion of the system. Drugs exposed to metabolic activity at the site of application, during the absorption process, or upon first pass through the liver risk further biotransformation upon entry into the lungs. The extensive capillary network in the lungs exposes the blood to an endothelial surface area of roughly 70 to 125 m^2. Large numbers of pinocytotic vesicles containing drug-metabolizing enzymes are found in lung tissues. On a mass basis, the lungs represent a smaller organ and contain proportionately more fibrous tissue than the liver. Blood flow to the lungs, however, is approximately three times that to the liver. Thus, while the intrinsic clearance of the lungs is normally smaller than that of the liver, total clearance by the lungs may be significant because of blood flow.[98]

The lungs have been implicated in the metabolism of a number of compounds. For example, benzphetamine, aminopyrine, ethylmorphine, and imipramine undergo demethylation, while ethoxycoumarin and coumarin undergo O-deethylation and aromatic hydroxylation, respectively. Reductive reactions in the lungs are not well understood, but dehydrogenation of steroids has been reported. The reduction of nitro groups to the corresponding amines is operative and is applicable for chloramphenicol. Hydrolytic enzymes are numerous in the lungs and play an important role in the metabolism of endogenous compounds. Their role in the metabolism of xenobiotics, however, is not well understood. The major conjugative enzyme systems detected in the lungs are glutathione S-transferase, UDP glucuronyltransferase, sulfotransferase, and N-acetyltransferase, with glutathione conjugation being most important.[99]

Other Tissues

Little is known about the presystemic metabolism of drugs that are administered intramuscularly, subcutaneously, nasally, or dermally; however, many of the enzymes identified in the liver, gut wall, or lungs may be present at these sites of application as well and could contribute to the presystemic elimination of agents so administered. The metabolic potential of the skin has been extensively evaluated.[100,101] The skin contains many of the same enzymes found in the liver and is capable of oxidative, reductive, hydrolytic, and conjugative-type reactions. Most of the enzyme activity appears to be localized in the epidermal layer, which constitutes only about 3% of the total skin. While enzyme activity in whole-skin homogenates is low compared to the liver, if the enzymes are concentrated in the epidermal layer, activities are actually close to those of liver enzymes. Such activity may result in first-pass metabolism (during absorption) of topically applied drugs that are intended for systemic action.

Physiologic Factors

The physiologic conditions at the site of drug application, the residence time of the drug at the site, and shunting through body fluids also influence drug entry into the systemic circulation.

Site of Application

The large effective surface area of the gastrointestinal tract exerts a great influence on the absorption of orally administered drugs. The gastrointestinal mucosal surface is a mass of folded tissue covered by projections of columnar epithelial cells called *villi* and *microvilli*. These structures increase the effective surface area of the intestinal tract 600-fold over its simple tube-like appearance. Surface area decreases in a distal direction, suggesting that passive drug absorption is less efficient as the drug migrates toward the colon. Active transport processes, more prevalent in the ileum than in the upper small intestine, may compensate for the decrease in passive absorption.

The buccal cavity is richly supplied with capillaries. Venous return bypasses the liver. Many of the chemical and metabolic processes encountered with oral administration are avoided when drugs are administered by the buccal route.

The rectal cavity has a surface area of 200 to 400 cm^2. In general, drugs absorbed in the lower region of the rectum enter directly into the systemic circulation. Those absorbed in the upper region pass through the liver first. Anastomoses among the rectal veins complicate this picture.[102]

The nasal mucosa represents a site of drug application that has absorption characteristics similar to those of intramuscular administration. An ample blood supply, neutral pH, and low enzymatic activity contribute to these characteristics.[103] If other than local effects are intended, drug potency is of prime concern since maintaining relatively large amounts of drug at the absorption site is difficult.

Until recently, dermal application of drugs was intended for local effects only. As transport of substances through skin is better understood, however, lipophilic drugs that are reasonably potent are being incorporated into transdermal dosage forms with the intent of establishing therapeutic blood levels of drug. Since skin on various portions of the body has been shown to have different permeability characteristics for a given drug, selection of a site of application is important. The rate of penetration depends on diffusion of drug in the vehicle to the skin surface, surface pH considerations, and diffusion through the stratum corneum and supportive tissues. Drug may also move along hair follicles, sweat glands, sebaceous glands, or aqueous channels.[104,105]

Bioavailability is usually good following intramuscular and subcutaneous drug administration. A large muscle mass is most often chosen for intramuscular injection. Muscle is richly supplied with blood, and absorption of drug is efficient. Though usually not a problem, the potential for metabolism at these injection sites exists. On the other hand, blood flow is more restricted in subcutaneous tissue; therefore, absorption from a subcutaneous injection is likely to be sustained.

Residence Time

The time for which a drug remains at its site of absorption may affect its bioavailability. The effect is minimal with intramuscular or subcutaneous injection, or with dermal application, since the drug is confined to the site of application. Drug may be available for absorption from these sites for a protracted period. Because of leakage, swallowing, or expectoration, absorption following the intranasal and buccal administration may be more variable and less complete.

Drugs taken orally enter the stomach, where gastric emptying regulates movement into the intestinal tract. Once drug has moved into the small intestine, transit should proceed unimpeded until drug reaches the colon. The mouth-to-cecum transit time in healthy humans has been shown to be as short as 1.5 to 3.5 hours.[106] Hence, within 3 hours of ingestion, drug may enter the large intestine, where absorption may be inherently less efficient or impeded by the presence of fecal material. Depending on the dosage form and the presence of food, however, the stomach and small intestine may not be completely clear of drug for up to 5 and 20 hours respectively.[107] The physicochemical nature of the drug, the type of formulation, and the sites of absorption along the gastrointestinal tract will determine the effect of delayed gastric emptying or decreased intestinal motility on drug bioavailability.

With regard to rectal drug administration, residence time in the rectal cavity is governed by leakage, defecation, or upward migration of the drug into the lower bowel. The first two factors would reduce or terminate drug absorption, while the latter would increase drug exposure to first-pass metabolism in the liver.

Shunting and Recycling

The plasma concentration profile of a drug may be altered by shunting, a process that may occur following drug administration. Shunting refers to the entry of a drug into a body fluid (other than blood) before or after entry into the systemic circulation. Depending on the route of administration and the efficiency of the shunting process, the drug might conceivably never appear systemically. Usually, however, the drug is recycled, through absorption or mixing, into the systemic circulation. One example of shunting involves secretion of the drug from blood into the parotid or submaxillary fluids.

The liver may also secrete the drug from blood into bile. Bile is then stored in the gallbladder, which empties periodically, albeit irregularly, into the small intestine. Drug may then be reabsorbed, and the process recurs. A notable example of this is the drug indomethacin, for which it has been estimated that 50 to 60% of a dose administered orally, rectally, or intravenously may be recycled through the bile.[108]

Finally, the lymphatic system is a pathway through which the drug, having been absorbed gastrointestinally or parenterally, may be shunted, only to reappear later in the systemic circulation. Nearly all tissues of the body have lymphatic channels that drain excess fluid directly from the interstitial spaces. The lymphatic system is a major pathway for absorption of fatty substances from the gastrointestinal tract. About one tenth of the fluid filtering from arterial capillaries enters the terminal lymphatic capillaries. This shunt is particularly important for substances with high molecular weight because lymphatic capillaries are much more permeable than venous capillaries. Lymph generated in the lower half of the body, and in the left half of the upper body, eventually re-enters the systemic circulation at the juncture of the left internal jugular and subclavian veins, whereas lymph from the right half of the upper body re-enters contralaterally. The flow of lymph is slow compared to blood flow dynamics.[109] Hence, the initial effect of drug shunting through the lymphatics is a reduction of drug concentrations in blood, followed later by a sustaining effect.

Product Development

Pharmacokinetic and biopharmaceutic concepts and techniques are used routinely throughout the life cycle of a drug. In the drug discovery phase, absorption, first-pass metabolism, active metabolites, and plasma half-lives are common criteria in the selection of candidates for safety assessment. In the post-marketing phase, pharmacokinetic bases for important clinical drug-drug interactions may be sought, while interchangeability among multisource drug products may be evaluated on the basis of their relative bioavailability. The remainder of this chapter pertains to the application of pharmacokinetics and biopharmaceutics in the product development phase, with particular emphasis on dosage form design and evaluation.

Preclinical Information

Pharmacology and Toxicology

When a drug candidate begins to undergo safety assessment, much is already known about its biochemical, pharmacologic, and/or anti-infective properties in vitro and in animals. Differences in potency between routes of administration provide initial clues on drug absorption and disposition. As a point of reference, data following the intravascular administration of the drug are preferred. Data from other parenteral routes, however (e.g., intramuscular, subcutaneous, or intraperitoneal), may suffice if experimental limitations exist (e.g., drug solubility). Similar ED_{50} values following parenteral and other routes suggest comparable bioavailability. A higher ED_{50} following oral administration may indicate poor absorption or the presence of luminal, gut wall, or hepatic inactivation. A lower ED_{50} following a nonintravascular route may indicate the presystemic formation of active metabolites.

Similar clues can be derived from toxicologic studies in animals. Comparative LD_{50} values in the assessment of acute toxicity may be used in the same manner as ED_{50} data. Dosages needed to induce lethality, however, may be such that capacity limits in absorption, protein binding, and biotransformation are approached or exceeded. For example, the fraction that is bioavailable may initially increase with dose because of saturation in first-pass metabolism and may subsequently decrease because of saturation in transport.

Changes in apparent potency or toxicity on repeated administration of drug by the same route suggest drug accumulation, enzymatic induction, or inhibition. Support may be found in results of studies on the effect of drug on hexobarbitol sleeping time or specific enzymatic systems in vitro. Specific disposition studies can be designed to evaluate drug or metabolite accumulation.

In the course of pharmacologic and toxicologic testing, the process and scale by which the compound is synthesized evolves continually. These tasks often involve different formulations as well. Since these differences are known, significant changes in physicochemical properties can be directly studied for their effect on absorption. The relative importance of process and formulation variables to the bioavailability of the test compound can be deduced from a systematic examination of changes in indices of activity and toxicity over time.

Biotransformation

Before a drug candidate is tested in humans, information on its disposition in several species of laboratory animals is usually available. A thorough knowledge of these preclinical data is necessary for the rational design of pharmacokinetic and bioavailability studies in humans. Typically, studies are performed in several species wherein radiolabeled drug is administered both intravenously and orally; urine, feces, blood, and possibly expired air are sampled and assayed radiometrically. Accountability of the administered dose (i.e., mass balance) in the excreta is determined, as is the profile of radioactivity in blood or plasma. Incomplete absorption or the presence of significant biliary excretion of the drug may be detected.

If such studies are coupled with a sensitive analytic method specific for unchanged drug, valuable information may also be obtained on oral bioavailability, first-pass metabolism, metabolic profile, routes of elimination of unchanged drug, plasma and renal drug clearances, and half-lives. Principal metabolites may also be isolated and identified. For compounds with a clear and measurable pharmacologic endpoint (e.g., diuretic/saluretic agents), concomitant measurements of pharmacologic responses in animal disposition studies may reveal correlations with drug concentration data and provide evidence for the presence of active metabolite(s). When metabolites contribute to the pharmacologic or toxicologic profile of the drug, sensitive and specific analytic methods must be developed for them prior to initiation of wide-scale clinical studies. Multiple-dose studies in animals to assess the degree of accumulation of drug and active metabolite, as well as the possibility of enzymatic induction or inhibition of the bioactivation process, may also be useful.

In general, drug disposition data in animals cannot be directly extrapolated to man. Species differences in metabolic pattern have been the subject of extensive investigation.[110] While routes of drug metabolism are often similar in laboratory animals and man, metabolic rates frequently differ.[110] In some cases, these quantitative differences among species can be reconciled on the basis of their intrinsic metabolic clearances.[111] Hence, animal disposition data provide the basis to design initial disposition studies in humans.

The following examples illustrate the application of preclinical metabolism data to product development.

Methyldopa. Methyldopa is an antihypertensive agent that is variably and incompletely absorbed from the gastrointestinal tract of man. A number of methyldopa esters were tested in the spontaneously hypertensive rat model to identify derivatives that had improved absorption characteristics and that were readily hydrolyzed to methyldopa in vivo.[112] Two compounds having a longer duration of action and an apparent antihypertensive potency approximately three times that of methyldopa were selected for further study: the pivaloyloxyethyl (POE) and succinimidoethyl (SIE) esters of methyldopa.

TABLE 9-5. *Disposition of Radioactivity after Oral Administration of Labeled Methyldopa or its Ester Progenitors*

Species	Compound Given*	Radioactivity Recovered (% Dose)		% Urinary Radioactivity	
		Urine	Feces	Methyldopa	Conjugated Methyldopa
Rat	SIE	77	12	51	—
	POE	61	33	65	—
	Methyldopa	29	71	—	—
Human	SIE	70.7	8.5	4.2	24.9
	POE	69.2	8.9	22.5	18.7

*Oral doses in terms of methyldopa equivalents were 40 mg/kg in rats and ~100 mg in man.
— Not measured.
Adapted from Vickers et al.[113]

When radiolabeled doses of either ester were administered orally to rats,[113] improved absorption characteristics were demonstrated: more of the label was excreted in urine and less in feces than after a comparable dose of methyldopa (Table 9-5); over half of the urinary radioactivity after either ester was due to methyldopa. A similar excretion pattern of radioactivity was observed[113] when the labeled esters were administered to humans (Table 9-5).

Since ~40% of a labeled oral dose of methyldopa is excreted in urine, and the remainder is recovered in feces as unchanged drug,[114,115] higher absorption of the esters from the gastrointestinal tract is indicated. Based on urinary recoveries of methyldopa, however, the bioavailability of methyldopa from the SIE ester is considerably lower than that from the POE ester (Table 9-5), or even from oral methyldopa.[114] A six-fold higher ratio of conjugated to free methyldopa in urine after the SIE ester compared to the POE ester suggests that the lower bioavailability is related to a greater first-pass conjugation after the SIE ester.

The POE ester labeled with ³H in the methyldopa moiety or ¹⁴C in the pivalic acid moiety was given orally to rats, dogs, and rhesus monkeys at doses of up to 300 mg/kg.[113] Profiles of ³H and ¹⁴C in the portal circulation differed, and negligible amounts of the intact ester were present in the portal plasma. When added to rat, dog, or human plasma, the ester is rapidly hydrolyzed.[113] These results indicate that the ester is hydrolyzed in the gut wall during the absorption process and that the active therapeutic moiety, methyldopa, is delivered to the portal circulation. Intact ester that may survive gut wall metabolism is subject to rapid hydrolysis by plasma esterases in the portal and systemic circulation.

The metabolic disposition of ³H- and ¹⁴C-labeled POE ester was also studied in man at doses equivalent to 500 mg of methyldopa.[116] More than 90% of either label was recovered in urine, indicating that absorption from the gastrointestinal tract was nearly complete. About 42% of the dose was excreted in urine as unchanged methyldopa. When methyldopa itself is given orally, ~25% of the dose is available to the systemic circulation (i.e., is bioavailable), and ~18% of the dose is excreted unchanged in urine.[117] The higher urinary recovery of methyldopa after the POE ester suggests that approximately 60% of the dose is bioavailable as methyldopa.

Different profiles were observed for the ³H and ¹⁴C labels in the systemic circulation, indicating that as in the animal studies, hydrolysis of the POE ester occurs presystemically. Plasma was collected in the presence of an esterase inhibitor to quench in vitro hydrolysis of any ester present and was assayed specifically for the intact compound.[118] No intact ester was detected, which confirms that hydrolysis occurs presystemically and is essentially complete. Only the initial 2-hour urine collection in one of four subjects contained the intact ester equivalent to <0.001% of the dose.[117] Since sampling of portal blood is not feasible, the site of hydrolysis in man cannot be ascribed exclusively to the gut wall; it may also include esterases in the portal blood and/or the liver.

The POE ester at doses equivalent to 500 and 1000 mg of methyldopa was compared to oral and i.v. doses of methyldopa in a bioavailability study in humans.[119] The average value for and range of bioavailability of methyldopa after administration of the 500-mg equivalent doses are compared in Table 9-6. The bioavailability of methyldopa from the ester is ~2.2 times higher and is much less variable than that from an

TABLE 9-6. *Mean Systemic Availability of Methyldopa After Oral Administration of Methyldopa or Its POE Ester Progenitor**

| Species | N | Systemic Availability of Methyldopa (% Dose) After | |
		Methyldopa	POE Ester Prodrug
Dog (beagle)	4	91.4 (74.6–103)†	97.1‡
Rhesus monkey	3	16.8 (10.9–28.5)	69.9 (66.8–75.1)
Cynomolgus monkey	3	19.4 (14.4–33.5)	39.7 (30.2–50.2)
Man	10	27.3 (11–59)	60.6 (53.3–69.7)

*Human data from Dobrinska et al.[117]
†Range.
‡Non-crossover study.

equivalent dose of methyldopa itself. Also summarized in Table 9-6 are results for bioavailability of the two compounds in several species of animals. Considerable variation exists among species. Results in the rhesus monkey are closest to those in man.

Levodopa/Carbidopa. Parkinsonism is a debilitating disease that is associated with a deficiency of dopamine in the brain. Levodopa is used to treat the disease because unlike dopamine, it readily crosses the blood-brain barrier, and it is decarboxylated in the brain to dopamine. Effective treatment requires large oral doses because levodopa bioavailability is limited by extensive metabolism. Presystemic and systemic decarboxylation to dopamine causes nausea and vomiting, which limits further increases in dose.

Studies in animals have established that presystemic elimination of levodopa occurs in the gastrointestinal lumen and/or gut wall rather than in the liver. In the dog and rat,[119,120] the AUC of levodopa in the systemic circulation is nearly identical after intravenous and intraportal administration (Table 9-7), which indicates that the liver does not contribute to first-pass elimination of the drug. After oral administration of ^{14}C-labeled levodopa to the dog, the label is completely absorbed,[119] but the AUC for intact drug is only ~40% that after an equivalent i.v. dose (Table 9-7). Thus, the low systemic bio-

TABLE 9-7. *Influence of Route of Administration on Systemic Plasma Concentrations of Levodopa*[119,120]

| Species | Mean AUC (μg min/ml) of Levodopa When Equivalent Doses are Administered | | |
	Intravenously	Intraportally	Orally
Dog	1392	1272	584
Rat	433	419	—

availability occurs because of prehepatic metabolism. Gastrointestinal metabolism of levodopa has also been demonstrated in humans,[121,122] and gastrointestinal side effects may be related to the presence of metabolic products in the stomach.[121]

Carbidopa is a dopa decarboxylase inhibitor that does not penetrate the blood-brain barrier. Coadministration of levodopa with carbidopa results in an increase in levodopa bioavailability and permits a significant reduction in dosage requirements; gastrointestinal side effects are correspondingly reduced. The effect of carbidopa pretreatment on the plasma concentrations of levodopa in humans are exemplified by the data in Table 9-8. Levodopa was administered as a single 250-mg dose alone or following pretreatment for 48 hours with 50 mg carbidopa three times a day. Levodopa bioavailability, expressed as the amount absorbed divided by its volume of distribution as given in equation (48), and the plasma $t_{\frac{1}{2}}$ of levodopa were compared between treatments. In the presence of carbidopa, $A(\infty)/V_1$ of levodopa is increased by a factor of 5 and $t_{\frac{1}{2}}$ is twice as long. The increase in bioavailability results from inhibition of presystemic decarboxylation by carbidopa, whereas the prolonged $t_{\frac{1}{2}}$ reflects the inhibition of decarboxylation of levodopa in the general circulation. Consequently, more levodopa is available for a longer period of time for transport into the brain, where it becomes a source of dopamine since carbidopa itself does not pass the blood-brain barrier.

Preformulation

Solubility

Most drugs are administered orally in solid dosage forms. Following administration of such dosages, the delivery of the active ingredient to the systemic circulation requires initial trans-

TABLE 9-8. *Effects of Carbidopa on Levodopa in Humans*

Treatment	Levodopa	
	$\dfrac{A(\infty)}{V_1}$ $(\mu g/ml)^*$	$t_{\frac{1}{2}}$ (h)
Levodopa 250 mg	$0.44 \pm 0.19\dagger$	0.94 ± 0.28
Levodopa 250 mg + carbidopa 50 mg t.i.d.	2.19 ± 1.32	2.15 ± 1.02

*Total amount of levodopa absorbed divided by volume of distribution,—see equation (48).
†Mean ± S.D.; N = 4

port through the gastrointestinal membrane. Solubility characteristics play an important role in this initial process. Hydrophilicity favors drug dissolution in the aqueous milieu of the gastrointestinal lumen, while lipophilicity favors subsequent penetration into the lipoidal membrane. For efficient absorption, a proper balance between these two opposing properties is required.

Because of the finite fluid volume within the gastrointestinal lumen, the efficiency of absorption is also affected by the size of the dose. For example, dexamethasone is only slightly soluble in water (0.1 mg/ml), but it is highly soluble in common organic solvents. Because of its relatively low dosage (<10 mg), it is well absorbed orally.[123] On the other hand, methyldopa requires a high dosage and is more soluble in water (10 mg/ml), but its bioavailability is poor. Partly because of its lipophobicity, methyldopa does not penetrate the gastrointestinal membrane efficiently.

For acidic or basic compounds that are poorly absorbed because of low solubility in both organic and aqueous media, improved absorption can be achieved by the formation of appropriate soluble salts. These salts in general show faster dissolution, with their water solubility being pH-dependent. For example, chlorpheniramine base is an oily liquid with low water solubility. Formation of the maleate salt, which is crystalline and easily handled at room temperature, allows its incorporation into solid dosage forms. Indomethacin is practically insoluble in water at neutral or acidic pH. When incorporated into osmotically controlled drug delivery systems, indomethacin itself is incapable of generating the required osmotic pressure. The formation of the soluble sodium salt enables the drug to be released from the dosage form at a predetermined rate.[124]

Formation of soluble ester derivatives is another approach to resolving the solubility issue. Injectable dosage forms of dexamethasone employ a sodium phosphate salt that has enhanced solubility. The greater solubility of the sodium salt also allows its incorporation in inhalation as well as in ophthalmic preparations. Similarly, an injectable dosage solution of methyldopa is formulated as the hydrochloride salt of its ethyl ester in order to increase solubility and stability. These ester derivatives are distinct chemical entities, however, with properties different from those of the parent compound. Competing biotransformational and excretory pathways may affect the quantitative in vivo hydrolysis to the active moieties. For example, while over 90% of the intravenously injected dexamethasone sodium phosphate is bioavailable as dexamethasone,[125] the bioavailability of methyldopa from injections of the ethyl ester hydrochloride is less than 20%.[126]

Decreasing aqueous solubility by the formation of insoluble esters may also be desirable under certain circumstances. A classic example is chloramphenicol palmitate, which minimizes the unpleasant taste of the drug in oral suspensions. Excessive suppression of solubility, however, may adversely affect bioavailability.

Polymorphism

Different crystal forms of a drug may be produced in the course of chemical synthesis, isolation, and purification. At a specific temperature and pressure, only one form has the strongest intermolecular forces and is the most thermodynamically stable. Metastable forms melt at lower temperatures are more soluble, and are less dense. Differences in these variables between polymorphs are measures of their relative stability. Less stable forms seek to revert to the more stable ones. Because of this tendency to revert on storage, the thermodynamically stable form is preferred in dosages forms. For example, there are at least five known polymorphs of cortisone acetate, the caking of which in aqueous suspensions has been attributed to polymorphic reversion.[127]

Polymorphism is not a concern if the drug is inherently well absorbed or if the energy differences among polymorphs are small. For example, diflunisal exists in two nonsolvated enantiotropic forms. At temperatures below 90°C, the more stable Form II has a lower aqueous solubility than Form I—0.014 versus 0.026 mg/ml at 25°C. Since both forms are equally well absorbed,[128] Form II is used in tablet formulations.

For drugs that are poorly absorbed because of solubility limitations, amorphous solids or metastable crystalline forms may be considered. For example, different polymorphs of chloramphenical palmitate are known to influence its bioavailability following oral administration.[85] If the enhancement in bioavailability were to be reproducibly maintained by these means, however, methods must be found to prevent spontaneous nucleation or reversion.

Design Variables

Mode of Administration

Oral administration, which provides convenient access of drug to the systemic circulation, is traditionally the preferred route of drug administration. The appropriateness of this route of administration for a given drug, however, is determined by such factors as rate and extent of gastrointestinal absorption, acid lability, first-pass metabolism, gastrointestinal transit time, and duration of action. Acid lability can be minimized or overcome by formulation. Buffering, however, usually adds considerable bulk to an oral dosage form, and enteric coating invariably delays the onset of drug absorption.

The feasibility of optimizing drug delivery by alternative modes of administration depends on the physicochemical and pharmacokinetic properties of the drug, its potency, and physiologic conditions at the alternate site of application. Most of the potential disadvantages of oral administration can be circumvented by controlled intravenous administration, provided that the drug is sufficiently soluble in a vehicle for injection; however, chronic intravenous drug administration is rarely considered. Usually, a compromise is made between patient acceptance and the technology that is available to deliver the drug reliably.

Much of the convenience of oral administration is negated if the duration of a drug's action is such that the frequency of administration is unacceptably high. Compounds with this characteristic are candidates for controlled delivery, which is discussed later in this chapter. Intramuscular and transdermal routes may also be considered. Both routes involve sites from which absorption may be the slowest and therefore the rate-limiting step. For rapidly eliminated drugs, intramuscular injection may sustain absorption sufficiently to permit a reduction in dosage frequency. This route of administration is a practical alternative for drugs that are not used chronically, such as antibiotics. Absorption through the skin may be similarly rate-limiting and thus suitable for chronic drug administration. The usefulness of transdermal drug delivery may be limited by local irritation and site variations in skin permeability. As with oral administration, both intramuscularly and transdermally administered drugs may be subject to degradation or metabolism at the site of application.

Hepatic first-pass metabolism can be avoided or minimized by directing drug input to the systemic circulation away from the oral route of administration. The buccal and sublingual routes of administration completely circumvent the liver and the gastrointestinal wall. These routes are suitable for potent drugs that are rapidly absorbed; however, if the drug is retained at the site of application for a protracted period of time, part of the dose may be swallowed and thus be subjected to presystemic hepatic metabolism. Rectal and intravaginal routes of administration provide at least partial avoidance of the liver in the first pass, and in addition, are useful for drugs whose unit dosage exceeds 1 g.

For drugs that are poorly absorbed by other routes, subcutaneous injection and intranasal instillation may be considered. Drug delivery to the lungs may be intended for local or systemic effects. The large surface area and rich blood supply of the lungs provide a rate of systemic drug availability approaching that of intravenous administration. Optimal drug delivery to the bronchi and lungs by aerosol or insufflation techniques requires a conscientious effort by the patient. Even so, drug losses to the alimentary canal are inevitable.

When drugs are administered topically for local rather than systemic effect, selective chemical or metabolic lability may be desirable. For example, topical steroids should ideally be rapidly biotransformed before reaching the systemic circulation; highly reactive antineoplastics may be injected into the arterial supply of a tumor; intraocular delivery of the prodrug dipivalyl epinephrine favors corneal penetration and reduces drug loss through the nasolacrimal duct, maximizing the local availability of the active agent epinephrine. In each case, the goal is to effect a greater separation of local activity in the target tissue from systemic side effects.

Finally, parenteral routes such as intra-articular, intrathecal, and intracardiac administration are available for selected drugs, but restricted to critical situations in which immediate access to a specific site is required.

Dosage Regimen

The goal in the design of dosage regimens is to achieve and maintain drug concentrations in plasma or at the site of action that are both safe and effective. Maximum safe concentration and minimum therapeutic concentration are schematically illustrated in Figure 9-27. Toxicity would result if doses were administered too frequently, whereas, effectiveness would wane if the dosage rate were too infrequent. The optimal regimens are combinations of dose and dosage frequency that would result in steady-state concentrations within the chosen limits.

Acceptable plasma concentration profiles at steady state can be devised with the aid of pharmacokinetic parameters derived from single-dose experiments. The important parameters are plasma clearance, half-life, and bioavailability. Suppose that the desired mean plasma concentration, $\overline{C}_1^{(ss)}$, for a drug is 2 μg/ml, and its plasma clearance is 125 ml/min. According to equations (58), or (73), the dosage rate by the intravenous route should be 250 μg/min, or 360 mg/day. The target concentration can be attained by either a constant infusion or intermittent boluses (see Fig. 9-14). The dose and dosage intervals need not be equally divided; a steady state may be obtained as long as the dosing pattern recurs in regular cycles (see Fig. 9-15). If the same drug is to be given by a nonintravascular route with a bioavailability of 50%, the same target concentration can be achieved with a dosage rate of 720 mg/day.

The peak and trough concentrations within a dosage cycle as well as the rate of approach to steady state depend on the half-life. The shorter the half-life is, the more the daily dose must be subdivided to maintain peak and trough concentrations within the chosen limits. Furthermore, approximately 7 half-lives in time must elapse to achieve a steady state. To hasten the approach to steady state, a loading dose of the drug may be given. An appropriate loading dose can be calculated based on the mode of administration by using the following equations.

For a continuous intravenous infusion, an initial loading bolus dose D* is administered:

$$D^* = C_1^{ss}V_1 \qquad (103)$$

This initial dose followed immediately by an infusion at a dosage rate prescribed by equation (58) results in the immediate attainment C_1^{ss} for a drug whose disposition is described by a one-compartment pharmacokinetic model (see Fig. 9-1). For drugs whose plasma concentration decays polyexponentially (see Fig. 9-9), a similar approach causes plasma concentrations to fall for a period of time before returning to C_1^{ss}. To compensate for this initial fall in C_1^{ss}, a loading bolus dose D* equal to or greater than that given by equation (104) may be considered:

$$D^* = \frac{C_1^{ss}CL}{\omega} \qquad (104)$$

where ω is the eigenvalue associated with the terminal slope. This dose is followed immediately by a continuous infusion at a rate prescribed by equation (58); however, this strategy results in initial plasma concentrations higher than C_1^{ss} and may be inappropriate for drugs having a narrow margin of safety.

For intermittent dosage at regular intervals, a loading dose (D*) could be chosen such that the mean plasma concentration following the first dosage interval, $\overline{C}_1^{(1)}$, would equal that at steady state, $\overline{C}_1^{(ss)}$. Combining equations (73) and (76) yields:

$$D^* = \frac{\tau \overline{C}_1^{(ss)}CL}{F} \qquad (105)$$

where F represents the bioavailability of the drug. Administration of D* followed by the maintenance dose given every τ hours immediately establishes steady state plasma concentrations.

Special consideration must be given to the design of dosage regimens when the disease

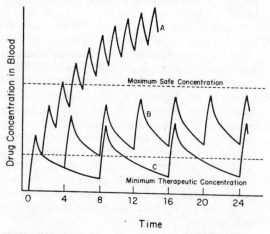

FIG. 9-27. *Effect on plasma concentration of too frequent (A), proper (B), and inadequate (C) frequencies of drug administration.*

state of the patient might affect drug disposition. In patients with less than normal cardiovascular function, tissue perfusion is decreased. If hepatic or renal function is compromised, drug elimination is decreased because of a decrease in metabolic or renal clearance, respectively. In each case, plasma clearance decreases and half-life is prolonged. These altered parameters should be used in equations (58), (73), (103), (104), and (105) to calculate the doses and dosage rates needed to achieve the desired C_1^{ss} in patients.

Controlled Delivery

The goals of controlled drug delivery are to conserve dose, maintain effective drug concentrations, eliminate nighttime dosage, improve compliance, and decrease side effects, thus optimizing drug therapy. Pharmacokinetic information is essential in determining the feasibility and design of a controlled delivery dosage form. Drugs with plasma half-lives of 6 hours or less, inactive metabolites, well-defined minimum therapeutic blood levels, and rapid absorption are the most likely candidates for controlled delivery. Dosages for drugs with longer half-lives can be calculated conventionally so that therapeutic blood levels are established and then self-sustained, allowing for twice-daily dosage or less. A narrow margin of safety complicates this approach, as does the fact that well-defined minimum therapeutic drug levels are difficult to establish even in the absence of active metabolites.[107]

A common approach has been to combine a rapid-release dose fraction with a fraction having pseudo-first-order release characteristics. When absorption is not rate-limiting, the ideal approach to this situation is zero-order delivery of drug to the absorption site. The amount of drug reaching the absorption site changes with time for first-order drug delivery, thus precluding the desired constant blood level profile. Following administration of a zero-order-input delivery system, steady-state blood levels (C_1^{ss}) of the drug are obtained:

$$C_1^{ss} = \frac{k_0}{V_1 k_{10}} \qquad (106)$$

where k_0 is the zero-order input rate. The dose D is a function of k_0, the dosage interval τ, and the bioavailability:

$$k_0 \tau = FD \qquad (107)$$

As indicated in equation (106), the C_1^{ss} attained with a zero-order input delivery system is a function of both the input rate and the CL of the drug. The time required to reach C_1^{ss} after the dose is administered, however, is governed primarily by the plasma half-life of the drug. Approximately 7 half-lives are required to approach C_1^{ss}. If more rapid attainment of the steady-state level is desired, then an immediate release drug fraction (loading dose) can be administered with the zero-order delivery system. Design strategies accompanying this approach, including the effects following multiple-dose administration, have been reviewed.[129]

While advantages of controlled-delivery dosage forms are readily apparent, limitations must also be addressed prior to and throughout the development process. A convenient once-a-day dosage form is precluded, for instance, for a drug that is bulky or where daily dosage requirements are high. The length of time that an oral controlled-delivery dosage unit remains functional within the gastrointestinal tract must be considered—functional in terms of transit time as well as the release of drug at the site of absorption. Certain drugs manifest "absorption windows" whereby absorption is limited to a specific region of the gastrointestinal tract. Others may be absorbed, albeit nonuniformly, along the entire intestinal length. Once the dosage unit is embedded in fecal matter, drug diffusion to the gut wall may become difficult.[130]

Controlled drug delivery systems for routes of administration other than oral are becoming increasingly popular. Topical dosage forms such as ophthalmic delivery devices (e.g., Ocusert) and dermal drug delivery patches are usually intended for local drug effects. Drugs with lipophilic characteristics may also be delivered transdermally for their systemic effect. Once the skin becomes saturated, the drug should enter the systemic circulation at a constant rate as long as drug activity at the skin surface remains at unity. The rate of drug entry into the systemic circulation is governed by the inherent flux of drug through the skin or by the combined effect of a rate-controlling membrane on the patch itself and the skin flux. With the further advantage of being able to keep a transdermal device in contact with the skin for days, this method may be an ideal approach to the goals of controlled drug delivery. Hence, complete pharmacokinetic characterization of the drug and the delivery device becomes even more critical.

Combinations[131]

Rational combination therapy may be divided into three general categories: (1) those combinations whereby the individual components are independently required in the treatment of a specific illness or symptom complex (e.g., an analgesic may be combined with an antipyretic or an antihistamine to alleviate the symptoms of influenza or allergy, while a β-blocker may be combined with a diuretic to control hypertension); (2) therapy whereby a second agent is needed to ameliorate an unwanted pharmacodynamic effect of the primary agent (e.g., anticholinergic/narcotic antidiarrheals reduce potential for narcotic abuse, while some diuretic combinations minimize potassium loss); and (3) combinations designed to effect an improvement in pharmacokinetic properties, (e.g., the coadministration of levodopa and a decarboxylase inhibitor greatly reduces dopamine formation in the gastrointestinal lumen and outside the central nervous system, the net result being a reduction in the dose and the dosing frequency of levodopa and in side effects associated with peripheral dopamine).

Fixed combinations are dosage forms designed to effect a planned interaction between the components or to provide convenience to the patient. Since each component is required for rational therapy, fixed combinations ensure compliance. Where the components interact, by design or otherwise, fixed combinations define the intensity and the duration of the net effect. In any event, clinical proof of safety and efficacy is needed to support the usefulness of a proposed combination.

For convenience dosage forms, the primary biopharmaceutic concern is to ensure that the bioavailability of each component in the fixed combination is equivalent to that following the concomitant administration of the single entities at the same dose by the same route. As long as there is proof of safety and efficacy, incidental pharmacokinetic interactions between the components should not be a concern, but may in fact be a strong argument for the fixed combination.

With planned pharmacokinetic interactions, biopharmaceutic considerations are to optimize the dose of the individual components, their ratio, and the dosage regimen of the combination. More often than not, the desired therapeutic activity resides with one of the components whose absorption or disposition characteristics are improved by a second agent. For example, carbidopa, a dopa decarboxylase inhibitor, is given in combination to maximize the availability of L-dopa for transport to the central nervous system and to minimize dopamine formation in the periphery. In designing this particular combination, it became evident that there is a minimum daily dose of carbidopa above which pe-

ripheral dopa decarboxylase activity is maximally inhibited. Above this threshold, a relatively large range in the ratio of L-dopa to carbidopa can be accommodated. Finally, the inhibitory effect of carbidopa requires one or two days of intermittent dosing to be fully manifested. The requirement is not a concern, however, since the combination is intended for chronic therapy.

In contrast, there are physical and pharmacokinetic arguments against fixed combination dosage forms of a β-lactam antibiotic and probenecid. Like carbidopa, a threshold dose of probenecid is required for maximal blockade of the renal secretory component of antibiotic elimination, and mainly because probenecid is usually given orally, some time must elapse before its effect is fully manifested. Since the optimal route for the antibiotic is often parenteral, however, and the effective dose of the components often exceeds 500 mg each, their combination in a single dosage form is not usually considered. Secondarily, pharmacokinetic considerations suggest pretreatment with probenecid to ensure maximal conservation of the antibiotic. This pretreatment is particularly relevant when only a single dose of the antibiotic is indicated, such as in the treatment of gonorrhea.

Divergent pharmacokinetic properties among individual components in fixed combinations of convenience are unimportant, even if incidental interactions exist. With planned interactions, on the other hand, the adjuvant (e.g., carbidopa and probenecid) should ideally be long-lived relative to the therapeutic moiety. This ensures a stable platform on which the pharmacokinetic behavior of the therapeutic moiety can be reproduced from one dose to the next. Without this stable platform, the kinetic behavior of the compound of primary interest may be difficult to assess.

Dosage Form Evaluation

The foregoing discussion pertains to factors that contribute to the evolution of pharmaceutical products. The final step is to design appropriate studies for evaluating the resultant dosage forms in vivo. The following discussion applies equally to verterinary and human health products.

Studies for evaluation of dosage forms in vivo are conducted in human subjects in a randomized complete-block design to minimize intersubject variations. The size of the study panel should be sufficient to produce statistically meaningful results. Determination of sample size is often based on pilot studies conducted in smaller test panels. Washout periods between treatments are incorporated into the study plan to avoid carryover effects from the previous treatment. The analytic method must be specific for the drug and validated with respect to sensitivity, reproducibility, and linearity.

Dose Dependence

To make reliable inferences based on blood and/or urine drug concentration data, some basic pharmacokinetic properties of the drug must be known. At the minimum, it is necessary to determine whether absorption and disposition kinetics are linear. Nonlinearity is indicated if absorption or disposition kinetics depend on the dose of drug administered. Proportionate increase in AUC and similarity of $t_{\frac{1}{2}}$ following gradated oral doses imply linearity in both absorption and disposition kinetics. Changes in $t_{\frac{1}{2}}$ or disproportionate increase in AUC with increased doses may be manifestations of nonlinearity in absorption or disposition. Intravenous administration of the drug avoids the influence of absorption, and any nonlinearity observed with gradated intravenous doses is attributable to disposition.

Bioavailability

Bioavailability is defined as the extent and the rate at which the active ingredient is delivered to the general circulation from the dosage form. Thus, by definition, intravenously administered drugs are completely bioavailable. The bioavailability F following a nonintravenous dose D^x is given by equation (46), which can also be expressed as:

$$FD^x = \frac{CL}{CL_r}U_\infty^x = \frac{U_\infty^x}{f_r} \qquad (108)$$

Estimation of the product FD^x requires knowledge of CL (or f_r), which is obtained in a separate treatment following an intravenous dose of the drug (i.e., F = 1). When intravenous use of the drug is precluded, an oral solution of the drug may serve as the reference standard for a solid oral dosage form. In principle, the bioavailability of the drug from an oral solution is the maximum to be expected from a solid oral dosage form. Ideally, a solid dosage form is compared to both an intravenous and an oral solution dose of the drug. In this manner, the effect of formulation as well as the absolute bioavailability can be determined. If bioavailability from the solid dosage form is lower than that from an oral solution, then the performance of the dosage form may be improved by reformulation. Low bioavailability from the oral solution, on the other hand, indicates that the drug is intrinsically poorly absorbed or is subject to significant first-pass metabolism and is not likely to be improved by formulation.

In all cases, bioavailability of a test dosage form x is obtained by comparison to a reference standard s, which may be an intravenous or oral solution, or in bioequivalence studies, another formulation of the same drug. Based on equation (46), the bioavailability of dosage form x relative to that of s is defined as:

$$\frac{F^x}{F^s} = \frac{D^s}{D^x}\frac{CL^x}{CL^s}\frac{AUC_\infty^x}{AUC_\infty^s}$$

$$= \frac{D^s}{D^x}\frac{CL^x}{CL^s}\frac{CL_r^s}{CL_r^x}\frac{U_\infty^x}{U_\infty^s} \qquad (109)$$

If the standard is an intravenous dose, then $F^s = 1$ and the absolute bioavailability of x is determined; otherwise, a relative bioavailability is obtained. In any event, an assumption must be made regarding body clearances between treatments before bioavailability can be assessed. Depending on the assumption, different procedures may be employed.

If the assumption of $CL^x = CL^s$ is adopted and substituted into equation (109), the relative bioavailability is given by the dose-corrected ratio of AUC values:

$$F^x/F^s = \frac{D^s}{D^x}\frac{AUC_\infty^x}{AUC_\infty^s} \qquad (110)$$

This method requires data defining the entire area under the plasma concentration time curve for both treatments.

On the other hand, for drugs excreted unchanged in the urine, bioavailability may be obtained assuming that the renal to plasma clearance ratio remains constant between treatments. Equation (109) is reduced to:

$$F^x/F^s = \frac{D^s}{D^x}\frac{U_\infty^x}{U_\infty^s} \qquad (111)$$

Thus, the bioavailability ratio equals the ratio of dose-corrected total urinary recoveries of the unchanged drug.

If both urine and AUC data are available, a third method may be employed.[132,133] This method assumes that the change in plasma clearance between two treatments is caused by that of the renal clearance only, and that the nonrenal clearance remains unchanged. The ratio of the two plasma clearances becomes:

$$\frac{CL^x}{CL^s} = \left(\frac{U_\infty^x}{AUC_\infty^x} + \frac{F^sD^s - U_\infty^s}{AUC_\infty^s}\right) \bigg/ \left(\frac{F^sD^s}{AUC_\infty^s}\right)$$

$$(112)$$

Substitution of equation (112) into equation (109) yields:

$$F^x/F^s = \frac{D^s}{D^x}\frac{AUC_\infty^x}{AUC_\infty^s}$$

$$+ \frac{1}{F^sD^x}\left(U_\infty^x - U_\infty^s\frac{AUC_\infty^x}{AUC_\infty^s}\right) \qquad (113)$$

Equation (113) differs from equation (110) in that it incorporates, in addition to the dose-corrected AUC ratio, a correction term to account for the assumed change in plasma clearance. When s is an intravenous dose, $F^s = 1$ and equation (113) reduces to:

$$F^x = (CL^s - CL_r^s + CL_r^x)\frac{AUC_\infty^x}{D^x} \qquad (114)$$

Thus, CL^x is calculated from the sum of CL_r^x and the nonrenal clearance observed in the i.v. treatment, that is, $CL^s - CL_r^s$. If the bioavailability of the reference standard is unknown, an approximate solution to equation (113) may be obtained by setting F^sD^x in the second term equal to D^x. The nature of this approximation has been defined, and an optimal solution suggested.[133]

A unique approach that obviates the need for assumptions concerning CL between treatments is to administer simultaneously an i.v. dose of the drug labeled with a stable radioisotope and the oral dose of the unlabeled drug.[134,135]

The foregoing methods of estimating the extent of bioavailability apply only to drugs that obey linear pharmacokinetics. For drugs following nonlinear pharmacokinetics, methodology should be developed on a case-by-case basis. For example, in the absence of first-pass metabolism, total urinary recovery is a measure of bioavailability if the unchanged drug and its metabolites are quantitatively excreted in the urine.

After a nonintravenous dose of the drug is administered, the time to reach the maximum plasma concentration, t_{max}, may be regarded as a qualitative measure of the rate of absorption, with the recognition that t_{max} is a function of not only absorption but also elimination of the drug. The preferred method is to use an intravenous dose as a reference standard and to isolate the absorption profile for the nonintravenous formulation by the use of deconvolution or model-dependent means such as the Wagner-Nelson or Loo-Riegelman methods given in equations (48) through (56).

Example

Test for Linearity. Simulated results for a subject in a typical dose-dependence pharmacokinetic study are used to illustrate the application of the methods described. The subject received single 250-, 500-, and 1000-mg i.v. boluses of the drug on separate occasions in a randomized, three-way crossover study. Serial plasma samples were collected over 12 hours, and total urine was collected in intervals through 48 hours after drug administration. Analytic results for the unchanged drug are given in Table 9-9.

Plasma drug concentration-time profiles, when plotted on semilogarithmic paper (Fig. 9-28), show a rapid initial decline and then become linear after ~6 hours. Upon curve-stripping, as given in equations (28) and (29), it is clear that the data are best described by biexponential functions. Estimates of A, B, α, and β can be obtained by curve-stripping, linear regression techniques,[136,137] or nonlinear regres-

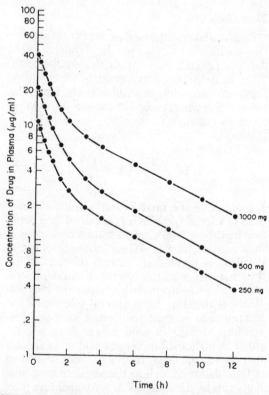

FIG. 9-28. *Typical plasma drug concentration profiles of drug in plasma following single intravenous doses.*

TABLE 9-9. *Analytic Results for a Subject in a Typical Dose-Dependence Pharmacokinetic Study of a Drug Given by Bolus Intravenous Injection at Doses of 250, 500, and 1000 mg*

	Plasma Drug Concentration (μg/ml)				Urinary Drug Excretion (mg)		
Time(h)	250 mg	500 mg	1000 mg	Time(h)	250 mg	500 mg	1000 mg
0(predrug)	0	0	0	−2 to 0 (predrug)	0	0	0
0.1	10.8	21.0	40.9	0–2	80.2	179.2	293.7
0.25	9.2	18.1	35.2	2–4	28.8	59.0	112.1
0.50	7.3	14.3	27.9	4–6	18.7	36.4	74.5
0.75	5.8	11.5	22.6	6–8	13.2	25.6	53.2
1.0	4.8	9.4	18.7	8–12	16.1	30.1	65.7
1.5	3.4	6.7	13.7	12–24	14.4	27.0	60.6
2.0	2.7	5.1	10.9	24–36	1.90	2.90	8.4
3.0	1.9	3.5	8.1	36–48	0	0.4	1.2
4.0	1.6	2.7	6.5				
6.0	1.1	1.8	4.6	Total	173.3	360.6	669.4
8.0	0.77	1.3	3.3				
10.0	0.55	0.91	2.4				
12.0	0.39	0.64	1.7				

sion methods.[138,139] Parameters given in Table 9-10 were used to generate the solid lines in Figure 9-28. These parameters are then used to calculate pharmacokinetic parameters for the drug; methods and results are also summarized in Table 9-10.

Half-lives, rate constants, and volume of distribution are similar among the three doses. As shown in Figure 9-29, AUC_∞ increases in proportion to dose, indicating that the drug obeys linear (first-order) disposition kinetics over the range of doses studied. Since $AUC_\infty = D_{iv}/CL$

according to equation (18), this finding also indicates that CL should be constant and independent of the dose. Some variation in CL is observed (Table 9-10) but there is no consistent trend as dose increases.

As indicated in Table 9-10, renal clearance of the drug is the major component of CL; about 70% of the dose is excreted unchanged in urine (f_r). The average CL_r differs somewhat between treatments, but as with CL, there is no consistent trend as the dose increases.

Bioavailability. Suppose the same drug is to

TABLE 9-10. *Pharmacokinetic Parameters Derived from Data in Table 9-9.*

Parameter	Units	D_{iv} 250 mg	D_{iv} 500 mg	D_{iv} 1000 mg	Equation in Text or Calculation Method
A	μg/ml	9.01	18.0	33.1	28
B	μg/ml	3.00	5.28	12.3	28
α	h^{-1}	1.39	1.28	1.39	28
β	h^{-1}	0.170	0.178	0.164	28
AUC_∞	μg · h/ml	24.1	43.7	98.8	$\dfrac{A}{\alpha}+\dfrac{B}{\beta}$
$t_{\frac{1}{2},\alpha}$	h	0.50	0.54	0.50	$0.693/\alpha$
$t_{\frac{1}{2},\beta}$	h	4.08	3.89	4.23	$0.693/\beta$
k_{10}	h^{-1}	0.498	0.531	0.460	41
k_{21}	h^{-1}	0.476	0.428	0.496	42
k_{12}	h^{-1}	0.589	0.497	0.596	43
V_1	L	20.8	21.5	22.0	40
CL	ml/min	173	190	169	44
CL_r	ml/min	120	137	113	12 or 14
CL_{nr}	ml/min	53	53	56	20
f_r	% dose	69.3	72.1	66.9	7

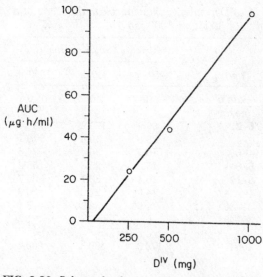

FIG. 9-29. *Relationship between AUC∞ and dosage.*

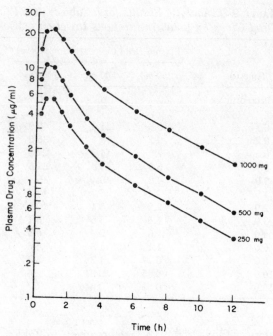

FIG. 9-30. *Typical plasma concentration profiles after oral administration of single doses of a drug.*

be marketed in tablet formulations containing 250-, 500-, and 1000-mg of the drug. The bioavailability of the drug and therefore whether the amount of drug absorbed is proportional to the administered dose (dose-proportionality) need to be determined. Since it is already established that the drug obeys linear disposition kinetics, both objectives can be met by comparing the three formulations with a single i.v. reference dose of the drug in a single-dose, randomized, four-way crossover study. A 500-mg intravenous dose is selected for the study since this is in the middle of the oral dose range.

Simulated results for drug assay in plasma and urine after the 250-, 500-, and 1000-mg oral

dose treatments are given in Table 9-11. For convenience, suppose that the 500-mg i.v. dose data are identical to those used in the previous example (Table 9-9). As before, the i.v. data are analyzed, and the resulting pharmacokinetic parameters for the 500-mg dose are as given in Table 9-10. Plasma drug profiles after the oral doses are compared in Figure 9-30. The drug is apparently rapidly absorbed, peak plasma concentrations are observed within an hour of each

TABLE 9-11. *Analytic Results for a Subject in a Typical Bioavailability Study Comparing Single 250-, 500-, and 1000-mg Oral Tablet Doses of a Drug*

	Plasma Drug Concentration (μg/ml)				Urinary Drug Excretion (mg)		
Time(h)	250 mg	500 mg	1000 mg	Time(h)	250 mg	500 mg	1000 mg
0	0	0	0	−2 to 0 (predrug)	0	0	0
0.25	4.0	7.9	14.7	0–2	66.2	136.3	256.1
0.5	5.4	10.7	20.8	2–4	32.7	63.2	137.3
1.0	5.4	10.1	21.7	4–6	18.5	35.5	77.6
1.5	4.2	7.8	17.9	6–8	12.7	24.1	53.4
2.0	3.2	5.9	14.1	8–12	15.5	28.8	65.4
3.0	2.1	3.7	9.1	12–24	13.8	24.7	59.7
4.0	1.5	2.7	6.7	24–36	1.8	3.0	8.1
6.0	1.0	1.8	4.4	36–48	0.27	0.30	1.1
8.0	0.71	1.2	3.1				
10.0	0.51	0.87	2.2	Total	161.5	315.9	658.7
12.0	0.36	0.61	1.6				

TABLE 9-12. *Summary of Results for a Subject in a Dose-Proportionality/Bioavailability Study Comparing 250-, 500-, and 1000-mg Oral Tablet Formulations With a 500-mg Intravenous Dose as the Standard*

Parameter	Units	D^{po} 250 mg	D^{po} 500 mg	D^{po} 1000 mg	D^{iv} 500 mg	Source or Method of Calculation
C_{max}	μg/ml	5.4	10.7	21.7	—	Table 9-11
t_{max}	h	0.5	0.5	1.0	—	Table 9-11
$t_{\frac{1}{2}}$	h	4.08	3.88	4.10		-0.693/terminal slope
					3.89	Table 9-10
CL_r	ml/min	125	135	120		Equation (12): $t_1 = 0, t_2 = 12$
					137	Table 9-10
AUC_∞	μg · h/ml	21.5	39.0	91.5		Equation (14): U_∞/CL_r
					43.7	Table 9-10
U_∞	% Dose	64.6	63.2	65.9		Table 9-11
					72.1	Table 9-10
F	% Dose	98.4	89.2	105		Equation (110)
		89.6	87.7	91.4		Equation (111)
		91.8	88.0	95.0		Equation (114)

dose and increase in proportion to the administered dose. After ~6 hours, plasma concentrations decline log-linearly with a terminal disposition half-life that is similar among all treatments, including the i.v. dose (Table 9-12).

The renal clearance of the drug is calculated by equation (12) where t_1 and t_2 are times corresponding to the beginning and the end of a urine collection interval; the area under the plasma concentration curve over the same time interval, $\int_{t_1}^{t_2} C_1 dt$, is evaluated by the trapezoidal method or by other suitable methods of interpolation.[132] The average CL_r observed in each oral dose treatment (i.e., 0 to 12 hours) is given in Table 9-12. Note that by design, urine collections are segmented into five discrete intervals over the time plasma is being sampled (Table 9-11), and plasma samples are included at the beginning and end of each urine collection period. Equation (12) can then be used to calculate CL_r for each of these intervals to compare these "incremental" values of CL_r with the average value. In the present example, CL_r is constant within a treatment (calculations not shown) and thereby is also independent of the plasma concentration of the drug. Typically, there is some variation in mean CL_r between treatments (Table 9-11).

Since CL_r^{po} is constant within a treatment, the total area under the curve, AUC_∞^{po}, can be obtained from the ratio of total urinary recovery, U_∞^{po} and CL_r^{po}, as given in equation (14). This method is model-independent and does not require extrapolation based on $t_{\frac{1}{2}}$ of the plasma profile after the last data point (12 hours) to obtain the total area under the curve. Dose-proportionality is observed with the three oral formulations because AUC_∞^{po} approximately doubles when the administered dose is doubled (Table 9-12).

Bioavailability estimates of the drug calculated under the three alternative assumptions expressed in equations (110), (111), and (114), regarding CL between treatments, are given in Table 9-12. Without evidence to the contrary, estimates based on equation (114) may be preferred on the basis that plasma clearance in the oral dose treatments is adjusted only for that portion that is experimentally observable, the renal clearance. The bioavailability of the drug, F, is independent of the dose, and the drug is nearly quantitatively absorbed over the 250- to 1000-mg dosage range.

To obtain the rate of absorption, the intravenous dose data (see Table 9-10) are used as the reference standard to define the disposition of the drug, and the absorption profile is constructed based on the Loo-Riegelman method, as given in equations (49) through (56). The absorption profiles for the oral dose treatments are given in Table 9-13. For this calculation, AUC_∞^{po} values were estimated by the trapezoidal method, and CL was adjusted for the observed change in CL_r between the i.v. and p.o. routes of administration consistent with the estimate of F. Absorption of the drug is rapid and is nearly over by 6 hours after the dose has been administered; by 12 hours, the total amount absorbed is nearly identical to that calculated by the model-independent methods (Table 9-12).

TABLE 9-13. *Absorption Profiles for Drug After Single Oral Doses of 250, 500, and 1000 mg*

Time (h)	Cumulative Amount of Drug Absorbed, A(t)					
	250 mg		500 mg		1000 mg	
	mg	% Dose	mg	% Dose	mg	% Dose
0	0	0	0	0	0	0
0.25	96.5	38.6	191.2	38.2	354.1	35.4
0.5	150.6	60.2	300.2	60.0	574.5	57.4
1.0	202.2	80.9	389.6	77.9	794.4	79.4
1.5	217.4	87.0	418.8	83.8	881.0	88.1
2.0	222.8	89.1	429.2	85.8	917.0	91.7
3.0	228.6	91.4	436.3	87.3	941.2	94.1
4.0	228.5	91.4	437.5	87.5	947.7	94.8
6.0	229.3	91.7	440.4	88.1	952.8	95.3
8.0	229.5	91.8	438.8	87.8	952.1	95.2
10.0	229.7	91.9	439.1	87.8	950.8	95.1
12.0	229.7	91.9	439.2	87.8	951.2	95.1

References

1. Riegelman, S., Benet, L. Z., and Rowland, M.: J. Pharmacokinet. Biopharm., 1:3, 1973.
2. Teorell, T.: Arch. Int. Pharmacodyn. Ther., 57:205, 1973.
3. Teorell, T.: Arch. Int. Pharmacodyn. Ther., 57:226, 1973.
4. Dost, F. H.: Der Blutspiegel. Konzentrations—Ablaüfe in der Kreishauffflussigkeit. Georg Thieme, Leipzig, 1953.
5. Hogben, C. A. M., Tocco, D. J., Brodie, B. B., and Schanker, L. S.: J. Pharmacol. Exp. Ther., 125:275, 1959.
6. Schanker, L. S.: J. Med. Pharm. Chem., 2:343, 1960.
7. Wagner, J. G.: J. Pharm. Sci., 50:359, 1961.
8. Ballard, B. E., and Nelson, E.: J. Pharmacol. Exp. Ther., 135:120, 1962.
9. Levy, G.: Biopharmaceutical considerations in dosage form design and evaluation. In Prescription Pharmacy. Edited by J. B. Sprowls. J. B. Lippincott, Philadelphia, 1963, p. 31.
10. Wilson, T. H.: Intestinal Absorption. W. B. Saunders, Philadelphia, 1962.
11. Riggs, D. S.: The Mathematical Approach to Physiological Problems. Williams & Wilkins, Baltimore, 1963.
12. Binns, T. B. (ed.): Absorption and Distribution of Drugs. Williams & Wilkins, Baltimore, 1964.
13. Ariens, E.J. (ed.): Physico-Chemical Aspects of Drug Action. Pergamon, Oxford, 1968.
14. Levine, R. R., and Pelikan, E. W.: Ann. Rev. Pharmacol., 4:69, 1964.
15. Swarbrick, J. (ed.): Current Concepts in the Pharmaceutical Sciences: Biopharmaceutics. Lea & Febiger, Philadelphia, 1970.
16. Wagner, J. G.: The role of biopharmaceutics in the design of drug products. In Drug Design. Vol. I. Edited by E.J. Ariens. Academic Press, New York, 1971, p. 451.
17. Van Rossum, J. M.: Significance of pharmacokinetics for drug design and the planning of dosage regimens. In Drug Design. Vol. I. Edited by E. J. Ariens. Academic Press, New York, 1971, p. 470.
18. Wagner, J. G.: Biopharmaceutics and Relevant Pharmacokinetics. Drug Intelligence Publications, Hamilton, IL, 1971.
19. LaDu, B. N., Mandel, H. G., and Way, E. L. (eds.): Fundamentals of Drug Metabolism and Drug Disposition. Williams & Wilkins, Baltimore, 1971.
20. Teorell, T., Dedrick, R. L., and Condliffe, P. G. (eds.): Pharmacology and Pharmacokinetics. Plenum Press, New York, 1974.
21. Brodie, B. B., and Heller, W. M. (eds.): Bioavailability of Drugs. S. Karger, Basel, 1972.
22. Swarbrick, J. (ed.): Current Concepts in the Pharmaceutical Sciences: Dosage Form Design and Bioavailability. Lea & Febiger, Philadelphia, 1973.
23. Benet, L. Z.: Biopharmaceutics as the basis for the design of drug products. In Drug Design. Vol. IV. Edited by E. J. Ariens. Academic Press, New York, 1973, p. 24.
24. Gillette, J. R., and Mitchell, J. R. (eds.): Concepts in Biochemical Pharmacology. Handbook of Experimental Pharmacology. Vol. XXVIII, Pt. 3. Springer-Verlag, Berlin, 1975.
25. Wagner, J.G.: Fundamentals of Clinical Pharmacokinetics. Drug Intelligence Publications, Hamilton, IL, 1975.
26. Van Rossum, J. M. (ed.): Kinetics of Drug Action. Springer-Verlag, Berlin, 1977.
27. Gilbaldi, M.: Biopharmaceutics and Clinical Pharmacokinetics. Lea & Febiger, Philadelphia, 1977.
28. Banker, G. S., and Rhodes, C. T. (eds.): Modern Pharmaceutics. Marcel Dekker, New York, 1979.
29. Blanchard, J., Sawchuk, R., and Brodie, B. B. (eds.): Principles and Perspectives in Drug Bioavailability. S. Karger, New York, 1979.
30. Rowland, M., and Tozer, T. N.: Clinical Pharmacokinetics: Concepts and Applications. Lea & Febiger, Philadelphia, 1980.
31. Notari, R. E.: Biopharmaceutics and Clinical Pharmacokinetics. Marcel Dekker, New York, 1980.
32. Gibaldi, M., and Perrier, D.: Pharmacokinetics. Marcel Dekker, New York, 1982.

33. Yeh, K. C., and Kwan, K. C.: J. Pharmacokinet. Biopharm., 6:79, 1978.
34. Pang, R. S., and Gillett, J. M.: J. Pharmacokinet. Biopharm., 7:275, 1979.
35. Wagner, J. G., and Nelson, E.: J. Pharm. Sci., 52:610, 1963.
36. Loo, J. C. K., and Riegelman, S.: J. Pharm. Sci., 57:918, 1968.
37. Wagner, J. G., Northam, J. I., Alway, C. D., and Carpenter, D. S.: Nature, 207:1301, 1965.
38. Yeh, K. C., and Kwan, K. C.: J. Pharm. Sci., 65:512, 1976.
39. Anton, A. H., and Solomon, H. M. (eds.): Acad. Sci., 226:1, 1973.
40. Goldstein, A.: Pharmacol. Rev., 1:102, 1949.
41. Jusko, W. J., and Gretch, M.: Drug Metab. Rev., 5:43, 1976.
42. Davison, C.: Protein binding. In Fundamentals of Drug Metabolism and Drug Disposition. Edited by B. N. LaDu, H. G. Mandel, and E. L. Way. Waverly Press, Baltimore, 1971, p. 63.
43. Rowland, M., and Tozer, T. N.: Clinical Pharmacokinetics: Concepts and Applications. Lea & Febiger, Philadelphia, 1980, p. 34.
44. Gibaldi, M., and McNamara, P. J.: J. Pharm. Sci., 66:1211, 1977.
45. Gibaldi, M., Levy, G., and McNamara, P. J.: Clin. Pharmacol. Ther., 24:1, 1978.
46. Tisher, C.: Anatomy of the kidney. In The Kidney. Vol. 1. Edited by B. M. Brenner and F. C. Rector, Jr. W. B. Saunders, Philadelphia, 1976, p. 3.
47. Ganong, W. F.: Review of Medical Physiology. 7th Ed. Lange Medical Publications, Los Altos, CA, 1975, p. 514.
48. Pitts, R. F.: Physiology of the Kidney and Body Fluids. Year Book Medical Publishers, Chicago, 1966.
49. Cafruny, E. J.: Renal excretion of drugs. In Fundamentals of Drug Metabolism and Disposition. Edited by B. N. LaDu, H. G. Mandel, and E. L. Way. Waverly Press, Baltimore, 1971, p. 119.
50. Smith, H. W.: Principles of Renal Physiology. Oxford University Press, New York, 1956, p. 3.
51. Weiner, I. M., and Mudge, G. H.: Am. J. Med., 36:743, 1964.
52. Rowland, M., and Tozer, T. N.: Clinical Pharmacokinetics: Concepts and Applications. Lea & Febiger, Philadelphia, 1980, p. 52.
53. Milne, M., Scribner, B. H., and Crawford, M. A.: Am. J. Med., 24:709, 1958.
54. Taggart, J. V.: Am. J. Med., 24:774, 1958.
55. Weiner, I. M.: Transport of weak acids and bases. In Handbook of Physiology. Sec. 8, Renal Physiology. Edited by J. Orloff, R. W. Berliner, and S. R. Geiger. American Physiological Society, Washington, D.C., 1973, p. 521.
56. Mudge, G. H., Silva, P., and Stibitz, G. R.: Med. Clin. North Am., 59:681, 1975.
57. Cohn, V. H.: Transmembrane movement of drug molecules. In Fundamentals of Drug Metabolism and Drug Disposition. Edited by B. N. LaDu, H. G., Mandel, and E. L. Way. Waverly Press, Baltimore, 1971, p. 3.
58. Neame, K. D., and Richards, T.G.: Elementary Kinetics of Membrane Carrier Transport, John Wiley and Sons, New York, 1972, p. 1.
59. Renick, B.: Ann. Rev. Pharmacol., 12:141, 1972.
60. Butler, T. C., and Waddell, W. J.: Neurology (Suppl. 1), 8:106, 1958.
61. Dobrinska, M. R., and Welling, P. G.: J. Pharm. Sci., 66:688, 1977.
62. Silber, B., Holford, N. H. G., and Riegelman, S.: J. Pharm. Sci., 71:699, 1982.
63. Rowland, M., Benet, L. Z., and Graham, G. G.: J. Pharmacokinet. Biopharm., 1:123, 1973.
64. Wilkinson, G. R., and Shand, D. G.: Clin. Pharmacol. Ther., 18:377, 1975.
65. Pang, K. S., and Rowland, M.: J. Pharmacokinet. Biopharm., 5:625, 1977.
66. Wilkinson, G. R.: Ann. Rev. Pharmacol., 15:11, 1975.
67. Duggan, D. E., Hooke, K. F., Noll, R. M., and Kwan, K. C.: Biochem. Pharmacol., 24:1749, 1975.
68. Duggan, D. E., Hooke, K. F., Noll, R. M., et al.: Biochem. Pharmacol., 27:2311, 1978.
69. Hucker, H. B., Stauffer, S. C., White, S. D., et al.: Drug Metab. Dispos., 1:721, 1973.
70. Dujovne, C. A., Pitterman, A., Vincek, W. C., et al.: Clin. Pharmacol. Ther., 33:172, 1983.
71. Dobrinska, M. R., Furst, D. E., Spiegel, T., et al.: Biopharm. Drug Dispos., 4:347, 1983.
72. Duggan, D. E., Hare, L. E., Ditzler, C. A., et al.: Clin. Pharmacol. Ther., 21:326, 1977.
73. Kwan, K. C., and Duggan, D. E.: Acta Rhum. Belg., 1:168, 1977.
74. Levy, G., Tsuchiya, T., and Amsel, L. P.: Clin. Pharmacol. Ther., 13:258, 1972.
75. Rowland, M., and Riegelman, S.: J. Pharm. Sci., 57:1313, 1968.
76. The Effect of Disease States on Drug Pharmacokinetics. Edited by L. Z. Benet. American Pharmaceutical Association, Washington, D.C., 1976.
77. Triggs, E. J., and Nation, R. L.: J. Pharmacokinet. Biopharm., 3:387, 1975.
78. Rone, A., and Tomson, G.: Eur. J. Clin. Pharmacol., 18:9, 1980.
79. George, C. F.: Br. J. Clin. Pharmacol., 9:94, 1980.
80. Weiss, P., and Hersey, R. M., Dujovne, C. A., and Bianchine, J. R.: Clin. Pharmacol. Ther., 10:401, 1969.
81. Welling, P. G., Craig, W. A., and Kunin, C. M.: Clin. Pharmacol., Ther., 18:45, 1975.
82. Thomson, P. D., Melmon, K. L., Richardson, J. A., et al.: Ann. Int. Med., 78:499, 1973.
83. Williams, R. L., Blaschke, T. F., Meffin, P. J., et al.: Clin. Pharmacol. Ther., 21:301, 1977.
84. Atkinson, R. M., Bedford, C., Child, K. J., and Tomich, E. G.: Antibiot. Chemother., 12:232, 1962.
85. Aguiar, A. J., Krc, J., Jr., Kinkel, A. W., and Samyn, J. C.: J. Pharm. Sci., 56:847, 1967.
86. Simmons, D. L., and Ranz, R. J.: Can. J. Pharm. Sci., 8:125, 1973.
87. Rowland, M., and Tozer, T. N.: Clinical Pharmacokinetics: Concepts and Applications. Lea & Febiger, Philadelphia, 1980, p. 20.
88. Nishibata, T., Tytting, H. J., and Higuchi, T.: J. Pharm. Sci., 70:71, 1980.
89. Renwick, A. G.: First-pass metabolism within the lumen of the gastrointestinal tract. In Clinical Pharmacology and Therapeutics 1—Presystemic Drug Elimination. Edited by C. F. George and D. G. Shand. Butterworth and Co., London, 1982, p. 3.
90. Goldman P.: Ann. Rev. Pharmacol. Toxicol., 18:523, 1978.

91. George, C. F.: Clin. Pharmacokinet., 6:259, 1981.
92. Caldwell, J., and Marsh, M. V.: Metabolism of drugs by the gastrointestinal tract. *In* Clinical Pharmacology and Therapeutics 1—Presystemic Drug Elimination. Edited by C. F. George and D. G. Shand. Butterworth and Co., London, 1982, p. 29.
93. Griffin, J. P.: J. Pharmac. Ther., 15:79, 1981.
94. George, C. F., and Shand, D. G.: Presystemic drug metabolism in the liver. *In* Clinical Pharmacology and Therapeutics 1—Presystemic Drug Elimination. Edited by C. F. George and D. G. Shand. Butterworth and Co., London, 1982, p. 69.
95. Ladu, B. N., Mandel, H. G., and Way, E. L.: Fundamentals of Drug Metabolism and Drug Disposition. Williams & Wilkins, Baltimore, 1972, p. 149.
96. Williams, R. T.: Detoxification Mechanisms. 2nd Ed. Chapman and Hall, London, 1959.
97. Williams, R. T.: Biochemic. Soc. Trans., 2:359, 1974.
98. Routledge, P. A., and George, C. F.: First-pass metabolism by the lung: Introduction. *In* Clinical Pharmacology and Therapeutics 1—Presystemic Drug Elimination. Edited by C. F. George and D. G. Shand. Butterworth and Co., London, 1982, p. 111.
99. Hook, G. E. R.: The metabolic potential of the lungs. *In* Clinical Pharmacology and Therapeutics 1-Presystemic Drug Elimination. Edited by C. F. George and D. G. Shand. Butterworth and Co., London, 1982, p. 117.
100. Pannatier, A., Jenner, P., Testa, B., and Etter, J. C.: Drug Metab. Rev., 8:319, 1978.
101. Wester, R. C., and Noonan, P. K.: Internat. J. Pharmaceut., 7:99, 1980.
102. deBoer, A. G., Moolenaar, F., deLeede, L. G. J., and Breimer, D. D.: Clin. Pharmacokinet., 7:285, 1982.
103. Hirai, S., Yashiki, T., Matsuzawa, T., and Mima, H.: Internat. J. Pharmaceut., 7:317, 1981.
104. Albery, W. J., and Hadgraft, J.: J. Pharm. Pharmacol., 31:65, 1979.
105. Roberts, M. S., Anderson, R. A., Swarbrick, J., and Moore, D. E.: J. Pharm. Pharmacol., 30:486, 1978.
106. Benmair, Y., Fischel, B., Frei, E. H., and Gilat. T.: Am. J. Gastroenterol., 68:475, 1977.
107. Boxenbaum, H. G.: Drug Develop. and Indust. Pharm., 8:1, 1982.
108. Kwan, K. C., Breault, G. O., Umbenhauer, E. R., et al.: J. Pharmacokinet. Biopharm., 4:255, 1976.
109. Guyton, A. C. The lymphatic system, interstitial fluid dynamics and edema. *In* Textbook of Medical Physiology. 3rd Ed. W. B. Saunders, Philadelphia, 1966, p. 446.
110. Parke, D. V., and Smith, R. L. (eds.): Drug Metabolism—From Microbe to Man. Taylor & Francis, London, 1977.
111. Boxenbaum, H.: J. Pharmacokinet. Biopharm., 8:165, 1980.
112. Saari, W. S., Freedman, M. B., Hartman, R. D., et al.: J. Med. Chem., 21:746, 1978.
113. Vickers, S., Duncan, C. A., White, S. D., et al.: Drug Metab. Disp., 6:640, 1978.
114. Stenbaek, Ø., Myhre, E., Rugstad, H. E., et al.: Eur. J. Clin. Pharmacol., 12:117, 1977.
115. Buhs, R. P., Beck, J. L., Speth, O. C., et al.: J. Pharmacol. Exp. Ther., 143:205, 1964.
116. Vickers, S., Duncan, C. A. H., Ramjit, H. G., et al.: Drug Metab. Dispos., 12:242, 1984.
117. Dobrinska, M. R., Kukovetz, W., Beubler, E., et al.: J. Pharmacokinet. Biopharm., 10:587, 1982.
118. Musson, D. G., Vincek, W. C., Dobrinska, M. R., et al.: J. Chromatogr., 308:251, 1984.
119. Cotler, S., Holazo, A., Boxenbaum, H. G., and Kaplan, S. A.: J. Pharm. Sci., 65:822, 1976.
120. Mearrick, P. T., Graham, G. G., and Wade, D. N.: J. Pharmacokinet. Biopharm., 3:13, 1975.
121. Rivera-Calimlim, L., Dujovne, C. A., Morgan, J. P., et al.: J. Clin. Invest., 1:313, 1971.
122. Bianchine, J. R., Calimlim, L. R., Morgan, J. P., et al.: Ann. N.Y. Acad. Sci., 179:126, 1971.
123. Duggan, D. E., Yeh, K. C., Matalia, N., et al.: Clin. Pharmacol. Ther., 18:205, 1975.
124. Theeuwes, F., Swanson, D., Wong P., et al.: J. Pharm. Sci., 72:253, 1983.
125. Hare, L. E., Yeh, K. C., Ditzler, C. A., et al.: Clin. Pharmacol. Ther., 18:330, 1975.
126. Janssen, H. J. L.: Ion-Pair Partition Chromatography of Catecholamines. Ph.D. Thesis. State University of Leiden, The Netherlands, 1981.
127. Macek, T. J.: Am. J. Pharm., 137:217, 1965.
128. Dresse, A., Gegard, M. A., Lays, A., et al.: Pharm. Acta. Helv., 53:177, 1978.
129. Welling, P. G., and Dobrinska, M. R.: Multiple dosing of sustained release systems. *In* Sustained and Controlled Release Drug Delivery Systems. Edited by J. R. Robinson. Marcel Dekker, New York, 1978.
130. Rogers, J. D., and Kwan, K. C.: Pharmacokinetic requirements for controlled release dosage forms. *In* Controlled Release Pharmaceuticals. Edited by J. Urquhart. American Pharmaceutical Association, Washington, D.C., 1981, p. 95.
131. Lasagna, L. (ed.): Combination Drugs, Their Use and Regulation. Stratton Intercontinental Medical Book Corp., New York, 1975.
132. Kwan, K. C., and Till, A. E.,: J. Pharm. Sci., 62:1494, 1973.
133. Hwang, S., and Kwan, K. C.: J. Pharm. Sci., 69:77, 1980.
134. Murphy, P. J., and Sullivan, H. R.: Ann. Rev. Pharmacol. Toxicol., 20:609, 1980.
135. Carlin, J. R., Rodger, J. D., Davies, R. O., et al.: Simultaneous Determination of the Intravenous and Oral Pharmacokinetics of Timolol. Proceedings of the 30th Annual Conference on Mass Spectrometry and Allied Topics. Honolulu, 1982, p. 159.
136. Yeh, K. C.: J. Pharm. Sci., 66:1688, 1977.
137. Yeh, K. C., and Kwan, K. C.: J. Pharm. Sci., 68:1120, 1979.
138. Nelder, J. A., and Mead, R.: Comput. J., 7:308, 1965.
139. Metzler, C. M., Elfring, G. L., and McEwen, A. J.: A Users Manual for NONLIN and Associated Programs. Upjohn Co., Kalamazoo, MI, 1974.

10

Statistical Applications in the Pharmaceutical Sciences

SANFORD BOLTON

Statisticians have become familiar faces in the research laboratories of industrial pharmaceutical companies. Part of this recent upsurge has been due to the recognition by research scientists that the application of statistics can be a useful tool in the design, analysis, and interpretation of experiments. Also, governmental agencies, principally the Food and Drug Administration (FDA) have promulgated rules and regulations that virtually necessitate the application of statistical techniques to fulfill the law or its recommendations.

The "Good Manufacturing Practices" (GMPs) and the "Good Laboratory Practices" (GLPs) are more recent examples of FDA regulations that recommend statistical usage, formally or implied, as part of the routine of careful implementation and record-keeping of research and manufacturing operations. For example, in section 211.166 of the GMPs, the following statement appears with regard to stability testing and expiration dating of pharmaceuticals: ". . . sample size and test intervals based on statistical criteria for each attribute examined to assure valid estimates of stability." In section 58.120 of the GLPs regarding the protocol for nonclinical laboratory studies, the following statement implies both a prior statistical input and the ultimate statistical analysis of the experimental results: "A statement of the proposed statistical methods to be used [is to be included in all protocols]. . . ."

Statistical input in sampling and testing for quality control, stability testing, process validation, design of preclinical protocols, including statistical methods and appropriate statistical analysis of the resulting data, are applications routinely applied by the pharmaceutical industry to satisfy both internal requirements and FDA recommendations. Both statistical treatment and interpretation of clinical data are requirements of all FDA submissions on new drugs or new dosage forms.

Applications of statistical techniques to pharmaceutical research are beginning to be more appreciated. Some statisticians and pharmaceutical researchers, alone or in collaboration, have had the foresight to recognize applications in this area, and recent publications in the areas of optimization and experimental design indicate the activity in formulation research.[1,2,3,4]

Since this book deals with pharmaceutical technology, a chapter on statistics cannot be expected to be in any way complete. Statisticians should be consulted for all but the simplest problems. Data from real experiments almost always have unexpected wrinkles that need special consideration. The interaction should allow both the statistician and the pharmaceutical scientist to learn and grow.

There will always be more than one way to examine, analyze, and interpret data. Statistics is not an exact science; given a set of data, two statisticians may analyze and present the results differently. Data that comes from a *well-designed experiment*, however, should lead the experimenter to the same conclusion, independent of the analyses. In fact, if this is not the case, something is amiss, and the data and/or analysis should be carefully re-examined.

Computations in the statistical analysis of data are not difficult, but can be complicated, especially for the novice. Statistical packages are readily available, and if the data are compatible with software programs, they should be used. Often, however, the analysis that should be used is not obvious except to the expert, and frequently, there are situations in which only a custom-made program can fit the data. In addition, the statistician must sometimes improvise, using creativity and ingenuity for a situation for which an analysis has yet to be devised. Nevertheless, anyone who uses statistics should practice some of the computations. This allows a "hands-on" appreciation of what is involved, helping the user to learn more about what he is doing.

Introductory Statistical Concepts

Statistics encompasses many areas of human endeavor, and within each area is a scientific field in itself. The statistical techniques most applicable to pharmaceutical experimentation can be categorized broadly as follows:

1. Descriptive statistics: Presentation of data including tabular and graphic representation

2. Hypothesis testing

3. Estimation

4. Experimental design

1. Although this chapter is mainly concerned with the latter three categories, *descriptive statistics* are important. Professional statisticians have expertise in this area, and collaboration between pharmaceutical scientist and statistician should be complementary, using to full advantage the knowledge and experience of both parties. One should carefully consider various alternatives, presenting "pictures" of the data in the most convincing manner.

2. The possible overuse of *hypothesis testing* in statistics has been debated, but at present it is certainly a popular standard statistical approach to decision making. Government agencies, the FDA in particular, rely on significance levels (5%) for drug-related claims.

3. *Estimation* of unknown parameters such as a population mean or the slope of a line is often the objective of a statistical investigation. This concept is illustrated and discussed in some detail in this chapter.

4. Statistical *experimental design* pervades all areas, and some designs commonly used in pharmaceutical experiments are presented. Poor or inadequate design can invalidate an otherwise carefully conducted experiment.

Statistical analysis does not yield unequivocal answers, nor can the analysis redeem a poor experiment. Good experimental design is essential. The statistics presented here are concerned with probability. Observations by their very nature are variable. By "variable," we mean that if an observation (an experiment) is repeated, the new outcome cannot be exactly predicted. Variability and unpredictability characterize most of our experience; here, the uncertainty is harnessed and put to work.

Choosing Samples

When 100 tablets are inspected for defects, or when 20 tablets are assayed for potency, only a small proportion of the potentially available data is being tested. Much of the work in statistics involves examining relatively small samples and then making inferences about the population from which the sample came. There are many reasons why the totality of data cannot always be observed or tested. For instance, 100% sampling may be precluded because of practical time and cost considerations. Situations in which 100% sampling cannot be accomplished practically are (1) destructive assays that may occur in analytical procedures and (2) cases in which the population definition precludes 100% sampling, as occurs in clinical studies in which the population may include *all* patients with a particular disease.

The proper selection of samples is an essential part of a good experiment and is a consequence of the experimental design. A *random sample* is one in which each of all possible experimental units have an *equal chance* of being included in the experiment or sample. Data derived from random samples yield fair, unbiased estimates of population parameters such as the mean. To sample tablets randomly from a batch for visual inspection or assay, each tablet should have an equal chance of being chosen. The method of "random sampling" clearly must be modified to apply to many real-life experimental situations. For example, if the experiment entails stratification, the random sampling is done within each stratum. To obtain a random sample, a number can be conceptually assigned to each potential candidate, and then a table of random numbers can be used to select those units or individuals to be included in the experiment or to be assigned to a particular treatment group. Alternatively, all possible experimental units can be thoroughly mixed (literally or figuratively), and samples can be chosen at random as in a lottery.

One must be aware that bias can easily be introduced into the selection of samples if care is not taken in randomization. Often, one must compromise between theory and practice. In a multicenter clinical trial where there is a choice of large numbers of patients from perhaps thousands of clinical sites, the sample chosen may be based more on convenience than randomness. If an effort is made, however, to choose sites based on relevant factors such as geographic location, for example, one might practically consider this a random sample. Certainly, choosing tablets for inspection cannot be done both conveniently and strictly at random. How would one identify the 1,565,387th tablet if it was to be included in the sample? An alternative is to select samples stratified over various time periods during the production run. Ingenuity can often be used to devise a "pseudorandom" sampling procedure that can be satisfactory in difficult situations.

Systematic sampling is often used as an improvement over random sampling. Every nth sample is chosen for inspection, testing, or analysis, which ensures a regular sampling throughout a process such as the manufacture of tablets. If the process is cyclic or periodic in nature, and if by chance the sampling corresponds to the period, this method of sampling can lead to erroneous conclusions.

Sampling for quality control should be carefully implemented to ensure that the samples selected are representative. A representative sample can be regarded as one that is carefully chosen, and perhaps subsequently treated or modified (e.g., by compositing in the case of bulk powders) so that the sample has the same characteristics as the bulk material (powder) if it were homogeneous. For example, sampling from the top of a large container might not be representative and can result in samples that are different from those that might have been obtained from the main bulk of material. It is not easy to define exactly (statistically) a representative sampling scheme for testing bulk materials. The amount of material to be inspected, as well as the number and kind of samples to be chosen, is often based on experience and empirical rules. One method of sampling bulk raw materials from drums, for example, is to sample $\sqrt{N}$ containers (add one container if there is a remainder) where N is the number of containers. The material may then be taken from different parts of the container using a *thief*, a sampling device that is basically a long hollow tube inserted into the powdered material. After collection, the various samples are often thoroughly mixed, and samples for assay are taken from this homogeneous mixture. If carefully implemented, such procedures for finished dosage forms or powdered raw materials and intermediates should result in representative samples for analysis.

Independence and Bias

Many analyses and interpretation of data assume that the sample data points are independent of one another, i.e., that the result of one observation does not influence the result of another concurrent, future, or past observation. Examples of dependent or correlated observations are (1) blood pressure of the same individual taken on two or more occasions, (2) assays

from the same small portion of material repeated over time, and (3) responses to a flavor preference from the same individual on multiple occasions. In these cases, the same experimental unit being used for more than one observation is responsible for the dependence, i.e., each observation has a common component as part of its variability. Note that in (2) the nature of the data is different if the assay is performed on different portions of material rather than on a single homogeneous portion.

The same data may be treated as independent in one situation and correlated in another. For example, to assess the stability of a product, a single bottle from a batch is assayed over time with duplicate assays at each time period. Are the duplicates assayed at a given time period independent? If they are analyzed concurrently, the duplicates are probably not independent because of the common conditions existing at the time of the assay. These common conditions could include, for example, the same analyst, the same reagents, and the same instrument standardized with the same standard material. Duplicates performed at two different laboratories by two different analysts or assays done at different points in time are probably independent if proper care is taken. Since the tablets come from a single bottle in which the material is more homogeneous than the batch as a whole, can any of the assays be considered independent? These are rhetorical questions and serve to illustrate the complexity of a seemingly simple concept. If observations are correlated, special analyses may be necessary to account for the correlation.

Bias is another term common to statistics. If samples are not carefully chosen, bias, which may not be obvious, can easily be introduced. Human beings cannot always be objective, and if some controls are not imposed, what is observed is often what one wishes to observe. Try to make up a series of "random" numbers from 0 to 9 or letters of the alphabet quickly, without too much thinking, and you will observe your own bias. Randomization and blinding are ways to overcome bias. In blinded experiments, the person observing and recording experimental results is not aware of the source of the data. This procedure is especially important in experiments with subjective evaluations. Some examples of how bias may enter an experiment may seem obvious to an objective outsider, but may often not be obvious to the scientist closely involved with his experiment. In an open (not blinded) clinical trial, the more severely affected patients may be selected for the treatment that the investigator feels (perhaps erroneously) is the better one. During duplicate assays, a knowledge of the results of the first assay may serve as a criterion for accepting or rejecting the second assay. Data used in curve fitting, e.g., as a function of time, may be rejected because the fit is not as good as expected.

Probability Distributions

Observations can be categorized as discrete or continuous. A discrete observation is one of a countable finite number, such as (1) a tablet categorized as either out of limits or within limits or (2) the number of tablets in a bottle whose label indicates 100 tablets. A continuous observation is one that can be measured more and more precisely according to the sensitivity of the measuring instrument. Weights of tablets and blood pressure are continuous measurements. Most of the statistical problems in pharmaceutical research can be dealt with using the binominal (discrete) and the normal (continuous) *probability distributions*. The data that at least approximate these distributions are not mysterious as suggested by the foregoing examples. These are the ordinary data that are observed in real-life experiments: weight, blood pressure, intact drug in a formulation, dissolution, blood level of a drug, proportion of tablets out of specification, tablet weights, or number of defective bottles. By defining distributions of hypothetical data, inferences can be made about samples of real data that are observed in the laboratory, the production area, or the clinic.

A probability distribution can be visualized as a frequency distribution constructed from a large number of observations. For example, the weights of 200 tablets can be summarized in a frequency distribution, as shown in Table 10-1. The number of tablets that fall into a given interval is the frequency for that interval. The frequency distribution for the 200 tablets approximates the true distribution. The weights of an entire batch of 1,000,000 tablets can be thought of as the *universe*, or true underlying distribution, from which the 200 tablets were selected. In Table 10-1, the tablets are placed in a discrete number (12) of class intervals. If the intervals were made small enough, resulting in a large number of intervals of equal width, a plot of the proportion of tablets in the batch falling into each interval (as in a histogram) would result in a smooth curve as the distinction between intervals disappears. Such a curve might look like one of the normal curves shown in Figures 10-1 or 10-2.

TABLE 10-1. *Frequency Distribution of Weights of 200 Tablets*

Interval*	Frequency (Number of Tablets)	Proportion of Tablets in Interval
176–180	3	0.015
180–184	6	0.03
184–188	12	0.06
188–192	17	0.085
192–196	26	0.13
196–200	33	0.165
200–204	36	0.18
204–208	23	0.115
208–212	22	0.11
212–216	11	0.055
216–220	7	0.035
220–224	4	0.02
TOTAL	200	1.000

*Tablets included from the lower weight in interval up to, but not including, the higher weight in interval.

Normal Distribution—A Continuous Distribution. Examples of two normal distributions are shown in Figure 10-1. The reader may find it helpful to visualize these distributions as frequency distributions of tablet weights, as has just been described. The two distributions in Figure 10-1 have certain similarities and differences. Both curves are symmetric about a central value designated as μ, the mean, and both are bell-shaped. This shape indicates that most of the values in the distribution are near the mean, and as values are further from the mean, they are less prevalent. Although theoretically the data comprising a normal distribution can take on values between $-\infty$ and $+\infty$, values sufficiently far from the mean have little chance of being observed. For example, if the mean weight of a batch of tablets were 200 mg, the chances of

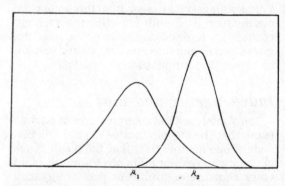

FIG. 10-1. *Examples of two normal curves with different means and variances. The curve on the right has a smaller variance and a larger mean.*

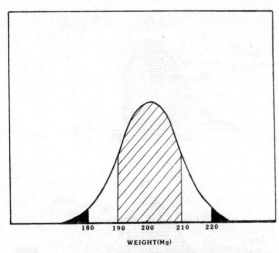

FIG. 10-2. *Distribution of tablet weights with mean =
200, and standard deviation = 10. The small shaded areas
in the tails each represent a probability of approximately
0.025.*

having a 100- or 300-mg tablet in a typical batch
would be small.

In addition to normal curves being distinguished by the mean or central value, they differ
in their "spread." The curve on the left-hand
side of Figure 10-1 is more spread out than the
one on the right, a consequence of its larger
standard deviation (σ). Normal curves are exactly defined by two parameters: the mean, a
measure of location, and the standard deviation,
a measure of spread.

The Greek letters μ and σ refer to the mean
and standard deviation of the universe or population. The population is the totality of data from
which sample data are derived. In the example
of 200 tablet weights, the 200 tablets are samples taken from a population of a batch of tablets
that may consist of 1,000,000 tablets or more. In
general, μ and σ are unknown and are estimated
from the data derived from the sample. The
sample mean, or average, $\bar{X}$, is an *unbiased* estimate of the true population mean μ. That is, although the average obtained from any single
experiment cannot be expected to equal μ, if an
experiment is repeated many times, and all the
$\bar{X}$'s are averaged, this overall average would
equal μ. The average is calculated as $\Sigma X_i/N$,
where ΣX_i is the sum of N data points. The average of the tablet weights in Table 10.1 is
200.32 mg. The average weight of the entire
batch of tablets is probably not equal to
200.32 mg. The sample mean, $\bar{X}$, however, is
the best estimate of the population mean, μ. The
standard deviation, S, is calculated as
$\sqrt{\Sigma(X_i - \bar{X})^2/(N - 1)}$. The sum of the squared

deviations of each value from the mean divided
by $(N - 1)$ is called the variance (S^2). The
square root of the variance is the standard deviation. The number of observations minus one
$(N - 1)$, is known as the *degrees of freedom*.
Many statistical calculations involve $\Sigma(X_i - \bar{X})^2$,
and this expression appears often in this chap-
ter, with examples of the calculations.*

As a simple illustration of the calculation of
the standard deviation, consider three data
points with values 2, 4, and 6. The mean is
$12/3 = 4$. The value for $\Sigma(X - \bar{X})^2$ is calculated
as follows:

X	$\bar{X}$	$(X - \bar{X})$	$(X - \bar{X})^2$
2	4	−2	4
4	4	0	0
6	4	2	4

$$\Sigma(X - \bar{X})^2 = 8$$

The standard deviation of the numbers 2, 4, and
6 is $\sqrt{8}/2 = 2$. The variance S^2 is the square of
the standard deviation and is equal to $2^2 = 4$ in
this example. The sample variance S^2 is an unbiased estimate of the population variance σ^2.
The use of $(N - 1)$ in the denominator of the
expression for S^2 ensures that the estimate is
unbiased. A shortcut and more accurate com-
puting formula for $\Sigma(X - \bar{X})^2$ is $\Sigma X^2 - (\Sigma X)^2/N$
equal to $2^2 + 4^2 + 6^2 - \frac{12}{3}^2 = 8$ in the above
example.

Another property of the normal distribution is
that the area under the normal curve as shown
in Figure 10-1, for example, is exactly one (1)
irrespective of the values μ and σ. *The area between any two points* (Figure 10-2), *e.g., 190 and
210, represents the probability of observing a
value between 190 and 210.* Because the theoretic normal curve comprises an infinite number
of values, the probability of observing any single
value is zero. However, in many statistical procedures, there is a need to compute the probability of observing values in some interval. For example, suppose that the distribution of tablet
weights approximates a normal distribution as
shown in Figure 10-2. The mean weight, μ, of
this batch of tablets is 200 mg, and the standard
deviation, σ, is 10. The proportion of tablets
weighing between 190 and 210 mg can be considered a measure of homogeneity of the batch
and is equivalent to the probability of choosing a
tablet at random that weighs between 190 and
210 mg. Probability can be conveniently thought

*Future use of summation notation in this chapter does
not include the subscript i, although its use is implied.

of as the proportion of times a value or range of values is observed after many observations.

This problem can be solved by referring to a table of "areas under the standard normal curve." Table 10-2 is a short version of such a table that gives the area between $-\infty$ and Z, where Z is a transformation that changes all normal curves into the *standard normal curve*, which has a *mean* of 0 and a *standard deviation* of 1. This transformation allows the use of a single table, which can be used to calculate the area between any two points for any normal curve. The transformation is:

$$Z = (X - \mu)/\sigma$$

To calculate the area between $-\infty$ and X, compute Z and find the area in Table 10-2. The reader may find it convenient to refer to Figures 10-2 and 10-3 in the following discussion, which describes the calculation for finding the area between 190 and 210.

1. Area between $-\infty$ and 210: $Z = (X - \mu)/\sigma = (210 - 200)/10 = 1$. Area between $-\infty$ and 210 = 0.84 from Table 10-2.

2. Area between $-\infty$ and 190: $Z = (190 - 200)/10 = -1$. Area between $-\infty$ and 190 = 0.16 from Table 10-2.

TABLE 10-2. *Short Table of Cumulative Areas Under the Standard Normal Curve*

$Z = (X - \mu)/\sigma$	Area From $-\infty$ to Z
-2.576^*	0.005
-2.326	0.01
-1.96^*	0.025
-1.645^*	0.05
-1.58	0.057
-1.28	0.10
-1.00	0.16
-0.50	0.31
0	0.50
0.50	0.69
1.00	0.84
1.28	0.90
1.58	0.943
1.645^*	0.95
1.96^*	0.975
2.326	0.99
2.576^*	0.995

$^*Z = \pm 2.576, \pm 1.96$, and ± 1.645 are the cutoff points used for a two-sided test at the 1%, 5%, and 10% levels respectively.

$Z = 1.645$ is the cutoff point for a one-sided test at the 5% level where H_0 is $\mu \le \mu_0$ and H_A is $\mu > \mu_0$.

$Z = -1.645$ is the cutoff point at the 5% level for a one-sided test where $H_0: \mu \ge \mu_0$ and $H_A: \mu < \mu_0$.

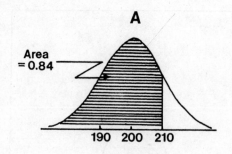
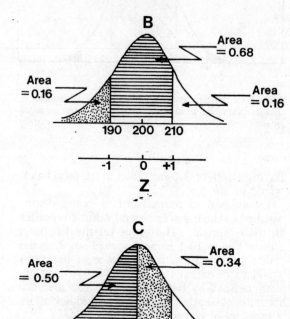

FIG. 10-3. A to C, *Calculation of areas under a normal curve with $\mu = 200$ and $\sigma = 10$ from table of areas under the standard normal curve (see Table 10-2).*

$$Z = (X - \mu)/\sigma.$$

3. Area between 190 and 210 = (Area between $-\infty$ and 210) − (Area between $-\infty$ and 190) = $0.84 - 0.16 = 0.68$.

This computation is illustrated in Figure 10-3.

These calculations may also be made based on the symmetry of the normal curve; the portion of the curve below the mean is the mirror image of that above the mean, and therefore the area above and below the mean each equal 0.5 by definition. In this case, the area between 210 and 200 (μ) is $0.84 - 0.5 = 0.34$. Therefore, the area between 190 and 210 is $2 \times 0.34 = 0.68$ (see Fig. 10-3C). Thus, 68% of the tablets weigh between 190 and 210 mg, or equivalently, the probability of choosing a single tablet at random that weighs between 190 and 210 mg is 0.68. (Chances are 68/100 that a tablet randomly taken from the batch will weigh between 190 and 210 mg.)

What are the chances of finding a tablet chosen at random that weighs 10% more or less than the mean weight? This question is equivalent to asking, "What is the probability that a tablet will weigh less than 180 mg or more than 220 mg?" As before, calculate Z for X = 220 and Z for X = 180. $Z_{220} = (220 - 200)/10 = 2$; the area is approximately 0.975. $Z_{180} = (180 - 200)/10 = -2$; the area is approximately 0.025. The area between 180 and 220 is $0.975 - 0.025 = 0.95$. Therefore, 5% of the tablets will weigh above 220 or less than 180 mg. By using the area between 180 and $-\infty$ (0.025), and the symmetric properties of the normal curve, the same result is obtained (see Fig. 10-2).

Another, slightly different question is also germane: "What is the probability that the *mean of 10 randomly chosen tablets* is between 195 and 205 mg?" An important result in statistical theory that relates to the distribution of *means*, the *central limit theorem*, must be considered before this question can be answered. This theorem states that for any probability distribution (with finite variance), the distribution of means of N randomly selected samples will tend to be normal as N becomes large. Thus, if a new distribution is formed, based not on the original data but on means of size N drawn from the original data, the distribution of means will tend to be normal. This consequence of the central limit theorem allows a comfortable application of normal curve theory when dealing with means. A natural question is, "What is meant by large N?" If the original data are normal, then means of any size N will be normal. The sample sizes needed to make means from non-normal distributions close to being normally distributed vary depending to a great extent on how aberrant the distribution of the original data is from a normal distribution. A good guess is that the means of sample sizes of 30 or more for the kind of data that are usually encountered will closely approximate a normal distribution.

The distribution of means of N observations will have the same mean as the original distribution, but the variance will be smaller, equal to σ^2/N where σ^2 is the variance of the original distribution. The means of many samples of size 10, for example, will tend to cluster more closely together than the individual data because extreme values will be compensated for by the other sample values composing the mean. Therefore, the mean of samples of size 10 from

the batch of tablets will have a normal distribution with a mean weight, μ, of 200 mg and a standard deviation, σ, equal to $\sqrt{\sigma^2/N} = \sqrt{100/10} = 3.16$. The value $\sigma_{\overline{X}}$ (or $S_{\overline{X}} = S/\sqrt{N}$, the sample estimate) is commonly known as the standard error of the mean. Figure 10-4 shows how the distribution of means (N = 10) compares with the original distribution.

To answer the foregoing question, the probability of the mean being less than 195 is calculated, as before, with $\mu = 200$ and with $\sigma = 3.16$. Thus, $Z = (195 - 200)/3.16 = -1.58$. From Table 10-2, the probability of $\overline{X}$ being between $-\infty$ and 195 is 0.057. Using the symmetry of the normal curve, the probability of an average weight of 10 tablets being above 205 is also 0.057, and the probability of $\overline{X}$ being below 195 or more than 205 is $0.057 + 0.057 = 0.114$. Therefore, the probability that the mean of ten tablets will be between 195 and 205 mg is $(1 - 0.114) = 0.886$.

The distribution of tablet weights cannot be identically equivalent to a normal distribution because there is some upper limit on tablet weight, and the lower limit must be greater than zero. Usually, real-life data does not conform exactly to theoretic distributions, and an exact analogy of the normal curve does not exist in real examples. This does not mean that we cannot make practical use of this well-known bell-shaped symmetric distribution. Much of the raw

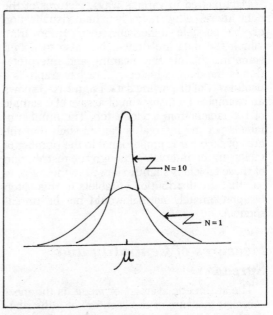

FIG. 10-4. *Normal distribution of single observations (N = 1) and means of size 10 (N = 10).*

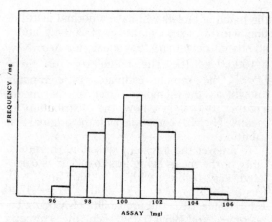

FIG. 10-5. *Histogram of assays of a sample of 100 tablets.*

or transformed data encountered in pharmaceutical sciences are close enough to normal distributions to allow adequate treatment, as if such data were normal. Usually, insufficient data are available to define the probability distribution exactly since only a sample, a small part of the totality of data, is available. There are quantitative methods of assessing if a sample of data is likely to belong to some known distribution, e.g., the normal distribution;[5] however, in this presentation, the true distribution underlying the relative small data sets that are often subjected to analysis will be assumed to be known, as a result of experience or other available information.

Data plotted in various ways, pictures of the data, are revealing, not only to help visualization of the possible underlying distribution from which the data are drawn, but also to obtain some insight into the meaning and interpretation of the data. A histogram, or bar graph, is a useful way of displaying data. Figure 10-5 shows an example of a histogram of assays of a sample of 100 tablets from a pilot batch. The number of tablets per mg interval is plotted such that the area of each bar is proportional to the number of tablets in the interval. Although the distribution of these tablets is slightly skewed to the right, to say that the distribution of tablets in this batch is approximately normal would not be unreasonable.

Measures of Centrality and Spread

The arithmetic average, or *mean,* is the most common measure of the "center" of a distribution and is equal to $\Sigma X/N$, as previously noted. Another often used measure of centrality is the *median.* The median, also known as the 50th percentile, is the value that splits the data in half, i.e., half of the observations are greater and half are less than the median value. With an even number of observations, the median may be considered to be the average of the two observations in the middle of the data set, the numbers having been ordered from lowest to highest. For example, if N = 10, the median is the average of the fifth and sixth values. If a distribution of data is perfectly symmetric (as in the normal curve), the median equals the mean. The *median* is often used to describe asymmetric distributions, e.g., the *median* income.

The *spread,* or dispersion of data, is commonly expressed as the standard deviation, $S = \sqrt{\Sigma(X - \bar{X})^2/(N - 1)}$. The larger the value of S, the greater is the spread of the data. Another common way of expressing the spread is the range, which is equal to the difference between the highest and lowest values in the data set. The coefficient of variation (C.V.) is a measure of relative variation and is equal to the standard deviation divided by the mean, σ/μ, or $S/\bar{X}$, the sample estimate.

Statistical Inference and Estimation

t Distribution

Practical examples of experiments in which data are derived from populations with a normal distribution are commonplace. The examples in which probabilities have been calculated thus far assume a prior knowledge of the parameters of the distribution, that is, the mean and variance are known. In the great majority of cases, population parameters are unknown. In fact, often the purpose of the statistical analysis is to estimate these unknown parameters based on the sample statistics. The sample mean and variance, $\bar{X}$ and S^2, are unbiased estimates of these parameters, and if the underlying distribution (or population) is normal, probabilities of events based on these estimates can be obtained from the t distribution in a manner similar to that described previously for the normal distribution.

The ratio $t = (\bar{X} - \mu)/(S/\sqrt{N})$ has a student's t distribution with $N - 1$ degrees of freedom (df), where N is the sample size. The value $\bar{X}$ is the mean of the N samples selected; μ is the mean of the underlying population distribution from which the samples were selected; and S is the sample standard deviation, $\sqrt{\Sigma(X - \bar{X})^2/(N - 1)}$. This formula for t is the

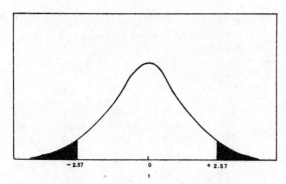

FIG. 10-6. *Illustration of "t" distribution with 5 degrees of freedom. The area in each of the shaded portions at t = ±2.57 is 0.025.*

same as that for Z for the normal distribution, where $Z = (\overline{X} - \mu)/(\sigma/\sqrt{N})$, except that for t, the sample standard deviation, S, is used in the denominator.

The t distribution is similar in shape to the normal distribution (Fig. 10-6), but is more spread out with more area in the tails, the extremities of the curve comprising the smaller and larger values. There are any number of t distributions, each defined by the degrees of freedom. The mean of the t distribution is zero and the spread depends on the degrees of freedom. With 1 df (N = 2), the curve is spread out, but as the degrees of freedom increase, the t distribution becomes tighter, with less spread, approximating more closely the standard normal distribution. When df = ∞ (i.e., the standard deviation is known), the t distribution is identical to the standard normal distribution. The t distribution is used to calculate probabilities when the standard deviation is unknown and estimated from the sample. The use of the t distribution is illustrated below in the testing of hypotheses involving continuous data derived from a normal distribution.

Hypothesis Testing (For Statistical Significance)

Testing of hypotheses is a traditional use of statistical methodology. Because many people have been trained to understand the meaning of these tests, hypothesis testing serves to communicate clearly certain experimental conclusions from a statistical point of view. This statistical procedure is important for assessing differences in treatment effects for government submissions involved with new drugs and dosage forms, including results from clinical trials and bioavailability studies.

The process involves a hypothesis about one or more parameters of a statistical model. An example of a hypothesis is that the mean, μ, of a population, e.g., a batch of tablets, is some value, μ_0, perhaps 200 mg. A sample is chosen, and the estimate of the parameter $\overline{X}$ is calculated. If the sample estimate is close to the hypothesized value, the hypothesis is accepted. If the sample estimate or statistic is sufficiently far from the hypothesized value, the hypothesis is rejected. Rejection implies that the sample estimate of the parameter is evidence that the population parameter is different from that hypothesized. The conclusion in this case is that a statistically significant difference exists between the hypothesized parameter and the true parameter estimated from the sample.

To illustrate this concept, suppose that a hypothesis states that the average 90% dissolution time of a tablet batch is 30 min or less. A dissolution test using 12 tablets from a new batch shows an average result of 33 min. Can one conclude that the average dissolution time of the batch is greater than 30 min? If the average result of the 12 tablets were 50 min, the conclusion might be reached more easily. Depending on the individual tablet results, the decision would be more or less equivocal. Such decisions as whether to accept or reject the hypothesis, based on the sample data, can be made using probabilities derived from the t distribution. The procedure followed in making such decisions, as well as sample computations, are given here for some simpler problems, and the reader is encouraged to try as many computations as possible to gain insight into the statistical process.

The procedure of hypothesis testing is exemplified by a simple test that compares a sample mean with a hypothesized mean.

1. Initially, the *hypothetical mean* against which the mean of the sample data points is to be compared is defined. This is the *null hypothesis*. Statistically, the question being asked is, "Does the mean being estimated from the sample come from a distribution described by the hypothetical mean?" The null hypothesis is traditionally written as:

$$H_0: \mu = \mu_0$$

where μ_0 is the hypothetical mean. Some examples of hypotheses follow. (a) The target weight of a batch of tablets is 325 mg (the specification weight). ($H_0: \mu = 325$ mg.) (b) An antihypertensive agent is hypothesized to lower the blood pressure by 10 mm Hg on the average. ($H_0: \Delta = 10$ mm Hg, where Δ is the blood pressure reduction.) (c) The specification for disintegration time of tablets is not more than 15 min. (H_0: $\mu \le 15$ min.)

2. The *alternative* to the null hypothesis should be stated, i.e., the domain of answers if H_0 is not true. This may be written as H_A: $\mu \ne \mu_0$. In the previous example (a), the alternative could be written as H_A: $\mu \ne 325$ mg, i.e., the mean weight of the batch is either less than or greater than 325 mg. This is a two-sided alternative. A one-sided alternative, H_A: $\mu < 325$ mg, suggests that if the true mean weight is not 325 mg (H_0), only values of the mean less than 325 mg are relevant or possible.

3. Having defined the hypothesis and alternative, a *level of significance* (the α, or Type I, error) is chosen, the probability of erroneous rejection of the null hypothesis. The statement that a result is statistically significant, e.g., $P < 0.05$ or "significant at the 5% level," refers to the α error. A hypothesis tested at the 5% level means that if the test shows significance (H_0 is rejected), there is a 5% chance that the decision to reject H_0 is incorrect. In quality control plans, the α error can be thought of as the manufacturer's or producer's risk. For example, at $\alpha = 0.05$, a good batch of material is erroneously rejected 5% of the time.

4. An appropriate *sample* is chosen, and the mean and standard deviation are calculated. This is a simple concept, yet more complex than it seems at first glance. What is an *appropriate* sample? *How many* observations should one make? (How many times should the experiment be replicated?) How are samples chosen? Are the observations independent? If a sample of 20 tablets is chosen from a batch, the mean weight represents the mean of the entire batch, perhaps a million or more tablets. A large burden is placed on these 20 tablets. In this situation, independence means that the selection and/or weighing of any one tablet is not influenced by or will not influence the weighing of the other tablets. Tablets should be selected at random or in a known "designed" way so that the statistical analysis will have a valid interpretation. One method of sampling might be to take the 20 tablets at regular intervals during the run. (Are there situations in which this method could lead to bias?) Selection of twenty consecutive tablets from any one part of a run would not be a good procedure. Why should 20 tablets be sampled rather than 10 or 30, for example? The sample size may be dictated by an official method, or by cost, or to obtain sufficient *power*. In the case of tablet weights, "power" might refer to the ability of the statistical test to correctly find a significant difference if the tablets are truly out of specification.

TABLE 10-3. *Short Table of Absolute Values of t Corresponding to Various Probability Levels in a Two-Sided Test**

Degrees of Freedom (DF)	P = 0.01	P = 0.02	P = 0.05	P = 0.10
1	63.66	31.82	12.71	6.31
2	9.93	6.97	4.30	2.92
3	5.84	4.54	3.18	2.35
4	4.60	3.75	2.78	2.13
5	4.03	3.37	2.57	2.02
7	3.50	3.00	2.36	1.89
10	3.17	2.76	2.23	1.81
11	3.11	2.72	2.20	1.80
12	3.06	2.68	2.18	1.78
13	3.01	2.65	2.16	1.77
15	2.95	2.60	2.13	1.75
19	2.86	2.54	2.09	1.73
25	2.79	2.49	2.06	1.71
40	2.70	2.42	2.02	1.68
∞	2.58	2.33	1.96	1.65

*For a one-sided test, use P/2. For example, at the 5% level, look in the column labeled $P = 0.10$.

5. The next step in the hypothesis testing procedure is to *compute the t statistic*, which leads to a *decision* of whether to accept or reject the null hypothesis.*

$$t = |\bar{X} - \mu|/(S/\sqrt{N})$$

The value of t determines whether or not the null hypothesis will be rejected, rejection leading to a declaration of *significance*. If t is small, the hypothesis is accepted. If t is large, that is, if $|\bar{X} - \mu|$ is large compared to the standard error of $\bar{X}$ ($S/\sqrt{N}$), then $\bar{X}$ is said to be significantly different from μ. To make this decision, the computed value of t is compared to the value in a "t" table under $N - 1$ d.f. at the stated α level, usually 5% (Table 10-3). If the absolute value of t is greater than the tabled value, the difference ($\bar{X} - \mu$) is statistically significant. Significance means that if the null hypothesis is true, the chances of observing a t value equal to or greater than that observed is less than α, or 5% in this case.

The following example illustrates the hypothesis testing procedure just described. Table 10-4 shows the weights of 20 randomly selected tablets arranged in ascending order. The null hypothesis is H_0: $\mu = 325$ mg, and the alternative

*This is a two-sided test. There is no reason to believe that the tablets will be either higher or lower in weight than the target value; hence, the absolute value is the numerator.

TABLE 10-4. *Tablet Weights (mg) of 20 Randomly Selected Tablets*

300	321
306	321
310	322
315	323
316	325
316	325
317	325
319	327
320	331
320	336

hypothesis is H_A: $\mu \neq 325$ mg. Since the sample size is 20, the degrees of freedom are 19 $(20 - 1)$. Calculations of the mean, standard deviation, and t statistic follow. The shortcut formula for the variance or standard deviation, previously illustrated, should always be used for speed and accuracy. Also, when computing by hand, it is important to retain as many decimal places as possible.

$$H_0: \mu = 325 \text{ mg}; \qquad H_A: \mu \neq 325 \text{ mg}$$

$$\bar{X} = (300 + 306 + \ldots 336)/20$$

$$= 319.75 \text{ mg}$$

$$S^2 = \Sigma(X - \bar{X})^2/(N - 1)$$

$$= [(300 - 319.75)^2 + \ldots (336 - 319.75)^2]/19$$

$$= 67.2$$

Shortcut formula for S^2

$$= [N(\Sigma X^2) - (\Sigma X)^2]/[N(N - 1)]$$

$$= [20(300^2 + 306^2 + \ldots 336^2)$$

$$\quad - (300 + 306 + \ldots 336)^2]/(20)(19)$$

$$= [20(2046079) - (6395)^2]/380 = 67.2$$

$$S = \sqrt{S^2} = \sqrt{67.2} = \underline{8.20}$$

$$t_{19} = |\bar{X} - \mu|/(S/\sqrt{N})$$

$$= |319.75 - 325|/(8.20/\sqrt{20}) = 2.86$$

From Table 10-3, for significance at $\alpha = 0.05$, t_{19} must be greater than or equal to 2.09. Since the observed t is 2.86, the decision is to reject

H_0. Large values of t lead to rejection of the null hypothesis; the test results in a decision of "significance."

Interpretation. The conclusion based on this sample of 20 tablets is that the average batch weight is approximately 319.75 mg, which is sufficiently far from the target weight of 325 mg to declare a significant difference. In such an experiment, one can never be certain that this conclusion is correct. The statement that the difference is significant at the 5% level means that if, in fact, the batch mean were 325 mg, the probability would be small ($P < 0.05$, or less than 1 chance in 20) that a result as small as 319.75 or less (or greater than 330.25) would be observed. The decision that the batch mean is not 325 mg may be incorrect, but the chance that this error will occur is 5% or less.

No matter how small or large the sample size is, a declaration of significance rings true. There is a small, but known, probability of erring in coming to the conclusion that a difference exists. On the other hand, a verdict of nonsignificance is not conclusive. A decision of nonsignificance can be virtually ensured by choosing a sufficiently small sample size, resulting in weak power, i.e., a weak ability to obtain a statistically significant difference. One should also be aware of the distinction between statistical and practical significance. Just as a small sample size can result in a large difference being statistically nonsignificant, a large sample size can result in a small difference being statistically significant, because the large sample size effectively reduces the variance ($S_{\bar{X}}^2 = S^2/N$). In this example, the difference of 5.25 mg (325 − 319.75 mg) from the target weight is statistically significant. The important question is, "Is the difference apt to cause a problem from a therapeutic or regulatory point of view?" If the difference is not sufficiently large to reject the batch, the next or other future batches should be closely monitored. The use of the 5% significance level has no basis other than tradition and the fact that the risk associated with the 5% level seems reasonable; *one time in twenty the null hypothesis will be erroneously rejected.*

The assumptions implicit in the t test, both in this and in other examples, are (1) that the data comes from a normal distribution, (2) that the observations are independent, and (3) that the variance of the observations is equal (weighing error in this case). In general, independence and equality of variance are more stringent assumptions than normality. The central limit theorem helps to overcome non-normality of data when using averages.

Comparison of Means of Two Independent Samples. An important class of problems in statistics is the comparison of the effects of two treatments or conditions on experimental outcomes. Examples of such experiments are (1) the comparison of the effects of two therapeutic treatments on blood pressure, (2) the comparison of two disintegrants on drug dissolution of tablets, and (3) the comparison of two analytical methods. In these problems, the variance is usually unknown and is estimated from the data. If the experimental units are not related, i.e., are independent, the statistical test is known as an independent two-sample t test.

In the case of a clinical trial in which two drugs are being compared, this statistical test would be applicable if all of the patients taking the two drugs are different. The null hypothesis and alternative hypothesis are:

$$H_0: \mu_1 = \mu_2 \qquad H_A: \mu_1 \neq \mu_2$$

The population means of the two treatments are assumed to be equal, and the null hypothesis is rejected only if the observed sample means are sufficiently different, based on the magnitude of the t statistic, which is computed as follows:

$$t = |\bar{X}_1 - \bar{X}_2|/(S_p\sqrt{1/N_1 + 1/N_2})$$

where N_1 and N_2 are the sample sizes associated with $\bar{X}_1$ and $\bar{X}_2$ respectively, and t has $(N_1 + N_2 - 2)$ degrees of freedom. The hypothesis of equal means is tested by comparing the value of the calculated t to tabled t values with appropriate df at the stated α level (Table 10-3).

To estimate σ^2, the common variance of the two groups, the variance of each sample is calculated, and the results are pooled, with the assumption that the true variances of the two groups are equal. (If the variances of the two groups are different, other statistical techniques are available.[6]) In general, to obtain an unbiased estimate of σ^2 when independent estimates of the common variance are available, a weighted average of the variance estimates is calculated with df $(N - 1)$ as the weights. In the case of two samples, the weighted average is:

$$S_p^2 = \frac{(N_1 - 1)S_1^2 + (N_2 - 1)S_2^2}{(N_1 - 1) + (N_2 - 1)}$$

which equals:

$$\frac{\left[-\sum_1 (X - \bar{X})^2 + \sum_2 (X - \bar{X})^2 \right]}{(N_1 + N_2 - 2)}$$

where the subscripts 1 and 2 refer to treatments 1 and 2 respectively. Note the following:

$$(N - 1)S^2 = (N - 1)[\Sigma(X - \bar{X})^2/(N - 1)]$$

$$= \Sigma(X - \bar{X})^2$$

The following example illustrates the independent two-sample t test. Two batches of tablets were prepared using disintegrating agents A or B. Dissolution was determined on randomly selected tablets with the following results: Disintegrant A: 45, 50, 47, 43, 41, 49, 35; $\bar{X} = 44.29$ and $S^2 = 26.9$. Disintegrant B: 38, 47, 42, 39, 32, 36, 41; $\bar{X} = 39.29$ and $S^2 = 22.57$. The variances are similar and are pooled to obtain an estimate of the common variance.

$$S_p^2 = [6(26.90) + 6(22.57)]/12 = 24.74$$

$$t = |44.29 - 39.29|/\sqrt{24.74(1/7 + 1/7)} = 1.88$$

The tabulated t at the 5% level with 12 df $(N_1 + N_2 - 2 = 12)$ is 2.18 (Table 10-3). Therefore, the difference is *not significant at the 5% level.* One may conclude that although the data are insufficient to prove an effect due to disintegrants, the results are equivocal $(P < 0.10)$, i.e., if the observed difference can be considered of practical significance, further testing is indicated. (Note that the tabulated t for significance at the 10% level with 19 df is 1.73.)

The sample sizes of the two groups need not be equal in this design, although maximum efficiency for discriminating two means is obtained by use of equal sample sizes, given a fixed total number of observations. Thus, $(1/N_1 + 1/N_2)$ is minimized, and the value of t is thereby maximized.

Comparison of Means of Paired Samples. Observations from two groups to be compared can often be paired in some natural way. The more alike the pairs are, the more precise the test is, and such pairing can be considered an example of a choice of experimental design. Rather than different experimental units being chosen at random for the two groups, pairs are chosen to be as alike as possible. Examples of pairing are (1) using the same individual for more than one treatment, (2) using twins or litter-mates for two or more treatments, and (3) providing similar samples of granulation for comparison of assay methods. If a difference between two groups exists and the pairs are chosen judiciously, the difference will be detected more readily than if distinct individuals are randomly chosen for both treatments (given the same number of observations). Calculations for the statistical test comparing means of paired data consist of first taking differences of the pairs and then performing a one-sample t test on the differences. The null hypothesis is:

$$H_0: \mu_1 = \mu_2 \quad \text{or} \quad \mu_1 - \mu_2 = \Delta = 0$$

A comparison of two analytic methods was made using five batches of material, and analysis was performed on each batch by each method. As shown in Table 10-5, the differences between methods for each batch is first computed, and the standard deviation of the differences is calculated, equal to 1.42. N is equal to 5 (there are 5 pairs). The calculated value of t is:

$$t = |0.50 - 0|/(1.42\sqrt{1/5}) = 0.79$$

Since the tabulated value of t with 4 df at the 5% level is 2.78, the difference is not significant at the 0.05 level.

One-Sided Tests. The tests described thus far have been two-sided tests. Values of the observed mean, or difference of means, that are either too small or too large lead to rejection of the null hypothesis. One-sided tests are used when the null hypothesis is rejected only for unidirectional differences of the observed mean(s). Care should be taken in using one-sided tests since this choice implies that the alternative (values either too high or too low) is not important or is of no interest. For example, in testing a new drug, H_0 might be rejected only if a positive effect is observed; however, if a negative response (opposite of the expected effect) is possible and of interest, a two-sided test might be more appropriate.

TABLE 10-5. *Comparison of Two Analytic Methods*

Batch	METHOD *mg active/g* A	B	Δ A–B
1	100.8	100.1	0.7
2	101.9	99.3	2.6
3	98.7	100.0	−1.3
4	101.3	101.4	−0.1
5	102.5	101.9	0.6
AVERAGE	101.04	100.54	0.50
S	1.46	1.07	1.42

Confidence Intervals

A confidence interval can be formed for a mean, μ, or the difference between two means, with confidence, $1 - \alpha$, as follows:

$$D \pm (t_{d.f.,\alpha})(S_{\overline{D}})$$

where D is a mean value or mean difference; $t_{d.f.,\alpha}$ is the tabulated t value with appropriate degrees of freedom (Table 10-3) at the α level of significance; and $S_{\overline{D}}$ is the standard error of the mean or mean difference.

This procedure is related to hypothesis testing in that *if the confidence interval covers zero,* the test of significance of the difference between two means is *not* significant at the α level (two-sided test). In the previous example, a 95% confidence interval for the mean difference between the two analytical methods is 0.50 ± 2.78 (1.42) ($\sqrt{1/5}$) or −1.26 to 2.26. A confidence interval of $1 - \alpha$ (e.g., 95% if $\alpha = 0.05$) means that the probability is 95% that such intervals cover the true mean value, or difference of means. *There is no guarantee that in any single experiment the true value will be covered;* however, on the average, the true value will be included in the confidence interval of 19 out of every 20 such experiments. A lower degree of confidence is associated with a smaller interval. The smaller the interval is, the less is the confidence that the true value is contained within the interval. The confidence interval is a useful way of defining the region that contains the true mean or difference; it is a statement having a probability associated with it.

In another example, a paired t test was used to analyze the data from a bioavailability study in which 12 volunteers were used to compare two dosage forms. The average areas under the time versus blood level curves were as follows: Formula A = 524; Formula B = 486. The variance computed from the 12 differences (A − B) was 94. A 95% confidence interval is calculated using the value 2.20 for t (see Table 10-3):

$$(524 - 486) \pm t_{11,0.05} (S\sqrt{1/N})$$
$$= 38 \pm 2.20(\sqrt{94/12}) = 31.8 \text{ to } 44.2$$

A 90% interval is $38 \pm t_{11,0.1} (S\sqrt{1/N})$
$$= 38 \pm 1.80(\sqrt{94/12}) = 33.0 \text{ to } 43.0$$

Some statisticians feel that in certain situations, such as bioavailability studies, confidence intervals are a better way of expressing results than stating only that one formula is or is not significantly different from the other. By providing upper and lower limits for the comparison, the confidence interval allows the user or prescriber of a product to make a judgment about the practical equivalency of two products.

Comparison of Variances

In some experimental situations, a test of the equality of two independent variance estimates, S_1^2 and S_2^2, is of interest. In a one-sided test where σ_1^2 is hypothesized to be equal to or less than σ_2^2 (H_0: $\sigma_1^2 \leq \sigma_2^2$; H_A: $\sigma_1^2 > \sigma_2^2$), the statistical test consists of forming the ratio S_1^2/S_2^2. If S_1^2 is smaller than S_2^2, H_0 is accepted as true. If S_1^2 is larger than S_2^2, a test of significance is performed using the F distribution. The ratio S_1^2/S_2^2 is compared to tabulated values of the F distribution with ν_1 and ν_2 degrees of freedom, where $\nu_1 = N_1 - 1$ and $\nu_2 = N_2 - 1$ (N_1 and N_2 are the sample sizes associated with S_1^2 and S_2^2, respectively). If the ratio exceeds the tabulated value at the specified α level, σ_1^2 is considered to be significantly greater than σ_2^2. The F distribution is a probability distribution that is completely described by degrees of freedom in the numerator and denominator of the F ratio (Fig. 10-7). The values tabulated in Table 10-6 are the upper cutoff points and are appropriate for a one-sided test (H_0: $\sigma_1^2 \leq \sigma_2^2$; H_A: $\sigma_1^2 > \sigma_2^2$).

For a two-sided test (H_0: $\sigma_1^2 = \sigma_2^2$; H_A: $\sigma_1^2 \neq \sigma_2^2$), form the ratio S_1^2/S_2^2 if S_1^2 is greater than S_2^2; if S_2^2 is the larger variance, form the ratio S_2^2/S_1^2. That is, the ratio is formed with the larger variance in the numerator and is always greater

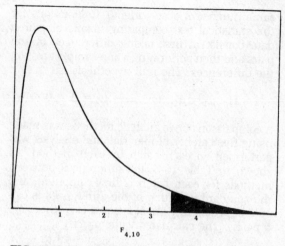

FIG. 10-7. *Illustration of "F" distribution with 4 and 10 degrees of freedom. The shaded portion represents values from 3.48 to ∞ and equals 5% of the area.*

than 1. The significance level using the cutoff points in Table 10-6 is 10% in this test because the ratio has been deliberately constructed with the larger variance in the numerator. In a two-sided test, if the ratio S_1^2/S_2^2 is formed whether or not S_1^2 is greater than S_2^2, tables with the lower cutoff points in addition to the upper points are necessary. When the ratio is intentionally formed with the larger variance in the numerator, the F tables used to assess significance are simplified.

An example follows to clarify the test procedure. The variances obtained from a formulation mixed in two different mixers will be compared. Five samples were analyzed from Mixer A with a

TABLE 10-6. *Short Table of Upper Points of the F Distribution at 5% Level of Significance*

Degrees of Freedom in Denominator	Degrees of Freedom in Numerator						
	1	*2*	*3*	*4*	*6*	*7*	*10*
3	10.10	9.55	9.28	9.12	8.94	8.89	8.79
4	7.71	6.94	6.59	6.39	6.16	6.09	5.96
5	6.61	5.79	5.41	5.19	4.95	4.88	4.74
7	5.59	4.74	4.35	4.12	3.87	3.79	3.64
8	5.32	4.46	4.07	3.84	3.58	3.50	3.35
10	4.96	4.10	3.71	3.48	3.22	3.14	2.98
13	4.67	3.81	3.41	3.18	2.92	2.83	2.67
20	4.35	3.49	3.10	2.87	2.60	2.51	2.35
40	4.08	3.23	2.84	2.61	2.34	2.25	2.08
120	3.92	3.07	2.68	2.45	2.18	2.09	1.91
∞	3.84	3.00	2.60	2.37	2.10	2.01	1.83

variance of 2; eight samples from Mixer B had a variance of 13. Does the use of the two mixers result in formulations of different homogeneity? This is a two-sided test, because a priori, it is not known which mixer will result in more variability, if a difference in variability exists.

$$H_0: \sigma_A^2 = \sigma_B^2$$
$$H_A: \sigma_A^2 \neq \sigma_B^2$$
$$\alpha = 0.10$$

In a two-sided test, $F = S_B^2/S_A^2 = 6.5$ (where S_B^2 is the larger variance estimate). Since 6.5 is greater than the tabulated value ($F_{7,4,0.05} = 6.09$), reject H_0 at the 10% level. If the variance from Mixer B is known a priori to be no less than that in Mixer A ($H_A: \sigma_B^2 > \sigma_A^2$), a one-sided test would be appropriate, and the difference would be significant at the 5% level.

Detection of Outliers

Although many rules have been proposed to detect aberrant values, or outliers, considerable judgment should be exercised before discarding suspect data. For example, if replicate values from an analysis were 5.10, 5.11, 5.09, and 5.30, the last value would immediately be suspected with or without a statistical test. When doubt arises, Table 10-7, "Dixon criteria for Testing an Extreme Mean," can be used to decide if an extreme value belongs with the rest of the data.[5] The data are first ordered numerically from low to high, $X_1, X_2, \ldots X_k$, where there are k values. For example, if k is between 3 and 7, and X_k is the extreme value, form the ratio $(X_k - X_{k-1})/(X_k - X_1)$. If this ratio is greater than the tabulated value, the extreme value is considered aberrant (Table 10-7).

In the foregoing example, 5.30 appears to be an outlier. Since $k = 4$, form the ratio $(5.30 - 5.11)/(5.30 - 5.09) = 0.9$. Table 10-7 shows that at the 5% level with $k = 4$, a value of 0.765 or greater is significant. The value 5.30 is deemed to be an outlier and is rejected.

An intelligent discussion dealing with outliers and various recommended procedures is presented in ASTM, E178-75.[7]

TABLE 10-7. *Dixon Criteria for Testing an Extreme Mean*

k		Significance Level 5 percent
3	$r_{10} = (X_2 - X_1)/(X_k - X_1)$ if smallest value	0.941
4	is suspected;	0.765
5	$= (X_k - X_{k-1})/(X_k - X_1)$ if largest value	0.642
6	is suspected.	0.560
7		0.507
8	$r_{11} = (X_2 - X_1)/(X_{k-1})$ if smallest value	0.554
9	is suspected;	0.512
10	$= (X_k - X_{k-1})/(X_k - X_2)$ if largest value	0.477
	is suspected.	
11	$r_{21} = (X_3 - X_1)/(X_{k-1} - X_1)$ if smallest value	0.576
12	is suspected;	0.546
13	$= (X_k - X_{k-2})/(X_k - X_2)$ if largest value	0.521
	is suspected.	
14	$r_{22} = (X_3 - X_1)/(X_{k-2} - X_1)$ if smallest value	0.546
15	is suspected;	0.525
16	$= (X_k - X_{k-2})/(X_k - X_3)$ if largest value	0.507
17	is suspected.	0.490
18		0.475
19		0.462
20		0.450
21		0.440
22		0.430
23		0.421
24		0.413
25		0.406

From Dixon, W.J.: Processing data for outliers. Biometrics, *9*:74–88, 1953. With permission from The Biometric Society.

Binomial Distribution

The normal distribution is an example of a continuous probability distribution. Although never exactly fitting this distribution, experimental data often approximate normality, and inferences based on this assumption are reasonably accurate. Often, however, data are clearly not continuous, and other distributions must be found to accommodate these situations. The binomial distribution is an example of a discrete probability distribution that can be used to describe the outcome of experiments common in the pharmaceutical sciences. It consists of dichotomous data, data that can have one of two possible outcomes. Examples of experiments with a binomial outcome are (1) preference for one of two formulations, (2) life or death (used to compute the LD_{50}), (3) acceptance or rejection of dosage units in quality control, and (4) improvement or worsening after treatment with a drug.

The binomial is a two-parameter distribution: (1) p, the probability of one of the two possible outcomes and (2) N, the number of trials or observations. If 100 tablets sampled from a batch have 5 rejects, p, the probability of rejection, is estimated as 0.05, and N = 100. Note that in this example, probability is equated with the proportion of rejects; the best estimate of the unknown probability is the sample proportion. If the entire batch were inspected, the *true probability* of a reject would equal the proportion of rejects in the batch.

An example of a binomial probability distribution for N = 18 and p = 0.3 is shown in Figure 10-8 and Table 10-8. The probability of observing *exactly* 5 successes in 18 trials, for example, is 0.202. A "success" is one of the two possible outcomes of a single binomial trial with probability p, and a "failure" is the other outcome (probability of a failure = 1 − p = q). In this example, p = 0.3 and q = 0.7. The sum of the probabilities of all N + 1 possible results from N binomial trials is one. There is a discrete number of possible results, (N + 1) in N trials. In 18 trials, 0, 1, 2 . . . or 18 successes are possible, but the probability of more than 10 successes is extremely small if p = 0.3. If a batch of tablets were assumed to have 30% defects (p = 0.3), the probability of observing 10 or more defective tablets (successes) in a random sample of 18 (N) tablets would be so small that such an observation would probably lead to the conclusion that the batch really had more than 30% defects. The distribution shown in Figure 10-8 looks somewhat symmetric. In fact, if Np *and* N (1 − p) = Nq are both greater than or equal to 5, the distribution is close enough to normal to allow use of normal curve probabilities to approximate the probability of binomial results.

As is the case for the normal distribution, the binomial can be parsimoniously presented in terms of its mean and standard deviation. The mean corresponds to the true probability of success, p, and the standard deviation (a function of p and N) is $\sigma = \sqrt{pq/N}$, where q = (1 − p). To compute probabilities of events using the binomial, one can refer to binomial tables,[8] using the normal approximation when appropriate (see next section, "Normal Approximation to the Binomial Distribution"), or calculate probabilities using the binomial formula. The binomial formula gives the probability of X successes in N trials.

$$P(X) = \binom{N}{X} P^X q^{N-X} \qquad (1)$$

TABLE 10-8. *Binomial Probabilities For N = 18 and p = 0.3*

Number of Successes	Probability
0	0.002
1	0.013
2	0.046
3	0.105
4	0.168
5	0.202
6	0.187
7	0.138
8	0.081
9	0.039
10	0.015
11	0.005
12	0.001

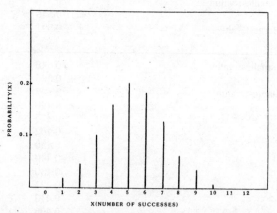

FIG. 10-8. *Binomial distribution with N = 18 and p = 0.3.*

where P(X) is the probability of observing X successes in N trials and $\binom{N}{X} = N!/(N - X)!(X!)$.

As an example of the use of the binomial formula, consider the following. According to the USP weight variation test for tablets weighing less than 130 mg, no single tablet out of 20 tablets weighed should differ by more than ±20% from the average weight. For a batch of 100 mg tablets, suppose 3% weigh less than 80 mg or more than 120 mg. What is the probability of finding at least one aberrant tablet in a random sample of 20 tablets? If the average weight is 100 mg, the probability of finding one or more bad tablets equals (1 − probability of finding 0 bad tablets out of 20). This probability equals:

$$\left[1 - \binom{20}{0}(0.03)^0 (0.97)^{20}\right] = 0.46$$

Note that $\binom{20}{0} = 20!/20!0! = 1$ because 0! equals 1 by definition.) Thus, there is a 46% chance that one would find at least one bad tablet in this test if 3% of the batch were outside the limits.

Normal Approximation to the Binomial Distribution. If Np and Nq are both equal to or greater than 5, cumulative binomial probabilities can be closely approximated by areas under the standard normal curve. The following example illustrates this concept. It is known from past experience that the incidence of a specific malignant tumor is 10% during the lifetime of a certain strain of normal rats. A drug is administered to 50 rats, and the tumor occurs in 9 (18%) of the animals. Is this an unlikely event if the drug is not carcinogenic? The probability of observing 9 or more afflicted animals can be computed if indeed the normal rate of 10% has not changed (H_0: $p_0 = 0.10$, where p_0 is the hypothesized proportion). The normal approximation can be used since both Np and Nq are equal to or greater than 5 (N = 50, p = 0.10, q = 0.90). Note that p_0, the hypothetical population value of p, is used for this calculation. The probability is computed using a normal curve with mean 0.10 and $\sigma = \sqrt{(0.1)(0.9)/50}$, calculating the area for values greater than 0.18.

$Z = (\overline{X} - \mu)/\sigma_{\overline{X}} = (p - p_0)/\sqrt{p_0 q_0/N}$ (where p is the observed proportion) = $(0.18 - 0.10)/\sqrt{(0.10)(0.90)/50} = 1.89$.

The interpretation depends on whether a one- or two-sided test is used. The one-sided test would be appropriate if the drug cannot truly decrease the proportion of cancerous events below 10%; that is, an observation of a tumor

incidence of less than 10% in the 50 rats would only be due to chance. A two-sided (two-tailed) test allows for the possibility of results both greater and smaller than 10%, suggesting that the drug might improve the carcinogenic profile. Since the value of Z is 1.89, less than 1.96, a two-sided test would fail to reach significance at the 5% level (see Table 10-2). Since Z is greater than 1.65, a one-sided test would be significant at the 5% level; the drug increases the tumor incidence. This example shows clearly that the choice of either one- or two-sided tests should be seriously considered and justified a priori.

The calculation of Z as described above approximates cumulative binomial probabilities, estimating the probability of 9 or more events in 50 animals if p = 0.10. A "continuity" correction suggested by Yates[6] improves the normal approximation resulting in less significance. The correction consists of subtracting 1/2N from the absolute difference of the numerator of Z. For a two-sided test, Conover describes an improved correction.[6] If the fractional part of $|N_p - Np_0|$ is greater than 0.5 but less than 1.0, the fractional part is replaced by 0.5. If the fractional part is greater than 0 but less than or equal to 0.5, the fractional part is deleted. If the value is an integer (i.e., the fractional part is 0), the value is reduced by 0.5, which is equivalent to the Yates correction. The adjusted value of $|Np - Np_0|$ is divided by N for the numerator of the Z ratio.

In the example, $|Np - Np_0|$ is equal to $|0.18 \times 50 - 0.10 \times 50| = 4.00$. According to the foregoing rule, the value is decreased by 0.50: 4.00 minus 0.50 = 3.50. The numerator of Z is 3.50/50 = 0.07.

$$Z = 0.07/\sqrt{p_0 q_0/N}$$
$$= 0.07/\sqrt{(0.1)(0.9)/50}$$
$$= 1.65$$

Now, a one-sided test is just significant at the 0.05 level.

Confidence Limits in the Binomial Case. Confidence limits can be constructed for binomial data in a manner similar to that for the normal distribution, as follows:

$$p \pm Z\sqrt{pq/N}$$

The value of Z (see Table 10-2) depends on the degree of confidence. Suppose that of 1000 tablets inspected, 25 were found to be defective. The proportion of good tablets in the sample is

0.975 (975/1000). A 99% confidence interval for the true proportion of good tablets is:*

$$0.975 \pm 2.58\sqrt{(0.025)(0.975)/1000}$$

$$= 0.975 \pm 0.013$$

The width of the confidence interval is dependent on p and N, the number of observations, and is independent of the size of the batch, provided the number of observations is small relative to the batch size. A proportion (or any parameter for that matter) can be estimated with any desired precision by appropriately increasing the sample size. Realistically, time, expense, and accuracy of observations are limiting factors.

Statistical Tests of Binomial Data

Tests of hypotheses in the binomial case have a form similar to normal distribution tests, as can be seen in the following examples.

Comparison of a Sample Proportion to a Known Proportion. Quality control (QC) data gathered from many batches showed that 4% of tablets manufactured with a target weight of 200 mg weighed more than 220 mg or less than 180 mg, the upper and lower QC limits. Examination of a new batch shows that 32 of 500 tablets (6.4%) are out of specifications. Is this result unexpected based on the previous history of the batch (4%, or 20 tablets, are expected to be out of limits)? As in the t test, the null hypothesis and the alternative hypothesis are stated. A "Z" ratio is then formed, using the continuity correction to compare the observed and hypothetical proportions:

$$H_0: p_0 = 0.04 \qquad H_A: p_0 \neq 0.04$$

$$Z = [|p - p_0| - 1/(2N)]/\sqrt{p_0 q_0/N}$$

$$Z \doteq (|0.064 - 0.040| - 1/1000)$$

$$\div \sqrt{(0.04)(0.96)/500}$$

$$= 2.62$$

The new batch has significantly more tablets out of limits than are normally observed (Table 10-2, P < 0.01). A 95% confidence interval on the true proportion of out-of-limit tablets in this batch is:

$$0.064 \pm 1.96\sqrt{(0.064)(0.936)/500}$$

$$= 0.064 \pm 0.021$$

*For 95% confidence limits, substitute 1.96 for 2.58.

Comparison of Two Proportions. When comparing the proportion of successes in two groups, the data are often presented in the form of a "fourfold" table as shown in Table 10-9. Diseased animals were treated with either placebo (control) or drug. Sixty-one of 75 of the control animals survived, whereas 69 of 75 animals given the drug survived. Is the drug more effective than the control in preventing death? The null and alternate hypotheses are stated as follows.

$$H_0: P_{drug} = P_{placebo}; \ H_A: P_{drug} \neq P_{placebo}$$

where P_{drug} is the probability that an animal will survive the drug treatment, and $P_{placebo}$ is the probability that an animal will survive placebo treatment.

This is the binomial analog of the independent groups two-sample t test. In the t test, the variances were pooled under the assumption of equal variability in the two groups. Here, *all the data are pooled to estimate a common p,* the best estimate of the true probability under the null hypothesis, which states that the two populations have the same proportion of survivors. The pooled $p = p_0 = 130/150 = 0.867$. (130 of 150 animals survived and the overall proportion of survivors is 0.867.) When the sample size (N) is equal in the two groups, the continuity correction in the test of significance consists of subtracting 1/N from the absolute value of the numerator. The Z ratio is computed as follows:

$$Z = [|p_1 - p_2| - 1/N]/\sqrt{p_0 q_0(1/N_1 + 1/N_2)}$$

$$Z = [|0.92 - 0.813| - 1/75]$$

$$\div \sqrt{(0.867)(0.133)(1/75 + 1/75)}$$

$$= 1.68$$

where $N_1 = N_2 = N$. As in the t test, the Z ratio is a "difference" divided by the variability of the difference, expressed as the standard deviation. In this case, the difference is significant at the 10% level, not significant at the usual 5% level.

TABLE 10-9. *Fourfold Table Showing Number of Animals Alive and Dead After Three Months*

	Alive	Dead	Total
CONTROL	61	14	75
DRUG	69	6	75
TOTAL	130	20	150

Does this mean that the drug and control do not differ? In all statistical tests, a nonsignificant difference does not imply sameness. The experiment may not have had sufficient sensitivity to pick up a difference that may have occurred with a larger sample size. A significant difference, no matter how small or large the experiment, means that a real difference probably exists (with odds of 19–1 at the 5% level). The practical meaning of any difference must be interpreted in context, with an understanding of the implications of decisions based on experimental results. In this example, if increase in survival due to the drug is small compared to comparable marketed drugs, there might be little interest no matter what the degree of significance. But if there is no drug on the market effective in this disease, these results might be a stimulus for further work.

Chi-Square Tests of Significance

Another way of testing for significance of the difference of two proportions is by means of the X^2 (chi-square) distribution. An example of this test is illustrated by a preclinical study performed to determine the carcinogenic potential of a new drug in which 100 control animals were compared to a group of 100 animals given the drug. At the end of the experiment, the animals were examined for tumors. Ten animals in the control group and eight in the drug group died of nondrug related causes before the experiment was completed, and these animals were not included in the final count. The results are summarized in Table 10-10.

The first step in the statistical analysis is to compute the numbers of animals that would be expected to be observed in each of the four "cells" of the table if the null hypothesis were true (i.e., if the treatments were the same). This is accomplished by multiplying the marginal totals for each cell and dividing by the grand total. For example, in the upper left cell (animals on drug with tumors) the expected number is $(32 \times 92)/182 = 16.18$. Theoretically, this means that if the treatments were identical and no variation occurred, "16.18" of 92 animals would develop tumors in the drug group. For the fourfold table, only one calculation is needed to obtain the expected values for each cell, since the cell totals must sum to the marginal totals as shown in Table 10-10. The expected numbers in row 1 must add to 92; therefore, the value in the second column must be 75.82. Similarly, the value in the second row, first column, must be 15.82 to ensure that the column total is 32, and so forth.

TABLE 10-10. *Actual and Expected* Number of Animals with Tumors After Drug Treatment and Placebo*

	Number with Tumors	Number without Tumors	Total
DRUG	18 (16.18)	74 (75.82)	92
PLACEBO	14 (15.82)	76 (74.18)	90
TOTAL	32	150	182

*Values in parentheses are expected values.

The chi-square statistic, which is used to assess significance, is calculated as $\Sigma(O - E)^2/(E)$, where O is the observed count and E is the expected count. In this example, chi-square is calculated as follows:

$$(1.82)^2/16.18 + (1.82)^2/75.82 + (1.82)^2/15.82$$

$$+ (1.82)^2/74.18$$

$$= 0.50$$

The chi-square distribution is a probability distribution defined by a single parameter, degrees of freedom. The chi-square test can also be used for experiments other than that described by the 2×2 table. If three drugs are being compared rather than two, a 3×2 table would describe the results for a dichotomous response. In an R × C (rows × columns) table, degrees of freedom equal $(R - 1) \times (C - 1)$. For the 2×2 table illustrated here, df = 1. The cutoff point for significance for chi-square with one df is equal to Z^2, where Z is the standard normal deviate previously discussed (see Table 10-2). At the 5% level, for example, X_1^2 must exceed $(1.96)^2 = 3.84$ for significance, since 1.96 is the cutoff point for a two-sided test at the 5% level. Therefore, in the previous example, the difference between drug and placebo is not significant. (Cutoff points for X^2 tests with more than one d.f. can be found in most standard texts.[5]) As is the case for the normal approximation to the binomial, the chi-square test is also approximate. The expected count (E) in each cell should be equal to or greater than 5 for the approximation to be valid. In this example, all four expected values are considerably greater than 5, as can be seen in Table 10-10.

As in the previously described binomial tests, a continuity correction can be used to improve the approximation. If the fractional portion of $|O - E|$ is greater than 0 but less than or equal to 0.5, delete the fractional portion (e.g., if

$|O - E| = 5.3$, replace 5.3 by 5.0). If the fractional portion is greater than 0.5 but less than 1.00, replace the fractional portion by 0.5 (e.g., if $|O - E| = 6.98$, replace 6.98 by 6.5). If the difference $|O - E|$ is an integer, decrease the value by 0.5. In the above example, $|O - E|$ is 1.82. Therefore, use 1.5 as the value of $|O - E|$, rather than 1.82. The recalculated value of X^2 is 0.34.

In this experiment, a comparison of the total number of tumors found in the two groups may also be of interest when tumors may be found in different organs, i.e., when a single animal may have more than one tumor. The analyses discussed here, however, would be inappropriate because of the lack of independence. Suppose in the above experiment that 18 animals on drug had at least one tumor with a total of 33 tumors, and that 14 animals on placebo had at least one tumor with a total of 16 tumors. Clearly, one would have to look carefully at both statistics: (1) the proportion of animals with tumors and (2) the total number, type, and location of tumors. However, the comparison of the total number of tumors, 16 versus 33, in the two groups must somehow take into account the number of animals with and without tumors.

The Sign Test

The sign test is a popular nonparametric test used to assess the significance of differences of paired data. The underlying distribution that represents the data need not be precisely defined, as opposed, for example, to the assumption of normality necessary for the t test. The sign test, however, has less power to differentiate the two treatments than a test in which the actual distribution of data is taken into account. This means that for a given set of data, the sign test may not result in a significant difference, whereas an appropriate parametric test (such as the t test) might show significance. The sign test has the advantage of using simple binomial calculations, and it is useful for a quick assessment of the results of an experiment. The procedure for performing the sign test follows:

1. The differences of each of the paired samples are tabulated, indicating only whether one treatment or factor has a higher or lower value than the other. For example, a positive difference means that the second treatment gives higher results, and a negative difference means that the first treatment gives higher results. In case of a tie, the difference is ignored. With continuous data, there should be no ties, but ties do occur because of limitations of measuring techniques and/or because the data are not really continuous.

2. After tabulation, the proportion of "wins" (positive differences, for example) is calculated. The observed proportion of "wins" is compared to that expected under the null hypothesis of equality of treatments (H_0: $p_0 = 0.5$), using a one-sample binomial test.

In the following example (Table 10-11), tablets were taken from two different punches of a tablet press at various times during a run because a difference in weight had been suspected. In 18 of 24 cases, the tablet from the left side had a higher weight than that on the right side (a positive difference for the left side minus right side). There is one tie (7:00), which is disregarded for the purposes of the statistical test. The observed proportion p is $18/24 = 0.75$, and the hypothetical proportion p_0 is 0.5.

$$Z = (|0.75 - 0.5| - 1/48)/\sqrt{(0.5)(0.5)/24} = 2.25$$

Since Z is greater than 1.96, the difference is significant at the 5% level. The tablets from the

TABLE 10-11. *Weight Differences of Tablets Taken From Right and Left Sides of Tablet Press*

Time	Right	Left	Δ	Time	Right	Left	Δ
1:00 PM	220	221	+1	4:15	218	219	+1
1:15	221	220	−1	4:30	222	223	+1
1:30	219	223	+4	4:45	226	228	+2
1:45	218	221	+3	5:00	217	227	+10
2:00	223	218	−5	5:15	219	220	+1
2:15	217	213	−4	5:30	215	218	+3
2:30	221	225	+4	5:45	220	224	+4
2:45	218	220	+2	6:00	219	220	+1
3:00	226	224	−2	6:15	223	221	−2
3:15	220	223	+3	6:30	216	220	+4
3:30	217	219	+2	6:45	222	226	+4
3:45	224	223	−1	7:00	221	221	0
4:00	222	225	+3				

left side tend to have higher weights than those from the right side, suggesting that an adjustment on the tablet press should be made.

Sampling for Attributes and Operating Characteristic Curves

The binomial distribution can be used to construct acceptance/rejection sampling plans in quality control. MIL STD 105D is an excellent document describing sampling plans for attributes.[9] These plans recommend the number of items to be inspected, and the number of rejects that are observed determine whether or not the lot will be accepted. The plans are more or less stringent depending on the seriousness of a defect and the risk of making a wrong decision. A wrong decision is either (1) to pass a poor lot or (2) reject a good lot.

As an example, Plan N from Mil Std 105D is devised such that if there are 0.25% defects in a lot, there is a good chance of passing the lot.[9] This corresponds to an acceptable quality limit (AQL) of 0.25. In this plan, 500 samples are taken at random, and if 3 or fewer defects are found, the lot passes; otherwise, the lot is rejected. If 0.25% of the lot is defective, the probability of the lot passing this inspection is equal to the probability of finding either 0, 1, 2, or 3 defects in the 500 samples inspected, since any one of these observations will result in a decision to pass the lot. This probability can be calculated using the binomial formula given in equation (1):

$$\sum_{X=0}^{X=3} \binom{N}{X} p^X q^{N-X} = P(0) + P(1) + P(2) + P(3)$$

where $P(0)$, $P(1)$, $P(2)$, and $P(3)$ are the probabilities of finding 0, 1, 2, and 3 defects, respectively. The sum of these four probabilities is $\binom{500}{0}(0.0025)^0 (0.9975)^{500} + \ldots \binom{500}{3}$ $(0.0025)^3 (0.9975)^{497} = 0.29 + 0.36 + 0.22 + 0.09 = 0.96$. Therefore, the probability of passing the lot is at least 0.96 if there are 0.25% or less rejects in the batch. Conversely, the probability of rejecting such a lot is 0.04 $(1 - 0.96)$. Four percent (0.04) is equivalent to the α error in hypothesis testing, if 0.25% or less defects characterize an acceptable lot.

What about the probability of accepting lots of bad quality? This is an important aspect of a sampling plan and is described by an operating characteristic (OC) curve as shown in Figure 10-9. The OC curve shows the probability of

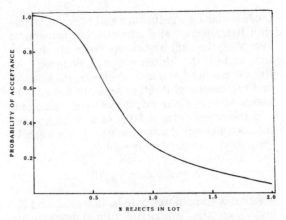

FIG. 10-9. *Operating characteristic curve (OC) for Plan N, AQL = 0.25. (MIL STD 105D.[9])*

accepting a lot for a specified plan, given the true percentage of defects in the lot. Note that the probability of rejecting a lot of specified quality is simply (1 − probability of acceptance of that lot). To construct the OC curve, it is sufficient to calculate the probabilities of acceptance at various "percent defective" values (as was done for 0.25%) and draw a smooth curve through these points. For example, if there are 1% rejects in the lot, the probability of acceptance can be calculated from equation (1).

$$\sum_{X=0}^{X=3} \binom{500}{0}(0.01)^X (0.99)^{N-X} = 0.26$$

Note that p = 0.01 (probability of observing a reject), and that q = 0.99 (1 − p). Since 0.26 is the probability of accepting such a lot using Plan N, the probability of rejecting the lot is (1 − 0.26) = 0.74. The interpretation is that a lot with 1% chipped tablets, for example, will be rejected about 3/4 of the time and will pass the test 1/4 of the time using this plan.

Sample Size

"What size sample do I need?" and "How many patients should I recruit?" are common questions that arise during planning of experiments. Estimation of the sample size needed to show a statistically significant difference (if at least some predetermined true difference exists) is an important problem in pharmaceutical and clinical studies. When testing means, the difference to be detected (d) under H_A, the α and β errors, and the sample size, N, are closely related. Given three of these values, the fourth is fixed. To calculate the sample size, one must specify (1) the variance; (2) α, the risk of erroneously declaring significance and rejection of the null hypothesis; (3) β, the risk of erroneously accepting the null hypothesis given an alternative, and (4) the "difference to be detected." As the experienced researcher knows, these risks and the meaningful differences are not easy to assess and are often a matter of good judgment.

If the sample size is large or if σ^2 is known, the computation of a sample size, N, for a single (or paired) sample experiment is:.

$$N = \sigma^2[(Z_\alpha + Z_\beta)/d]^2 \qquad (2)$$

where d is the difference to be detected, and Z_α and Z_β are the appropriate normal deviates for the α level and β level, respectively. For a two-sided test, Z_α is the value of Z above which $\alpha/2\%$ of the area is found in the normal curve (see Table 10-2). These are the same values used for hypothesis testing, e.g., 1.96 at the 5% level of significance, and 2.58 at the 1% level. Z_β is the value of Z above which β of the area is found in the upper tail. For example, for $\beta = 0.2$, $Z = 0.842$; for $\beta = 0.1$, $Z = 1.28$; and for $\beta = 0.05$, $Z = 1.645$. Although this may appear complicated, the examples that follow should clarify the use of this equation.

For example, a question regarding sample size may be posed as follows. It is important to detect a mean tablet weight that is 3 mg or more different from the target weight. If such a difference exists, there should be a 90% chance that a statistical test will show significance ($\beta = 0.10$; power $= 1 - \beta = 0.90$). The chance of concluding that a difference of 3 mg or more exists when in fact the batch is on target should be small, e.g., 5% ($\alpha = 5\%$). The difference, 3 mg, and the α and β risks described previously are not preordained. These values are a result of careful thought and experience, and are usually "ball-park" figures, unless legal or official requirements dictate exact limits and risks. If the standard deviation is 10, N is calculated from equation (2):

$$N = 10^2[(1.96 + 1.28)/3]^2 = 117$$

This means that 117 tablets should be sampled to determine the mean weight. A statistical test comparing the observed mean weight versus the target weight would then have α and β risks of 0.05 and 0.10, respectively. The values of 1.96 and 1.28 in the calculation of N refer to the standard normal deviate for $\alpha = 0.05$ and $\beta = 0.10$.

A variation of equation (2) gives the approximate sample size for binomial data, replacing σ^2 appropriately with pq.[6]

For small sample sizes and unknown σ, the problem is more difficult because the value of t changes considerably with changes in sample size (appropriate t values must be used in the above formula, replacing Z). If an arbitrary value of t is chosen based on a preliminary guess of df, and the calculated N is substantially different from the preliminary guess, the estimate of the sample size will be incorrect. Guenther has shown that increasing the sample size as calculated from equation (2) by 0.5 Z_α^2 gives a nearly correct value for the sample size.[10] Davies provides tables for the sample size needed for t tests given α, β, and d/σ.[11]

As an example of this calculation, consider a bioequivalency study in which the areas under the blood level versus time curves (AUC) for two formulations are to be compared. What sample size would be needed to detect a difference in the AUCs of ± 20 hour $\cdot$ mcg/ml with a power of 90% at the 5% level in a situation in which the average area is expected to be about 100 and the standard deviation is estimated to be 25? Bioequivalency tests are usually designed so that each subject receives each formulation on separate occasions (a paired design). According to equation (2), the sample size needed is:

$$N = (25)^2[(1.96 + 1.28)/20]^2 = 16.4$$

Since σ^2 is unknown, add 0.5 Z_α^2 to 16.4:

$$(0.5) \cdot (1.96)^2 + 16.4 = 18.3$$

Nineteen subjects will satisfy the requirements for this study.

The above calculations are for a single-sample or paired-sample test. The calculations for a two-sample test are slightly different. The sample size for the two-sample case, where $N_1 = N_2 = N$, (N_1 and N_2 are the sample sizes for the groups to be compared), is calculated as follows:

$$N = 2\sigma^2[(Z_\alpha + Z_\beta)/d]^2 \qquad (3)$$

If σ^2 is unknown, add 0.25 Z_α^2 to N.[10]

For example, time to dissolution (50%) is to be compared for two formulations of the same drug. How many tablets of each formulation should be used if a true difference of 15 min or more is to be detected with a power of 80% at the 10% level of significance (two-sided test)? The standard deviation is approximately 10. In comparison with the previous example, the experimenter is willing to take greater risks of making errors of the first and second kinds (α and β are 0.1 and 0.2, respectively). When the risks of making these errors are larger, the sample size needed to meet these criteria is smaller. Using equation (3), the sample size is:

$$N = 2(10)^2[(1.645 + 0.842)/15]^2 = 5.5$$

Adding $0.25\, Z_\alpha^2 (0.25 \times 1.65^2 = 0.7)$ to N results in 6.2. Seven tablets from each formulation should be sufficient to satisfy the above conditions.

For one-sided tests, the same formulas are used, but Z_α has $\alpha\%$ of the area in the upper tail (e.g., at the 5% level, $Z_\alpha = 1.645$, and at the 10% level, $Z_\alpha = 1.28$). In the previous example, if a one-sided test were appropriate, using equation (3) results in the following calculation of N:

$$N = 2(10)^2[(1.282 + 0.842)/15]^2$$

$$+ 0.25(1.282)^2$$

$$= 4.4$$

Five tablets of each formulation would be adequate.

Power

The power of a test is its ability to detect a difference if such a difference truly exists. The power can be calculated solving for Z_β from equations (2) or (3), specifying values for N, α, and "d". In the one-sample (or paired-sample) test, for example, from equation (2):

$$Z_\beta = d \cdot \sqrt{N/\sigma^2} - Z_\alpha \qquad (4)$$

If N is small, substitute appropriate values of t for Z, or make the inverse adjustment for N as discussed previously, i.e., make the computations using Z, but subtract $0.5\, Z_\alpha^2$ from N.

Consider a bioavailability study in which the average of the ratios of AUC of a tablet formulation and solution of the same drug is to be assessed. If the bioavailabilities of the tablet and solution are the same, the ratios of the areas should be equal to 1, on the average. Therefore, the null hypothesis is H_0: Ratio = 1. The two-sided alternative is H_A: Ratio $\neq$ 1. The FDA is interested in knowing the power of such tests because small sample sizes that result in nonsignificant differences may have little power. What is the power of the test with a sample size of 12 in which protection is to be provided against erroneous acceptance of alternatives for which the true ratio differs from 1 by 0.2 (20%) or more? The test is performed at the 5% level, and the s.d. is approximately 0.25. Since N is small, subtract $0.5\, Z_\alpha^2$ from N ($Z_\alpha = 1.96$;

$12 - 0.5\, Z_\alpha^2 \sim 10$), and use this value in equation (4). (This is the inverse of the procedure used previously in calculating the sample size.) The calculation using equation (4) follows:

$$Z_\beta = 0.2\sqrt{10/0.25^2} - 1.96 = 0.57$$

$\beta = 0.285$ and the power is 71.5% as determined from Table 10-2.

In a two-sample test, the following is used:

$$Z_\beta = d\sqrt{N/2\sigma^2} - Z_\alpha \qquad (5)$$

Suppose, in a two-sample, two-sided test, $N_1 = N_2 = 10$, $\alpha = 0.05$, $d = 2$, and $\sigma^2 = 3$. Again, subtracting $0.25 \cdot Z_\alpha^2$ from N as before ($10 - 1 = 9$), and using equation (5):

$$Z_\beta = 2\sqrt{9/(2)(3)} - 1.96 = 0.49$$

Z_β is 0.49 and the power is approximately 69% (Table 10-2). This means that if a statistical test (t test) is performed comparing the means of the two groups at the 5% level with 10 experimental units in each group, if the true difference (d) between the group means is 2 or more, the statistical test will show a significant result with a probability of at least 69%. The calculation of power is discussed more fully in Pharmaceutical Statistics by Bolton (see General References).

Consumer Acceptance Testing

Before a product is introduced to the market, it may be advisable to assess patient or consumer acceptability of one or more formulation attributes, such as taste, color, packaging, and physical characteristics (e.g., viscosity of a liquid suspension or thickness of an ointment). The formulation section is often involved in implementing and evaluating these tests, and a familiarity with common designs such as monadic tests, paired comparisons, and triangle tests is important.

Monadic or Single-Product Test

In this test, the attributes of two or more products are compared, and each individual evaluates only a single product. To analyze the resulting data, some quantitative measurement must be associated with the test since such tests are often qualitative in nature. A number or score may be assigned to a descriptive term related to the attribute being assessed. For example, "excellent" = 1; "good" = 2; "fair" = 3; and "poor" = 4; or "I would buy this product" = 3, "I might buy this product" = 2; and "I would not buy this product" = 1. The scoring systems are often arbitrary, but research on the development of such scoring schemes considers the following: (1) How many choices should be given to the test panelist? (2) How should the evaluation statements be expressed? (3) Are the intervals between adjacent statements equal? For example, is the difference between "poor" and "fair" the same as the difference between "fair" and "good"? Usually, an arbitrary equi-interval linear scale is used despite its theoretical shortcomings.

Use of six or seven reasonably spaced evaluation statements with a sufficiently large panel (30 or more) results in data that can be reliably analyzed. Snedecor and Cochran discuss such scaled data and conclude that the ordinary t test is applicable (with a small continuity correction) provided a reasonable sample size is used.[6] The test for two products can be analyzed using a two-sample t test. For more than two products, analysis of variance is used. The design, analysis, and interpretation of such experiments are the same as for other similar tests described in this chapter, e.g., *comparison of two drugs in independent groups.* Consider the following example.

An antacid product is reformulated with a new less expensive flavoring agent. Fifty subjects, users of this product, were randomly divided into two groups of 25 each, with each subject evaluating either the new or old formula. A "thermometer" scale (Fig. 10-10) was used, and the results are shown in Table 10-12. Testing the hypothesis of equality of means, $H_0: \mu_1 = \mu_2$, use the t test for two independent groups at the 5% level. The procedure and calculations have been described in the section "Hypothesis Testing for Statistical Significance" for the case of the independent two-sample t test.

$$t_{47} = |\bar{X}_1 - \bar{X}_2 - 0|/(S_p\sqrt{1/N_1 + 1/N_2})$$

$$S_p = \sqrt{24(1.94)^2 + 23(1.90)^2]/47} = 1.917$$

$$t_{47} = |7.44 - 6.88|/[1.917\sqrt{1/25 + 1/24}] = 1.02$$

Although the old product received a higher rating, the two formulations are not significantly different. The t value needed for significance is 2.01 (see Table 10-3).

The action based on these results depends on many factors, including common sense. In this situation, the new product might be marketed because of the "nonsignificant" difference and the decreased production costs. Alternatively, the marketing group might feel that the existing

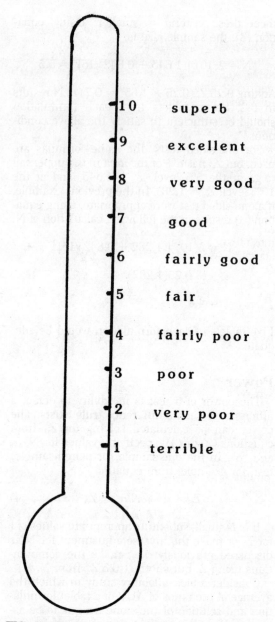

FIG. 10-10. *Typical thermometer scale for evaluating consumer products.*

TABLE 10-12. *Comparison of Flavor Using Thermometer Scale*

	Old Product	New Product
NUMBER OF SUBJECTS	25	24*
AVERAGE SCORE	7.44	6.88
STANDARD DEVIATION	1.94	1.90

*One subject was ill and could not evaluate the product.

franchise is so good that any product that is conceivably not as good (as in the case here), or different in any way for that matter, would not be a viable substitute. In the latter case, an experiment designed to test if products are distinguishable might be preferred.

The independent two-sample t test described in this section, sometimes known as a "monadic" test, may lack sensitivity because of large intersubject variability. Nevertheless, this test is often preferred, depending on product type as well as on cost and time restraints. Such tests can be completed more quickly than paired tests in which each subject evaluates two products. Also, the procedure used in this test may be more realistic when related to how products are actually used in the marketplace.

Paired Tests

A paired test in which each subject compares two or more products is often desirable because of convenience and the improved sensitivity resulting from the intrasubject comparison. Products may be evaluated by (1) preference whereby the subject notes which product is preferred, (2) a ranking procedure, or (3) a scoring or rating system as discussed under "monadic" tests. If more than one product is to be compared, "round robin" tests can be used, whereby each subject tests each and every possible pair of products. A variation is the incomplete block design, in which a balanced subset of the products are tested by each individual.[11,12] In repeat tests, products are evaluated sequentially, and sufficient time should be allowed between assessments for the subject to return to his normal state. For example, in taste or smell tests, the sensory organs can be overstimulated and a recovery period should be part of the experimental design. Order effects occur often in such tests because of unconscious bias as well as sensory fatigue, and principles of good design including blinding and randomization are particularly important. Testing using a response scale (e.g., 1 to 10) can be analyzed by paired t test procedures or by a two-way analysis of variance.

If the number of subjects is small and the experimenter feels that assumptions such as normality that underly the statistical analysis are not valid, suitable nonparametric techniques (such as ranking tests) can be used (these tests are described at the end of this chapter). As an example consider a test in which 60 subjects were asked to use two variations of a formula, A and B. Preference was indicated based on the formula's "feel" in the mouth, and the results were the following:

Prefer Formula A	Prefer Formula B	No Preference
32	16	12

The question of what to do with "no preference" decisions is controversial. Should subjects be forced to state a preference? Although there is no definitive answer, it appears best to allow subjects to give a "no preference" decision, but not to include this data in the statistical analysis. Certainly, the "no preference" data should not be ignored when the recommended action is finally made. It would certainly make a difference, for example, whether either 90% or 10% of the subjects made a "no preference" decision, regardless of statistical significance.

These data can be analyzed by *chi-square or equivalent binomial techniques*. The hypothesis to be tested is that among the subjects who express a preference, there is equal preference for the two formulas.

$$H_0: p = 0.5 \qquad H_A: p \neq 0.5$$

Percentage preferring A = 32/48 = 66.7%

$$Z = [|p_A - 0.5| - 1/(2N)]/\sqrt{pq/N}$$

$$= (0.667 - 0.5 - 1/96)/\sqrt{(0.5)(0.5)/48}$$

$$= 2.17$$

There is a significant preference (P < 0.05) for Formula A among those who express a preference. As just explained, when the results of such an experiment are reported, the number of consumers who had no preference should be acknowledged. In this example, the conclusion is that of 48 subjects who expressed a preference, 2/3 preferred Formula A (P < 0.05), and there were 12 subjects who had no preference.

Triangle Tests

Preference tests are primarily designed to predict the proportion of the consumer population that will prefer one preparation to another. However, consumers may perceive two formulas as being very different, but they could be segmented into two equal groups, each of which prefers the alternate product. Thus, equality of preferences does not distinguish between two possible situations: (1) the existence of two distinct but equal groups, each of which prefers one or the other product and (2) one homogeneous group that simply cannot differentiate the products.

The triangle test is designed to assess if products are in fact distinguishable. Three samples, similar in appearance, are submitted for testing, two of one product and one of another. The consumer is asked to choose the product that is different from the other two (optionally, a preference can also be requested). If there is a "significant" number of correct guesses, the products are considered distinguishable, and preference data, if requested, may be analyzed to determine the preferred product.

Order effects are important in such a test, and the order of presentation should be randomized or balanced. There are six possible ways of presenting three products of which two are identical. If the products are called A and B, they can be presented in the following orders. (The products should be labeled in some random manner, and the six orders should be randomized.)

Subject	1st	2nd	3rd
1	A	B	B
2	A	A	B
3	B	B	A
4	B	A	A
5	B	A	B
6	A	B	A

If order effects are present (e.g., the choice by the panelist of the odd, or different, product tends to be the second product tested), the balanced design protects against bias.

Carry over effects cause a problem. For example, in a taste test, if one or more products has so strong a taste as to numb the taste buds, this would influence the evaluation of the subsequent products. Sufficient recovery time in between assessments would be an important part of the design. On the other hand, too long a time interval between tastes could involve a "memory" factor, thus introducing excess variation. One could, however, reason that this situation is more realistic in that consumers do not normally compare products side by side. These are all valid arguments to be individually assessed for each product and marketing situation.

Suppose that a variation of the base of a marketed ointment is made to improve its kinesthetic properties and that 30 panelists are to compare the "feel" of the old and new products using a triangle test design. After proper randomization of the products, 15 of the 30 panelists make the correct choice, i.e., choose the correct "different" product.

The statistical analysis is based on a test of the following hypothesis:

$$H_0: p = 1/3$$
$$H_A: p > 1/3$$

This means that if there is no difference, the correct product will be chosen one third of the time by chance. This is a good example of a one-sided test, i.e., a difference can be tested for significance only if correct choices are made by more than one third of the panelists. If less than one third choose the odd product, this result can be due only to chance. If the experiment results in significantly less than one-third correct choices, the experimental procedure should be questioned. The test of hypothesis uses the binomial distribution with $p = 1/3$ and $N = 30$. The test statistic is:

$$Z = [|p_{obs} - 1/3| - 1/(2N)]/\sqrt{(1/3)(2/3)/N}$$

where p_{obs} is the observed proportion of correct choices, and N is the number of responses. For this example:

$$p_{obs} = 15/30 = 0.50$$

and

$$Z = (|1/2 - 1/3| - 1/60)/\sqrt{(2/9)/30} = 1.74$$

At the 5% level (one-sided test), a value of Z equal to or greater than 1.65 is significant (see Table 10-2). In this example, the conclusion is that the products are distinguishable at the 5% level.

Other Tests

Other designs used in consumer testing include round-robin, sequential, and repeat paired preference tests.[13] The round-robin used for more than two products compares all preparations in all possible pairs. The sequential design is based on the idea that results can be analyzed sequentially after each preference, so that if large enough differences exist, a smaller sized panel can be used to come to a decision more quickly than if a fixed sample size is chosen in advance. The advantage of this design depends on many factors, including anticipated differences, the nature of the products, and the setting of the test. Repeat paired comparison tests consist of a paired preference test repeated on a second occasion. The analysis can result in a segmenting of the population into two groups preferring each product as well as a group who cannot distinguish the products. This test may be physically difficult to implement, however, and the data are sensitive to deviations from the model.

Analysis of Variance and Experimental Design

Analysis of variance (ANOVA) is inextricably connected to experimental design. Experiments that are conceived to compare, estimate, and test such effects as drug treatments, formulation differences, and analytical methods can be designed to yield an optimal return for effort expended. The experimental results may then be analyzed by ANOVA techniques. A good experiment speaks for itself; the conclusions are often obvious without complicated mathematical treatment. With sophisticated calculators and computers readily available, however, most experiments, if designed properly, can be easily analyzed. In a poorly designed experiment, on the other hand, more than one factor may contribute to an experimental result with no way of untangling the effects of the factors. (This is called "confounding.") Examples of obvious confounding are (1) a clinical study in which patients are allowed to take various concomitant drugs other than the test drug that affect the condition being treated; and (2) a comparison of a new tablet formulation to the former formulation for dissolution, with the tablets prepared on two different tablet presses, one formulation on each press. Differences in the performance of the presses (pressure, for example) can contribute to differences in dissolution in addition to differences due to formulation changes.

Analysis of variance separates the total variation in the data into parts, each of which represents variation caused by factors imposed on the experiment. A properly designed experiment allows a clear unconfounded estimate of such variation or, at least, can identify the confounding factors, if present. Consider an experiment to assess the effects of lubricating agent and disintegrating agent on the dissolution of a tablet. The final analysis of variance would separate the effects of these factors by computing that part of the total variation attributable to the lubricating and disintegration agents isolated from that variation due to experimental error. This separation serves as a basis for testing statistical hypotheses.

One-Way Analysis of Variance

One-way ANOVA can be considered an extension of the independent two-sample t test to more than two groups. In the t test, the following statistic compares the difference of two sample means to the standard deviation of the difference (the denominator of the t statistic):

$$(\bar{X}_1 - \bar{X}_2)/\sqrt{S_p^2(1/N_1 + 1/N_2)}$$

The pooled variance, S_p^2, depends on the variability *within* each of the two groups. If the two means come from the same normal distribution, the difference between these means (suitably weighted) should also be a measure of the variability of the data. Since the variance of a mean, $S_{\bar{X}}^2$, is equal to S^2/N, then S^2 is equal to $N(S_{\bar{X}}^2)$. A comparison of the the estimate of S^2 from the difference of the two (or more) means to the *within group* variability (S^2 pooled) is a measure of the difference between means. If these two estimates of variation are similar, one may conclude that the means of the groups do not differ, i.e., that the difference between the means can be accounted for by ordinary variability. If the variability due to the difference between means is "significantly" larger than that within groups, one can conclude that the means of the groups differ.

A large variability of the means is associated with large differences between the means. Since as noted previously, the variance of a mean is σ^2/N (where N is the sample size), the sample variance of the mean is weighted by N to obtain an estimate of σ^2. Thus, a statistic that can be used to test treatment (group) differences is formed by the following ratio:

$$\sum \frac{N_i(\bar{X}_i - \bar{X}_0)^2/(G - 1)}{S^2} = F$$

where the numerator is the variability (variance estimate) due to the different means, and the denominator is the pooled within group variance. $\bar{X}_i$ is the mean of the *ith* group, $\bar{X}_0$ is the overall mean of all the groups, and G is the number of groups.

The distribution of this F ratio under the hypothesis that the group means are equal is the same F probability distribution previously mentioned when testing for the equality of two variances. The F distribution has ν_1 and ν_2 degrees of freedom, where ν_1 is the degrees of freedom associated with the numerator (G − 1), and ν_2 is the *degrees of freedom* associated with the denominator equal to $\Sigma(N_i)$ − G. For two groups, analysis of variance results in exactly the same probability level as the two-sample t test. (The F statistic with 1 df in the numerator, which is the case for two groups, is the *square* of the t statistic with degrees of freedom equal to that in the denominator of the F ratio.) The following example should clarify some of the foregoing concepts and computations.

In a preclinical study, animals were treated with two antihypertensive experimental drugs and a control drug, with 12 animals randomly assigned to the three groups, four per group. One animal died from a nondrug related cause and was lost to the experiment. The results (change in blood pressure from baseline) are shown in Table 10-13. Are the treatment means different, or do the observed differences merely reflect the inherent variation of the animals' response to such treatments? Under the assumptions that the *variances within each group are equal*, and that the data are *independent* and *normally distributed*, a test for equality of means can be performed using analysis of variance. The reader should refer to Table 10-13 as an aid in following the calculations needed for the ANOVA.

The overall mean is:

$$\bar{X}_0 = 156/11 = 14.18$$

The Between Treatment Mean Square (BMS) is:

$$\Sigma N_i(\bar{X}_i - \bar{X}_0)^2/(G - 1)$$

$$= [4(14.25 - 14.18)^2$$

$$+ 4(10.25 - 14.18)^2$$

$$+ 3(19.33 - 14.18)^2]/2$$

$$= 70.74$$

The Within Treatment Mean Square (WMS) is the variance *pooled* from within each group.

$$[3(S_1^2) + 3(S_2^2) + 2(S_3^2)]/(N_t - 3) = 102.167/8$$

$$= 12.77$$

where $N_t = \Sigma N_i = 11$.

The F ratio with 2 and 8 df, a test of differences among treatment means, is BMS/WMS.

$$F_{2,8} = 70.74/12.77 = 5.54$$

If the hypothesis that all three means are the same is true, the ratio BMS/WMS should be equal to 1, on the average. If the computed F ratio is less than 1, the means are not significantly different. If the F ratio is greater than 1, an F table should be used to determine if the

TABLE 10-13. *Change Of Blood Pressure in Preclinical Study Comparing Two Drugs and Control*

	Drug 1	Drug 2	Control
	15	8	
	12	14	16
	19	13	20
	11	6	22
SUM	57	41	58
MEAN ($\bar{X}$)	14.25	10.25	19.33
S	3.59	3.86	3.06

ratio is sufficiently large to declare significance. The cutoff point for significance at the 5% level for $F_{2,8}$ is 4.46 (see Table 10-6). Since the calculated $F(5.54)$ is larger than 4.46, the conclusion is that at least two of the means differ from each other at the 5% level.

Computations for ANOVA, when done by hand, routinely use shortcut formulas, and the results are presented in an analysis of variance table. For the above example, the calculations can be simplified as shown below (refer to Table 10-13 to help in following the calculations).

Total Sum $(\Sigma X) = 156$

$$(\Sigma X)^2/N_t = \text{Correction Term (C.T.)}$$

$$= 156^2/11$$

$$= 2212.36$$

$$\Sigma X^2 = 2456$$

Total Sum of Squares = TSS

$$= \Sigma X^2 - \text{C.T.}$$

$$= 2456 - 2212.36$$

$$= 243.64$$

Between Treatment Sum of Squares

$$= \text{BSS}$$

$$= \Sigma T_i^2/N_i - \text{C.T.}$$

$$= \frac{57^2}{4} + \frac{41^2}{4} + \frac{58^2}{3} - 2212.36$$

$$= 141.47$$

ANALYSIS OF VARIANCE (ANOVA) TABLE

SOURCE	DF	SUM OF SQUARES (SS)	MEAN SQUARE (MS)
Between Groups	2 (G − 1)	141.47	70.74 $F_{2,8}$ = 5.54
Within Groups	8 (N − 3)	102.17	12.77
Total	10 (N − 1)	243.64	

where T_i is the total sum of data in *ith* treatment group.

Within Treatment Sum of Squares

$$= WSS = TSS - BSS$$

$$= 102.17$$

The analysis is typically presented in an "analysis of variance (ANOVA) table."

The total variation is $\Sigma(X - \overline{X})^2$ and is separated into two parts, that due to differences of the means of the groups, and that due to the pooled variation within the groups. If the groups are not different, the variation among different groups should be no greater than that due to variation among individuals within groups, the "within" variation.

In general, there are "G" groups with replicate measurements in at least one of the groups. Although calculations are simplified and efficiency is usually optimal when comparing means if the number of observations in each group is equal, this is not a necessary condition for this analysis. In many experiments, especially in those involving humans, the original plan usually provides for equal numbers in each group, but life circumstances intervene, resulting in dropouts and lack of a symmetric design. The imbalance presents no problem, however, in the analysis of this one-way design.

Consider another example of this design in which an analytical method is tested by sending the same (blinded) sample to each of seven laboratories from the same company, located at different sites. Each of laboratories 1 through 6 has three analysts perform the analysis. Laboratory 7 reports only two results because only two analysts are available. In this experiment, a problem would result if one of the two analysts in laboratory 7 does a third analysis to present three results, since then the data for that laboratory would not be independent. Independence, in this example, refers to the fact that within each laboratory, analysts perform their analyses independently. The results are shown in Table 10-14. The computation is identical to that described in the previous example.

Total Sum of Squares = ΣX^2 − C.T.

$$= 1408 - 1280$$

$$= 128$$

Between Labs Sum of Squares

$$= \frac{(\text{Sum Column 1})^2}{3} + \frac{(\text{Sum Column 2})^2}{3}$$

$$\ldots + \frac{(\text{Sum Column 7})^2}{2} - \text{C.T.}$$

$$= \frac{24^2}{3} + \frac{33^2}{3} \ldots + \frac{22^2}{2} - 1280$$

$$= 102$$

Within Labs Sum of Squares

$$= \text{Total SS} - \text{Between SS}$$

$$= 128 - 102$$

$$= 26$$

Table 10-6 shows $F_{6,13}$ = 2.9 at the 5% level. Therefore, the ratio 8.5 is significant, and at least two of the laboratories are considered to be different ($P < 0.05$).

Confidence limits on the overall average can be constructed to give a range for the true mean of the analysis: $\overline{X}_0 \pm t(S_{\overline{X}_0})$. For 95% confidence

TABLE 10-14. *Assay Results for Seven Laboratories*

	LABORATORY						
	1	2	3	4	5	6	7
	9	11	6	10	5	7	12
	8	9	9	10	3	7	10
	7	13	9	7	4	7	—
AVERAGE	8	11	7	9	4	7	11
	OVERALL AVERAGE = 8.0						

ANOVA

Source	DF	SS	MS	
Between Labs	6	102	17	$F_{6,13} = 8.5$
Within Labs	13	26	2	
Total	19	128		

limits, the value of t is 2.16 and $S_{\bar{x}_0}^2 = 2/20$. (From the ANOVA Table, df = 13 and $S^2 = 2$; the total number of observations is 20.) The 95% confidence limits are $8 \pm 2.16\sqrt{2/20} = 8 \pm 0.7$. Note that the variance estimate for the computation is the *within error,* or *variance.* This is the correct error term because *all* of the laboratories of interest were included in the experiment (a *fixed model*). If the laboratories were only a sample of many possible laboratories, then the correct error term would be the between mean square with $(C - 1)$ degrees of freedom. (This is known as a *random model.*) In general, the between mean square is larger and has less degrees of freedom than the within mean square, and confidence limits are wider in this case. This less precise estimate is to be expected, because in the random case, not all members of the population have been sampled. The overall mean is estimated from a small sample of the possible laboratories. In the fixed model, each of all of the possible laboratories (7) have been sampled with replicate determinations (analysts) obtained from each laboratory. If the number of observations in each group is not equal in the random model, construction of a confidence interval for the overall mean is difficult.

Multiple Comparisons

With more than two treatments, if the F test is significant in the analysis of variance, one must determine which of the treatments differ. If a separate test is done comparing each pair of treatments, the chances of finding significance when the treatments are really identical are greater than that indicated by the α level. If the α level is 0.05, by definition, one time in twenty a difference will be found to be significant when the treatments are truly identical. If more than one pair of treatments are tested for significance in the same experiment, significant differences are found in more than 5% of such experiments, if treatments are truly identical. This concept may be better understood if one thinks of a large experiment in which 20 independent comparisons are to be made at the 5% level. On the average, one significant difference would be expected in each experiment of this kind, if the hypothesis of equal treatment means is true.

The problem of multiple comparisons is complex, and many solutions have been proposed.

The simplest method of dealing with multiple comparisons gives more significant results than would be expected from the ANOVA α level. A t test is constructed for differences between means using the degrees of freedom and mean square error from the ANOVA. If the sample sizes are the same in each group, a single least significant difference (LSD) can be constructed:

$$LSD = t_{df,\alpha}\sqrt{S^2(2/N)}$$

where t is the tabled value of t with appropriate df at the α level of significance. Any difference exceeding the LSD can be considered to be significant. The LSD test should be used *only if the F test from the ANOVA is significant.*

In the above example of seven laboratories, comparisons of laboratories with three observations (Laboratories 1 through 6) would result in an LSD equal to $2.16\sqrt{2(2/3)} = 2.49$, where 2.16 is the value of t with 13 df at the 0.05 level, and 2 is the within mean square. Laboratories 1 and 2 are significantly different from each other, the difference of their means $(11 - 8 = 3)$ exceeding the LSD (2.49). Laboratories 1 and 3, for example, are not significantly different. In comparing any of laboratories 1 through 6 to laboratory 7, an ordinary two-sample t test is used. For example, the comparison of laboratories 1 and 7 is performed as follows:

$$t = (11 - 8)/\sqrt{2(1/3 + 1/2)} = 2.32$$

Since the calculated t (2.32) is greater than the tabulated t at the 5% level with 13 df (2.16), the difference is significant.

Other tests take into account the multiplicity of comparisons and impose a penalty so that differences greater than that calculated for the t test are required for significance. One commonly used method is Tukey's multiple range method:

$$\text{Compute } |\text{Difference}|/\sqrt{S^2/N} = q \qquad (6)$$

Table A15 in the text by Snedecor and Cochran shows significant values of q depending on the number of treatments, df and α level.[6]

From equation (6) the minimum difference for significance for any pair of treatments is $q\sqrt{S^2/N}$. Strictly speaking, when using this formula, N should be the same for each treatment. In the laboratory example, laboratory 7 has two observations, compared to three observations in the other 6 laboratories. A slight adjustment for N would be necessary in this example,[6] but for purposes of illustration, assume that there are three observations for all laboratories (N = 3).

For this example at the 5% level, q equals 4.88, and the minimum difference needed for significance is:

$$4.88\sqrt{2/3} = 3.98$$

This difference is larger than that computed by the LSD procedure. Laboratories 1 and 2 are not significantly different using this method. Laboratory 5 is significantly different from all the other laboratories except for laboratories 3 and 6. Significant difference in laboratory results may require an action to determine and correct the cause; or, perhaps, it might be important just to know that differences exist.

Another commonly used method is Duncan's multiple range test, which is considered to have excellent properties.[14]

Two-Way Analysis of Variance (Randomized Blocks)

The two-way model is an extension of the paired t test in which more than two groups or treatments are compared. As in the paired t test, each individual (often referred to as a "block") is subjected to every treatment. Sometimes this model is described as a design in which each individual acts as his own "control."

In general, the order in which treatments are assigned to individuals is randomized unless a special design such as a crossover is used, which is discussed in a subsequent section of this chapter. A table of random numbers can be used to randomize the order of treatments to be tested on each individual or experimental unit.

The analysis of the two-way design is similar to the one-way ANOVA except that an additional source of variation is present, that due to the differences among the blocks. For example, if three assay methods are to be compared on six batches of granular material, the variation due to blocks (the batches) is associated with the differences in concentration of active material in the six batches.

The following example should clarify the design and data analysis. The time to 10% decomposition at accelerated conditions was compared

TABLE 10-15. *Stability of Five Batches of Tablets Using Three Kinds of Packaging Material*

Batches	Packaging Material			Mean
	A	B	C	
1	96	101	89	95.33
2	89	99	80	89.33
3	82	88	83	84.33
4	94	94	90	92.67
5	93	90	89	90.67
Mean	90.8	94.4	86.2	

for five batches of tablets using three different kinds of packaging material, with the results shown in Table 10-15. The computations for the ANOVA are shown below on page 274. Note that the computation of the between batch and between packages sum of squares is performed in the same way as the one-way analysis of variance. The difference between the *total sum of squares* and the *sum of the between packages and between batches sum of squares* is the *error sum of squares*.

In this design, the error sum of squares is less than that which would be computed from the same data without the "blocking" factor of batches. If the batches sum of squares were not included in the analysis, the error sum of squares would be increased by that amount. The inclusion of the batch, or blocking factor, usually results in a smaller mean square for error, and thus a more precise experiment.

Total SS

$$= \Sigma X^2 - \text{C.T.}$$

$$= 96^2 + 101^2 + \ldots + 89^2$$

$$- \frac{(96 + 101 + \ldots + 89)^2}{15}$$

$$= 123{,}259 - 122{,}763.27$$

$$= 495.73$$

Between Package SS

$$= R\Sigma(\bar{C}_i)^2 - \text{C.T.}$$

$$= 5(90.8^2 + 94.4^2 + 86.2^2)$$

$$- 122{,}763.27$$

$$= 168.93$$

where R is the number of rows (batches), and $\bar{C}_i$ is the column (packages) means.

Between Batch SS

$$= C\Sigma(\bar{R}_i)^2 - C.T.$$

$$= 3(95.33^2 + 89.33^2 + \ldots + 90.67^2)$$

$$- 122,763.27$$

$$= 202.40$$

where C is the number of columns (packages), and $\bar{R}_i$ is the row (batch) means.

Error SS = Total SS − Package SS − Batch SS
$$= 495.73 - 168.93 - 202.40$$
$$= 124.40$$

As in the case of the one-way ANOVA, F ratios are referred to in F Table (see Table 10-6) with appropriate degrees of freedom for tests of significance. The F ratio for packages, with 2 and 8 df, is 5.43 (Between Packages MS/Error MS), which is significant at the 5% level. Therefore, at least two of the packages differ. The least significant difference (LSD) is $t\sqrt{S^2(2/N)} = 2.31\sqrt{15.55(2/5)} = 5.76$. In this case, packages B and C are significantly different, with package B resulting in the least degradation.

The Question of a Fixed or Mixed Model

The F ratio for batches, with 4 and 8 df, is 3.25, which is significant at the 10% level but not at the 5% level (see Table 10-6). A relevant question is, "Is the fact that these batches may differ from each other with regard to their stability an important consideration, or are the five batches being used merely as a means of obtaining replication for the assessment of the three packages?" If the batches were somehow special, perhaps prepared so that they differed in some known way, it would be of interest to know if the stability of these batches were different. In these cases, "batches" is considered a *fixed* effect, i.e., there is a concern in the results of *only* these five special batches (or the method by which each was prepared), and all the batches of interest have been tested. Inferences about future batches made under unknown conditions are not of current interest.

If the batches are chosen randomly merely to provide replication, however, then the batch differences *per se* are not of primary concern. In this case, the ANOVA is referred to as a *mixed* model: the *batches are random* and the *packages are fixed*, i.e., in this experiment, possible differences among the three packages are of interest, and inferences about other yet untested packages are of no concern. If batches are random, the F test for batches described previously may be incorrect in the presence of batch X package interaction. Interaction, in this example, would be evident if package differences depended on which batch was being tested. A more correct error term (the denominator of the F ratio) for batch differences would come from replicate determinations within each batch, e.g., a repeat determination obtained by assaying a duplicate separate package. In any event, if batches are *random*, serving only as replicates for assessing package differences, there is usually little interest in whether or not batches differ. In fact, batch differences are known to exist, and that is why each package is tested on the different batches.

The two-way design is used in preclinical and clinical studies in which two or more drugs and/or placebos are to be compared. In these cases, animals or humans represent the rows or blocks that are considered to be random, i.e., the subjects are chosen as a means of replication to estimate the error in the experiment. The question of mixed and fixed effects models is an important consideration in the analysis of multicenter clinical trials. Suppose a clinical study comparing the effect of an antihypertensive drug to placebo included 20 patients (10 on drug and 10 on placebo) at each of eight clinical sites, with results shown in Table 10-16. The difference between treatments is not quite significant at the 5% level as indicated by the (Treatment)/(Sites × Treatment) ratio of 4.68. An F ratio of 5.59 with 1,7 df is needed for significance.

ANOVA

Source	DF	SS	MS	
Between Batches (Rows)	R − 1 = 4	202.40	50.6	$F_{4,8} = 3.25$
Between Packages (Columns)	C − 1 = 2	168.93	84.5	$F_{2,8} = 5.43$
Error (Row × Column)	(R − 1)(C − 1) = 8	124.40	15.55	
Total	14	495.73		

TABLE 10-16. *Multicenter Trial Of An Antihypertensive Drug and Analysis of Variance*

	Average Blood Pressure Change (mm Hg)	
Site	Placebo	Active
1	−2.6	−9.3
2	0.8	−6.4
3	−5.9	−5.4
4	−3.2	−8.4
5	2.5	−1.2
6	−8.2	−4.2
7	−0.9	−6.8
8	−10.0	−10.4
	−3.44	−6.51

In this example, there is replication in each cell of the two-way design. (A cell is defined as the intersection of a row and column, e.g., site 3 and placebo in the 8×2 table, Table 10-16.) Each cell consists of ten patients. There are now two error terms in the analysis of variance, the interaction term and the within error term, the variability estimate from replicate determinations within each cell. The variation due to replicates (within mean square) can be estimated by pooling the variance between patients within each treatment group at each center ($N = 10$). This estimate has 144 df, 9 df within each treatment and 18df from each of the eight centers.

If interaction is present, the "interaction" variance is a composite of the "within" variance and the interaction of sites and drug treatments, and thus is greater than the "within" error.* The interaction represents the degree to which the sites differ in their ability to differentiate the drugs. Interaction is great if some sites favor drug and others favor placebo. *If a sites × treatment interaction exists,* "within" error is the correct error term for treatments if sites are considered to be *fixed;* that is, the correct F ratio for treatments in the fixed model is

*Sampling variation can result in occasionally larger "within" error *estimates.*

$37.82/5.49 = 6.89$. This F has 1 and 144 df and is significant at the 1% level. Which, then, is the correct F test? Is the drug significantly better than the placebo or not? With the assumption that the interaction variance is not zero, (that is, interaction is present), the answer depends on whether clinical sites are *fixed* or *random.* If fixed, the result is highly significant; if random, the result misses significance at the 5% level, an important significance level for governmental acceptance of data for a drug submission.

Practically speaking, the sites are not randomly selected; on the other hand, they may not be considered fixed. A *"fixed"* effect means that all members of the population have been sampled. In the present case, is not the purpose of the experiment to make inferences to other clinical sites? Although rhetorical, this dilemma is real, and two points should be carefully considered and understood: (1) An assumption of a *fixed model* makes it *easier to obtain a significant difference between drug and placebo,* and (2) If the *mixed model* shows no significance and the *fixed model* shows *significance,* the possibility exists that a significant interaction is present. A significant interaction means that clinical sites do not differentiate treatments equally, an important consideration if some clinical sites favor one treatment, and others favor the other treatment (as opposed to interaction in which one treatment is consistently favored, and only the *degree of difference is different*). The implication of interaction in this context is that the effect of the treatment is not consistent but depends on the clinic, patient population, and so forth.

Missing Values

Although data may be inadvertently lost from any experiment, human clinical trials are particularly susceptible to data loss. Even the most well-designed, well-intentioned study cannot enforce exact adherence to the plan, owing to the usual vagaries of life. Patient dropouts due to noncompliance, adverse effects, and missed visits due to illness or forgetfulness are part of al-

ANOVA

SOURCE	DF	SS	MS	F
Sites	7	137.05	19.58	
Treatments	1	37.82	37.82	$F_{1,7} = 4.68$
Sites X Treatments (interaction)	7	56.52	8.07	$F_{7,144} = 1.47$
Within Sites*	144	780.56	5.49*	

*Between subject variance (see text), within sites and treatments, is adjusted to be comparable to other terms in the ANOVA.

most every clinical study. In cross-classified designs—e.g., two-way, factorial—the usual analysis is not valid when pieces of data are missing. Various options for the analysis exist depending on the design, the quantity of missing data, and the nature of the data. Alternatives include estimation of the missing data, curve fitting, and the use of special complex computer programs, which make adjustments for the unbalanced design. The analyses are usually not simple and often are difficult to interpret. Herein lies much of the art of statistics, and an experienced statistician should be consulted in such matters.

Bioavailability and Crossover Designs

Evaluation and analysis of bioavailability and pharmacokinetic parameters are important considerations for the pharmaceutical scientist. Usually, a finished dosage form is compared to some preliminary formulation or marketed formulation regarding relative absorption. The usual method of comparison consists of a clinical study in normal volunteers in which single doses of the experimental and comparative formulations are taken in a crossover design. In this design, half of the subjects are randomly chosen to take either one or the other of two formulations on the first experimental occasion (also known as period, leg, or visit), and the remaining formulation on the second occasion. A sufficient period of time should intervene between the two periods so that "all" of the drug is eliminated before the second dose is administered. It is important that power considerations be taken into account when determining sample size; the FDA recommends that the experiment be of sufficient sensitivity to have 80% power to detect a difference of 20% or more between formulations at the 5% level. Usually, 12 to 24 subjects satisfy these conditions using a crossover design.

Various parameters can be considered in the comparison of formulas for bioavailability, including (1) total amount of drug absorbed (from area under the blood level versus time curve, for example), (2) peak blood level, and (3) time to peak. Analysis of the results at each plasma (or urine) sampling time should be discouraged because the multiplicity of tests and correlation of data at proximal time points lead to confusion regarding the true significance level of such tests.[15] Also, interpretation is difficult. Other analyses for bioavailability data have been proposed that may be more relevant depending on the drug under consideration.[16] Although these alternative analyses have much merit, bioavailability data are usually reduced at present to the comparison of the three parameters just mentioned; this procedure is acceptable to the FDA in most cases.

The simplest analysis of bioavailability comparisons uses an analysis of variance for a crossover design. Statistical tests of hypotheses may be done separately for each parameter, e.g., relative absorption, time to peak, and peak plasma level. This method involves the easiest computation and interpretation but does not take into account multiple statistical tests and correlation of the parameters. Thus, although a multivariate test may be more appropriate, it may often be difficult to interpret. Some statisticians have suggested that hypothesis testing is not appropriate in bioavailability tests, because acceptance of the null hypothesis cannot logically lead to the conclusion that two formulations are exactly the same, since two different formulations cannot be *identically* equivalent. Rather, confidence intervals provide more useful information.[17,18] For example, if two formulas can be said to be within 25% of each other with a high degree of confidence, the clinician can then decide whether the two formulations are similar from a practical point of view.

The following example concerns the analysis of only a single parameter for purposes of illustration. The bioavailability of a tablet formulation of a new drug is to be compared to an equivalent amount of drug given in solution. The values in Table 10-17 for area under the blood level versus time curve were obtained from 12 subjects in a crossover design. The analysis of

TABLE 10-17. *Results of Bioavailability Study—Area Under Blood Level vs. Time Curve*

Subject	Tablet	Solution	Order of Administration
1	76	83	T-S*
2	59	54	T-S
3	84	95	S-T
4	96	81	T-S
5	50	64	S-T
6	61	66	S-T
7	48	57	S-T
8	68	61	T-S
9	74	70	S-T
10	86	79	T-S
11	91	88	S-T
12	57	68	T-S
AVERAGE	70.83	72.17	

*T-S = Tablet first, solution second.

variance accounts for *order of administration* with 1 df as well as "subject" and 'formulations" variance. The error sum of squares is the total sum of squares minus the sum of squares due to order, subjects, and formulations. Otherwise, the computations are similar to those previously described:

Between Subject SS

$$= \Sigma R_i^2/2 - C.T.$$

$$= \frac{(159^2 + 113^2 + \ldots 125^2)}{2}$$

$$- \frac{1716^2}{24}$$

$$= 4225$$

Between Formulation SS

$$= \frac{\Sigma C_i^2}{12} - C.T.$$

$$= \frac{(850^2 + 866^2)}{12} - 122,694$$

$$= 10.67$$

$$\text{Order SS} = \frac{\Sigma O_i^2}{12} - C.T.$$

$$= \frac{882^2 + 834^2}{12} - 112,694$$

$$= 96$$

where O_1 is the sum of results of first visit and O_2 is the sum of results for second visit.

$$\text{Total SS} = \Sigma X_i^2 - C.T.$$

$$= 127,402 - 122,694$$

$$= 4708$$

Error SS = Total SS − Subject SS

$$- \text{Formulation SS} - \text{Order SS}$$

$$= 4708 - 4225 - 10.67 - 96$$

$$= 376.33$$

The F tests for formulations and order of administration are not significant ($F_{1,10}$ is 4.96 at the 5% level), suggesting that the values of total absorption from both formulations are similar. A significant order effect would occur if the average results of the first visit differed from the average results of the second visit. Such a difference could be caused by systematic differences in the experimental procedure, the assay procedure, or the state of the subjects. A significant order effect does not invalidate the experiment. The design separates the variability due to order of administration from the residual experimental error.

The crossover design is a special case of the Latin square design, and the same deficiencies (and advantages) are present in both. A discussion of Latin square designs can be found in standard texts on experimental design. (See "General References.") If differential carryover effects exist (i.e., the effect of one drug preceding the other has a carryover effect different from that which occurs if the order of administration is reversed), the treatment effects are confounded and inferences can be misleading. In this case, confounding is interpreted as a confusion of treatment differences with differences due to the different carryover effects. Also, if interactions exist, the error is inflated, and interpretation of the results is unclear. Therefore, if either carryover effects or interactions are suspected, crossover designs should not be used. Special Latin square designs can be used to estimate and account for carryover effects,[19] or a simple parallel group (one-way) design can be used.

The advantage of the crossover design as compared with a parallel group design is that the sensitivity of the experiment is increased, owing

ANOVA

Source	DF	SS	MS	
Subjects	11	4225	384.1	
Formulations	1	10.67	10.67	$F_{1,10} = 0.3$
Order	1	96	96	$F_{1,10} = 2.6$
Error	10	376.33	37.63	
Total	23	4708		

to the use of within subject variance as the error in the crossover design, which is smaller than the between patient variance measured in the parallel groups design. Grizzle has proposed an analysis that detects carryover effects.[20] If such effects are present, the data from only the first visit are used and then analyzed as a one-way ANOVA, disregarding the data obtained from the second visit. (In the case of two treatments, this analysis is the same as an independent two-sample t test.)

Incomplete block designs may be used for bioavailability studies when more than two formulations are to be compared. For example, if three formulations are included in a study, a full crossover would require three visits. An incomplete block design would have each subject take only two of the possible three formulations in a symmetric pattern. For formulations A, B, and C, six subjects taking A-B, A-C, B-C, B-A, C-A, and C-B, in the order specified, results in an incomplete block design, balanced for order. Elementary discussions of incomplete block designs can be found in the works of Davies and Cox.[11,12]

Bioavailability data are often analyzed by using a log transformation or by computing a ratio of parameter estimates (e.g., $AUC_{tablet}/AUC_{solution}$) as the test statistic. These techniques usually result in similar conclusions although the use of the log transformation results in an asymmetric confidence interval when the antilog is calculated to back transform the data.[21] An advantage of using ratios is that the statistic may be more easily interpreted by the clinical scientist. As previously noted, use of confidence intervals may be a more appropriate way of expressing the difference between two formulations with regard to a given parameter.[16,18] For the example shown in Table 10-17, 95% confidence limits on the difference between the formulations for "area under the curve" can be constructed as follows (t with 10 df = 2.23):

$$(72.17 - 70.83) \pm 2.23\sqrt{37.63(1/12 + 1/12)}$$

$$= 1.34 \pm 5.58$$

$$= (-4.24 \text{ to } 6.92)$$

The true difference between the AUCs for the two formulations lies between -4.24 and 6.92 with a probability of 95%.

Transformations

Data analysis can often be improved by means of transformations, which result in a better fit of the data to the statistical model, or an improvement in properties that satisfy the test assumptions, such as variance homogeneity.

Probably the most frequently used transformation is the logarithmic transformation, obviously restricted to data with positive values. Examples in which the log transformation is recommended include the following situations. (1) The data have a log-normal distribution. (The transformation results in normally distributed data.) (2) The coefficient of variation ($S/\bar{X}$) of the observations, X, is constant. (Log X has approximately constant variance.) (3) If the data consist of a simple exponential function of the independent variable X (that is, $Y = Ae^{BX}$), then log Y is linear with respect to X. One should consider the effects of the log transformation on the variance as well as on the distribution of the data. The transformation may make skewed data appear more normal, but at the same time, it may result in nonhomogeneity of variance, heteroscedasticity. Ideally, the transformation results in satisfying both the normality and variance homogeneity assumptions implicit in the usual tests. Fortunately, this transformation often results in data that approximately satisfy both of these assumptions.

Other useful transformations are the arcsin transformation, which is used for proportions, and the square root transformation, which stabilizes the variance if the variance is proportional to the mean.[5]

Regression

Regression is a form of curve fitting that can be used for descriptive or predictive purposes. The theory of regression analysis allows equations relating variables to be established; it also aids in understanding the behavior (reliability) of the estimated equation parameters.

Simple Linear Regression

Simple linear regression is concerned with the fitting of straight lines, $Y = A + BX$, where A and B are the parameters of the line, the intercept, and slope, respectively. The dependent variable Y is a response that is the outcome of an experiment and is variable, i.e., its outcome cannot be exactly predicted. The independent variable is considered to be known precisely. For example, if blood pressure is the dependent variable, any or all of the following may be independent variables, depending on the objective of the experiment: dose of drug, length of treatment, and weight of patient. Some examples in which regression analysis would be appropriate are (1) cholesterol lowering as a function of dose, (2) log plasma concentration as a function of time, (3) optical density as a function of concentration, (4) dissolution as a function of stearate concentration, and (5) tablet assay as a function of tablet weight.

The objective of linear regression analysis is to fit the best straight line, $Y = a + bX$, from the experimental data, using least squares. The least squares line is defined as the line that makes $[\Sigma(\text{Observed Y} - \text{calculated Y})^2]$ a minimum, where the "calculated Y" is obtained from the least squares line. From the methods of calculus, it can be shown that:

$$\text{The slope, } b = [\Sigma(X - \bar{X})(Y - \bar{Y})]/[\Sigma(X - \bar{X})^2]$$

$$\text{The intercept, } a = \bar{Y} - b\bar{X}$$

Various significance tests may be performed on the estimates of the parameters a and b if the following assumptions are met:

1. X is measured without error. (If both X and Y are subject to error, line fitting may be accomplished by other minimizing techniques.[22])

2. Y is a variable with a normal distribution at each X, and the observed Ys are statistically independent.

3. The variance of Y is the same at each X.

4. The *true* relationship between X and Y is a straight line.

With these assumptions, the least squares fit can be used to estimate the variance; the variance of the slope; the variance of the intercept; a predicted value of Y; and confidence limits at a new value of X. It can also be used to determine if the relationship is a straight line. (Multiple observations of Y at at least one value of X are needed for the latter test.) All of the statistical tests and confidence intervals are based on normal curve theory. If the data are normal, it can be shown that estimates of the parameters a and b have normal distributions. The procedure for fitting straight lines and some relevant statistical tests are presented, using data derived from stability studies for illustrative purposes.

Fitting Lines to Stability Data

Because federal regulations now require expiration dating of pharmaceutical products, statistical procedures play an important role in the analysis of stability data. The fitting of data to straight line models and determination of variability allow inferences and predictions of future potency, as well as of the time to a given level of degradation, to be made with probability qualifications. Proper design of such studies is extremely important. Design considerations include the number of points in time at which the drug will be analyzed, various storage conditions, the number of samples to be analyzed at each point in time, and the source of these replicates. FDA statisticians recommend that three batches at ambient conditions be used to estimate stability characteristics.[23] Tablets should be taken from more than one bottle at each time period, especially during early development or marketing stages. Recommendations regarding an optimal choice of time periods for assay to reduce the variability of the regression line have appeared in the literature; however, in practice, the choice of time points seems to involve more than just this kind of optimality.[24] Designs should include appropriate observation intervals to reveal possible lack of linearity in the stability plots.

Table 10-18 shows the concentration of intact drug in tablets as a function of time at 25°C. Three "randomly" selected tablets from a single batch were assayed at each sample time. (In the case of tablets taken from each of three batches, the statistical analysis would take the different batches into account, and would be more complex than what is presented here.) The results are plotted in Figure 10-11.

Some pertinent questions are: (1) Do these data represent a straight line? (Does the decomposition follow zero-order kinetics?) (2) If so, at what time will the product be 10% decomposed? (3) How much intact drug will be present in one year? To answer these questions, estimates of the slope (b) and intercept (a) that define the straight line, and the variance estimate are ob-

TABLE 10-18. *Stability Data With Triplicate Assays From A Single Batch*

Time	Concentration (% of Label)
0 weeks	102,102,104
8 weeks	100,99,101
16 weeks	98,99,98
24 weeks	94,97,96
32 weeks	97,95,93
$\Sigma X = 240^*$	$\Sigma Y = 1473$
$\Sigma(X - \bar{X})^2 = 1920$	$\Sigma(Y - \bar{Y})^2 = 137.33$

*Note that the sum of "time" values (X) equals $3 \times 80 = 240$ because each "time" appears 3 times, one for each value of the concentration (Y).

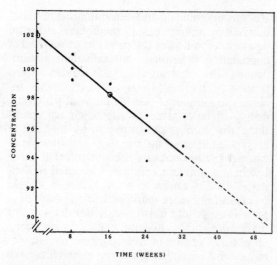

FIG. 10-11. *Stability plot showing loss of drug with time in a tablet formulation.*

tained using the least squares procedure as follows (see also Table 10-18).

The sample estimate of the *slope*, b, is:

$$b = \Sigma(X - \bar{X})(Y - \bar{Y})/\Sigma(X - \bar{X})^2$$

A shortcut computing formula for b is:

$$b = (N\Sigma XY - \Sigma X\Sigma Y)/[N\Sigma X^2 - (\Sigma X)^2]$$

$$= \frac{15 \cdot [0(102) + 0(102) + \ldots 32(93)] - (240)(1473)}{[(15)(0^2 + 0^2 + \ldots 32^2) - (240)^2]}$$

$$= (346{,}920 - 354{,}000)/(86{,}400 - 57{,}600) = 0.246$$

The sample estimate of the *intercept*, a, is:

$$a = \bar{Y} - b\bar{X} = 98.33 - (-0.246)(16) = 102.27$$

Therefore, the *equation of the fitted line* is:

$$C_T = 102.27 - 0.246T \tag{7}$$

where C_T is the concentration of drug at time T. The *variance* estimate, S^2, is:

$$S^2 = [\Sigma(Y - (a + bX))^2]/(N - 2)$$

A shortcut formula is:

$$S^2 = [\Sigma(Y - \bar{Y})^2 - b^2\Sigma(X - \bar{X})^2]/(N - 2)$$

$$= [137.33 - (-0.246)^2(1920)]/13 = 1.638$$

The variance, as computed here, is an estimate of the error in the line fitting, which includes tabletting variation (weight variation, mixing heterogeneity, and other random errors) and assay error, as well as variation due to the fact that a straight line might not be an accurate representation of the data. In the present example, an independent estimate of the tablet variation is available from the replicates at each observation point. A one-way ANOVA of these data is the first step in separating the sum of squares into its various components. There are five observation times with three replicates at each time.

The Between Times sum of squares can be further subdivided into two parts.

The *regression* sum of squares is calculated as:

$$b^2\Sigma(X - \bar{X})^2 = (-0.246)^2 \times (1920)$$

and is the sum of squares due to the slope of the line. A slope of zero would result in a zero regression sum of squares; a large slope results in a large sum of squares. The *deviations* sum of squares is equal to between times sum of squares minus regression sum of squares, $(119.33 - 116.03)$, and represents the variance due to the deviations of the average results at each time period from the fitted line.

Test For Linearity. The F test for linearity has 3 and 10 degrees of freedom ($F_{3,10}$) and is equal to Deviations MS/Within Times MS, or

ANOVA

Source	DF	SS	MS
Between Times	4	119.33	29.83
Within Times	10	18.00	1.80
Total	14	137.33	

Source	DF	SS	MS
Regression	1	116.03	116.03
Deviations from Regression	3	3.30	1.10

1.10/1.80 = 0.61. This is not significant ($F_{3,10}$ = 3.71 at the 5% level. See Table 10-6). There is no evidence for lack of linearity. The nonsignificant test for linearity in this context suggests that the use of a straight line as a model for these data is reasonable. The F ratio compares the deviations of the means of the observations from the fitted line at each time period to the error determined from replicates within each time period. If this ratio is small, there is no reason to believe that the relationship is not linear. A lack of linearity would result in an inflated deviations mean square, because the data representing a nonlinear function would be far removed from the least squares line.

Test of Slope. It is of interest to test if the slope differs from zero, i.e., the drug is indeed degrading. A zero slope means that no degradation is occurring. The test compares the sample estimate of the slope to its variance using a t test. The variance estimate of a slope is $S^2/\Sigma(X - \bar{X})^2$.

$$H_0: B = 0 \qquad H_A: B \neq 0$$

$$t_{13} = |b - 0|/\sqrt{S^2/\Sigma(X - \bar{X})^2}$$

$$= 0.246/\sqrt{1.638^*/1920}$$

$$= 8.416$$

(Equivalently, $F_{1,13}$ = Regression MS/Error MS = 70.84 = t^2.) The slope is significant (see Table 10-3); the drug is degrading.

Test of Intercept. Although it may not be of special interest in this example, a test for the significance of the intercept may also be performed. In this example, one might wish to test if the intercept is different from 100. A t test is performed comparing the difference between the intercept estimate, a, and 100 to its standard deviation.

$$H_0: A = 100 \qquad H_A: A \neq 100$$

$$t_{13} = |a - 100|/\sqrt{S^2[1/N + \bar{X}^2/\Sigma(X - \bar{X})^2]}$$

$$= (2.27)/\sqrt{1.638(1/15 + 256/1920)}$$

$$= 3.97$$

Thus, the intercept, 102.27, (potency at time 0) is significantly greater than 100, P < 0.05 (see Table 10-3).

*1.638 is the variance estimated from the original least squares fit. A safer estimate of error is the within mean square with 10 df equal to 1.80.

Prediction. Based on the data, the best prediction for the time at which 10% of the drug is decomposed (or when 90% of the intact drug is present) is determined by rearranging equation (7).

$$T_{90} = (90 - 102.27)/(-0.246) = 49.9 \text{ weeks}$$

where C_T is 90 and T_{90} is the time when 10% of the drug is degraded.

The amount of active drug predicted to be present after one year is calculated from equation (7):

$$C_{52} = 102.27 - 0.246(52) = 89.5\%$$

The estimates of both T_{90} and C_{52} just described are variable and have error associated with them. The error of a predicted value of Y (concentration, C_{52}, for example), where a *predicted value is an actual observation at time X,* depends on the magnitude of the variance, and how far away the new time is from the mean of the time values ($\bar{X}$) used to compute the least squares equation. The further the new value of X is from $\bar{X}$, the more variable is the estimate of the predicted value. The variance of a predicted value is:

$$S_p^2 = S^2(\text{Predicted Value})$$

$$= S^2[1 + 1/N + (X_T - \bar{X})^2/\Sigma(X - \bar{X})^2]$$

where X_T is the time of prediction. The predicted value, an assay actually determined at the time of prediction, has a variance that consists of the error due to the estimation involved in the line fitting *plus* the error associated with the new assay at the predicted time. A 95% confidence interval for a single assay performed at 52 weeks can be computed once the variance estimate of the predicted value is calculated. A 95% confidence interval equals $C_{52} \pm t_{df,0.05}(S_p)$. In the example, the confidence interval is:

$$89.5 \pm t_{13,0.05}\sqrt{1.638[1 + 1/15 + (52 - 16)^2/1920]}$$

$$= 89.5 \pm 2.16\sqrt{2.85} = 89.5 \pm 3.65$$

A confidence interval for the "true" potency at 52 weeks (a sample would not actually be assayed at this point) is:

$$C_{52} \pm t_{13,0.05}\sqrt{S^2[1/N + (X_T - \bar{X})^2/\Sigma(X - \bar{X})^2]}$$

$$= 89.5 \pm 2.38$$

The time at which 90% remains, for example, is known as *inverse prediction,* or a linear calibration problem, in which it is of interest to estimate the time, $T = (C_T - C_0)/b$, with an associated confidence interval. It can be shown that the confidence interval for T is:

$$[(T - g\bar{T}) \pm (tS/b)$$

$$\times \sqrt{[(N + 1)/N](1 - g) + (T - \bar{T})^2/\Sigma(T - \bar{T})^2}$$

$$\div [(1 - g)] \qquad (8)$$

where $g = (t^2)(S^2)/[b^2\Sigma(T - \bar{T})^2]$ and t is the appropriate tabled "t" value for the confidence interval. In the present example, the time for 10% decomposition, T_{90}, is 49.9 weeks. For a 95% confidence interval:

$$g = (2.16)^2(1.638)/(0.246)^2(1920) = 0.0658$$

$$(t_{13} \text{ for } \alpha = 0.05 \text{ is } 2.16)$$

(Note that if the slope b is not significantly different from zero, g will be greater than 1 and confidence limits cannot be obtained.) A 95% confidence interval for T_{90}, the time for 10% decomposition, using equation (8) is:

$$[48.85 \pm (2.16 \times 1.28/0.246)$$

$$\times \sqrt{(16/15)(0.9342) + (49.9 - 16)^2/1920}]$$

$$\div [0.9342] = 37.1 \text{ to } 67.5$$

Thus, the time for 10% decomposition probably occurs between 37.1 and 67.5 weeks. A conservative expiration date based on the time for 10% decomposition is 37.1 weeks, according to the lower limit of the confidence interval.

Allocation of X. The slope is estimated better if the X values are maximally spread apart. This can be seen from inspection of the variance of the slope, which is equal to σ^2 divided by $\Sigma(X - \bar{X})^2$. This quantity is maximized if the assay points are equally divided between points at zero time and the last assay time. This is not usually done, however, because considerations are important in addition to this "optimal" allocation. For example, in stability testing, data are usually obtained at intermediate points to observe the functional relationship between concentration and time.

Weighting in Regression. If the reaction is first order, a least squares procedure is followed using log C for concentration. This transforms the exponential equation, $C = C_0e^{-kt}$, to a linear function, $\log C = \log C_0 - kt/2.303$. If the data are log-normal, i.e., if log C is normal, then the variance homogeneity assumption is satisfied as

a result of the log transformation if the coefficient of variation, $S/\bar{X}$, of the original untransformed data is approximately constant. If a log transformation is inappropriate (as in zero-order reactions), and the variance is not constant but depends on the magnitude of the value (e.g., the coefficient of variation is constant), a weighting procedure should be used when fitting the least squares line, with weights equal to the inverse of the variance.[25]

The weighting procedure is used for any least squares fit in which the variance is not constant, but the procedure is more complex than the examples considered here. When fitting lines to the Arrhenius relationship, $\log k = -H_A/T + K$, a weighted least squares procedure should be used, because in general, the log k's do not have equal variance. A nonlinear approach to the statistical analysis of stability data combining the first order and Arrhenius equations has recently been described.[26]

Correlation

Figure 10-12 is a scattergram showing the relationship of change in blood pressure after treatment and the pretreatment blood pressure measurement. If both variables are subject to error and are distributed bivariately normal, a correlation coefficient r can be computed and tested for significance:

$$r = \Sigma(X - \bar{X})(Y - \bar{Y})/\sqrt{\Sigma(X - \bar{X})^2\Sigma(Y - \bar{Y})^2}$$

where the X's and Y's are paired values, e.g., change of blood pressure and baseline blood pressure values. The value of r lies between +1 and −1 and measures the linear relationship between two variables, X and Y. A correlation

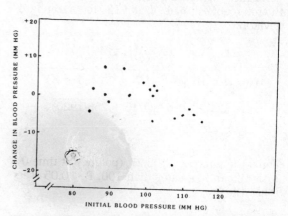

FIG. 10-12. *Scattergram showing the relationship of post-treatment change in blood pressure to pretreatment blood pressure.*

coefficient of +1 and −1 indicates that all points fall *exactly* on a straight line of positive slope or negative slope, respectively. A correlation of 0 indicates independence of the two variables, a zero slope (if they are bivariately normal). In practice, an exact fit ($r = \pm 1$) or a zero correlation rarely occur, and one must decide if the observed r is large enough to be taken seriously. The test of the correlation coefficient ($H_0: \rho = 0$) is a t test: $t = r/\sqrt{(1 - r^2)/(N - 2)}$ with $N - 2$ df. For data in Figure 10-12, where $N = 19$ and $r = 0.478$, the test of significance (17 df), $t = (0.478 - 0)/\sqrt{(1 - 0.228)/(17)} = 2.24$, shows a significant correlation at the 5% level (see Table 10-3).

Correlations should be carefully considered since a significant correlation does not necessarily indicate cause and effect. For example, a strong correlation between plasma uric acid increase and potassium decrease in patients on diuretics does not mean that one causes the other. Also, it should be appreciated that a small, perhaps meaningless, correlation coefficient may be statistically significant when dealing with large sample sizes. In general, one should interpret correlations with caution and use such results as clues for further experiments.

Empiric Models and Optimization

For the last 30 years in the chemical industry, relatively simple empiric equations associated with optimizing techniques have been used to describe otherwise complicated response relationships. Recently, these techniques have been shown to be useful in developing pharmaceutical dosage forms.[1-4] Usually, least squares procedures are used to obtain an empirical polynomial equation from experimental data that adequately describes the system within the range of the test variables, the levels of which are fixed in advance. Predictions and optimization are then based on the polynomial equation. Any set of data can be fit exactly by a polynomial of sufficient degree. For example, an equation of the form $y = a + bx + cx^2$ can be fit exactly to three points (x,y pairs). This does not mean that such an equation has physical meaning in describing the system or that it will accurately predict responses at extra-design points, i.e., combinations of factors not included in the experiment. These procedures usually result, however, in equations that closely approximate the response as a function of the variables being studied, and although the procedure may seem chancy, it has good predictive properties if used cautiously and intelligently. This approach is further elucidated in the following discussion of the simplex method, one of several techniques used in formulation optimization procedures, which are useful in designing dosage forms.

Simplex Lattice

This procedure may be used to determine the relative *proportion* of ingredients that optimizes a formulation with respect to a specified variable(s) or outcome.[27] A common problem in pharmaceutics occurs when the components of a formulation are varied in an attempt to optimize its performance with respect to such variables as drug solubility, dissolution time, and hardness. Application of a simplex design can be used to help solve this problem.[28,29] The method is illustrated using data estimated from a publication by Fonner and co-workers, in which a different approach, a constrained optimization, is described.[2] In the present example, three components of the formulation will be varied—stearic acid, starch, and dicalcium phosphate—with the restriction that the sum of their total weight must equal 350 mg. The active ingredient is kept constant at 50 mg; the total weight of the formulation is 400 mg. The formulation can be optimized for more than one attribute, but for the sake of simplicity, only one effect, dissolution rate, is considered.

The arrangement of the three variable ingredients in a simplex is shown in Figure 10-13. Note that this simplex is represented by a triangle. With more than three ingredients, the representation of the simplex is more difficult. The simplex, in general, is represented by an equilateral figure, such as a triangle for the three-component mixture and a tetrahedron for a four-component system. Each *vertex* repre-

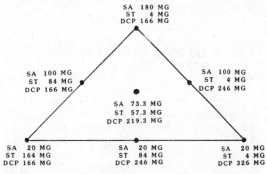

FIG. 10-13. *Special cubic simplex design for a three-component mixture. Each point represents a different formulation. SA = stearic acid; ST = starch; DCP = dicalcium phosphate.*

sents a formulation containing either (1) a pure component or (2) the maximum percentage of that component, with the other two components absent or at their minimum concentration. The choice of upper (maximum) and lower (minimum) concentrations of the variable ingredients is usually based on judgment, experience, or data from preliminary experiments, and represents concentrations within which a viable product can be manufactured. In this example, the vertices represent mixtures of all three components, with each vertex representing a formulation with one of the ingredients at its maximum concentration. The reason for not using pure components is that a formulation containing only one of the three components (350 mg of only starch, for example) would result in an unacceptable product. Careful preliminary thought must be given to the choice of the upper and lower concentrations of the three ingredients, under the constraint that the *total weight of the components is fixed*. In this case, the lower and upper limits are stearic acid 20 to 180 mg (5.7 to 51.4%[*]); starch 4 to 164 mg (1.1 to 46.9%); dicalcium phosphate 166 to 326 mg (47.4 to 93.1%). Thus, as shown in Figure 10-13, the vertex associated with the maximum percentage of starch would be represented by a formulation containing 164 mg of starch (46.9%), 166 mg of dicalcium phosphate (47.4%), and 20 mg of stearic acid (5.7%).

Various formulations can be studied in this triangular simplex space. One basic simplex design includes formulations at each vertex, halfway between the vertices, and at one center point as shown in Figure 10-13. Note that a formulation represented by a point halfway between two vertices contains the average of the minimum and maximum concentration of the

two ingredients represented by the two vertices. The composition of these seven formulas in the present example, a three-component system, is shown in Table 10-19.

If the vertices in the design are *not* single pure substances (100%), as is the case in this example, the computation is made easier if a simple transformation is initially performed to convert the maximum percentage of a component to 100%, and the minimum percentage to zero (0%), as follows.

Transformed %

$$= \frac{(\text{Actual \%} - \text{Minimum \%})}{(\text{Maximum \%} - \text{Minimum \%})}$$

In the case of stearic acid, for example, the transformation is (Actual % − 5.7)/(51.4 − 5.7). An actual concentration of stearic acid of 28.6% is transformed to a concentration of 50%, using this formula. Figure 10-13 shows that the simplex points nicely cover the space in a symmetric fashion. This simplex arrangement allows easy construction of an equation that exactly fits the resulting data, a polynomial equation with seven terms.

$$\text{Response} = b_1X_1 + b_2X_2 + b_3X_3 + b_{12}X_1X_2$$
$$+ b_{13}X_1X_3 + b_{23}X_2X_3 + b_{123}X_1X_2X_3 \quad (9)$$

where X_1, X_2, and X_3 represent transformed percentage concentrations of stearic acid, starch, and dicalcium phosphate, respectively. This empirical equation represents the data in the confines of the simplex space, and the coefficients can be calculated as simple linear combinations of the responses as follows, using ln Y, the response variable recommended by Fonner.[2] As shown in Table 10-19, the responses are Y(1), Y(2), and so forth where, for example, Y(1) is the

[*]The percentage is based on a total of 350 mg of excipients, and the total percentage of the three ingredients must necessarily equal 100%.

TABLE 10-19. *Seven Formulas To Be Tested—Actual and (Transformed) Values*

Stearic Acid %	Starch %	DCP %	Response (min)	ln Response
51.4 (100)	1.1 (0)	47.4 (0)	292 Y(1)	5.68
5.7 (0)	46.9 (100)	47.4 (0)	5.6 Y(2)	1.72
5.7 (0)	1.1 (0)	93.1 (100)	50.4 Y(3)	3.92
5.7 (0)	24.0 (50)	70.2 (50)	15.6 Y(2,3)	2.75
28.6 (50)	24.0 (50)	47.4 (0)	25.6 Y(1,2)	3.24
28.6 (50)	1.1 (0)	70.2 (50)	124.5 Y(1,3)	4.82
20.9 (33)	16.4 (33)	62.6 (33)	37 Y(1,2,3)	3.61

response for the formulation with X_1 (stearic acid) at a maximum concentration.

$$b_1 = Y(1) = 5.68$$

$$b_2 = Y(2) = 1.72$$

$$b_3 = Y(3) = 3.92$$

$$b_{12} = 4Y(1,2) - 2Y(1) - 2Y(2) = -1.83$$

$$b_{13} = 4Y(1,3) - 2Y(1) - 2Y(3) = 0.10$$

$$b_{23} = 4Y(2,3) - 2Y(2) - 2Y(3) = -0.30$$

$$b_{123} = 27Y(1,2,3) - 12\,[Y(1,2) + Y(1,3)$$

$$+ Y(2,3)] + 3[Y(1) + Y(2) + Y(3)]$$

$$= 1.71$$

Substituting these values of the coefficients into equation (9), the following response equation is obtained.

Dissolution Time

$$= Y$$

$$= 5.68X_1 + 1.72X_2 + 3.92X_3$$

$$- 1.83X_1X_2 + 0.10X_1X_3$$

$$- 0.30X_2X_3 - 1.71X_1X_2X_3$$

$$(10)$$

This is an empirical equation that should represent the response surface in the simplex space. Its adequacy can be tested by running one or more experiments at other experimental points (different formulations from those in the simplex) and noting if the equation accurately predicts the results. In the analysis of their experiment, Fonner and co-workers included data from four experiments not covered by the simplex.[2] Using equation (10), the prediction of the results for these four formulations is good, as can be seen in Table 10-20. The last point in Table 10-20 represents a formulation outside of the region of the simplex, and the prediction is good in this case. In general, predictions outside of the simplex space might not be reliable, and caution should be exerted when extrapolating into extra-design regions. When possible, replication is recommended in simplex experiments to estimate the variance, which can be used to assess the "fit" of the model by comparing the predicted and actual results from extra-design points.

Computer programs can be used to construct contour maps and identify optimal regions once the response equation has been established.

Nonparametric Statistics

Most of the statistical tests described in this chapter are based on an assumption that the underlying distribution of the data is known (binomial or normal, for example). Although tests based on the normal distribution give valid results in face of a moderate degree of non-normality, especially when inferences about means are made, situations arise in which data should be analyzed with limited assumptions about the data distribution. One such nonparametric test has already been described, the sign test. Many nonparametric tests assume only that the underlying distribution is continuous. In addition, analysis of data using nonparametric methods has the advantage of using simple calculations that are often based on ordering or ranking procedures. Thus, these methods can be used to

TABLE 10-20. *Prediction of Dissolution Results of Extra-Design Points Using Equation Derived From Simplex Experiment*

Extra-Design Formulations (Transformed)			Observed Dissolution	Dissolution Predicted from Eq (10)
Stearic Acid (%)	Starch (%)	DCP (%)		(antilog)*
20.4	21.6	58.2	33.4	38.9
20.4	65.3	14.4	12.9	12.7
64.1	21.6	14.4	72.8	72.9
64.1	65.3	−29.3	19.9	22.1

*Fonner and associates recommend use of ln (response) for the optimization using their method. This transformation is used here.

obtain a quick look before a full-fledged analysis is undertaken.

A disadvantage is that these tests lack power compared with corresponding parameteric tests; nevertheless, some nonparametric tests are surprisingly powerful. (As noted previously, power is the ability of a test to find significance, should a true difference exist.) Also, in more complex designs, nonparametric tests may not give the variety of analyses and interpretations given by parametric analyses. Several popular methods of analysis are presented in this discussion; more detail is given by Wilcoxon and Wilcox.[30]

Wilcoxon Rank Sum Test

This test is used to compare the averages of two treatments and has excellent power compared with the more powerful t test if the data are normally distributed. Consider the example in Table 10-21 showing changes in weight of control animals compared with animals given an anorexic drug. Values for drug and control groups are ranked in order of magnitude. A rank is assigned to each value; *average ranks* are assigned in case of *ties*. The ranks are then summed within each treatment group. In most cases, a significance test may be used based on an approximation to the normal distribution:

$$Z = [T - E(T)]/\sqrt{S_T^2}$$

has a distribution that is approximately normal with variance equal to 1.

$$E(T) = N_1(N_1 + N_2 + 1)/2 \text{ and}$$

$$S_T^2 = N_1 N_2(N_1 + N_2 + 1)/12$$

N_1 = Smaller sample size

N_2 = Larger sample size

T = Sum of ranks for smaller sized sample

In this example:

$$E(T) = (8)(8 + 9 + 1)/2 = 72$$

$$S_T^2 = (8)(9)(8 + 9 + 1)/12 = 108$$

For a two-sided test:

$$Z = [|94 - 72|]/\sqrt{108} = 2.12$$

According to Table 10-3, a value greater than 1.96 is needed for significance at the 5% level. Therefore, the drug is significantly different from the control ($P < 0.05$); the drug group showed a greater weight loss. Wilcoxon and Wilcox provide a table that can be used to assess significance, given the sample sizes of the two groups and the rank sum.[30]

For paired data, the non-zero differences (zero differences are not included in the analysis) of the pairs are first ranked in order, *disregarding sign*. Then, the sum of the ranks of the positive differences and the sum of the ranks of the negative differences are computed and tested for significance. The data in Table 10-22 were obtained from a bioavailability study using 15 subjects. The peak serum concentration is compared for the two products. The sum of the positive ranks is 68.5, and the sum of the negative ranks is 36.5. An approximate "normal" test is:

$$Z = [T - (N)(N + 1)/4]/\sqrt{N(N + 1)(2N + 1)/24}$$

TABLE 10-21. *Weight Change in Drug and Control Groups and Ranks*

Control		Drug	
Weight Change	Rank	Weight Change	Rank
0	14	−2	10.5
−3	9	−8	3
+9	17	+1	15
−1	12.5	−19	1
−4	7.5	−4	7.5
+3	16	−2	10.5
−1	12.5	−11	2
−5	5.5	−5	5.5
		−7	4
Sum of Ranks =	94	Sum of Ranks =	59

TABLE 10-22. *Results of Bioavailability Comparison Peak Height of Serum Concentration*

Subject	Test Product	Control Product	Difference	Rank
1	9.6	9.4	+0.2	1.5
2	3.3	3.3	0	Omit
3	2.8	2.4	+0.4	5.5
4	5.0	4.1	+0.9	10
5	6.4	4.7	+1.7	14
6	2.8	3.5	−0.7	8
7	4.0	3.7	+0.3	3.5
8	3.2	3.0	+0.2	1.5
9	4.3	3.3	+1.0	11
10	4.7	6.2	−1.5	13
11	3.3	2.9	+0.4	5.5
12	4.6	3.8	+0.8	9
13	4.0	5.1	−1.1	12
14	5.9	5.3	+0.6	7
15	3.6	3.9	−0.3	3.5

where N is the number of pairs, and T is the sum of the ranks (either positive or negative).

$$Z = [68.5 - (14)(15)/4]/\sqrt{(14)(15)(29)/24}$$

$$= 1.00$$

Since Z is less than 1.96, the test product is not significantly different from the control at the 5% level. Wilcoxon and Wilcox have a table for significance testing,[30] and for small sample sizes, this table rather than the foregoing approximate formula should be used.

One-Way and Two-Way Designs

Nonparametric tests are available for one- and two-way ANOVA type designs. In the case of more than two independent groups arranged in a one-way design, the data are first ranked in order over all groups, disregarding group designation. The sum of the ranks for each group is then calculated. A statistic with an approximate X^2 distribution can be computed as shown in the following example, in which the hardness of tablets of three different formulations of the same drug are compared (Table 10-23). The replicates are randomly selected tablets. The X^2 test, with $C - 1 = 3 - 1 = 2$ df, is:

$$X^2_{C-1} = [12/N(N + 1)]\Sigma R^2_i/N_i - 3(N + 1)$$

where C is the number of treatments, R_i is the sum of ranks in ith treatment, N_i is the number of observations in ith treatment, and N is the total number of observations.

In this example:

$$X^2_2 = [12/(10)(11)][208.33 + 65.33 + 64.0]$$

$$- (3)(11)$$

$$= 3.84$$

For significance at the 5% level, a X^2 value with 2 degrees of freedom must exceed 5.99.[5] Therefore, the differences among the three formulations are not significant at the 5% level.

Friedman's Two-Way Analysis. Friedman's analysis for related samples with more than two groups is also based on ranking of data.[31] This test is analogous to a two-way ANOVA.

Four batches of tablets were produced on three tablet presses (machines), and the average weight of the tablets was estimated as the mean of 20 randomly selected tablets. To test for machine differences, the machines are ranked

TABLE 10-23. *Hardness (Rank) of Tablets From Three Formulations*

	Formula		
	1	2	3
	8.3 (6)	7.9 (4)	8.4 (7)
	10.0 (10)	7.1 (2)	8.0 (5)
	9.7 (9)	8.5 (8)	6.5 (1)
			7.3 (3)
$R_i = \Sigma$Ranks	25	14	16
$(\Sigma R^2_i)/N_i$	208.33	65.33	64.0

TABLE 10-24. *Data Showing Comparison of Tablet Weights From Four Machines Using Three Batches With Ranks*

| | Machine | | | | | |
| | 1 | | 2 | | 3 | |
Batch	Weight	Rank	Weight	Rank	Weight	Rank
1	202	(3)	199	(2)	197	(1)
2	203	(3)	199	(2)	198	(1)
3	205	(3)	200	(2)	196	(1)
4	202	(3)	197	(1)	198	(2)

within each batch as shown in Table 10-24. An approximate X^2 test can be used to assess significance using the following formula.

$$X^2_{C-1} = [12/(RC(C + 1))]\Sigma C_j^2 - 3R(C + 1)$$

where C is the number of groups (machines), R is the number of blocks (batches), and C_j is the sum of ranks in the *jth* group.

In this example:

$$X^2_2 = [12/(4 \cdot 3 \cdot 4)] \cdot 218 - (12)(4) = 6.5$$

Since 6.5 is greater than the tabulated value of X^2_2 (5.99) at the 5% level,[5] the result is significant; the first machine shows the higher average weight. (Wilcoxon and Wilcox provide a discussion of comparisons that involve more than two groups.[30])

The tests described in this section, as well as other nonparametric tests, are described in more detail by Siegel,[31] Wilcoxon and Wilcox,[30] and Hollander and Wolfe.[32] Tables for tests of significance are also provided by these sources.

References

1. Schwartz, J. B., Flamholz, J. R., and Press, R. H.: J. Pharm. Sci., 62:1165, 1973.
2. Fonner, D. E., Buck, J. K., and Banker, G. S.: J. Pharm. Sci., 59:1587, 1976.
3. Dincer, S., and Ozdurmus, S.: J. Pharm. Sci., 66:1070, 1978.
4. Bolton, S.: J. Pharm. Sci., 72:362, 1983.
5. Dixon, W. J., and Massey, F. J., Jr.: Introduction to Statistical Analysis. 3rd Ed. McGraw-Hill, New York, 1969.
6. Snedecor, G. W., and Cochran, W. G.: Statistical Methods. 7th Ed. Iowa State Univ. Press, Ames, IA, 1980.
7. American Society for Testing Materials (ASTM), E 178-75, Standard Recommended Practice for Dealing with Outlying Observations. April 1975, p. 183.
8. Tables of the Binomial Distribution. National Bureau of Standards, U.S. Government Printing Office, Washingon, DC, 1952.
9. MIL STD 105D, Military Sampling Procedures and Tables for Inspection by Attributes. U.S. Government Printing Office, Washington, DC, 1963.
10. Guenther, W. C.: The American Statistician, 35:243, 1981.
11. Davies, O.: Design and Analysis of Industrial Experiments. Hafner, New York, 1963.
12. Cox, D. R.: Planning of Experiments. John Wiley and Sons, New York, 1965, p. 221.
13. Ferris, G.: Biometrics, 14:39, 1958.
14. Steele, R. G. D., and Torre, J. H.: Principle and Procedures of Statistics. McGraw-Hill, New York, 1960, p. 107.
15. Albert, K. S. (Ed.): Drug Absorption and Disposition: Statistical Considerations. Am. Pharm. Assoc., Washington, DC, 1980.
16. Westlake, W. J.: Int. J. Clin. Pharmacol., 11:342, 1975.
17. Westlake, W. J.: J. Pharm. Sci., 61:1340, 1972.
18. Shirley, E. J.: J. Pharm. Pharmacol., 28:312, 1976.
19. Cochran, W. G., and Cox, G. M.: Experimental Designs. 2nd Ed. John Wiley and Sons, New York, 1957, p. 117.
20. Grizzle, J. E.: Biometrics, 21:467, 1965.
21. Westlake, W. J.: Biometrics, 32:741, 1976.
22. Mandel, J.: The Statistical Analysis of Experimental Data. Interscience, New York, 1964, p. 288.
23. O'Neill, R. T., and Schuirmann, D. J.: Presentation at meeting of Am. Statistical Assoc. Meeting, Washington, DC, August 13–16, 1979.
24. Tootill, J. P. R.: J. Pharm. Pharmacol. (Suppl.), 13:75T, 1961.
25. Williams, E. W. J.: Regression Analysis. John Wiley and Sons, New York, 1964.
26. King, S. P., Kung, M., and Fung, H.: J. Pharm. Sci., 73:657, 1984.
27. Gorman, J. W., and Hinman, J. E.: Technometrics, 4:463, 1962.
28. Shek, E., Ghani, M., and Jones, R.: J. Pharm. Sci., 69:1135, 1980.
29. Anik, S. T., and Sukamer, L.: J. Pharm. Sci., 70:897, 1981.
30. Wilcoxon, F., and Wilcox, R.: Some Rapid Approximate Statistical Procedures. Lederle Labs., Pearl River, NY, 1964.
31. Siegel, S.: Non-Parametric Statistics for the Behavioral Sciences. McGraw-Hill, New York, 1956, p. 166.
32. Hollander, M., and Wolfe, D. A.: Nonparametric Statistical Methods. John Wiley and Sons, New York, 1973.

General References

Albert, K. S. (Ed.): Drug Absorption and Disposition, Statistical Considerations. Am. Pharm. Assoc., Washington, DC, 1980.

Bolton, S.: Pharmaceutical Statistics. Marcel Dekker, New York, 1984.

Buncher, C. R., and Tsay, J. (Eds.): Statistics in the Pharmaceutical Industry. Marcel Dekker, New York, 1981.

Cox, D. R.: Planning of Experiments. John Wiley and Sons, New York, 1965.

Davies, O. (Ed.): Design and Analysis of Industrial Experiments. Hafner, New York, 1963.

Dixon, W. J., and Massey, F. J., Jr.: Introduction to Statistical Analysis. 3rd Ed. McGraw-Hill, New York, 1969.

Siegel, S.: Nonparametric Statistics for the Behavioral Sciences. McGraw-Hill, New York, 1956.

Snedecor, G. W., and Cochran, W. G.: Statistical Methods. 7th Ed. Iowa State Univ. Pres, Ames, IA, 1980.

Pharmaceutical Dosage Forms

11

Tablets

GILBERT S. BANKER *and* NEIL R. ANDERSON

Role in Therapy

The oral route of drug administration is the most important method of administering drugs for systemic effects. Except in cases of insulin therapy, the parenteral route is not routinely used for self-administration of medication. The topical route of administration has only recently been employed to deliver drugs to the body for systemic effects, with two classes of marketed products: nitroglycerin for the treatment of angina and scopolamine for the treatment of motion sickness. Other drugs are certain to follow, but the topical route of administration is limited in its ability to allow effective drug absorption for systemic drug action. The parenteral route of administration is important in treating medical emergencies in which a subject is comatose or cannot swallow, and in providing various types of maintenance therapy for hospitalized patients. Nevertheless, it is probable that at least 90% of all drugs used to produce systemic effects are administered by the oral route. When a new drug is discovered, one of the first questions a pharmaceutical company asks is whether or not the drug can be effectively administered for its intended effect by the oral route. If it cannot, the drug is primarily relegated to administration in a hospital setting or physician's office. If patient self-administration cannot be achieved, the sales of the drug constitute only a small fraction of what the market would be otherwise.

Of drugs that are administered orally, solid oral dosage forms represent the preferred class of product. The reasons for this preference are as follows.

Tablets and capsules represent unit dosage forms in which one usual dose of the drug has been accurately placed. By comparison, liquid oral dosage forms, such as syrups, suspensions, emulsions, solutions, and elixirs, are usually designed to contain one dose of medication in 5 to 30 ml. The patient is then asked to measure his or her own medication using a teaspoon, tablespoon, or other measuring device. Such dosage measurements are typically in error by a factor ranging from 20 to 50% when the drug is self-administered by the patient.

Liquid oral dosage forms have other disadvantages and limitations when compared with tablets. They are much more expensive to ship (one liquid dosage weighs 5 g or more versus 0.25 to 0.40 g for the average tablet), and breakage or leakage during shipment is a more serious problem with liquids than with tablets. Taste masking of the drug is often a problem (if the drug is in solution even partially). In addition, liquids are less portable and require much more space per number of doses on the pharmacist's shelf. Drugs are in general less stable (both chemically and physically) in liquid form than in a dry state and expiration dates tend to be shorter. Careful attention is required to assure that the product will not allow a heavy microbiologic burden to develop on standing or under normal conditions of use once opened (preservation requirements). There are basically three reasons for having liquid dosage forms of a drug: (1) The liquid form is what the public has come to expect for certain types of products (e.g., cough medicines). (2) The product is more effective in a liquid form (e.g., many adsorbents and antacids). (3) The drug(s) are used fairly commonly by young children or the elderly, who have trouble swallowing the solid oral dosage forms.

Advantages

Of the two oral solid dosage forms commonly employed in this country, the tablet and the capsule, the tablet has a number of advantages. One of the major advantages of tablets over capsules, which has recently proved significant, is that the tablet is an essentially tamperproof dosage form. In recent episodes of tampering with pharmaceutical products, products have been altered after leaving the manufacturer and the wholesaler or distributor. A number of deaths and serious injuries have resulted from such tampering, with the result that the FDA has found it necessary to impose new standards for tamper-resistant packaging.[1] The major advantage of capsules—their ability to hide their contents from sight and to mask or hide the taste or odor of their contents—makes them the most vulnerable to tampering of all dosage forms. In contrast, any adulteration of a tablet after its manufacture is almost certain to be observed. Addition of any liquid to a tablet would produce disintegration if the liquid is aqueous, or would produce visible changes if the liquid is nonaqueous. Addition of extraneous powder to a tablet is not readily feasible. Even though improved packaging provides some consumer protection for such dosage forms as capsules, which are susceptible to tampering, *no* packaging is completely tamperproof.

A major disadvantage of capsules over tablets is their higher cost. Capsules, whether hard gelatin or soft elastic capsules, employ a capsule shell to contain the drug contents. The cost of this shell is approximately several tenths of a cent or more, depending on whether the capsule is banded, printed with identification, or otherwise treated. In addition to this is the cost of filling. This filling cost is higher than the typical total cost of tablet production, now that direct compression methods of tablet manufacture exist, since the capsule filling operation is far slower than the tablet compression operation.

In consideration of these few comparisons to capsules, the following may be cited as the primary potential advantages of tablets.

1. They are a unit dose form, and they offer the greatest capabilities of all oral dosage forms for the greatest dose precision and the least content variability.

2. Their cost is lowest of all oral dosage forms.

3. They are the lightest and most compact of all oral dosage forms.

4. They are in general the easiest and cheapest to package and ship of all oral dosage forms.

5. Product identification is potentially the simplest and cheapest, requiring no additional processing steps when employing an embossed or monogrammed punch face.

6. They may provide the greatest ease of swallowing with the least tendency for "hang-up" above the stomach, especially when coated, provided that tablet disintegration is not excessively rapid.

7. They lend themselves to certain special-release profile products, such as enteric or delayed-release products.

8. They are better suited to large-scale production than other unit oral forms.

9. They have the best combined properties of chemical, mechanical and microbiologic stability of all the oral forms.

The development pharmacist should know fully what the potential advantages of tablets are as a dosage form class. If these general advantages together with the specific criteria specifications for the product are not met, an optimum or even near-optimum product may not have been achieved.

Disadvantages

The disadvantages of tablets include the following.

1. Some drugs resist compression into dense compacts, owing to their amorphous nature or flocculent, low-density character.

2. Drugs with poor wetting, slow dissolution properties, intermediate to large dosages, optimum absorption high in the gastrointestinal tract, or any combination of these features may be difficult or impossible to formulate and manufacture as a tablet that will still provide adequate or full drug bioavailability.

3. Bitter-tasting drugs, drugs with an objectionable odor, or drugs that are sensitive to oxygen or atmospheric moisture may require encapsulation or entrapment prior to compression (if feasible or practical), or the tablets may require coating. In such cases, the capsule may offer the best and lowest cost approach.

In summary of the foregoing advantages and disadvantages of tablets in comparison to other oral dosage forms, tablets do provide advantages to the pharmacist, in minimal storage space requirements as well as ease of dispensing and possibly control; to the patient in convenience of use, optimum portability, and lowest cost; and to the physician in flexibility of dosage (with bisected tablets), and in accuracy and precision of dosage in general.

Challenges in Product Design, Formulation, and Manufacture

As a class, tablets are one of the most challenging of all pharmaceutical products to design and manufacture. The difficulty of achieving full and reliable drug bioavailability for drugs with poor wetting and slow dissolution, for example, has previously been mentioned, as has the difficulty of achieving good cohesive compacts of amorphous or flocculent drugs. However, even for drugs with good compression characteristics, good dissolution, and no bioavailability problems, tablet product design and manufacture can be challenging because of the many competing objectives of this dosage form. That is, any action that is taken to improve one objective or set of objectives may cause another objective or set of objectives to degrade. For example, tablets should have a smooth surface, good appearance, and perhaps some surface gloss, and be cohesive and compact so that they do not undergo friability, powdering, or chipping in the bottle during shipping or handling. Whatever step is taken to achieve this first set of objectives, whether it is using more binder or adhesive, increasing compression pressure or punch dwell time, or using precompression, it may be expected to have a negative effect on another set of objectives, tablet disintegration time, drug dissolution rate, and possibly bioavailability. Depending on a drug's degree of compressibility, its dose, its solubility and solubility rate, its site of absorption along the GI tract, and other factors, finding a satisfactory compromise between competing sets of objectives may be simple or extremely complex.

When finding the correct compromise is not straightforward and simple, the pharmaceutical scientist should seriously consider use of optimization procedures to design the best compromise product.[2-4] Trial and error methods of formulation do not allow the formulator to know how close any particular formulation is to the optimum solution, and without a model to define the relationships between formulation and manufacturing variables, and levels of values for the quality features of the product, it is not possible to investigate play-off decisions between objectives. Once the product is mathematically/statistically modeled, one can compute how much a secondary objective or set of objectives suffers or gains if a primary objective specification is slightly relaxed (or tightened). As a result of the various competing objectives that are encountered in tablet product design, the formulation and manufacture of this product class are ideal for a mathematical optimization approach. Whether or not such an approach may be warranted depends on how simple and straightforward the design/manufacturing processes appear to be; however, using statistical experimental design procedures readily available today, the generation of a model for the system may be little additional work, if any, especially with computer assistance. It is preferable to stumbling through three or four levels of trial and error experimentation.

The Pharmaceutical Tablet Dosage Form

Properties

The objective of the design and manufacture of the compressed tablet is to deliver orally the correct amount of drug in the proper form, at or over the proper time and in the desired location, and to have its chemical integrity protected to that point. Aside from the physical and chemical properties of the medicinal agent(s) to be formulated into a tablet, the actual physical design, manufacturing process, and complete chemical makeup of the tablet can have a profound effect on the efficacy of the drug(s) being administered.

A tablet (1) should be an elegant product having its own identity while being free of defects such as chips, cracks, discoloration, contamination, and the like; (2) should have the strength to withstand the rigors of mechanical shocks encountered in its production, packaging, shipping, and dispensing; and (3) should have the chemical and physical stability to maintain its physical attributes over time. Pharmaceutical scientists now understand that various physical properties of tablets can undergo change under environmental or stress conditions, and that physical stability, through its effect on bioavailability in particular, can be of more significance and concern in some tablet systems than chemical stability.

On the other hand, the tablet (1) must be able to release the medicinal agent(s) in the body in a predictable and reproducible manner and (2) must have a suitable chemical stability over time so as not to allow alteration of the medicinal agent(s). In many instances, these sets of objectives are competing. The design of a tablet that emphasizes only the desired medicinal effects may produce a physically inadequate product. The design of a tablet emphasizing only the physical aspects may produce tablets of limited and varying therapeutic effects. As one example of this point, Meyer and associates present information on 14 nitrofurantoin products, all of which passed the compendial physical requirements, but showed statistically significant bioavailability differences.[5]

Evaluation

To design tablets and later monitor tablet production quality, quantitative evaluations and assessments of a tablet's chemical, physical, and bioavailability properties must be made. Not only could all three property classes have a significant stability profile, but the stability profiles may be interrelated, i.e., *chemical* breakdown or interactions between tablet components may alter *physical* tablet properties, greatly changing the *bioavailability* of a tablet system.

General Appearance. The general appearance of a tablet, its visual identity and overall "elegance," is essential for consumer acceptance, for control of lot-to-lot uniformity and general tablet-to-tablet uniformity, and for monitoring trouble-free manufacturing. The control of the general appearance of a tablet involves the measurement of a number of attributes such as a tablet's size, shape, color, presence or absence of an odor, taste, surface texture, physical flaws and consistency, and legibility of any identifying markings.

Size and Shape. The size and shape of the tablet can be dimensionally described, monitored, and controlled. A compressed tablet's shape and dimensions are determined by the tooling during the compression process. The thickness of a tablet is the only dimensional variable related to the process. At a constant compressive load, tablet thickness varies with changes in die fill, with particle size distribution and packing of the particle mix being compressed, and with tablet weight, while with a constant die fill, thickness varies with variations in compressive load. Tablet thickness is consistent batch to batch or within a batch only if the tablet granulation or powder blend is adequately consistent in particle size and size distribution, if the punch tooling is of consistent length, and if the tablet press is clean and in good working order.

The crown thickness of individual tablets may be measured with a micrometer, which permits accurate measurements and provides information on the variation between tablets. Other techniques employed in production control involve placing 5 or 10 tablets in a holding tray, where their total crown thickness may be measured with a sliding caliper scale. This method is much more rapid than measurement with a micrometer in providing an overall estimate of tablet thickness in production operations, but it does not as readily provide information on variability between tablets; however, if the punch and die tooling has been satisfactorily standardized and the tablet machine is functioning properly, this method is satisfactory for production work.

Tablet thickness should be controlled within a $\pm5\%$ variation of a standard value. Any variation in tablet thickness within a particular lot of tablets or between manufacturer's lots should not be apparent to the unaided eye for consumer acceptance of the product. In addition, thickness must be controlled to facilitate packaging. Difficulties may be encountered in the use of unit dose and other types of packaging equipment if the volume of the material being packaged is not consistent. A secondary packaging problem with tablets of variable thickness relates to consistent fill levels of the same product container with a given number of dosage units.

The physical dimensions of the tablet, along with the density of the materials in the tablet formulation and their proportions, determine the weight of the tablet. The size and shape of the tablet can also influence the choice of tablet machine to use, the best particle size for the granulation, production lot sizes that can be made, the best type of tablet processing that can be used, packaging operations, and the cost to produce the tablet. The shape of the tablet alone can influence the choice of tablet machine used. Shaped tablets requiring "slotted punches" must be run at slower speeds than are possible with round tablets, using conventional punches. Because of the nonuniform forces involved within a tablet during compression, the more convex the tablet surface, the more likely it is to cause capping problems, forcing the use of a slower tablet machine or one with precompression capabilities.[6]

Unique Identification Markings. Pharmaceutical companies manufacturing tablets often use some type of unique markings on the tablet in addition to color, to aid in the rapid identification of their products. These markings utilize some form of embossing, engraving, or printing. A look into the product identification section of the current Physician's Desk Reference (PDR),[7] provides a quick reference to the multitude of marking variations, both artistic and informational, that can be produced.

The type of informational markings placed on a tablet usually includes the company name or symbol, a product code such as that from the National Drug Code (NDC) number, the product name, or the product potency. In the future, these identifying marks, in conjunction with a greater diversity of tablet sizes and shapes, may provide the sole means of identification of tablets, if the pharmaceutical industry continues to lose the use of approved Food, Drug, and Cosmetic (FD&C) colors.

Organoleptic Properties. Many pharmaceutical tablets use color as a vital means of rapid identification and consumer acceptance. The color of a product must be uniform within a single tablet (nonuniformity is generally referred to as "mottling"), from tablet to tablet, and from lot to lot. Nonuniformity of coloring not only lacks esthetic appeal but could be associated by the consumer with nonuniformity of content and general poor quality of the product.[8]

The eye cannot discriminate small differences in color nor can it precisely define color. The eye has limited memory storage capability for color, and the storage of visually acquired data is difficult, which results in people perceiving the same color differently and a single person describing the same color differently at different times. In addition, visual color comparisons require that a sample be compared against some color standard. Color standards themselves are subject to change with time, thus forcing their frequent redefinition, which can lead to a gradual and significant change in acceptable color.[8] Efforts to quantitate color evaluations have used reflectance spectrophotometry, tristimulus colorimetric measurements, and the use of a microreflectance photometer to measure the color uniformity and gloss on a tablet surface.[8–10]

The presence of an odor in a batch of tablets could indicate a stability problem, such as the characteristic odor of acetic acid in degrading aspirin tablets; however, the presence of an odor could be characteristic of the drug, (vitamins have a characteristic odor), added ingredients (flavoring agents have pleasant odors), or the dosage form (film-coated tablets usually have a characteristic odor).

Taste is important in consumer acceptance of chewable tablets. Many companies utilize taste panels to judge the preference of different flavors and flavor levels in the development of a product. Owing to the subjectiveness of "taste" preference, however, the control of taste in the production of chewable tablets is often simply the presence or absence of a specified taste.

A tablet's level of flaws such as chips, cracks, contamination from foreign solid substances (e.g., hair, drops of oil, and "dirt"), surface texture ("smooth" versus "rough"), and appearance ("shiny" versus "dull") may have a zero-defect

specification, but the visual inspection techniques used for detecting or evaluating these characteristics are subjective in nature. Electronic devices that are currently being developed hold promise for making inspection a more quantitative and reproducible operation.

Hardness and Friability. Tablets require a certain amount of strength, or hardness and resistance to friability, to withstand mechanical shocks of handling in manufacture, packaging, and shipping. In addition, tablets should be able to withstand reasonable abuse when in the hands of the consumer, such as bouncing about in a woman's purse in a partially filled prescription bottle. Adequate tablet hardness and resistance to powdering and friability are necessary requisites for consumer acceptance. More recently, the relationship of hardness to tablet disintegration, and perhaps more significantly, to the drug dissolution release rate, has become apparent. The monitoring of tablet hardness is especially important for drug products that possess real or potential bioavailability problems or that are sensitive to altered dissolution release profiles as a function of the compressive force employed.

Historically, the strength of a tablet was determined by breaking it between the second and third fingers with the thumb acting as a fulcrum. If there was a "sharp" snap, the tablet was deemed to have acceptable strength. More recently, however, tablet hardness has been defined as the force required to break a tablet in a diametric compression test. To perform this test, a tablet is placed between two anvils, force is applied to the anvils, and the crushing strength that just causes the tablet to break is recorded. Hardness is thus sometimes termed the *tablet crushing strength*. Several devices operating in this manner have been and continue to be used to test tablet hardness: the Monsanto tester, the Strong-Cobb tester, the Pfizer tester, the Erweka tester, and the Schleuniger tester.[11–15]

One of the earliest testers to evaluate tablet hardness was the Monsanto hardness tester, which was developed approximately fifty years ago. The tester consists of a barrel containing a compressible spring held between two plungers. The lower plunger is placed in contact with the tablet, and a zero reading is taken. The upper plunger is then forced against a spring by turning a threaded bolt until the tablet fractures. As the spring is compressed, a pointer rides along a gauge in the barrel to indicate the force. The force of fracture is recorded, and the zero force reading is deducted from it. To overcome the manual nature of the Monsanto tester and the minute or longer time required to make an individual test, the Strong-Cobb tester was developed about twenty years later. The original design employed a plunger activated by pumping a lever arm, which forces an anvil against a stationary platform by hydraulic pressure. The force required to fracture the tablet is read from a hydraulic gauge. Later modifications of the Strong-Cobb tester were built with the force applied by air-pressure rather than by a manual pump.

Approximately one decade later, the Pfizer tester was developed and made available to the industry. This tester operates on the same mechanical principle as a pair of pliers. As the plier's handles are squeezed, the tablet is compressed between a holding anvil and a piston connected to a direct force reading gauge. The dial indicator remains at the reading where the tablet breaks and is returned to zero by depressing a reset button. The Pfizer tester became extensively used in comparison to the earlier testers, based on its simplicity, low cost, and the rapidity with which it could be used.

Two testers have been developed to eliminate operator variation. In the Erweka tester, the tablet is placed on the lower anvil, and the anvil is then adjusted so that the tablet just touches the upper test anvil. A suspended weight, motor driven, moves along a rail, which slowly and uniformly transmits pressure to the tablet. A pointer moving along a scale provides the breaking strength value in kilograms. As shown in Figure 11-1, the Schleuniger tester operates in a horizontal position. An anvil driven by an electric motor presses the tablet at a constant load rate against a stationary anvil until the tablet breaks. A pointer moving along a scale indicator provides the breaking strength value. The instrument reads in both kilograms and Strong-Cobb units. This instrument is currently the most widely employed and has the advantage of being both fast and reproducible.

Unfortunately, these testers do not produce the same results for the same tablet. Studies have shown that operator variation, lack of calibration, spring fatigue, and manufacturer variation contribute greatly to the lack of uniformity. Even those testers designed to eliminate operator variability have been found to vary.[15,16]

Operators must be aware of these variations, especially when the tablets are to be evaluated by other persons or in other labs. For accurate comparison, each instrument should be carefully calibrated against a known standard.

The hardness of a tablet, like its thickness, is a function of the die fill and compression force. At a constant die fill, the hardness values increase and thickness decreases as additional compression force is applied. This relationship holds up to a maximum value for hardness and a mini-

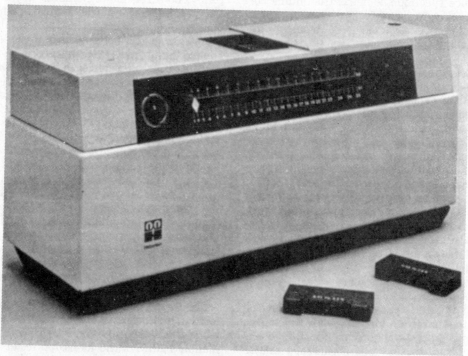

FIG. 11-1. *The Schleuniger tablet hardness tester. (Courtesy of Vector Corporation, Marion, IA.)*

mum value for thickness, beyond which increases in pressure cause the tablet to laminate or cap, thus destroying the integrity of the tablet. At a constant compression force (fixed distance between upper and lower punches), hardness increases with increasing die fills and decreases with lower die fills.

When uniform tooling is used, the die-fill/force relationship makes control of tablet hardness a useful method of physically controlling tablet properties during a production operation, particularly when this measurement is combined with measurements of tablet thickness. The fill/force relationship is also the basis for instrumenting tablet machines.

In general, tablets are harder several hours after compression than they are immediately after compression. Lubricants can affect tablet hardness when they are used in too high a concentration or mixed for too long a period. Large tablets require a greater force to cause fracture and are therefore "harder" than small tablets. For a given granulation, a flat beveled tool produces a tablet harder than a deep cup tool.

Tablet hardness is not an absolute indicator of strength since some formulations, when compressed into very hard tablets, tend to "cap" on attrition, losing their crown portions. Therefore, another measure of a tablet's strength, its friability, is often measured. Tablets that tend to powder, chip, and fragment when handled lack elegance and consumer acceptance, and can create excessively dirty processes in such areas of manufacturing as coating and packaging. They can also add to a tablet's weight variation or content uniformity problems.

The laboratory friability tester is known as the Roche friabilator.[17] This device, shown in Figure 11-2, subjects a number of tablets to the combined effects of abrasion and shock by utilizing a plastic chamber that revolves at 25 rpm, dropping the tablets a distance of six inches with each revolution. Normally, a preweighed tablet sample is placed in the friabilator, which is then operated for 100 revolutions. The tablets are then dusted and reweighed. Conventional compressed tablets that lose less than 0.5 to 1.0% of their weight are generally considered acceptable. Some chewable tablets and most effervescent tablets undergo high friability weight losses, which accounts for the special stack packaging that may be required for these types of tablets. When capping is observed on friability testing, the tablet should not be considered for commercial use, regardless of the percentage of loss seen.

When concave and especially deep concave punches are used in tabletting, and especially

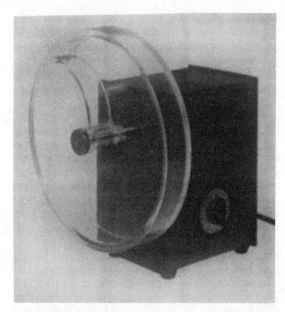

FIG. 11-2. *The Roche type friabilator. (Courtesy of Van-Kel Industries, Chatham, NJ.)*

when the punches are in poor condition or worn at their surface edges, the tablets produced result in "whiskering" at the tablet edge. Such tablets have higher than normal friability values because the "whiskers" are removed in testing. Tablet friability may also be influenced by the moisture content of the tablet granulation and finished tablets. A low but acceptable moisture level frequently acts as a binder. Very dry granulations that contain only fractional percentages of moisture often produce more friable tablets than do granulations containing 2 to 4% moisture. For this reason, the manufacture of chemically stable tablets that contain some hydrolyzable drugs that are mechanically sound is difficult.

The traditional hardness and friability evaluations performed on tablets involve only a small sample of tablets. How the tablets withstand the mechanical shocks of a production environment is related to the large number of tablets involved, the production equipment used, and the skill of the production personnel. Rough handling tests can be performed to give an indication of how well a tablet will hold up in its specified package and shipping container during shipment. Rough handling tests usually include a vibration test, a drop test, and an incline plane impact test.[18] Some investigators have actually shipped bottled products across the country and back again to estimate the strength of the new tablet product in shipment.

Drug Content and Release. As mentioned

earlier, a physically sound tablet may not produce the desired effects. To evaluate a tablet's potential for efficacy, the amount of drug per tablet needs to be monitored from tablet to tablet and batch to batch, and a measure of the tablet's ability to release the drug needs to be ascertained.

Weight Variation. With a tablet designed to contain a specific amount of drug in a specific amount of tablet formula, the weight of the tablet being made is routinely measured to help ensure that a tablet contains the proper amount of drug. In practice, composite samples of tablets (usually 10) are taken and weighed throughout the compression process. The composite weight divided by 10, however, provides an average weight but contains the usual problems of averaged values. Within the composite sample that has an acceptable average weight, there could be tablets excessively overweight or underweight. To help alleviate this problem the United States Pharmacopeia (USP)/National Formulary (NF) provides limits for the permissible variations in the weights of individual tablets expressed as a percentage of the average weight of the sample.[19] The USP weight variation test is run by weighing 20 tablets individually, calculating the average weight, and comparing the individual tablet weights to the average. The tablets meet the USP test if no more than 2 tablets are outside the percentage limit and if no tablet differs by more than 2 times the percentage limit. The weight variation tolerances for uncoated tablets differ depending on average tablet weight (Table 11-1).

The weight variation test would be a satisfactory method of determining the drug content uniformity of tablets if the tablets were all or essentially all (90 to 95%) active ingredient, or if the uniformity of the drug distribution in the granulation or powder from which the tablets were made were perfect. For tablets such as aspirin, which are usually 90% or more active ingredient, the ±5% weight variation should come close to defining true potency and content uniformity (95 to 105% of the label strength) if the

TABLE 11-1. *Weight Variation Tolerances for Uncoated Tablets*

Average Weight of Tablets (mg)	Maximum Percentage Difference Allowed
130 or less	10
130–324	7.5
More than 324	5

Copied from USP XX—NF XV, © 1980, U.S. Pharmacopeial Convention, Inc. Permission granted.

average tablet weight is close to the theoretic average weight. The weight variation test is clearly not sufficient to assure uniform potency of tablets of moderate- or low-dose drugs, in which excipients make up the bulk of the tablet weight.

The potency of tablets is expressed in terms of grams, milligrams, or micrograms (for some potent drugs) of drug per tablet and is given as the label strength of the product. Official compendia or other standards provide an acceptable potency range around the label potency. For highly potent, low-dose drugs such as digitoxin, this range is usually not less than 90% and not more than 110% of the labeled amount. For most other larger-dose drugs in tablet form, the official potency range that is permitted is not less than 95% and not more than 105% of the labeled amount.

In general, official potency analytic methods require that a composite sample of the tablets be taken, ground up, mixed, and analyzed to produce an average potency value. In composite assays, individual discrepancies can be masked by use of the blended sample. Even though the average assay result looks acceptable, it could mask a wide variation in potency, with the result that a patient could be variably underdosed or overdosed. With such a drug as digitoxin, in which the safe and effective level and the toxic level are close (or even overlapping), exceeding the official or accepted potency range is not only undesirable, but possibly dangerous.

Three factors can directly contribute to content uniformity problems in tablets: (1) nonuniform distribution of the drug substance throughout the powder mixture or granulation, (2) segregation of the powder mixture or granulation during the various manufacturing processes, and (3) tablet weight variation. As noted in the previous section, the use of weight cannot be used as a potency indicator, except perhaps when the active ingredient is 90 to 95% of the total tablet weight. In tablets with smaller dosages, a good weight variation does not ensure good content uniformity, but a large weight variation precludes good content uniformity.

To assure uniform potency for tablets of low-dose drugs, a content uniformity test is applied.[19] In this test, 30 tablets are randomly selected for the sample, and at least 10 of them are assayed individually. Nine of the 10 tablets must contain not less than 85% or more than 115% of the labeled drug content. The tenth tablet may not contain less than 75% or more than 125% of the labeled content. If these conditions are not met, the tablets remaining from the 30 must be assayed individually, and none may fall outside of the 85 to 115% range. In evaluating a particular lot of tablets, several samples of tablets should be taken from various parts of the production run to satisfy statistical procedures.

The *purity* of official tablets is usually assured by utilizing raw materials, both active drug and all excipients, that meet official or other rigid specifications. Extraneous substances present in a raw material or a drug that are not specifically allowed by compendial specifications or well-defined manufacturer's specifications may render the product unacceptable for pharmaceutical use. These extraneous substances may be toxic on acute or long-term use or may have an unpredictable or deleterious effect on product stability or efficacy. Certain well-defined impurities often appear in the specification of raw materials or drug substances, or if they are the product of unavoidable decomposition of the drug, they may be listed with an upper tolerance limit. For example, aspirin tablets as specified by the USP may contain no more than 0.15% of free salicylic acid relative to the amount of aspirin present.

Disintegration. A generally accepted maxim is that for a drug to be readily available to the body, it must be in solution. For most tablets, the first important step toward solution is breakdown of the tablet into smaller particles or granules, a process known as *disintegration*. The time that it takes a tablet to disintegrate is measured in a device described in the USP/NF.[19] Wagner has written an excellent review of the disintegration test,[20] to which the reader is referred for a more detailed study.

Research has established that one should not automatically expect a correlation between disintegration and dissolution. However, since the dissolution of a drug from the fragmented tablet appears to control partially or completely the appearance of the drug in the blood, disintegration is still used as a guide to the formulator in the preparation of an optimum tablet formula and as an in-process control test to ensure lot-to-lot uniformity.

The USP device to test disintegration uses 6 glass tubes that are 3 inches long, open at the top, and held against a 10-mesh screen at the bottom end of the basket rack assembly (Fig. 11-3). To test for disintegration time, one tablet is placed in each tube, and the basket rack is positioned in a 1-L beaker of water, simulated gastric fluid, or simulated intestinal fluid, at 37°C ± 2°C, such that the tablets remain 2.5 cm below the surface of the liquid on their upward movement and descend not closer than 2.5 cm from the bottom of the beaker. A standard motor-driven device is used to move the basket

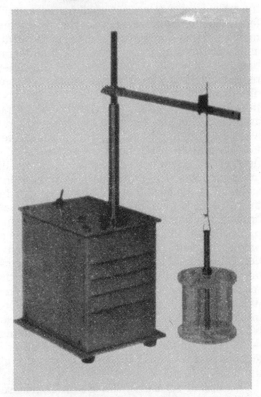

FIG. 11-3. *Tablet disintegration tester. (Courtesy of Van-Kel Industries, Chatham, NJ.)*

assembly containing the tablets up and down through a distance of 5 to 6 cm at a frequency of 28 to 32 cycles per minute. Perforated plastic discs may also be used in the test. These are placed on top of the tablets and impart an abrasive action to the tablets. The discs may or may not be meaningful or impart more sensitivity to the test, but they are useful for tablets that float.

To be in compliance with the USP standards, the tablets must disintegrate, and all particles must pass through the 10-mesh screen in the time specified. If any residue remains, it must have a soft mass with no palpably firm core. Procedures are stated for running disintegration times for uncoated tablets, plain-coated tablets, enteric coated tablets, buccal tablets, and sublingual tablets. Uncoated USP tablets have disintegration time standards as low as 5 min (aspirin tablets), but the majority of the tablets have a maximum disintegration time of 30 min. Enteric coated tablets are to show no evidence of disintegration after 1 hour in simulated gastric fluid. The same tablets are then tested in simulated intestinal fluid and are to disintegrate in 2 hours plus the time specified in the monograph.

Dissolution. The original rationale for using tablet disintegration tests was the fact that as the tablet breaks down into small particles, it offers a greater surface area to the dissolving media and therefore must be related to the availability of the drug to the body. The disintegration test, however, simply identifies the times required for the tablet to break up under the conditions of the test and for all particles to pass through a 10-mesh screen. The test offers no assurance that the resultant particles will release the drug in solution at an appropriate rate. For this reason, dissolution tests and test specifications have now been developed for nearly all tablet products. The rate of drug absorption for acidic drug moieties that are absorbed high in the GI tract is often determined by the rate of drug dissolution from the tablet. If the attainment of high peak blood levels for the drug is a product objective, obtaining rapid drug dissolution from the tablet is usually critically important. The rate of dissolution may thus be directly related to the efficacy of the tablet product, as well as to bioavailability differences between formulations. Therefore, an evaluation as to whether or not a tablet releases its drug contents when placed in the environment of the gastrointestinal tract is often of fundamental concern to the tablet formulator.

The most direct assessment of a drug's release from various tablet formulations or products is accomplished through in vivo bioavailability measurements. The use of in vivo studies is restricted, however, for several reasons: the length of time needed to plan, conduct, and interpret the study; the highly skilled personnel required for human studies; the low precision and high variability typical of the measurements; the high cost of the studies; the use of human subjects for "nonessential" research; and the necessary assumption that a perfect correlation exists between diseased patients and the healthy human subjects used in the test. Consequently, in vitro dissolution tests have been extensively studied, developed, and used as an indirect measurement of drug availability, especially in preliminary assessments of formulation factors and manufacturing methods that are likely to influence bioavailability. As with any in vitro test, it is critically important that the dissolution test be correlated with in vivo bioavailability tests.

Two objectives in the development of in vitro dissolution tests are to show (1) that the release of the drug from the tablet is as close as possible to 100% and (2) that the rate of drug release is uniform batch to batch and is the same as the release rate from those batches proven to be bioavailable and clinically effective. Since 1970, the United States Pharmacopeia and the National Formulary have provided procedures for dissolution testing. They determine compliance with the limits on dissolution as specified in the individual monograph for a tablet (or a capsule). The USPXX/NFXV, Supplement 3, specifies that either of two apparatuses be used for determining dissolution rates.[21]

Apparatus 1. In general, a single tablet is placed in a small wire mesh basket fastened to the bottom of the shaft connected to a variable speed motor (Fig. 11-4A). The basket is immersed in the dissolution medium (as specified in the monograph) contained in a 100-ml flask. The flask is cylindric with a hemispherical bottom. The flask is maintained at 37°C ± 0.5°C by a constant temperature bath. The motor is adjusted to turn at the specified speed, and samples of the fluid are withdrawn at intervals to determine the amount of drug in solution.

Apparatus 2. The same equipment as in apparatus 1 is used, except that the basket is replaced by a paddle, formed from a blade and a shaft, as the stirring element (Fig.4B). The dosage form is allowed to sink to the bottom of the flask before stirring. Dosage forms may have a "small, loose piece of nonreactive material such as not more than a few turns of wire helix" attached to prevent them from floating.[20] Description of a dissolution test in a USP/NF monograph specifies the dissolution test medium and volume, which apparatus is to be used, the speed (rpm) at which the test is to be performed, the time limit of the test, and the assay procedure. The test tolerance is expressed as a percentage of the labeled amount of drug dissolved in the time limit. For example, for methyldopa tablets, the dissolution test calls for a medium of 900 ml of 0.1N HCl, apparatus 2 turning at 50 rpm, and a time limit of 20 min. The accepted amount dissolved in 20 min is not less than 80% of the labeled amount of methyldopa (based on the cited assay procedure).

Dissolution testing and interpretation can be continued through three stages if necessary. In stage $1(S_1)$, six tablets are tested and are acceptable if all of the tablets are not less than the monograph tolerance limit (Q) plus 5%. If the tablets fail S_1, an additional six tablets are tested (S_2). The tablets are acceptable if the average of the twelve tablets is greater than or equal to Q and no unit is less than Q minus 15%. If the tablets still fail the test, an additional 12 tablets are tested. The tablets are acceptable if the average of all 24 tablets is greater than or equal to Q and if not more than 2 tablets are less than Q minus 15%.

Industrial pharmacists routinely test their formulations for dissolution. Their results are plotted as concentration versus time. Values for

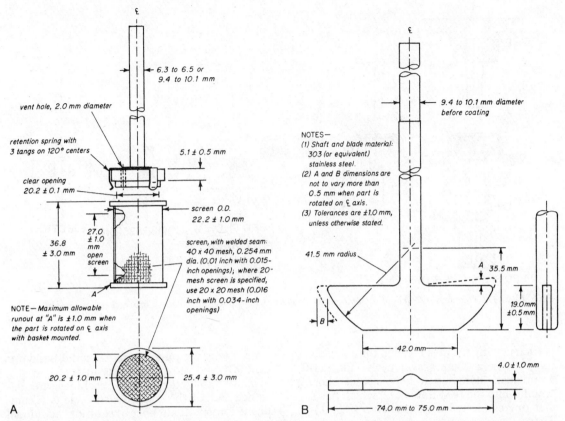

FIG. 11-4. A, *USP dissolution apparatus 1. B, USP dissolution apparatus 2. (Reproduced from the Third Supplement to USP XX-NF XV, © 1982, USP Convention, pages 310 and 311. Permission granted.)*

$t_{50\%}$, $t_{90\%}$, and the percentage dissolved in 30 min are used as guides. The value for $t_{50\%}$ is the length of time required for 50% of the drug to go into solution. A value for $t_{90\%}$ of 30 min is often considered satisfactory and is an excellent goal since a common dissolution tolerance in the USP/NF is not less than 75% dissolved in 45 min.

Tablet Compression Operation

Tablet Compression Machines

Tablets are made by compressing a formulation containing a drug or drugs with excipients on stamping machines called *presses.* Tablet compression machines or tablet presses are designed with the following basic components:

1. Hopper(s) for holding and feeding granulation to be compressed.

2. Dies that define the size and shape of the tablet.

3. Punches for compressing the granulation within the dies.

4. Cam tracks for guiding the movement of the punches.

5. A feeding mechanism for moving granulation from the hopper into the dies.

Tablet presses are classified as either single-punch or multi-station rotary presses. Figure 11-5 illustrates in cross-section the compression process on a single punch machine. Note that all of the compression is applied by the upper punch, making the single punch machine a "stamping press."

Multi-station presses are termed *rotary* because the head of the tablet machine that holds the upper punches, dies, and lower punches in place rotates. As the head rotates, the punches are guided up and down by fixed cam tracks, which control the sequence of filling, compression, and ejection. The portions of the head that hold the upper and lower punches are called the upper and lower turrets respectively, and the

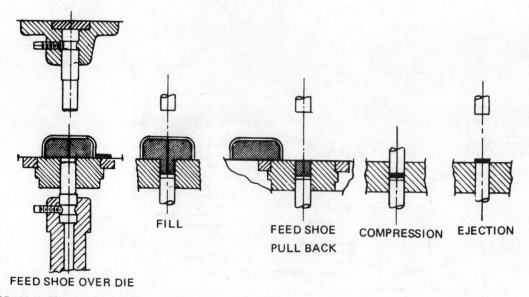

FILL

FEED SHOE
PULL BACK

COMPRESSION

EJECTION

FEED SHOE OVER DIE

FIG. 11-5. *The compression cycle of a single-punch tablet press. (Courtesy of Vector Corporation, Marion, IA.)*

portion holding the dies is called the *die table*. At the start of a compression cycle (Fig. 11-6), granulation stored in a hopper (not shown), empties into the feed-frame (A), which has several interconnected compartments (Fig. 11-7). These compartments spread the granulation over a wide area to provide time for the dies (B) to fill (Fig. 11-6). The pull-down cam (C) of Figure 11-6 guides the lower punches to the bottom of their vertical travel, allowing the dies to overfill. The punches then pass over a weight-control cam (E), which reduces the fill in the dies to the desired amount. A wipe-off blade (D) at the end of the feed-frame removes the excess granulation and directs it around the turret and back into the front of the feed-frame. Next, the lower punches travel over the lower compression roll (F) while simultaneously the upper punches ride beneath the upper compression roll (G). The upper punches enter a fixed distance into the dies, while the lower punches are raised to squeeze and compact the granulation within the dies. To regulate the upward movement of the lower punches, the height of the lower pressure roll is changed. After the moment of compression, the upper punches are withdrawn as they follow the upper punch raising cam (H); the lower punches ride up the cam (I), which brings the tablets flush with or slightly above the surface of the dies. The exact position is determined by a threaded bolt called the *ejector knob*. The tablets strike a sweep-off blade affixed to the front of the feed-frame (A) and slide down a chute into a receptacle. At the same time, the lower punches re-enter the pulldown cam (C), and the cycle is repeated.

Many production tablet machines are designed so that the compression cycle is accomplished more than once (requiring additional granulation hoppers, feed frames, cam tracks, and compression rolls) while the machine head makes a single revolution.

All other parts of a tablet press are designed to control the functioning of the components just listed. Such features as capacity, speed, maximum weight, and pressure vary with the design of the equipment, but the basic elements remain essentially the same.

Although tablet compressing machinery has undergone numerous mechanical modifications over the years, the compaction of materials between a pair of moving punches within a stationary die has remained unchanged. The principal modification from earlier equipment has been an increase in production rate rather than any fundamental change in the process. Better control and simplification have been corollary benefits.

In recent years, there has been a change by manufacturers from activities concerned with production rate to problems of process improvement and control. Growth of governmental and pharmacopeia tests related to intertablet weight and potency variation, as noted earlier in the chapter, have created some of the new requirements for tablet compressing machinery. As tablet production rates have increased with modern equipment, for example, the need for automatic

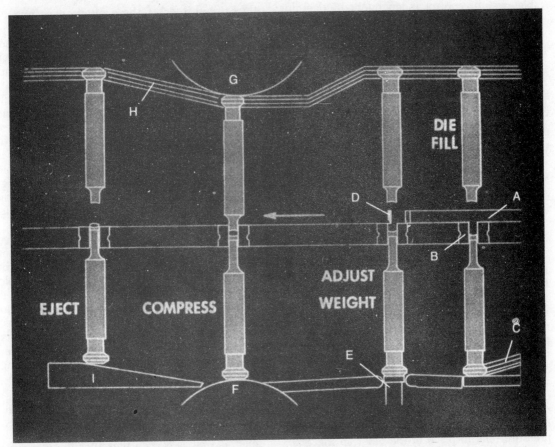

FIG. 11-6. *The compression cycle of a rotary tablet press. (See text for explanation of lettered labels.) (Courtesy of Thomas Engineering, Hoffman Estates, IL.)*

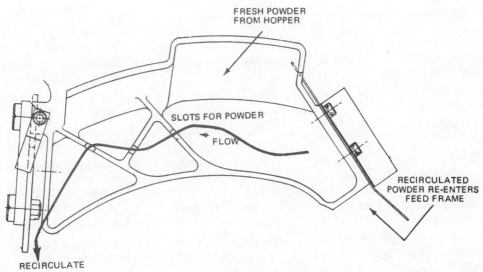

FIG. 11-7. *Granulation flow in an open feed frame of a rotary tablet press. (Courtesy of Vector Corporation, Marion, IA.)*

tablet weight control independent of operator vigilance has become a matter of increasing concern. This topic is discussed later, in the section "Auxiliary Equipment."

Tabletting presses vary principally in the number of tooling stations available for compression and in special application features. Table 11-2 tabulates the maximum and minimum tablet manufacturing output capable within the various press models of several manufacturers.

A tablet machine's output is regulated by three basic characteristics of its design:

Number of tooling sets

Number of compression stations

Rotational speed of the press

In general, all rotary presses are engineered for fast and economical production of all kinds of tablets. Larger machines can readily produce several million tablets each in a working day, and their performance can be geared to continuous low-maintenance operation. Figure 11-8 is an example of a modern high-speed tabletting machine.

There are many modifications and options that can be obtained from various manufacturers. One modification, which is found on most modern high-speed tablet presses, is the use of hydraulic or pneumatic pressure to control the pressure rolls in place of the older spring type pressure. Either of these alternatives gives a smoother pressure or compressive load force over a longer period of time. Hydraulic or pneumatic pressure is much more accurate and can be set with closer tolerances, which do not change with time or fatigue.

Special adaptations of tablet machines allow for the compression of "layered" tablets and coated tablets. Precompression stations are also available to help in compressing difficult granulations. Available with certain Fette machines is a device that chills the compression components to allow for the compression of low-melting-point substances such as waxes, thereby making it possible to compress products with low melting points, such as suppositories.

There are many basic and optional features available in tablet machines, including some not mentioned in this text. Manufacturers' brochures should be closely checked for available features. One should attend equipment shows, if possible, to obtain up-to-date information on equipment developments. In some instances, test runs on machinery may be made before a final decision to purchase new high-speed tablet equipment or specialized granulation or drying equipment.

Compression Machine Tooling

As mentioned earlier, the size and shape of a tablet as well as certain identification markings

TABLE 11-2. *Selected Rotary Tablet Press Characteristics*

Manufacturer	Number of Stations Available		Rated Output, Tablets per Minute (TPM)		U.S. Representative
	Min	Max	Min	Max	
Colton	12	90	480	16,000	Vector Corp. Marion, IA 52302
Wilhelm Fette, Gmbh Hamburg, W. Germany	20	55	300/900	3300/8250	Raymond Automation Company, Inc. Norwalk, CT 06856
Kilian & Co., Gmbh Koln, W. Germany	14	67	140/383	1083/10,000	INPPEC Fairfield, CT 06430
Manesty Machines Ltd. Liverpool, England	16	69	600/1500	3330/10,000	Thomas Engineering Hoffman Estates, IL 60172
Stokes-Merrill	33	65	1200/3300	3500/10,000	Stokes-Merrill Division Penwalt Corp. Oak Brook, IL 60521
Korsch Maschinenfabrik Berlin, W. Germany	20	55	540/1100	1640/5500	Aeromatic East Towaco, NJ 07082
Hata Ironworks Hori Engineering Co., Osaka, Japan	28	71	420/1420	1960/7100	Elizabeth-Hata International Inc. McKeesport, PA 15132

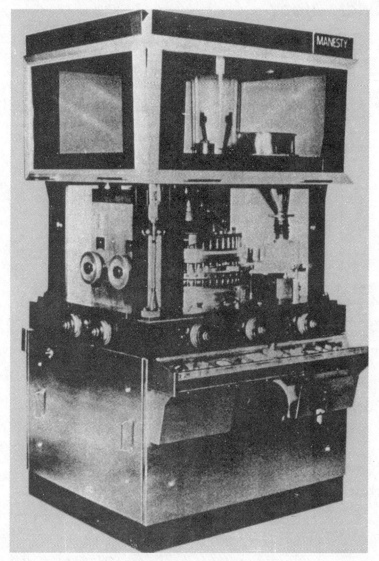

FIG. 11-8. *The Manesty Nova rotary tablet press. (Courtesy of Thomas Engineering, Hoffman Estates, IL.)*

are determined by the compression machine tooling. Each tooling set consists of a die and upper and lower punches. Since each tablet is formed by a tooling set, the tooling must meet many requirements to satisfy the needs of dosage uniformity, production efficiency, and esthetic appearance.

The terminology used with tooling is illustrated in Figure 11-9. The most common tools employed are referred to as BB tooling and are 5.25 inches in length, and have a nominal barrel diameter of 0.75 inches and 1-inch head diameter. B tooling is identical to the BB type except that the lower punch is only 3%16 inches long. D tooling is popular for large tablets, utilizing a 1-inch barrel diameter, 1¼-inch head diameter, and 5.25-inch length. The dies that are used with the above punches are either a 0.945-inch outside diameter (OD) die capable of making a 7/16-inch round tablet or 9/16-inch capsule-shaped tablet; or a 1³/16-inch OD die capable of handling a 9/16-inch round or ¾-inch capsule shaped tablet.

Several types of steel are normally used in the manufacture of compression tooling. These steels differ in toughness, to withstand the cyclic compacting forces (ductility), and in wear resistance. Unfortunately, no single steel type has a high resistance to abrasive wear and a high ductility. Therefore, the selection of the

PUNCH BODY

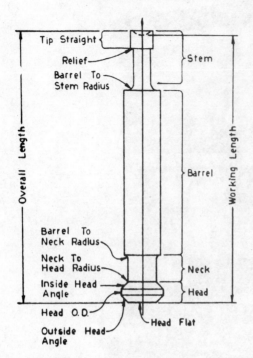

Tip Straight
Relief
Barrel To Stem Radius
Stem
Overall Length
Working Length
Barrel
Barrel To Neck Radius
Neck To Head Radius
Inside Head Angle
Neck
Head
Head O.D.
Head Flat
Outside Head Angle

PUNCH TIP

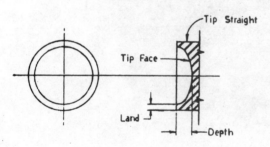

Tip Straight
Tip Face
Land
Depth

DIE

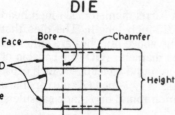

Face   Bore   Chamfer
O D
Die Groove
Height
I.D.

FIG. 11-9. *Tablet press tooling nomenclature. (Courtesy of Thomas Engineering, Hoffman Estates, IL.)*

best steel for a specific application must be based on experience and an accumulated history of the product being tabletted. In the selection of the proper steel for a specific use, one should also consider the shape of the punch tip, whether or not debossing is to be employed on the tooling, the expected compression forces involved, and whether the materials to be processed are abrasive or corrosive.

The size, shape, and contour of a tablet is almost unlimited within the given limits of the specified die size. A survey of the PDR Product Identification section reveals numerous variations on tablet size and shape.[4] In addition, tooling can be made with certain other information to aid in producing a visibly unique tablet product. Company names or symbols, trade names, dosage strength, or National Drug Code (NDC) numbers can be cut or engraved into a punch face, or the punches may be scored, to produce uniquely embossed or engraved tablets. Even though tooling design would appear to be limitless, certain practical aspects do limit design implementation. Because of the movement of tooling during a compression operation, certain tablet shapes or contour configurations perform better than others. Round tablets perform better than irregularly shaped tooling since they do not require "keying" to maintain the proper upper punch orientation with the die. When the tip on an upper punch is not round, it must not rotate, or it will strike the edge of the die hole as it descends for compression. To prevent this, a slot is cut longitudinally into the barrel of the punch, and a key is inserted. This key protrudes a short distance so that it engages a similar slot cut into the upper punch guides on the tablet press. Lower punches do not need keys because their tips remain within the die bore, which controls the axial movement of the punch. Because keyed punches cannot rotate, wear is distributed unevenly, and punch life is shortened.

When a press is set up with keyed punches, the upper punches are inserted first to determine the placement of the dies. Once the dies are properly aligned and seated, they are locked in place, and the lower punches are inserted. The more curvature that is built into a tablet contour, the more difficult it is to compress, especially if the tablet tends to laminate or cap. The engraving or embossing on a tablet must be designed to be legible, must not add to compression problems, and must fit on the tablet surface. Many considerations, at close tolerances, must be incorporated in tooling design to produce tablets that are uniform and esthetic. Manufacturing specifications for tooling have been standardized by the Industrial Pharmaceutical

Technology Section of the Academy of Pharmaceutical Sciences in its Standard Specifications of Tabletting Tools.[22]

Because of its hard steel structure, tablet tooling may appear to be indestructible. During normal use, however, the punches and dies become worn, and the cyclic application of stress can cause the steel to fatigue and break. Improper storage and handling can readily result in damage that necessitates discarding of an entire tooling set. The punch tips are especially delicate and susceptible to damage if the tips make contact with each other, the dies, or the press turret upon insertion or removal of the tools from the tablet machine. A good tool control system must be employed to maintain the history of each tool set, not only to maintain a constant surveillance of critical tolerances altered by wear, but also to eliminate product mixups by preventing the wrong tooling from being used for a product.

To avoid tooling damage, compressive loads or pressures at the pressure rolls must be translated into a calculation of pressure at the punch tips. As tablet punch diameter decreases, less force is required to produce the same pressure at the punch face, since the face represents a smaller fraction of a unit area (square inch). The formula for the area of a circle is πr^2 where r is the radius of the circle. Given a flat punch face, the area of a ¼-inch-diameter punch would thus be $3.14 \times (\frac{1}{8})^2$ or $3.14 \times \frac{1}{64}$, or approximately ½₀ square-inch. If a 1-ton load is being applied by the pressure roll, this area is translated as 2000 pounds on ½₀ square inch, or 40,000 pounds on 1 square inch, a gross overload.

The following are manufacturers of tablet compression tooling:

Thomas Engineering, Hoffman Estates, IL

Stokes, Warminster, PA

Natoli Engineering Company, Chesterfield, MO

Elizabeth Carbide Die Co., McKeesport, PA

Key Industries, Englishtown, NJ

Advance Engineering and Manufacturing Co., St. Louis, MO

Aeromatic Inc., Somerville, N.J.

Carle and Montanari Inc., Hackensack, NJ

I. Holland Ltd., Nottingham, U.K.

Auxiliary Equipment

There are some common auxiliary pieces of equipment that increase the efficiency of the tablet compression operation. In many cases, the speed of the die table is such that the dwell time of a die under the feed frame is too short to allow for adequate or consistent gravity filling of the die with granulation. Improper filling of the dies with granulation results in unsatisfactory weight variation and content uniformity of the resulting tablets. A similar result can occur with a poorly flowing granulation. To help alleviate these problems, mechanized feeders can be employed to force granulation into the dies (Fig. 11-10).

The high tablet output rates of modern presses demand that the granulation hoppers be refilled at frequent intervals; the larger the tablet is, the more frequently the hopper needs to be replenished. Allowing a tablet machine to run "dry" results in a series of rapidly degenerating and unacceptable events. First, low-weight tablets and tablets with poor weight variation are produced. Then, the soft granulation is unable to be formed into tablets. Finally, the tooling is usually ruined, particularly with thin tablets, by the punches being forced together without any granulation between them. Because of the relatively low volume of press hoppers, the filling of hoppers by hand on high-speed presses is inefficient, increases the risk of punch damage, and can contribute to weight variation problems. Therefore, mechanized equipment has been developed to load granulation into the press hoppers.

A popular method of handling large quantities of material is to place bulk granulation containers directly above tabletting machines to gravity-feed the granulation into hoppers. This can be accomplished by several means. Bulk granulation containers can be placed on floors above a tablet machine, and granulation can then be directed through openings in the floor into the hoppers. In a similar fashion, granulation containers can be held on mezzanines above tablet machines. If such overhead room is unavailable, hoists and mechanical lifts can be used to elevate granulation containers or material transfer devices directly in position above the press. Granulation level sensors can be used to stop the press automatically when the granulation level drops to a critical level in the hopper.

The high rate of tablet output with modern presses calls for a higher frequency or even continuous monitoring of tablet weight. Electronic monitoring devices, such as the Thomas Tablet Sentinel (Fig. 11-11), Pharmakontroll, and the Kilian Control System-MC, monitor the force at each compression station, which correlates with tablet weight. These monitors are also capable of initiating corrective actions, altering the amount

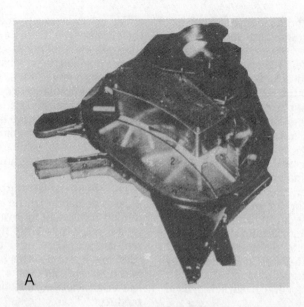

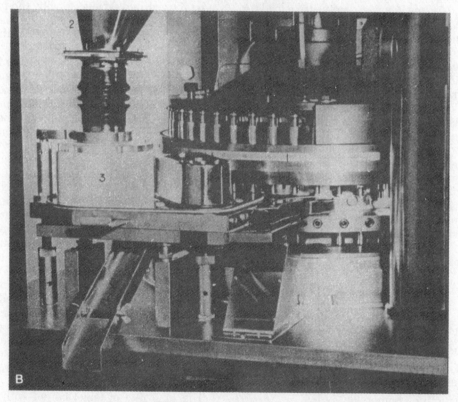

FIG. 11-10. A, *Manesty granulation feeding device. (1) Granulation input port from tablet machine feed hopper. (2) Rotating feed fingers. (3) Compressed tablet scrape-off blade. B, Manesty granulation feeding device mounted on a rotary tablet machine. (1) Tablet machine turret. (2) Tablet machine hopper. (3) Feeding device. (4) Compressed tablet output chute. (Courtesy of Thomas Engineering, Hoffman Estates, IL.)*

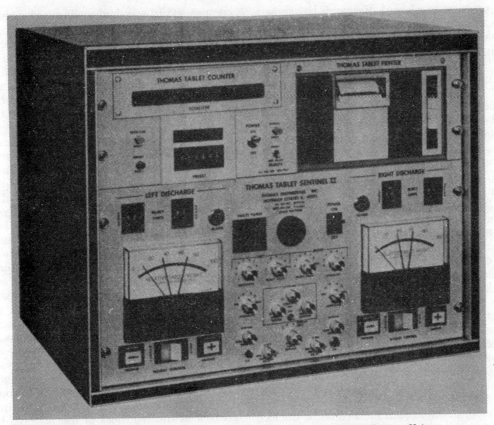

FIG. 11-11. *Thomas Table Sentinel II. (Courtesy of Thomas Engineering, Hoffman Estates, IL.)*

of die fill to maintain a fixed force, ejecting tablets that are out of specification, counting, and documenting the machine operation throughout the run.

In almost all cases, tablets coming off a tablet machine bear excess powder and are run through a tablet deduster to remove that excess.

In-Process Quality Control

During the compression of tablets, in-process tests are routinely run to monitor the process, including tests for tablet weight, weight variation, hardness, thickness, disintegration, and various evaulations of elegance. The in-process tests are performed by production and/or quality control (QC) personnel. In addition, many in-process tests are performed during product development by the formulator. Such testing during development has become increasingly important in recent years for process validation purposes. The data supplied by the formulator is usually employed by QC personnel to establish the test limits. At the start-up of a tablet compression operation, the identity of the granula-

tion is verified, along with the set-up of the proper tabletting machine and proper tooling.

Processing Problems

In the normal process of developing formulations, and in the routine manufacture of tablets, various problems occur. Sometimes, the source of the problem is the formulation, the compression equipment, or a combination of the two.

Capping and Lamination. *Capping* is a term. used to describe the partial or complete separation of the top or bottom *crowns* of a tablet from the main body of the tablet. *Lamination* is the separation of a tablet into two or more distinct layers. Usually, these processing problems are readily apparent immediately after compression; however, capping and lamination may occur hours or even days later. Subjecting tablets to the friability test described earlier is the quickest way of revealing such problems. Capping and lamination have in the past been attributed to air entrapment. During the compression process, air is entrapped among the particles or granules and does not escape until the compression pressure is released. Research has shown, however, that capping and lamination are due to the deformational properties of the formulation during and immediately following compression.[6,23]

During compaction, particles undergo sufficient plastic deformation to produce die-wall pressures greater than can be relieved by elastic recovery when the punch pressure is removed. In some materials, this die-wall pressure causes enough internal stress to cause a crack to propagate and initiate fracture of the compact in the die. If the excess stresses do not initiate fracture upon decompression in the die, the compact may laminate or cap upon ejection from the die. As the compact is ejected, the die-wall pressure falls to zero. The emerging portion of the compact expands while the confined portion cannot, thus concentrating shear stresses at the edge of the die and causing a break to develop. Tablets that do not fracture have the ability to relieve the shear stresses developed during decompression and/or ejection by plastic deformation. This stress relaxation is time-dependent; therefore, the occurrence of tablet fracture is also time-dependent. Intact tablets of acetaminophen, methenamine, and erythromycin can be made if the decompression is extended for several hours. Rapid decompression results in tablets that fracture. Stress relaxation could be the explanation for some practical tabletting problems. Tablet lamination or capping problems are often eliminated by precompression, slowing the tabletting rate, and reducing the final compression pressure. As the stress relaxation time is increased, the amount of stress needing to be relieved is reduced, allowing an intact compact to be formed.

Often, deep concave punches produce tablets that cap. The curved part of such tablets expands radially while the body of the tablet cannot, which establishes a shear stress that produces the fracture. Flat punches may eliminate this additional shear stress.

A certain percentage of moisture is often essential for good compaction. A granulation that is too dry tends to cap or laminate for lack of cohesion. For moisture-critical granulations, the addition of a hygroscopic substance, e.g., sorbitol, methylcellulose, or polyethylene glycol 4000, can help to maintain a proper moisture level. Capping and lamination may also be encountered in direct compression product development. Some powder or fine particulate materials may not be compressible or may have poor compression properties. Relative compressibility of various materials may be reflected by their degree of consolidation (crown thickness) when compressed in standard tooling under identical compression conditions.

Tablet tooling can also be a cause of capping. The concave or beveled edge faces of punches gradually curve inward with use and form a "claw" that can pull off the crowns of a tablet. Wear in the upper punch guides accelerates this claw formation by permitting the punch tips to strike the edges of the die holes. Also, the greater the radius of curvature of the punch face, the greater is the force exerted on the edges and the less on the center of the tablet at the moment of compression.

Dies develop a wear "ring" in the area of compression. As the ring develops, and enlarges, the tablets that are compressed in the rings have a diameter that is too large to pass easily through the narrower portion of the die above the ring. Upon ejection, this constriction causes the tablet to cap or laminate. A simple solution of this particular problem is to turn the die over so that compression occurs in an unworn area above the ring. On some presses, the depth of penetration of the upper punch can be regulated so that compression may be performed over some range of locations within the die. There are also dies available with tungsten carbide inserts. The carbide is so durable that the casing wears out before the insert does. Wear on tablet tooling increases as the hardness of the material being compressed increases. Most organic materials are soft; certain inorganic materials such as magnesium trisilicate are relatively hard and abrasive.

Another cause of capping is an incorrect setup at the press. When a compressed tablet is ejected from a die, the lower punch must rise flush with or protrude slightly above the face of the die at the point where the tablet strikes the sweep-off blade. If the punch remains below the face of the die, the sweep-off blade cuts off the tablet, leaving the bottom in the die. A less severe result of this incorrect adjustment is that the edge of the tablet catches on the die and chip. An incorrect adjustment of the sweep-off blade can also result in tablet fracture. If the blade is adjusted too high, tablets can start to travel under it, become stuck, and break off. The resulting broken pieces of tablets then enter the feed frame; if they are large enough, they can cause a disruption of the granulation feed, as well as affect the weight and hardness of subsequent tablets.

Picking and Sticking. "Picking" is a term used to describe the surface material from a tablet that is sticking to and being removed from the tablet's surface by a punch. Picking is of particular concern when punch tips have engraving or embossing. Small enclosed areas such as those found in the letters "B," "A," and "O" are difficult to manufacture cleanly. Tablet materials that stick to the punches can accumulate to the point of obliterating the tip design. "Sticking" refers to tablet material adhering to the die wall. When sticking occurs, additional force is required to overcome the friction between the tablet and the die wall during ejection. Serious sticking at ejection can cause chipping of a tablet's edges and can produce a rough edge. Also, a sticking problem does not allow the lower punches free movement and therefore can place unusual stresses on the cam tracks and punch heads, resulting in their damage. Sticking can also apply to the buildup of material on punch faces.

These flaws have many remedies. Lettering should be designed as large as possible, particularly on punches with small diameters. The tablet can perhaps be reformulated to a larger size. Plating of the punch faces with chromium is a method for producing a smooth, nonadherent face.

In some cases, colloidal silica added to the formula acts as a polishing agent and makes the punch faces smooth so that material does not cling to them. On the other hand, the frictional nature of this material may require additional lubrication to facilitate release of the tablet from the die. Sometimes, additional binder or a change in binder may make the granules more cohesive, and therefore less adherent, than before.

Low-melting-point substances, either active ingredients or additives such as stearic acid and polyethylene glycol, may soften sufficiently from the heat of compression to cause sticking. Dilution of the active ingredient with additional higher-melting-point materials and a consequent increase in the size of the tablet may help. The level of low-melting-point lubricants may be reduced, or higher-melting-point replacements may be substituted. When a low-melting-point medicament is present in high concentration, refrigeration of the granulation and the press may be in order. Excessive moisture may be responsible for sticking, and further drying of the granulation is then required.

Mottling. Mottling is an unequal distribution of color on a tablet, with light or dark areas standing out in an otherwise uniform surface. One cause of mottling is a drug whose color differs from the tablet excipients or a drug whose degradation products are colored. The use of colorants may solve the above problem but can create others. A dye can cause mottling by migrating to the surface of a granulation during drying. To overcome this difficulty, the formulator may change the solvent system, change the binder system, reduce the drying temperature, or grind to a smaller particle size. The use of colorants in direct compression formulations can lead to mottling if the dye is not well dispersed or if its particle size is too large.

Certain colored adhesive gel solutions may not be distributed well because they must be hot when added to much cooler powder mixtures. The adhesive then precipitates from solution and carries most of the color with it. Further wetting, even overwetting, is needed to disperse the binder and the color. The additional mixing and increased activation of the binder, however, may result in tablets with increased disintegration times. Therefore, a better practice may be to incorporate fine powder adhesives such as acacia and tragacanth into the product before adding the granulating fluid, or to disperse a dry color additive during the powder blending step.

Weight Variation. In previous sections, weight variation of tablets has been mentioned as an important in-process control measurement, and weight variation specifications have been given. The weight of a tablet being compressed is determined by the amount of granulation in the die prior to compression. Therefore, anything that can alter the die-filling process can alter tablet weight and weight variation.

Granule Size and Size Distribution Before Compression. Variations in the ratio of small to large granules and in the magnitude of difference between granule sizes influence how the void spaces between particles are filled. Thus, although the apparent volume in the die is essentially the same, different proportions of large and small particles may change the weight of fill in each die. Furthermore, if large granules are being used to fill a small die cavity, relatively few granules are required, and the difference of only a few granules around the average may represent a high percentage weight variation. If hundreds of granules are required on the average for die fill, a variation of a few granules around the average would produce a minor weight variation, given a narrow particle size range.

Poor Flow. The die-fill process is based on a continuous and uniform flow of granulation from the hopper through the feed frame. When the granulation does not flow readily, it tends to move spasmodically through the feed frame so that some dies are incompletely filled. Similarly, dies are not filled properly when machine speed is in excess of the granulation's flow capabilities. With poor flow, the addition of a glidant such as talcum or colloidal silica, or an increase in the amount already present, may be helpful.

Also available are induced die feeders, which mechanically "force" the granulation down into the die cavities as they pass beneath the feed frame.

Poor flow through the feed frame is usually a sign that the granulation is not flowing properly out of the hopper. As particulate solids move under the force of gravity through progressively smaller openings, they are subjected to uneven pressures from the mass above and alongside. Depending on the geometry of the hopper, this situation may give rise to one or another of two causes for poor flow: "arching" or "bridging," and "rat-holing." Figure 11-12 illustrates these phenomena. When poor hopper flow occurs, it may be controllable with vibrators attached to the hopper sides to induce the granulation flow.

Devices designed to improve poor flow characteristics of materials often introduce another problem, however. Since most tablet granulations consist of materials with a range of particle sizes, the vibration or mixing action of the flow-promoting devices may induce segregation and stratification of the particles. The larger particles tend to drift upward while the smaller particles sift downward. Not only can the resulting "classification" of particle sizes cause appreciable changes in tablet weight and weight variation as described earlier, but it can also lead to poor content uniformity, since drug is often not uniformly distributed between the larger and smaller particles. Poor particulate flow may be caused not by the granulation, but by poor design of the granulation hopper, which can be exaggerated by dents that effectively cut off the flow. Poor weight variation can also be caused by surges of excessive flow. Direct compression granulations fed through typical wet-granulation hoppers and feed frames are prone to this type of flow. Often, restricting the flow out of the hopper corrects the problem. Recently, a patent was issued for a new feed frame design that accommodated excessive flow from the hopper without compromising uniform weight variation.[24]

Poor Mixing. Sometimes, the lubricants and glidants are not thoroughly distributed. The flow of particles is then impaired, and the granules do not move efficiently into the dies. There is a tendency to minimize the mixing time during lubricant addition to prevent or reduce granule friability; however, inadequate mixing at this stage can result in unsatisfactory granulation flow.

Punch Variation. When lower punches are of unequal lengths—the difference may be only a few thousandths of an inch—the fill in each die varies because the fill is volumetric. Only a good punch and die control program can provide tooling of uniform dimensions.

Hardness Variation. Hardness variation is a problem that has the same causes as weight variation. Hardness depends on the weight of material and the space between the upper and lower punches at the moment of compression. If the volume of material or the distance between punches varies, hardness is likewise inconsistent.

Double Impression. A last problem for discussion is that of double impression. This involves only punches that have a monogram or other engraving on them. At the moment of compression, the tablet receives the imprint of the punch. On some machines, the lower punch is free to drop and then travel uncontrolled for a short distance before it rides up the ejection cam to push the tablet out of the die. During its free travel, it rotates. At this point, the punch may make a new, although lighter, impression on the bottom of the tablet, resulting in a double imprint. Similar problems can be encountered with engraved upper punches and tablet machines that utilize two compression stages to compress a tablet. The first stage, *precompression,* uses a lower compaction force than the final compression stage, but the tablet does receive the imprint of the punch. If the upper punch is uncontrolled, it can rotate during the short travel to the final compression stage and thus create a double imprint. The newer presses have antiturning devices as an integral part of their design and construction.

Tablet Granulations

Basic Characteristics

The characteristics of a tablet that make it a popular dosage form, e.g., compactness, physical stability, rapid production capability, chemical stability, and efficacy, are in general dictated primarily by the qualities of the granulation from which it is made. Basically stated, materials intended for compaction into a tablet must

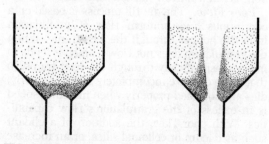

FIG. 11-12. *Bridging (left); rat-holing (right).*

possess two characteristics: fluidity and compressibility. To a great extent, these properties are required by the compression machine design. As previously discussed, good flow properties are essential for the transport of the material through the hopper, into and through the feed frame, and into the dies. Tablet materials should therefore be in a physical form that flows smoothly and uniformly. The ideal physical form for this purpose is spheres, since these offer minimum contact surfaces between themselves and with the walls of the machine parts. Unfortunately, most materials do not easily form spheres; however, shapes that approach spheres improve flowability. Therefore granulation is in part the pharmaceutical process that attempts to improve the flow of powdered materials by forming spherelike or regularly shaped aggregates called *granules*. The need to assess the shape of particles and their relative regularity or approximation to spheres has led to the development of equations whereby certain "factors" can be calculated to provide quantitative comparisons of different particle shapes. By measuring particle surface area (S), volume (V) and a projected equivalent diameter (d_p), a volume shape factor (α_v), a surface shape factor (α_s), and a shape coefficient (α_{vs}) can be calculated using equations (1) to (3) for quantitative work.[25]

$$\alpha_s = \frac{S}{d_p^z} \tag{1}$$

$$\alpha_v = \frac{V}{d_p^z} \tag{2}$$

$$\alpha_{vs} = \frac{\alpha_s}{\alpha_v} \tag{3}$$

The shape coefficient for a sphere is 6. As a particle becomes more irregular in shape, the value of α_{vs} increases. For a cube, α_{vs} is equal to 6.8.

The other desirable characteristic, compressibility, is the property of forming a stable, compact mass when pressure is applied. The requisite physical properties and the forces that hold the tablet together are discussed in Chapter 4, "Compression and Consolidation of Powdered Solids." The consideration of compressibility in this discussion is limited to stating that granulation is also the pharmaceutical process that converts a mixture of powders, which have poor cohesion, into aggregates capable of compaction.

Granulation Properties

There are many formulation and process variables involved in the granulation step, and all of these can affect the characteristics of the granulations produced. Therefore, methods to measure certain granulation characteristics have been developed to monitor granulation suitability for tabletting.

Particle Size and Shape. The particle size of a granulation is known to affect the average tablet weight, tablet weight variation, disintegration time, granule friability, granulation flowability, and the drying rate kinetics of wet granulations.[26–28] The exact effect of granule size and size distribution on processing requirements, bulk granulation characteristics, and final tablet characteristics depends upon the formulation ingredients and their concentrations, as well as the type of granulating equipment and processing conditions employed. Therefore, the formulator should determine for each formulation and manufacturing process the effects of granule size and size distribution on processability and tablet quality features. The methods for measuring and interpreting particle size and particle size distribution are discussed in Chapter 2, "Milling."

Surface Area. The determination of the surface area of finely milled drug powders may be of value for drugs that have only limited water solubility. In these cases, particle size, and especially the surface area of the drug, can have a significant effect upon dissolution rate. The determination of the surface area of granulations is not a common practice. In general, if one is interested in effects of granulation surface upon measurable properties of the final dosage form, particle size of the granulation is measured. An inverse relationship normally exists between particle size and surface area; however, granulations can have convoluted structures with considerable internal surface. Technology available for determining the surface area of coarse powders or agglomerates (granulations) is not as advanced as that available for fine powders. The two most common methods for determining surface area of solid particles are gas adsorption and air permeability. In the first method (gas adsorption), the amount of gas that is adsorbed onto the powder to form a monolayer is measured and then used to calculate the surface area of the powder sample. Air permeability, the rate at which air permeates a bed of powder, is used to calculate the surface area of the powder sample. These methods are described in Chapter 4.

Density. Granule density may influence compressibility, tablet porosity, dissolution, and other properties. Dense, hard granules may require higher compressible loads to produce a cohesive compact, let alone tablets of acceptable appearance that are free from visible granule boundaries. The higher compression load, in turn, has the potential of increasing the tablet disintegration and drug dissolution times. Even if the tablets disintegrate readily, the harder, denser granules may dissolve less readily. At the same time, harder, denser granules are usually less friable. Basically, two methods are used to determine granule density. Both involve the use of a pycnometer. In one, the intrusion fluid is mercury, and in the other, it is a solvent of low surface tension (e.g., benzene) in which the granules are not soluble. The accuracy of these pycnometer methods depends on the ability of the intrusion fluids to penetrate the pores of the granules. Density is calculated from the volume of intrusion fluid displaced in the pycnometer by a given mass of granulation:[25]

$$D = M/V_p - V_i \qquad (4)$$

where D is density, V_p is the total volume of the pycnometer, and V_i is the volume of intrusion fluid containing that mass of granules (M) that is required to fill the pycnometer.

The term *bulk density* refers to a measure used to describe a packing of particles or granules. The equation for determining bulk density (ρ_b) is:[25]

$$\rho_b = \frac{M}{V_b} \qquad (5)$$

where M is the mass of the particles and V_b is the total volume of packing. The volume of the packing can be determined in an apparatus consisting of a graduated cylinder mounted on a mechanical tapping device that has a specially cut rotating cam. An accurately weighed sample of powder or granulation is carefully added to the cylinder with the aid of a funnel. Typically, the initial volume is noted, and the sample is then tapped until no further reduction in volume is noted. The volume at this tightest packing is then used in equation (1) to compute bulk density ρ_b. A sufficient number of taps should be employed to assure reproducibility for the material in question. The tapping should not produce particle attrition or a change in the particle size distribution of the material undergoing testing. See Chapter 4 for further details.

An important measure that can then be obtained from bulk density determinations is the percent compressibility, C, which is defined as follows:[25]

$$C = \frac{\rho_b - \rho_u}{\rho_b}(100) \qquad (6)$$

where ρ_u is the untapped bulk density (often called *loose* or *aerated* bulk density). In theory, the more compressible a bed of particulates is, the less flowable the powder or granulation will be. Conversely, the less compressible a material is, the more flowable it will be.

Bulk density largely depends on particle shape. As the particles became more spherical in shape, bulk density is increased. In addition, as granule size increases, bulk density decreases. The smaller granules are able to form a close, more intimate packing than larger granules.

Strength and Friability. A granule is an aggregation of component particles that is held together by bonds of finite strength. The strength of a wet granule is due mainly to the surface tension of liquid and capillary forces. These forces are responsible for initial agglomeration of the wet powder. Upon drying, the granule has strong bonds resulting from fusion or recrystallization of particles and curing of the adhesive or binder. Under these conditions, van der Waals forces are of sufficient strength to produce a strong, dry granule. Measurements of granule strength are therefore aimed at estimating the relative magnitude of attractive forces seeking to hold the granule together. The resultant strength of a granule depends, of course, on base material, the kind and amount of granulating agent used, the granulating equipment used, and so forth. Factors affecting granule strength are discussed in this section.

Granule strength and friability are important, as they affect changes in particle size distribution of granulations, and consequently, compressibility into cohesive tablets. When determining a relative measure of granule strength, two distinct types of measurements can be made. Perhaps, the one most commonly used is that of compression strength. In this test, a granule is placed between anvils, and the force required to break the granule is measured.[29,30] Other common methods of studying granule strength are those that relate to friability measurements. Most of these methods are variations of the American Society for Testing Materials (ASTM) tumbler test for the friability of coal, and provide a means of measuring the propensity of granules to break into smaller pieces when subjected to disruptive forces.[31]

Flow Properties. The flow properties of a material result from many forces. Solid particles attract one another, and forces acting between particles when they are in contact are predominately surface forces. There are many types of forces that can act between solid particles: (1) frictional forces, (2) surface tension forces, (3) mechanical forces caused by interlocking of particles of irregular shape, (4) electrostatic forces, and (5) cohesive or van der Waals forces. All of these forces can affect flow properties of a solid. They can also affect granule properties such as particle size, particle size distribution, particle shape, surface texture or roughness, residual surface energy, and surface area. With fine powders ($\leq 150 \mu$m), the magnitude of the frictional and van der Waals forces usually predominate. For larger particles ($\geq 150 \mu$m) such as granules produced by a wet granulation technique, frictional forces normally predominate over van der Waals forces. Also, as particles increase in size, mechanical or physical properties of particles and their packings become important. While an evaluation of some of the fundamental properties of particles discussed earlier (e.g., shape and bulk density) is important, there are tests that can be employed as flow measurements of the effect of all the interparticulate forces acting at once. Two of the most common methods are (1) repose angle, and (2) hopper flow rate measurements.

Repose Angle. The fixed funnel and free-standing cone methods employ a funnel that is secured with its tip at a given height, H, above graph paper that is placed on a flat horizontal surface. Powder or granulation is carefully poured through the funnel until the apex of the conical pile just touches the tip of the funnel. Thus, with R being the radius of the base of the conical pile:

$$\tan \alpha = \frac{H}{R} \qquad (7)$$

or

$$\alpha = \arctan\frac{H}{R} \qquad (8)$$

where α is the angle of repose. The fixed cone method establishes the diameter of the cone base by using a circular dish with sharp edges. Powder is poured onto the center of the dish from a funnel that can be raised vertically until a maximum cone height, H, is obtained. The repose angle is calculated as before. In the tilting box method, a rectangular box is filled with powder and tipped until the contents begin to slide. In the revolving cylinder method, a cylinder with a transparent end is made to revolve horizontally when half filled with powder. The maximum angle that the plane of powder makes with the horizontal surface on rotation is taken as the angle of repose. The angle determined by these first three methods is often referred to as the

static angle of repose, and the angle arrived at in the last method is commonly called the *kinetic* or *dynamic angle of repose.* Values for angles of repose $\leq 30°$ usually indicate a free-flowing material and angles $\geq 40°$ suggest a poorly flowing material. As mentioned previously, flow of coarse particles is also related to packing densities and mechanical arrangements of particles. For this reason, a good auxiliary test to run in conjunction with the repose angle test is the compressibility test, discussed previously. From the angle of repose and compressibility values, a reasonable indication of a material's inherent flow properties should be possible.

Hopper Flow Rates. Hopper flow rates have been used as a method of assessing flowability. Instrumentation to obtain hopper flow rates continually monitors the flow of material out of conical hoppers onto a recording balance device. Instrumentation of this kind is quite simple, and results are easy to interpret, making the method attractive from a pragmatic standpoint. Unfortunately, the two methods used for studying flow, hopper tests and repose angles, do not correlate well.

Compaction. The process of consolidating and compacting powder or granule materials to form a tablet is complex, owing to the numerous internal events that act simultaneously (see Chap. 4). The basic tool that has been developed for studying the compression process is the instrumented tablet press. Tablet presses are instrumented by affixing transducers to measure the forces applied during the compression process. The signals produced by the transducer system are then monitored by some means—most recently, by computer. Properly instrumented and monitored tablet presses have been shown to be of great assistance in studying the mechanism of compaction, the relationship of compaction mechanism to tablet properties, and various formulation evaluations. Such studies have also allowed for the development of compression profile references for comparison, the development of automatic control systems, and the monitoring of tooling wear.[32]

Manufacture of Granulations

Dry Manufacturing Methods

The manufacture of granulations for tablet compression may follow one or a combination of three established methods: the dry methods of direct compression, compression granulation, and wet granulation. Table 11-3 compares the type and number of processing steps commonly required with each technique. A consideration of the important aspects of these processes illustrates the advantages and disadvantages of each.

Direct Compression. There are a few crystalline substances, such as sodium chloride, sodium bromide, and potassium chloride, that may be compressed directly. The vast majority of medicinal agents are rarely so easy to tablet, however. In addition, the compression of a single substance may produce tablets that do not disintegrate. If disintegration is a problem, other components are needed, which in turn may interfere with the compressibility of the active ingredient and thus minimize the usefulness of the method. Most materials possess relatively weak intermolecular attraction or are covered with films of adsorbed gases that tend to hinder compaction. Thus, most large-dose drugs do not lend themselves to this process. With many other drugs having small doses, uniform blends of the drug and coarser direct compression diluents cannot be achieved, which makes this process impractical. However, the use of compressible diluents with many moderate-dose drugs makes this process the most streamlined method of tablet manufacture (Table 11-3).

A directly compressible diluent is an inert substance that may be compacted with little difficulty and may compress even when quantities of drugs are mixed with it. Compression capacity is still maintained when other tablet materials necessary for flow, disintegration, and so forth are blended in. Directly compressible vehicles are examined in detail later in this chapter. Direct compression materials, in addition to possessing good flow and compressibility, must be inert, tasteless, reworkable, able to disintegrate, and inexpensive.

Even though direct compression has some important advantages (low labor input, a dry process, fewest processing steps) there are some limitations to the technique.

1. Differences in particle size and bulk density between the drug and diluent may lead to stratification within the granulation. The stratification may then result in poor content uniformity of the drug in the compressed tablet. The stratification and resultant content uniformity problems are of special concern with low-dose drugs.

2. A large-dose drug may present problems with direct compression if it is not easily compressible by itself. To facilitate compression, noncompressible large-dose drugs, which are usually restricted to about 30% of a direct compression formula, could require an amount of diluent so large that the resultant tablet is costly and difficult to swallow.

3. In some instances, the direct compression diluent may interact with the drug. A good example of such a reaction is that which occurs between amine compounds and spray-dried lactose, as evidenced by a yellow discoloration.

4. Because of the dry nature of direct compression, static charge buildup can occur on the drug during routine screening and mixing, which may prevent a uniform distribution of the drug in the granulation.

The equipment and procedures used in direct compression are basically screening or milling and mixing. These topics are covered in Chapter 1, "Mixing," and Chapter 2, "Milling."

Compression Granulation. Compression granulation has been used for many years, and is a valuable technique in situations where the effective dose of a drug is too high for direct compaction, and the drug is sensitive to heat, moisture, or both, which precludes wet granulation. Many aspirin and vitamin formulations are prepared for tabletting by compression granulation.

Compression granulation involves the compaction of the components of a tablet formulation by means of a tablet press or specially designed machinery, followed by milling and screening, prior to final compression into a tablet. When the initial blend of powders is forced into the dies of a large-capacity tablet press and is compacted by means of flat-faced punches, the compacted masses are called *slugs*, and the process is referred to as "slugging." The slugs are then screened or milled to produce a granular form of tabletting material, which now flows more uniformly than the original powder mixture. When a single slugging process is insufficient to confer the desired granular properties to the material, the slugs are sometimes screened, slugged again, and screened once more.

TABLE 11-3. *Processing Steps Commonly Required in the Various Tablet Granulation Preparation Techniques*

Processing Step	Wet	Dry	Direct
Raw material	X	X	X
Weigh	X	X	X
Screen	X	X	X
Mix	X	X	
Compress (slug)		X	
Wet mass	X		
Mill	X		
Dry	X		
Mill	X	X	
Mix	X	X	
Compress	X	X	X

Slugging is just an elaborate method of subjecting a material to increased compression time. The act of slugging followed by screening and subsequent compression of the particles is roughly equivalent to an extended dwell time during compression in a tablet machine. The two or more times that the material is subjected to compaction pressures causes a strengthening of the bonds that hold the tablet together. The resultant granules also increase the fluidity of these powder mixtures, which by themselves do not flow well enough to fill the dies satisfactorily.

As shown in Table 11-3, the compression granulation method requires less equipment and space than other methods, and eliminates the addition of moisture and the application of heat, as found in the wet massing and drying steps of the wet granulation method.

On a large scale, compression granulation can also be performed on a specially designed machine called a *roller compactor*. Roller compactors are capable of producing as much as 500 kg per hour or more of compacted ribbon-like material, which can then be screened or milled into a granulation suitable for compression into tablets.

Roller compactors, utilize two rollers that revolve toward each other (Fig. 11-13). By means of a hydraulic ram forcing one of the rollers against the other, the machine is capable of exerting known fixed pressures on any powdered material that flows between the rollers. Powdered material is fed between the rollers by a screw conveyor system. After passing through the rollers, the compacted mass resembles a thin wide ribbon that has fallen apart into large segments. These are equivalent to the slugs produced by the slugging process. The segments are then screened or milled for the production of granules.

The compaction force of the roller compactor is controlled by three variables: (1) the hydraulic pressure exerted on the compaction rolls, (2) the rotational speed of the compaction rolls, and (3) the rotational speed of the feed screws. The roll speed and the feed-screw speed have the greatest effect on the compaction process. The feed screws on most modern compactors consist of a variable-speed horizontal and vertical screw. The horizontal screw picks up the powder from the hopper and maintains a continuous flow to the vertical screw. The vertical screw delivers the powder to the compaction rolls. The vertical screw speed is critical for uniform compaction. It serves to deaerate the powder and maintains a constant flow onto the compaction rolls. Any variation in deaeration or load causes extreme

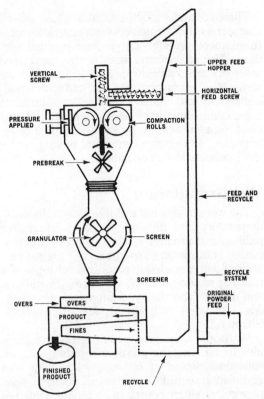

FIG. 11-13. *Schematic diagram of a Chilsonator roller compactor in a granulation production system. (Courtesy of the Fitzpatrick Company, Elmhurst, IL.)*

changes in the compact. The vertical feed screw is usually set so that it delivers more material than the compaction rolls accept, assuring constant loading during the compaction process. The speed of the compaction rolls controls the pressure dwell time, which has a great effect on the density and hardness of the compact.

A standard procedure for testing compaction uniformity and machine capacity is to select a hydraulic pressure in the mid-ranges of the equipment. Set the compaction roll at the slowest speed, and set the feed screw at the highest speed. If the powders are compactible in the first pass, the machine will overload. When this happens, the compaction roll speed should be increased until the loading is constant. Maximum throughput is achieved at this setting for the material being tested. If no overloading occurs, the powder should be passed through a second time, using the same procedure. The roller compactor offers the advantages over the slugging process of increased production capacity, greater control of compaction pressure and dwell time, and no need for excessive lubrication of the powder.

There are many modifications available on roll compactors. Roll designs cover a complete range from smooth to sign curves and serrated surfaces. The shapes and sizes of the screw feed assembly are available in a wide range of designs. Most compactors can be fitted with liquid-cooled rolls and chambers. All manufacturers of roller compactors have pilot plant facilities and offer complete testing programs. Trial runs are advisable, so that the compactor is suitable for the materials to be compacted.

Wet Granulation

The wet granulation technique uses the same preparatory and finishing steps (screening or milling, and mixing) as the two previously discussed granulation techniques. The unique portions of wet granulation process involve the wet massing of the powders, wet sizing or milling, and drying. The theory, equipment, and methods associated with drying are discussed in Chapter 3.

Methods. Wet granulation forms the granules by binding the powders together with an adhesive, instead of by compaction. The wet granulation technique employs a solution, suspension, or slurry containing a binder, which is usually added to the powder mixture; however, the binder may be incorporated dry into the powder mix, and the liquid may be added by itself.

The method of introducing the binder depends on its solubility and on the components of the mixture. Since, in general, the mass should merely be moist rather than wet or pasty, there is a limit to the amount of solvent that may be employed. Therefore, when only a small quantity is permissible, the binder is blended in with the dry powders initially; when a large quantity is required, the binder is usually dissolved in the liquid. The solubility of the binder also has an influence on the choice of methods, since the solution should be fluid enough to disperse readily in the mass.

The liquid plays a key role in the granulation process. Liquid bridges are developed between particles, and the tensile strength of these bonds increases as the amount of liquid added is increased. These surface tension forces and capillary pressure are primarily responsible for initial granule formation and strength. Once the granulating liquid has been added, mixing continues until a uniform dispersion is attained and all the binder has been activated. During granulation, particles and agglomerates are subjected to consolidating forces by action of machine parts and of interparticulate forces. Granulation in large blenders requires 15 min to an hour. The length of time depends on the wetting properties of the powder mixture and the granulating fluid, and upon the efficiency of the mixer. A rough way of determining the end point is to press a portion of the mass in the palm of the hand; if the ball crumbles under moderate pressure, the mixture is ready for the next stage in processing, which is wet screening.

The wet screening process involves converting the moist mass into coarse, granular aggregates by passage through a hammer mill or oscillating granulator, equipped with screens having large perforations. The purpose is to further consolidate granules, increase particle contact points, and increase surface area to facilitate drying. Overly wet material dries slowly and forms hard aggregates, which tend to turn to powder during subsequent dry milling. There are many instances in which wet milling may be omitted, with a considerable saving of time. The formulator should be alert to these opportunities and not follow the old method blindly.

A drying process is required in all wet granulation procedures to remove the solvent that was used in forming the aggregates and to reduce the moisture content to an optimum level of concentration within the granules. During drying, interparticulate bonds result from fusion or recrystallization and curing of the binding agent, with van der Waals forces playing a significant role.

After drying, the granulation is screened again. The size of the screen depends upon the grinding equipment used and the size of the tablet to be made.

The use of volatile or inflammable solvents for wet granulation creates other problems. Safety considerations demand that at a minimum, the work areas be well-ventilated to reduce direct toxic effects or to keep the solvent vapor concentration below explosion limits. Also, all equipment should be electrically grounded to prevent sparks that could initiate explosions. Explosion-proof or explosion-resistant motors may also be required. If solvent granulating systems are to be used, the entire process should be thoroughly discussed, and the facilities should be inspected by the company's safety engineer.

Exhausting solvent vapors or drying granulations made with solvents also requires special precautions. Environmental Protection Agency (EPA) regulations limit the amount of solvent vapors that can be exhausted into the atmosphere. Such EPA limits could require recovery or burning of the solvent vapors, which are expensive operations. Ovens employed for drying granulations wetted with explosive solvents should employ high airflow rates, to stay well below vapor explosive limit concentrations in air. Such ovens should also contain appropriate controls to prevent explosions due to accumulation of vapors following a power outage or during later resumption of power.

Equipment. When traditional equipment is used in the conventional wet granulation scheme (Table 11-4), the entire process is labor-intensive and time-consuming. The equipment used for granulation is not highly effective for dry mixing. Therefore, in many instances, a different mixer is used for dry mixing prior to granulating. Examples are sigma blade and planetary mixers. Granulating mixers are slow, are generally poor powder mixers, and require care for even addition of granulating liquids. Also, considerable time is needed to distribute the binder properly throughout the mass.

While some tablets are still made in the traditional manner, newer equipment has been developed that can accomplish both dry mixing and wet granulation efficiently and in much less time. These new mixers are classified as high-speed mixer/granulators.

TABLE 11-4. *Some Common Tablet Excipients*

Diluents	
Lactose USP	Mannitol USP
Lactose USP, anhydrous	Sorbitol
Lactose USP, spray-dried	Sucrose USP powder
Directly compressible starches	Sucrose-based materials
Hydrolyzed starches	Calcium sulfate dihydrate NF
Microcrystalline cellulose NF	Dextrose
Other cellulose derivatives	
Dibasic calcium phosphate dihydrate NF	

Binders and Adhesives	
Acacia	Starch, pregelatinized
Cellulose derivatives	Sodium alginate and alginate
Gelatin	derivatives
Glucose	Sorbitol
Polyvinylpyrrolidone (PVP)	Tragacanth
Starch, paste	

Disintegrants	
Starch	Cellulose derivatives
Starch derivatives	Alginates
Clays	PVP, cross-linked
Cellulose	

Lubricants	
Stearic acid	Polyethylene glycols
Stearic acid salts	Surfactants
Stearic acid derivatives	Waxes
Talc	

Glidants and Flow Promoters	
Silica derivatives	
Talc	
Cornstarch	

Colors, Flavors and Sweeteners	
FD & C and D & C dyes and lakes	
Spray-dried and other flavors	
Natural sweeteners	
Artificial sweeteners	

The Littleford Lodige mixer was one of the first high-shear powder blenders capable of rapidly blending pharmaceutical powders and wet massing within the same equipment. With some formulations, the equipment may also be capable of producing agglomerated granular particles that are ready for fluid bed or other drying methods without further processing. Figure 11-14 illustrates a conventional Lodige mixer and describes the various assemblies of the unit. The unit consists of a horizontal cylindric shell equipped with a series of plow-shaped mixing tools and one or more high-speed blending chopper assemblies mounted at the rear of the mixer. When the chopper blades are operated during dry mixing, dry lumps of powder are effectively dispersed so that sieving is no longer an essential prerequisite of powder blending when this type of equipment is employed. For the addition of liquids, an injection tube terminating in one or more spray nozzles is provided. The nozzles are located immediately above the chopper assembly.

In operation, the plow-shaped mixing tools may be revolved at variable speeds to maintain the contents of the mixer in an essentially fluid-ized condition and provide a high-volume rate of transfer of material back and forth across the blender. When liquid granulating agents are added to dry powders, the liquid enters the mixer under pressure through the liquid nozzle immediately above the chopper assembly, or assemblies, and is immediately dispersed.

Using this type of high-shear powder mixing equipment, complete mixing may be obtained in as little as 30 to 60 sec. A temperature rise of 10 to 15° may be expected if dry blending is continued over a period of 5 to 10 min. When a high-speed, high-shear mixer of the Litteford Lodige type is used for wet granulation, the power used by the mixer increases as the powder mass becomes increasingly wet. Power usage is often reflected in the readings of an ammeter or watt-meter mounted on the equipment and may be useful in helping to identify the proper end point for the wet granulation process.

The Diosna mixer/granulator is another type of high-speed powder mixer and processor (Fig. 11-15). The mixer utilizes a bowl (1) mounted in the vertical position. A high-speed mixer blade (2) revolves around the bottom of the bowl. The blade fits over a pin bar at the bottom of the mix-

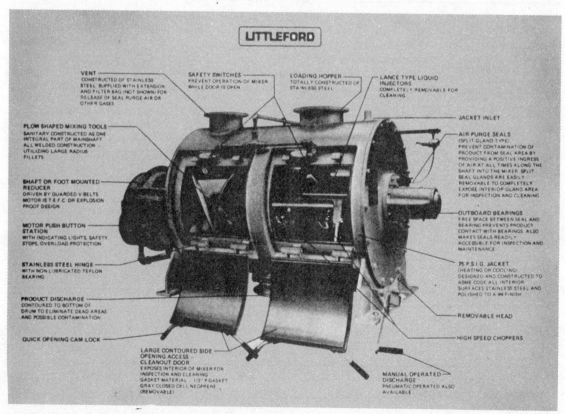

FIG. 11-14. *The Littleford Lodige mixer. (Courtesy of Littleford Brothers, Florence, KY.)*

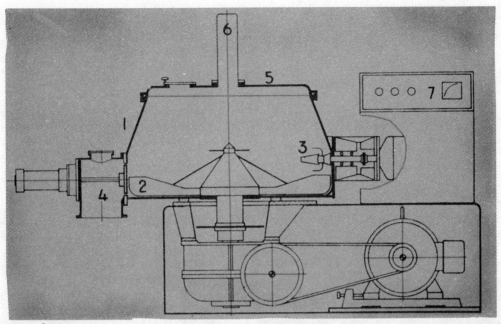

FIG. 11-15. *Schematic diagram of the Diosna mixer. (1) Mixer bowl. (2) High-speed mixer blade. (3) High-speed chopper blade. (4) Pneumatic discharge port. (5) Mixed lid. (6) Exhaust air sleeve. (7) Mixer control panel. (Courtesy of Dierks and Sohne, Osnabrück, West Germany.)*

ing bowl, which powers the blade. The blade is specially constructed to discourage material from getting under it. The mixer also contains a high-speed chopper blade (3), which functions as a lump and agglomerate breaker. A pneumatic discharge port (4) provides the unit with automatic discharge. The unit is provided with a lid (5) and the larger units employ a counterweight to assist in raising and lowering the lid. The lid has three openings: one to accommodate a spray nozzle, a second larger opening for an air exhaust sleeve (6), and a third opening for a viewing port. The units are also equipped with an ammeter on the control panel, (7) which may be employed to determine the end point of granulation operations. Typical time sequences for the use of a Diosna mixer are as follows: mixing, 2 min or less; granulating, 8 min or less; discharge, 1 min with the discharge capable of being preset when the pneumatic discharge system is in place.

Figure 11-16 describes the Littleford MGT mixer/granulator, which has been developed to meet granulation needs more specifically. For comparison, the horizontal configuration of the Lodige unit (Fig. 11-15) has been rotated 90° to a vertical configuration, the drum assembly has been converted to a bowl assembly, and a discharge port has been added to facilitate emptying and cleaning of the bowl. The principle of

operation, however, is the same as that described previously for the Diosna mixer.

When a high-shear solids mixer is used in a production operation, mounting the mixer in a position that allows the bowl from a fluid bed dryer to be placed under the mixer facilitates materials transfer. Most fluid bed dryers for production operations have wheeled assemblies to facilitate materials transfer to and from the fluid bed unit. Since wet granular material may resist transfer by air conveyor systems such as the Vacumax, a gravity type of transfer provision may be especially helpful. The need to raise the equipment to an appropriate working height in order to discharge directly into a bowl of a fluid bed dryer is not regarded as a major disadvantage, provided that powder can be conveniently charged into the unit when it is in a raised position.

Figure 11-17 illustrates the Gral mixer/ granulator. This equipment is a modification of the industrial planetary mixers. The difference between the Gral mixer/granulator and a standard planetary mixer is that the new unit contains two mixing devices. A large mixing arm is shaped to the rounded configuration of the bowl and provides the large-scale mixing motion on the powder. A smaller chopper blade enters off-center from the mixing arm and is located above it. The larger mixing blade and a second-

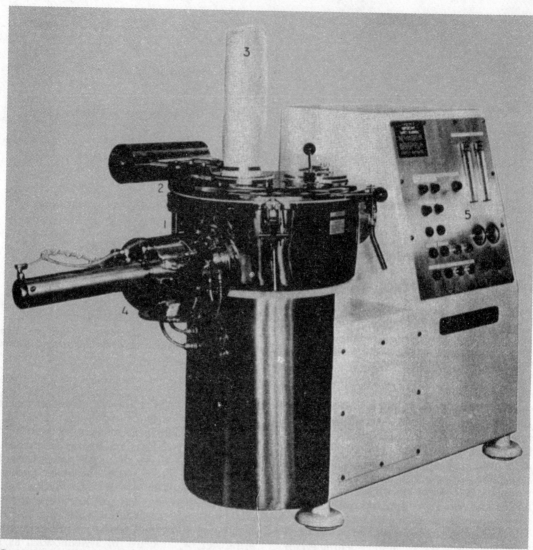

FIG. 11-16. *The Littleford MGT mixer-granulator. (1) Bowl. (2) Lid with counter weight. (3) Exhaust sleeve. (4) Discharge port. (5) Control panel. (Courtesy of Littleford Brothers, Florence, KY.)*

ary chopper blade system is therefore similar to the Lodige and Diosna units previously described. The difference, however, is that the Gral unit has the configuration of a planetary top-entering mixer. The mixing bowl may be loaded at floor level, as in Figure 11-17, and then raised to the mixing position by the hydraulic bowl elevator cradle. The bowl is brought into contact with a cover providing a tight seal. An advantage of the unit is that it may be discharged by its hydraulic port while in the raised position, offering sufficient space for a container to be placed beneath the discharged port. The entire mixer unit does not have to be elevated to provide this vertical discharge distance as is

necessary with the two previously mentioned high-shear mixers. Another advantage of the unit is that the main mixing blade is not a part of the bowl, thus making cleanup easier. Fluid may be injected into the mixer bowl. The equipment is available with time control.

Tablet Design and Formulation

The three basic methods of tablet manufacture have been previously detailed, the desirable properties and required features of granulations and tablets defined, and the interrelationships between many of these properties and the processing and machine variables noted. Regardless

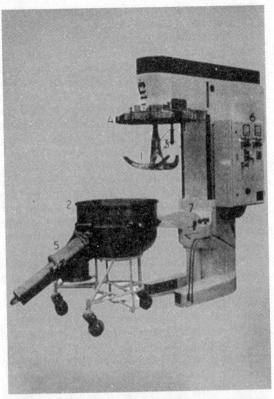

FIG. 11-17. *The Gral mixer-granulator. (1) Mixing arm. (2) Bowl. (3) Chopper blade. (4) Bowl cover. (5) Hydraulic discharge port. (6) Mixer control panel. (7) Bowl elevator cradle. (Courtesy of Machines Collette, Wheeling, IL.)*

of how tablets are manufactured, conventional oral tablets for ingestion usually contain the same classes of components in addition to the active ingredients, which are one or more agents functioning as (1) a diluent, (2) a binder or an adhesive, (3) a disintegrant, and (4) a lubricant. Some tablet formulations may additionally require a flow promoter. Other more optional components include colorants, and in chewable tablets, flavors and sweeteners. All nondrug components of a formula are termed excipients.

Diluents

Diluents are fillers designed to make up the required bulk of the tablet when the drug dosage itself is inadequate to produce this bulk. The dose of some drugs is sufficiently high that no filler is required (e.g., aspirin and certain antibiotics). Round tablets for ingestion are usually in a size range of 3/16 to 1/2 inch. Tablets below 3/16 inch may be difficult for the elderly to handle, and those larger than 1/2 inch become difficult to swallow. This provides a tablet weight range of

perhaps 120 to 700 mg for standard density organic materials. By using oval tablets, which may be easier to swallow, tablets weighing up to 800 mg or more may be produced. Tablet formulations may contain a diluent for secondary reasons: to provide better tablet properties such as improved cohesion, to permit use of direct compression manufacturing, or to promote flow.

Regardless of why a diluent is selected, diluents and *all* other tablet excipients must meet certain criteria in the formulation. These include the following:

1. They must be nontoxic and acceptable to the regulatory agencies in all countries where the product is to be marketed.

2. They must be commercially available in an acceptable grade in all countries where the product is to be manufactured.

3. Their cost must be acceptably low.

4. They must not be contraindicated by themselves (e.g., sucrose) or because of a component (e.g., sodium) in any segment of the population.

5. They must be physiologically inert.

6. They must be physically and chemically stable by themselves and in combination with the drug(s) and other tablet components.

7. They must be free of any unacceptable microbiologic "load."

8. They must be color-compatible (not produce any off-color appearance).

9. If the drug product is also classified as a food, (certain vitamin products), the diluent and other excipients must be approved direct food additives.

10. They must have no deleterious effect on the bioavailability of the drug(s) in the product.

There are cited cases of pharmaceutical manufacturers actually producing products in which an excipient reduced the bioavailability of a drug, or in which chemical incompatibilities existed. The former situation occurred with the marketing of an antibiotic that utilized a calcium salt as the diluent. The tetracycline product made with a calcium phosphate filler had less than half the bioavailability of the standard product.[33] Divalent and trivalent cations form insoluble complexes and salts with a number of amphoteric or acid functionality antibiotics, which greatly reduces their absorption (which is also why milk should not be coadministered with these drugs). A classic case of a chemical incompatibility that went unrecognized for several years was the interaction of certain amine drugs with the commonly used diluent lactose, in the presence of a metal stearate lubricant (such as magnesium stearate); the resulting tablets were gradually discolored with time.[34-35] Tablet formulators should remember that physical and chemical interactions between formulation components may be promoted by the intimate contact between potential reactants that are tightly compressed together in a tablet compact. Thus, materials that are capable of forming a eutectic mixture, for example, may pose no problem when loosely packed as a powder in a capsule, while the same formulation when compressed in a tablet forms a compact that quickly softens and becomes unacceptable.

Table 11-4 lists some of the commonly used tablet diluents. Note that several of the diluents listed exist as hydrates (dibasic calcium phosphate and calcium sulfate). Diluents that exist in their common salt form as hydrates, containing appreciable bound water as water of crystallization, may nevertheless be excellent for very water-sensitive drugs, provided that the bound water is not released under any elevated storage condition to which the product might be exposed. Dibasic calcium phosphate and calcium sulfate have the advantages of possessing low concentrations of unbound moisture and having a low affinity for atmospheric moisture. These are required features for any excipient material to be combined with a water-sensitive drug. The bound water of calcium sulfate is not released until a temperature of approximately 80°C is reached. Such bound water is usually unavailable for chemical reaction. Such excipients containing tightly bound water but having a low remaining moisture demand may be vastly superior to an anhydrous diluent, which has a moderate to high moisture demand.

Lactose is the first diluent listed in Table 11-4 because it is still the most widely used diluent in tablet formulation. Lactose is an excipient that has no reaction with most drugs, whether it is used in the hydrous or anhydrous form. Anhydrous lactose has the advantage over lactose in that it does not undergo the Maillard reaction, which can lead to browning and discoloration with certain drugs, as noted previously. The anhydrous form, however, picks up moisture when exposed to elevated humidity. Such tablets may have to be carefully packaged to prevent moisture exposure. When a wet granulation process is employed, the hydrous form of lactose should generally be used. Two grades of lactose are commonly available commercially: a 60- to 80-mesh (coarse) and an 80- to 100-mesh (regular) grade. In general, lactose formulations show good drug release rates, their granulations are readily dried, and the tablet disintegration times of lactose tablets are not strongly sensitive to variations in tablet hardness. Lactose is a low-cost diluent, but it may discolor in the presence of amine drug bases or salts of alkaline compounds.

Spray-dried lactose is one of several diluents now available for direct compression following mixing with the active ingredient, and possibly, a disintegrant and a lubricant. If this form of lactose is allowed to dry out and the moisture content falls below the usual 3% level, the material loses some of its direct compressional characteristics. In addition to its direct compression properties, spray-dried lactose also has good flow characteristics. It can usually be combined with as much as 20 to 25% of active ingredient without losing these advantageous features. Spray-dried lactose is especially prone to darkening in the presence of excess moisture, amines, and other compounds, owing to the presence of a furaldehyde. A neutral or acid lubricant should be used when spray-dried lactose is employed.

Starch, which may come from corn, wheat or potatoes, is occasionally used as a tablet diluent. The USP grade of starch, however, has four flow and compression characteristics and possesses a high typical moisture content of between 11 and 14%. Specially dried types of starch that have a standard moisture level of 2 to 4% are available, but at a premium price. Use of such starches in wet granulation is wasteful since their moisture levels increase to 6 to 8% following moisture exposure.

Various directly compressible starches are now available commercially. Sta-Rx 1500 is one such free-flowing, directly compressible starch; it may be used as a diluent, binder, and/or disintegrating agent. Since it is self-lubricating, it may be compressed alone, but when combined with as little as 5 to 10% of drug, it typically requires addition of a lubricant, and possibly a flow promoter such as 0.25% of a colloidal silicone dioxide. Sta-Rx 1500 contains about 10% moisture and is reportedly prone to softening when combined with excessive amounts (more than 0.5%) of magnesium stearate.

Two hydrolyzed starches are Emdex and Celutab, which are basically 90 to 92% dextrose and about 3 to 5% maltose. They are free-flowing and directly compressible. These materials may be used in place of mannitol in chewable tablets because of their sweetness and smooth feeling in the mouth. These materials contain about 8 to 10% moisture and may increase in hardness after compression.

Dextrose is also used as a tablet diluent. It is available from one supplier under the name Cerelose and comes in two forms: as a hydrate, and in anhydrous form for when low moisture contents are required. Dextrose is sometimes combined in formulation to replace some of the spray-dried lactose, which may reduce the tendency of the resulting tablets to darken.

Mannitol is perhaps the most expensive sugar used as a tablet diluent, but because of its negative heat of solution, its slow solubility, and its pleasant feeling in the mouth, it is widely used in chewable tablets. It is relatively nonhygroscopic and can be used in vitamin formulation, in which moisture sensitivity may be a problem. Mannitol formulations typically have poor flow characteristics and usually require fairly high lubricant levels.

Sorbitol is an optical isomer of mannitol and is sometimes combined in mannitol formulations to reduce diluent cost; however, sorbitol is hygroscopic at humidities above 65%. Both of these sugars have a low caloric content and are noncariogenic.

Sucrose, or sugar, and various sucrose-based diluents are employed in tablet making. Some manufacturers avoid their use in products that would subject a diabetic to multiple gram quantities of sugar. Some of the sucrose-based diluents have such tradenames as Sugartab (90 to 93% sucrose plus 7 to 10% invert sugar), DiPac (97% sucrose plus 3% modified dextrins), and Nu Tab (95% sucrose and 4% invert sugar with a small amount of corn starch and magnesium stearate). All of these diluents are available for direct compression, and some are also employed, with or without mannitol, in chewable tablets. All have a tendency to pick up moisture when exposed to elevated humidity.

Microcrystalline cellulose, often referred to by the tradename Avicel, is a direct compression material. Two tablet grades exist: PH 101 (powder) and PH 102 (granules). The flow properties of the material are generally good, and the direct compression characteristics are excellent. This is a somewhat unique diluent in that while producing cohesive compacts, the material also acts as a disintegrating agent. It is, however, a relatively expensive material when used as a diluent in high concentration and is thus typically combined with other materials. As in the case of starch, microcrystalline cellulose is often added to tablet formulation for several possible functions. It is a commonly employed excipient.

While a careful search of the literature reveals over 50 chemicals that have been evaluated and advocated as tablet diluents, those listed in Table 11-4 probably represent 80 to 90% of currently used diluents.

Binders and Adhesives

These materials are added either dry or in liquid form during wet granulation to form granules or to promote cohesive compacts for directly compressed tablets. Acacia and tragacanth are natural gums (listed in Table 11-4), and are employed in solutions ranging from 10 to 25% concentration, alone or in combination. These materials are much more effective when they are added as solutions in the preparation of granulations than when they are added dry to a direct compression formula. These natural gums have the disadvantage of being variable in their composition and performance based on their natural origin, and they are usually fairly heavily contaminated with bacteria. When these materials are used, their wet granulation masses should be quickly dried at a temperature above 37° to reduce microbial proliferation.

Gelatin is a natural protein and is sometimes used in combination with acacia. It is a more consistent material than the two natural gums, is easier to prepare in solution form, and forms tablets equally as hard as acacia or tragacanth. Starch paste has historically been one of the most common granulating agents. It is prepared by dispersing starch into water, which is then heated for some prescribed time. During the heating, the starch undergoes hydrolysis to dextrin and to glucose. A properly made paste is translucent rather than clear (which would indicate virtually complete conversion to glucose) and produces cohesive tablets that readily disintegrate when properly formulated. Liquid glucose, which is a 50% solution in water, is a fairly common wet granulating agent. Its properties are similar to those of sucrose solutions, which are commonly employed in concentrations between 50 and 74%. These sugar solutions are capable of producing wet granulations, which when tabletted, produce hard but somewhat brittle compacts. These materials have the advantage of being low-cost adhesives. Unless the sugar solutions are highly concentrated, bacterial proliferation may be a problem.

Modified natural polymers, such as the alginates and cellulose derivatives (methylcellulose, hydroxypropyl methylcellulose, and hydroxypropyl cellulose), are common binders and adhesives. Used dry for direct compression, they have some binder capabilities, while their aqueous solutions have adhesive properties. Hydroxypropyl cellulose may also be used as an alcohol solution to provide an anhydrous adhesive. Ethylcellulose may be used only as an alcoholic solution, and it may be expected to retard disintegration and dissolution time of drugs in the resulting tablets when wet granulation is employed. Polyvinylpyrrolidone is a synthetic polymer that may be used as an adhesive in either an aqueous solution or alcohol. It also has some capabilities as a dry binder.

Disintegrants

A disintegrant is added to most tablet formulations to facilitate a breakup or disintegration of the tablet when it contacts water in the gastrointestinal tract. Disintegrants may function by drawing water into the tablet, swelling, and causing the tablet to burst apart. Such tablet fragmentation may be critical to the subsequent dissolution of the drug and to the attainment of satisfactory drug bioavailability. Starch USP and various starch derivatives are the most common disintegrating agents. They also have the lowest cost. Starch is typically used in a concentration range of 5 to 20% of tablet weight. Such modified starches as Primogel and Explotab, which are low substituted carboxylmethyl starches, are used in lower concentrations (1 to 8%, with 4% usually reported as optimum). Various pregelatinized starches are also employed as disintegrants, usually in a 5% concentration.

Clays such as Veegum HV and bentonite have been used as disintegrants at about a 10% level. Such use of these materials is limited unless the tablets are colored, since the clays produce an off-white appearance. The clays are typically less effective as disintegrants than some of the newer modified polymers and starches, which can increase in volume in the presence of water by 200 to 500%. The disintegrating characteristics of microcrystalline cellulose have been reported previously in this chapter; however, in the cellulose class, a new material known as Ac-Di-Sol is now available and is effective in low concentration levels. It is an internally cross-linked form of sodium carboxymethylcellulose. Another cross-linked polymer that is available as a disintegrant is cross-linked polyvinylpyrrolidone.

Lubricants, Antiadherents, and Glidants

These three classes of materials are typically described together because they have overlapping functions. A material that is primarily described as an antiadherent is typically also a lubricant, with some glidant properties as well. The differentiation between these terms is as follows: Lubricants are intended to reduce the friction during tablet ejection between the walls of the tablet and the walls of the die cavity in which the tablet was formed. Antiadherents have the purpose of reducing sticking or adhesion of any of the tablet granulation or powder to the faces of the punches or to the die wall. Glidants are intended to promote flow of the tablet granulation or powder materials by reducing friction between the particles.

In addition to the lubricants listed in Table 11-4, hydrocarbon oils such as mineral oil have been employed by application to granulation as a fine spray, either directly or in a solvent solution. The problem with using this type of lubricant is the production of oil spots. The most widely used lubricants have been stearic acid and various stearic acid salts and derivatives. Calcium and magnesium stearate are the most common salts employed. Stearic acid is a less effective lubricant than these salts and also has a lower melting point. Talc is probably the second most commonly used tablet lubricant, historically. Most talc samples are found to contain trace quantities of iron, and talc should be considered carefully in any formulation containing a drug whose breakdown is catalyzed by the presence of iron. The higher-molecular-weight polyethylene glycols and certain polymeric surfactants have been used as water-soluble lubricants. These materials are much less effective as lubricants, however, than the materials previously cited. Since lubrication is basically a coating process, the finer the particle size of the lubricant, the more effective the lubricant action is likely to be.

As previously noted, most of the materials listed as lubricants, with the possible exception of those that are water-soluble, also function as antiadherents. Talc, magnesium stearate, and starch as well as starch derivatives possess antiadherent properties. In addition, various colloidal silicas have been used as antiadherents.

Materials used as glidants, or flow promoters, are typically talc at a 5% concentration, corn starch at a 5 to 10% concentration, or colloidal silicas such as Cab-O-Sil, Syloid, or Aerosil in 0.25 to 3% concentrations.

Colors, Flavors and Sweeteners

The use of colors and dyes in tablet making has served three purposes over the years: disguising of off-color drugs, product identification, and production of a more elegant product. With the continual decertification of many synthetic dyes, pharmaceutical manufacturers are becoming quite concerned as to how future tablet formulations will be colored. The availability of natural vegetable colors is limited, and these colors are often unstable. Two forms of color have typically been used in tablet preparation. These are the FD&C and D&C dyes—which are applied as solutions, typically in the granulating agent—and the lake forms of these dyes. Lakes are dyes that have been absorbed on a hydrous oxide and usually are employed as dry powders for coloring. In addition to concerns regarding possible delisting in the future, several other precautions should be considered when colors are employed. When using water-soluble dyes, pastel shades usually show the least mottling from uneven distribution in the final tablet. When wet granulation is employed, care should be taken to prevent color migration during drying. In any colored tablet, the formulation should be checked for resistance to color changes on exposure to light. Various artificial light sources are available that simulate the ultraviolet spectrum of sunlight. Methods of quantifying color are given earlier in the chapter under the heading, "Organoleptic Properties."

Flavors are usually limited to chewable tablets or other tablets intended to dissolve in the mouth. In general, flavors that are water-soluble have found little acceptance in tablet making because of their poor stability. Flavor oils are added to tablet granulations in solvents, are dispersed on clays and other absorbents, or are emulsified in aqueous granulating agents. Various dry flavors for use in pharmaceutical products are also available from flavor suppliers. Usually, the maximum amount of oil that can be added to a granulation without influencing its tabletting characteristics is 0.5 to 0.75%.

The use of sweeteners is primarily limited to chewable tablets to exclude or limit the use of sugar in the tablets. Various sugars used as tablet excipients have been described earlier. Mannitol is reportedly about 72% as sweet as sucrose. Until recently, saccharin was the only artificial sweetener available. This material is about 500 times sweeter than sucrose. Its major disadvantages are that it has a bitter aftertaste and has been reported to be carcinogenic. A new artificial sweetener that is expected to largely replace saccharin is aspartame. The primary disadvantage of aspartame is its lack of stability in the presence of moisture. When aspartame is used in a formulation, e.g., a chewable tablet with hygroscopic components, it will be necessary to determine its stability under conditions in which the product can adsorb atmospheric moisture.

Examples of tablet formulations are shown in the Appendices to this chapter. Not only do the formulations illustrate the use of common ingredients, but they also illustrate the use of the ingredients in tablets to be made by wet granulation, dry granulation, and direct compression processes.

It has previously been noted that while the excipients are the inactive part of a tablet formulation, they have a direct influence on the quality and effectiveness of the final product. Figure 11-18 describes, for example, the influence of compression force on disintegration time for various direct compression materials. Some materials have a maximum disintegration time of no higher than 200 to 250 sec, regardless of the compression force applied over the range studied. One material rapidly increased in disintegration time to over 500 sec at a compression force of less than 1000 kg. Similar relationships between important tablet properties and processing characteristics can be shown for many other tablet excipients.

Another important consideration that many pharmaceutical formulators must consider in tablet formulation is the worldwide acceptability of their formulation components. An excipient used in the United States, for example, may not be permitted in a major market area such as Japan or Europe, or vice-versa. Companies with major international markets strive to have tablet formulations that are equally acceptable around the world and that contain components that are not likely to be delisted in any country.

Types and Classes of Tablets

Tablets are classified by their route of administration or function, by the type of drug delivery system they represent within that route, and by their form and method of manufacture. Table 11-5 lists the various classes of tablets, with the primary classification being the route of administration or function.

Tablets Ingested Orally

Well over 90% of the tablets manufactured today are ingested orally. Orally ingested tablets are designed to be swallowed intact, with the exception of chewable tablets. .

Compressed Tablets or Standard Compressed Tablets. This category refers to standard uncoated tablets made by compression and employing any of the three basic methods of manufacture: wet granulation, double compaction, or direct compression. Tablets in this category are usually intended to provide rapid disin-

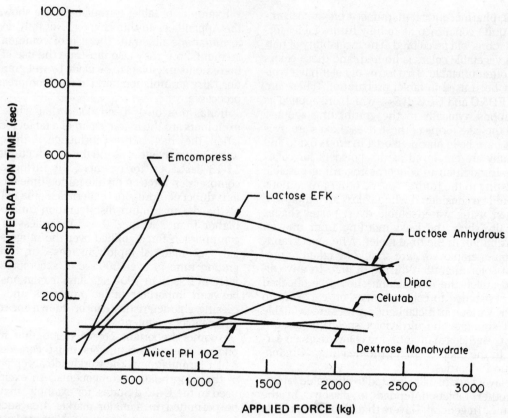

FIG. 11-18. *Disintegration time vs. applied force for tablets prepared from various direct compression diluents. (Reprinted from Banker, G. S., Peck, G. E., and Baley, G.: Tablet formulation and design. In Pharmaceutical Dosage Forms: Tablets. Vol. 1. Edited by H. Lieberman and L. Lachman. Marcel Dekker, New York, 1980, p. 75, by courtesy of Marcel Dekker, Inc.)*

tegration and drug release. Most tablets containing drugs intended to exert a local effect in the gastrointestinal tract are of this type. These drugs are typically water-insoluble and include such therapeutic categories as the antacids and adsorbents. Other drugs in this group are intended to produce a systemic effect. These drugs have some aqueous solubility, dissolve from the tablet and disintegrated tablet fragments in GI contents, and are then absorbed and distributed in the body. As described earlier in this chapter, proper disintegration of the tablet and deaggregation of the tablet fragments or granular particles are often critical to the proper performance of the dosage form. The locally acting drugs mentioned perform in accordance with their state of deaggregation, since adsorbents and antacids both involve surface activity that increases as their surface area increases. Dissolution is also a surface-related phenomenon, with dissolution rates increasing as a drug's surface area is increased. Thus, tablet breakup and particle deaggregation is also important for

drugs designed to produce systemic effects. As the solubility of the drug decreases, especially with acidic drug moieties that are absorbed best in the upper GI tract, rapid tablet disintegration becomes increasingly important, even critical, for this tablet category.

Multiple Compressed Tablets. There are two classes of multiple compressed tablets: layered tablets and compression-coated tablets. Both types may be either two-component or three-component systems: two- or three-layer tablets, a tablet within a tablet, or a tablet within a tablet within a tablet. Both types of tablets usually undergo a light compression as each component is laid down, with the main compression being the final one. Tablet machine production speeds for multiple compressed tablets are appreciably slower than for standard compressed tablets, especially in the case of compression-coated tablets.

Tablets in this category are usually prepared for one of two reasons: to separate physically or chemically incompatible ingredients, or to pro-

TABLE 11-5. *Types and Classes of Tablets*

Oral Tablets for Ingestion

Compressed tablets or standard compressed tablets (CT)
Multiple compressed tablets (MCT)
    Layered tablets
    Compression-coated tablets
Repeat-action tablets
Delayed-action and enteric coated tablets
Sugar- and chocolate-coated Tablets
Film-coated tablets
Chewable tablets

Tablets Used in the Oral Cavity

Buccal tablets
Sublingual tablets
Troches and lozenges
Dental cones

Tablets Administered by Other Routes

Implantation tablets
Vaginal tablets

Tablets Used to Prepare Solutions

Effervescent tablets
Dispensing tablets (DT)
Hypodermic tablets (HT)
Tablet triturates (TT)

---

duce repeat-action or prolonged-action products. In some cases, a two-layer tablet may provide adequate surface separation of reactive ingredients; if complete physical separation is required for stability purposes, the three-layer tablet may be employed. The layered tablet is preferred to the compression-coated tablet; surface contact between layers is lessened, and production is simpler and more rapid.

Multiple compressed tablets readily lend themselves to repeat-action products, wherein one layer of the layered tablet or the outer tablet of the compression-coated tablet provides the initial dose, rapidly disintegrating in the stomach. The other layer or the inner tablet is formulated with components that are insoluble in gastric media but are released in the intestinal environment. The shortcoming of this category of dosage form for repeat-action products is that its performance is highly dependent on gastric emptying. If the second layer or core tablet quickly leaves the stomach following release of the initial fast-release dose, an entirely different blood level profile results than if there is a several-hour or longer delay before the second fraction is emptied. It is probably for this reason that

relatively few repeat-action or controlled-release products using this approach are marketed.

Repeat-Action Tablets. The mode of operation of repeat-action tablets, and their limitations based on uncontrolled and unpredictable gastric emptying, have just been mentioned. In addition to multiple compressed tablets being used for this effect, sugar-coated tablets may also be employed. The core tablet is usually coated with shellac or an enteric polymer so that it will not release its drug load in the stomach. The second dose of drug is then added in the sugar coating, either in solution in the sugar syrup or as a part of the dusting powder added for rapid coat buildup. More uniform drug addition occurs if the drug is in solution or fine suspension in the sugar solution, especially if an automated-spray sugar-coating operation is employed. Even so, the coating operation will probably require interruption one or more times while the partially coated tablets are assayed to establish that the correct amount of drug has been applied in the coating.

Delayed-Action and Enteric Coated Tablets. The delayed-action tablet dosage form is intended to release a drug after some time delay, or after the tablet has passed through one part of the GI tract into another. The enteric coated tablet is the most common example of a delayed-action tablet product. All enteric coated tablets (which remain intact in the stomach but quickly release in the upper intestine) are a type of delayed-action tablet. Not all delayed-action tablets are enteric or are intended to produce the enteric effect. In veterinary product development, tablets may be designed to pass through the stomach (or several stomachs) of an animal or through all or most of the small intestine before releasing—or even into the cecum or large bowel, as in the case of treating worm parasites located in this lower region. In a human drug application, a product may be designed to pass through the stomach intact and then release gradually for several hours or longer in the intestines.

The compendial specifications for an enteric coated tablet are that all of the six tablets placed in separate tubes of the USP disintegration apparatus (using discs) remain intact after 30 min of exposure in simulated gastric fluid at $37°C \pm 2°C$ and then disintegrate within the time specified for that product's monograph, plus 30 min. If one or two tablets fail to disintegrate completely in the intestinal fluid, the test is repeated on 12 additional tablets; not less than 16 of the total 18 tablets tested must disintegrate completely. Prior to gastric exposure, the tablets are immersed in water at room temperature for 5 minutes.

The coatings that are used today to produce enteric effects are primarily mixed acid functionality and acid ester functionality synthetic or modified natural polymers. Cellulose acetate phthalate has the longest history of use as an enteric coating. More recently, polyvinyl acetate phthalate and hydroxypropyl methylcellulose phthalate have come into use. All three polymers have the common feature of containing the dicarboxylic acid, phthalic acid, in partially esterfied form. These polymers, being acid esters, are insoluble in gastric media that have a pH of up to about 4; they are intended to hydrate and begin dissolving as the tablets leave the stomach, enter the duodenum (pH of 4 to 6), and move further along the small intestine, where the pH increases to a range of 7 to 8. The primary mechanism by which these polymers lose their film integrity, thereby admitting intestinal fluid and releasing drug, is ionization of the residual carboxyl groups on the chain and subsequent hydration. The presence of esterases in the intestinal fluid that break down ester linkages of the polymer chains may also play some role, as may surface activity effects of bile salts and other components in bile that enter the upper small intestine via the bile duct.

Enteric coatings are employed for a number of therapeutic, safety, and medical reasons. Some drugs are irritating when directly exposed to the gastric mucosa, including aspirin and strong electrolytes such as NH_4Cl. While for most people the occasional aspirin tablet may not cause irritation, those on daily doses of aspirin, such as arthritics, may find gastric upset a major problem. Enteric coating is one method of reducing or eliminating irritation from such drugs. There are other drugs that if released in the stomach may produce nausea and vomiting. The low pH of the stomach destroys other drugs (for example, erythromycin), and hence enteric coating may be necessary to bring the drug through that environment to the more neutral intestinal contents. Yet another reason for enteric coating may be the desire to release the drug undiluted and in the highest concentration possible within the intestine. (Examples are intestinal antibacterial or antiseptic agents and intestinal vermifuges.) As in the case of repeat-action and other controlled-release dosage forms, the influence of altering the release profile of the drug on total drug bioavailability, distribution, and pharmacokinetics must be investigated.

Sugar- and Chocolate-Coated Tablets. Chocolate-coated tablets are nearly a thing of the past. They are too easily mistaken for candy by children. Sugar-coated tablets suffer the same disadvantage. Their primary historical role was to produce an elegant, glossy, easy-to-swallow tablet dosage form. Also, they permit separation of incompatible ingredients between coating and core, and this fact has been widely utilized in preparing many multivitamin and multivitamin mineral combinations. The process as originally developed was time-consuming and required skilled coating artisans to be conducted properly. Earlier sugar coatings typically doubled tablet weight. Today, water-soluble polymers are often incorporated in the sugar solution, automated-spray coating equipment is employed, and high-drying-efficiency side-vented coating pans are used. The result is that the coatings are more elastic and mechanically stable, coat weight may be 50% or less of the core weight, and the process may be completed in a day or less.

Film-Coated Tablets. Film-coated tablets were developed as an alternative procedure to the preparation of coated tablets in which drug was not required in the coating. The initial film-coating compositions employed one or more polymers, which usually included a plasticizer for the polymer and possibly a surfactant to facilitate spreading, all delivered to the tablets in solution from an organic solvent. The film-coating process was an attractive tablet coating method since it permitted the completion of the tablet coating operation in a period of one or two hours. An airless spray coating procedure was typically employed for such film-coating compositions, using either conventional coating pans or side-vented equipment. During the decade of the 1970s, several factors began to make solvent-based film coating less attractive. These factors were the increase in cost of the organic solvents, OSHA restrictions on worker exposure to solvent vapors, and EPA limitations on solvent vapor discharge to the atmosphere. As a result of these influences, many companies have now converted their earlier film-coating process to a totally aqueous-based procedure. Polymers such as hydroxypropyl cellulose and hydroxypropyl methylcellulose, which are dissolved in water with an appropriate plasticizer, are now widely used to produce immediate-release film coatings. The recent development of a colloidal dispersion of ethylcellulose in water also makes it possible to produce slow- or controlled-release film coatings without the use of organic solvents. A 30% ethylcellulose dispersion is marketed under the trade name Aquacoat by the FMC Corporation.

Film-coated tablets offer a number of advantages over sugar-coated tablets. These advantages include better mechanical strength of the coating based on the elasticity and flexibility of the polymer coating, little increase in tablet weight, the ability to retain debossed markings on a tablet through the thin film coating, the avoidance of sugar, which is contraindicated in the diets of a significant segment of the population, and the employment of a process that may be continuous, or that readily lends itself to automation. The primary disadvantage of film coating compared with sugar coating is that it is difficult to produce film-coated tablets that match the physical appearance and elegance of the sugar-coated product. Film coating in the future will assume increasing importance as a means of controlling drug delivery release rates from both tablets and bead particles as well as from drug crystals. Film-coated tablets, which are basically tasteless, also offer the advantage over sugar-coated tablets of being less likely to be mistaken for candy.

Chewable Tablets. Chewable tablets are intended to be chewed in the mouth prior to swallowing and are not intended to be swallowed intact. The purpose of the chewable tablet is to provide a unit dosage form of medication which can be easily administered to infants and children or to the elderly, who may have difficulty swallowing a tablet intact. The types of sugars and other components employed in chewable tablets have been designated in this chapter under the heading "Table Design and Formulation." The most common chewable tablet on the market is the chewable aspirin tablet intended for use in children. Bitter or foul-tasting drugs are not good candidates for this type of tablet, and this fact restricts the use of the chewable tablet dosage form. Many antacid tablet products are of the chewable type. The chewable tablet offers two major advantages to the delivery of a solid antacid dosage form. First, the dose of most antacids is large, so that the typical antacid tablet would be too large to swallow. Second, as noted previously, the activity of an antacid is related to its particle size. If the tablet is chewed prior to swallowing, better acid neutralization may be possible from a given antacid dose.

Tablets Used in the Oral Cavity

Buccal and Sublingual Tablets. These two classes of tablets are intended to be held in the mouth, where they release their drug contents for absorption directly through the oral mucosa. These tablets are usually small and somewhat flat, and are intended to be held between the cheek and teeth or in the cheek pouch (buccal tablets), or beneath the tongue (sublingual tablets). Drugs administered by this route are intended to produce systemic drug effects, and consequently, they must have good absorption properties through the oral mucosa. Drug absorption from the oral mucosa into the bloodstream leads directly to the general circulation. Drug absorption from the gastrointestinal tract leads to the mesenteric circulation, which connects directly to the liver via the portal vein. Thus, drug absorption from the oral cavity avoids first-pass metabolism. The oral route of administration from these two classes of tablet dosage form thus offers several possible advantages: The gastric environment, where decomposition may be extensive (for certain steroids and hormones), may be avoided for drugs that are well absorbed in the mouth. A more rapid onset of drug action occurs than for tablets that are swallowed (an advantage with vasodilators given by this route). The first-pass effect may be avoided as noted previously, and for certain drugs (e.g., methyltestosterone), the nausea produced when the product is swallowed is avoided.

Buccal and sublingual tablets should be formulated with bland excipients, which do not stimulate salivation. This reduces the fraction of the drug that is swallowed rather than being absorbed through the oral mucosa. In addition, these tablets should be designed not to disintegrate but to slowly dissolve, typically over a 15- to 30-min period, to provide for effective absorption.

Troches and Lozenges. These are two other types of tablets used in the oral cavity, where they are intended to exert a local effect in the mouth or throat. These tablet forms are commonly used to treat sore throat or to control coughing in the common cold. They may contain local anesthetics, various antiseptic and antibacterial agents, demulcents, astringents, and antitussives. Lozenges were originally termed pastilles, but are more commonly called cough drops. They are usually made with the drug incorporated in a flavored hard-candy sugar base. Lozenges may be made by compression but are usually formed by fusion or by a candy-molding process. Troches, on the other hand, are manufactured by compression as are other tablets. These two classes of tablets are designed not to disintegrate in the mouth but to dissolve or slowly erode over a period of perhaps 30 min or less.

Dental Cones. Dental cones are a relatively minor tablet form that are designed to be placed in the empty socket remaining following a tooth extraction. Their usual purpose is to prevent the multiplication of bacteria in the socket following such extraction by employing a slow-releasing antibacterial compound, or to reduce bleeding by containing an astringent or coagulant. The usual vehicle of these tablets is sodium bicarbonate, sodium chloride, or an amino acid. The tablet should not be formulated with a component that might provide media for bacterial proliferation. The tablet should be formulated to dissolve or erode slowly in the presence of a small volume of serum or fluid, over a 20- to 40-min period, when loosely packed in the extraction site.

Tablets Administered by Other Routes

Implantation Tablets. Implantation or depot tablets are designed for subcutaneous implantation in animals or man. Their purpose is to provide prolonged drug effects, ranging from one month to a year. They are usually designed to provide as constant a drug delivery release rate as possible. These tablets are usually small, cylindric, or rosette-shaped forms, and are typically not more than 8 mm in length. Since there are two major safety problems with this form of drug administration, this class of dosage form has achieved little use in humans. The safety problems include the need for a surgical technique to discontinue therapy, and tissue toxicity problems in the area of the implantation site. A special injector utilizing a hollow needle and plunger (the Kern injector) may be used to administer rod-shaped tablets. Surgical techniques may be required for administering tablets of other shapes. Implantation tablets have been largely replaced by other dosage forms, such as diffusion-controlled silicone tubes filled with drug or biodegradable polymers that contain entrapped drug in a variety of forms. The primary application of current implantation tablets and depot forms is to the administration of growth hormones to food-producing animals. In this case, the implant or depot should be made in an animal structure that is not consumed. The ear of the animal is typically used, and appropriate drug release to the animal from the ear site must be achieved.

Vaginal Tablets. Vaginal tablets or inserts are designed to undergo slow dissolution and drug release in the vaginal cavity. The tablets are typically ovoid or pear-shaped to facilitate retention in the vagina. This tablet form is used to release antibacterial agents, antiseptics, or astringents to treat vaginal infections, or possibly to release steroids for systemic absorption. The tablets are often buffered to promote a pH

favorable to the action of a given antiseptic agent. The buffer pH, however, should not be greatly removed from physiologic pH. The vehicle of these tablets is typically a slowly soluble material similar to agents described for the preparation of buccal and sublingual tablets. The tablets should be designed to be compatible with some type of plastic tube inserter, which is usually employed to place the tablet in the upper region of the vaginal tract.

Tablets Used to Prepare Solutions

Effervescent Tablets. Effervescent tablets are designed to produce a solution rapidly with the simultaneous release of carbon dioxide. The tablets are typically prepared by compressing the active ingredients with mixtures of organic acids—such as citric acid or tartaric acid—and sodium bicarbonate. When such a tablet is dropped into a glass of water, a chemical reaction is initiated between the acid and the sodium bicarbonate to form the sodium salt of the acid, and to produce carbon dioxide and water. The reaction is quite rapid and is usually completed within one minute or less. In addition to having the capability of producing clear solutions, such tablets also produce a pleasantly flavored carbonated drink, which assists in masking the taste of certain drugs. For many years, various saline cathartics were prepared as effervescent mixtures and powders. The most widely produced effervescent tablet today is one that contains aspirin. If a clear solution is to be produced, the drug that is incorporated in the tablet must be soluble at a neutral or slightly alkaline pH, and any lubricant or other additive employed to facilitate tablet compression must be water-soluble.

The advantage of the effervescent tablet as a dosage form is that it provides a means of extemporaneously preparing a solution containing an accurate drug dose. As in the case of aspirin, this dosage form may provide other advantages as well. The solution produced by the most widely marketed effervescent aspirin tablet has a pH of about 8. If the volume of the solution and the pH of the solution are adequate to raise the gastric contents to neutral or near-netural pH, the aspirin remains in solution and is rapidly available upon emptying from the stomach. Some literature has been published to indicate that this form of aspirin is less irritating to the stomach mucosa. In addition, neutralization of gastric contents may be rapidly obtained from solutions of this type of tablet. The product does, however, represent a "systemic" antacid effect, with an appreciable dose of sodium or potassium, and thus does not represent a recommended method of producing routine gastric neutralization.

The disadvantage of the effervescent tablet, and one reason for its somewhat limited utilization, is related to the difficulty of producing a chemically stable product. Even the moisture in the air during product preparation may be adequate to initiate effervescent reactivity. During the course of the reaction, water is liberated from the bicarbonate, which autocatalyzes the reaction. Providing adequate protection of effervescent tablets in the hands of the consumer is another problem. The moisture to which tablets are exposed after opening the container can also result in a rapid loss of product quality in the hands of the consumer. It is for this reason that effervescent tablets are specially packaged in hermetic-type foil pouches or are stack-packed in cylindric tubes with minimal air space. Another reason for such packing is the fact that the tablets are usually compressed to be soft enough to produce an effervescent reaction that is adequately rapid.

A number of investigators have looked at alternative effervescent components in recent years in an attempt to produce a more chemically stable system. Such studies have included investigation of malic acid, fumaric acid, and various acid anyhdrides, in combination with newer carbonate sources such as sodium glycine carbonate and various sesquicarbonates. If, in the future, more chemically stable effervescent mixtures are identified that continue to provide rapid reactivity in water, the effervescent tablet system may expand as a method of producing extemporaneous drug-containing solutions.

Dispensing Tablets (DT). Dispensing tablets are intended to be added to a given volume of water by the pharmacist or the consumer, to produce a solution of a given drug concentration. Materials that have been commonly incorporated in dispensing tablets include mild silver proteinate, bichloride of mercury, merbromin, and quaternary ammonium compounds. The dispensing tablet must typically comprise totally soluble components, and the excipient ingredients of the tablet must not produce deleterious effects in the intended application of the solution or undesirable physical or chemical interactions with the active agent. In some cases, as in applications where the solution is to be used in contact with mucous membranes or on wounds, the tablet may also contain components to provide buffering or isotonicity. Dispensing tablets are less commonly used than formerly, since they cannot be employed on a routine basis with

water of known quality to produce sterile solutions. Another difficulty with dispensing tablets is that some of the components previously used in this dosage form are highly toxic and are extremely hazardous, and even lethal, if mistakenly swallowed. Great care must be taken in the packaging and labeling of such tablets to attempt to prevent their oral consumption. In the past, bichloride of mercury was usually prepared in coffin-shaped tablets, with an embossed skull and crossbones to emphasize its toxicity.

Hypodermic tablets (HT). Hypodermic tablets are composed of one or more drugs with other readily water-soluble ingredients and are intended to be added to sterile water or water for injection. Such extemporaneous preparation of an injectable solution was once widely used in medicine, because the physician, especially the rural physician, could carry many vials of such tablets in his bag with only one bottle of sterile water for injection, to prepare a great many types of injectable medications as the need arose. Hypodermic tablets are little used today in this country because their use increases the likelihood of administering a nonsterile solution, even though portable sterile filtration equipment exists to help assure the sterility and freedom from particulate matter in such a product. Furthermore, since physicians today practice most of their medicine from an office or a hospital, the advantage of portability of tablets for injection is far outweighed by the hazards and disadvantages of this dosage form in most medical situations.

Tablet Triturates (TT). Tablet triturates are small, usually cylindric, molded, or compressed tablets. Though rarely used today, they provided an extemporaneous method of preparation by the pharmacist. The drugs employed in such products were usually quite potent and were mixed with lactose and possibly a binder, such as powdered acacia, after which the mixture was moistened to produce a moldable, compactable mass. This mass was forced into the holes of a mold board fabricated from wood or plastic, after which the tablets were ejected using a pegboard, whose pegs matched the holes in the mold. The tablets were then allowed to dry and were available for dispensing. Since virtually every conceivable drug that would be useful in a tablet dosage form is available in that form, or in capsule form, there is virtually no need today for pharmacists to prepare tablets extemporaneously. Since in preparing this form of molded tablet, alcohol was commonly used to wet the powder mass to expedite drying of the tablets, tablet triturates were usually soft and quite friable. Many of the drugs employed in these tablets were highly potent, and drug migration could occur as the alcohol evaporated, so content uniformity of such tablets was often questionable. Because of these problems and the question of producing bioavailable dosage forms from such extemporaneous preparations, the tablet triturate is rarely seen today.

Future Trends

Formulation and Product Trends

Uncoated Tablets. Future design, formulation, and manufacture of conventional uncoated tablets will follow the existing trend to more efficient processing, combining or eliminating processing steps where possible, reducing handling, reducing processing variables, minimizing production time, and further reducing total production costs. Where possible, direct compression will continue to expand as a preferred method of tablet manufacture, and new and improved excipient materials that are especially compatible with direct compression and extend its utility, reliability, or simplicity as a process will find favor in pharmaceutical solid dosage form development. Where direct compression is not the process of choice, use of high-shear mixer/granulators will continue to expand, followed by efficient and rapid fluid-bed drying of the agglomerates. More progressive companies willoptimize formulations and processing conditions to produce the highest-quality agglomerates (granulations) at the lowest cost, employing regression and other mathematical approaches. Optimizing binder efficiency and processing conditions for reliable production of consistent agglomerates in a single high-shear mixer/granulator will be a major goal in such studies. Automation and computer control will rapidly expand in monitoring and controlling tablet production operations and entire tablet production facilities. Some type of continuous system to monitor tablet weight, utilizing instrumented tablet presses or high-speed electro-balances tied in to press operation, will become routine good manufacturing practice for high-speed tablet production.

Excipient Materials. New and improved excipients will continue to be developed to meet the needs of advancing tablet manufacturing technology. In recent years, new improved disintegrants have been marketed that are extremely efficient in lower concentrations, and that have good compressional properties. New direct compression diluents have also become available, as noted in the previous section on tablet design and formulation. A number of these newer excipient materials are polymeric, such as the cross-linked form of carboxymethylcellulose, which is sold under the trade name Ac-Di-Sol. It is predicted that the majority of the new future excipients will be polymers, based on their ability to produce a wide range of materials and properties according to molecular structural alterations. The majority of these polymer derivatives are of natural origin, based on their better regulatory approval status.

Coatings. Solvent-based film coating will continue to decline, based on high solvent costs and EPA and OSHA restrictions. They will be virtually replaced by completely water-based systems. Polymer solutions in water may be used to produce water-soluble film coatings. Colloidal dispersions of polymers (such as the 30% ethylcellulose dispersion marketed as Aquacoat), which produce dense films by particle coalescence, not only will make the formation of water-soluble film coating a highly efficient process, (virtually equal to earlier solvent-based methods), but will show the way to produce totally water-based enteric and sustained-release coatings. Side-vented coating pans, and pan designs with improved drying efficiencies will virtually replace the conventional solid-pan design. Improved methods of fabricating small spherical drug-containing particles will continue to develop, as will more reproducible methods of coating such particles. Air suspension coating will continue to play a role in coating such small particles; it is not likely that air suspension coating will grow appreciably as a tablet coating method.

Controlled-Release Tablets. Theoretically, tablets offer the lowest-cost approach to sustained- and controlled-release solid dosage forms. Currently, the vast majority of such products are coated pellets placed in capsules. This particulate approach to sustained release has offered several advantages: metered particle emptying from the stomach, utilization of a plurality of coatings, and several release profiles for the various populations of coatings, thereby permitting an immediate release fraction followed by a sustaining fraction. Matrix slow-releasing tablets cannot match these characteristics. For this reason, and based on public expectations (or those of marketing specialists) that controlled-release products are expected to be beads in a capsule, relatively few sustained-release oral products have been in tablet form.

A major recent break in that trend is the highly successful sustained-release theophylline product of Key Pharmaceuticals, Inc., Theo-

Dur. This is a unique type of sustained-release tablet that overcomes some of the limitations of earlier matrix tablets. Under gastric pH conditions, the Theo-Dur tablet slowly erodes; however, at a pH corresponding to the upper small intestine, the tablet disintegrates rapidly to release coated particles, which in turn slowly release drug. Two different release mechanisms are operative, neither of which is zero-order—erosion and decreasing surface area, and dissolution of coated particles—but the overall tablet release profile comprising the two mechanisms in sequence is nearly linear for most of the dose in the tablet. The result is the ability to control theophylline blood levels in a narrow range, above the minimum effective level and below the toxic level. This type of sustained-release tablet has clearly shown the potential of the tablet as a reliable sustained-release dosage form with good release profile precision.[36,37] More sustained-release tablet forms of this type are sure to follow.

A prolonged gastric retention coated tablet system has been reported.[38] The tablet utilizes a cross-linked polymer coating that has the capacity to swell greatly and rapidly in the stomach and be restricted there by physical size. Gastric fluid that penetrates the hydrated swollen film dissolves the drug within the sac enveloping the tablet, and drug is released from solution by diffusion across the hydrated membrane/film. Drug release is at a constant rate so long as the concentration of drug within the sac exceeds the capacity of the membrane to deliver the drug, and the film/membrane is thus providing the rate-limiting step. If the dimension of the fluid-filled sacs exceeds approximately 2 cm, these dosage units consistently remain in the stomach for at least 6 to 8 hours, releasing drug in solution to the gastric contents at a constant rate. This gastric retention tablet dosage form reflects the type of innovation to control not only the rate of drug release, but also the site of release, that will undoubtedly continue in the years ahead to further improve and enhance drug delivery capabilities.

The Oros product of the Alza Corporation is another new zero-order sustained-release tablet product; it is based on osmotic pressure as the rate-controlling process. This concept will also expand the use of tablet dosage forms in controlled release. The first such products are already being marketed in Europe, and the drug indomethacin is about to be marketed in the United States in an Oros system, at the time of this writing.

Film coatings that may be applied to tablets to provide diffusion-controlled "membranes" for constant drug release rate profiles as the tablet dosage form moves along the GI tract are also under active development. Such a system offers the potential ultimate dosage form as a simple, low-cost, and reproducible physicochemical approach to oral controlled and sustained drug release.

Manufacturing Improvements

Basic Improvement Areas. Wet granulation has traditionally been a highly labor-intensive and time-consuming process (see Table 11-3). In the last 20 years, however, significant improvements in tablet manufacturing efficiency have taken place. These can be attributed to four basic areas: the elimination or combination of processing steps, the improvement of specific unit operations, the design of new equipment specifically oriented to granulation objectives, and the improvement of materials handling techniques and systems. Illustrating the use of these improvement areas, Table 11-6 compares the processing steps of Lederle's old tablet-manufacturing process to its new tablet-manufacturing process.

Elimination or Combination of Steps. Tables 11-3 and 11-6 indicate the processing steps that may be omitted on conversion from wet granulation to direct compression. As noted, new mixer/granulators allow several processes of wet granulation to be conducted in rapid succession or to be combined in one piece of equipment.

Unit Operation Improvement. The efficiency of new tablet manufacturing methods, as exemplified by the new process, was achieved by enhancing the efficiency of three specific unit operations. First, material blending was improved by replacing slow-speed planetary type mixers with high-speed mixer/granulators. Second, the tablet compression operation was improved by replacing old single-fill-station, gravity-fed compression machines with newer high-speed, multi-station presses, with induced die feed and automated weight control. Third, the coating operation was brought into better compliance with EPA standards by switching from organic-solvent based systems to aqueous systems, which were further aided by side-vented coating equipment having greatly improved drying efficiencies.

Materials Handling. A major labor-saving change made in equipment designs allowed material to be moved by gravity. A granulation gravity feed system was designed that eliminated the manual feeding of granulation into the presses.

TABLE 11-6. *Unit Processing of Solid Dosage Forms (Tablet Manufacturing)—Lederle Laboratories*

Old Process (Wet Granulation)	New Process (Direct Compression)
Raw Materials	Raw materials
Weighing and measuring	Weighing and measuring (automatic weigher and recording system)*
Screening	Gravity feeding
Manual feeding	Blending (Littleford blender)
Blending (slow-speed planetary mixer)	Gravity feeding from the storage tank*
Wetting (hand addition)	Compression (high-speed rotary press)*
Subdivision (comminutor)	Aqueous coating (Hi-Coater)
Drying (fluid bed dryer)	
Subdivision (comminutor)	
Premixing (barrel roller)	
Batching and lubrication (ribbon blender)	
Manual feeding	
Compression (Stokes rotary press)	
Solvent film coating (Wurster column)	
Tablet inspection (manual)	

*In planning phase, to be installed later.
Courtesy of Lederle Laboratories, Pearl River, NY.

With use of similar techniques, even wet granulation operations have been made more efficient, and a hypothetical state-of-the-art processing scheme is presented in the flow chart in Figure 11-19. All processing steps including drying might be combined in a single processor in the wet granulation method of the future. Such equipment will minimize materials handling, labor requirement, and human variables.

Equipment. Various equipment improvements that would combine several of the wet granulation processing steps are being investigated. One such method is the use of the sprayer dryer. The components of the formula-diluent,

binder, disintegrant, and lubricant may be suspended and/or dissolved in a suitable vehicle according to their nature. The solids should represent at least 50 to 60% of the suspension. Under constant stirring to maintain good distribution, the slurry is pumped to an atomizing wheel, which whirls the material into a stream of hot air. The heat removes the liquid carrier, and the solids fall to the bottom of the dryer as fine, spherical granules ranging from as low as 10 to as high as 250 microns in diameter, the size depending on the speed of the wheel and the flow rate of the feed. The drug may be mixed with this "base" in proportions as high as 1:1. If

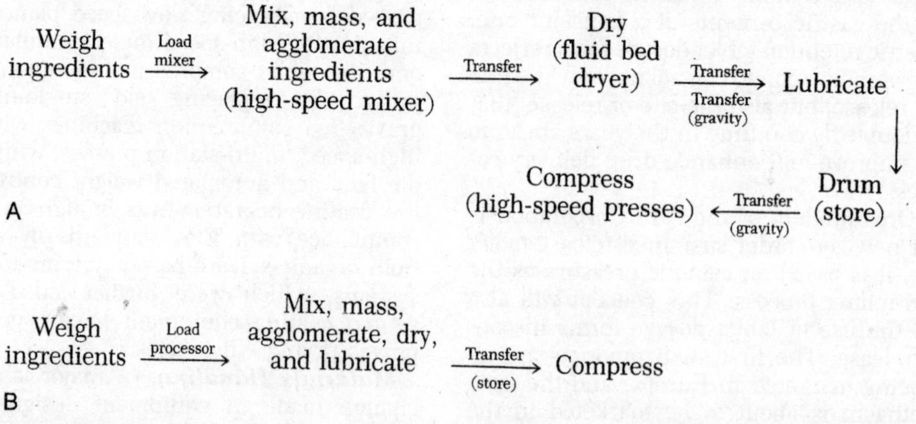

FIG. 11-19. *Flow charts depict state-of-the-art wet granulation processing of the 1980s (A), and projected wet granulation processing methods of the future—1990 and beyond (B). (Adapted from Anderson, N.R., Banker, G.S., and Peck, G.E.: Principles of improved tablet production system design. In Pharmaceutical Dosage Forms: Tablets. Vol. 3. Edited by H. Lieberman and L. Lachman. Marcel Dekker, Inc., New York, 1982, p. 14, by courtesy of Marcel Dekker, Inc.)*

the drug remains stable with the temperatures and solvents used, it may also be included in the slurry.

Fluid Bed Spray Granulators. The first equipment reported in the pharmaceutical literature to provide continuous-batch wet granulation was fluid bed drying equipment, which was modified by the addition of spray nozzles or fluid injectors to provide addition of liquid binding and adhesive agents to dry-powdered materials for powder agglomeration, followed by drying in the same equipment.

Figure 11-20 presents a schematic cross-section of such a fluid bed spray granulator. The airflow necessary for fluidization of these powders is generated by a suction fan mounted in the top portion of the unit, which is directly driven by an electric motor. The air used for fluidization is heated to the desired temperature by an air heater, after first being drawn through prefilters to remove any impurities. The material

to be processed is shown in the material container just below the spray inlet. The liquid granulating agent is pumped from its container and is sprayed as a fine mist through a spray head onto the fluidized powder. The wetted particles undergo agglomeration through particle-particle contacts. Exhaust filters are mounted above the product retainer to retain dust and fine particles. After appropriate agglomeration is achieved, the spray operation is discontinued, and the material is dried and discharged from the unit.

The advantages of such rapid wet massing, agglomeration, and drying within one unit are obviously attractive. Excluding equipment cleanup, the process may readily be sequentially completed within 60 to 90 min or less.

There are several difficulties in the fluid bed spray granulating process. Fluid bed systems may not provide adequate mixing of powder components. In fact, there is a tendency for

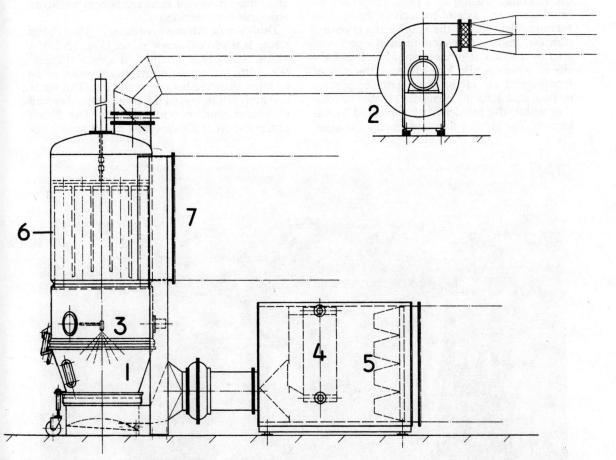

FIG. 11-20. *Schematic diagram of a fluid bed granulator dryer. (1) Material container. (2) Air suction fan. (3) Fluid spray head. (4) Inlet air heater. (5) Inlet air filter. (6) Exhaust air filters. (7) Explosion relief panels. (Courtesy of Aeromatic, Iowaco, NJ.)*

demixing to occur when there are disparities in particle size or density in the materials being processed. Particles with granulating agents on their surfaces tend to stick to the equipment filters, reducing the effective filter surface area, causing product loss, and increasing cleanup difficulties. Special attention is also needed for safety in any fluid bed processor. Dust explosions can occur in a fluid bed dryer, with flammable solvents or with dry materials that develop static charges, and all production size fluid bed equipment must contain explosion relief panels.

Double-Core and Twin-Shell Blenders With Liquid Feed and Vacuum-Drying Capabilities. A number of manufacturers of both double-cone and twin-shell blenders have produced equipment modifications that provide the potential for sequencing the operations of powder mixing, wet massing, agglomeration, and drying. The specialized equipment typically includes a liquid feed through the trunnion of the machine, leading to a spray dispenser located above the axis of rotation of the unit; a vacuum inlet through the same or the opposing trunnion leading to a vacuum intake port covered by a nylon or other appropriate fine-filter sleeve, which is also located above the axis of rotation and out of the direct path of powder motion; and agitating elements capable of rotation within the powder mass contained in the blender. The blender may also employ a double-wall construction to provide circulation of a heating medium; in other cases, the systems are designed to operate at room temperature and use vacuum as the sole source of water or liquid removal.

Figure 11-21 provides a cutaway view of a double-cone mixer-dryer processor. As in any vacuum-drying operation, equipment and drying costs are relatively high. Drying times are considerably longer than with the fluid bed granulator processor. The double-cone or twin-shell processor would be considerably easier to clean, however. The attractiveness today of the double-cone or twin-shell mixer, granulator, and dryer as a continuous-batch processor of wet granulation products hinges on the use of nonaqueous granulating liquids. Standard auxiliary equipment is available to condense solvent vapors and provide substantially complete solvent recovery. This is important from two standpoints: solvent vapors are not discharged to the atmosphere, an environmental consideration, and efficient solvent recovery is achievable, an economic consideration.

Day-Nauta Mixer-Processor. The Nauta mixer is a vertical screw mixer (Fig. 11-22). A screw assembly is mounted in a conical chamber, with the screw lifting the powder to be blended from the bottom to the top. The screw assembly orbits around the conical chamber wall to ensure more uniform mixing. The Nauta mixer was originally designed not as a wet gran-

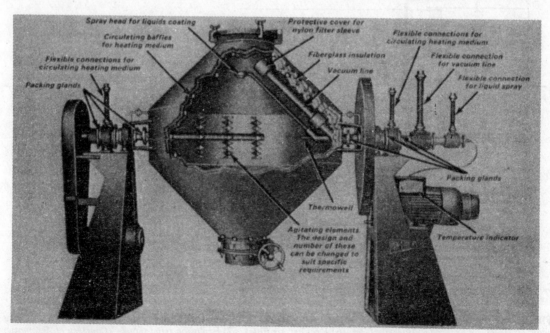

FIG. 11-21. *A cutaway view of a double-cone mixer-dryer processor. (Courtesy of Paul O. Abbe, Little Falls, NJ.)*

breaker, which may be attached at the bottom of the conical chamber; a temperature monitor; a nuclear, noncontact density gauge; an ammeter or wattmeter; an infrared moisture analyzer; and a sampling system.

Topo Granulator. The Topo granulator was developed in Austria for the preparation of granules and coated particles under high vacuum. The machine is illustrated in Figure 11-23. The material to be granulated or coated is placed in the chamber, which may be accomplished by dust-free suction. A granulating compartment is then loaded by vacuum, and each granulating fluid or addition product (liquid or solid) is added as desired by imploding the added ingredient(s) upon the components already in the chamber. When granulating agents are thus added to the chamber under vacuum, the granulation forces are reportedly greatly increased to produce the necessary compaction. The resultant agglomerated particles can then be dried under vacuum in the chamber. Some of the advantages reported for this granulation process are a reduction in the required volume of granulating fluid; a unique agglomeration mechanism

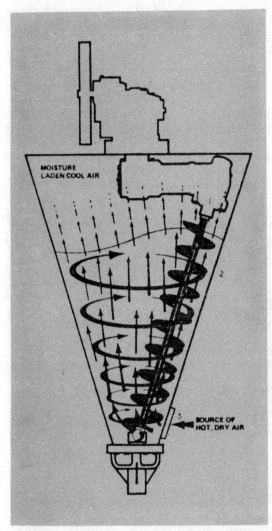

FIG. 11-22. *Schematic diagram of the Nauta processor. (1) Screw assembly. (2) Conical chamber. (3) Source of hot, dry air. Hot air moves up through the material (vertical arrows), which is kept in motion by the orbiting screw assembly (circular arrows). (Courtesy of Day Mixing, Cincinnati, OH.)*

ulation mixer-granulator but as a powder and semisolids mixer. The basic operation following power mixing includes incorporation of the liquid-granulating agent, wet massing, and drying as hot, dry air is passed through the wet material. The hot air moves up through the material, which is kept in a state of motion by the orbiting screw assembly. It dries the granulation and exits the top of the processor. If additional help is required for particular drying needs, the Nauta can be constructed to utilize vacuum drying. Accessory equipment designed to monitor and control processor operation includes a lump

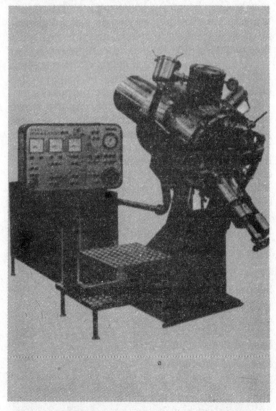

FIG. 11-23. *The Topo granulator. (Courtesy of Machines Collette, Wheeling, IL.)*

for the granulation process as it occurs under vacuum; a reduction in the amount of excipient materials that may be required to produce a satisfactory granule, owing to the intensified compaction of the granulation process; and generation of a granulation that produces tablets of exceptional hardness and stability.

By imploding coating materials on existing granulations, coating within the unit is reportedly possible. It has also been reported that by alternately imploding various drug and excipient materials, the equipment is capable of effectively separating incompatible drugs or of producing effervescent products of improved stability to moisture. Unfortunately, little published scientific or technical information is available regarding products produced by this equipment.

CF Granulator. The CF granulator utilizes a cylindric bowl with a rotating base plate (Fig. 11-24). Passing through the space between the bowl and base plate is fluidizing and drying air. A feeding device feeds powders, granules, or other solids into the machine. The rotating base and air form the material into rounded particles, a doughnut-like ring along the wall of the chamber, in a twisted-rope motion. While the material is thus formed, binding or coating solutions and powders can be sprayed onto the material. Operating in this fashion, materials can be granulated, agglomerated or coated, and dried within a reasonably limited time. The equipment is also used to produce spherical beads of drug applied to sugar beads, which may then be coated in the equipment for controlled-release purposes.

Computer Process Control. As the tablet manufacturing processes continue to be improved in the four areas indicated, human worker involvement will continue to decline. As human involvement requirements are reduced, computer control of the process is inevitable. There are many good reasons for implementing computer process control.

Rigid control enforcement

Operational information

Documentation of the process

Security of the process and its control

Increased consistency

Increased flexibility

Increased reliability

Increased productivity

Merck, Sharp and Dohme's computer-controlled Aldomet plant has shown that tablet production

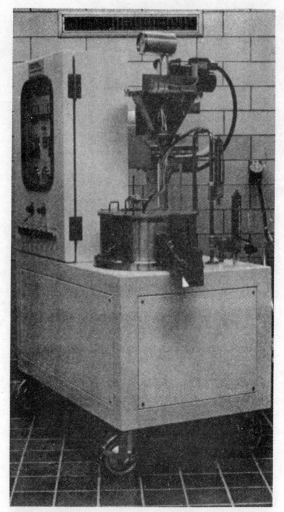

FIG. 11-24. *The CF granulator. (Courtesy of Vector Corporation, Marion, IA.)*

under computer control with limited human intervention is possible in a continuous mode.

In the common batch mode of tablet production, individual unit operations such as coating processes, fluid bed dryers and tablet press monitors are becoming automated by microcomputers. There are obstacles to computer control, including the need for smaller and more powerful computer devices, better process interfacing sensors, particularly of the "composition" type, and better man/machine interfacing. Therefore, as the price and size of computers continue to decrease, as the availability of sensors increases, and as our knowledge of tablet processes increases, the computer control of tablet batch operations will rapidly grow in the future.

Appendices

Appendix A

Common Tablet Ingredients in Wet Granulation Formulas

Phenobarbital Tablets

Ingredient	Quantity per Tablet	Quantity per 10,000 Tablets
Phenobarbital	65 mg	650 g
Lactose (fine powder)	40 mg	400 g
Starch (paste)	4 mg	40 g
Starch (dry)	10 mg	100 g
Talc	10 mg	100 g
Mineral oil, 50 cps	4 mg	40 g

Mix the phenobarbital and lactose, and moisten with 10% starch paste to proper wetness. Granulate by passing through a 14-mesh screen, and dry at 140°F. When dry, pass through a 20-mesh screen; add the dry starch and talc; mix well. Finally, add the mineral oil, mix again, and compress using 9/32-in. standard cup punches.

Reprinted from reference 39, p. 109, by courtesy of Marcel Dekker, Inc.

Aminophylline Tablets

Ingredient	Quantity per Tablet	Quantity per 10,000 Tablets
Aminophylline	100 mg	1.0 kg
Tricalcium phosphate	50 mg	0.5 kg
Pregelatinized starch	15 mg	0.15 kg
Water	q.s.	q.s.
Talc	30 mg	0.3 kg
Mineral oil, light	2 mg	0.02 kg

Mix the aminophylline, tricalcium phosphate, and starch; moisten with water. Pass through a 12-mesh screen, and dry at 100°F. Size the dry granules through a 20-mesh screen; add the talc and mix. Add the mineral oil, mix for 10 min, and compress using 5/16-in. deep cup punches for enteric coating.

Reprinted from reference 39, p. 109, by courtesy of Marcel Dekker, Inc.

Chewable Antacid Tablets

Ingredient	Quantity per Tablet	Quantity per 10,000 Tablets
Aluminum hydroxide (dried gel)	400 mg	4.0 kg
Magnesium hydroxide (fine powder)	80 mg	0.8 kg
Sucrose (confectioner's)	20 mg	0.2 kg
Mannitol (fine powder)	180 mg	1.8 kg
Polyvinylpyrrolidone (10% solution)	30 mg	0.3 kg

Mix the first four ingredients, and moisten with a 10% PVP solution in 50% ethanol. Granulate by passing through a 14-mesh screen. Dry at 140 to 150°F. Size through a 20-mesh screen, add the oil of peppermint mixed with the Cab-O-Sil and finally the magnesium stearate; mix well and compress using ½-in. flat-face beveled-edge punches.

Reprinted from reference 39, p. 109, by courtesy of Marcel Dekker, Inc.

Chewable Laxative Tablets

Ingredient	Quantity per Tablet	Quantity per 10,000 Tablets
Phenolphthalein	64 mg	0.64 kg
Powdered sugar	750 mg	7.5 kg
Powdered cocoa (defatted)	350 mg	3.5 kg
Gelatin (10% solution)	q.s.	q.s.
Calcium stearate	12 mg	0.12 kg
Talc	60 mg	0.60 kg

Mix the phenolphthalein, sugar, and cocoa, and moisten with the gelatin solution. Pass through an 8-mesh screen, and dry in a tray oven at 120 to 130°F. When dry, reduce granule size by passing through a 16-mesh screen. Mix the calcium stearate and talc, pass through a 100-mesh screen, add to the granulation, and compress to weight using 5/8-in. flat-face punches.

Reprinted from reference 39, p. 109, by courtesy of Marcel Dekker, Inc.

Ferrous Sulfate Tablets

Ingredient	Quantity per Tablet	Quantity per 10,000 Tablets
Ferrous sulfate (dried)	300 mg	3.0 kg
Corn starch	60 mg	0.60 kg
20% Sugar solution	q.s.	q.s.
Explotab	45 mg	0.45 kg
Talc	30 mg	0.30 kg
Magnesium stearate	4 mg	0.04 kg

Mix the ferrous sulfate and cornstarch; moisten with sugar syrup to granulate through a 12-mesh screen. Dry in a tray oven overnight at 140 to 150°F. Size through an 18-mesh screen; add the Explotab, talc, and magnesium stearate, and compress to weight using 3/8-in. deep cup punches in preparation for sugar-coating.

Reprinted from reference 39, p. 109, by courtesy of Marcel Dekker, Inc.

Appendix B

Common Tablet Ingredients in Dry Granulation Formulas

Aspirin Tablets (5-Grain)

Ingredient	Quantity per Tablet	Quantity per 10,000 Tablets
Aspirin (20-mesh)	325.0 mg	3.250 kg
Starch USP (dried	32.5 mg	0.325 kg
Cab-O-Sil	0.1 mg	0.010 kg

Combine the aspirin, starch, and Cab-O-Sil, and mix in a P-K twin-shell blender for 10 min. Compress into slugs using 1-in. flat-face punches. Reduce the slugs to granulation by passing through a 16-mesh screen in a Stokes Oscillating Granulator or through a Fitzpatrick Mill with a #2B screen, at medium speed, and with knives forward. Transfer the granulation to a tablet machine hopper, and compress into tablets using 13/32-in. standard concave punches.

Note: All operations should be carried out in a dehumidified area at a relative humidity of less than 30% at 70°F.

Reprinted from reference 39, p. 109, by courtesy of Marcel Dekker, Inc.

Effervescent Aspirin Tablets (5-Grain)

Ingredient	Quantity per Tablet	Quantity per 10,000 Tablets
Sodium bicarbonate (fine granular)	2.050 g	20.500 kg
Citric acid (fine granular)	0.520 g	5.200 kg
Fumaric acid (fine granular)	0.305 g	3.050 kg
Aspirin (20-mesh, granular)	0.325 g	3.250 kg

Mix the above ingredients in a P-K twin-shell blender for 20 min; transfer to a tablet machine equipped with 1¼-in. flat-face punches, and compress slugs to approximately ⅜-in. thick. Grind the slugs through a 16-mesh screen. Mix for 5 min in a twin-shell blender, and compress into tablets using ⅞-in. flat-face beveled-edge punches.

Note: All operations should be carried out in a dehumidified area at a relative humidity of less than 30% at 70°F.

Reprinted from reference 39, p. 109, by courtesy of Marcel Dekker, Inc.

Appendix C

Common Tablet Ingredients in Direct Compression Formulas

Acetaminophen Tablets (USP)

Ingredient	Quantity per Tablet	Quantity per 10,000 Tablets
Acetaminohpen USP (granular or large crystal)*	325.00 mg	3.25 kg
Avicel PH 101	138.35 mg	1.3835 kg
Stearic acid (fine powder)	1.65 mg	0.0165 kg

*If smaller crystalline size acetaminophen is desired to improve dissolution, it is necessary to use a higher proportion of Avicel, to use PH 102 in place of PH 101, and to use a glidant. All lubricants should be screened before being added to blender.

Blend the acetaminophen and Avicel PH 101 for 25 min. Screen in the stearic acid, and blend for an additional 5 min. Compress tablets using 7/16-in. standard concave or flat beveled tooling.

Reprinted from reference 39, p. 109, by courtesy of Marcel Dekker Inc.

Vitamin B₁ Tablets (Thiamine Hydrochloride USP; 100 mg)

Ingredient	Quantity per Tablet	Quantity per 10,000 Tablets
Thiamine hydrochloride USP	100.00 mg	1.0 kg
Avicel PH 102	83.35 mg	0.8335 kg
Lactose (anhydrous)	141.65 mg	1.4165 kg
Magnesium stearate	6.65 mg	0.0665 kg
Cab-O-Sil	1.65 mg	0.0165 kg

Blend all ingredients except the magnesium stearate for 25 min. Screen in the magnesium stearate and blend for an additional 5 min. Compress using 13/32-in. standard concave tooling.

Note: Anhydrous lactose could be replaced with Fast Flo lactose with no loss in tablet quality. This would reduce the need for a glidant (which is probably present in too high a concentration in most of these formulations). Usually, only 0.25% is necessary to optimize fluidity.

Reprinted from reference 39, p. 109, by courtesy of Marcel Dekker, Inc.

Chlorpromazine Tablets USP (100 mg)

Ingredient	Quantity per Tablet	Quantity per 10,000 Tablets
Chlorpromazine hydrochloride USP	100.00 mg	1.0 kg
Avicel PH 102	125.00 mg	1.25 kg
Dicalcium phosphate (unmilled) or Emcompress	125.00 mg	1.25 kg
Cab-O-Sil	1.74 mg	0.0174 kg
Magnesium stearate	5.25 mg	0.0525 kg

Blend all ingredients except the magnesium stearate for 25 min. Screen in the magnesium stearate, and blend for an additional 5 min. Compress into tablets using ¹¹⁄₃₂-in. tooling.

Reprinted from reference 39, p. 109, by courtesy of Marcel Dekker, Inc.

References

1. Federal Register, 47(Nov. 5):50441, 1982.
2. Fonner, D. E., Buck, J. R. and Banker, G. S.: J. Pharm. Sci., 59:1578, 1970.
3. Schwartz, J. B.: Optimization techniques in pharmaceutical formulation and processing. In Modern Pharmaceutics. Edited by G. Banker and C. Rhodes. Marcel Dekker, New York, 1978.
4. Buck, J. R., Peck, G. E., and Banker, G. S.: Drug Develop. Commun., 1:89, 1974/1975.
5. Meyer, M. C., Slyka, G. W. A., Dann, R. E., and Whyatt, P. L.: J. Pharm. Sci., 63:1693, 1974.
6. Hiestand, E. N., Well, J. E., Pool, C. B., and Ocks, J. F.: J. Pharm. Sci., 66:510, 1977.
7. Physician's Desk Reference. 36th Ed. Medical Economics, Oradell, NJ, 1982, p. 403.
8. Matthews, B. A., Matsumota, S., and Shibata, M.: Drug Dev. Commun., 1:303, 1974/1975.
9. Bogdansky, F. M.: J. Pharm. Sci., 64:323, 1975.
10. Goodhart, F. W., Everhand, M. E., and Dickcius, D. A.: J. Pharm. Sci., 53:338, 1964.
11. Smith, F. D., and Grosch, D.: U. S. Patent 2,041,869 (1936).
12. Albrecht, R.: U.S. Patent 2,645,936 (1953).
13. Michel, F.: U.S. Patent 2,975,630 (1961).
14. Brook, D. B., and Marshall, K. J.: Pharm. Sci., 57:481, 1968.
15. Goodhart, F. W., Draper, J. R., Dancz, D., and Ninger, F. C.: J. Pharm. Sci., 62:297, 1973.
16. Newton, J. M., and Stanley, P.: J. Pharm. Pharmacol., 29:41P, 1977.
17. Shafer, E. G. E., Wollish, E. G., and Engel, C. E.: J. Am. Pharm. Assoc., Sci. Ed., 45:114, 1956.
18. Annual Book of ASTM Standards. Part 20. American Society for Testing and Materials, Philadelphia, 1978, (D775) p. 180, (D880) p. 229, (D999) p. 282.
19. The United States Pharmacopeia XX/National Formulary XV. U. S. Pharmacopeial Convention, Rockville, MD, 1980, pp. 958, 990.
20. Wagner, J. G.: Biopharmaceutics and Relevant Pharmacokinetics. Drug Intelligence Publications, Hamilton, IL, 1971, p. 64.
21. The United States Pharmacopeia XX/National Formulary XV. Supplement 3. U.S. Pharmacopeial Convention, Rockville, MD, 1982. p. 310.
22. Tabletting Specification Manual, Industrial Pharmaceutical Technology Standard Specifications for Tabletting Tools. 1981 revision. American Pharmaceutical Association, Washington, D.C.
23. Hiestand, E. N.: Paper presented at the International Conference on Powder Technology and Pharmacy, Basel, Switzerland, 1978.
24. White, G.: U.S. Patent 4,157,148 (1979).
25. Fonner, D. E., Anderson, N. R., and Banker, G. S.: Granulation and tablet characteristics. In Pharmaceutical Dosage Forms: Tablets. Vol. 2. Edited by H. Lieberman and L. Lachman. Dekker, New York, 1982, p. 202.
26. Marks, A. M., and Sciarra, J. J.: J. Pharm. Sci., 57:497, 1968.
27. Forlano, A. S., and Chavkin, L.: J. Am. Pharm. Assoc., Sci. Ed., 49:67, 1960.
28. Pitkin, C., and Carstensen, J.: J. Pharm. Sci., 62:1215, 1973.
29. Harwood, C. F., and Pilpel, N.: J. Pharm. Sci., 57:478, 1968.
30. Gold, G., Duvall, R. N., Palarmo, B. J., and Hurtle, R. L.: J. Pharm. Sci., 60:922, 1971.
31. Fonner, D. E., Banker, G. S., and Swarbrick, J.: J. Pharm. Sci. 51:181, 1966.
32. Schwartz, J. B.: Pharm. Tech., 5:102, 1981.
33. Boger, W. P., and Gavin, J. J.: New Engl. J. Med., 261:827, 1959.
34. Costello, R., and Mattocks, A.: J. Pharm. Sci., 51:106, 1962.
35. Duvall, R. N., et al.: J. Pharm. Sci. 54:607, 1965.
36. Jonkman, J.H.G., Schoenmaker, R., Grunberg, N., and DeZeeuw, R.: Internat. J. Pharm. 8:153, 1981.
37. McGinity, J. W., Cameron, C. G., and Cuff, G. W.: Drug Develop. and Ind. Pharm., 9:57, 1983.
38. Banker, G.: Bioadhesive Polymers for Oral and Rectal Administration in Sumposium Proceedings on "Emploi des Polymeres dans L'elaboration de Nouvelles Formes Medicamenteuses," p. 129, School of Pharmacy, University of Geneve, 1980.
39. Seth, B. B., Bandelin, F. S., and Shangraw, R. F.: Compressed tablets. In Pharmaceutical Dosage Forms: Tablets. Vol. 1. Edited by H. Lieberman and L. Lachman. Marcel Dekker, New York, 1980.

12

Tablet Coating

JAMES A. SEITZ, SHASHI P. MEHTA, *and* JAMES L. YEAGER

Historical Perspective

No discussion on tablet coating would be complete without a brief historical review of pharmaceutical coating to provide an appropriate perspective to the evolutions in the coating process that have occurred over the past thousand years.

One of the earliest references to coated solid dosage forms appears in early Islamic drug literature, where coated pills were mentioned by Rhazes (850–923).[1] The use of coating on drugs was probably an adaptation from early food preservation methods, and French publications in the 1600s described coating as a means of masking the taste of medicines. Sugar coating of pills was developed to a considerable extent by the French in the mid-1800s, and patents issued in 1837 and 1840 utilized sugar compositions for coated pills of cubeb and copaiba. Subsequently, there was rapid acceptance of sugar-coated pills as the preferred solid dosage form for both prescription and patent medicines in Europe and the United States. It soon was recognized that quality sugar coating on a large scale could be accomplished more readily in coating pans, and several early pharmaceutical companies in the United States were established, with coated pills as a major part of their product line.

Except for the substitution of compressed tablets for pills, the sugar coating equipment and process remained essentially unchanged for the next 75 years. In 1953, a dramatic change was made in tablet coating when Abbott Laboratories marketed the first film-coated pharmaceutical tablet. Concurrently, in the early 1950s, Dr. Dale Wurster, a professor at the University of Wisconsin, patented an air suspension coater that efficiently applied film coating compositions.[2–4] This stimulated renewed interest in tablet coating technology, and for the next 12 to 15 years, several hundred patents and research papers on the subject were published. The invention by Dr. Wurster showed the merits of high airflow in the coating process, and eventually, a series of perforated coating pans (Accela-Cota,* Hi-Coater,† Driacoater‡) were developed as replacements for the coating pans of the 30s and 40s (Figs. 12-1, 12-2, and 12-3).

In this chapter, the current state of tablet coating and the opportunities for continued improvement are presented.

Tablet Coating Principles

The application of coating to tablets, which is an additional step in the manufacturing process, increases the cost of the product; therefore, the decision to coat a tablet is usually based on one or more of the following objectives:

1. To mask the taste, odor, or color of the drug.

2. To provide physical and chemical protection for the drug.

3. To control the release of the drug from the tablet.

4. To protect the drug from the gastric environment of the stomach with an acid-resistant enteric coating.

5. To incorporate another drug or formula adjuvant in the coating to avoid chemical incompatibilities or to provide sequential drug release.

6. To improve the pharmaceutical elegance by use of special colors and contrasting printing.

* Thomas Engineering, Hoffman Estates, IL.
† Vector Corporation, Marion, IA.
‡ Driam Metallprodukt GmbH & Co. KG, Eriskirch, West Germany.

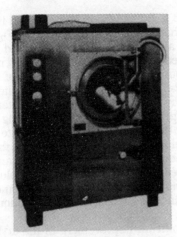

FIG. 12-1. *Accela-Cota system. (Courtesy of Thomas Engineering Inc., Hoffman Estates, IL.)*

The coating process can best be described by initially discussing the key factors that it comprises and then showing their complex interactions. There are three primary components involved in tablet coating:

1. Tablet properties.

2. Coating process.
   Coating equipment.
   Parameters of the coating process.
   Facility and ancillary equipment.
   Automation in coating processes.

3. Coating compositions. (Specific examples are

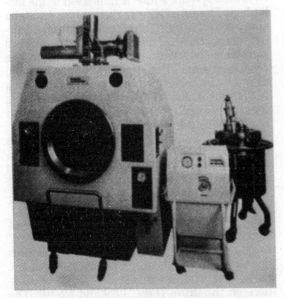

FIG. 12-2. *Hi-Coater system. (Courtesy of Vector Corporation, Marion, IA.)*

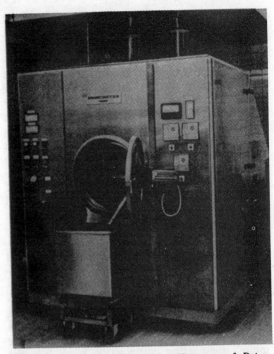

FIG. 12-3. *Driacoater system. (Courtesy of Driam Metallprodukt GmbH & Co. KG, Eriskirch, West Germany.)*

discussed in the section entitled "Tablet Coating Processes.")

Tablet Properties. Tablets that are to be coated must possess the proper physical characteristics. In the coating process, the tablets roll in a coating pan or cascade in the air stream of an air suspension coater as the coating composition is applied. To tolerate the intense attrition of tablets striking other tablets or walls of the coating equipment, the tablets must be resistant to abrasion and chipping. Tablet surfaces that are brittle, that soften in the presence of heat, or that are affected by the coating composition tend to become rough in the early phase of the coating process and are unacceptable for film coating. Film coatings adhere to all exposed surfaces, so that any surface imperfection is coated and not eliminated. The quality of thin film coatings applied to compressed tablets usually depends much more on the quality of the starting tablet than on the time at which sugar coatings are applied. Sugar coatings, with their high solids content, dry more slowly and can fill many of the minor tablet surface imperfections that may occur in the early phase of the coating process.

In addition to a smooth surface, the physical shape of the tablet is important. When a coating composition is applied to a batch of tablets in a coating pan, the tablet surfaces become covered with a tacky polymeric film. Before the tablet surface dries, the applied coating changes from a sticky liquid to a tacky semisolid, and eventually to a nontacky dry surface. The tablets must be in constant motion during the early drying phase or tablet agglomeration can occur. The ideal tablet shape for coating is a sphere, which allows tablets to roll freely in the coating pan, with minimal tablet-to-tablet contact. The worst shape is a square flat-faced tablet, in which case coating materials would collect between the surfaces to glue them together, like a stack of dominos or poker chips. For this reason, coated tablets have rounded surfaces; the more convex the surface is, the fewer difficulties will be encountered with tablet agglomeration.

A compressed tablet formulation includes many ingredients besides the active drug to provide a readily compressible, resilient, and rapidly dissolving dosage form. The resulting surface properties of the tablet depend on the chemical nature of the ingredients utilized in the formulation. For the coating to adhere to the tablet, the coating composition must wet the surface. Hydrophobic tablet surfaces are difficult to coat with aqueous-based coatings that do not wet the surface. The composition of the coating formulation can be adjusted, however, through the addition of appropriate surfactants to reduce the surface tension of the coating composition and improve coating adhesion.

Coating Process. The principles of tablet coating are relatively simple. Tablet coating is the application of a coating composition to a moving bed of tablets with the concurrent use of heated air to facilitate evaporation of the solvent. The distribution of the coating is accomplished by the movement of the tablets either perpendicular (coating pan) or vertical (air suspension coater) to the application of the coating composition.

Equipment. Most coating processes use one of three general types of equipment: (1) the standard coating pan, (2) the perforated coating pan, or (3) the fluidized bed (air suspension) coater. The general trend has been toward energy-efficient, automated systems to shorten the total coating time and reduce operator participation in the coating process. In addition, several pharmaceutical companies have developed their own coating equipment or made modifications in standard equipment to accommodate their particular coating processes. Most of the systems, however, are based on three basic designs.

Conventional Pan System. The standard coating pan system consists of a circular metal pan mounted somewhat angularly on a stand. The

pan is 8 to 60 inches in diameter and is rotated on its horizontal axis by a motor (Fig. 12-4). Heated air is directed into the pan and onto the tablet bed surface, and is exhausted by means of ducts positioned through the front of the pan (Fig. 12-5). Coating solutions are applied to the tablets by ladling or spraying the material onto the rotating tablet bed. Use of atomizing systems to spray the liquid coating material onto the tablets produces a faster, more even distribution of the solution or suspension. Spraying can significantly reduce drying time between solution applications in sugar coating processes and allows for continuous application of the solution in film coating.

A significant improvement in the drying efficiency of the standard coating pan is achieved by the Pellegrini pan (Fig. 12-6), the immersion-sword (Fig. 12-7), and the immersion-tube systems (Fig. 12-8). The Pellegrini system has a baffled pan and a diffuser that distributes the drying air uniformly over the tablet bed surface. Newer models are completely enclosed, which further increases their drying efficiency and facilitates automated control. With the immersion-sword system, drying air is introduced through a perforated metal sword device that is immersed in the tablet bed. The drying air flows upward from the sword through the tablet bed. Since the air is more intimately mixed with the wetted tablets, a more efficient drying environment is provided. Coating solutions are applied by an atomized spray system directed to the surface of the rotating tablet bed. With the immersion-tube system, a tube is immersed in the tablet bed. The tube delivers the heated air, and a spray nozzle is built in the tip of the tube. During this operation, the coating solution is applied simultaneously with the heated air from the immersed tube. The drying air flows upward through the tablet bed and is exhausted by a conventional duct. Relatively rapid processing times have been reported for both film and sugar coating with this system.[5]

Both the immersion-sword and the immersion-tube systems have been introduced in Europe, and they are adaptable to conventional coating pans.

Perforated Pan Systems. In general, all equipment of this type consists of a perforated or partially perforated drum that is rotated on its horizontal axis in an enclosed housing. In the Accela-Cota and Hi-Coater systems, drying air is directed into the drum, is passed through the tablet bed, and is exhausted through perforations in the drum (Figs. 12-9 and 12-10). The Driacoater introduces drying air through hollow perforated ribs located on the inside periphery of

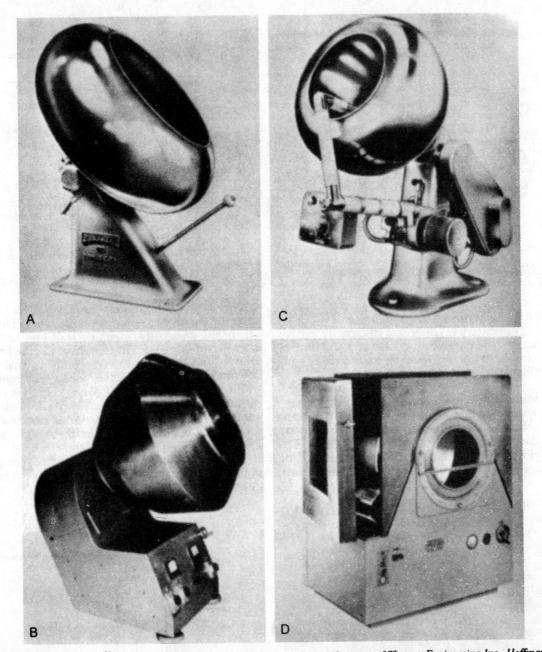

FIG. 12-4. *Standard coating pans.* A, B, *Pan shapes.* C, D, *Air sources.* (*Courtesy of Thomas Engineering Inc., Hoffman Estates, IL.*)

the drum (Fig. 12-11). As the coating pan rotates, the ribs dip into the tablet bed, and drying air passes up through and fluidizes the tablet bed. Exhaust is from the back of the pan.

The Glatt coater is the latest perforated pan coater to be introduced in the industry (Fig. 12-11A). In the Glatt coater, drying air can be directed from inside the drum through the tablet

bed and out an exhaust duct; alternatively, with an optional split-chambered plenum, drying air can be directed in the reverse manner up through the drum perforations for partial fluidization of the tablet bed. Several airflow configurations are possible.

In all four of these perforated pan systems, the coating solution is applied to the surface of the

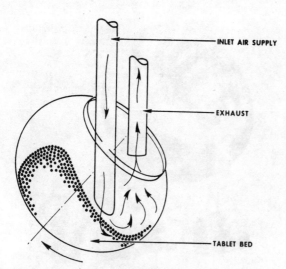

FIG. 12-5. *Diagram of standard coating pans.*

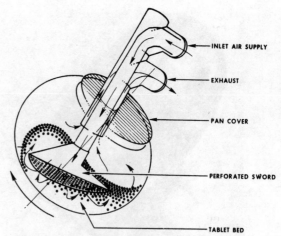

FIG. 12-7. *Simplified diagram of Glatt immersion-sword system.*

rotating bed of tablets through spraying nozzles that are positioned inside the drum.

Perforated pan coaters are efficient drying systems with high coating capacity, and can be completely automated for both sugar coating and film coating processes.

Fluidized Bed (Air Suspension) Systems. Fluidized bed coaters are also highly efficient drying systems. Fluidization of the tablet mass is achieved in a columnar chamber by the upward flow of drying air (Figs. 12-12 and 12-13). The airflow is controlled so that more air enters the center of the column, causing the tablets to rise in the center. The movement of tablets is upward through the center of the chamber. They then fall toward the chamber wall and move downward to re-enter the air stream at the bottom of the chamber. In some units, a smaller column(s) is used to direct tablet movement within the main column. Coating solutions are continuously applied from a spray nozzle located at the bottom of the chamber or are sprayed onto the top of the cascading tablet bed by nozzles located in the upper region of the chamber.

Tablet cores that are friable and prone to chipping and edge abrasion may be difficult to coat even under optimum conditions in the fluidized

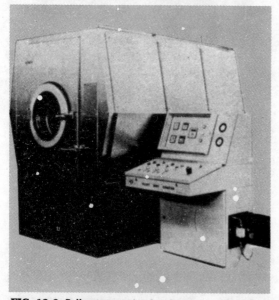

FIG. 12-6. *Pellegrini pan (enclosed) system. (Courtesy of Nicomac, Milan, Italy.)*

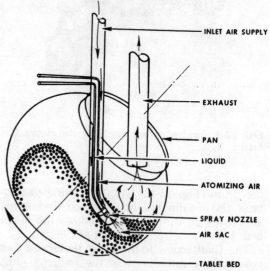

FIG. 12-8. *Diagram of immersion-tube system. (From Demmer et al.[5])*

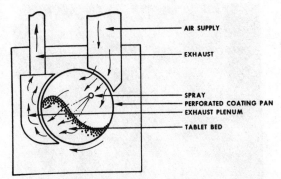

FIG. 12-9. *Simplified diagram of Accela-Cota system.*

bed systems, owing to the relatively rough tablet-to-tablet impact and tablet-chamber contact.

*Spray Application Systems.** The two basic types of systems used to apply a finely divided (atomized) spray of coating solutions or suspensions onto tablets are (1) high-pressure, airless and (2) low-pressure, air-atomized. The principal difference in the two types is the manner in which atomization of the liquid is achieved.

In the airless spray system, liquid is pumped at high pressure (250 to 3000 pounds per square

*Suppliers of spray application systems include (1) Spraying Systems Co., Wheaton, IL; (2) Graco Inc., Minneapolis, MN; (3) Vector Corp., Marion, IA; (4) Binks Manufacturing Co., Franklin Park, IL; (5) Nordson Corp., Amherst, OH.

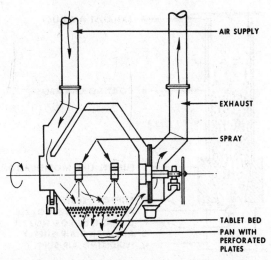

FIG. 12-10. *Simplified diagram of Hi-Coater system.*

inch gauge (psig)) through a small orifice (.009 inch to .020 inch id) in the fluid nozzle (Fig. 12-14), which results in a finely divided spray. The degree of atomization and the spray rate are controlled by the fluid pressure, orifice size, and viscosity of the liquid. Because of the small orifice, suspended solids in the coating composition must be finely milled or filtered to prevent orifice blockage.

In the low-pressure air-atomized system, liquid is pumped through a somewhat larger orifice (0.020 inch to 0.060 inch id) at relatively low

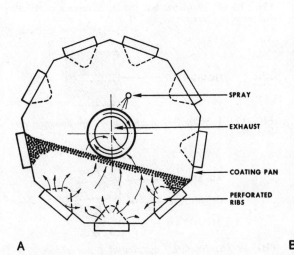

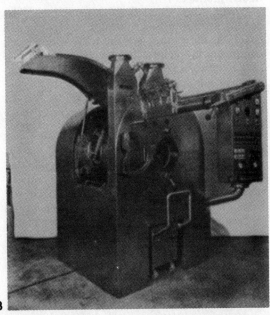

A **B**

FIG. 12-11. A, *Diagram of Driacoater pan.* B, *Glatt coater. (Courtesy of Glatt Air Techniques Inc., Ramsey, NJ.)*

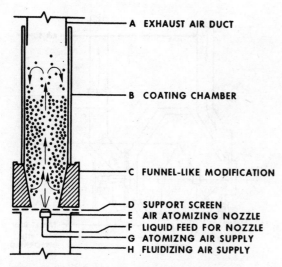

A — EXHAUST AIR DUCT

B — COATING CHAMBER

C — FUNNEL-LIKE MODIFICATION

D — SUPPORT SCREEN
E — AIR ATOMIZING NOZZLE
F — LIQUID FEED FOR NOZZLE
G — ATOMIZNG AIR SUPPLY
H — FLUIDIZING AIR SUPPLY

FIG. 12-12. *Diagram of a fluidized bed coater.*

pressures (5 to 50 psig) (Fig. 12-15). Low-pressure (10 to 100 psig) air contacts the liquid stream at the tip of the atomizer, and a finely divided spray is produced. The degree of atomization is controlled by the fluid pressure, fluid cap orifice, viscosity of the liquid, air pressure, and air cap design.

Both airless and air atomizing systems can be used effectively. Originally, airless systems were primarily used in air suspension coaters, but now the choice depends on the coating solution formula and on the process developed for a particular product.

Parameters. The following discussion of the coating process focuses primarily on perforated coating pans, as they are the most widely used equipment in the industry. However, the principles of the coating pan method are equally applicable to air suspension coating, with the exception that a portion of the air in the air suspension coater is used to suspend or move the tablets.

During the coating process, the tablets move through an application zone in which a portion of the tablets receive some coating. Outside this zone, a portion of the applied coating composition may be physically transferred from the coated tablets to adjacent ones, or even to the surface of the coating equipment. Most of the time, the tablets are in a drying mode moving away from the application zone and are recycled repeatedly through the application zone. The coating application and heated airflow can be continuous or intermediate, depending on the coating composition and drying conditions. In a continuous coating operation, the coating opera-

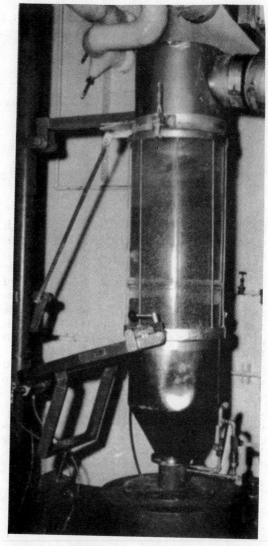

FIG. 12-13. *Fluidized bed coater. (Courtesy of Abbott Laboratories, North Chicago, IL.)*

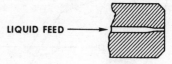

LIQUID FEED →

FIG. 12-14. *Simplified diagram of a high-pressure, airless nozzle.*

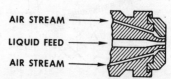

AIR STREAM →
LIQUID FEED →
AIR STREAM →

FIG. 12-15. *Simplified diagram of a low-pressure, air-atomized nozzle.*

tion is maintained essentially at equilibrium, where the rate of application of the coating composition equals the rate of evaporation of the volatile solvents. Deviation from this equilibrium results in serious coating problems. Mathematical modeling of the aqueous coating process has been accomplished by Stetsko and associates,[6] and by Reiland and associates.[7] These basic studies have formed the basis for the automated coating systems described later in the chapter.

A better appreciation of the balancing act that must be maintained in the coating process can be visually shown as follows:

$$\textit{Inlet } A(T_1, H_1) + C_1(S) + pSA_1$$
$$\xrightarrow{E} A\ (T_2, H_2) + C_2 + pSA_2\ \textit{Exhaust}$$

where $A(T, H)$ is the air capacity, $C(S)$ is the coating composition, pSA is the tablet surface area, and E is the equipment efficiency.

Air Capacity, $A(T, H)$. This value represents the quantity of water or solvent that can be removed during the coating process, which depends on the quantity of air flowing through the tablet bed (CFM), the temperature of the air (T), and the quantity of water that the inlet air contains (H). This relationship can best be illustrated by using a psychrometric chart from an engineering handbook. The chart graphically shows the relationship between air temperatures and the quantity of water that air can contain at various relative humidities (RH).

For example, if the temperature of the inlet air is 100°F at about 10% RH it contains 30 g H_2O per pound of dry air. During the coating operation, water is evaporated from the applied aqueous coating solution, and the air temperature falls. The temperature of the exit air depends on the amount of water it contains. If the exit temperature is 75°F, the fall in temperature of 25°F is primarily due to evaporation of water, and the exit air contains 70 g of H_2O per pound of dry air (about 55% RH). Saturating the exit air yields a wet bulb temperature of 63.5°F.

Given the operating conditions, it is possible to know if the application rate is approaching the capacity of the drying system. Only a small portion of the tablet bed (pSA) receives coating at any given time; the exit temperature therefore measures the average of temperature conditions associated with tablets that are completely dry to those of tablets partially coated with the coating composition.

Coating Composition, $C(S)$. The coating contains the ingredients that are to be applied on the tablet surface and the solvents, which act as carriers for the ingredients. These solvents are essentially removed during the coating process. The inlet air provides the heat to evaporate the water. The exhaust air becomes cooler and contains more water, owing to the evaporation of the solvent from the coating composition (see preceding example). If water is applied to a nonpenetrating surface, the relationship between inlet air (temperature/humidity) and exhaust air at a given spray rate can be clearly demonstrated. Tablet surfaces are permeable to the applied coating solution, which can cause coating difficulties. Most of the coating composition is solvent, so that rapid removal is necessary to prevent adverse effects on tablet integrity; however, high temperatures needed to achieve rapid drying may be detrimental to the stability of the drug in the tablet and may prevent partial distribution of the coating that occurs with movement of the tablets outside the application zone. The drying characteristic of the film must also be considered in determining the rate of application. In general, more viscous, aqueous-based coating compositions use movement of the tablets outside the application zone to produce partial distribution of the coating; longer drying periods are required so that intermittent coating application may be used. Thin, rapidly drying formulations dry quickly on the tablet surface, allowing constant application by efficient atomization of the coating solution.

Tablet Surface Area, pSA. The quality of the tablets needed for coating has already been considered, but the size of the tablet and the presence of debossed features also affect the coating conditions. The total surface area per unit weight decreases significantly from smaller to larger tablets. Application of a film with the same thickness requires correspondingly less coating composition. For example, when film coating a small pan load (20 kg) of tablets, a 0.281-inch round convex tablet that has a thickness of 0.114 inch requires 40% more coating than when the same coating thickness is applied to a 0.438-inch round convex tablet of 0.202-inch thickness.

In the coating process, only a portion of the total surface area (pSA) is coated. The balance consists of partially coated tablets being dried or dried tablets to be further coated in the application zone. Continuous partial coating and recycling eventually results in fully coated tablets.

The addition of small product identity markings or intagliations further complicates the coating process. The size of the atomized coating droplet must be smaller and better controlled as the features to be coated become smaller.

Equipment Efficiency, E. Tablet coaters use the expression "coating efficiency," a value obtained by dividing the net increase in coated tablet weight by the total nonvolatile coating weight applied to the tablets. Ideally, 90 to 95% of the applied film coating should be on the tablet surface. Any quantity less than that suggests that improvements in the coating operation should be sought. Coating efficiency for conventional sugar coating is much less, and 60% would be acceptable. This significant difference in coating efficiency between film and sugar coating relates to the quantity of coating material that collects on the pan walls. With an efficient film coating process, little coating material accumulates on the wall, but with sugar coating, the pan walls become thickly covered with coating. A common cause of low film coating efficiency is that the application rate is too slow for the coating conditions (large tablet surface area, high airflow, and high temperature). This results in drying part of the coating composition before it reaches the tablet surfaces, so that it is exhausted as dust.

Facility and Ancillary Equipment.
The facility required for any coating operation should be designed to meet the requirements of current Good Manufacturing Practices (GMPs) as set forth in the latest revision of the Code of Federal Regulations, Title 21, Part 211. Adequate space is needed not only for the coating equipment, but also for solution preparation and in-process storage. The specific safety requirement for coating areas depends on the nature of the solvent. Where explosive or toxic concentrations of organic solvent could occur, during either solution preparation or the coating operation, electrical explosion-proofing and specialized ventilation are required.

Treatment of the exhaust air from the coating operation may be desired to recover expensive organic solvents or to prevent solvents and particulate from entering the atmosphere. Local, state, and federal Environmental Protection Agency (EPA) regulations define the limits of organic solvent and particulate allowed in the atmosphere.

Compliance with the regulations can be extremely expensive, and this cost factor should be considered in developing a new coating. A major advantage of totally aqueous-based film coating is that all direct and indirect expenses relating to the purchase, handling, and environmentally acceptable removal of the organic solvent are circumvented.

Other equipment is needed to support the coating operation. Solution preparation requires tanks, filters, and mixers. A colloid mill or ball mill may be needed for the homogeneous dispersion of insoluble solids in the liquid coating mixture. Jacketed tanks may be needed for keeping some solutions at an elevated temperature.

The coating liquid can be supplied to the nozzle system of the coating equipment by means of portable pressure tanks or various pumping systems.

Automation.
There is little published information providing details of automated coating processes. A review article by Thomas discusses details of a programmable controller for pan coating systems.[8] Within the last 6 to 8 years, automation has been achieved in sugar coating and film coating (nonaqueous and aqueous) systems. Through a series of sensors and regulating devices for temperature, airflow, spray rate and pan speed, a feedback control of the process is maintained. Precise automated control of such a dynamic process is possible only with the help of the programmable controller. As in all automated processes, a manual bypass should be built into the system to accommodate any special applications or equipment malfunctions. For process automation, the perforated pans are preferred over the old conventional coating pans because of their better efficiency. Figure 12-16 represents a completely automated system used for film or sugar coating. As new tablet manufacturing plants are built by major pharmaceutical companies, varying degrees of automation are built into the tablet coating process. These automated coating systems are either designed by coating equipment manufacturers or developed by individual companies and tailored to their specific equipment and/or products. A detailed description of such a system is provided by V. Sharma et al.[9].

Tablet Coating Processes

In most cases, the coating process is the last critical step in the tablet production cycle. The successful application of the coating solution formula to a tablet provides the visual characteristics for the product; thus, the quality of the product may be judged on this final production step. The type of process chosen depends on the type of coating that is to be applied, the durability (toughness) of the tablet core, and the economics of the process. Because of the ever-increasing cost of energy and labor, the cost of organic solvents, and the associated environmental constraints, the economics of the process is receiving greater emphasis. Sugar coating is still a widely used coating process because of the excellent tablet appearance it achieves.

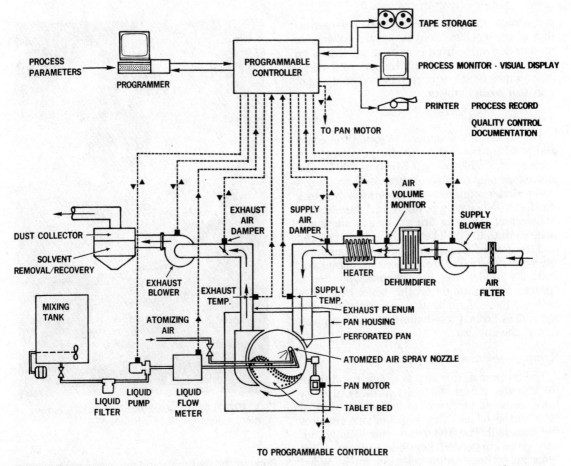

FIG. 12-16. *Diagram of an automated coating system.*

Sugar Coating

The sugar coating process involves several steps, the duration of which ranges from a few hours to a few days. A successful product greatly depends on the skill of the coating operator. This is especially true in the pan-ladling method, in which the coating solutions are poured over the tablet cores. The operator determines the quantity of solution to add, the method and rate of pouring, when to apply drying air, and how long or how fast the tablets should be tumbled in the pan. Newer techniques utilize spraying systems and varying degrees of automation to improve coating efficiency and product uniformity. Regardless of the methods used, a successful sugar coating process yields elegant, highly glossed tablets.

The basic sugar coating process involves the following steps: (1) sealing, (2) subcoating, (3) syruping (smoothing), (4) finishing, and (5) polishing.

The tablet cores preferably have deep convex surfaces with thin rounded edges to facilitate sugar coating. Since sugar coating tends to be long and vigorous, the cores should be relatively resistant to breakage, chipping, and abrasion.

Seal Coating

To prevent moisture penetration into the tablet core, a seal coat is applied. This is especially needed in pan-ladling processes, in which localized overwetting of a portion of the tablet bed occurs. Without a seal coat, the overwetted tablets would absorb excess moisture, leading to tablet softening or disintegration and affecting the physical and chemical stability of the finished product. In spray processes, it is possible to adjust the application of the subcoats and further coats so that localized overwetting does not occur. This adjustment thus eliminates the seal coating step. Shellac is an effective sealant, but tablet disintegration and dissolution times tend to lengthen on aging because of the polymerization of the shellac. Zein is an alcohol-soluble protein derivative from corn that has also been used as an effective sealant. Lengthening dissolution times have not been reported on aging of zein seal coated tablets.

Subcoating

The subcoating is applied to round the edges and build up the tablet size. Sugar coating can increase the tablet weight by 50 to 100%. The subcoating step consists of alternately applying a sticky binder solution to the tablets followed by a dusting of subcoating powders and then drying. Subsequent subcoats are applied in the same manner until the tablet edges have been covered and the desired thickness is achieved. For spray processes, a subcoating suspension containing both the binder and the insoluble powder is sprayed intermittently on the tablet bed. With both methods of application, control of the drying rate is critical to obtaining a rapid application of the subcoat.

Syrup (Smoothing/Color) Coating

The purpose of this step is to cover and fill in the imperfections in the tablet surface caused by the subcoating step, and to impart the desired color to the tablet. This step perhaps requires the most skill. The first syrup coats usually contain some suspended powders and are called "grossing syrups." Dilute colorants can be added to this phase to provide a tinted base that facilitates uniform coloring in later steps. In general, no color is added until the tablets are quite smooth; premature application to rough tablets can produce a mottled appearance in the final coated tablets. In subsequent syruping steps, syrup solutions containing the dye are applied until the final size and color are achieved. In the final syruping or finishing step, a few clear coats of syrup may be applied.

Polishing

The desired luster is obtained in this final step of the sugar coating process. The tablets can be polished in clean standard coating pans, or canvas-lined polishing pans (Fig. 12-17), by carefully applying powdered wax (beeswax or carnauba) or warm solutions of these waxes in naphtha or other suitable volatile solvents.

Example*

The basic sugar coating process is illustrated in this example. An infinite number of varia-

*See Table 12-1 for formulations used in this process.

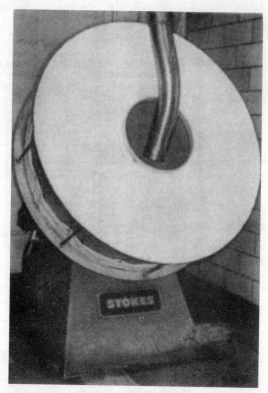

FIG. 12-17. *Canvas-lined polishing pan. (Courtesy of Warner-Lambert Co., Morris Plains, NJ.)*

tions in the materials and processes are possible; however, the complexity of the process can be appreciated by the following example.

I. Materials and Equipment

Coating pans—Stainless steel, 40 inches in diameter, with variable speed control; or 48-inch Accela-Cota, with 2 to 3 air atomizing nozzles. Nozzles should have a fluid orifice of .040 to .060 inch. Set atomizing air to 30 to 40 psig.

Tablet cores—55 to 70 kg of 3/8-inch standard convex tablets.

NOTE: If desired, coating solutions may be poured or ladled onto the tablets. If this method is chosen, apply the solutions in a steady flow, with even distribution over the rotating tablet bed.

II. Process

A. Seal Coat

1. The specific advantage of using a spray system described in this example is that a faster and more even distribution of the coating materials is obtained. Start the tablets rolling (pan speed: 10 rpm). Set supply air to 30°C.

TABLE 12-1. *Formulations Used in Sugar Coating*

Seal Coating Solutions	Formula Variation	
	I	II
Cellulose acetate phthalate		175 g
Zein	480 g	
Oleic acid, USP	60 g	
Propylene glycol, USP		52.5 g
Polyethylene glycol 4000	144 g	
Methylene chloride	480 ml	840 ml
Alcohol SD 3A 200-proof	q.s. to 2.4 L	q.s. to 1.75 L

Subcoating Solutions	Formula Variation			
	I	II	III	IV
Gelatin	60 g	5.4 kg		60 g
Acacia	60 g	2.7 kg	450 g	60 g
Sugar, cane	1500 g	53.7 kg		1500 g
Syrup, corn			450 g	
Syrup, USP			3.785 L	
Water, distilled	1.0 L	44.3 kg		1.0 L

Subcoating Powders	Formula Variation						
	I	II	III	IV	V	VI	VII
Kaolin		225 kg					
Dextrin		112 kg	185 kg				
Cocoa powder		60 kg					
Calcium carbonate, pptd			480 kg		7.72 kg		8.62 kg
Sugar, cane, powdered	4.1 kg	112 kg	240 kg	40 kg	0.9 kg	180 g	0.86 kg
Acacia, powdered	0.12 kg			6 kg		1 g	
Starch, corn	1.35 kg				0.9 kg	60 g	
Talc, USP	0.23 kg					1 g	
Calcium sulfate, NF							8.62 kg

Syrup Solutions	Grossing Syrups			Heavy Syrups		Regular Syrups	
	I	II	III	I	II	I	II
Colorant	q.s. ad	q.s. ad	q.s. ad	q.s. ad	q.s. ad	q.s. ad	q.s. ad
Subcoating powder	22.7 kg						
Calcium carbonate, light		7.75 kg	69 g				
Sugar, cane, powder	136 kg	22.7 kg	572 g	2.73 kg	181 kg	85 g	1.2 kg
Starch, corn		1.36 kg	69 g				
Syrup, USP		22.7 L		3.785 L	256 kg		
Water, distilled	76 kg		290 ml			q.s. 100 ml	1.0 L

Polishing Solutions	Formula Variation	
	I	II
Wax, carnauba, yellow	0.09 kg	10 g
Beeswax, white	0.09 kg	90 g
Wax, paraffin	0.02 kg	
Naphtha	3.785 L	1.0 L

Apply 3 applications of zein solution (see Table 12-1), 800 ml per application. Allow 15 to 20 min between applications to ensure that the tablets are dry. If tablets become tacky between applications, apply just enough talc to prevent sticking to the pan and to each other. Make sure that the solution is well distributed. Additional mixing by hand may be necessary to achieve this if pan design and baffling are inefficient.

B. *Subcoat*

Use any of the gelatin/acacia solutions and subcoating powders listed in Table 12-1.

1. Turn heat and inlet air off. Use exhaust only. Start pan speed at 10 rpm.
2. Apply 3 to 9 coats. Use 1.5 L of warm-gelatin/acacia solution for the first coat. Reduce subsequent amounts accordingly to obtain the correct thickness. Be sure that edges are covered. Thickness is checked volumetrically.
3. Allow at least 20 min between coats to permit adequate drying. Be sure the solution is rapidly and uniformly dispersed in the tablet bed. Dust with subcoating powder when tackiness develops. Apply subcoating powder until tablets roll freely and show no signs of tackiness.
4. After the last coat, jog the pan periodically for at least 2 to 4 hours to ensure dryness.

C. *Syrup (Smoothing/Color) Coat*

The syruping coat usually involves three basic phases: grossing syrup (a syrup solution with subcoating powders dispersed in it), heavy syrup, and regular syrup. Apply each step in the sequence outlined.

1. Remove excess dust in pan before starting. Turn on exhaust outlet air. Set inlet air temperature to provide an exhaust temperature of 45 to 48°C. Set pan speed at 12 rpm.
2. Apply 5 to 15 coats of the grossing syrup, just enough to wet the entire bed. Because this solution dries relatively quickly, uniform, rapid distribution must be provided. Apply successive amounts of grossing syrup immediately after each preceding application is drying and slightly dusty.
3. Apply several heavy-colored syrup coats in a similar manner until a specific tablet volume is attained.

4. Turn off heat, and reduce inlet and exhaust air.
5. Apply several coats of the regular-colored syrup solution to achieve a final smoothness, size, and color development.
6. Each coat of regular-colored syrup is applied as soon as the tablets exhibit a slightly frosted appearance. Do not allow them to become dusty.

D. *Finishing*

1. Make sure that the pan is clean.
2. Operate pan with the heat turned off, no supply, and greatly reduced exhaust air. Set pan speed at 12 rpm.
3. Apply 3 or 4 coats of regular-colored syrup rapidly, without permitting the tablet bed to frost or become dusty.
4. The last coats of regular syrup can be applied without colorant. This gives "depth" to the color and enhances the elegance of the coat.
5. Shut off exhaust air before applying the last coat. Apply coat; mix uniformly and shut off pan while the tablets are still damp. A quick jog every few minutes prevents sticking. After 15 to 30 min, stop jogging and leave tablets in pan to dry slowly overnight.

E. *Polishing*

Polishing can be done in the same pan as the sugar coating, but better results are obtained in canvas-lined pans.

1. Supply air, exhaust air, and heat should be turned off. Pan speed 12 rpm.
2. Apply 3 to 4 coats of warm polishing solution, approximately 300 ml per application.
3. Let solvent evaporate completely between coats.

Tablet coatings achieve their luster during the polishing phase. In the canvas-lined pans, the lining is used to transfer the waxes to the tablet surface and to provide a buffing action. The wax polishing solutions are usually poured onto the canvas, and the tablets pick up the wax shine as they tumble in the pan. The waxes can also be dusted onto the tablets. Care must be exercised to distribute the wax evenly to avoid wax spots on some tablets. Application of warm air can facilitate distribution.

The techniques used to obtain the desired product, especially in the pan-ladling process, are complex and can only be learned through practice. The beginner is advised to consult the listed literature for specific techniques, materials, and precautions of the sugar coating processes.[10–15] The use of modern efficient automated systems is rapidly making manual techniques obsolete. Several automated processes have been described in the literature.[8,16–18]

Through the addition of cellulosic polymers, and other coating ingredients normally associated with film coating, much thinner sugar coatings have been attained.[19,20]

Film Coating

Since film coating originated from the pan sugar coating era, it is not surprising that the film coating process today still contains some of the process features associated with the early work. With the possible exception of the air suspension coater, film coating and sugar coating share the same equipment and process parameters.

Pan-Pour Methods

Pan-pour methods have been used for many years for film coating, but they have been supplanted by newer coating techniques that are faster and more reproducible. Coating compositions used in the earlier pan-pour methods were usually too viscous to be sprayed effectively. Tablets coated by pan-pour methods are subjected to alternate solution application, mixing and drying steps similar to pan-pour sugar coating. The method is relatively slow and relies heavily on the skill and technique of the operator to balance the steps to produce an acceptable product. Tablets that are film coated by pan-pour processes almost always require additional drying steps to remove latent solvents. Aqueous-based film coatings are not suitable for this method of application because localized overwetting inherent with the pan-pour process causes numerous problems ranging from surface erosion to product instability due to unacceptably high latent moisture content in the cores.

Pan-Spray Methods

The introduction of spraying equipment was the next evolution in improving the efficiency of film coating processes. Spraying lends versatility to the process and allows for automated control of liquid application. Spray patterns are selected to provide a continuous band across the tablet bed surface. Broad, flat spray patterns are usually chosen by selection of appropriate nozzle systems so that the entire width of the tablet bed can be covered by the spray from 1 to 5 nozzles.

Process Variables

Whether the coating process is in a conventional pan system or in one of the perforated pan systems previously described, certain elements of the process need to be controlled to ensure consistent product quality. The process is as important as the coating solution formulation; consequently development of a well-defined and well-controlled process should be a major concern of the formulator.

The variables to be controlled in pan-spray film coating processes are:

1. *Pan Variables*
   pan design/baffling
   speed
   pan load

2. *Process Air*
   air quality
   temperature
   airflow rate/volume/balance

3. *Spray Variables*
   spray rate
   degree of atomization
   spray pattern
   nozzle-to-bed distance

Since each listed variable is important to the overall success of the coating, further discussion is warranted.

Pan Variables. Pan shape, baffling, rotational speed, and loading all affect the mixing of the tablet mass. Uniform mixing is essential to depositing the same quantity of film on each tablet. The tablet coating adds an approximate increase in weight of only 2 to 5% to the tablet. Unacceptable color uniformity or enteric film integrity is encountered if the tablets are inadequately coated because of poor tablet movement in the coating pan.

Tablet shape can also affect mixing. Some tablet shapes may mix freely while other shapes may require a specific baffling arrangement to ensure adequate mixing. Baffles, however, provide a source for chipping and breakage if they are not carefully selected and used.

Pan speed affects not only mixing, but also the velocity at which the tablets pass under the spray. Speeds that are too slow may cause localized overwetting, resulting in the tablets sticking to each other or to the pan. Speeds that are too high may not allow enough time for drying before the same tablets are reintroduced to the spray; again, this results in a rough coating appearance on the tablets. Pan speeds of 10 to 15 rpm are commonly used in the large pan coaters for nonaqueous film coating. Slower pan speeds (3 to 10 rpm) are used for aqueous film coating primarily to accommodate slower application rate and drying of the coating liquid. Selection of pan operating conditions depends on the equipment availability, type of tablets being coated, and the characteristics of the coating solution.

Spray Variables. The spray variables to be controlled are the rate of liquid application, the spray pattern, and the degree of atomization. These three variables are interdependent. In the airless, high-pressure system, all three variables are directly affected by fluid pressure and nozzle design. In the air-atomized, low-pressure system, the rate of liquid flow is most directly affected by the liquid pressure and liquid orifice size. The degree of atomization and spray pattern are most directly affected by atomizing air pressure, air volume, and the shape and design of the air jets in relation to the fluid stream.

The proper rate at which the coating solution should be applied depends on the mixing and drying efficiency of the system, in addition to the coating formula and core characteristics. There is a range in which the coating rate must operate to achieve the desired product quality or processing time. Overwetting and underwetting must be avoided in all coating operations.

A band of spray should be spread evenly over the tablet mass. In larger pans, more nozzles must be added to cover the tablet bed width. A spray pattern that is too wide could result in the application of coating directly to the pan surface, producing lower coating efficiency and wasted material. If the spray pattern is too narrow, localized overwetting may result, and the tablet-to-tablet coating uniformity will be poor. Thus, tablets need to make many more passes through the spraying area to be adequately coated. During the coating operation, the spray width can be adjusted by moving the nozzles closer or farther away from the tablet bed. In the air-atomized, low-pressure systems, adjusting the air pressure and/or direction accomplishes the same effect. The distance that the nozzle is from the tablet bed affects not only the spray width, but also the quantity of coating applied to individual tablets per pass under the spray.

Atomization is the process whereby the liquid stream is finely subdivided into droplets. The degree of atomization—the size and size distribution of the droplets—obtained from the spray nozzle is not an easily controllable parameter.

The relationships between the orifice size, nozzle configuration, fluid pressure, atomizing air pressure, air volume, and fluid viscosity vary with each coating formulation. Manufacturing literature may provide the droplet size range expected from a particular nozzle type based on water; however, this type of data is inadequate for optimizing the nozzle performance in relation to the variety of solutions and suspensions used to coat tablets.

The degree of atomization, at present, can only be controlled empirically. Adjustments of either the fluid pressure on the airless high-pressure systems or the atomizing air pressure and air volume on the low-pressure systems change the degree of atomization. Higher pressures yield greater atomization. Atomization that is too fine causes some droplets to dry before reaching the tablet bed. This "spray-drying" effect can be readily detected as roughness on the tablet surface, especially in intagliations or as excess dust in the pan. Insufficient atomization may result in droplets that are too large reaching the tablet surface and causing localized overwetting, which could lead to sticking, picking, or a rough "orange-peel" effect.

Process Air Variables. The temperature, volume, rate, quality, and balance are parameters of the process air that need to be controlled to obtain an optimum drying environment for a particular coating process. The sensitivity of the film former and product core to heat largely determines the upper temperature at which the coating process is successful. In general, higher tablet bed and coating chamber temperatures are more conducive to rapid solvent evaporation, and consequently to faster coating rate. The limits to the air volume and rate depend on the overall design of the air-handling system and coating equipment. The upper end of the system's range is used most often. The more efficient the equipment design, the less air volume is needed for drying.

Supply air should have some degree of dehumidification. Seasonal fluctuations in the moisture content of incoming air can alter coating and drying conditions and possibly have adverse affects on the quality of the coating.

The balance between supply and exhaust airflow should be such that all dust and solvent are contained within the coating system.

Fluidized Bed Process

The fluidized bed systems have been successfully used for rapid coating of tablets, granules, and capsules. The coating solution formulations used with these processes are similar to those used for the pan processes. Since air is used to move the tablets in the coating process, there are some specific process controls unique to air suspension coaters.

The chamber design, together with the process air, controls the fluidization pattern. Tablet shape, size, density, and quantity of load affect the ability of the tablet mass to be fluidized.

Adequate fluidization and drying depend on the volume and rate of the process air. Control of the process air is achieved by adjusting a variable speed blower or by using dampers to keep the tablet mass in a constant "fluid" motion inside the chamber. Too high an airflow results in excess tablet attrition and breakage. If the airflow rate is too low, the mass does not move fast enough through the spray region, and overwetting may occur. Fluidization may also be affected by the increase in weight or by changes in the frictional characteristics of the tablets during coating application. Consequently, periodic adjustment of the rate and volume will be necessary to maintain optimum fluidization.

During the coating operation, both the inlet and exhaust air temperatures are monitored. Evaporation of the solvent causes the exhaust air temperature to be cooler than the inlet. Any change in the rate of application of the coating solution can be monitored by the difference between the inlet and exit air temperatures.

Examples

Representative examples of organic and aqueous-based film coating formulations for use in laboratory perforated coating pan are provided.

I. Materials and Equipment
Standard 24-inch Accela-Cota with 2 baffles.
Spray system—Air-atomized spray nozzle with a .040-inch fluid orifice and a flat spray air cap.
Pumping system—Pressure tanks.
Coating materials—Description to follow (see example 1).
Pan load—12 kg of 1/2-inch standard convex tablets.
Operating conditions—Set pan speed at 12 to 15 rpm. Adjust supply air temperature to give an exhaust air temperature of 30°C during spray application. Use 40 to 50°C for the aqueous coating systems. Atomizing air pressure should equal 30 to 50 psig.

II. Process
1. Load tablets into pan. Attach and adjust the spray nozzle to spray on upper half of tablet bed.
2. Turn on heat, drying air, exhaust, and atomizing air.
3. Intermittently jog the pan while tablets are warming.
4. When exhaust temperature reaches 30°C, start spraying.
5. Apply 3.0 to 4.0 L of color solution at a rate of 70 to 100 ml/min. Adjust rate downward if tablets become tacky.
6. Apply 1.5 to 2.5 L of clear solution at a rate of 70 to 100 ml/min. Adjust rate downward if tablets become tacky. Allow tablets to dry in pan with air and heat on for 5 to 10 min.

One of the simplest film compositions would have all of the ingredients solubilized in the solvents, as in example 1.

Example 1: Hydroxypropyl Methylcellulose Nonaqueous Formula

(This formula can be applied by spraying or pouring systems.)

Hydroxypropyl methylcellulose 2910, USP, 15 cps	4%
Propylene glycol, USP	1.2%
Ethyl alcohol 200-proof	45%
Methylene chloride	q.s. ad 100%

The polymer is gradually added to the ethyl alcohol while the solvent is continuously agitated. A portion of the methylene chloride is added to this suspension, to solubilize the polymer. The propylene glycol is then added, and the remainder of the methylene chloride is added to obtain the proper volume.

The addition of insoluble colorants, opaquants, or flavors requires a milling step to facilitate their adequate dispersal.

Example 2: Cellulose Acetate Phthalate/Carbowax Nonaqueous Formula

(This formula should be poured, or diluted with appropriate solvents for spraying.)

Nonenteric Formula

Cellulose acetate phthalate, NF	5.0%
Polyethylene glycol 8000, NF	15.0%
Sorbitan monooleate, NF	0.3%
Dye yellow, D&C Lake #5	0.05%
Titanium dioxide	0.5%
Vanillin	0.1%
Castor oil	0.25%
Ethyl alcohol 200-proof	12.0%
Acetone	q.s. ad 100.0%

The cellulose acetate phthalate is dissolved in

the ethyl alcohol, sorbitan monooleate, and part of the acetone. To ensure proper dispersion, the dye, titanium dioxide, and vanillin are milled in a ball or high-energy mill, or are dispersed in acetone using a colloid mill. After the particle size reduction or dispersion has occurred, the colorants are added to the solution containing the polymer. The polyethylene glycol 8000 is melted and added with the castor oil to the polymer dispersion. The composition is brought to proper volume with acetone. This preparation must be kept slightly warm and must be properly agitated to assure proper distribution of the polyethylene glycol 8000 and the colorants in suspension.

Examples 3, 4, 5, and 6: Cellulose Aqueous Formula

(Aqueous systems should be sprayed.)

	3	4	5	6
Hydroxypropyl methylcellulose 2910, 15 cps	4.0%		2.0%	5.0%
Hydroxypropyl methylcellulose, 6 cps		6.0%	4.0%	
Hydroxypropyl cellulose				1.0%
Propylene glycol, USP	1.0%	1.0%		
Polyethylene glycol 400		0.5%	2.0%	1.0%
Water q.s.	100.0%	100.0%	100.0%	100.0%

These polymers are soluble in water. Slowly add the polymer(s) to vigorously stirred water. Continue the agitation until the polymer(s) are solubilized, add propylene glycol or polyethylene glycol or both, then bring to proper volume with water. Colorants and pigments may be added after milling or dispersion in water.

Cellulose acetate phthalate was the primary synthetic enteric polymer used in the industry for many years. Now enteric acrylic resins and phthalate derivatives of polyvinyl acetate or hydroxypropyl methylcellulose are also available.

Example 7: Cellulose Acetate Phthalate Enteric Solution

(This system could be sprayed or poured.)

Cellulose acetate phthalate, NF	12.0%
Propylene glycol	3.0%
Sorbitan monooleate, NF	1.0%
Ethyl alcohol 200-proof	45.0%
Acetone	q.s. ad 100.0%

This solution is prepared in a manner similar to example 2. The cellulose acetate phthalate is dissolved in solvent mixture, and acetone is added to obtain the proper volume after polymer solvation is obtained.

The literature available from pharmaceutical polymer manufacturers provides numerous coating formulas utilizing their particular polymers. These formulas require the effective utilization of the favorable properties of the various polymers, plasticizers, and additives in the final coating composition to acquire a quality coated tablet.

Development of Film Coating Formulations

The decision to coat a tablet is usually the simplest one in the sequence that converts a compressed tablet to a coated tablet. The following questions must be answered concurrently with the decision to coat.

1. What is the purpose of the coating? Is it necessary to mask objectionable taste, color, or odor, or is it necessary to control drug release?

2. What tablet size, shape, or color constraints must be placed on the developmental work?

In the pharmaceutical industry, the color, shape, and size of the final coated tablet is important to marketing, and these properties have a significant influence on the decisions. Quality assurance is another function that exercises control over the product appearance. Quality assurance personnel evaluate the properties of the new product against the characteristics of existing products. In general, companies avoid marketing different products with the same appearance. There are a relatively limited number of colors available to the formulator, so that the product lines of many major pharmaceutical companies contain several coated tablets with various shades of red, yellow, green, and blue. Fortunately, tablet sizes and shapes can be easily varied; thus, the ability to select a tablet with a distinctive appearance is unlimited.

An experienced formulator usually takes the pragmatic approach and develops a coating formulation as a modification of one that has performed well in the past. The inexperienced coater or the formulator seeking a better coating system needs to start from a more basic position and essentially builds his coating composition from a primary film former. The effect of the addition of plasticizers, opaquants, colorants, and the solvent system can then be individually and collectively assessed.

Film formulations can be preliminarily screened by spraying or casting films. Through the preparation of a series of films with slight changes in formula ingredients, it is possible to eliminate the obvious physical incompatibilities and poor film combinations rather quickly. One should recognize that this is only a screening study. Cast films and sprayed films can have different characteristics. In fact, some coating compositions yield poor cast films yet are effective tablet coatings.

Cast films can be prepared by spreading the coating composition on a Teflon, glass, or aluminum foil surface using a spreading bar to get a uniform film thickness. Many cast films adhere so well to glass that the film cannot be removed intact, but glass is certainly suitable for evaluating the appearance of the film. Many investigators who conducted water vapor permeability studies prepared their films by pouring their coating composition on mercury in petri dishes. This is convenient, as the surface area is constant, and the film can be readily removed from the liquid surface.

Sprayed films can be obtained by mounting a plastic-coated surface in a spray hood or coating pan. Care must be used in spraying the film to obtain a uniform film representative of the type achieved in tablet coating.

The physical appearance of these films can provide evidence of potential colorant or opaquant separation. Lack of color uniformity within the film could suggest that the insoluble additives have not been properly suspended or that some interaction has occurred between the ingredients. In addition, the films can be submitted for the following tests.

Water Vapor Permeability

If the coating is going to be used as a seal coat or to provide some physical protection for a tablet containing a water-unstable drug, then knowledge of the film's water vapor permeability should be assessed. (Detailed descriptions of the test procedure can be found in the literature.[21-24])

Film Tensile Strength

Strips of the film are tested on a tensile-strength tester by applying a known force at a constant rate. The elasticity and tensile strength/breaking stress of the films are evaluated. This test is particularly good when the effect of varying the concentration of a series of plasticizers or additives is being evaluated. Coating compositions that yield brittle films must be plasticized to obtain a more flexible film that is acceptable for tablet coating. Tensile-strength testing is one of the better ways to optimize the level of additives in the formulation.

Coated Tablet Evaluations

Once the preliminary screening of formulation variables has been accomplished, the candidate coating must now be studied under tablet coating conditions. Frequently, these studies are conducted on placebo tablets or on a group of placebo tablets with a limited number of drug tablets. The drug tablets must be of essentially the same shape, size, and density as the placebos, so that their patterns of movement in the coating pan are comparable. Obviously, there should be some distinctive tablet feature to permit separation of the tablets and allow evaluation of the two coated tablets. The technique of coating two different tablets at the same time has merit only if the surface properties of the two are equivalent. If two formulations, one having a hydrophilic surface and the other a hydrophobic surface, are aqueous-coated, the coating may preferentially adhere to one of the formulations.

Evaluation of the quality of coating on a tablet involves studying not only the film per se, but also the film-tablet surface interactions. A number of test methods can be employed.

1. Adhesion tests with tensile-strength testers have been used to measure the force required to peel the film from the tablet surface.[25-27] Rowe has been a prolific investigator in the area of film coating evaluation and the factors affecting film strength.[28,29]

2. Diametral crushing strength of coated tablets can be determined with a tablet hardness tester. Obviously, the resistance of the uncoated tablet to crushing will be a major factor in the test results. With this test, one is seeking information on the relative increase in crushing strength provided by the film and the contribution made by changes in the film composition.

3. The rate of coated tablet disintegration and/or dissolution must also be assessed. Unless the coating is intended to control drug release, the coating should have a minimal effect on tablet disintegration or dissolution.

4. Stability studies must be conducted on coated tablets to determine if temperature and humidity changes will cause film defects. Exposure of coated tablets to elevated humidity and measurement of tablet weight gain provide rela-

tive information on the protection provided by the film.

5. Some investigators have attempted to quantify film surface roughness, hardness, and color uniformity through instrumental means, but in general, visual inspection is sufficient to define relative coated tablet quality. A practical qualitative measure of the resistance of a coated tablet to abrasion can be obtained by merely rubbing the coated tablet on a white sheet of paper. Resilient films remain intact, and no color is transferred to the paper; very soft coatings are readily "erased" from the tablet surface to the paper.

Coating Formula Optimization

Optimization is usually associated with minor modifications in a basic formula. As discussed earlier, the basic or starting formula is obtained from past experience or from various sources in the literature. Modifications on this basic formula may be necessary to improve adhesion of the coating to the core; to decrease bridging of intagliations; to increase coating hardness; or to improve any property of the coating that the formulator deems deficient. Colorant and opaquant concentrations are usually fixed to achieve a predetermined shade. Changes of the polymer(s)-to-plasticizer ratio, however, or the addition of different plasticizers or polymers, are common modifications made in optimization of the coating.

This type of experimentation can be best achieved by conducting a fractional factorial type of study,* in which the concentration of a few plasticizers or polymers are evaluated in the same general coating formulation. Factorial studies allow evaluation of more variables with fewer experiments. The evaluation of each coating composition, however, must be conducted by a readily quantifiable criterion. For example, if the coating compositions are to be applied to tablets, can the coating conditions be effectively repeated? Can the properties of the film be measured by an objective testing system? The conditions used in the coating process frequently have as great an effect on the quality of the tablet coating as the coating composition. Studies on free films are much easier to conduct because there are test methods that can be used to evaluate changes in film properties with modifications in coating composition. Bonding of a film to a tablet surface or bridging of an intagliation can be measured, but the experimental error is much higher. Optimization of a particular property in free films should always be confirmed by the performance and appearance of the coated tablet.

The literature and patents cite numerous film coating compositions. The selection of a specific formulation depends on the coating equipment and conditions available, the intended purpose of the coating, and total solid load desired in the coating.

Materials Used in Film Coating

The coating materials may be a physical deposition of the material on the tablet substrate, or they may form a continuous film with a wide variety of properties depending upon the composition of the coating formulations. Examples of physical deposition of the coating materials are the techniques of sugar,[10,11] shellac,[30] and wax coatings.[31] During the last 40 years, a wide variety of polymers have been evaluated and are being used commercially for tablet coating. Further discussion of coating materials in this chapter is limited to synthetic polymers, solvents, plasticizers, colorants, opaquant-extenders, and miscellaneous coating solution components.

An ideal film coating material should have the following attributes:

1. Solubility in solvent of choice for coating preparation.

2. Solubility required for the intended use, e.g., free water-solubility, slow water-solubility, or pH-dependent solubility (enteric coating)

3. Capacity to produce an elegant looking product.

4. Stability in the presence of heat, light, moisture, air, and the substrate being coated. The film properties should not change with aging.

5. Essentially no color, taste or odor.

6. Compatibility with common coating solution additives.

7. Nontoxicity with no pharmacologic activity, and ease of application to the particles or tablets.

8. Resistance to cracking, and provision of adequate moisture, light, odor, or drug sublimation barrier when desired.

9. No bridging or filling of the debossed tablet surfaces by the film former.

10. Ease of printing procedure on high-speed equipment.

*Plackett-Burman statistical method.

No commercially available material fulfills all requirements of an ideal coating material. A pharmaceutical scientist usually formulates a coating solution to achieve certain desired properties for the film-coated product. The available film formers can be classified into nonenteric and enteric materials.

Film Formers

Nonenteric Materials

It is not possible to mention all polymers that have been investigated for filmcoating. The following discussion describes only some of the materials most commonly used by the pharmaceutical industry and is intended as a guide for the student or pharmaceutical scientist.

HYDROXYPROPYL METHYLCELLULOSE, USP

The polymer is prepared by reacting alkali-treated cellulose first with methyl chloride to introduce methoxy groups and then with propylene oxide to introduce propylene glycol ether groups. The resulting products are commercially available in different viscosity grades. This polymer is a material of choice for air suspension and pan-spray coating systems. The reasons for its widespread acceptance include (1) solubility characteristics of the polymer in gastrointestinal fluid, and in organic and aqueous solvent systems, (2) noninterference with tablet disintegration and drug availability, (3) flexibility, chip resistance, and absence of taste or odor, (4) stability in the presence of heat, light, air, or reasonable levels of moisture, (5) ability to incorporate color and other additives into the film without difficulty. The interaction of this polymer with colorants is rare.[32] Hydroxypropyl methylcellulose closely approaches the desired attributes of an ideal polymer for film coating. When used alone, the polymer has the tendency to bridge or fill the debossed tablet surfaces. A mixture of hydroxypropyl methylcellulose with other polymers or plasticizers is used to eliminate bridging or filling problems. This polymer is also used considerably in glossing solutions.[33]

METHYL HYDROXYETHYLCELLULOSE

This polymer is prepared by reacting alkali-treated cellulose first with methyl chloride and then with ethylene oxide. A wide variety of viscosity grades are available. Because of its structural similarity to hydroxypropyl methylcellulose, this polymer is expected to have similar properties. It is marketed in Europe, but because it is soluble in fewer organic solvents, it is not used as frequently as hydroxypropyl methylcellulose.

ETHYLCELLULOSE, NF

Ethylcellulose is manufactured by the reaction of ethyl chloride or ethyl sulfate with cellulose dissolved in sodium hydroxide. Depending on the degree of ethoxy substitution, different viscosity grades are obtained and available commercially. This material is completely insoluble in water and gastrointestinal fluids, and thus cannot be used alone for tablet coating. It is usually combined with water-soluble additives, e.g., hydroxypropyl methylcellulose, to prepare films with reduced water solubility properties. A combination of ethylcellulose with water-soluble additives has been widely used in preparing sustained-release coatings of fine particles and tablets. The polymer is soluble in a wide variety of organic solvents and is nontoxic, colorless, odorless, tasteless, and quite stable to most environmental conditions. Unplasticized ethylcellulose films are brittle and require film modifiers to obtain an acceptable film formulation. Banker and co-workers from Purdue University have developed aqueous polymeric dispersions utilizing ethylcellulose.[34] These pseudolatex systems are high-solids, low-viscosity compositions that have coating properties quite different from the regular ethylcellulose solutions. The material is commercially available through FMC Corporation as Aquacoat.*

HYDROXYPROPYLCELLULOSE, FCC

This material is manufactured by treatment of cellulose with sodium hydroxide, followed by a reaction with propylene oxide at an elevated temperature and pressure. It is soluble in water below 40°C (insoluble above 45°C), gastrointestinal fluids, and many polar organic solvents. This polymer is extremely tacky as it dries from a solution system and may be desirable for a subcoat, but not for a color or gloss coat. The polymer yields very flexible films. It is usually not used alone, but it is used in combination with other polymers to improve the film characteristics.

POVIDONE, USP

Povidone is a synthetic polymer consisting of linear 1-vinyl-2-pyrrolidinone groups. The degree of polymerization results in materials of

---

*FMC Corporation, 2000 Market Street, Philadelphia, PA 19103.

various molecular weight range. Povidone is usually available in four viscosity grades identified by their K values, which approximate K-15, K-30, K-60, and K-90. The average molecular weight of these grades are 10,000, 40,000, 160,000, and 360,000 respectively. The most common uses of povidone in pharmaceuticals (frequently K-30) are as a tablet binder and a tablet coating. It has excellent solubility in a wide variety of organic solvents, in water, and in gastric and intestinal fluids. When dry, povidone films are clear, glossy, and hard. The material is extremely tacky, but it is possible to modify the polymer properties by use of appropriate plasticizers, suspended powders, or other polymers. Although povidone is soluble in both acidic and basic fluids, it can be cross-linked with other materials to produce films with enteric properties. Povidone has been used to improve the dispersion of colorants in coating solutions to obtain a more uniformly colored film.

SODIUM CARBOXYMETHYLCELLULOSE, USP

This material is a sodium salt of carboxymethylcellulose and is manufactured by the reaction of soda cellulose with the sodium salt of monochloroacetic acid. It is available in low, medium, high, and extra high viscosity grades. Sodium carboxymethylcellulose is easily dispersed in water to form colloidal solutions, but it is insoluble in most organic solvents, and therefore is not a material of choice for coating solutions based on organic solvents. Films prepared with sodium carboxymethylcellulose are brittle, but adhere well to tablets. Partially dried films are tacky, however, so coating compositions must be modified with additives. Conversion to aqueous-based film coating with high coating efficiency equipment probably increases the usefulness of this polymer in coating systems.

POLYETHYLENE GLYCOLS

Polyethylene glycols (PEG) are manufactured by the reaction of ethylene glycol with ethylene oxide in the presence of sodium hydroxide at elevated temperature and under pressure. In addition to their other uses in formulations, they are used in film coating for which a wide variety of molecular weights are available. The materials with low molecular weights (200 to 600 series) are liquid at room temperature and are used as plasticizers for coating solution films. The materials with high molecular weights (series 900 to 8,000) are white, waxy solids at room temperature. These polymers are used in combination with other polymers to modify film properties. Combinations of polyethylene glycol waxes with cellulose acetate phthalate provide films that are soluble in gastric fluids. Such systems constituted one of the first commercially used nonenteric film coating processes.[35] Coats produced with the use of high-molecular-weight PEGs can be hard, smooth, tasteless, and nontoxic, but are somewhat sensitive to elevated temperatures.

ACRYLATE POLYMERS

A series of acrylate polymers is marketed under the trademark Eudragit.* Eudragit E is a cationic copolymer based on dimethylaminoethyl methacrylate and other neutral methacrylic acid esters, and is the only Eudragit material that is freely soluble in gastric fluid up to pH 5, and expandable and permeable above pH 5. This material is available as (1) organic solution (12.5%) in isopropanol/acetone, (2) solid material, or (3) 30% aqueous dispersion. Eudragit RL and RS are copolymers synthesized from acrylic and methacrylic acid esters with a low content of quaternary ammonium groups. These are available only as organic solutions and solid materials. These polymers produce films for the delayed-action (pH-independent) preparations similar to ethylcellulose formulations. These materials are widely used in Europe, but have limited use so far in the United States.

Enteric Materials

Enteric coating of pills and compressed tablets has existed for more than a century.[36] Some of the most important reasons for enteric coating are as follows:

1. To protect acid-labile drugs from the gastric fluid, e.g., enzymes and certain antibiotics.

2. To prevent gastric distress or nausea due to irritation from a drug, e.g., sodium salicylate.

3. To deliver drugs intended for local action in the intestines, e.g., intestinal antiseptics could be delivered to their site of action in a concentrated form and bypass systemic absorption in the stomach.

4. To deliver drugs that are optimally absorbed in the small intestine to their primary absorption site in their most concentrated form.

5. To provide a delayed-release component for repeat-action tablets.

*Rohm and Haas Co. Inc., Pharma. Gmbh., Germany.

An ideal enteric coating material should have the following properties:

1. Resistance to gastric fluids.

2. Ready susceptibility to or permeability to intestinal fluids.

3. Compatibility with most coating solution components and the drug substrates.

4. Stability alone and in coating solutions. The films should not change on aging.

5. Formation of a continuous (uninterrupted) film.

6. Nontoxicity.

7. Low cost.

8. Ease of application without specialized equipment.

9. Ability to be readily printed or to allow film to be applied to debossed tablets.

Pharmaceutical formulators have a wide choice of materials for use in developing an enteric coated granule, pellet, or tablet product. These materials range from water-resistant films to pH-sensitive materials. Some are digested or emulsified by intestinal juices, and some slowly swell and fall apart when solvated. Many formulators use a combination of the actions just listed to achieve the desired objective. Most commercially available enteric materials fail to display two or more of the ideal properties of an enteric coating material. The following section discusses some of the difficulties encountered in enteric formulations.

The United States Pharmacopeia (USP) disintegration test for enteric coated tablets requires that the tablets tolerate agitation in simulated gastric fluid test solution at $37 \pm 2°C$ (no discs). After 1 hour of exposure in simulated gastric fluid, tablets should show no evidence of disintegration, cracking, or softening. Then a disc is added to each tube, and the test is continued using simulated intestinal fluid maintained at $37 \pm 2°C$ as the immersion fluid, for a period of time equal to 2 hours or to the time limit specified in the individual monograph. If all the tablets disintegrate, the product passes the test. If 1 or 2 tablets fail to disintegrate completely, the test is repeated on 12 additional tablets. To pass the disintegration test, at least 16 out of 18 tablets should disintegrate.

All enteric coated tablets must meet these requirements. Passing the USP enteric test does not guarantee optimal bioavailability of a particular dosage form. Several situations complicate the absorption of drug from enteric coated tablets. The pH of the stomach contents may vary from 1.5 to 4.0, with about 10% of the patients having achlorhydria. The amount of gastric fluid may vary between individuals, and for the same individual from time to time. Gastric residence time for the dosage form may range from less than half an hour to more than 4 hours depending on the time of its administration, whether it was consumed with food, and if so, the type and quantity of food. The USP disintegration test does not require a qualitative or quantitative test for the active drug after agitation in artificial gastric fluid for 1 hour. Several commercially available enteric products passed the USP enteric test, but released varying amounts of drugs in simulated gastric fluid.[37] Most acid-labile drugs need protection between pH values 1 and 5. The pH of material approaching pylorus is expected to be about 5. An ideal enteric polymer should dissolve or become permeable near and above pH 5.

A common problem associated with the retardant type of polymers (non-pH dependent solubility), which act by mechanical hydrophobicity, is that to provide enteric effect, the film might be so thick that if the dosage form travels too fast through the gastrointestinal tract, solubilization in intestinal fluids may never be achieved. Commercial products have failed the enteric test both for lack of gastric protection and for lack of solubility in intestinal fluids.[38,39] Many others passed these in vitro tests, but failed to perform adequately when studied in vivo.[40]

A review of tablet coating by Porter summarizes the commercially available enteric polymers.[41]

CELLULOSE ACETATE PHTHALATE (CAP)

CAP has been widely used in the industry. It has the disadvantage of dissolving only above pH 6, and possibly delaying the absorption of drugs. It is also hygroscopic and relatively permeable to moisture and gastric fluids, in comparison with some other enteric polymers. CAP films are susceptible to hydrolytic removal of phthalic and acetic acids, resulting in a change of film properties. CAP films are brittle and usually formulated with hydrophobic-film forming materials or adjuvants to achieve a better enteric film. FMC Corporation has developed a patented aqueous enteric coating called Aquateric.[42] Aquateric coating is a reconstituted colloidal dispersion of latex particles (not a solvent solution coating system). It is composed of solid or semisolid polymer spheres of cellulose acetate phthalate ranging in size from 0.05 to 3 microns with an average particle size of 0.2 micron. This material is currently being offered for potential industrial applications.

ACRYLATE POLYMERS

Two forms of commercially available enteric acrylic resins are Eudragit L and Eudragit S. Both resins produce films that are resistant to gastric fluid. Eudragit L and S are soluble in intestinal fluid at pH 6 and 7, respectively. Eudragit L is available as an organic solution (Isopropanol), solid, or aqueous dispersion. Eudragit S is available only as an organic solution (Isopropanol) and solid.

HYDROXYPROPYL METHYLCELLULOSE PHTHALATE*

Shin-Etsu Chemical Company has made three enteric polymers available commercially. These are derived from hydroxypropyl methylcellulose, N.F., by esterification with phthalic anhydride, and are marketed as HPMCP 50, 55, and 55S (also known as HP-50, HP-55, and HP-55-S). HPMCP is the trade name for hydroxypropyl methylcellulose phthalate. These polymers dissolve at a lower pH (at 5 to 5.5) than CAP or acrylic copolymers, and this solubility characteristic may result in higher bioavailability of some specific drugs.[43] For general enteric preparations, HP-55 is recommended by Shin-Etsu; HP-50 and HP-55S are recommended for special situations. These polymers are quite stable compared with CAP because of their absence of labile acetyl groups.

POLYVINYL ACETATE PHTHALATE (PVAP)†

PVAP is manufactured by the esterification of a partially hydrolyzed polyvinyl acetate with phthalic anhydride. This polymer is similar to HP-55 in stability and pH-dependent solubility. It is supplied as ready-to-use or ready-to-disperse enteric systems.

Solvents

The primary function of a solvent system is to dissolve or disperse the polymers and other additives and convey them to the substrate surface. All major manufacturers of polymers for tablet coating provide basic physical-chemical data on their polymers. These data are usually helpful to a formulator. Some important considerations for an ideal solvent system are as follows:

* Distributed by Biddle Sawyer Corporation, 2 Penn Plaza, New York, NY 10121.
† Supplied by Colorcon, Inc., West Point, PA 19486.

1. It should either dissolve or disperse the polymer system.

2. It should easily disperse other coating solution components into the solvent system.

3. Small concentrations of polymers (2 to 10%) should not result in an extremely viscous solution system (>300 cps), creating processing problems.

4. It should be colorless, tasteless, odorless, inexpensive, nontoxic, inert, and nonflammable.

5. It should have a rapid drying rate (the ability to coat a 300 kg load in 3 to 5 hours).

6. It should have no environmental impact.

The most widely used solvents, either alone or in combination are water, ethanol, methanol, isopropanol, chloroform, acetone, methylethylketone, and methylene chloride. Because of environmental and economic considerations, water is the solvent of choice; however, several polymers cannot be applied from aqueous systems. Drugs that readily hydrolyze in the presence of water can be more effectively coated with nonaqueous-solvent-based coatings. Such a process might require applying an initial sealing coat from an organic-based subcoating, followed by aqueous color and gloss coating. The use of organic-solvent-based film coatings will undoubtedly decrease as better aqueous systems are developed. It is unlikely, however, that organic solvents will be entirely supplanted.

Plasticizers

The quality of a film can be modified by the use of "internal" or "external" plasticizing techniques. Internal plasticizing pertains to the chemical modification of the basic polymer that alters the physical properties of the polymer. This aspect has been discussed earlier under different polymeric materials. By controlling the degree of substitution, the type of substitution, and the chain length, polymer properties can be altered significantly. Most often, the formulator uses external plasticizers as additives to the coating solution formula so that the desired effects are achieved for the film. An external plasticizer can be a nonvolatile liquid or another polymer, which when incorporated with the primary polymeric film former, changes the flexibility, tensile strength, or adhesion properties of the resulting film.

As the solvent is removed, most polymeric materials tend to pack together in three-dimensional honeycomb arrangements.[44] The choice of plasticizer depends upon the ability of plasticizer material to solvate the polymer and alter the polymer-polymer interactions. When used in correct proportion to the polymer, these materials impart flexibility by relieving the molecular rigidity. The type of plasticizer(s) and its ratio to the polymer can be optimized to achieve the desired film properties. One should also consider the viscosity of the plasticizer; its influence on the final coating solution; its effect on film permeability, tackiness, flexibility, solubility, and taste; and its toxicity, compatibility with other coating solution components, and stability of the film and the final coated product.

A combination of plasticizers may be needed to achieve the desired effect. The concentration of the plasticizers depends on many factors, including the polymer chemistry, method of application, and the other components present in the system. Even changes in the drying rate or use of elevated temperatures may alter the influence of the plasticizer in the coating process. The presence of titanium dioxide, colorants, flavors, and other additives also affect the film former. Most film formers tolerate only a certain additive load, and beyond that limit, the film properties are adversely affected.

The amount and type of plasticizers to be used for any given polymer can be based on the polymer manufacturer's recommendations. Optimization of the plasticizer concentration must be based on the presence of the other additives. Concentration of a plasticizer is expressed in relation to the polymer being plasticized. Recommended levels of plasticizers range from 1 to 50% by weight of the film former. Some of the commonly used plasticizers are castor oil; propylene glycol; glycerin; low-molecular-weight polyethylene glycols of 200 and 400 series; and surfactants, e.g., polysorbates (Tweens), sorbitan esters (Spans), and organic acid esters. With the increasing interest in aqueous coating, water-soluble plasticizers, e.g., polyethylene glycols and propylene glycol, are used. Conversely, castor oil and Spans are used primarily for organic-solvent-based coating solutions. For an external plasticizer to be effective, it should be soluble in the solvent system used for dissolving the film former and plasticizer. The plasticizer and the film former must be at least partially soluble or miscible in each other.

Colorants

Coating solution formulations may contain a wide variety of components in addition to the film former, solvents, and plasticizers. Colorants may be soluble in the solvent system or suspended as insoluble powders. They are used to provide distinctive color and elegance to a dosage form. To achieve proper distribution of suspended colorants in the coating solutions requires the use of fine-powdered colorants (<10 microns). Repetitive production of colored coating solutions from different lots of the same colorant can be particularly difficult if colorant lots have different dye content, crystal form of dye, or particle size distribution. In general, the suspended colorants must be milled in the coating solvent or solution to attain a uniform dispersion of the colorants. Color variation in a product can be readily detected by the pharmacist and patient; therefore, the colors must be reproducible and stable.

The most common colorants in use are certified Food Drug and Cosmetic (FD&C) or Drug and Cosmetic (D&C) colorants. These are synthetic dyes or lakes of dyes. Lakes are derived from dyes by precipitating with carriers, e.g., alumina or talc. Lakes have become the colorants of choice for sugar or film-coating systems, as more reproducible tablet colors are attainable. Most commercially available lakes contain 10 to 30% of the pure dye content, but some lakes approach up to 50%. An occasional problem with the lake system might be the use of a solvent system that dissolves the dye, thereby establishing a time- and temperature-dependent equilibrium for leaching the dye from the lake system. Use of pure dye is recommended in such cases.

The concentration of colorants in the coating solutions depends on the color shade desired, the type of dye (i.e., dye versus the lake of the dye), and the concentration of the opaquant-extenders. If a very light shade is desired, a concentration of less than 0.01% may be adequate. On the other hand, if a dark color is desired, a concentration of more than 2.0% may be required. Since lakes contain less colorant, a larger concentration in solution is generally required.

The inorganic materials (e.g., iron oxides) and the natural coloring materials (e.g., anthocyanins, caramel, carotenoids, chlorophyll, indigo, flavones, turmeric, and carminic acid) are also used to prepare coating solutions.

A new line of colorants is being developed.[45] These colorants are nonabsorbable in the biologic system. This is accomplished by attaching dyes to polymers that are too large to be absorbed in the gastrointestinal tract and yet are resistant to degradation in the gastrointestinal tract. A magenta red dye is projected to be the first dye to be cleared for use.

A variety of products that are commercially available permit preparation of coating solution without additional milling equipment.* Some examples are:

Opalux—Opaquant color concentrate for sugar coating.

Opaspray—Opaque color concentrate for film coating.

Opadry—Complete film coating concentrate.

All of these concentrates are promoted as achieving less lot-to-lot color variation.

Opaquant-Extenders

These are very fine inorganic powders used in the coating solution formulations to provide more pastel colors and increase film coverage. These opaquants can provide a white coating or mask the color of the tablet core. Colorants are much more expensive than these inorganic materials, and effectively less colorant is required when opaquants are used. The most commonly used material for this purpose is titanium dioxide. Some other materials are silicates (talc, aluminum silicate), carbonates (magnesium carbonate), sulfates (calcium sulfate), oxides (magnesium oxide), and hydroxides (aluminum hydroxide).

Rowe and associates have observed differences in the refractive indices of polymer film formers, pigments, and other additives commonly used for film coating.[46,47] These observations have implications for the use of pigments and additives in the production of opaque films with good hiding power and film-coated tablets with highlighted intagliations.

Miscellaneous Coating Solution Components

To provide a dosage form with a unique characteristic, special materials may be incorporated into the coating solution. Flavors or sweeteners are added to mask objectionable odors or to enhance a desired taste. Surfactants are used to solubilize otherwise immiscible or insoluble ingredients, or to facilitate faster dissolution of the coating. Antioxidants are incorporated to stabilize a dye system to oxidation and color change. Antimicrobials are added to prevent microbial growth in the coating composition during its preparation and storage, and on the coated tablets. Some aqueous cellulosic coating solutions

---

*Colorcon, Inc., West Point, PA 19486.

are particularly prone to microbial growth, and prolonged storage of the coating composition should be avoided.

Quality Control

After coating, the tablets should be inspected and tested for appearance and performance. Inspection should include checks for color (both hue and continuity), size, appearance, and any physical defects in the coating, which could affect the performance or stability of the product.

The in vitro performance of the coated product is evaluated by disintegration and dissolution testing. A standard disintegration test measures the time required for the tablet to break up into particles small enough to fall through a 10-mesh screen. Dissolution testing measures the amount of active drug in solution over time. A description of the standard equipment and methods used for each test is given in the USP/NF. Standards of acceptance for drug products can be found in the USP/NF or the Code of Federal Regulations, Title 21.

To be a valid quality control method, the in vitro test should be discriminating. This means that it should be sufficiently sensitive to reflect variation in the product caused by improper processing or by the effects of storage and aging. For this reason, modifications of the test media and rates of agitation are commonly adjusted to accommodate each specific product.

Ideally, the in vitro performance should reflect in vivo performance. This correlation is rare, owing to the difficulty of devising an in vitro testing method to mimic the complex and dynamic nature of the physiologic system. Drug availability can be affected by apparently minor changes in the concentration of ingredients in either the core or film formulation. Therefore, for most drug products, bioavailability testing remains the only valid assessment of the product's in vivo performance.

Additional testing of coated tablets may also include tests for mechanical strength and for resistance to chipping and cracking during handling. Methods and devices for these tests are similar to those used for uncoated tablets.

Stability Testing

Stability testing is conducted to determine the effect of time and storage conditions on the physical and chemical stability of the coated product. The stability program should be designed to determine the shelf-life or expiry dating of the coated product under normal storage conditions in its intended package. As a rule, tablet products should have at least a two-year expiration date, which means that the product must conform to all standards of performance and potency for at least two years after manufacture.

The testing program may also be designed to test the product's stability at elevated or accelerated storage conditions. This type of program may help to establish acceptable storage conditions for the product in relation to temperature, humidity, and light exposure, or it may help to study the rate of degradation of the active ingredient under various conditions. Potency data from tablets stored at elevated temperatures can be evaluated by using the Arrhenius relationship to project a degradation rate for the active ingredient and to project an expiration date for the product stored under ambient conditions.

In the development stage, the stability program may be used to test variations in the formulation or process. On aging, or under various conditions of storage, a particular variation may result in physical instability of the film, color changes, or chemical degradation of the active ingredient.

Film Defects

Variations in formulation and processing conditions may result in unacceptable quality defects in the film coating. The source of these defects and some of their probable causes are described in the following sections.

Sticking and Picking. Overwetting or excessive film tackiness causes tablets to stick to each other or to the coating pan. On drying, at the point of contact, a piece of the film may remain adhered to the pan or to another tablet, giving a "picked" appearance to the tablet surface and resulting in a small exposed area of the core. A reduction in the liquid application rate or increases in the drying air temperature and air volume usually solve this problem. Excessive tackiness may be an indication of a poor formulation.

Roughness. A rough or gritty surface is a defect often observed when the coating is applied by a spray. Some of the droplets may dry too rapidly before reaching the tablet bed, resulting in deposits on the tablet surface of "spray-dried" particles instead of finely divided droplets of coating solution. Moving the nozzle closer to the tablet bed or reducing the degree of atomization can decrease the roughness due to "spray-drying." Surface roughness also increases with

pigment concentration and polymer concentration in the coating solution.[48]

Orange-Peel Effects. Inadequate spreading of the coating solution before drying causes a bumpy or "orange-peel" effect on the coating. This indicates that spreading is impeded by too rapid drying or by high solution viscosity. Thinning the solution with additional solvent may correct this problem.

Bridging and Filling. During drying, the film may shrink and pull away from the sharp corners of an intagliation or bisect, resulting in a "bridging" of the surface depression. This defect can be so severe that the monogram or bisect is completely obscured. This mainly represents a problem with the formulation. Increasing the plasticizer content or changing the plasticizer can decrease the incidence of bridging.[49] Filling is caused by applying too much solution, resulting in a thick film that fills and narrows the monogram or bisect. In addition, if the solution is applied too fast, overwetting may cause the liquid to quickly fill and be retained in the monogram. Judicious monitoring of the fluid application rate and thorough mixing of the tablets in the pan prevent filling.

Blistering. When coated tablets require further drying in ovens, too rapid evaporation of the solvent from the core and the effect of high temperature on the strength, elasticity, and adhesion of the film may result in blistering. Milder drying conditions are warranted in this case.

Hazing/Dull Film. This is sometimes called *bloom*. It can occur when too high a processing temperature is used for a particular formulation. Dulling is particularly evident when cellulosic polymers are applied out of aqueous media at high processing temperatures. It can also occur if the coated tablets are exposed to high humidity conditions and partial solvation of film results.

Color Variation. This problem can be caused by processing conditions or the formulation. Improper mixing, uneven spray pattern, and insufficient coating may result in color variation. The migration of soluble dyes, plasticizers, and other additives during drying may give the coating a mottled or spotted appearance. The use of lake dyes eliminates dye migration. A reformulation with different plasticizers and additives is the best way to solve film instabilities caused by the ingredients.

Cracking. Cracking occurs if internal stresses in the film exceed the tensile strength of the film. The tensile strength of the film can be increased by using higher-molecular-weight polymers or polymer blends.[50] Internal stresses in the film can be minimized by adjusting the plasticizer type and concentration, and the pigment type and concentration.[51]

Specialized Coatings

Compression Coating. This type of coating requires a specialized tablet machine. The finished product is a tablet within a tablet, as described in Chapter 11. Compression coating is not widely used, but it has advantages in some cases in which the tablet core cannot tolerate organic solvents or water and yet needs to be coated for taste masking, or to provide delayed or enteric properties to the product. In addition, incompatible ingredients can be conveniently separated by this process.

Electrostatic Coating. Electrostatic coating is an efficient method of applying coating to conductive substrates. A strong electrostatic charge is applied to the substrate. The coating material containing conductive ionic species of opposite charge is sprayed onto the charged substrate. Complete and uniform coating of corners and intagliations on the substrate is achieved. The adaptability of this method to such relatively nonconductive substrates as pharmaceutical tablets is limited, although one process has been proposed.[52]

Dip Coating. Coating is applied to the tablet cores by dipping them into the coating liquid. The wet tablets are dried in a conventional manner in coating pans. Alternate dipping and drying steps may be repeated several times to obtain the desired coating. This process lacks the speed, versatility, and reliability of spray-coating techniques. Specialized equipment has been developed to dip-coat tablets, but no commercial pharmaceutical application has been obtained.

Vacuum Film Coating. Vacuum film coating is a new coating procedure that employs a specially designed baffled pan.[53] The pan is hot water jacketed, and it can be sealed to achieve a vacuum system. The tablets are placed in the sealed pan, and the air in the pan is displaced by nitrogen before the desired vacuum level is obtained. The coating solution is then applied with an airless (hydraulic) spray system. The evaporation is caused by the heated pan, and the vapors are removed by the vacuum system. Because there is no high-velocity heated air, the energy requirements are low and coating efficiency is high. Organic solvents can be effectively used with this coating system with minimal environmental or safety concerns.

Future Tablet Developments

Much progress has been achieved in tablet coating through significant equipment improvements. The expanded use of microprocessors for process control and improved spraying systems are likely.

The advent of the pseudo-latex coating systems has shown that high solids containing coating formulations are attainable. Most film coating formulations still are primarily volatile solvents. Reducing the quantity of solvent that must be removed in the coating process would dramatically improve coating efficiency.

With the exception of the polymers used for enteric coating, most polymers available for pharmaceuticals were primarily developed for nonpharmaceutical use. There is a need for polymers developed specifically to meet the pharmaceutical coating requirements. Polymers that can be applied in high concentration from aqueous-based solvents would be desirable. Their films should be flexible, adhere well to all tablet surfaces, and be nontacky.

References

1. Sonnedecker, G., et al.: Pharm. Technol., 4:77, 1980.
2. Wurster, D.E. (Wisconsin Alumni Research Foundation): U.S. Patent 2,648,609 (1953).
3. Wurster, D.E. (Wisconsin Alumni Research Foundation): U.S. Patent 2,799,241 (1957).
4. Wurster, D.E.: J. Am. Pharm. Assoc., Sci. Ed., 48:451, 1959.
5. Demmer, F., et al.: Drugs Made in Germany, 24:30, 1981.
6. Stetsko, G., et al.: Pharm. Technol., 7:50, 1983.
7. Reiland, T., et al.: Drug Dev. Ind. Pharm., 9:945, 1983.
8. Thomas, R.: Pharm. Eng. 1:16, 1981.
9. Sharma, V.K., Lippmann, I., and Mangold, G.W.: The Aster Guide to Tablet Coating Automation. Aster Publishing, Springfield, OR, 1984.
10. Lachman, L.: Manuf. Chem. Aerosol News, 37:35, 1966.
11. Tucker, S.S., et al.: J. Am. Pharm. Assoc., Sci. Ed., 49:738, 1960.
12. Abbott Laboratories: Brit. Patent 760,403 (1956).
13. Rowell, T.R.: Drug Cosmet. Ind., 64:300, 1949.
14. Martin, E.W.: Remington's Pharmaceutical Sciences. 13th Ed. Mack Publishing, Easton, PA, 1965, p. 595.
15. Ellis, J.R., Prillig, E.B., and Amann, A.H.: Tablet coating. In The Theory and Practice of Industrial Pharmacy. 2nd Ed. Edited by L. Lachman et al. Lea & Febiger, Philadelphia, 1976, pp. 386–388.
16. Krause, G.M., et al.: J. Pharm. Sci., 57:1223, 1968.
17. Heyd, A., et al.: J. Pharm. Sci., 59:1171, 1970.
18. Kunze, K- H., Drugs Made in Germany, 9:42, 1966.
19. Cretu, G.Y., Radulescu, N.K., Sirbu, C., et al.

(Institutui de Cercetari Chimico-Farmaceutice): Rom. Patent RO 81576B (1983).
20. Shin-Etsu Chemical Industry., Ltd., Jpn. Kokai Tokkyo Koho Japanese Patent 58/201724 A2 [83/201724] (1983).
21. The American Society for Testing and Materials, Test No. E96-66.
22. Parker, J.W., et al.: J. Pharm. Sci., 63:119. 1974.
23. Woodruff, C.W., et al.: J. Pharm. Sci., 61:1956, 1972.
24. Porter, S.: Pharm. Technol., 4:67, 1980.
25. Wood, J.A., et al.: Can. J. Pharm. Sci., 5:18, 1970.
26. Nadkarni, P.D., et al.: J. Pharm. Sci., 64:1554, 1975.
27. Fisher, D.G., et al.: J. Pharm. Pharmacol., 28:886, 1976.
28. Rowe, R.C.: Acta Pharm. Terchnol., 29:205, 1983.
29. Rowe, R.C.: Int. J. Pharm. Technol. Prod. Manuf., 3:67, 1982.
30. Wruble, M.S.: Am. J. Pharm., 102:318, 1980.
31. Gans, E.H., et al.: J. Am. Pharm. Assoc., Sci. Ed., 43:483, 1954.
32. Prillig, E.B.: J. Pharm. Sci., 58:1245, 1969.
33. Singiser, R.E. (Abbott Laboratories): U.S. Patent 3,256,111 (1966).
34. Banker, G.S., et al.: Pharm. Technol., 5:54, 1981.
35. Endicott, C.J., Dallavis, A.A., and Dickinson, H.M.N. (Abbott Laboratories): U.S. Patent 2,881,085 (1959).
36. Am. J. Pharm., 39:467, 1867.
37. Madan, P.L.: Indian J. Pharm. Sci., 41:99, 1979.
38. Payne, M.: Pharm. J., 196:657, 1966.
39. Couvreur, A., et al.: Modern Coating of Tablets and Pills. A partial translation distributed by Distillation Products Industries, Div. of Eastman Kodak Co., Rochester, New York, 1958.
40. Maney, P.V., et al.: Manuf. Chem., 36:55, 1965.
41. Porter, S.C.: Drug Cosmet. Ind. 128:44, 1981.
42. McGinley, E.J., and Tuason, D.C. (FMC Corp.): U.S. Patent 4,462,839 (1984).
43. Kriesel, D., and Mehta, S.P. (Abbott Laboratories): U.S. Patent 4,340,582 (1982).
44. Doolittle, A.K.: The Technology of Solvents and Plasticizers. John Wiley and Sons, New York, 1954, p. 869.
45. Meggos, H.N.: Pharm. Technol. 5:41, 1981.
46. Rowe, R.C.: J. Pharm. Pharmacol. 35:43, 1983.
47. Rowe, R.C., et al.: J. Pharm. Pharmacol. 35:205, 1983.
48. Rowe, R.C.: J. Pharm. Pharmacol., 30:669, 1978.
49. Rowe, R.C., et al.: J. Pharm. Pharmacol. 33:174, 1981.
50. Rowe, R.C., et al.: J. Pharm. Pharmacol. 32:583, 1980.
51. Rowe, R.C.: J. Pharm. Pharmacol., 33:423, 1981.
52. Tanabe, S., et al.: Brit. Patent 1,075,404 (1967).
53. Wehrle, K.: Drugs Made in Germany, 25:66, 1982.

13

Capsules

<table>
<tr><td>

PART ONE

Hard Capsules

VAN HOSTETLER

</td></tr>
</table>

Mothes and Dublanc, two Frenchmen, are generally credited with the invention of the gelatin capsule. Their patents, granted in March and December of 1834, covered a method for producing single-piece, olive-shaped, gelatin capsules, which were closed after filling by a drop of concentrated warm gelatin solution. The two-piece telescoping capsule, invented by James Murdock of London (1848), was patented in England in 1865.

In addition to having the advantages of elegance, ease of use, and portability, capsules have become a popular dosage form because they provide a smooth, slippery, easily swallowed, and tasteless shell for drugs; the last advantage is particularly beneficial for drugs having an unpleasant taste or odor. They are economically produced in large quantities and in a wide range of colors, and they generally provide ready availability of the contained drug, since minimal excipient and little pressure are required to compact the material, as is necessary in tabletting.

Capsules are not usually used for the administration of extremely soluble materials such as potassium chloride, potassium bromide, or ammonium chloride since the sudden release of such compounds in the stomach could result in irritating concentrations. Capsules should not

Some of the material in this chapter has been retained from the previous edition, to which Mr. J. Q. Bellard contributed.

be used for highly efflorescent or deliquescent materials. Efflorescent materials may cause the capsules to soften, whereas deliquescent powders may dry the capsule shell to excessive brittleness. In some cases, this dehydration may be retarded or prevented by the use of small amounts of inert oils in the powder mixture.

Materials

Telescoping capsules are made principally of gelatin blends and may contain small amounts of certified dyes, opaquing agents, plasticizers, and preservatives. Capsules have been made with methylcellulose, polyvinyl alcohols, and denatured gelatins to modify their solubility or produce an enteric effect. They are formed by dipping cool stainless steel mold pins into a gelatin solution, a process described in this chapter. Other methods, such as centrifugal casting, have been used, but the pin method is the only one used in large-scale commercial production.

Gelatin is a heterogeneous product derived by irreversible hydrolytic extraction of treated animal collagen, and as such, it never occurs naturally. Its physical and chemical properties are mainly functions of the parent collagen, method of extraction, pH value, thermal degradation, and electrolyte content. Common sources of collagen are animal bones, hide portions, and frozen pork skin. Bone and skin gelatins are readily available in commercial quantities in most areas of the world.

Type A gelatin is derived from an acid-treated precursor and exhibits an isoelectric point in the region of pH 9, whereas type B gelatin is from an alkali-treated precursor and has its isoelectric zone in the region of pH 4.7. Although capsules may be made from either type of gelatin, the usual practice is to use a mixture of both types as dictated by availability and cost considerations. Differences in the physical properties of finished capsules as a function of the type of gelatin used are slight.

Blends of bone and pork skin gelatins of relatively high gel strength are normally used for hard capsule production. The bone gelatin produces a tough, firm film, but tends to be hazy and brittle. The pork skin gelatin contributes plasticity and clarity to the blend, thereby reducing haze or cloudiness in the finished capsule.

An abbreviated flowchart for the manufacture of gelatin for use in capsules is presented in Figure 13-1.

Two recent developments have taken place in the gelatin supply area. First, "green" (fresh) bones are being used commercially as a source of Type B gelatin. Aside from additional pretreatment to remove residual tissues and fat, the processing coincides with that used for aged bones, and the gelatins obtained are indistinguishable from each other in practical use.

The second development is the processing of an "acid-bone" gelatin prepared from bone by techniques essentially comparable to those for Type A gelatins. The resulting gelatin shows an altered isoelectric point (pH 5.5–6.0), and generally, intermediate physical characteristics for the film. The acid extraction technique for bones is valuable to processors of gelatin because of the decreased extraction time required.

Both of the aforementioned materials are commercially available and are used in hard capsule production.

Method of Production

The three major suppliers of empty gelatin capsules are Eli Lilly and Company, Indianapolis, IN; Capsugel, Greenwood, SC; and the R. P. Scherer Corporation, Troy, MI. Several smaller volume suppliers exist throughout the world, some of which process for their own use only.

The completely automatic machine most commonly used for capsule production consists of mechanisms for automatically dipping, spinning, drying, stripping, trimming, and joining the capsules. The stainless steel mold pin (Fig. 13-2), on which the capsule is formed, controls some of the final critical dimensions of the capsule, and tolerances must be held within fractions of a thousandth of an inch.

One hundred and fifty pairs of these pins are dipped, as shown in Figure 13-2, into a gelatin sol of carefully controlled viscosity to form caps and bodies simultaneously. As shown in Figure 13-3, the pins are usually rotated to distribute the gelatin uniformly (1), during which time the gelatin may be set or gelled by a blast of cool air (2). The pins are moved through a series of controlled air drying kilns for the gradual and precisely controlled removal of water (3 to 6). The capsules are stripped from the pins by bronze jaws and trimmed to length by stationary knives (7) while the capsule halves are being spun in

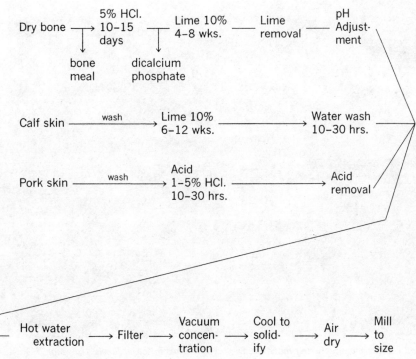

FIG. 13-1. *The process of manufacturing gelatin used in capsules.*

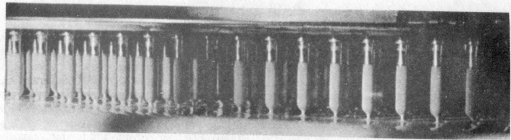

FIG. 13-2. *Mold pin dipping.*

chucks or collets. After being trimmed to exact length, the cap and body sections are joined and ejected from the machine. The entire cycle of the machine lasts approximately 45 min.

Thickness of the capsule wall is controlled by the viscosity of the gelatin solution and the speed and time of dipping. Other matters critical to the final dimensions are mold pin dimensions, precise drying, and machine control relating to cut lengths. Precise control of drying conditions is essential to the ultimate quality of the cast film.

At the least, in-process controls include periodic monitoring, and adjustment when required, of film thickness, cut lengths of both cap and body, color, and moisture content.

Recent strides have been made in several areas to provide computer control of viscosity (and consequent wall thickness) during either machine operations or gelatin solution make-up.

Inspection processes—to remove imperfect capsules—which historically have been done visually, have recently been automated following the development and patenting of a practical electronic sorting mechanism by Eli Lilly and Company. This equipment mechanically orients the capsules and transports them past a series of optical scanners, at which time those having detectable visual imperfections are automatically rejected.

Empty capsules are subject to size variation as a result of moisture content variation. This can be caused by exposure to extreme variations in absolute humidity or elevated temperature.

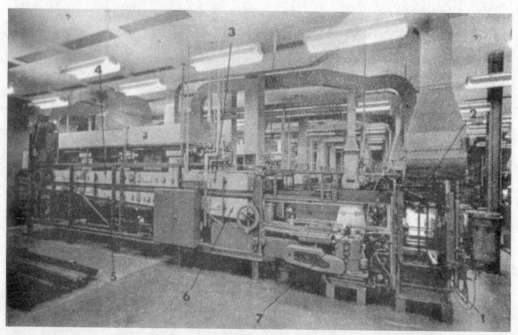

FIG. 13-3. *Hard capsule manufacturing machine. See text for explanation of labels 1 through 7.*

Unopened shipping containers are usually adequate protection against these changes, but storage in unopened containers should not be subjected to temperature conditions of over 100°F. Open storage under either high or low humidity conditions should be minimized. Empty capsules as usually received range in moisture content between 12% and 15%. Below 10% moisture content, they become brittle and may shrink to the point of not fitting into the filling equipment. Above 16% moisture content, they may cause size problems in the filling equipment, plus a loss of mechanical strength. Exposure to either heat or moisture extremes can distort empty capsules to the extent that they cannot be handled by automatic filling equipment.

Filling Equipment

At present, at least nine manufacturers of capsule filling equipment are either located in or selling their products within the United States. Most of the units manufactured outside the United States have local representatives. The nine individual companies are:

Eli Lilly and Company, Indianapolis, IN

Farmatic SNC, Bologna, Italy

Höfliger and Karg, Waiblingen, Germany

Macofar SAS, Bologna, Italy

mG2 S.p.A., Bologna, Italy

Osaka, Osaka, Japan

Parke-Davis and Company, Detroit, MI

Perry Industries, Green Bay, WI

Zanasi Nigris, S.p.A., Bologna, Italy

Each machine type is briefly discussed in the following sections, but no attempt is made to quantify or compare weight variation figures among the various types because of obvious dependence on such factors as the conditions of the equipment, formulas, methods of operation, operator competence, machine rates, and sizes of capsules. Along with suitable consideration of all other details, adequate statistical weight checks or the use of 100% check-weighing should be employed to ensure compliance with regulatory requirements.

The largest number of total machines are supplied by Lilly and Parke-Davis. Since the machines of both manufacturers have essentially the same method of operation, only one description is given.

Lilly/Parke-Davis

Each of these capsule filling machines requires an individual operator and may achieve a daily output of up to 200,000 capsules.

The Lilly machine is shown in Figure 13-4. The empty capsules are fed from the storage hopper (1) and through the rectifying unit (2), into the two-piece filling ring (3A and 3B). Rectification is based on dimensional differences between the outside diameters of the cap and body portions of the capsule. As the ring (3A and 3B) is rotated, a vacuum is applied on its underside. This vacuum seats the bodies into the lower half of the ring, while the caps are retained in the upper portion. The two pieces of the ring are separated, and the cap-containing portion is placed aside. The body-containing portion of the ring is placed on a variable speed turntable and is mechanically rotated under the powder hopper (4), which contains an auger for the forced delivery of the powder. After one (or more) complete rotations of the ring, the powder hopper (4) is removed, and the two segments of the ring (3A and 3B) are rejoined. The intact ring is positioned in front of the peg ring (5), and the closing plate (6) is pivoted to a position approximately 180 degrees from that shown in Figure 13-4. Pneumatic pressure is applied to the peg

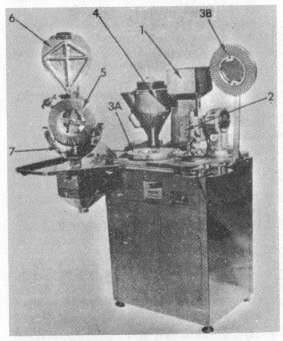

FIG. 13-4. *Lilly capsule filling machine. See text for explanation of labels 1 through 7. (Courtesy of Eli Lilly & Co., Indianapolis, IN.)*

ring (5), which forces the capsule body into the cap, and the closing plate (6) holds the caps in position. Ejection of the filled capsules from the rings cannot occur with the plate in the closing position. For ejection of the capsules, the pressure is released, the closing plate is restored to its original position, and the capsules are expelled through the upper portion of the ring. Normal closing and ejection occur with the peg ring in a vertical position, as shown in Figure 13-4, with the filled capsules being collected through a chute (7) into a collection chamber.

In this equipment, the powder is filled to the upper surface of the body-containing ring, and the fill is therefore primarily volumetric. Although changes in the total amount of powder can be caused by changes in the rotational speed of the turntable (which changes the amount of time for which each hole is under the auger), there is no way to produce a partially filled capsule consistently. Although slower speeds usually produce less weight variation, they also usually result in heavier total fill weights, which may not be economical because of the resultant decrease in productivity.

Minimum total fill weights (but usually maximum weight variation) are achieved with the highest turntable speed.

Maximum total fill weights (but generally minimum weight variation) are achieved at the lowest rotational speed.

Some of the variables that must be properly controlled in order to achieve minimum weight variation and proper uniformity of the finished capsules are given in the following list:

1. The body-containing ring (3A) must be flat across its surface to avoid creating volumetric differences from one area of the ring to another.

2. The powder hopper (4) must be properly positioned during the filling operation to avoid uneven powder distribution from the auger. The proper location includes consideration of both the centering of the auger over the ring holes and the parallelism between the lower surface of the hopper and the upper surface of the ring.

3. Extreme variations in powder level in the filling hopper (4) can cause uneven powder flow, resulting in excessive fill weight variation.

4. The individual rods in the peg ring must fit the rings being used, be of uniform length, and be perpendicular to the closing plate (6).

5. Flow properties of the powder being filled

must be such that a constant amount of powder is available for delivery from the auger. Diluents and glidants should be selected with this phase of the operation in mind.

Pelletized or granular materials may be readily filled using this equipment. It is desirable to remove the auger to avoid crushing. It may also be desirable to perform the closing operations in a position other than the vertical position usually used for powder. In a vertical position, pellets or granules may escape from the body ring, and this may cause damage to the capsules.

Since filling is best accomplished without an auger in these cases, minimal change in fill weight can be achieved by alteration of rotational speed. Additional ring rotations do not increase the fill, but usually cause actual damage to the pellets or granules.

In addition to the semiautomatic machines described previously, a relatively high-speed, automatic, continuous-motion machine called the ROTOFIL is available from Eli Lilly and Company (Fig. 13-5). This machine is specifically designed to fill pellets.

The machine uses a rotary rectification system, which orients the capsules into a turret. After the capsules are seated, the blocks containing the caps are retracted, and the bodies are gravity-filled from the recirculating bed of pellets.

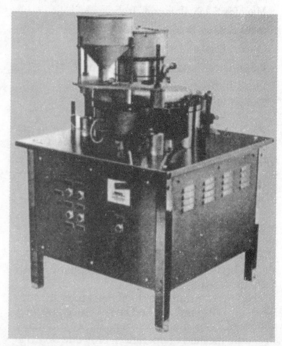

FIG. 13-5. *Lilly ROTOFIL capsule filling machine. (Courtesy of Eli Lilly & Co., Indianapolis, IN.)*

The excess pellets are rolled from the surface of the turret and are transported back to the hopper by vacuum. The cap blocks are realigned over the turret, and a simple continuous cam motion provides the closing action. Filled capsules are ejected by compressed air, and both cap and body cavities are cleaned by compressed air and vacuum prior to the next use. Fill weight may be adjusted while the machine is in operation.

The machine is rated as filling 1200 capsules per minute.

Farmatic

Farmatic offers three models of filling equipment for sale: 2000/15, 2000/30, and 2000/60, with rated outputs of up to 40,000, up to 80,000, and up to 160,000 capsules per hour, respectively. A Farmatic capsule filling machine is presented in Figure 13-6.

The machines feature continuous motion with dosator-type powder feeding units, and are totally enclosed for dust and noise control. Adjustable vacuum is used for separating the cap-

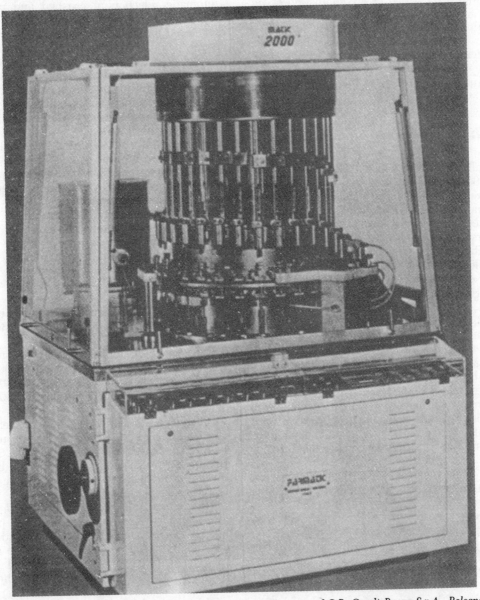

FIG. 13-6. *Farmatic Model 2000/60 capsule filling machine. (Courtesy of G.B. Gundi Bruno S.p.A., Bologna, Italy.)*

sules after rectification, and any defective or unopened capsules are automatically rejected.

Powder is moved from the product hopper by a screw conveyor to the operating tower, where its level is continuously monitored.

Dosators measure and deliver the powder as a slug to the capsules. A digital display indicates the status of the weight and compression. Adjustments are made externally.

The powder slug is ejected into the capsule body, after which the capsule is closed. In the case of a missing capsule, the slug is ejected in such a way as to avoid its being carried into the completed capsules. Following ejection, all bushings are cleaned by a combination of vacuum and air.

Various options are available, including automatic feeders for both capsules and powder, counters, and automatic sampling with feedback to the closing units to adjust incorrect weights.

Farmatic does not have U.S. representation.

Höfliger and Karg

The Höfliger and Karg (H & K) line consists basically of four machines—Models GKF-303, GKF-602, GKF-1500, and GKF-2500; the numbers represent the approximate output of filled capsules per minute. All models can be modified to accept powders, pellets, or tablets. In addition, the first three models may be equipped to handle the filling of thixotropic liquids into hard gelatin capsules, at some reduction of output.

Labels appearing in Figure 13-7, which depicts H & K Model GKF-602, signify the following: 1, empty capsule storage hopper; 2, rectifier; 3, bulk powder storage hopper; 4, capsule body transport segment; 5, closing station; and 6, filled capsules ejection station.

In Models GKF-602, GKF-1500, and GKF-2500, capsules are handled 6, 15, and 25, at one time, according to the respective model number. The empty capsule feed provides for the removal of faulty capsules, and is checked by a vacuum system, which provides a signal upon feed interruption. The rectified empty capsules are inserted into individual cap and body segments bolted to the transport wheel. The segments are then transported to the various work stations carrying the caps and bodies. Thus, only these segments, along with the rectifier and the tamps, require replacement for size change.

Removal of capsule bodies to the carrier is mechanical with a vacuum assist, to ensure gentle handling of the capsules. After separation of cap and body, the cap segment is lifted before retraction of the segment to remove the possibil-

ity of shearing off long or improperly seated bodies.

Powder is auger-fed from the supply hopper to the filling chamber, which completely surrounds the filling disc and in which the powder height is level-controlled. Tamping of powder into the holes of the filling disc is performed at five successive stations. Tamps are externally adjustable at each individual station while the machine is in operation. An additional station is available for the insertion of tablets or pellets, so that mixed fills can be achieved.

Safety features built into the system include an empty capsule feed interruption signal with automatic rejection of crushed and unjoined capsules, and automatic clearance of empty capsule feed tubes after a predetermined number of cycles. If no body is present in the body segment, the powder is discharged through the segment into a collecting container.

Closing of filled capsules is performed in two successive operations to allow for slower closing. Closing is accomplished by the use of both upper and lower closing rods.

Figure 13-8 shows Model GKF-1200/1500, and Figure 13-9 shows Model GKF-2400.

All Höfliger and Karg machines are completely automatic and require only compressed air and a power for operation.

Höfliger and Karg is represented in the United States by Robert Bosch Packaging Machinery Division, Piscataway, NJ.

Macofar

The Macofar line of capsule filling equipment consists of three models: MT-12, MT-13/1, and MT-13/2. Model MT-12 is shown in Figure 13-10. All three models are low-to-medium-capacity machines, ranging from 5,000 filled capsules per hour (MT-13/1) and 10,000 capsules per hour (MT-13/2) to over 35,000 capsules per hour (MT-12).

All units are based upon a similar method of rectification and filling. The empty capsules are rectified into bushings in a central plate. Separation of cap from body is accomplished by vacuum, and the body-carrying bushings are positioned under the dosator unit.

The dosator units pick up powder to a predetermined level from a level-controlled powder hopper. The powder is lightly tamped within the dosators, following which the units are raised, the body-carrying bushing is aligned under them, and the powder is ejected into the open bodies.

The body bushings are retracted to the central

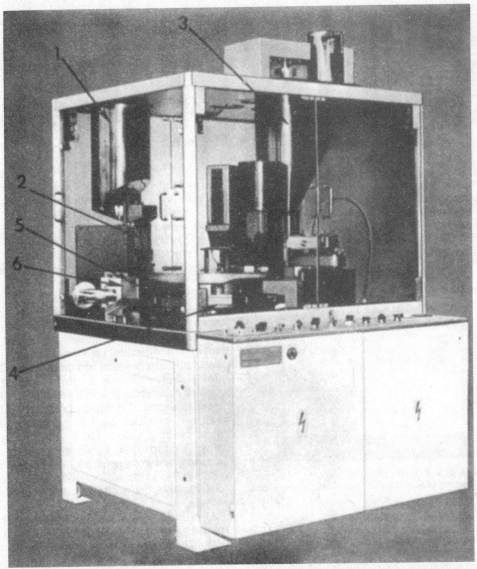

FIG. 13-7. *H & K Model 602 capsule filling machine. See text for explanation of labels 1 through 6. (Courtesy of Robert Bosch GmbH, Waiblingen, West Germany.)*

plate beneath the cap blocks, and closing of the capsule occurs. Prior to reuse, the capsule-holding bushings are cleaned of powder by means of air/vacuum.

Various filling options are available for materials other than powders.

The distributor for Macofar in the United States is Production Equipment, Inc., Rochelle Park, NJ.

mG2

Five models of continuous-motion filling machines are currently offered by mG2. Model G36/4 is rated at 150 capsules per minute, G36/2 at 300, G36 at 600, G37N at 1600, and G38 at 1000. All models utilize the same general methods for both powder and capsule handling. In the following section, Models G36, G37N, and G38 are briefly discussed.

The following identifications apply to the labels in the illustration of Model G36 (Fig. 13-11): 1, empty capsule hopper and rectifier; 2, cap holder removal station; 3, cleaning station; 4, powder dosing head; 5, bulk powder hopper; 6, cap holder replacing station; 7, capsule closing and ejection station.

In Model G36, the capsules are fed from the

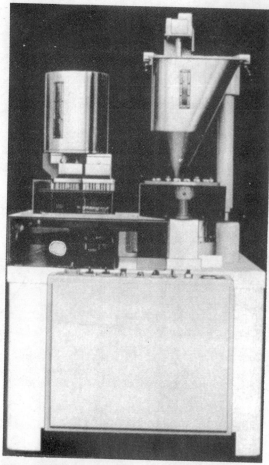

FIG. 13-8. *K & K Model 1200/1500 capsule filling machine. (Courtesy of Robert Bosch GmbH, Waiblingen, West Germany.)*

neously to all dosing units while the machine is in operation. The cap container is repositioned over the body block (6), and closing is accomplished by both upper and lower closing pins (7). Ejection is accomplished by compressed air.

Each-station is equipped with a safety device that automatically stops the machine in the event of an irregularity. Capsule carrying holders are cleaned by air prior to being returned to the rectifier station.

Model G37 has recently been modified (G37N) to provide several new and/or improved features: the handling of empty capsules has been improved, the powder handling system has been modified to lessen powder dusting, several noise-reduction features have been incorporated, and both cleanup and size changing have been simplified. Adjustments of weight control and powder compression can be made externally while the unit is operating.

Model G37N, shown in Figure 13-12, is a continuous-motion turret machine that provides approximately two and one-half times the filling rate of the G36. As indicated previously, it also employs a different capsule handling mechanism. It is composed of two main units. The first unit provides capsule feeding, rectifying, and opening in a manner similar to that of the G36, but with a greater number of elements. The second unit provides capsule separation, dosage, closure, and ejection. The higher output is obtained by providing 40 dosing nozzles and 40 pairs of capsule transfer holders. Dosage adjustment is the same as for Model G36, providing simultaneous control of the position of all dosing pistons.

Model G38 (Fig. 13-13) is a newly introduced machine that is slightly slower than the G37N (with 20 filling tubes versus 40), but is totally enclosed. As with the G37N, all weight adjustments can be made through external controls with the machine in operation. Several features have been added to allow machine jogging, powder-level control, and photoelectric shutoff (if more than three successive unopened capsules are encountered), as well as automatic ejection of certain other empty capsule defects.

All mG2 models either run or can be fitted with attachments to allow them to run with powders, granules, or pellets. Models G37N and G38 can be supplied with auxiliary equipment to provide for presorting of the empty capsules, automatic sampling of filled capsules, and an inspection unit, based upon weight, for filled capsules.

The representative for mG2 in the United States is Supermatic Packaging Machinery, Inc., Fairfield, NJ.

storage hopper through individual tubes and rectified (1) into individual two-piece side holders on a continuous chain. The capsules are separated within the two-piece holders by applying vacuum to the lower portion, which pulls the body into it while the cap is retained in the upper holder. As the chain and retaining blocks progress through the cycle, the cap-containing upper holder (2) is moved aside to a recess at the outer end of the conveying holder, exposing the lower holder containing the body. The powder is continuously mixed within the powder hopper (5) and is maintained at a constant level prior to discharge. The body-carrying units now are carried under a series of 12 volumetric dosing nozzles (4), each of which picks up the product from a rotating container, first compressing and then ejecting the powder into the capsule bodies. Precise weight adjustments may be made simulta-

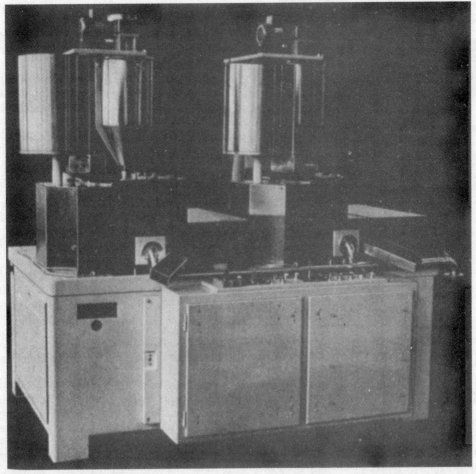

FIG. 13-9. *H & K Model 2400 capsule filling machine. (Courtesy of Robert Bosch GmbH, Waiblingen, West Germany.)*

Osaka

The Osaka filling machine is a high-capacity, continuous-motion machine recently introduced in the United States. The only model currently available is the R-180 (Fig. 13-14), which has a rated capacity of 70,000 to 165,000 capsules per hour. The unit handles either powder or granular materials.

The unit is totally enclosed, with external access to the capsule and powder hoppers.

The powder-filling principle utilized is unique in that vibration is used to move the powder from the powder hopper to powder shoes and from the powder shoes into the capsule bodies. Capsule bodies pass under the powder-filling area in two rows. Each row is fed by two vibratory units. The vibrators are externally controlled so that fill-weight adjustments can be made during machine operation. Because of this method of powder feed, correct powder formulations are essential, and limitations exist in the possible amounts with which to fill a given size capsule.

Provision is made to remove unjoined capsules during the rectification process and empty or broken capsules after filling.

The Osaka equipment can be supplemented with several pieces of auxiliary equipment, including a cleaner/polisher unit that has a rated capacity of up to 400,000 capsules per hour.

The Osaka distributor in the United States is the Sharples-Stokes Division of the Pennwalt Corporation, Warminster, PA.

Perry

The Model CF ACCOFIL machine offered by Perry utilizes the well-established ACCOFIL

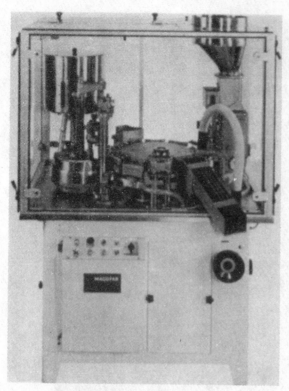

FIG. 13-10. *Macofar Model MT-12 capsule filling machine. (Courtesy of Macofar, Bologna, Italy.)*

method of powder dose control, which is unique in capsule filling (Fig. 13-15). The machine is a continuous-motion rotary machine with a rated output of up to about 60,000 capsules per hour; it fills powder mixtures only.

Capsules are rectified from 24 vertical tubes, and are cammed into a body downward position in a plate, from which they are dropped with a vacuum assist into a conveyor chain of two parts, the lower containing the bodies and the upper containing the caps. A sensor system is present, which provides for rejection of un-separated capsules and prevents ejection of powder in the absence of a capsule body. The cap-containing portion is caused to swing away from the body portion by a guide rail. Filling is accomplished while the cap links are displaced, following which the chain links are repositioned over each other.

Powder is supplied from a bulk supply hopper to a powder pan via a screw feeder. The level in the pan is controlled to a constant level. In the continuously rotating powder turret, 24 vertically operating, cam-controlled empty needles are immersed into the powder, and a vacuum is applied, sucking the powder up (in a predetermined amount) into the needle. Excess powder

is doctored from the sides and tips of the needles. The vacuum is held as the needle is positioned over an empty body, at which time the vacuum is broken and a light surge of air is applied to expel the powder.

Following filling, the chain links are properly realigned, and the body is moved into the cap by the slow cam action of the 24 closing pins. Following closing, the capsule is ejected by air from the conveyor, at which time it is counted, and the count is recorded by a digital readout on the front panel. Cleaning of all bushings, as well as the powder needles, is accomplished by high-pressure air.

The Model CF ACCOFIL machine is available through Perry Industries, Inc., Green Bay, WI.

Zanasi

The line of Zanasi equipment currently available includes nine different units in four model lines. With suitable change parts, all may be capable of handling powders, pellets, or tablets. Some models may be purchased with attachments to allow the insertion of smaller capsules, and some may be capable of paste or liquid filling.

Two models, the LZ-64 (Fig. 13-16) and AZ-20 (Fig. 13-17), retain the familiar intermittent operation of past Zanasi machines. The LZ-64 is rated at about 4,000 capsules per hour, while the AZ-20 speed is variable—from approximately 9,000 to 20,000 capsules per hour.

Two newer series consist of continuous-motion machines, but retain the dosator principle. The BZ series consists of four machines: BZ-40 (30,000/hour), BZ-72 (60,000/hour), BZ-110 (110,000/hour), and BZ-150 (150,000/hour). The BZ-40 and BZ-72 can handle powders, pellets, and tablets, while the BZ-110 handles only powders and granules. The BZ-150 handles powders only. A variety of auxiliary equipment is available with the BZ series of machines, including an empty capsule presorter, a powder recovery system, a filled-capsule sampling system, and a check weighing system.

Zanasi's newest series is the Z-5000 (Fig. 13-18), consisting of the Z-5000-R1, rated at up to 70,000 capsules per hour; the Z-5000-R2, rated at up to 110,000 capsules per hour; and the Z-5000-R3, rated at up to 150,000 capsules per hour. With change parts, all are capable of filling powders, granules, and tablets. Special attention has been paid to safety devices and acoustical treatments for operator protection.

Zanasi equipment is available in the United States from Z-Packaging Systems, Monsey, NY.

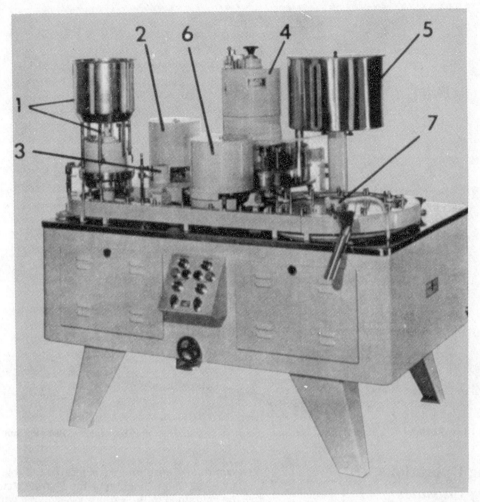

FIG. 13-11. *mG2 Model G36 capsule filling machine. See text for explanation of labels 1 through 7. (Courtesy of mG2 Macchine Automatiche, Bologna, Italy.)*

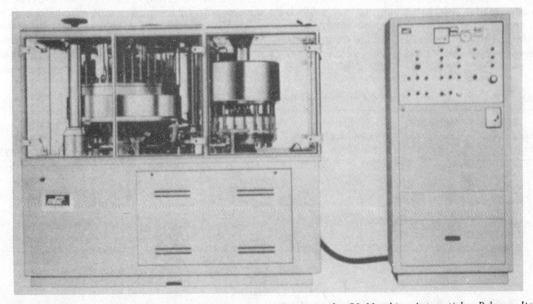

FIG. 13-12. *mG2 Model G37N capsule filling machine. (Courtesy of mG2 Macchine Automatiche, Bologna, Italy.)*

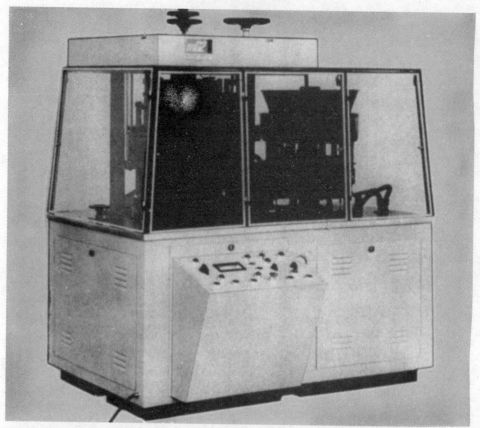

FIG. 13-13. *mG2 Model G38 capsule filling machine. (Courtesy of mG2 Macchine Automatiche, Bologna, Italy.)*

Filling Operations

Empty Capsules

Empty capsules are sold by sizes. The ones most commonly employed for human use range from size 0, the largest, to size 5, the smallest. Size 00 capsules may occasionally be required because of the volume of material to be filled, but this size is not used commercially in large volume. Although capsules change dimensions to some extent with varied moisture content and conditions encountered before use, Table 13-1 gives an approximation of the volume that may be contained in the various sizes, along with the amounts of some powders that can be contained in these sizes. The powder weights listed are approximate and vary with the amount of pressure employed in hand filling, or with the type of equipment utilized in machine filling.

Much consideration should be given to techniques for handling and storage of empty capsules in any production facility. This is of great

TABLE 13-1. *Filling Capacity of Empty Capsules*

Capsule Size	Approx. Volume (ml)	Quinine Sulfate (g)	Sodium Bicarbonate (g)	Acetyl- salicylic Acid (g)	Bismuth Subnitrate (g)
0	0.75	0.33	0.68	0.55	0.8
1	0.55	0.23	0.55	0.33	0.65
2	0.4	0.2	0.4	0.25	0.55
3	0.3	0.12	0.33	0.2	0.4
4	0.25	0.1	0.25	0.15	0.25
5	0.15	0.07	0.12	0.1	0.12

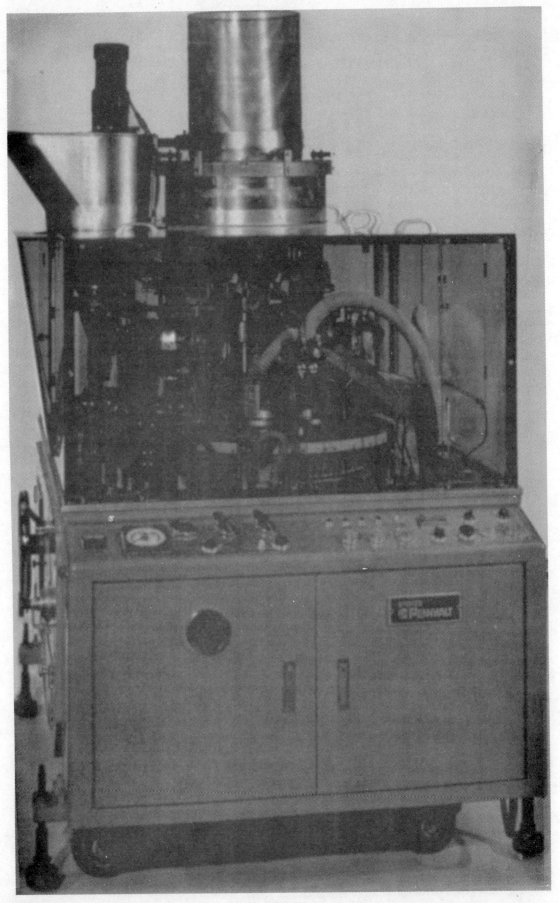

FIG. 13-14. *Osaka Model 180 capsule filling machine. (Courtesy of Sharples-Stokes, Warminster, PA.)*

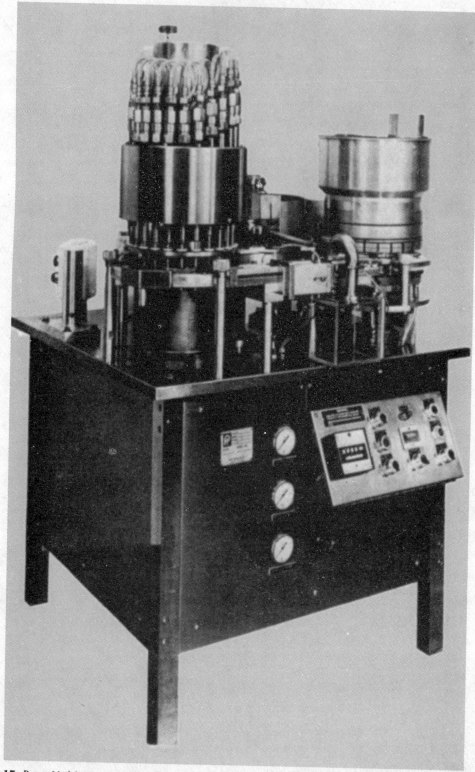

FIG. 13-15. *Perry Model CF ACCOFIL capsule filling machine. (Courtesy of Perry Industries, Green Bay, WI.)*

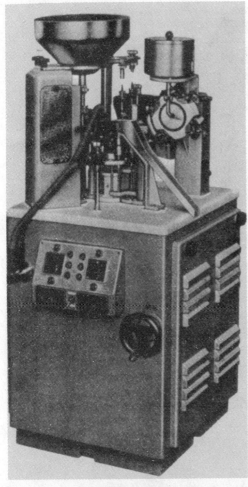

FIG. 13-16. *Zanasi Model LZ-64 capsule filling machine. (Courtesy of Zanasi, S.p.A., Bologna, Italy.)*

importance when use rates are high, as when high-speed filling equipment is used.

Capsules as received from the supplier generally have moisture content between 12 and 15%, and these levels are maintained during storage in the original container. Storage under high-temperature conditions (above 100°F) must not be prolonged. Exposure to extremely high or extremely low humidity conditions for extended periods after the containers are opened causes the capsules to either gain or lose moisture. At high moisture levels, the capsules absorb moisture, and may soften and become tacky. In severe cases, the capsules may absorb sufficient moisture to cause them to deform under their own weight. At low moisture levels, they become brittle and suffer dimensional changes, which may cause handling problems in the filling equipment.

Regarding the empty capsules only, handling is ideally carried on in areas within the relative humidity range of approximately 30 to 45%, since major moisture content changes do not occur within these limits. If conditions drier than these are necessitated because of the ingredients being filled, exposures of the empty capsules prior to filling should be minimized. Strong consideration should be given to the use of air-conditioned facilities to control both temperatures and humidity when high-speed filling equipment is being operated.

Formulations

The problems encountered in handling powders during mixing and filling operations are so diverse as to preclude any but general comments. Although some problems are common to all types of filling equipment, certain machines themselves represent unique situations. Among the general problems, two major ones can be listed.

1. After the powder ingredients have been homogeneously blended by any suitable technique, the flow of the resultant mixture must be adequate to ensure delivery of sufficient powder to the capsules at the time of filling. De-mixing must not occur during the powder handling in the filling equipment itself.

2. Physical incompatibilities between active ingredients, between diluents, or between active ingredients and/or diluents and the capsule shell may create problems.

The capsule seldom contains only the active ingredient(s); most capsule formulations require the use of some diluent material. Because of the wide range of materials encapsulated, no attempt can be made to outline specific criteria for the choice of suitable diluents. The following are three major general considerations.

1. The powder mix must provide the type of flow characteristics required by the equipment. In the case of the Lilly, Parke-Davis, Höfliger and Karg, Osaka, and Perry machines, powders must be free flowing. In the case of Zanasi, Macofar, Farmatic, and mG2 equipment, the powder must have sufficient cohesiveness to retain its slug form during delivery to the capsules. For example, when one is filling with acetylsalicylic acid, an excipient such as a flowable cornstarch allows filling in the former case, whereas compactible excipients such as microcrystalline cellulose are required in the latter case. In all cases, the powder mixture must retain its homogeneous composition without de-mixing during the machine handling operations. Lubricants, such as a metallic stearate,

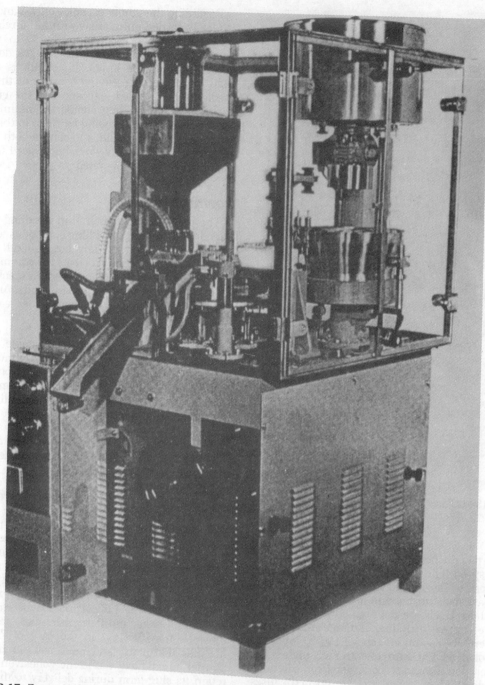

FIG. 13-17. *Zanasi Model AZ-20 capsule filling machine. (Courtesy of Zanasi, S.p.A., Bologna, Italy.)*

may be used in the former case; binders, such as mineral oil, are sometimes used in the latter. Particle sizes and powder densities of all ingredients should be matched as closely as possible to assist in the prevention of de-mixing.

2. Potential incompatibilities should be antic-ipated with each new mixture of materials. Reactions at elevated temperatures and humidities should be studied, for effects not only on the contained powder mixture, but also on the gelatin capsules. Studies such as these should include an evaluation in the presence of probable

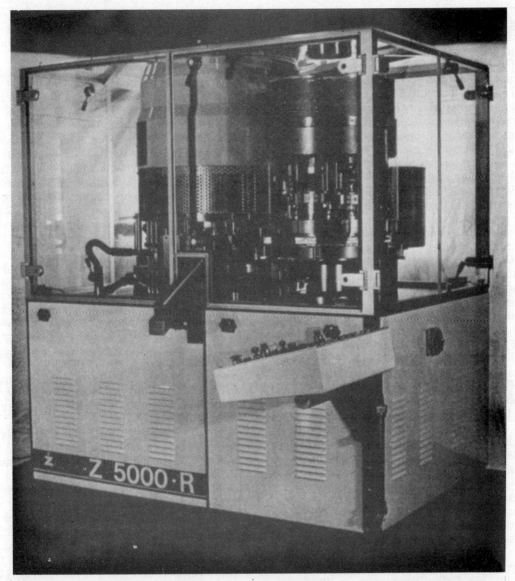

FIG. 13-18. *Zanasi Model Z-5000 capsule filling machine. (Courtesy of Zanasi, S.p.A., Bologna, Italy.)*

packaging materials. Evaluation of any test procedure should be based on sound statistical techniques.

3. The choice of excipients should be made with a view toward current Food and Drug Administration (FDA) regulations as they apply to Investigational New Drug and New Drug applications. Any applicable foreign regulations also should be considered. Some materials that may be useful as excipients are bentonite, calcium carbonate, lactose, mannitol, magnesium carbonate, magnesium oxide, silica gel, starch, talc, and tapioca powder.

If it is desirable for any reason to consider materials other than the aforementioned, first consideration should be given to materials that are given a "Generally Recognized As Safe" designation by the FDA. Obtaining approval of materials that are not in this category can be an expensive and time-consuming process, although there are occasions when it cannot be avoided.

Materials that may be considered for improvement of flow characteristics (glidants and/or lubricants, as indicated earlier) may include the following: glycol esters, silicones, silicon dioxide, metallic stearates, stearic acid, and talc.

Oils that may be considered for use in assisting in the control of dusting, as well as in providing additional cohesiveness to a powder mix, could include any inert, edible, FDA-approved material.

The determination of amounts of diluents to be used is based on (1) the total amount of material that can possibly be put in the capsule in relation to the amount of active ingredients to be supplied by the capsule, and (2) the amounts of lubricant and/or oil (generally in the order of 2% or less) that can be used. Experimentation with the actual materials is the only positive way to arrive at these figures.

Serious consideration should be given to the choice of suitable control procedures for the filling operations. In addition, it may be desirable to provide 100% weight checking after filling. The control procedures must ensure that the finished, filled capsules meet the appropriate current regulatory tests, e.g., weight variation, content uniformity, solubility, and/or disintegration. Current legal requirements should be adequately explored since there are wide differences between countries. The weight variation test in USP XX has been replaced in USP XXI with the Uniformity of Dosage Units Tests. However, the weight variation test, as official in USP XX, is still useful in machine set-up and evaluation.

The *weight variation* test defined by USP XX is a sequential test, in which 20 intact capsules are individually weighed and the average weight is determined. The test requirements are met if none of the individual weights are less than 90%, or more than 110%, of the average. If the original 20 do not meet these criteria, the individual *net weights* are determined. These are averaged, and differences are determined between each individual net content and the average. The test requirements are met (1) if not more than two of the individual differences are greater than 10% of the average, or (2) if in no case any difference is greater than 25%.

If more than 2 but less than 6 net weights determined by the test deviate by more than 10% but less than 25%, the net contents are determined for an additional 40 capsules, and the average is calculated for the entire 60 capsules. Sixty deviations from the new average are calculated. The requirements are met (1) if the difference does not exceed 10% of the average in more than 6 of the 60 capsules, and (2) if in no case any difference exceeds 25%.

Two new pieces of equipment determine the weight of individual capsules, providing for the automatic rejection of overfilled and underfilled capsules. These machines may be used in-line to reclaim portions of a batch as it is processed, or off-line to weigh and sort a complete batch that has been shown statistically to have unacceptable weight variation.

The ROTOWEIGH is a high-speed capsule weighing machine sold by Eli Lilly and Company (Fig. 13-19). The capsules are gravity-fed onto vacuum pins for presentation to a unique weight detection system, which measures the reflected energy (backscatter) of a low power x-ray beam directed at each capsule. This reflected energy is proportional to the weight of the filled capsule, permitting automatic rejection of any individual capsule above or below preset weights. The machine operates at 73,000 capsules per hour, and its accuracy is more than adequate to assure compliance with the USP weight requirements.

The second unit is the Vericap 1200 machine (Fig. 13-20), which is sold by Modern Controls, Inc., Elk River, MN. It operates by detecting capacitance variation as filled capsules are propelled at high speed by compressed air between two charged plates. The measured change in dielectric constant thus produced is correlated to the weight of the capsule. Capsules that are overweight or underweight are then automatically separated from the acceptable capsules. The machine operates at a rate of 73,000 capsules per hour.

A second test in USP XX that may apply to capsules is that for *content uniformity,* which is performed when specified by individual monographs. In this case, 30 capsules are selected, 10 of which are assayed by the specified procedure. The requirements are met if 9 of the 10 are within the specified potency range of 85 to 115%, and the tenth is not outside 75 to 125%.

If more than 1, but less than 3, of the first 10 capsules fall outside the 85 to 115% limits, the remaining 20 are assayed. The requirements are met if all 30 capsules are within 75 to 125% of the specified potency range, and not less than 27 of the 30 are within the 85 to 115% range.

Broad generalizations about stability test programs cannot be made, since the question has to be answered according to each user's criteria. The tests should be based on adequate statistical design, however, and should include evaluation of not only active ingredient stability, but also visual and mechanical aspects of the finished dosage form. These tests must include extended storage at various elevated temperatures with different humidity levels. Tests should include the filled capsules, both by themselves and in the presence of all contemplated packaging materials.

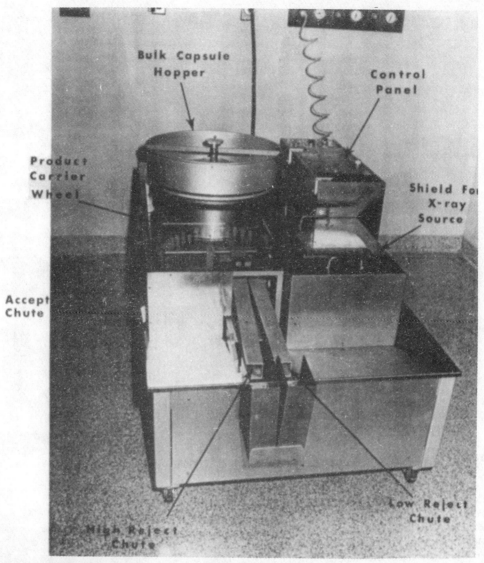

FIG. 13-19. *ROTOWEIGH capsule weighing machine. (Courtesy of Eli Lilly & Co., Indianapolis, IN.)*

Finishing

Finished capsules from all filling equipment require some sort of dusting and/or polishing operation before the remaining operations of inspection, bottling, and labeling are completed. Dusting or polishing operations vary according to the type of filling equipment used, the type of powder used for filling, and the individual desires for the finished appearance of the completed capsules. The following are the methods most commonly used, based on desired output, formulation, required final appearance, and so on.

1. *Pan polishing.* Because of its unique design (primarily in the area of airflow), the Accela-Cota tablet coating pan may be used to dust and polish capsules. A polyurethane or cheese cloth liner is placed in the pan, and the liner is used to trap the removed dust as well as to impart a gloss to the capsules.

2. *Cloth dusting.* In this method, the bulk-filled capsules are rubbed with a cloth that may or may not be impregnated with an inert oil. This procedure is a hand operation, but one that can handle reasonable volumes, and that results in a positive method for removal of resistant

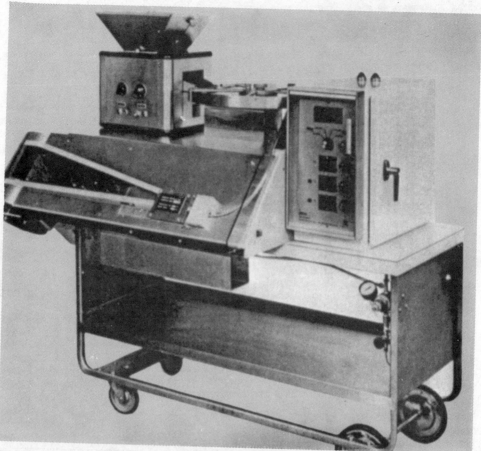

FIG. 13-20. *Vericap 1200 capsule weighing machine. (Courtesy of Modern Controls, Elk River, MN.)*

materials. In addition, it imparts a somewhat improved gloss to the capsules.

3. *Brushing.* In this procedure, capsules are fed under rotating soft brushes, which serve to remove the dust from the capsule shell. This operation must be accompanied by a vacuuming for dust removal. Some materials are extremely difficult to remove by brushing, even to the point of impregnating the brushes and causing scratches or deformation of the capsules.

Commercial capsule sort/polish equipment has become available. Some of the units, in addition to the Accela-Cota pan, are as follows.

ROTOSORT is a new filled capsule sorting machine sold by Eli Lilly and Company (Fig. 13-21). It is a mechanical sorting device that removes loose powder, unfilled joined capsules, filled or unfilled bodies, and loose caps. It can handle up to 150,000 capsules per hour, and it can run directly off a filling machine or be used separately.

The Erweka KEA dedusting and polishing machine for hard gelatin capsules is sold in the

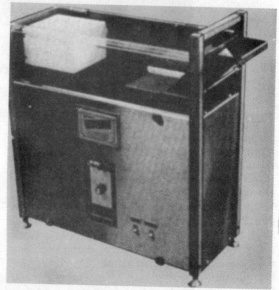

FIG. 13-21. *ROTOSORT capsule sorting machine. (Courtesy of Eli Lilly & Co., Indianapolis, IN.)*

United States by Key Industries, Englishtown, NJ (Fig. 13-22). The unit is designed to handle the output from any capsule filling machine. It moves the capsules between soft plastic tassels against a perforated plastic sleeve, under vacuum. Any residual powder is removed by the vacuum.

Seidenader Equipment, Totowa, NJ, offers two units that may be used separately or may be combined in the finishing of filled gelatin capsules. A belt is available that presents capsules for visual inspection, and it may include a vacuum system to automatically remove unfilled capsules. Cleaning and polishing machine PM60 (Fig. 13-23) may be used to polish finished capsules. It consists of two lamb's wool belts moving in opposite directions. The capsules are carried on the lower belt, and both belts are under suction.

Special Techniques

Some special techniques that may be applied to the capsules as a dosage form include the following.

1. Imprinting is a convenient method by which company and/or product identification information can be placed upon each capsule. The imprinting operation is best performed on the empty capsules, although filled capsules can be printed. The preference for imprinting empty

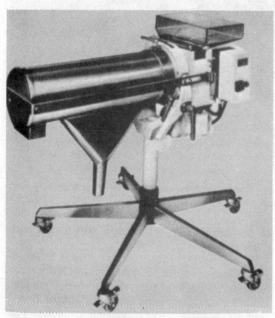

FIG. 13-22. *Erweka KEA capsule dedusting and polishing machine. (Courtesy of Erweka-Apparatebau, Heusenstamm, West Germany.)*

capsules arises from the fact that the imprinting operation may occasionally damage some capsules. When filled capsules are imprinted, contamination, poor print quality, and actual damage to the imprinting equipment result. Various types and capacities of equipment are commercially available for this purpose in the United States. The three major suppliers of this equipment are Ackley Machine Corporation, Moorestown, NJ, R. W. Hartnett Company, Philadelphia, PA; and the Markem Machine Company, Keene, NH.

Hartnett offers a variety of machines with outputs as high as 500,000 capsules per hour (model B, Fig. 13-24). Also available is a unit that prints around the circumference of the capsules, as opposed to a longitudinal imprint; however, this machine operates at a slower rate. A lower-capacity unit (up to 250,000 capsules per hour) allows printing on both sides of the capsule, in different colors if desired.

Markem offers three models, which range from approximately 60,000 to 250,000 capsules per hour (Model 280A, Fig. 13-25). All three models allow for two-sided printing, but not circumferential.

Ackley offers a straight-line imprinter with an output rate of about 500,000 capsules per hour, and has recently announced a new circumferential printer rated at about the same output.

In addition, several firms, including the major empty capsule suppliers, offer custom imprinting services.

All imprinting machines operate on a rotogravure process, and a wide variety of colors of edible inks, both water- and solvent-based, are commercially available.

2. Special purpose capsules are capsules to which a special treatment has been given in an attempt to retard the solubility in some manner. This may be done in an attempt to delay absorption of the active ingredient, or to provide enteric properties. Normal solubility for gelatin capsules, either empty or filled, is not defined by the USP XX. However, the General Service Administration, in Federal Specification #U-C-115b (2/10/58), defines solubility limits for empty capsules as follows: (a) water resistance—fails to dissolve in water at 20 to 30°C in 15 min; (b) acid solubility—dissolves in less than 5 min in 0.5% aqueous HCl (w/w) at 36 to 38°C.

None of the following is used for any commercial products as far as is known and cannot be seriously recommended except for experimental purposes, because of generally unpredictable results.

a. Formalin treatment has been employed to modify the solubility of gelatin capsules. Expo-

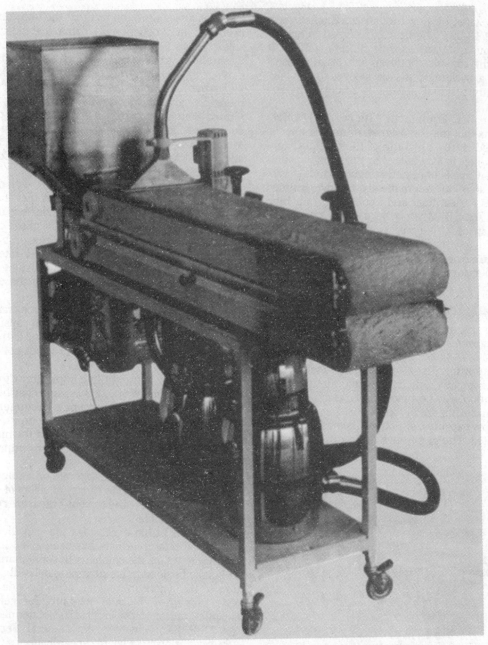

FIG. 13-23. *Seidenader Model PM60 capsule polishing machine. (Courtesy of Seidenader Maschinenbau München, West Germany.)*

sure to formalin vapors or treatment with aqueous formalin results in an unpredictable decrease in solubility of the gelatin film, owing to cross-linkage of the gelatin molecule initiated by the aldehyde. This result may also be noted if the product being filled contains aldehydic materials, or if aldehyde flavorants are added. Because of the nature of the reaction initiated in this manner, it is difficult to control the degree of insolubilization, or indeed, to prevent ultimate complete insolubility.

b. Various coatings have been used in an effort to provide similarly modified solubility characteristics. These coatings include salol, shellac, cellulose acetate phthalate, and certain resins that have usually been applied by usual pan coating techniques.

Gelatin capsules do, however, provide a con-

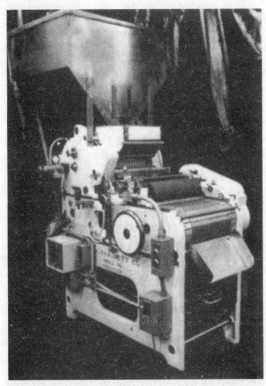

FIG. 13-24. *Hartnett Model B capsule imprinting machine. (Courtesy of R. H. Hartnett Co., Philadelphia, PA.)*

venient way to deliver pellets or granular material when delayed or prolonged release properties have been incorporated in all or portions of the material to be filled.

3. Separation of incompatible materials (a technique used for some commercial products) is carried out by the use of a two-phase fill in the capsule. One phase consists of either a soft capsule, a smaller hard capsule, a pill, or a suitably coated tablet that is filled into each capsule. Following this as a second phase, a powder fill is added in the usual manner. If this technique is used on commercial filling equipment, modifications must be made to the filling cycle of the machine. These changes would include, at minimum, the necessary changes in the machine operation to allow materials to be loaded at two points during the filling cycle. Tamp type powder filling machines require the disabling of the tamp cycle.

4. Recently, there has been a revival of interest in the filling of conventional two-piece gelatin capsules with liquids and semisolids. Hard gelatin capsules were commonly used as early as the 1890s for oils, ethereal extracts, and pill masses,[1] but the ability to fill the capsules on semiautomatic and automatic equipment is a recent development. The formulations used for filling are usually semisolids at ambient temper-

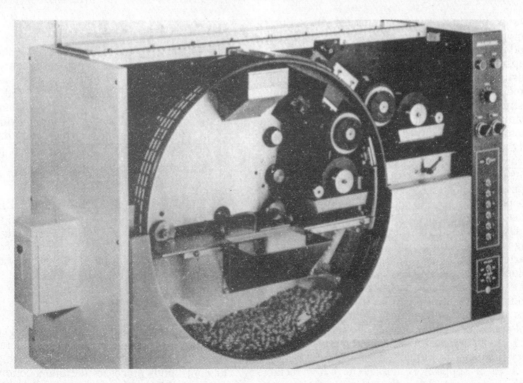

FIG. 13-25. *Markem Model 280A capsule imprinting machine. (Coursety of Markem Co., Keene, NH.)*

atures, which are melted to allow filling.[2] Or they are thixotropic formulations in which the shear developed in filling allows pumping, but whose high viscosity when shear is absent prevents leakage after filling. Quantitative assessment of the gastric emptying of hard gelatin capsules filled with thixotropic liquids can be made in terms of the lag time prior to emptying, and the slope of the first order emptying curve. Results have shown that the viscosity of the fill has no significant influence on the emptying characteristics of these dosage forms.[3] Machines for filling semisolid materials are currently available from Robert Bosch GmbH, Elanco, Harro Hofliger, and Zanasi.

5. A recent series of developments—primarily in Europe—have resulted in allowing the use of a liquid fill into two-piece hard capsules. The fills are either thermosetting (and filled warm) or thixotropic. Modified commercial equipment is available for filling.

References

1. Francois, D., and Jones, B.E.: Man. Chem. Aerosol News, 37:37, 1979.
2. Hunter, E., Fell, J.T., Sharma, H., and McNeilly, A.M.: Die Pharm. Ind., 44:90, 1982.
3. Hunter, E., Fell, J.T., Sharma, H., and McNeilly, A.M.: Die Pharm. Ind., 45:443, 1983.

PART TWO

Soft Gelatin Capsules

J. P. STANLEY

Many pharmaceutical companies have the equipment and facilities for the development and production of tablets, liquids, and hard-shell capsule products, but they usually depend upon custom manufacturers for the development and production of soft gelatin capsules. The custom manufacturers are specialists in this field, owing primarily to economic, patent, and technologic factors. Although few become directly involved in the manufacture of soft capsules, pharmaceutical chemists must be prepared to investigate this dosage form and to participate in its development, either in their own laboratories or in cooperation with the technical personnel of a custom manufacturer.

Owing to their special properties and advantages, soft gelatin capsules are used in a wide variety of industries, but they are used most widely in the pharmaceutical industry. Billions of capsules are made each year in various sizes and shapes (Fig. 13-26), and in a variety of colors and color combinations. Their pharmaceutical applications are:

1. As an oral dosage form of ethical or proprietary products for human or veterinary use.
2. As a suppository dosage form for rectal use,[1] or for vaginal use. Rectal dosage forms are becoming more acceptable for pediatric and geriatric use. Vaginal use is confined to applications that require the medication to be inserted at bedtime. Because of the action of the sphincter muscle, rectal use is not similarly limited.
3. As a specialty package in tube form, for human and veterinary single dose application of topical, ophthalmic, and otic preparations, and rectal ointments.

In the cosmetic industry, these capsules may be used as a specialty package for breath fresheners, perfumes, bath oils, suntan oils, and various skin creams.

Methods of Manufacture

Soft gelatin capsules have been available since the middle of the nineteenth century. Originally, they were made one at a time; leather molds—and later, iron molds—were used for shaping the capsule. The capsules were filled by medicine dropper and sealed by hand with a "glob" of molten gelatin. Since those early days, many methods of capsulation have been proposed and patented, but this discussion is confined to equipment of commercial significance in present use.

As technology advanced, the individual iron molds gave way to multiple molding units, and these eventually led to sets of plates containing die pockets. The *plate process* is the oldest commercial method of manufacture, but today this equipment can no longer be purchased, and consequently, only a few companies still use this process. The plate process—a batch process that requires two or three operators for each machine—has given way to the more modern continuous processes, which require considerably less manpower for operation.

The continuous processes became a commercial reality in 1933, when the late R. P. Scherer

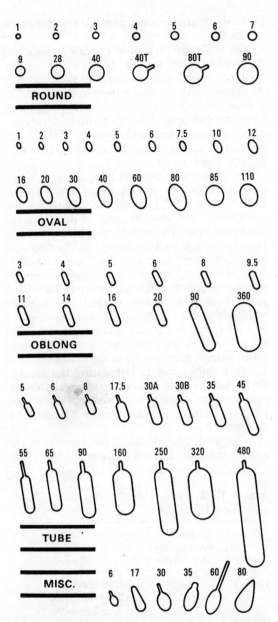

FIG. 13-26. *Sizes and shapes of soft gelatin capsules (1 cc = 16.23 m). Numbers represent the nominal capacity in minims. (Courtesy of R.P. Scherer Corporation, Troy, MI.)*

invented the rotary die process. Prior to this invention, soft gelatin capsules were not looked on favorably by the pharmaceutical industry, owing to the relatively large amount of the capsulated material (15 to 20%) lost during manufacture, and to the variation in the net content of the capsule (possibly 20 to 40%). The rotary die process reduced manufacturing losses to a negligible figure and content variation to less than

±3%. The Scherer machine cannot be purchased or leased, but the Scherer organization provides plant and laboratory facilities for the manufacture of this dosage form in the United States and nine foreign locations.

The early success of the rotary die process led others to develop continuous methods of soft gelatin capsule manufacture. One such method, known as the *reciprocating die process,* was announced in 1949 and was developed by the Norton Company, Worchester, MA. Another continuous process, also announced in 1949, was developed by the Lederle Laboratories Division of the American Cyanamid Company and has been used solely in the manufacture of that company's products. This equipment, known as the *Accogel machine,* is unique in that it is the only equipment that accurately fills powdered dry solids into soft gelatin capsules.

A discussion of the comparative advantages and disadvantages of the foregoing four processes—plate, rotary die, reciprocating die, and Accogel machine—is beyond the scope of this chapter and would have little instructive value, since the pharmaceutical chemist seldom has the opportunity to choose between the four types of equipment. One must consider, however, that for maximum production efficiency, the continuous processes demand almost 24 hours per day, 5 (preferably 7) days per week, of continuous operation. Thus, medicament formulations must be so designed as to maintain their desired physical characteristics during this period of operation as well as during periods of weekend shutdowns, should they occur. The production capacity of each of these machines is determined by (1) die size, which determines the number of die pockets on the standard-sized die plate, rotary die, or reciprocating die; (2) the speed of the machine (of the operators for the plate process); and (3) the physical characteristics of the material to be capsulated. Formulations are designed to achieve maximum production capacity consistent with maximum physical and ingredient stability and therapeutic efficacy.

All of the aforementioned equipment is limited to the production of gelatin capsules. Other films and film-forming polymers have not as yet been successfully adapted for use on these machines. An interesting review of the patent literature, covering capsule technology, has been published.[2]

The Nature of the Capsule Shell

The capsule shell is basically composed of gelatin, a plasticizer, and water; it may contain additional ingredients such as preservatives, coloring and opacifying agents, flavorings, sugars, acids, and medicaments to achieve desired effects.

Gelatin's chemical, physical, and physiological properties make it an ideal substance for the capsulation of pharmaceutical products.[3-6] The *gelatin* is USP grade with additional specifications required by the capsule manufacturer. The additional specifications concern the Bloom strength, viscosity, and iron content of the gelatins used.

The *Bloom* or *gel strength* of gelatin is a measure of the cohesive strength of the cross-linking that occurs between gelatin molecules and is proportional to the molecular weight of the gelatin. Bloom is determined by measuring the weight in grams required to move a plastic plunger that is 0.5 inches in diameter 4 mm into a 6⅔% gelatin gel that has been held at 10°C for 17 hours. Bloom may vary with the requirements of the individual custom manufacturer but ranges from 150 to 250 g. In general, with all other factors being equal, the higher the Bloom strength of the gelatin used, the more physically stable is the resulting capsule shell. The cost of gelatin is directly proportional to its Bloom or gel strength and thus is an important factor in the cost of soft capsules. Consequently, the higher Bloom gelatins are only used when necessary to improve the physical stability of a product or for large capsules (over 50 minims), which require greater structural strength during manufacture.

Viscosity of gelatin, determined on a 6⅔% concentration of gelatin in water at 60°C, is a measure of the molecular chain length and determines the manufacturing characteristics of the gelatin film. The desired film characteristics are usually based on standard gelatin formulations, which allow production at a set sealing temperature and definite drying conditions, and produce a firm, nontacky, nonbrittle, pharmaceutically elegant product. The viscosity for gelatin can range from 25 to 45 millipoise, but the individual manufacturer sets a narrow range, e.g., 38 ± 2 millipoise, for a particular type of gelatin, to make use of a standard formulation and thus conform to standard production conditions.

Low-viscosity (25 to 32 millipoise), high-Bloom (180 to 250 g) gelatins are used in conjunction with the capsulation of hygroscopic vehicles or solids, and standard gelatin formulas can be modified so as to require up to 50% less water for satisfactory operation on the capsulation machine. These modified formulas afford less opportunity for the hygroscopic fill materials to attract water from the shell and thereby improve the ingredient and physical stability of the product.[7]

Iron is always present in the raw gelatin, and its concentration usually depends on the iron content of the large quantities of water used in its manufacture. Gelatins used in the manufacture of soft gelatin capsules should not contain more than 15 ppm of this element, because of its effect on Food, Drug, and Cosmetic (FD&C) certified dyes and its possible color reactions with organic compounds.

The *plasticizers* used with gelatin in soft capsule manufacture are relatively few. Glycerin USP, Sorbitol USP, Pharmaceutical Grade Sorbitol Special, and combinations of these are the most prevalent. The ratio by weight of dry plasticizer to dry gelatin determines the "hardness" of the gelatin shell, assuming that there is no effect from the capsulated material. (Some examples of glycerin/gelatin ratios are shown in Table 13-2 along with their typical usage.) The ratio by weight of water to dry gelatin can vary from 0.7 to 1.3 (water) to 1.0 (dry gelatin) depending on the viscosity of the gelatin being used. For most formulations, however, it is approximately 1 to 1. Since only water is lost during the capsule drying process, the percentage of plasticizer and gelatin in the shell is increased, but the important plasticizer to gelatin ratio remains unchanged.

In general, the additional *components* of the gelatin mass are limited in their use by (1) the

TABLE 13-2. *Typical Shell "Hardness" Ratios and Their Uses*

Hardness	Ratio Dry Glycerin/ Dry Gelatin	Usage
Hard	0.4/1	Oral, oil-based, or shell-softening products and those destined primarily for hot, humid areas.
Medium	0.6/1	Oral, tube, vaginal oil-based, water-miscible-based, or shell-hardening products and those destined primarily for temperate areas.
Soft	0.8/1	Tube, vaginal, water-miscible-based or shell-hardening products and those destined primarily for cold, dry areas.

amounts required to produce the desired effect; (2) their effect on capsule manufacture; and (3) economic factors. Examples of ingredients falling into the first two categories are shown in Table 13-3.

The addition of medicaments to the gelatin mass usually is not recommended, for economic reasons, since only 50% of the gelatin mass is incorporated into the capsules. This results in a 50% loss of the added medicament. However, certain highly active, relatively inexpensive compounds such as benzocaine (3 mg/capsule shell) in chewable cough capsules may be used successfully.

Additional comments relative to the color of the gelatin shell are in order, since color is such an important aspect of all products. This is particularly true of soft gelatin capsules, in which the color of the capsule can be definitely affected by the color or type of material capsulated. As a general policy, the color of the capsule shell should never be lighter in hue than the capsulated material.

More specifically, darker colors are more appropriate for large-size (14 to 20 minim oblong) oral products, since they will not accentuate the size. Also, before a color is chosen, mixtures should be checked in the laboratory by addition of water to ascertain if reactions take place to cause the mixture to darken, as in the case of ascorbic acid and iron salts in vitamin and mineral formulations, or as in the case of reactions between iron and compounds of a phenolic nature. Since iron is present in gelatin, dark spots may occur in the shell owing to the migration of water-soluble iron-sensitive ingredients from the fill material into the shell. As a rule, clear colors usually are employed with clear type fill materials, and opaque colors are used with suspensions, but the reverse of this rule can be chosen to achieve a particular appearance or for ingredient stability purposes. For special effects or identification purposes, two colors, both opaque or one opaque and one clear, may be chosen since the manufacturing process involves two gelatin films.

A publication by Hom and co-workers describes a gelatin disk method for the determination of the effects of agitation, temperature, dissolution medium, and shell composition on the dissolution rate of soft gelatin capsules.[8] This information should be helpful in the formulation of gelatin capsules for various purposes.

From the foregoing discussion on the gelatin shell, one may conclude that the pharmaceutical chemist must rely heavily on the experience of the custom capsule manufacturer. However, in order to choose the proper gelatin, gelatin formula, and color, the custom manufacturer must rely on the technical and product information designed and developed by the pharmaceutical chemist. With such mutual cooperation and free exchange of information, new products or dosage forms can be efficiently developed.

The Nature of the Capsule Content

Soft gelatin capsules can be used to dispense a variety of liquids and solids. Requirements and specifications of these materials vary, depending on the equipment of the manufacturer, but there are basic precepts that may be used as a guide for the formulation and production of commercially and therapeutically acceptable capsules, regardless of method of capsulation. The formulation of the capsule content for each product is individually developed to fulfill the specifications and end-use requirements of the product.

Except for the Accogel process, which is primarily concerned with the capsulation of dry

TABLE 13-3. *Additional Components of the Gelatin Mass*

Ingredient	Concentration	Purpose
Category I		
Methylparaben, 4 parts; Propylparaben, 1 part	0.2%	Preservative
FD&C and D&C water-soluble dyes, certified lakes, pigments, and vegetable colors, alone or in combination	q.s.	Colorants
Titanium dioxide	0.2 to 1.2%	Opacifier
Ethyl vanillin	0.1%	Flavoring for odor and taste
Essential oils	to 2%	Flavoring for odor and taste
Category II		
Sugar (sucrose)	to 5%	To produce chewable shell and taste
Fumaric acid	to 1%	Aids solubility; reduces aldehydic tanning of gelatin

powders, the content of a soft gelatin capsule is a liquid, or a combination of miscible liquids, a solution of a solid(s) in a liquid(s), or a suspension of a solid(s) in a liquid(s). All such materials for capsulation are formulated to produce the smallest possible capsule consistent with maximum ingredient and physical stability, therapeutic effectiveness, and production efficiency. Once the smallest capsule size is determined, personnel in the sales or marketing departments usually choose the color, shape, and ultimate size of the retail product, unless there is a technical or production reason for the development chemist to specify a particular size, shape, and color. The maximum capsule size and shape for convenient oral use in humans is the 20 minim oblong, the 16 minim oval, or the 9 minim round as shown in Figure 13-26.

Liquids are an essential part of the capsule content. Only those liquids that are both water-miscible and volatile cannot be included as major constituents of the capsule content since they can migrate into the hydrophilic gelatin shell and volatilize from its surface. Water, ethyl alcohol, and, of course, emulsions fall into this category. Similarly, gelatin plasticizers such as glycerin and propylene glycol cannot be major constituents of the capsule content, owing to their softening effect on the gelatin shell, which thereby makes the capsule more susceptible to the effects of heat and humidity. As minor constituents (up to about 5% of the capsule content), water and alcohol can be used as cosolvents to aid in the preparation of solutions for capsulation. Also, up to 10% glycerin and/or propylene glycol can be used as cosolvents with polyethylene glycol or other liquids that have a shell-hardening effect when capsulated alone.

There are a large number of liquids that do not fall into the foregoing category and thus can function as active ingredients, solvents, or vehicles for suspension-type formulations. These liquids include aromatic and aliphatic hydrocarbons, chlorinated hydrocarbons, and high-molecular-weight alcohols, esters, and organic acids. Many of these are used in veterinary, cosmetic, and industrial products. For human use, however, the pharmaceutical chemist is often limited in his selection or use of a particular liquid because of government regulations, product performance specifications, ingredient incompatibilities, and liquid-solid adsorption characteristics. The most widely used liquids for human use are oily active ingredients (clofibrate), vegetable oils (soybean oil), mineral oil, nonionic surface active agents (polysorbate 80), and polyethylene glycols (400 and 600), either alone or in combination. Such active ingredient oils as fish oil may also function as a solvent, or as the suspending medium for one or more additional active ingredients, as in vitamin capsules.

All liquids, solutions, and suspensions for capsulation should be homogeneous and air-free (vide infra), and preferably should flow by gravity at room temperature, but not at a temperature exceeding 35°C at the point of capsulation, since the sealing temperature of the gelatin films is usually in the range of 37 to 40°C. In general, liquids ranging in *viscosity* from ethyl ether (0.222 cp at 25°C)[9] to heavy adhesive mixtures (exceeding 3000 cp at 25°C) may be encapsulated, but there are some exceptions since the property of viscosity alone is not the sole criterion. Liquids that exhibit the rheologic property of tack or tackiness, such as glycerin (954 cp at 25°C),[9] are exceptions, since such liquids can eventually cause the binding of slide valves and pumps in the capsule filling mechanism. Also, preparations for encapsulation should have a pH between 2.5 and 7.5, since preparations that are more acidic can cause hydrolysis and leakage of the gelatin shell, and preparations that are more alkaline can tan the gelatin and thus affect the solubility of the shell.

The capsulation of water-immiscible liquids is the simplest form of soft gelatin capsulation and usually requires little or no formulation. The minimum size capsule depends on the dosage desired, the minimum fill volume being calculated from the specific gravity of the liquid. A die size and shape may then be chosen from those shown in Figure 13-26. The nearest die size above the calculated fill volume may be used, or any larger die may be chosen if the active ingredient is to be diluted for some reason. For example, a 25,000-unit vitamin A capsule using vitamin A palmitate (1,000,000 units A/g) as a source for the vitamin A would have a minimum fill volume of about 0.45 minims, and thus could be diluted to any size capsule desired. On the other hand, the same potency capsule using fish oil (50,000 units A/g) as a source for the vitamin A would have a minimum fill volume of about 8.8 minims.

The minimum fill volume for water-miscible, nonvolatile liquids, such as polysorbate 80, is determined in the same manner. Because of their hygroscopic nature, however, they cause water to migrate from the gelatin shell into the fill material. This migration is rapid and could amount to 20% of the weight of the miscible liquid. During the drying period of the capsule, most of this water returns to and passes through the gelatin shell, but up to 7.5% of the original water can remain in the fill material, depending on the hydrophilic properties of the liquid. Thus, for liquids of this type, a safety factor must be used in establishing the minimum fill volume and in choosing the die.*

Although oily liquids do not retain moisture, water does pass from the shell of the capsule into the rill material and out again during the manufacture and drying of these capsules. This is important for the formulator to remember, since such water transfer can and does have a bearing on formulations in which oily liquids are used as solvents or as vehicles for suspensions. If such suspensions contain hydrophuic solids, water may be retained up to 3% by weight of the hydrophilic material.

Combinations of miscible liquids often are used to produce desired physiological results such as increased or more rapid absorption of active ingredient (vitamin A and polysorbate 80); or to produce desired physiochemical results, such as improved flow properties (dilution or partial substitution with a thinner liquid), or improved solubility (steroid with oil and benzyl alcohol).

Except for when the Accogel process is used, solids are filled into soft gelatin capsules, in the form of either a solution or a suspension. The preparation of a suitable solution of a solid medicament should be the first goal of the pharmaceutical chemist. Usually, a solution is more easily capsulated and exhibits better uniformity, stability, and biopharmaceutical properties than does a suspension. For oral products, the medicament must have sufficient solubility in the solvent system so that the necessary dose is contained in a maximum fill volume of 16 to 20 minims (1 to 1.25cc).

Solids that are not sufficiently soluble in liquids or in combinations of liquids are capsulated as suspensions. Most organic and inorganic solids or compounds may be capsulated. Such materials should be 80 mesh or finer in particle size, owing to certain close tolerances of the capsulation equipment and for maximum homogeneity of the suspension. Many compounds cannot be capsulated, owing to their solubility in water and thus their ability to affect the gelatin shell, unless they are minor constituents of a formula or are combined with a type of carrier

*For example, a capsule to contain 500 mg of Polysorbate 80 would have a calculated $\left(\dfrac{0.5g \times 16.23 \text{ minim}}{1.08g}\right)$ fill volume of about 7.5 minims. Assuming, however, that there is 5% residual water in the dry capsule, the final fill volume would be about 8 minims $\left(\dfrac{.525g \times 16.23 \text{ minim}}{1.08g}\right)$

(liquid or solid) that reduces their effect on the shell. Examples of such solids are strong acids (citric), strong alkalies (sodium salts of weak acids), salts of strong acids and bases (sodium chloride, choline chloride), and ammonium salts. Also, any substance that is unstable in the presence of moisture (e.g., aspirin) would not exhibit satisfactory chemical stability in soft gelatin capsules.

The capsulation of *suspensions* is the basis for the existence of a large group of products. Again, the design of suspension type formulations and the choice of the suspending medium are directed toward producing the smallest size capsule having the characteristics previously described, i.e., maximum production capacity consistent with maximum physical and ingredient stability and therapeutic efficacy.

The formulation of suspensions for capsulation follows the basic concepts of suspension technology. Formulation techniques, however, can vary depending on the drug substance, the desired flow characteristics, the physical or ingredient stability problems, or the biopharmaceutical properties desired. In most instances, these techniques must be developed through the ingenuity of the formulating chemist; however, in the formulation of suspensions for soft gelatin encapsulation, certain basic information must be developed to determine minimum capsule size.

One laboratory tool for this purpose is known as the "base adsorption" of the solid(s) to be suspended. Base adsorption is expressed as the number of grams of liquid base required to produce a capsulatable mixture when mixed with one gram of solid(s). The base adsorption of a solid is influenced by such factors as the solid's particle size and shape, its physical state (fibrous, amorphous, or crystalline), its density, its moisture content, and its oleophilic or hydrophilic nature.

In the determination of base adsorption, the solid(s) must be completely wetted by the liquid base. For glycol and nonionic type bases, the addition of a *wetting agent* is seldom required, but for vegetable oil bases, complete wetting of the solid(s) is not achieved without an additive. Soy lecithin, at a concentration of 2 to 3% by weight of the oil, serves excellently for this purpose, and being a natural product, is universally accepted for food and drug use. Increasing the concentration above 3% appears to have no added advantage.

A practical procedure for determining base adsorption and for judging the adequate fluidity of a mixture is as follows. Weigh a definite amount (40 g is convenient) of the solid into a

150-ml tared beaker. In a separate 150-ml tared beaker, place about 100 g of the liquid base. Add small increments of the base to the solid, and using a spatula, stir the base into the solid after each addition until the solid is thoroughly wetted and uniformly coated with the base. This should produce a mixture that has a soft ointment-like consistency. Continue to add liquid and stir until the mixture flows steadily from the spatula blade when held at a 45-degree angle above the mixture. The flow is even and continuous, and not in "globs." Attention also should be given to the nature of the "cut-off" quality of the mixture. As the mixture tends to stop flowing, proper cut-off is exhibited when the stream contracts rapidly upward toward the spatula blade rather than "stringing out" in intermediate flow.

At the conclusion of the foregoing test, the base adsorption is obtained by means of the following formula:

$$\frac{\text{Weight of Base}}{\text{Weight of Solid}} = \text{Base Adsorption}$$

The base adsorption mixture is milled or homogenized, and deaerated (a desiccator under vacuum is suitable), and the specific gravity is taken. The specific gravity is the weight of mixture (W) per cubic centimeter or per 16.23 minims (V). As in the case of liquids and solutions, the specific gravity may be used to determine the die size required for a given quantity of the particular mixture.

The base adsorption is used to determine the "minim per gram" factor (M/g) of the solid(s). The minim per gram factor is the volume in minims that is occupied by one gram (S) of the solid plus the weight of liquid base (BA) required to make a capsulatable mixture. The minim per gram factor is calculated by dividing the weight of base plus the gram of solid (BA + S) by the weight of mixture (W) per cubic centimeter or 16.23 minims (V). A convenient formula is:

$$\frac{(\text{BA} + \text{S}) \times \text{V}}{\text{W}} = \text{M/g}$$

Thus, the lower the base adsorption of the solid(s) and the higher the density of the mixture, the smaller the capsule will be. This also indicates the importance of establishing specifications for the control of those physical properties of a solid mentioned previously that can affect its base adsorption.

The BA and M/g data need not be obtained on any material that is to be capsulated alone at concentrations of 50 mg or less, since the smallest capsules can accommodate such quantities. If such material is to be used in combination, however, the data become necessary to allow for its inclusion in the formulation. The convenience of using M/g factors is particularly evident in the vitamin field, where there may be many ingredients and numerous combinations. Since the minim per gram factors are additive, they can be used for a more rapid calculation of capsule size than can be given by the preparation of the many possible mixtures in the laboratory. See Table 13-4 for BA and M/g data on some typical solids.

The final formulation of a suspension invariably requires a *suspending agent* to prevent the settling of the solids and to maintain homogeneity prior to, during, and after capsulation. The nature and concentration of the suspending agent vary, depending on the job to be done. Also, a rather delicate balance must be achieved between the requirement for a stable suspension and the requirement for the mixture to have the proper flow characteristics. There is evidence, too, that the proper suspending agent coats the suspended solids, imparting a certain lubricity to them and thereby aiding capsulation. Also, the coating can prevent contact with possible incompatible components in the mixture. Of the examples shown in Table 13-5, the most widely used suspending agent for oily bases is wax mixture, and in nonoily bases, the polyethylene glycols 4000 and 6000.

In all instances, the suspending agent used is melted in a suitable portion of the liquid base, and the hot melt is added slowly, with stirring, into the bulk portion of the base, which has been preheated to 40°C prior to the addition of any solids. The solids are then added, one by one, with sufficient mixing between additions to ensure complete wetting. Incompatible solids are added as far apart as possible in the mixing order to prevent interaction prior to complete wetting by the base.

Additional aids to formulation involve the physical and ingredient stability of the capsules. There should be little concern with oxidation or the effects of light as a cause of ingredient instability, since the gelatin shell is an excellent oxygen barrier and may be opacified.[10,11]

Most ingredient stability problems are associated with the available moisture from the gelatin shell, which when absorbed into the capsule content, can cause areas of high concentration of water-soluble solids, leading to ionization and interaction of the solids. Such problems may be alleviated or eliminated by employing a less soluble salt (procaine penicillin instead of potas-

TABLE 13-4. *BA and M/g Factors of Some Typical Solids*

Ingredient	Base*	BA	M/g
Acetaminophen	Veg. oil	0.76	25.97
Acetaminophen	PEG 400	0.75	23.07
Ascorbic acid	Veg. oil	0.60	20.60
Ascorbic acid	Polysorbate 80	1.10	26.92
$Al(OH)_3$—$MgCO_3$ (FMA 11)	Veg. oil	1.90	41.30
$Al(OH)_3$—$MgCO_3$ (FMA 11)	PEG 400	2.44	42.10
Danthron	Veg. oil	1.30	33.75
Danthron	Glyceryl monooleate	1.39	33.94
Danthron	Polysorbate 80	1.38	31.28
Danthron	PEG 400	1.60	33.62
Danthron	Triacetin	1.83	36.02
Ephedrine SO_4	Veg. oil	1.30	36.80
Ferrous SO_4 exsiccated	Veg. oil	0.30	10.60
Ferrous SO_4 exsiccated	Polysorbate 80	0.47	12.90
Guaifenesin	Veg. oil	1.28	34.68
Lactose	Veg. oil	0.75	23.87
Desiccated liver	Veg. oil	0.80	25.70
Mephenesin	Veg. oil	2.50	57.38
Mephenesin	PEG 400	2.13	44.77
Meprobamate	Veg. oil	1.59	42.55
Meprobamate	PEG 400	1.30	32.52
Niacinamide	Veg. oil	0.80	25.63
Neomycin sulfate	Veg. oil	0.60	20.66
Phenobarbital	Veg. oil	1.20	33.60
Procaine penicillin G	Veg. oil	0.91	28.63
Sodium ascorbate	Veg. oil	0.76	22.40
Salicylamide	Veg. oil	0.80	25.80
Sulfathiazole	Veg. oil	0.43	17.90
Sulfanilamide	Veg. oil	1.03	28.55
Tetracycline (amphoteric)	Veg. oil	0.61	21.63

*Vegetable oil bases contain 3% soy lecithin.

sium), employing coatings (gelatin-coated B_{12}), adjusting pH with appropriate small quantities of citric, lactic, or tartaric acids or with less restrictive quantities of sodium ascorbate or magnesium oxide, or salting-out with appropriate small quantities of sodium chloride or sodium acetate.

Usually, the *physical stability* of a product is associated primarily with the type of gelatin and gelatin formulation used but can be aided by proper fill formulation. If a particular solid may have a deleterious action on the gelatin shell, the form of the solid that is least water-soluble and the most oleophilic would be the form of

TABLE 13-5. *Typical Suspending Agents*

Type	Concentration of Oily Base (%)	Type	Concentration of Nonoily Base (%)
White wax, NF	5	Polyethylene glycol 4000 and 6000	1–15
Paraffin wax, NF	5	Solid nonionics	10
Animal stearates	1–6	Solid glycol esters	10
Wax mixture*	10 and 30	Acetylated monoglycerides	5
Aluminum monosterate, NF†	3–5		
Ethocel (100 cps)†	5–10		

*1 part hydrogenated soybean oil; 1 part yellow wax, NF; 4 parts vegetable shortening (melting point 33 to 38°C); used at 10% on the adsorption oil and at 30% on any filler oil required.

†Used with volatile organic liquids such as butyl chloride; toluene; tetrachlorethylene; benzene.

choice for an oil-based suspension. An example would be the use of calcium salicylate rather than the sodium or magnesium salts. Also, the type of liquid base used can have an effect on physical stability. For example, the proteolytic effect of chloral hydrate on the gelatin shell is greatly reduced when a polyethylene glycol base is used in place of an oily base.

With the proper selection of materials and formulation techniques, the pharmaceutical chemist can prepare solutions or suspensions for comparisons of stability and dissolution rate with formulations of other solid dosage forms. By accurately filling two-piece gelatin capsules with such formulations, comparative absorption, urinary excretion, and metabolic studies can be made prior to the actual preparation of the soft gelatin capsule dosage form. Today the product development laboratory must evaluate all potential formulations for a new drug substance or for product improvement.

Capsule Manufacture, Processing, and Control

Although this aspect of soft gelatin capsules is the primary responsibility of the custom manufacturer, the pharmaceutical chemist should have an understanding of the materials and equipment involved in the capsule's manufacture, processing, and quality control. The several methods of capsulation referred to in the early part of this chapter, although differing somewhat in mechanical principles, do require the use of similar materials, processing steps, and equipment, and the use of equivalent control procedures.

Except for the gelatin preparation department, the manufacturing areas of a typical plant are air-conditioned to assure the proper conditioning of the gelatin films, the proper drying of the capsules, and the consistent low moisture content of raw materials and mixtures. The temperature is usually in the range of 20 to 22°C, and the humidity is controlled to a maximum of 40% in the operating areas and a range of 20 to 30% in the drying areas.

In the *gelatin preparation* department of a typical manufacturer, the gelatin is weighed on printomatic scales and mixed with the accurately metered (printomatic) and chilled (7°C) liquid constituents in suitable equipment, such as a Pony Mixer. The resultant fluffy mass is transferred to melting tanks and melted under vacuum (29.5″ Hg) at 93°C. The mixing process requires about 25 min for 270 kg of mass, and the melting procedure requires about 3 hours. A sample of the resulting fluid mass is visually compared with a color standard, and additional colorants are blended into the mass if adjustments are required. The mass is then maintained at a temperature of 57 to 60°C before and during the capsulation process.

The *materials preparation* department will have a weigh-off and mixing area containing the necessary equipment and facilities for the preparation of the variety of mixtures that may be capsulated. Typical equipment would include printomatic scales for exacting measurements and control records; stainless-steel jacketed tanks for handling from 10- to 450-gallon batches of mix; and mixers, such as the Cowles, for the initial blending of solids with the liquid base. After the initial blending is completed, the mixture is put through a *milling* or *homogenizing* process, using equipment such as the homoloid mill, stone mill, hopper mill, or the Urschel Comitrol. The purpose of the milling operation is not to reduce particle size, but to break up agglomerates of solids and to make certain that all solids are "wet" with the liquid carrier, so as to achieve a smooth and homogenous mixture.

Following the milling operation, all mixtures are subjected to *deaeration,* and particularly so if the capsulation machine is equipped with a positive displacement pump. Deaeration is necessary to achieve uniform capsule fill weights; it also protects against loss of potency through oxidation prior to and during capsulation. When small amounts of volatile ingredients are included in a formulation, they are carefully added and blended into the bulk mixture after deaeration. Most liquids and suspensions may be deaerated by means of equipment designed to expose thin layers of the material continuously to a vacuum (29.5″ Hg) and at the same time transfer the material from the mixing tank to the container that will be used at the capsulation machine. Suspensions or liquid mixtures containing volatile liquids or liquid surface active agents as chief constituents of the formula may be deaerated by subjection to temperatures up to 60°C for the period required to achieve the results desired. After deaeration, the mixture is ready to be capsulated.

At this point, samples of the mixture are often sent to the quality control laboratory for various tests, such as ingredient assays and specific gravity, and tests for homogeneity of suspension, moisture content, or air entrapment. This in-process quality control step may or may not be routine, depending on the product or anticipated problems, but should always occur with new products until the process is validated.

Owing to space limitations, a detailed description of each capsulation process is not possible. A schematic drawing of the rotary die process is presented, however, to acquaint the pharmaceutical chemist with the fundamental aspects of capsulation (Fig. 13-27). The gelatin mass is fed by gravity to a metering device (spreader box), which controls the flow of the mass onto air-cooled (13 to 14°C) rotating drums. Gelatin ribbons of controlled (±10%) thickness are formed. The wet shell thickness may vary from 0.022 to 0.045 inch, but for most capsules, it is between 0.025 and 0.032 inch. Thicker shells are used on products requiring greater structural strength. Product cost is directly proportional to shell thickness. The ribbons are fed through a mineral oil lubricating bath, over guide rolls, and then down between the wedge and the die rolls.

The material to be capsulated flows by gravity into a positive displacement pump. The pump accurately meters the material through the leads and wedge and into the gelatin ribbons between the die rolls. The bottom of the wedge contains small orifices lined up with the die pockets of the die rolls. The capsule is about half sealed when the pressure of the pumped material forces the gelatin into the die pockets, where the capsules are simultaneously filled, shaped, hermetically sealed, and cut from the gelatin ribbon. The sealing of the capsule is achieved by

mechanical pressure on the die rolls and the heating (37 to 40°C) of the ribbons by the wedge.

During manufacture, capsule samples are taken periodically for seal thickness and fill weight checks. The seals are measured under a microscope, and changes in ribbon thickness, heat, or die pressure are made if necessary. Acceptable seal thickness is one half to two thirds of the ribbon thickness. Fill weight checks are made by weighing the whole fresh capsule, slitting it open, and expressing the contents. The shell is then washed in a suitable solvent (petroleum ether), and the empty shell is reweighed. If necessary, adjustments in the pump stroke can be made to obtain the proper fill weight.

Immediately after manufacture, the capsules are automatically conveyed through a naphtha wash unit to remove the mineral oil lubricant. The washed capsules may be automatically subjected to a preliminary infrared drying step, which removes 60 to 70% of the water that is to be lost, or may be manually spread directly on trays. Capsules from the infrared dryer are also spread on trays, and all capsules are allowed to come to equilibrium with forced air conditions of 20 to 30% relative humidity at 21 to 24°C.

Capsules at equilibrium with 20 to 30% RH at 21 to 24°C are considered "dry," and the shell of such a capsule contains 6 to 10% water, depending on the gelatin formula used. The moisture content of the shell is determined by the toluene distillation method, collecting the distillate over a period of one hour. Additional water may be removed from "dry" capsules by further heating, e.g., at 40°C, but such a manufacturing step has not been found to be practical or necessary.

After drying, the capsules are transferred to the inspection department and held until released by the quality control department. The *inspection and quality control* steps in the processing of capsules are much the same as with other dosage forms and must conform to good manufacturing practice. Control tests specifically applicable to the quality of soft gelatin capsules may involve seal thickness determinations, total or shell moisture tests, capsule fragility or rupture tests, and the determination of freezing and high temperature effects.

Also, capsules may be sent after drying to a finishing department for heat branding or ink printing for purposes of identification.

Final physical control processing and packaging may be accomplished by the following in-line continuous operations.

1. A capsule diameter sorter allows to pass to the next unit any capsule within ±0.020 inch of the theoretic diameter of the particular capsule being tested. Overfills, underfills, and "foreign"

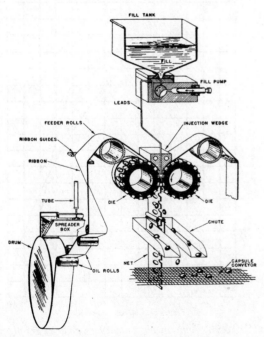

FIG. 13-27. *Schematic drawing of rotary die process. (Courtesy of R.P. Scherer Corporation, Troy, MI.)*

capsules are discarded. The unit is fed from a hopper, and the capsules are passed through a final naphtha washing unit just prior to the sorter. The unit employs a syntron vibrator, which is a series of divergent wire lanes, and can be used for capsule diameters ranging from 0.200 to 0.500 inch.

2. A capsule color sorter is the next unit in line. The capsules are fed to it automatically from the diameter sorter by a pneumatic conveyor. In this unit, any capsule whose color does not conform to the reference color standard for that particular product is discarded, while satisfactory capsules pass immediately to an electronic counting and packaging unit.

3. The electronic counting unit can count as many as 8,000 capsules per minute (depending upon size) directly into the bulk shipping carton. A printout of the content of each carton and a printout of the number of cartons are automatically produced and made a part of the production record. Following this step, the cartons are labeled, sealed, and palletized and are then ready for shipment.

Capsule Physical Stability and Packaging

Unprotected soft gelatin capsules (i.e., capsules that can breathe) rapidly reach equilibrium with the atmospheric conditions under which they are stored. This inherent characteristic warrants a brief discussion of the effects of temperature and humidity on these products, and points to the necessity of proper storage and packaging conditions and to the necessity of choosing an appropriate retail package. The variety of materials capsulated, which may have an effect on the gelatin shell, together with the many gelatin formulations that can be used, makes it imperative that physical standards are established for each product.

General statements relative to the effects of temperature and humidity on soft gelatin capsules must be confined to a control capsule that contains mineral oil, with a gelatin shell having a dry glycerin to dry gelatin ratio of about 0.5 to 1 and a water to dry gelatin ratio of 1 to 1, and that is dried to equilibrium with 20 to 30% RH at 21 to 24°C. The physical stability of soft gelatin capsules is associated primarily with the pick-up or loss of water by the capsule shell. If these are prevented by proper packaging, the above control capsule should have satisfactory physical stability at temperatures ranging from just above freezing to as high as 60°C.

For the unprotected control capsule, low humidities (<20% RH), low temperatures (<2°C) and high temperatures (>38°C) or combinations of these conditions have only transient effects. The capsule returns to normal when returned to optimum storage conditions. The transient effects are primarily brittleness and greater susceptibility to shock, requiring greater care in handling or a return to proper storage conditions prior to further handling.

As the humidity is increased, within a reasonable temperature range, the shell of the unprotected control capsule should pick up moisture in proportion to its glycerin and gelatin content in accordance with the curves shown in Figure 13-28. The total moisture content of the capsule shell, at equilibrium with any given relative humidity within a reasonable temperature range, should closely approximate the sum of the moisture content of the glycerin and the gelatin when held separately at the stated conditions. For example, the shell of the described control capsule contains 400 mg of dry gelatin and 200 mg of dry glycerin per gram. At equilibrium with 30% RH at room temperature (21 to 24°C), the curves show that the gelatin should retain about 12% (48 mg) of water, and the glycerin 7% (14 mg) of water. Thus, the "dry" shell

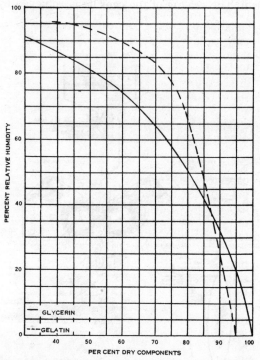

FIG. 13-28. *Equilibrium content by weight of dry glycerin (20 to 100°C) and dry gelatin (25°C) at various relative humidities.*[12,13]

would contain about 9.4% water (62 mg HgO/662 mg of shell).

If the conditions are changed to 60% RH (21 to 24°C), the moisture content should be approximately 17.4%. In actual practice, however, such calculated moistures are considered maximum, since moisture assays (toluene distillation method) of the shells of oil-filled capsules give results somewhat lower than the theoretical values. The deviation most likely is due to an interaction between the plasticizer and gelatin, partially satisfying their respective water-binding capacities and thereby causing a lower moisture content than would be theoretically expected. Nevertheless, the curves serve to illustrate the hygroscopic nature of capsule shells, the relative effect of changes in the glycerin to gelatin ratio on the hygroscopicity of the shell, and the potential effects of humidity on the chemical and physical stability of the product.

High humidities (>60% RH at 21 to 24°C) produce more lasting effects on the capsule shell, since as moisture is absorbed, the capsules become softer, tackier, and bloated. The capsules do not leak unless the increased moisture has allowed a deleterious ingredient in the capsule content to attack the gelatin. On return to optimum storage conditions, the capsules are dull in appearance and most likely inseparably stuck together. An increase in temperature (>24°C), together with humidity (>45%), results in more rapid and pronounced effects and may even cause the unprotected capsules to melt and fuse together. Capsules containing water-soluble or miscible liquid bases may be affected to a greater extent than oil-based capsules, owing to the residual moisture in the capsule content and to the dynamic relationship existing between capsule shell and capsule fill during the drying process.

The capsule manufacturer routinely conducts accelerated physical stability tests on all new capsule products as an integral part of the product development program. The following tests have proved adequate for determining the effect of the capsule content on the gelatin shell. The tests are strictly relevant to the integrity of the gelatin shell and should not be construed as stability tests for the active ingredients in the capsule content. The results of suc tests are used as a guide for the reformulation of the capsule content or the capsule shell, or for the selection of the proper retail package. The test conditions are (1) 80% RH at room temperature in an open container; (2) 40°C in an open container; (3) 40°C in a closed container (glass bottle with tight screw-cap). The capsules at these stations are observed periodically for 2 weeks. Both gross and subtle effects of the storage conditions on the capsule shell are noted and recorded. The control capsule should not be affected except at the 80% RH station, where the capsule would react as described under the effects of high humidity.

In the case of a newly developed product, the gross effects such as disintegration, leakers, unusual brittleness or softening, apparent color fading, or discoloration are obvious. The more subtle changes may be the loss of a volatile ingredient as detected by slight capsule indentation, or the slight darkening or widening of the capsule seams, or slight changes in color hue. Capsules often show a "soft spot" at the site at which they lie next to the tray or against another capsule. This spot is the result of slower drying and is of no consequence in the control capsule, since such areas firm up and are not flaws in the capsule shell. On the other hand, if such areas do not become firm, usually because of action by the capsule content, then physical stability problems can be anticipated during the shelf-life of the product. Such defects must be corrected before the product can be considered for production. Correction of such defects depends upon identifying their cause. Most defects can be corrected by appropriate changes in gelatin or fill material formulations, but in some cases, different colorants, machine speeds, and machine dies may have to be used. The experience and mature judgment of the custom manufacturer is invaluable in the solution of such problems.

Chemists conducting the physical stability tests in their own laboratories should keep two important points in mind: (1) Prior to testing, the capsules should be equilibrated to known atmospheric conditions, preferably 20 to 30% RH at 21 to 24°C. (2) Evaluation of the results of the previously described heat tests should be made only after the capsules have returned to equilibrium with room temperature.

After the capsules have passed the shell integrity tests, additional physical studies should be conducted using the various types of retail packages being considered for the product. These latter tests should be designed to determine the shelf-life of the product and may conform to most of the standard testing procedures employed by a company for its other solid dosage forms. Exceptions may involve those tests conducted at temperatures exceeding 45°C for time periods exceeding a month.

The soft gelatin capsule manufacturer takes great care in the production of capsules to meet the specifications of the product set forth by the customer. When *bulk shipments* of capsules are made by the manufacturer, they are temporarily protected from normal changes in humidity by a suitable moisture barrier such as a 0.003-inch polyethylene bag within a standard fiber board carton. Since such packaging is not a permanent moisture barrier, the capsules should be retail packaged as soon as possible after receipt. If immediate packaging is not practical, the bulk capsules in their original unopened cartons should be stored in an air-conditioned area in which the humidity does not exceed 45% RH at 21 to 24°C. The retail packaging of these capsules should be done under similar conditions, for the maximum physical and chemical stability of the product.

Soft gelatin capsules may be *retail packaged* using any modern packaging equipment, including the electronic type. Capsules may be packaged in glass or plastic containers or may be strip-packaged, so long as such packaging involves tight closures and plastics having a low moisture vapor transfer rate. Suppliers of rigid plastics and plastic films can be of immeasurable service in suggesting the proper types of packaging for testing. Since strip packaging usually is done by specialists in this field, their advice should be solicited, and test strips should be made and tested for adequacy.

Pharmaceutical Aspects

The pharmaceutical chemist should be cognizant of the inherent properties of soft gelatin capsules. Essentially, these capsules are solid dosage forms containing liquid medication and therefore offer certain advantages:

1. They permit liquid medications to become easily portable.

2. Accuracy and uniformity of dosage, capsule to capsule and lot to lot, are predominant advantages. These capsules easily pass the appropriate compendial tests and surpass other solid dosage forms in this respect, because liquid formulations can be more accurately and precisely compounded, blended, homogenized, and measured or dispensed than can dry solid formulations.

3. The pharmaceutical availability of drugs formulated for this dosage form, as measured by disintegration time,[14] or by dissolution rate,[15,16] often shows an advantage over other solid dosage formulations.

In the dissolution rate studies of twenty drugs, presented previously, which included a wide variety of chemical types and pharmacologic classes, the authors showed that in the majority of cases, the drugs were more rapidly and completely available from the soft gelatin capsule than from the commercial tablets or capsules.

For these studies, the NF XII (second supplement, 1967) rotating-bottle method was used.

A rationale for using a rotating-bottle method for dissolution studies on soft gelatin capsules is expressed, and examples are given by Withey and Mainville.[17] Their dissolution studies on thirteen brands of commercial chloramphenicol capsules, using their modified USP apparatus, showed the soft gelatin capsule brand to release only 22.3 to 24.8% of its chloramphenicol content in 30 min, while hard-shell capsule brands B_2 and D released 100.7% and 87.2% respectively. Upon change to a rotating-bottle method, the 30-min recoveries were 100% from the soft gelatin capsule brand, 82% from brand B_2, and 70% from brand D. None of these studies have been correlated with bioavailability data, and thus, the significance of the difference in results between the two dissolution methods is not clear. The difference could be attributed to greater agitation by the bottle method and less opportunity for the capsule to adhere to the sides or bottom of the apparatus. The effect of several variables on capsule dissolution is discussed by Hom and associates,[8] who indicate that the degree of agitation, the pH of the dissolution medium, and the presence or absence of pepsin in the medium are important to the dissolution of soft gelatin capsules.

4. The physiologic availability of drugs is often improved since these capsules contain the drug in liquid form, i.e., as a liquid drug substance, drug in solution, or drug in suspension. Nelson, in his review,[18] points out that the availability of a drug for absorption, from various types of oral formulations, usually decreases in the following order: solution, suspension, powder-filled capsule, compressed tablet, coated tablet. A study by Wagner and co-workers seems to confirm both Nelson's observation and the effective absorption from soft gelatin capsules.[19] Their study involved the effect of dosage form on the serum levels of indoxole (solubility in water 0.1 $\mu g/ml$) and showed the serum level decreased in the following order: emulsion $\simeq$ soft gelatin capsule (drug in polysorbate 80 solution), aqueous suspension, powder-filled capsule.

Maconachie, in his review article on soft gelatin capsules,[20] gives some specific examples of how this dosage form can improve drug absorption. His examples involve acetaminophen,[1] chlormethiazole,[21] and temazepam.[22] The 4-hour urinary recovery of acetaminophen from three soft gelatin rectal suppository formulations (oil base and water-miscible type base) was found to be five to eight times greater than from the traditional fatty type suppository formulation. The switch from a tablet to a soft gelatin capsule form not only improved the stability of chlormethiazole by protecting the drug from oxidation, but increased its bioavailability as evidenced by comparative blood levels and by earlier onset of a minor side effect (nose tingling). Major side effects of the tablet dosage form were also eliminated or ameliorated. The capsule formulation allowed the use of the liquid drug substance (chlormethiazole base) rather than the solid derivatives used in the tablet formulations. A temazepam soft gelatin formulation, when compared with hard gelatin capsule formulations of temazepam, nitrazepam, amobarbital sodium, and a placebo, gave superior bioavailability as indicated by "onset of sleep." Furthermore, this was achieved at a lower dosage (20 mg per soft capsules versus 30 mg per hard capsule).

In an article on soft gelatin capsules,[23] Ebert discusses and reports on the bioavailability and content uniformity of digoxin solutions in soft gelatin capsules. The capsulated solutions were 0.05 mg, 0.10mg and 0.20 mg of digoxin dissolved in a base consisting of polyethylene glycol 400, USP (89.4% w/w); alcohol, USP (6.5% w/w); propylene glycol, USP (3.4% w/w); and purified water, USP (0.6% w/w). These capsules were tested by various investigators for bioavailability in comparison with brand name tablets, digoxin solution, and digoxin elixir.[24,31] In all studies, the bioavailability of the soft gelatin capsule formulation was found to be superior to the commercially available tablets. The most surprising finding of all these studies, according to Ebert, was that the capsulated solution exhibited a more rapid and complete absorption than did the same solution not encapsulated. The commercially available tablets contain 20% more drug than the capsulated solutions. Thus, the capsule dosage form allows for a significant reduction in dose for this relatively toxic drug.

Another comparative bioavailability study of digoxin soft gelatin capsules and tablets was reported by Astorri and co-workers.[32] They found that in heart patients using digoxin, the absorption of digoxin from the capsulated solution was 36% higher than from the tablet, while in healthy volunteers absorption from the capsule was 20% higher than from the tablets.

The bioavailability of theophylline from soft gelatin capsules in comparison to a commercially available liquid aminophylline preparation and to a nonalcoholic ammophylhne solution was studied by Ebert,[33] and by Lesko and co-workers.[34] Both studies found that the two dosage forms were bioequivalent as measured by the area under the plasma-level-time curves.

This is an example of the capsule providing a convenient portable dosage form for a liquid medication. The capsule also effectively masked the bitter taste of theophylline.

Papaverine hydrochloride bioavailability from soft gelatin capsules was studied by Arnold et al.[35] These authors found that the peak blood level and area under the blood-level-time curve from soft gelatin capsules were equal to those obtained from an elixir and superior to those from a sustained release hard-shell capsule formulation. Healthy volunteers were used in this study. Lee et al. found not only high blood levels of papaverine 120 min after a 150-mg dose in soft gelatin capsules, but a higher degree of vasodilation after four doses (150 mg × 4) of the soft capsule dosage form when compared with equivalent doses from a sustained-release dosage form.[36] Patients with severe arteriosclerosis obliterans were used in the study. Both studies conclude that the soft gelatin capsule dosage form shows significant advantage over the sustained release tablet form of the drug.

The bioavailability of diazepam (structurally similar to that of temazepam, mentioned previously) was studied by Yamahira et al.[37] They compared diazepam, capsulated in soft gelatin using a medium-chain triglyceride base, with a tablet dosage form. They report that when these dosage forms were repeatedly orally administered to an individual subject, the capsule dosage form showed a tendency toward faster drug absorption and superior reproducibility of the plasma-level-time curve than the tablet dosage form. This suggests that capsule dosage forms have a more uniform drug absorption rate than tablets. The authors suggest that diazepam, though it is a weak base, was emptied from the stomach while mostly retained in the lipid, and this was affected by the movement of the triglyceride in the gastrointestinal tract.

5. The pharmaceutical chemist should certainly consider the bioavailability potential of soft gelatin formulations. The biopharmaceutical characteristics of such formulations can be altered or adjusted more easily than those of other solid dosage forms. Through the selection and use of liquids and combinations of liquids that range from water-immiscible through emulsifiable to completely water-miscible, and by altering the type or quantity of thickening or suspending agents, capsule formulations allow the formulating chemist more flexibility in the design of a dosage form to fit the biopharmaceutical specifications of a particular therapeutic agent.

6. Orally administered drugs, particularly if used chronically, can be irritating to the stom-

ach. The dosage form of such drugs can affect gastric tolerance, as indicated by the studies of Caldwell et al.[38] These authors compared the degree of irritation or ulcerogenic potential of soft gelatin capsule formulations of dexamethasone with a tablet formulation of the drug. Several liquid formulations and tablet formulations were administered to rats, and both ulcerogenic potential and bioavailability were determined. The authors concluded that the liquid or capsule formulations had a reduced ulcerogenic potential when compared to the tablet formulation, and that this effect is apparently not a reflection of reduced bioavailability.

References

1. Widmann, A.: Drugs Made in Germany, 3:167, 1960.
2. Gutches, M.: Capsule Technology and Microencapsulation. Noyes Data Corp., Park Ridge, NJ, 1972.
3. Idson, B., and Braswell, E.: Advances in Food Research. Vol. VII. Academic Press, New York, 1957, p. 235.
4. Gelatin. Gelatin Manufacturer's Institute of America, New York, 1962.
5. Traub, W., and Piez, K.: Advances in Protein Chemistry. Chemistry and Structure of Collagen. Vol. 25. Academic Press, New York, 1971.
6. Ramachandvan, G. N.: Treatise on Collagen. Chemistry of Collagen. Vol. 1. Academic Press, New York, 1967.
7. Stanley, J. P., and Bradley, C. W.: U.S. Patent 2,870,062, January 20, 1959.
8. Hom, F. S., Veresh, S. A., and Miskel, J. J.: J. Pharm. Sci., 62:1001, 1973.
9. Handbook of Chemistry and Physics. 44th Ed. Chemical Rubber Publishing Co., Cleveland, OH, 1963.
10. Lieberman, E. R., Gilbert, S. G., and Srinvasa, V.: Trans. N.Y. Acad. Sci., 34:694, 1972.
11. Hom. F. A., Veresh, S. A., and Ebert, W. R.: J. Pharm. Sci., 64:851, 1975.
12. Miner, C. A., and Dalton, N. N.: Glycerol. ACS Monograph Series No. 117. Reinhold, New York, 1953, p. 269.
13. Bull, H. B.: J. Am. Chem. Soc., 66:1949, 1944.
14. Eckert, V. T., Widmann, A., and Seidel, R.: Arz. neim-Forsch, 19:821, 1969.
15. Hom, F. S., and Miskel, J. J.: J. Pharm. Sci., 59:827, 1970.
16. Hom, F. S., and Miskel, J. J.: Lex Et. Scienta, 8:18, 1971.
17. Withey, R. J., and Mainville, C. A.: J. Pharm. Sci., 58:1120, 1969.
18. Nelson, E.: Clin. Pharmacol. Ther., 3:673, 1962.
19. Wagner, J. G., Gerard, E. S., and Kaiser, D. G.: 7:610, 1966.
20. Maconachie, S.: Mfg. Chemist and Aerosol News, Aug. 1977, p. 35.
21. Frisch, E. P., and Ortengren, B.: Acta Psych. Scand., 42(Suppl.):35, 1969.
22. Hindmarch, I.: Arzneimittel-Forsch., 25:1836, 1975.
23. Ebert, W. R.: Pharm. Tech., 1:44, 1977.
24. Binnion, P. F., and Klopp, R. W.: Lancet, 1:1422, 1975.
25. Mallis, G. I., Schmidt, D. H., and Lindenbaum, J.: Clin. Pharmacol. Ther., 18:761, 1975.
26. Marcus, F. I., Dickerson, J., Pippin, S., et al.: Clin. Pharmacol. Ther., 20:253, 1976.
27. Binnion, P. F.: J. Clin. Pharmacol., 16:461, 1976.
28. Johnson, B. J., Bye, C., Jones, G., and Sabey, G. A.: Clin. Pharmacol. Ther., 19:746, 1976.
29. Ghirardi, P., Catenazzo, G., Mantero, O., et al.: J. Pharm. Sci., 66:267, 1977.
30. Lindenbaum, J.: Clin. Pharmacol. Ther., 21:278, 1977.
31. Johnson, B. F., Smith, G., and French. J.: Br. J. Clin. Pharmacol., 4:209, 1977.
32. Astorri, E., Bianchi, G., La Canna, G., et al.: J. Pharm. Sci., 68:104, 1979.
33. Ebert, W. R.: Pharm. Tech., 3:61, 1979.
34. Lesko, L. J., Canada, A. T., Eastwood, G., et al.: J. Pharm. Sci., 68:1392, 1979.
35. Arnold, J. D., Baldridge, J., Riley, B., and Brody, G.: J. Clin. Pharmacol., 15:230, 1977.
36. Lee, B. Y., Sakamoto, H., Trainor, F., et al.: J. Clin. Pharmacol., 16:32, 1978.
37. Yamahira, Y., Noguchi, T., Takenaka, H., and Maeda, T.: Chem. Pharm. Bull., 27:1190, 1979.
38. Caldwell, L., Cargill, R., Ebert, W. R., and Windheuser, J. J.: Pharm. Tech., 3:52, 1979.

PART THREE

Microencapsulation

J. A. BAKAN

Microencapsulation is a rapidly expanding technology. As a process, it is a means of applying relatively thin coatings to small particles of solids or droplets of liquids and dispersions. For the purpose of this chapter, microencapsulation is arbitrarily differentiated from macrocoating techniques in that the former involves the coating of particles ranging dimensionally from several tenths of a micron to 5000 microns in size.

As the technology has developed, it has become apparent that the concept offers the industrial pharmacist a new working tool. Microencapsulation provides the means of converting liquids to solids, of altering colloidal and surface properties, of providing environmental protection, and of controlling the release characteristics or availability of coated materials. Several of these properties can be attained by macropackaging techniques; however, the uniqueness of microencapsulation is the smallness of the coated particles and their subsequent use and adaptation to a wide variety of dosage forms and product applications, which heretofore might not have been technically feasible. Because of the smallness of the particles, drug moieties can be widely distributed throughout the gastrointestinal tract, thus potentially improving drug sorption. Figure 13-29 shows microencapsulated barium sulfate being released from a dissolving gelatin capsule shortly after ingestion.[1] Figure 13-30 shows the microcapsules distributed throughout the intestines.[1]

The applications of microencapsulation might well include sustained-release or prolonged-action medications, taste-masked chewable tablets, powders and suspensions, single-layer tablets containing chemically incompatible ingredients, and new formulation concepts for creams, ointments, aerosols, dressings, plasters, suppositories, and injectables. Pharmaceutically related areas, such as hygiene, diagnostic aids, and medical equipment design, also are amenable to microencapsulation applications.

This new technology does not exclude problem areas; for instance, no single microencapsulation process is adaptable to all core material candidates or product applications. Dif-

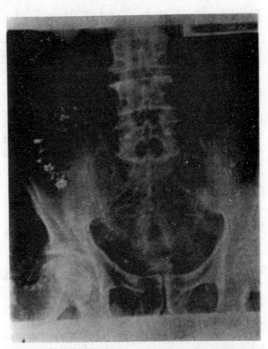

FIG. 13-30. *After a few hours, the same microencapsulated barium sulfate pellets as in Fig. 13-29 broadly distributed throughout intestines. (From Galeone, M., et al.: Current Therapeutic Research, 31:456, 1982.*

ficulties, such as incomplete or discontinuous coating, inadequate stability or shelf-life of sensitive pharmaceuticals, nonreproducible and unstable release characteristics of coated products, and economic limitations often are encountered in the attempt to apply a particular microencapsulation method to a specific task. Many times, successful adaptation is, in part, a result of the technical ingenuity of the investigators.

Microencapsulation is receiving considerable attention fundamentally, developmentally, and commercially. In view of this interest, it is the purpose of this chapter to present a description of the more prominent microencapsulation methods and some of their capabilities and limitations. The microencapsulation methods to be discussed are air suspension, coacervation-phase separation, spray drying and congealing, and polymerization techniques. A survey of the ever-expanding patent and published literature reveals that not all microencapsulation techniques are included within the methods cited in this chapter; however, the methods described represent the currently established, most highly developed and widely used commercial processes, although some may not be applicable to pharmaceuticals at this time.

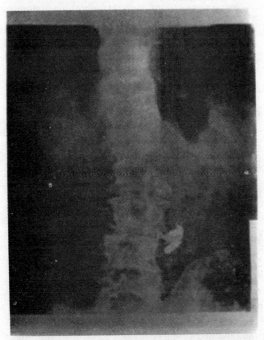

FIG. 13-29. *Microencapsulated barium sulfate releasing from hard gelatin capsules a few minutes after ingestion. (From Galeone, M., et al.: Current Therapeutic Research, 31:456, 1982.)*

Fundamental Considerations

The realization of the potential that microencapsulation offers involves a basic understanding of the general properties of microcapsules, such as the nature of the core and coating materials, the stability and release characteristics of the coated materials, and the microencapsulation methods. One should note, however, that the method employed in the manufacture of microcapsules may well result in products of varied composition, quality, and utility.

Core Material

The *core material*, defined as the specific material to be coated, can be liquid or solid in nature. The composition of the core material can be varied, as the liquid core can include dispersed and/or dissolved material. The solid core can be a mixture of active constituents, stabilizers, diluents, excipients, and release-rate retardants or accelerators. The ability to vary the core material composition provides definite flexibility and utilization of this characteristic often allows effectual design and development of the desired microcapsule properties.

It is not possible to discuss, or even list, all of the potential core materials and product applications that are or may be amenable to microencapsulation. However, to aid in illustrating the diversity of the materials and their applications, some of these products are listed in Table 13-6.

TABLE 13-6. *Properties of Some Microencapsulated Core Materials*

Core Material	Characteristic Property	Purpose of Encapsulation	Final Product Form
Acetaminophen	Slightly water-soluble solid	Taste-masking	Tablet
Activated charcoal	Adsorbent	Selective sorption	Dry powder
Aspirin	Slightly water-soluble solid	Taste-masking; sustained release; reduced gastric irritation; separation of incompatibles	Tablet or capsule
Islet of Langerhans	Viable cells	Sustained normalization of diabetic condition	Injectable
Isosorbide dinitrate	Water-soluble solid	Sustained release	Capsule
Liquid crystals	Liquid	Conversion of liquid to solid; stabilization	Flexible film for thermal mapping of anatomy
Menthol/methyl salicylate camphor mixture	Volatile solution	Reduction of volatility; sustained release	Lotion
Progesterone	Slightly water-soluble solid	Sustained release	Varied
Potassium chloride	Highly water-soluble solid	Reduced gastric irritation	Capsule
Urease	Water-soluble enzyme	Permselectivity of enzyme, substrate, and reaction products	Dispersion
Vitamin A palmitate	Nonvolatile liquid	Stabilization to oxidation	Dry powder

Coating Materials

The selection of a specific coating material from a lengthy list of candidate materials presents the following questions to be considered by the research pharmacist.

1. What are the specific dosage or product requirements—stabilization, reduced volatility, release characteristics, environmental conditions, etc?

2. What coating material will satisfy the product objectives and requirements?

3. What microencapsulation method is best suited to accomplish the coated product objectives?

The selection of the appropriate coating material dictates, to a major degree, the resultant physical and chemical properties of the microcapsules, and consequently, this selection must be given due consideration. The coating material should be capable of forming a film that is cohesive with the core material; be chemically compatible and nonreactive with the core material; and provide the desired coating properties, such as strength, flexibility, impermeability, optical properties, and stability. The coating materials used in microencapsulation methods are amenable, to some extent, to in situ modification. For example, colorants may be added to achieve product elegance or masking, or coatings may be plasticized or chemically altered through cross-linking, for instance, to achieve controlled dissolution or permeability. A partial listing of typical coating materials commonly used in the various microencapsulation methods is suggested in Table 13-7.

It is not within the scope of this discussion to describe the physical and chemical properties of coatings per se. It is pointed out, however, that typical coating properties such as cohesiveness, permeability, moisture sorption, solubility, stability, and clarity must be considered in the selection of the proper microcapsule coating material. The selection of a given coating often can be aided by the review of existing literature and by the study of free or cast films, although practical use of free-film information often is impeded for the following reasons.

1. Cast or free films prepared by the usual casting techniques yield films that are considerably thicker than those produced by the microencapsulation of small particles; hence, the results obtained from the cast films may not be extrapolatable to the thin microcapsule coatings.

2. The particular microencapsulation method employed for the deposition of a given coating produces specific and inherent properties that are difficult to simulate with existing film-casting methods.

3. The coating substrate or core material may have a decisive effect on coating material properties.

Hence, the selection of a particular coating material involves consideration of both classic free-film data and applied results.

As previously stated, the uniqueness of microcapsules in their properties and use involves their characteristic smallness. Consequently, the protective coatings that are applied are quite thin. Although the active content of many microencapsulated products can be varied from a few percent to over 99%, the effective coating thickness that can be realized, regardless of the method of application employed, varies from tenths of a micron to a few hundred microns, depending on the coating-to-core ratio and the particle size (surface area) of the core material. Figure 13-31 illustrates the theoretic film thickness that can be applied to small spherical particles.[2] The thinness of microencapsulation coatings, although not necessarily limiting, must be of prime consideration. Just as the smallness of microcapsules allows unique properties and formulations to be accomplished, the thinness of the resultant coatings also can present unique

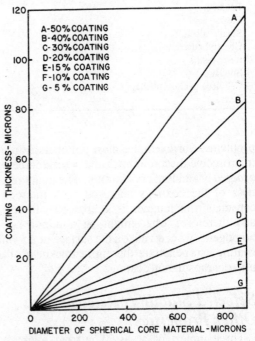

FIG. 13-31. *Theoretic coating thickness for spherical core material having various amounts of coating. (From Herbig.[2] Courtesy John Wiley and Sons.)*

TABLE 13-7. *Representative Coating Materials and Applicable Microencapsulation Process*

Coating Materials	Multiorifice—Centrifugal	Phase Separation—Coacervation	Pan Coating	Spray Drying and Congealing	Air Suspension	Solvent Evaporation
Water-soluble resins						
Gelatin	X	X	X	X	X	X
Gum arabic		X	X	X	X	X
Starch		X	X	X	X	
Polyvinylpyrrolidone	X	X	X	X	X	
Carboxymethylcellulose		X	X	X	X	
Hydroxyethylcellulose		X	X	X	X	
Methylcellulose		X	X	X	X	X
Arabinogalactan		X	X	X	X	
Polyvinyl alcohol	X	X	X	X	X	
Polyacrylic acid	X	X	X	X	X	X
Water-insoluble resins						
Ethylcellulose		X	X	X	X	X
Polyethylene	X				X	X
Polymethacrylate		X	X	X	X	X
Polyamide (Nylon)					X	X
Poly [Ethylene-Vinyl acetate]	X	X	X	X		X
Cellulose nitrate	X	X	X	X		X
Silicones			X	X		
Poly (lactide-co-glycolide)		X	X			X
Waxes and lipids						
Paraffin	X	X	X	X	X	
Carnauba			X	X	X	
Spermaceti		X	X	X	X	
Beeswax			X	X	X	
Stearic acid			X	X		
Stearyl alcohol			X	X	X	
Glyceryl stearates			X	X	X	
Enteric resins						
Shellac		X	X	X	X	
Cellulose acetate phthalate		X	X	X	X	X
Zein		X			X	

problems. For example, most polymers exhibit microscopic discontinuities and some degree of ordered or random crystalltnity. The total thickness of the coatings achieved with microencapsulation techniques is microscopic in size, and therefore, what might be a minor non-homogeneity occurring on the surface of a 5-mil coating can penetrate the entire thickness of a microencapsulation coating.

Selected Stability, Release, and Other Properties

Three important areas of current microencapsulation application are the stabilization of core materials, the control of the release or availability of core materials, and separation of chemically reactive ingredients within a tablet or powder mixture.

The following examples illustrate the concept of improved stabilization. Microencapsulation of certain vitamins to retard degradative losses has been practiced for many years. The potency retention properties of a microencapsulated vitamin A palmitate oil are illustrated in Figure 13-32.[3] The conversion of volatile liquids to dry, free-flowing powders with subsequent retention of the liquid core material during extended storage is another example of stabilization. Figure 13-33 depicts typical microcapsule stabilities of an anthelmintic (carbon tetrachloride), methyl sahcylate, and a flavor.[4] An example of stability enhancement, accomplished by microen-

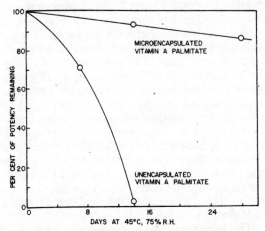

FIG. 13-32. *Stability of a microencapsulated vitamin A palmitate corn oil prepared by phase-separation/coacervation technique, compared with an unencapsulated control. (From Bakan.[3])*

capsulation of incompatible admixed constituents, is given in Figure 13-34. Compared in the graph is the formation of the aspirin hydrolysis product, salicylic acid, occurring with a mixture of aspirin and chlorpheniramine maleate.[3]

The release properties of microencapsulated materials require detailed consideration, as the

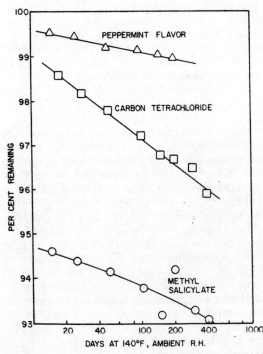

FIG. 13-33. *Stability of microencapsulated volatile liquids, prepared, by phase-separation/coacervation techniques. (From The NCR Corporation.[4])*

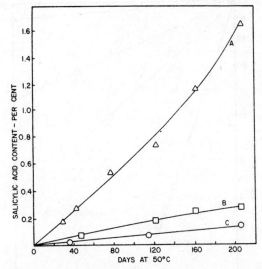

FIG. 13-34. *Stability enhancement of incompatible aspirin mixture by microencapsulation. A, Aspirin hydrolysis of chlorpheniramine maleate-aspirin mixture; B, aspirin hydrolysis of microencapsulated mixture; and C, hydrolysis of aspirin control. (From Bakan.[3])*

coated material must be released in a predictable and reproducible manner. A wide variety of mechanisms is available to release encapsulated core materials. Disruption of the coating can occur by pressure, shear, or abrasion forces, any of which affords a release mechanism. Other mechanisms involve permeability changes brought about enzymatically. Also, release can be achieved from inert coatings by diffusion or leaching of a permeant fluid. The rate of release is a function of the permeability of the coating to the extraction fluid; the permselectivity, if any, of the coating to core material solute; the dissolution rate of the core material; the coating thickness; and the concentration gradient existing across the coating membrane.

Prolonged-action or sustained-release formulations are obvious examples of controlled release from microencapsulated products, and Figures 13-35 and 13-36 demonstrate the versatility of two diverse microencapsulation processes and coating materials. The in vitro release patterns achieved by applying varied amounts of an ethylcellulose coating to small aspirin crystals using coacervation phase-separation encapsulation techniques are shown in Figure 13-35. Release of the aspirin is accomplished in this case by a leaching or diffusion mechanism from the inert, pH-insensitive ethylcellulose coating. Depicted in Figure 13-36 are the in vitro release responses of amphetamine sulfate pellets, that have been microencapsulated with varying amounts of a wax-fat coating applied by a pan-

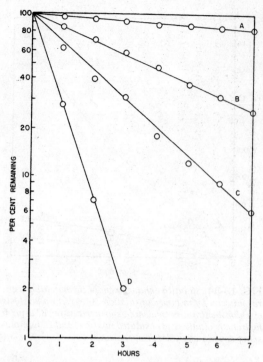

Fig. 13-35. *In vitro release patterns of crystalline aspirin coated with various amounts of ethylcellulose using phase-separation/coacervation techniques. A, 52% coating; B, 29% coating; C, 16% coating; D, 13% coating. (From The NCR Corporation.[4])*

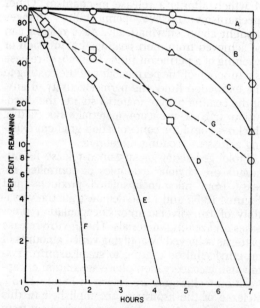

FIG. 13-36. *In vitro release patterns of amphetamine sulfate pellets pan coated with various amounts of a fat-wax coating. A, 17% coating; B, 15% coating; C, 13% coating; D, 11% coating; E, 9% coating; F, 7% coating; G, selected blend of uncoated pellets and coated pellets. (From the data of Rosen et al.[5] Courtesy Am. Pharmaceut. Assoc.)*

coating process.[5] Figure 13-36 illustrates the release rate effects of varied amounts of coating as well as the enteric nature of the coatings when subjected to the simulated gastrointestinal extraction conditions. The nonlinearity of the release curves plotted semilogarithmically suggests that the release of the amphetamine is accomplished initially by a leaching action through a gastric fluid-resistant coating followed by release from a dissolvable or disintegratable coating accomplished by the action of simulated intestinal fluid. Also shown in Figure 13-36 is the resultant release pattern (segmented curve) for an appropriate sustained release blend of two of the coated materials and a noncoated fraction of the amphetamine.

The in vitro release properties of the microencapsulated product forms already described—a rapidly disintegrating tablet containing coated particles, a microencapsulated powder, and a blend of coated pellets—all illustrate, in vitro, apparent first-order release kinetics, although diverse mechanisms are involved. Consequently, the rate of release of the drugs from these examples is proportional to the amount of drug remaining $-da/dt = k_r a$, or after integration, $a = a_0 e^{-k_r t}$ or $\ln (a/a_0) = -k_r t$, where a_0 is the total dose in the preparations, a is the fraction of the total dose remaining in the coated preparation at time t (if a_0 is unity), and k_r is the apparent first-order release constant. For sustained-release preparations formulated to release a fraction (f_i) of the dose immediately, and another fraction (f_r) exponentially as equated previously, the amount of drug release (a_r) by any time thereafter is therefore:

$$a_r = a_0 f_i + a_0 f_r (1 - e^{-k_r t})$$

Many sustained-release products release all or part of their drug content exponentially according to the first-order rate equation.[6] Improved gastrotolerability of drugs can be obtained by microencapsulation while good bioavailability is maintained.[7] To prove the tolerability of the microencapsulated product, one study of gastrointestinal bleeding was done with Cr-labeled red blood cells in 20 subjects treated for 3 months with microencapsulated KCl in the amount of 3 g daily. The daily blood loss in the feces of 20 subjects after administration of microencapsulated KCl was practically nil, mean values ranging from 0.432 to 0.596 ml in any 24-hour period, as opposed to 0.1 to 2.2 ml blood loss with raw KCl. In a study by McMahon et al., healthy male volunteers who had had no previous evidence of gastrointestinal disease were examined by endoscopy after ingestion of microencapsulated KC1 and wax matrix KC1 tablets.[8] The results of the study indicated that microcapsules had minimal endoscopically discernible lesions when compared with wax matrix tablets.

Equipment and Processing

The equipment required to conduct microencapsulation varies from complex machines designed specifically for microencapsulation to rather simple processing equipment common to many laboratories. The variation of microencapsulation equipment is evidenced by the descriptions included in the following methodology section.

Microcapsules as bulk materials, in either dry powder or dispersed form, can be processed into final product applications using common equipment such as V-blenders, tablet machines, granulators, homogenizers, kneaders, hard-gelatin capsule filling machines, or coating equipment if deposition onto a substrate is desired. The specific processing equipment employed depends on the final product form desired and on the microcapsule properties. All processing and formulation operations must be conducted with continual caution to avoid possible adverse effects (rupture, attrition, or dissolution) upon the thin microcapsule coating.

Methodology

Microencapsulation methods that have been or are being adapted to pharmaceutical use include air suspension, coacervation-phase separation, spray drying and congealing, pan coating, and solvent evaporation techniques. Methods not currently applicable to pharmaceutical preparations are vacuum deposition and polymerization techniques.

The physical nature of the core materials and the particle size ranges applicable to each process are given in Table 13-8.

Air Suspension

Microencapsulation by air suspension techniques is generally ascribed to the inventions of Professor Dale E. Wurster during his tenure at the University of Wisconsin.[9-16] Basically, the Wurster process consists of the dispersing of solid, particulate core materials in a supporting air stream and the spray-coating of the air-suspended particles. Figure 13-37 depicts a type of the Wurster air suspension encapsulation unit. Within the coating chamber, particles are suspended on an upward moving air stream as

TABLE 13-8. *Microencapsulation Processes and Their Applicabilities*

Microencapsulation Process	Applicable Core Material	Approximate Particle Size (μm)
Air suspension	Solids	35–5000*
Coacervation-phase separation	Solids & liquids	2–5000*
Multiorifice centrifugal	Solids & liquids	1–5000*
Pan coating	Solids	600–5000*
Solvent evaporation	Solids & liquids	5–5000*
Spray drying and congealing	Solids & liquids	600

*The 5000-μm size is not a particle limitation. The methods are also applicable to *macrocoating*, i.e., particles greater than 5000-μm in size.

indicated in the drawing. The design of the chamber and its operating parameters effect a recirculating flow of the particles through the coating zone portion of the chamber, where a coating material, usually a polymer solution, is spray-applied to the moving particles. During

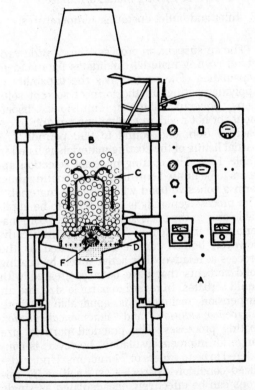

FIG. 13-37. *Schematic drawings of Wurster Air Suspension Apparatus: A, control panel; B, coating chamber; C, particles being treated; D, process airflow; E, air distribution plate; F, nozzle for applying film coatings. (Courtesy of Wisconsin Alumni Research Foundation.)*

each pass through the coating zone, the core material receives an increment of coating material. The cyclic process is repeated, perhaps several hundred times during processing, depending on the purpose of microencapsulation, the coating thickness desired, or whether the core material particles are thoroughly encapsulated. The supporting air stream also serves to dry the product while it is being encapsulated. Drying rates are directly related to the volume temperature of the supporting air stream.[17]

Processing variables that receive consideration for efficient, effective encapsulation by air suspension techniques include the following:

1. Density, surface area, melting point, solubility, friability, volatility, crystallinity, and flowability of the core material.

2. Coating material concentration (or melting point if not a solution).

3. Coating material application rate.

4. Volume of air required to support and fluidize the core material.

5. Amount of coating material required.

6. Inlet and outlet operating temperatures.

The air suspension process offers a wide variety of coating material candidates for microencapsulation. The process has the capability of applying coatings in the form of solvent solutions, aqueous solutions, emulsions, dispersions, or hot melts in equipment ranging in capacities from one pound to 990 pounds.[17] A partial listing of the coating materials is listed in Table 13-7. The coating material selection appears to be limited only in that the coating must form a cohesive bond with the core material.[18] The process generally is considered to be applicable only to the encapsulation of solid core materials as indicated in Table 13-8. Indirectly, however, liquids can be encapsulated by the process at relatively low active levels by coating solid sorbents that have been pretreated with liquid sorbates. In regard to particle size, the air suspension technique is applicable to both *microencapsulation* and *macroencapsulation* coating processes. The practical particle size range for microencapsulation, however, is considered to be in excess of 74 microns. Under idealized conditions, particles as small as 37 microns can be effectively encapsulated as single entities. Core materials comprised of micron or submicron particles can be effectively encapsulated by air suspension techniques, but agglomeration of the particles to some larger size is normally achieved.[17]

Coacervation-Phase Separation

Microencapsulation by coacervation-phase separation is generally attributed to The National Cash Register (NCR) Corporation* and the patents of B. K. Green et al.[19-28] The general outline of the processes consists of three steps carried out under continuous agitation: (1) formation of three immiscible chemical phases; (2) deposition of the coating; and (3) rigidization of the coating (Fig. 13-38).

Step 1 of the process is the formation of three immiscible chemical phases: a liquid manufacturing vehicle phase, a core material phase, and a coating material phase. To form the three phases, the core material is dispersed in a solution of the coating polymer, the solvent for the polymer being the liquid manufacturing vehicle phase. The coating material phase, an immiscible polymer in a liquid state, is formed by utilizing one of the methods of phase separation-coacervation, that is, by changing the temperature of the polymer solution; or by adding a salt, nonsolvent, or incompatible polymer to the polymer solution; or by inducing a polymer-polymer interaction. These general modes of effecting liquid-liquid phase separation are discussed in more detail later in this chapter.

Step 2 of the process consists of depositing the liquid polymer coating upon the core material. This is accomplished by controlled, physical mixing of the coating material (while liquid) and the core material in the manufacturing vehicle. Deposition of the liquid polymer coating around the core material occurs if the polymer is adsorbed at the interface formed between the core material and the liquid vehicle phase, and this adsorption phenomenon is a prerequisite to effective coating. The continued deposition of the coating material is promoted by a reduction in the total free interfacial energy of the system, brought about by the decrease of the coating material surface area during coalescence of the liquid polymer droplets.

Step 3 of the process involves rigidizing the coating, usually by thermal, cross-linking, or desolvation techniques, to form a self-sustaining microcapsule.

Because of the latitude in the material sys-

*The NCR Corporation's diversified microencapsulation patents and technology are now owned by Eurand America Inc.

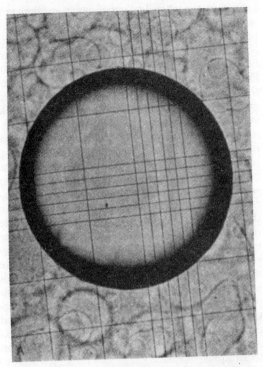

Step 1. Core and Liquid Coating in Manufacturing Vehicle

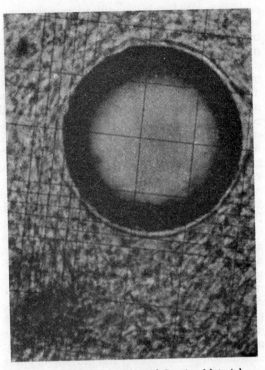

Step 2. Deposition of Liquid Coating Material

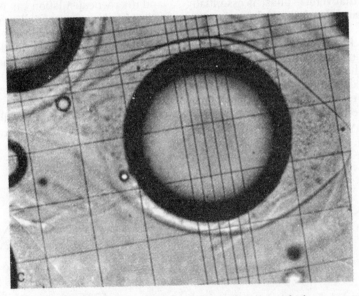

Step 3. Completed Capsules in Manufacturing Vehicle

FIG. 13-38. *Photomicrographs showing coating formation during phase-separation/coacervation process. A, Step 1. Core and liquid coating manufacturing vehicle. B, Step 2. Deposition of liquid coating material. C, Step 3. Completed manufacturing vehicle. ×300 magnification. (From Bakan.[28])*

tems associated with the utilization of this general scheme of accomplishing microencapsulation, a representative example to illustrate each method is given here.

Temperature Change. Figure 13-39 illustrates a general temperature-composition phase diagram for a binary system comprised of a polymer and a solvent. A system having an overall composition, represented as point X on the abscissa, exists as a single-phase, homogeneous solution at all points above the phase-boundary or binodal curve, FEG. As the temperature of the system is decreased from point *A* along the arrowed line *AEB,* the phase boundary is crossed at point *E*, and the two-phase region is entered. Phase separation of the dissolved polymer occurs in the form of immiscible liquid droplets, and if a core material is present in the system, under proper polymer concentration, temperature, and agitation conditions, the liquid polymer droplets coalesce around the dispersed core material particles, thus forming the embryonic microcapsules. The phase-boundary curve indicates that with decreasing temperature, one phase becomes polymer-poor (the microencapsulation vehicle phase) and the second phase (the coating material phase) becomes polymer-rich. At point *B*, for instance, the segmented tie-line suggests that vehicle phase is essentially pure solvent, point *C*, whereas the coexisting phase, point *D*, is a concentrated polymer-solvent mixture. In practice, the loss of solvent by the polymer-rich phase can constitute gelatin of polymer, and hence rigidization or solidification of the microcapsule polymeric coating.

The following example illustrates a microencapsulation procedure that utilizes the phase-separation/coacervation principle. Ethylcellu-

lose, a water-insoluble polymer, is applied to a water-soluble core material, N-acetyl p-aminophenol, by utilizing the temperature-solubility characteristics of the polymer in the hydrocarbon solvent cyclohexane. The etherified cellulosic, containing a relatively high ethoxyl content (high degree of substitution), is insoluble in cyclohexane at room temperature, but is soluble at elevated temperatures. Consequently, a working example involves dispersing ethylcellulose in cyclohexane to yield a polymer concentration of 2% by weight.[23] The mixture is heated to the boiling point to form a homogeneous polymer solution. The core material, finely divided crystalline N-acetyl p-aminophenol, is dispersed in the solution with stirring at a coating-to-core material (dry) ratio of 1:2. Allowing the mixture to cool, with continued stirring, effects phase-separation/coacervation of the ethyl-cellulose and microencapsulation of the core material. Allowing the mixture to cool further to room temperature accomplishes gelation and solidification of the coating. The microencapsulated product can then be collected from the cyclohexane by filtration, decantation, or centrifugation techniques.

Incompatible Polymer Addition. Liquid phase separation of a polymeric coating material and microencapsulation can be accomplished by utilizing the incompatibility of dissimilar polymers existing in a common solvent. Microencapsulation using this phenomenon is best described by considering the process in conjunction with the general phase diagram shown in Figure 13-40. The diagram illustrates a ternary system consisting of a solvent, and two polymers, X and Y. If an immiscible core material is dispersed in a solution of polymer Y (point *A* in

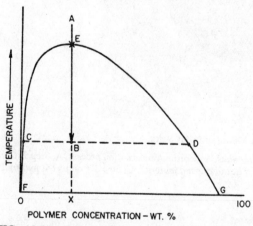

FIG. 13-39. *General phase diagram—coacervation induced thermally. (From Bakan.*[28]*)*

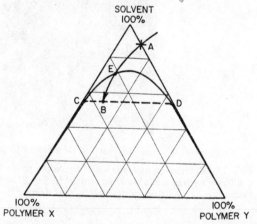

FIG. 13-40. *General phase diagram of phase-separation/coacervation induced by the addition of an incompatible polymer. (From Bakan.*[28]*)*

Figure 13-40) and polymer X is added to the system, denoted by the arrowed line, the phase boundary will be crossed at point E. As the two-phase region is penetrated with the further addition of polymer X, liquid polymer, immiscible droplets form and coalesce to form embryonic microcapsules. The coating of the microcapsules existing at point B, for example, consists of a concentrated solution of polymer Y dispersed in a solution comprised principally of polymer X, as indicated by the segmented tie-line and the phase-boundary intercepts C and D. The polymer that is more strongly adsorbed at the core material-solvent interface, in this case polymer Y, becomes the coating material.

In practice, solidification of the coating material is accomplished by further penetration into the two-phase region, chemical cross-linking, or washing the embryonic microcapsules with a liquid that is a nonsolvent for the coating, polymer Y, and that is a solvent for polymer X.

The microencapsulation of methylene blue hydrochloride with ethylcellulose by this mode of phase separation (incompatible polymer addition) is described as follows. Ethylcellulose is dissolved in toluene to yield a polymer concentration of 2% by weight. Crystalline methylene blue hydrochloride, being essentially insoluble in toluene, is dispersed, with stirring, in the polymer solution at a ratio, for instance, of 4 parts methylene blue hydrochloride to 1 part ethylcellulose. Phase-separation/coacervation is accomplished by slowly adding liquid polybutadiene in sufficient quantity to yield a ratio of 25 parts polybutadiene to 1 part ethylcellulose.[24] The polybutadiene, being quite soluble in toluene and incompatible with ethylcellulose, effects the demixing of the ethylcellulose from the polybutadiene toluene solution, and subsequent microencapsulation of the dispersed core material results. The ethylcellulose coating is solidified by adding a nonsolvent for the coating polymer, ethylcellulose, such as hexane. Also, the polybutadiene, being soluble in hexane, is washed from the mixture by decantation and by additional hexane wash cycles. The resultant product, crystalline methylene blue hydrochloride coated with ethylcellulose, is collected by standard filtration and drying techniques.

Nonsolvent Addition. A liquid that is a nonsolvent for a given polymer can be added to a solution of the polymer to induce phase separation, as indicated by the general phase diagram given in Figure 13-41. The resulting immiscible, liquid polymer can be utilized to effect microenipsulation of an immiscible core material as illustrated in the following example. A 5%, weight to volume, methyl ethyl ketone solution of cellu-

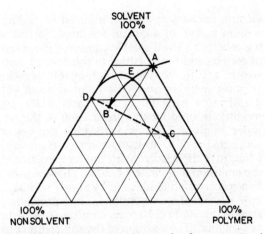

FIG. 13-41. *General phase diagram for phase-separation/coacervation induced by the addition of a nonsolvent. (From Bakan.[28])*

lose acetate butyrate is prepared, and in it, micronized methylscopolamine hydrobromide is dispersed with stirring. A core-material to coating-material ratio (methylscopolamine) hydrobromide to cellulose acetate butyrate) of about 2:1 is used. The resulting mixture is heated to 55°C, and isopropyl ether, a nonsolvent for the coating polymer, is added slowly to effect phase-separation/coacervation and microencapsulation of the suspended core material. The system is slowly cooled to room temperature, and the microencapsulated particles are separated by centrifugation, washed with isopropyl ether, and dried in vacuo.[25]

Salt Addition. Soluble inorganic salts can be added to aqueous solutions of certain water-soluble polymers to cause phase separation (Fig. 13-42). The following example of an oil-soluble

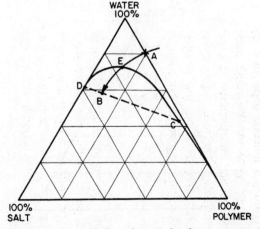

FIG. 13-42. *General phase diagram for phase-separation/coacervation induced by salt addition. (From Bakan.[28])*

vitamin microencapsulation induced by adding sodium sulfate to a gelatin solution illustrates the concept.[26] An oil-soluble vitamin is dissolved in corn oil and is emulsified to the desired drop size in a 10% solution of high-quality pigskin gelatin having an isoelectric point at about pH 8.9. Twenty parts oil to 100 parts water, by weight, are used for the preparation of the oil/water emulsion. The emulsification process is conducted at 50°C, well above the gelation temperature of the gelatin. With the temperature of the emulsion maintained at 50°C, phase-separation/coacervation is induced by slowly adding a 20% solution of sodium sulfate. The salt solution is added in a ratio of 10 parts emulsion to 4 parts salt solution. The addition of the salt solution to the continuously stirred emulsion effects the microencapsulation of the oil droplets with a uniform coating of gelatin. The resultant protein coating is rigidized by transferring the mixture into a sodium sulfate solution that is 7% by weight and is maintained at 19°C, with continued agitation. The gelatin salt solution comprises a volume approximately ten times that of the microencapsulation mixture volume. The microencapsulated product is collected by filtration, washed with water, chilled below the gelation temperature of the gelatin (to remove the salt), and voided of water by standard drying techniques such as spray drying.

Polymer-Polymer Interaction. The interaction of oppositely charged polyelectrolytes can result in the formation of a complex having such reduced solubility that phase separation occurs. Figure 13-43 illustrates the phase diagram for a ternary system comprised of two dissimilarly charged polyelectrolytes and the solvent, water. In the dilute solution region, interaction of the

oppositely charged poly electrolytes occurs, inducing phase separation within the phase-boundary curve ABA. The segmented tie-lines indicate that a system, having an overall composition within the two-phase region (point C for example), consists of two phases, one being polymer poor, point A, and one containing the hydrated, liquid complex, Pe⁺ and Pe⁻, point B.

As in the case of the previously described phase-separation/coacervation phenomena, microencapsulation can be accomplished by polymer-polymer interaction. Gelatin and gum arable are typical polyelectrolytes that can be caused to interact. Gelatin, at pH conditions below its isoelectric point, possesses a net positive charge, whereas the acidic gum arable is negatively charged. Under the proper temperature, pH, and concentrations, the two polymers can interact through their opposite electrical charges, forming a complex that exhibits phase-separation/coacervation. The following method for microencapsulating the water-immiscible liquid, methyl salicylate, is an example of this process.[27] Aqueous solutions of gum arable and pigskin gelatin (isoelectric point 8.9) are prepared, each being 2% by weight in concentration. The homogeneous polymer solutions are mixed together in equal amounts, diluted to about twice their volume with water, adjusted to pH 4.5, and warmed to 40 to 45°C. The oppositely charged macromolecules interact at these conditions and undergo phase-separation/coacervation. While maintaining the warm temperature conditions, the liquid core material, methyl salicylate, is added at a weight ratio of, for instance, 25 parts methyl salicylate to one part gelatin-gum arable (dry). The core material is emulsified by stirring to yield the desired drop size. The mixture is then slowly cooled to 25°C, with continued stirring, over a period of about one hour. During the cooling cycle, phase-separation/coacervation is further enhanced, resulting in the microencapsulation of the core material with the gelatin-gum arable complex. The coating is rigidized for drying purposes by cooling the mixture to about 10°C.

Owing to the fact that core materials are microencapsulated while being dispersed in some liquid manufacturing vehicle, subsequent drying operations may be required. Typical drying methods such as spray, freeze, fluid bed, solvent, and tray drying techniques are amenable to the microencapsulated products. The phase-separation/coacervation processes are conducted as batch operations using common production equipment in the manner illustrated in Figure 13-44. A wide variety of liquids, solids, or suspensions can be microencapsulated in various

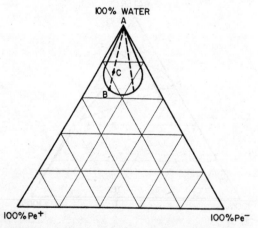

100% WATER

100% Pe⁺

100% Pe⁻

FIG. 13-43. *Phase diagram for phase-separation/coacervation by polymer interaction. (From Bakan.[28])*

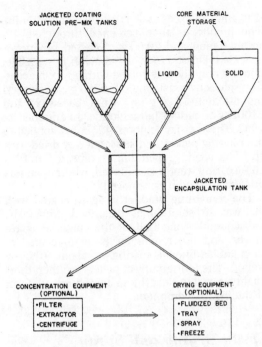

FIG. 13-44. *Flow diagram of a typical phase-separation/
coacervation process. (From Bakan.[28])*

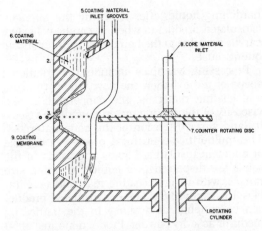

FIG. 13-45. *Sectional diagram of multiorifice-centrifugal
microencapsulation apparatus. (From Mattson.[30] Courtesy Conover-Mast Publications, Inc.)*

sizes (see Table 13-8) having a variety of coatings (see Table 13-7). Microcapsules are being
manufactured in vessels up to 2000 gallons in
capacity, at a multimillion pound per annum
rate.

Multiorifice-Centrifugal Process

The Southwest Research Institute (SWRI)
has developed a mechanical process for producing microcapsules that utilizes centrifugal forces
to hurl a core material particle through an enveloping microencapsulation membrane, thereby
effecting mechanical microencapsulation.[29] The
apparatus, illustrated cross-sectionally in Figure
13-45, depicts a rotating cylinder, 1, a major and
essential portion of the device. Located within
the cylinder are three circumferential grooves,
2, 3, and 4. Countersunk in the intermediate
groove, 3, are a plurality of orifices spaces closely
and circumferentially around the cylinder. The
upper and lower grooves, also located circumferentially around the cylinder, carry the coating
material in molten or solution form, via tubes, 5,
to the respective grooves. The ridges of the coat-
" ing material grooves, 2 and 4, serve as a weir
over which the coating material overflows when
the volume of the upper and lower grooves is
exceeded by the volume of material pumped into

the system. The coating material, 6, under centrifugal force imparted by the cylinder rotation,
flows outward along the side of the immediate
groove into the countersunk portion and forms a
film across the orifice. A counter rotating disc, 7,
mounted within the cylinder, atomizes or disperses the core material fed through the centrally located inlet, 8. The rotating disc flings the
particulate core material (liquid) droplets or
solid particles) toward the orifices. The core
material arrives at the orifices and encounters
the coating material membrane. The impact and
centrifugal force, generated by the rotating cylinder, hurls the core material through the enveloping coating membrane, 9, which is immediately regenerated by the continually overflowing
coating material.

The embryonic microcapsules, upon leaving
the orifices, are hardened, congealed, or voided
of coating solution by a variety of means. For
example, the microcapsules can be flung into a
heated, countercurrent air stream to harden or
congeal coatings containing residual solvent.
Also, the microcapsules can be forced into a rotating hardening or congealing bath. The coating material, if a melt, can be hurled into a cool
liquid (nonsolvent for the coating material) decreasing the temperature below the melting
point of the coating. Also, the hardening bath
can contain a coating nonsolvent that is capable
of extracting the coating solution solvent. The
rotating hardening bath not only provides a coating desolvation or congealing function, but
serves as a means of removing the microcapsules from their impact points, thus reducing
agglomeration tendencies. It also provides a
means of accumulating the coated product. The

hardening liquid, after removing the microencapsulated product to where it can be collected, can be recycled to the hardening bath for subsequent reuse.

Processing variables include the rotational speed of the cylinder, the flow rate of the core and coating materials, the concentration and viscosity of the coating material, and the viscosity and surface tension of the core material.[30] The multiorifice-centrifugal process is capable of microencapsulating liquids and solids (if the solids are dispersed in a liquid) of varied size ranges, with diverse coating materials (see Tables 13-7 and 13-8). The encapsulated product can be supplied as a slurry in the hardening media or as a dry powder. Production rates of 50 to 75 pounds per hour have been achieved with the process.

Pan Coating

The macroencapsulation of relatively large particles by pan methods has become widespread in the pharmaceutical industry, and the topic is covered in depth in Chapter 12 of this text. With respect to microencapsulation, solid particles greater than 600 microns in size are generally considered essential for effective coating, and the process has been extensively employed for the preparation of controlled-release beads (see Chap. 14). Medicaments are usually coated onto various spherical substrates such as nonpareil sugar seeds, and then coated with protective layers of various polymers.

In practice, the coating is applied as a solution, or as an atomized spray, to the desired solid core material in the coating pan. Usually, to remove the coating solvent, warm air is passed over the coated materials as the coatings are being applied in the coating pans. In some cases, final solvent removal is accomplished in a drying oven.

Blythe describes a method of preparing sustained-release pellets in which nonpareil seeds are coated initially with dextroamphetamine sulfate, and then with a release-rate retarding wax-fat coating.[31] Nonpareil seeds (sugar pellets), 15.5 kg and 12 to 40 mesh in size, are placed in a rotating, 36-inch coating pan. USP syrup, 240 ml, is slowly poured onto the pellets to wet them evenly. An 80/20 mixture (750 g) of dextroamphetamine and calcium dihydrate are sprinkled onto the wetted nonpareil seeds. The pellets were dried with warm air. This coating operation is repeated three times. The fifth coating, talc, is accomplished by wetting the product with 240 ml of syrup followed by dusting 600 g of talc on the seeds. The pellets are rolled until

dry, and the excess talc is removed by vacuum. The product is then screened through a 12-mesh screen and 20.0 kg of coated product is collected. One quarter of the batch is set aside, and the remainder is coated with a wax-fat coating solution consisting of 6300 g of glyceryl monostearate, 700 g of white beeswax, and 2100 ml of carbon tetrachloride, maintained at 70°C. The wax-fat solution, 425 ml is applied to the rotating pellets and subsequently dried with air. The coating operation is repeated until a 10% coating weight is achieved, whereupon one third of the batch is removed.

The remaining product is again coated with the wax-fat solution as described previously. Subsequently, one half of the material is removed and the remainder is again coated to yield an additional coating of about 10% by weight. The four groups of pellets are then thoroughly mixed to yield the sustained-release form of the sympathomimetic.

Spray Drying and Spray Congealing

Spray-drying and spray-congealing methods have been used for many years as microencapsulation techniques. Because of certain similarities of the two processes, they are discussed together.

Spray-drying and spray-congealing processes are similar in that both involve dispersing the core material in a liquefied coating substance and spraying or introducing the core-coating mixture into some environmental condition, whereby relatively rapid solidification (and formation) of the coating is effected. The principal difference between the two methods, for the purpose of this discussion, is the means by which coating solidification is accomplished. Coating solidification in the case of spray drying is effected by rapid evaporation of a solvent in which the coating material is dissolved. Coating solidification in spray congealing methods, however, is accomplished by thermally congealing a molten coating material or by solidifying a dissolved coating by introducing the coating-core material mixture into a nonsolvent. Removal of the nonsolvent or solvent from the coated product is then accomplished by sorption, extraction, or evaporation techniques.

In practice, microencapsulation by spray *drying* is conducted by dispersing a core material in a coating solution, in which the coating substance is dissolved and in which the core material is insoluble, and then by atomizing the mixture into an air stream. The air, usually heated, supplies the latent heat of vaporization required to remove the solvent from the coating material, thus forming the microencapsulated product. The equipment components of a standard spray dryer include an air heater, atomizer, main spray chamber, blower or fan, cyclone and product collector, as described in detail in Chapter 3.

Process control variables include feed material properties such as viscosity, uniformity, and concentration of core and coating material, feed rate/method of atomization, and the drying rate, which is normally controlled by the inlet and outlet temperatures and the air stream solvent concentration. The process produces microcapsules approaching a spherical structure in the size range of 5 to 600 microns (Table 13-8). Characteristically, spray drying yields products of low bulk density, owing to the porous nature of the coated particles. Low active contents are normally required to provide the necessary protection desired. For instance, the adequate retention of volatile, liquid core materials is difficult to achieve without maintaining low active content levels, perhaps below 20%.

Many coating materials (see Table 13-7) can be applied to liquid and solid core materials by spray drying coating solutions containing the dispersed core material. The process is commonly employed in the microencapsulation of liquid flavors yielding dry, free-flowing powders for use in foods and pharmaceuticals.

Microencapsulation by spray congealing can be accomplished with spray drying equipment when the protective coating is applied as a melt. General process variables and conditions are quite similar to those already described, except that the core material is dispersed in a coating material melt rather than a coating solution. Coating solidification (and microencapsulation) is accomplished by spraying the hot mixture into a cool air stream. Waxes, fatty acids and alcohols, polymers and sugars, which are solids at room temperature but meltable at reasonable temperatures, are applicable to spray-congealing techniques. Typically, the particle size of spray-congealed products can be accurately controlled when spray drying equipment is used,[32] and has been found to be a function of the feed rate, the atomizing wheel velocity, dispersion of feed material viscosity, and other variables.

Solvent Evaporation

This technique has been used by companies including The NCR Company, Gavaert Photo-Production NV, and .Fuji Photo Film Co., Ltd. to produce microcapsules.[33-36] The processes are carried out in a liquid manufacturing vehicle.

The microcapsule coating is dissolved in a volatile solvent, which is immiscible with the liquid manufacturing vehicle phase. A core material to be microencapsulated is dissolved or dispersed in the coating polymer solution. With agitation, the core coating material mixture is dispersed in the liquid manufacturing vehicle phase to obtain the appropriate size microcapsule. The mixture is then heated (if necessary) to evaporate the solvent for the polymer. In the case in which the core material is dispersed in the polymer solution, polymer shrinks around the core. In the case in which the core material is dissolved in the coating polymer solution, a matrix-type microcapsule is formed. Once all the solvent for the polymer is evaporated, the liquid vehicle temperature is reduced to ambient temperature (if required) with continued agitation. At this stage, the microcapsules can be used in suspension form, coated on to substrates or isolated as powders.

Process variables would include, but not be limited to, methods of forming dispersions, evaporation rate of the solvent for the coating polymer, temperature cycles, and agitation rates. Important factors that must be considered when preparing microcapsules by solvent evaporation techniques include choice of vehicle phase and solvent for the polymer coating, as these choices greatly influence microcapsule properties as well as the choice of solvent recovery techniques.

The solvent evaporation technique to produce microcapsules is applicable to a wide variety of liquid and solid core materials. The core materials may be either water-soluble or water-insoluble materials. A variety of film-forming polymers can be used as coatings as exemplified in Table 13-7.

Polymerization

A relatively new microencapsulation method utilizes polymerization techniques to form protective microcapsule coatings in situ. The methods involve the reaction of monomeric units located at the interface existing between a core material substance and a continuous phase in which the core material is dispersed. The continuous or core material supporting phase is usually a liquid or gas, and therefore the polymerization reaction occurs at a liquid-liquid, liquid-gas, solid-liquid, or solid-gas interface.

The polymerization method most applicable, perhaps, to pharmaceutical or medical use is that developed by Chang[37-41] in his research at McGill University. Chang has been able to accomplish permselective membrane properties for microcapsules having coatings of nylon formed by interfacial polymerization, or collodion formed by phase-separation/coacervation techniques. The membranes, typically about 200 angstroms thick, have an equivalent aqueous pore radius of about 16 angstroms. The microcapsules have been shown to be permselective in that protein and enzyme core materials, for instance, do not transfer out of the microcapsule, whereas smaller molecules such as enzyme substrates and resultant reaction products can permeate the membrane.[41]

Chang's interfacial polymerization method for forming polyamide (nylon) membranes involves the reaction occurring at the liquid-liquid interface existing between an aqueous solution of an aliphatic diamine and a water-immiscible organic solution of a dicarboxylic acid halide. The polymerization reaction depends on the fact that acid halides, such as sebacoyl chloride, are nearly water-insoluble, and diamines, such as hexanediamine, have an appreciable partition coefficient toward the water-immiscible organic phase. Hence, the hexanediamine diffuses to the organic sebacoyl chloride phase, and the polycondensation reaction occurs forming the polyamide. Because the chemical reaction rate exceeds the diffusion rate of the diamine into the nonaqueous phase, the polyamide is deposited almost entirely at the interface existing between the two solutions.[40]

Using this phenomenon, Chang prepares microcapsules containing protein solutions by incorporating the protein in the aqueous diamine phase. Chang has demonstrated the permselectivity of microcapsules containing the enzyme, urease, by their ability to convert blood urea to ammonia, the enzyme remaining within the microcapsules when incorporated within an extracorporeal shunt system. Numerous groups are utilizing polymerization techniques to accomplish microencapsulation. Examples are the National Lead Corporation, Union Carbide Corporation, Pennwalt Corporation, Eurand America Inc., Appleton Papers Inc., and Moore Business Forms, Inc. The processes are not discussed in this chapter, however, nor is microencapsulation that is effected by electrostatic and vacuum deposition techniques.[42-59]

References

1. Galeone, M., et al.: Current Therapeutic Research, 31:3, 1982.
2. Herbig, J.A.: Encyclopedia of Polymer Science and Technology. Vol. 8. John Wiley and Sons, New York, 1968.
3. Bakan, J.A., and Sloan, F.D.: Drug and Cosmetic Ind., March 1972.
4. The National Cash Register Company. Unpublished data. Dayton, OH.
5. Rosen, E., Ellison, T., Tannenbaum, P., et al.: J. Pharm. Sci., 56:365, 1967.
6. Wiegand, R.G., and Taylor, J.D.: Drug Standards, 27:165, 1959.
7. Clanchi, M.: Eurand Studies on Some Advantages of Drug Microencapsulation. Third International Symposium on Microencapsulation, Tokyo, Japan, 1976.
8. McMahon, F., et al.: Lancet, November 13, 1982, p. 1059.
9. Wurster, D.E.: U.S. Patent 2,648,609 (1953).
10. Wurster, D.E.: U.S. Patent 2,799,241 (1957).
11. Wurster, D.E.: U.S. Patent 3,089,824 (1963).
12. Wurster, D.E., and Lindlof, J.A.: U.S. Patent 3,117,027 (1964).
13. Wurster, D.E., and Lindlof, J.A.: U.S. Patent 3,196,827 (1965).
14. Wurster, D.E., Battista, J.V., and Lindlof, J.A.: U.S. Patent 3,207,824 (1965).
15. Wurster, D.E., and Lindlof, J.A.: U.S. Patent 3,241,520 (1966).
16. Wurster, D.E.: U.S. Patent 3,253,944 (1966).
17. Hinkes, T.M.: The Wurster Process for Encapsulation. Presented at Microencapsulation Course, Center for Professional Advancement, Somerville, New Jersey, September 1972.
18. Harvard Business School: Report on Microencapsulation. Management Reports, 38 Commington Street, Boston, 1963.
19. Green, B.K.: U.S. Patent 2,712,507 (1955).
20. Green, B.K., and Schleicher, L.: U.S. Patent 2,730,456 (1956).
21. Green, B.K.: U.S. Patent 2,800,457 (1957).
22. Miller, R.E., and Anderson, J.L.: U.S. Patent 3,155,590 (1964).
23. Miller, R.E., Fanger, G.O., and McNiff, R.G.: Union of So. Africa Patent 4211-66 (1967).
24. The National Cash Register Co.: Gr. Br. Patent 907,284 (1963).
25. Heistand, E.N., Wagner, J.G., and Knoechel, E.L.: U.S. Patent 3,242,051 (1966).
26. Green, B.K.: U.S. Patent Re 24,899 (1960).
27. Brynko, C., Bakan, J.A., Miller, R.E., and Scarpelli, J.A.: U.S. Patent 3,341,466 (1967).
28. Bakan, J.A.: Microencapsulation of Foods and Related Products. Food Technology, 7:34, 1973.
29. Somerville, G.R., Jr.: U.S. Patent 3,015,128 (1962).
30. Mattson, H.W.: Int. Sci. Technol., 40:66, 1965.
31. Blythe, R.H.: U.S. Patent 2,738,303 (1956).
32. Scott, M.W., Robinson, M.J., Pauls, V.F., and Lantz, R.S.: J. Pharm. Sci., 53:670, 1964.
33. Herbig, J.A., and Hanny, J.F.: U.S. Patent 3,732,172 (1973).
34. Vrancken, M.N., and Claeys, D.S.: U.S. Patent 3,523,906 (1970).
35. Matsukana, H.: U.S. Patent 3,660,304 (1972).
36. Yoshida, N.H.: U.S. Patent 3,657,144 (1972).
37. Chang, T.M.S.: Science, 146:524, 1964.
38. Chang, T.M.S., and MacIntosh, F.C.: Pharmacologist, 6:198, 1964.
39. Chang, T.M.S.: Ph.D. Thesis, McGill University, Montreal, Canada, 1965.
40. Chang, T.M.S., MacIntosh, F.C., and Mason, S.G.: Canad. J. Physiol. Pharmacol., 44:415, 1966.
41. Chang, T.M.S.: Trans Am. Soc. Artif. Int. Organs, 12:13. 1966.

42. Brynko, C.: U.S. Patent 2,969,330 (1961).
43. Brynko, C., and Scarpelli, J.A.: U.S. Patent 2,969,331 (1961).
44. Orsino, J.A., Herman, D.F., and Brancato, J.J.: U.S. Patent 3,121,698 (1964).
45. Orsino, J.A., and Mandel, C.E.: U.S. Patent 3,121,658 (1964).
46. Herman, D.F., and Dunlap, I.R.: TAPPI, 48:418, 1965.
47. Gorham, W.F., and Chappaqua, W.: U.S. Patent 3,330,332 (1967).
48. Chem. Week, February 27, 1965, p. 59.
49. Vandegaer, J.E., and Meier, F.G.: U.S. Patent 3,464,926 (1969).
50. Vandegaer, J.E., and Meier, F.G.: U.S. Patent 3,355,882 (1971).
51. Vandegaer, J.E.: U.S. Patent 3,577,515 (1971).
52. Moore Business Forms, Inc.: Gt. B. Patent 1,046,409 (1966).
53. Langer, G., and Yamate, G.: U.S. Patent 3,294,704 (1966).
54. Berger, B.B., Miller, C.D., Langer, W., and Langer, G.: U.S. Patent 3,208,951 (1965).
55. Baer, C.W., and Steeves, R.W.: U.S. Patent 2,846,971 (1958).
56. Chem. Eng. News, June 26, 1961.
57. Kiritani, M., et al.: U.S. Patent 3,981,821 (1976).
58. Foris, P.L., et al.: U.S. Patent 4,001,140 (1977).
59. Speiser, P., et al.: U.S. Patent 4,021,364 (1977).

General References

Bungenberg de Jong, H.G., and Kruyt, H.R.(eds.): Colloid Science. Vol. II. Elsevier Publishing Company, Amsterdam, 1949.
Chang, T.M.S.: Artificial Cells. Charles C Thomas, Springfield, IL, 1972.
Chang, T.M.S. (ed.): Microencapsulation and Artificial Cells. Humana Press, New York, 1984.
Deasy, P.: Microencapsulation and Related Drug Processes. Marcel Dekker, New York, 1984.
Eurand Lectures to International Symposia, Eurand Internation. Viale Monza, Milano, Italy, 1977.

Gutcho, M.: Microcapsules and Other Capsules—Advances Since 1975. Noyes Data Corporation, Ridge Park, NJ, 1979.
Gutcho, M.: Microcapsules and Microencapsulation Techniques. Noyes Data Corporation, Ridge Park, NJ, 1976.
Gutcho, M.: Capsule Technology and Microencapsulation. Noyes Data Corporation, Ridge Park, NJ, 1972.
Journal of Controlled Release. Elsevier Science Publishers, The Netherlands, began issuing 1984.
Journal of Microencapsulation. Taylor and Francis Ltd., London, England, began issuing 1984.
Kondo, T.: Microencapsulation. Techno Inc., Tokyo, Japan, 1979.
Kydonieus, A. (ed.): Controlled Release Technologies: Methods, Theory and Applications. Vols. I and II. CRC Press, Boca Raton, FL, 1980.
Lim, F. (ed.): Biomedical Applications of Microencapsulation. CRC Press, Boca Raton, FL, 1983.
Luzzi, L.A.: J. Pharm. Sci., 59:1367, 1970.
Merory, S.: Food Flavorings, Composition, Manufacture and Use. Avi Publishing, Westport, CT, 1960.
Nixon, J.R. (ed.): Microencapsulation—Drugs and Pharmaceutical Sciences. Vol. 3. Marcel Dekker, New York, 1976.
Roseman, T., and Mansdorf, Z. (eds.): Controlled Release Delivery Systems. Marcel Dekker, New York, 1983.
Sirine, G.: Drug and Cosmetic Ind., September 1969.
Sparks, R.E., Salemme, R.M., Meier, P.M., et al.: Trans. Am. Soc. Artif. Int. Organs, 14:353, 1969.
Sprowls, J.B., Jr.(ed.): Prescription Pharmacy. 2nd Ed. J.B. Lippincott, Philadelphia, 1970.
Swintosky, J.V.: Ind. J. of Pharm., 25:360. 1963.
Vandegaer, J.E. (ed.): Microencapsulation—Processes and Applications. Plenum Press, New York, 1974.

Acknowledgment

The author would like to express his sincere appreciation to J. L. Anderson, Appleton Papers, Inc., for his historical contribution to the preparation of this chapter.

14

Sustained Release Dosage Forms

NICHOLAS G. LORDI

With many drugs, the basic goal of therapy is to achieve a steady-state blood or tissue level that is therapeutically effective and nontoxic for an extended period of time. The design of proper dosage regimens is an important element in accomplishing this goal. A basic objective in dosage form design is to optimize the delivery of medication so as to achieve a measure of control of the therapeutic effect in the face of uncertain fluctuations in the in vivo environment in which drug release takes place. This is usually accomplished by maximizing drug availability, i.e., by attempting to attain a maximum rate and extent of drug absorption; however, control of drug action through formulation also implies controlling bioavailability to reduce drug absorption rates. In this chapter, approaches to the formulation of drug delivery systems, based on the deliberate control of drug availability, are considered with emphasis on peroral dosage forms.

The Sustained Release Concept

Sustained release, sustained action, prolonged action, controlled release, extended action, timed release, depot, and repository dosage forms are terms used to identify drug delivery systems that are designed to achieve a prolonged therapeutic effect by continuously releasing medication over an extended period of time after administration of a single dose. In the case of injectable dosage forms, this period may vary from days to months. In the case of orally administered forms, however, this period is measured in hours and critically depends on the residence time of the dosage form in the gastrointestinal (GI) tract. The term "controlled release" has become associated with those systems from which therapeutic agents may be automatically delivered at predefined rates over a long period of time. Products of this type have

been formulated for oral, injectable, and topical use, and include inserts for placement in body cavities as well.[1]

The pharmaceutical industry provides a variety of dosage forms and dosage levels of particular drugs, thus enabling the physician to control the onset and duration of drug therapy by altering the dose and/or mode of administration. In some instances, control of drug therapy can be achieved by taking advantage of beneficial drug interactions that affect drug disposition and elimination, e.g., the action of probenicid, which inhibits the excretion of penicillin, thus prolonging its blood level. Mixtures of drugs might be utilized to potentiate, synergize, or antagonize given drug actions. Alternately, drug mixtures might be formulated in which the rate and/or extent of drug absorption is modified. Sustained release dosage form design embodies this approach to the control of drug action, i.e., through a process of either drug modification or dosage form modification, the absorption process, and subsequently drug action, can be controlled.

Physicians can achieve several desirable therapeutic advantages by prescribing sustained release forms. Since the frequency of drug administration is reduced, patient compliance can be improved, and drug administration can be made more convenient as well. The blood level oscillation characteristic of multiple dosing of conventional dosage forms is reduced, because a more even blood level is maintained. A less obvious advantage, implicit in the design of sustained release forms, is that the total amount of drug administered can be reduced, thus maximizing availability with a minimum dose. In addition, better control of drug absorption can be attained, since the high blood level peaks that may be observed after administration of a dose of a high-availability drug can be reduced by formulation in an extended action form. The safety margin of high-potency drugs can be increased, and the incidence of both local and systemic adverse side effects can be reduced in sensitive patients. Overall, administration of sustained release forms enables increased reliability of therapy.[2]

In evaluating drugs as candidates for sustained release formulation, the disadvantages of such formulations that must be considered include the following: (1) Administration of sustained release medication does not permit the prompt termination of therapy. Immediate changes in drug need during therapy, such as might be encountered if significant adverse effects are noted, cannot be accommodated. (2) The physician has less flexibility in adjusting dosage regimens. This is fixed by the dosage form design. (3) Sustained release forms are designed for the normal population, i.e., on the basis of average drug biologic half-lives. Consequently, disease states that alter drug disposition, significant patient variation, and so forth are not accommodated. (4) Economic factors must also be assessed, since more costly processes and equipment are involved in manufacturing many sustained release forms.

Not all drugs are suitable candidates for formulation as prolonged action medication. Table 14-1 lists specific drug characteristics that would preclude formulation in peroral sustained release forms. Drugs with long biologic half-lives (e.g., digoxin—34 hours) are inherently long-acting and thus are viewed as questionable candidates for sustained release formulation. For some drugs in this group, however, a properly designed sustained release formulation may be advantageous. Because single doses capable of producing equally prolonged effects often yield significant concentration peaks immediately after each dosing interval, control of drug release may be indicated if toxicity or local gastric irritation is a hazard. Drugs with narrow requirements for absorption (e.g., drugs dependent on position in the GI tract for optimum absorption) are also poor candidates for oral sustained release formulation, since absorption must occur throughout the length of the gut. Very insoluble drugs whose availability is controlled by dissolution (e.g., griseofulvin) may not benefit from formulation in sustained release forms since the amount of drug available for absorption is limited by the poor solubility of the compound.

Before proceeding with the design of a sustained release form of an appropriate drug, the formulator should have an understanding of the pharmacokinetics of the candidate, should be assured that pharmacologic effect can be correlated with drug blood levels, and should be knowledgeable about the therapeutic dosage range, including the minimum effective and maximum safe doses.

Theory

Design

To establish a procedure for designing sustained release dosage forms, it is useful to examine the properties of drug blood-level-time profiles characteristic of multiple dosing therapy of immediate release forms. Figure 14-1 shows typical profiles observed after administration of equal doses of a drug using different dosage schedules: every 8 hours (curve A), every 3 hours (curve B), and every 2 hours (curve C). As the dosage interval is shortened, the number of doses required to attain a steady-state drug level increases, the amplitude of the drug level oscillations diminishes, and the steady state average blood level is increased. As a first approximation, the optimum dosage interval can be taken to be equal to the biologic half-life, in this case, 3 hours. Curve D represents a profile in which the first or loading dose is made twice that of all subsequent doses administered, i.e., the maintenance doses. This dosing regimen allows the relation between the loading (Di) and maintenance (Dm) doses to be determined as follows:

$$Di = Dm(1 - \exp(-0.693\tau/t_{\frac{1}{2}}))$$

TABLE 14-1. *Characteristics of Drugs Unsuitable for Peroral Sustained Release Forms*

Characteristics	Drugs
Not effectively absorbed in the lower intestine.	Riboflavin, ferrous salts
Absorbed and excreted rapidly; short biologic half-lives (<1 hr).	Penicillin G, furosemide
Long biologic half-lives (>12 hr).	Diazepam, phenytoin
Large doses required (>1 g).	Sulfonamides
Cumulative action and undesirable side effects; drugs with low therapeutic indices.	Phenobarbital, digitoxin
Precise dosage titrated to individual is required.	Anticoagulants, cardiac glycosides
No clear advantage for sustained release formulation.	Griseofulvin

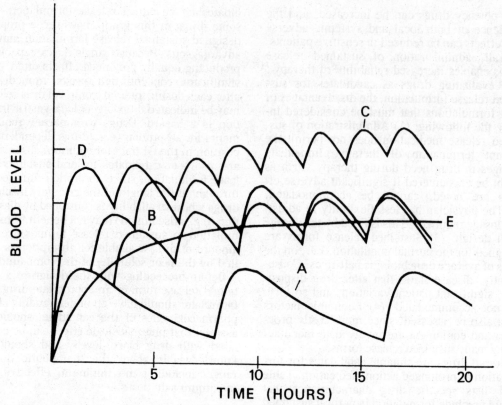

FIG. 14-1. *Multiple patterns of dosage that characterize nonsustained peroral administration of a drug with a biologic half-life of 3 hr and a half-life for absorption of 20 min. Dosage intervals are: A, 8 hr; B, 3 hr; C, 2 hr; and D, 3 hr (loading dose is twice the maintenance dose). E, Constant rate intravenous infusion.*

where τ is the dosing interval and $t_{\frac{1}{2}}$ is the biologic half-life. If $t_{\frac{1}{2}} = \tau$, Di = 2Dm. Selection of the proper dose and dosage interval is a prerequisite to obtaining a drug level pattern that will remain in the therapeutic range.

Elimination of drug level oscillations can be achieved by administration of drug through constant-rate intravenous infusion. Curve E in Figure 14-1 represents an example whereby the infusion rate was chosen to achieve the same average drug level as a 3-hour dosage interval for the specific case illustrated. The objective in formulating a sustained release dosage form is to be able to provide a similar blood level pattern for up to 12 hours after oral administration of the drug.

To design an efficacious sustained release dosage form, one must have a thorough knowledge of the pharmacokinetics of the drug chosen for this formulation. Figure 14-2 shows a general pharmacokinetic model of an ideal sustained release dosage form. For the purposes of this discussion, measurements of drug blood level are assumed to correlate with therapeutic effect and drug kinetics are assumed to be ade-

quately approximated by a one-body-compartment model. That is, drug distribution is sufficiently rapid so that a steady state is immediately attained between the central and peripheral compartments, i.e., the blood-tissue transfer rate constants, k_{12} and k_{21}, are large.

Under the foregoing circumstances, the drug kinetics can be characterized by three parameters: the elimination rate constant (ke) or biologic half-life ($t_{\frac{1}{2}} = 0.693/ke$), the absorption rate constant (ka), and the apparent distribution volume (Vd), which defines the apparent body space in which drug is distributed. A large Vd value (e.g., 100 L) means that drug is extensively distributed into extravascular space: a small Vd value (e.g., 10 L) means that drug is largely confined to the plasma. It is best interpreted as a proportionality factor which when multiplied by the blood level gives the total amount of drug in the body. For the two-body-compartment representation of drug kinetics, Vc is the volume of the central compartment, including both blood and any body water in which drug is rapidly perfused.

A diagrammatic representation of a dosage

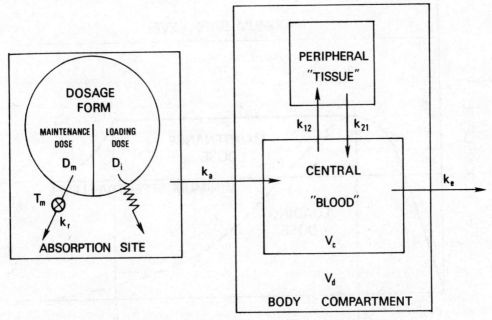

FIG. 14-2. *A general pharmacokinetic model of an ideal peroral sustained release dosage form.*

form, which identifies the specific parameters that must be taken into account in optimizing sustained release dosage form designs, is shown in Figure 14-2 at the absorption site. These are the loading or immediately available portion of the dose (Di), the maintenance or slowly available portion of the dose (Dm), the time (Tm) at which release of maintenance dose begins (i.e., the delay time between release of Di and Dm), and the specific rate of release (kr) of the maintenance dose.

Figure 14-3 shows the form of the body drug-level time profile that characterizes an ideal peroral sustained release dosage form after a single administration. Tp is the peak time, and h is the total time after administration in which the drug is effectively absorbed. Cp is the average drug level to be maintained constantly for a period of time equal to (h - Tp) hours; it is also the peak blood level observed after administration of a loading dose. The portion of the area under the blood level curve contributed by the loading and maintenance doses is indicated on the diagram. To obtain a constant drug level, the rate of drug absorption must be made equal to its rate of elimination. Consequently, drug must be provided by the dosage form at a rate such that the drug concentration becomes constant at the absorption site.

Detailed theoretic treatments of a number of sustained release dosage form designs have been reported. These include systems in which drug is released for absorption by zero-order and first-order processes with and without loading doses. In the former case, designs based on both immediate and delayed release of maintenance dose have been described. The following general assumptions have been made in developing these designs: (1) Drug disposition can be described by a one-compartment open model. (2) Absorption is first-order and complete. (3) Release of drug from the dosage form, not absorption, is rate-determining, i.e., the effect of variation in absorption rate is minimized (ka > ke).

Zero-Order Release Approximation

The profile shown in Figure 14-3 can most nearly be approximated by a design consisting of a loading dose and a zero-order release maintenance dose, as described by Robinson and Eriksen.[3] If a zero-order release characteristic can be implemented in a practical formulation, the release process becomes independent of the magnitude of the maintenance dose and does not change during the effective maintenance period. Table 14-2 lists the expressions that can be used to estimate the design parameters for an optimized zero-order model, for both simultaneous and delayed release of maintenance dose. Their application is illustrated using procaina-

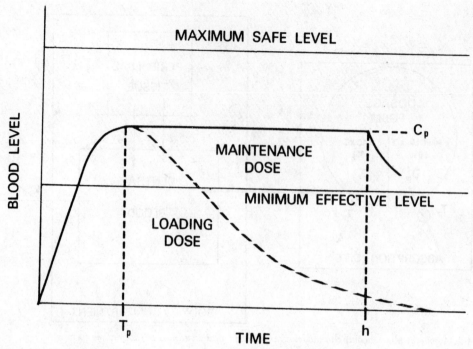

FIG. 14-3. *A blood-level time profile for an ideal peroral sustained release dosage form.*

mide, an important antiarrhythmic agent, as an example.

Table 14-3 lists the pharmacokinetic parameters characterizing the disposition of procainamide, which is described by a two-body-compartment open model, in an average patient based on data reported by Manion et al. for 11 subjects.[4] Conventional formulations are administered every 3 hours for maintenance of therapy, resulting in a maximum-to-minimum blood level ratio >2 at the steady state. Sustained release formulations have been shown to have advantages as an alternate dosage form. A comparison is made between estimates based on three cases: (1) the one-compartment model assumption with delayed release of maintenance dose, (2) the actual two-compartment fit of procainamide pharmacokinetic data with delayed release of maintenance dose, and (3) the two-compartment model with simultaneous release

TABLE 14-2. *Expressions Useful for Estimation of Design Parameters for Zero-Order Sustained Release Dosage Form Models*

Parameter	Equation	
Maximum body drug content to be maintained	$Am = CpVd$	Eq. (1)
Zero-order rate constant	$kr_0 = keAm$	Eq. (2)
Peak time	$Tp = (2.3/(ka - ke))\log(ka/ke)$	Eq. (3)
Bioavailability factor	$F = (AUC)oral/(AUC)iv$	Eq. (4)
Fraction of dose (Di) at peak (F = 1)	$f = \left(\dfrac{ka}{ke}\right)^{\frac{ke}{ke - ka}}$	Eq. (5)
Maintenance dose	$Dm = kr_0(h - Tm)/F$	Eq. (6)
Loading dose (Tm = Tp)	$Di = Am/fF$	Eq. (7)
Loading dose (Tm = 0)	$Di = (Di - kr_0Tp)$	Eq. (8)

Table 14-3. *Pharmacokinetic Parameters for Procainamide in an Average Subject (Weight: 75 kg)*

Parameter	Value	Parameter	Value
β	0.21 hr	k_{12}	3.15 hr
$t_{\frac{1}{2}}$	3.4 hr	k_{21}	1.4 hr
ke	0.97 hr	Vc	59 L
ka	2.0 hr	Vd	205 L
F	0.83	Tp	0.5 hr

From Manion, C.V., et al., J. Pharm. Sci., 66:981, 1977. Reproduced with permission of the copyright owner, the American Pharmaceutical Association.

of loading and maintenance doses. In all cases, the blood level is assumed to be maintained at 1 μg/ml for 8 hours, i.e., Cp = 1 mg/L, and h − Tp = 8. Table 14-4 summarizes the results of the calculation of sustained release design parameters for procainamide, assuming zero-order release kinetics. The following steps are required to estimate the design parameters listed in the table. (Equation numbers refer to equations in Table 14-2.)

1. Estimation of kr_0. Equation (2) is derived by considering that at the steady state the rate of absorption is constant and equal to the rate of elimination, that is: Rate Absorption = ka · Xa = Rate Elimination = ke · Xb where Xa is the amount of drug at the absorption site, and Xb is the body drug content, which is set equal to Vd · Cp, or Am in equation (1), the body drug content to be maintained constant. If absorption of the loading dose is effectively complete, $kaXa = kr_0$. For case 1 in Table 14-4, ke = 0.21 (the beta disposition constant), since the biologic half-life is estimated from the terminal part of the blood level curve if a one-compartment model is used to approximate blood level data. For cases 2 and 3, ke = 0.97. The apparent volume of the central compartment, Vc, rather than

Table 14-4. *Estimated Sustained Release Design Parameters for Procainamide (Cp = 1 μg/ml, h − Tm = 8 hours)*

Parameter	Case 1	Case 2	Case 3
Am (mg)	205	59	59
kr_0 (mg/hr)	43	57	57
Tm	1.2	0.5	0
Dm (mg)	414	549	549
f	0.768	0.274	0.274
Di (mg)	322	259	(Di) 224
Dm/Di	1.28	2.12	2.45
Dm + Di (mg)	736	808	773

Vd, is used to calculate Am for the two-compartment model, i.e., Am = CpVc. For example:

Case 1:
$$kr_0 = 0.21 \times 1 \times 205$$
$$= 43 \text{ mg/hr}$$

Cases 2 and 3:
$$kr_0 = 0.97 \times 1 \times 59$$
$$= 57 \text{ mg/hr}$$

2. Estimation of Tm. Release of maintenance dose is set at the peak time for the loading dose (cases 1 and 2). Equation (3) is used to calculate the peak time from known value absorption (2 hr^{-1}) and elimination (0.21 hr^{-1}) rate constants. Since equation (3) applies only to the one-compartment model, Tm, which is actually 0.5 hours, is significantly overestimated. For example:

Case 1: $Tm = Tp$ (Eq. 3) $= \dfrac{2.3 \times \log(2/0.21)}{2 - 0.21}$
$$= 1.2 \text{ hr}$$

Case 2: Tm = Tp (actual value) = 0.5 hr

Case 3: Tm = 0

3. Estimation of Dm. The maintenance dose is estimated as the product of release rate and maintenance time (equation 6), corrected for the bioavailability factor, F (equation 4), which is the fraction of the administered dose absorbed from a reference nonsustained release dosage form. The F-value is estimated as the ratio of the area under the plasma level curve (AUC-value) measured after oral administration to the AUC-value observed after intravenous administration of the same dose of drug. In the example, F < 1, since procainamide is subject to the first-pass effect, in which a small portion of the absorbed dose is metabolized in the liver. Dm is also a function of the loading dose and an inverse function of the biological half-life, i.e., Dm = 0.693f(h − Tm) Di/$t_{\frac{1}{2}}$, a relation obtained by combining equations (2), (6), and (7). Practically, h is not likely to exceed 10 to 12 hours, depending on the residence time in the small intestine. For drugs that are not efficiently absorbed in the stomach, such as procainamide, the gastric emptying rate is an uncertain variable that contributes to Tm. For example:

Case 1: Dm = 43 × 8/0.83 = 414 mg

Cases 2 and 3: Dm = 57 × 8/0.83 = 549 mg

Significant increases in dose size are required for drugs with short biologic half-lives, e.g., Dm is doubled if the biologic half-life is halved. For case 1, Dm would be 228 mg for $t_{\frac{1}{2}} = 6$ hr, 456 mg for $t_{\frac{1}{2}} = 3$ hr, and 685 mg for $t_{\frac{1}{2}} = 2$ hr.

4. Estimation of Di. The loading dose is that portion of the total dose that is initially released as a bolus and is therefore immediately available for absorption. It results in a peak blood level equal to the desired level to be maintained. Equation (7) allows estimation of Di if Dm is delayed (cases 1 and 2). If release of Dm is not delayed (case 3), the loading dose calculated using equation (7) is adjusted for the quantity of drug provided by the zero-order release process in time Tm as shown by equation (8). For example:

Case 1: Di = 205/(0.768 × 0.83) = 327 mg

Case 2: Di = 59/(0.274 × 0.83) = 259 mg

Case 3: Di = (259 − 57 × 0.5) = 224 mg

Figure 14-4 shows the simulated blood level profiles that result from administration of theoretic sustained release dosage forms of procainamide to the average subject for the three cases

listed in Table 14-4. Curve A is the profile observed after administration of the loading dose calculated for case 2. Calculations based on the assumption of a one-compartment model (curve B) fail to approximate the desired profile adequately. The procedure suggested for estimation of kr_0, however, based on the actual two-compartment model that fits procainamide data, gives a reasonable approximation of the optimum profile (curve C). A formulation designed to release loading and maintenance doses simultaneously (case 3) results in a profile (curve D) that does not significantly differ from case 2. The total dose required to maintain a blood level of 1 μg/ml for 8 to 10 hours is about the maximum (<1 g) that can be formulated in a reasonably sized solid peroral dosage form. The usual minimum therapeutic level required for procainamide is 3 to 4 μg/ml. Multiple units of a sustained release procainamide would have to be administered at each dosing interval to attain a therapeutic level.

Computer simulation provides a valuable tool for evaluating the performance of sustained release dosage form designs. Curve E in Figure 14-4 demonstrates another application of simu-

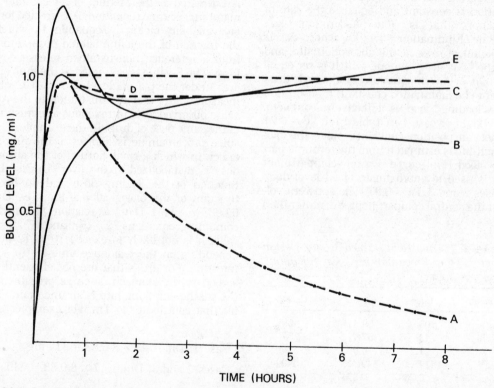

FIG. 14-4. *Simulated blood level profiles observed after administration of theoretic sustained release formulations of procainamide hydrochloride to an average patient. A, Case 2—loading dose; B, Case 1; C, Case 2; D, Case 3; E, Case 2—patient differs from average.*

lation, that is, to examine the performance of the dosage form in a patient in which the disposition of the drug (procainamide in the example) differs significantly from the average. In this subject, the pharmacokinetic parameters were as follows: $ka = 1.2$, $ke = 0.47$, $k_{12} = 0.8$, $k_{21} = 0.77$, $Vc = 101$, and $F = 0.7$. Lower blood levels are observed initially, and higher blood levels are observed at the end of the maintenance period, since the absorption rate was lower and the biologic half-life higher (approximately 4 hours) than average in this patient. Overall, the difference in response of this patient to the dosage form is not significant.

First-Order Release Approximation

The rate of release of drug from the maintenance portion of the dosage form should be zero-order if the amount of drug at the absorption site is to remain constant. Most currently marketed sustained release formulations, however, do not release drug at a constant rate, and consequently do not maintain the relative constant activity implied by Figure 14-3. Observed blood levels decrease over time until the next dose is administered. In many instances, the rate of appearance of drug at the absorption site can be approximated by an exponential or first-order process in which the rate of drug release is a function only of the amount of drug remaining in the dosage form. Table 14-5 lists the expressions that can be used to estimate the design parameters for optimized first-order release models. Three different designs are considered: Dm not delayed. Dm delayed where $Tm = Tp$, and Dm delayed where $Tm > Tp$. Table 14-6

lists the parameters calculated for a drug fitted by a one-body-compartment model, and Figure 14-5 shows the resulting profiles for each example considered. Doses listed in Table 14-6 are expressed as fractions of loading dose, using the calculation for a zero-order model (case 1, Table 14-4) as a reference.

Method 1. Simultaneous release of Dm and Di. The *crossing time,* Ti, is the time at which the blood level profiles produced by administration of separate loading and maintenance doses intersect. The closest approximation to the ideal profile is obtained if the crossing point is made at least equal to the desired maintenance period $(h - Tp)$. Equation (9) shown in Table 14-5, is an approximation of equation (11) where $ke > kr_1$. The maintenance dose is estimated from the initial release rate, i.e., $kr_1 Dm = keAm = kr_0$. The loading dose is estimated by correcting the immediate release dose required to achieve the maintenance level for the quantity of drug delivered by the maintenance dose in the time Tp. For example:

$$Ti = 9.2 - 1.2 = 8 \text{ hr}$$

$$kr_1 = 0.23 \exp(-0.23 \times 8) = 0.055 \text{ hr}$$

$$Dm = 0.173/0.055 = 3.1$$

$$Di = (0.75/0.75 \times 1) - 0.173 \times 1.2 = 0.8$$

Method 2. Delayed release of Dm: Tm = Tp. If Dm is large and kr is made small, maintenance dose may be released as a pseudo-zero-order process. As a first approximation, kr_1 may be estimated as the reciprocal of the maintenance time. Dm is then calculated as in method 1. Better approximation of a zero-order response can be obtained if Dm is increased and kr_1 is reduced to maintain the product $kr_1 DM$ con-

TABLE 14-5. *Expressions Useful for Estimation of Design Parameters for First-Order Sustained Release Dosage Form Models*

Parameter	Method 1	Method 2	Method 3
Tm	0	Tp (Eq. 3)	$4.6/ka$ (Eq. 10)
Ti	$(h - Tp)$	—	$(h - Tp)/2$
kr_1	$ke(\exp(-keTi))$ (Eq. 9)	$1/(h - Tp)$	$Ti = \dfrac{2.3\log(kr_1/ke)}{(kr_1 - ke)}$ (Eq. 11)
Dm	kr_0/kr_1	kr_0/kr_1	$Dm = \dfrac{ke(Am - Ai)}{kr_1} \exp(kr_1(2Ti - Tm)$ (Eq. 12) $Ai = \dfrac{Dika}{(ka - ke)} \exp(-ke(Ti + Tm))$ (Eq. 13)
Di	$CpVd/fF - kr_0Tp$	$CpVd/fF$	$CpVd/fF$

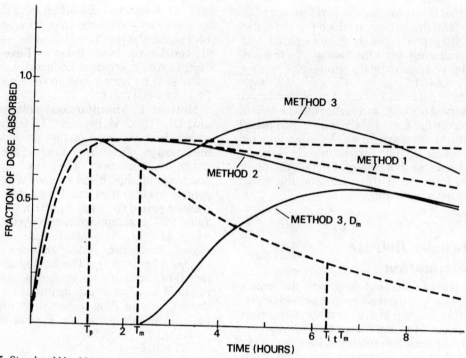

FIG. 14-5. *Simulated blood level profiles observed after administration of a theoretic sustained release dosage form to an average patient based on different first-order release models. Blood level is plotted as the fraction of dose absorbed (CpVd/FDi).*

stant. For example:

$$Tm = Tp = 1.2 \text{ hr}$$

$$kr_1 = 1/(9.2 - 1.2) = 0.125 \text{ hr}$$

$$Dm = 0.173/0.125 = 1.4$$

$$Di = 0.75/0.75 \times 1 = 1$$

Since $kr_1 Dm = 0.173$, then kr_1 should be reduced to 0.86 if Dm is increased to 2.0, to maintain this product constant.

Method 3. Delayed release of Dm: Tm > Tp. Increasing the delay time, Tm, allows the use of faster release rates. A period equal to the time at

which 99% of the loading dose has been absorbed is selected using equation (10) in Table 14-5. The release rate constant is iteratively calculated from equation (11) such that a peak is obtained from the maintenance dose at the midpoint of the maintenance time. The amount of drug required to produce a second peak at this time is the maintenance dose, calculated from equations (12, 13). For example:

$$Tm = 4.6/2.0 = 2.3 \text{ hr}$$

$$Ti = (9.2 - 1.2)/2 = 4 \text{ hr}$$

$$4 = 2.3 \times \log(kr_1/0.23)/(kr_1 - 0.23)$$

TABLE 14-6. *Estimated Design Parameters for a First-Order Sustained Release Model**

Parameter	Zero-Order	Method 1	Method 2	Method 3
Tm hr	1.2	0	1.2	2.3
Ti hr	—	8	—	4
kr_1 hr	($kr_0 = 0.173$)	0.055	0.125	0.27
Dm/Di	1.4	3.1	1.4	1.45
Di	1.0	0.8	1.0	1.0
(Di + Dm)/Di	2.4	3.9	2.4	2.45

*Drug Characteristics: One-Compartment Model

$t_{\frac{1}{2}} = 3$ hr	ka = 2 hr	ke = 0.23 hr	f = 0.75
Tp = 1.2 hr	h = 9.2 hr	F = 1	CpVd = 0.75

(Solve this expression iteratively by finding the value of kr_1 that satisfies the equality: in this case, $kr_1 = 0.27$.)

$$Di = 0.75/0.75 \times 1 = 1$$

$$Ai = (1 \times 2)\exp(-0.23(4 + 2.3))/(2.0 - 0.23) = 0.267$$

$$Am = kr_0/ke = 0.173/0.23 = 0.74$$

$$Dm = (0.23/0.27)(0.74 - 0.267)\exp(0.27(2 \times 4 - 2.3)) = 1.45$$

Methods 1 and 2 have the disadvantage that large maintenance doses are required, resulting in a significant loss of drug available for absorption. In the examples plotted in Figure 14-5, 50% of the dose calculated using method 1 and 30% of the dose calculated using method 2 were not available after 10 hours. Method 1 represents a design that is least efficient in terms of the dose required to achieve the design objective. Drugs characterized by large loading doses and small biologic half-lives could not be practically formulated in these designs. In spite of the fluctuation observed in the profile characterizing method 3, a reasonably average level is maintained with a minimum maintenance dose. Furthermore, only 15% of the dose remains unreleased after 10 hours. The maximum dose, which usually should be formulated in a sustained release dosage form, should not exceed the total dose administered by conventional forms during the maintenance period. If the total dose is released all at once, it should not result in a blood level exceeding the maximum safe level.

Optimization of sustained release dosage form design requires minimization of the total dose delivered and maximization of the duration of drug release. In the case of the zero-order model, adjustment of the maintenance dose is a function only of the duration time. Designs based on simultaneous release of Dm and Di require the minimum total dose (e.g., case 3, Table 14-4). Optimum first-order designs are those in which Dm is delayed beyond the peak obtained from the loading dose (e.g., method 3, Fig. 14-5).

From a practical point of view, the procedures summarized here provide a starting point for implementation. The use of mean values for parameters and the inherent variation in the population using the dosage form often lead to larger variations than the errors resulting from the approximate nature of these calculations. Where therapeutic effect cannot be correlated with measured body drug content, or where such measurements cannot be obtained, a clinically determined dosage regimen can be used as a basis for estimation of Dm-values. One may assume that Dm equals the sum of the maintenance doses ordinarily administered in the desired maintenance time. For example, for a drug administered 4 times a day, Di is the single dose, and Dm the sum of two doses for a maintenance period of 12 hours. As a rule of thumb, the total drug dose can be reduced from 5 to 10%.

Multiple Dosing

Like conventional dosage forms, peroral sustained release forms are administered as multiple dosing regimens in which the objective is to maintain the required average drug level for the duration of therapy with a minimal fluctuation between doses. If the dosing interval is made equal to (or less than) the total anticipated drug release time (Fig. 14-6, curve A), accumulation results from formulations designed with loading doses. Significant blood level peaks may be observed with the zero-order release model; however, minimal fluctuation between administered doses can be obtained if the dosing interval is set equal to $(h + t_i)$, as shown by curve B (Fig. 14-6). Increasing the dosing interval further while diminishing the peak also deepens the trough in the drug level profile, defeating one of the objectives of the dosage form design. Even with the zero-order model, multiple dosing therapy can result in non-ideal drug level profiles.

In sustained release therapy, only the dosing interval is adjustable. If two units are initially administered followed by single-unit subsequent doses, as is common in therapy with nonsustained forms, a slow fall in overall drug level occurs after several doses to the average level determined by the dosage form design. Welling has described several strategies for attaining approximations of the ideal profile in the multiple dosing of different sustained release designs based on both cumulative and noncumulative approaches.[5]

Alternately, administration of formulations designed without loading doses can result in minimal fluctuation during long term therapy. In Figure 14-6, curve C shows the result of this type of multiple dosing regimen where a zero-order based design consisting only of the slow release maintenance dose is administered at intervals of h hours. If absorption is consistent, profiles obtained are equivalent to those resulting from administration of drug by constant rate infusion (curve E, Fig. 14-1), with one dosing interval required to attain near-steady-state drug levels. Accumulation does not take place unless

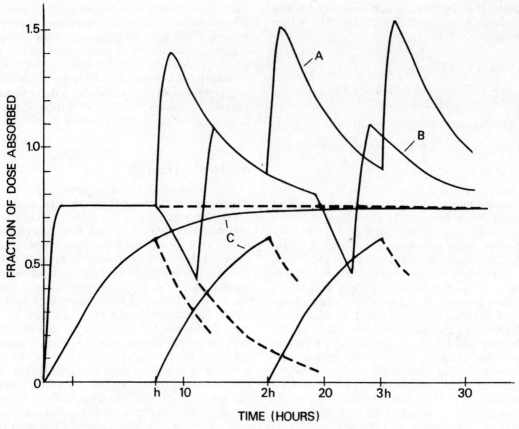

FIG. 14-6. *Multiple patterns of dosage of sustained release dosage forms where ka = 2 hr, ke = 0.23 hr, (t = 3 hr), F = 1, and H = 8 hr. Dosage intervals are: A, 8 hr; B, 12 hr; and C, 8 hr with no loading dose.*

the dosing interval is made less than the effective maintenance time.

Implementation of Designs

Approaches Based on Drug Modification

Two general sets of methods have been developed for implementation of practical sustained release dosage form designs: methods based on modification of the physical and/or chemical properties of the drug and methods based on modification of the drug release rate characteristics of the dosage that affect bioavailability. The physicochemical properties of a drug may be altered through complex formation, drug-adsorbate preparation, or prodrug synthesis. These techniques are possible only with drug moieties containing appropriate functional groups (e.g., acidic or basic). The principal advantage of this approach to sustained release is that it is independent of the dosage form design. Drugs so

modified may be formulated as liquid suspensions, capsules, or tablets. Loading doses of unmodified drug may also be incorporated in formulations that are ordinarily formulated to release both unmodified and modified drugs without significant delay.

Figure 14-7 identifies the mechanisms involved in controlling the release of drug from complexes, adsorbates, and prodrugs. In the case of drug complexes, the effective release rate is a function of two processes: the rate of dissolution of the solid complex into the biologic fluids and the rate of dissociation or breakdown of the complex in solution. In general, the dissolution step may be described by the following expression:

Rate Dissolution = ks(Solubility)(Surface Area)

where ks is the dissolution rate constant, a function of the hydrodynamic state as well as factors influencing the diffusion process (e.g., viscosity).

The formulator has the option of altering sur-

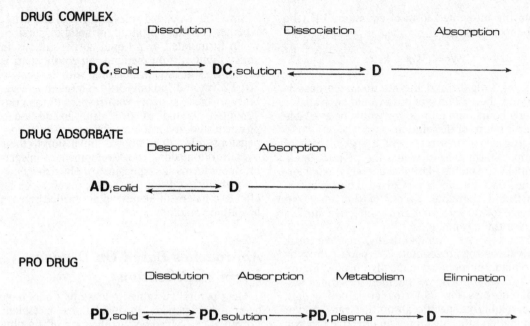

DRUG COMPLEX

Dissolution   Dissociation   Absorption

$$DC,\text{solid} \rightleftarrows DC,\text{solution} \rightleftarrows D \longrightarrow$$

DRUG ADSORBATE

Desorption   Absorption

$$AD,\text{solid} \rightleftarrows D \longrightarrow$$

PRO DRUG

Dissolution   Absorption   Metabolism   Elimination

$$PD,\text{solid} \rightleftarrows PD,\text{solution} \longrightarrow PD,\text{plasma} \longrightarrow D \longrightarrow$$

FIG. 14-7. *Mechanisms of sustained release based on drug modification.*

face area through particle size control and/or solubility of the drug complex through selection of the complexing agent. While both processes are dependent on the pH and composition of the gastric and intestinal fluids, the dissociation step is critically so, since its rate may be pH-dependent, may be determined by the ionic composition of the fluid, and may be affected by the natural digestive processes including enzymatic and bile salt action. The formulator should select the appropriate complex for preparation with knowledge of the specific in vivo processes involved in the control of drug release from the complex. For example, tannate complexes of bases are hydrolyzed in both acidic and basic media, the dissociation of the complex being more rapid at the gastric pH. Drug release from cationic ion-exchange resin complexes depends on sodium ion concentration in GI fluids, and although a stearate salt of a weak base resists the action of gastric fluid, natural digestive processes in the intestine act to dissociate the complex.

If the rate of dissolution is greater than the rate of dissociation, a zero-order release pattern might be realized, because the concentration of complex is maintained at its saturation point if the solubility of the complex is sufficiently low so that excess solid complex is present during most of the effective maintenance time. In this case, high specific surface material should be prepared to promote dissolution. On the other

hand, if the rate of dissociation is greater than the rate of dissolution, the dissolution of the complex is rate-determining. Particle size of the complex should be adjusted to establish the most appropriate rate of release. With sufficient excess solid phase, a zero-order release may also be approximated. The complex may be viewed in this instance as simply a means of reducing the solubility of the drug in order to reduce its availability.

Equation (14) describes the rate (R) at which drug is made available through dissolution under conditions of diminishing surface:

$$R = \frac{4.85 DCs\, W^{\frac{2}{3}}}{h\rho^{\frac{2}{3}}} = ks'W^{\frac{2}{3}} \qquad (14)$$

where D is the diffusion coefficient, h is the thickness of the diffusion layer, Cs is the solubility, ρ is the density, and W is the weight of undissolved solid. This expression has been derived assuming that the simple diffusion-layer model applies, that the particles are spherical in form, and that a near sink condition is maintained with respect to dissolved complex. Consequently, the rate of drug availability, expressed as the rate of decrease in mass of undissolved complex, diminishes during the effective maintenance period if the surface area decreases as drug is dissolved and absorbed. The amount of drug available at any time can be calculated from the integrated form of equation (14) (the cube-root law):

$$W^{\frac{1}{3}} = (Wo^{\frac{1}{3}} - ks't) \qquad (15)$$

If $ks' = 3$ mg$^{\frac{1}{3}}$/hr and the maintenance dose is 900 mg, then 324 mg of drug would be available after 4 hours, and only 36 mg would be available after 8 hours of dissolution.

Drug adsorbates represent a special case of complex formation in which the product is essentially insoluble. Drug availability is determined only by the rate of dissociation (desorption), and therefore, access of the adsorbent surface to water as well as the effective surface area of the adsorbate.

Prodrugs are therapeutically inactive drug derivatives that regenerate the parent drug by enzymatic or nonenzymatic hydrolysis. Figure 14-7 shows the scheme that identifies the potential processes for achieving sustained action. The solubility, specific absorption rate, and/or elimination rate constant of an effective prodrug should be significantly lower than that of the parent compound. Kwan has described the pharmacokinetics of a prodrug in which the sustained blood level is determined by the metabolic rate, i.e., by formation of the active moiety after absorption.[6] If the solubility of a drug has been significantly reduced by the formation of prodrug, and if breakdown of the prodrug takes place at the absorption site, then availability is limited by dissolution rate, and the same arguments as in the case of an insoluble drug complex apply. Examples of drugs from which prodrugs designed for prolonged action have been synthesized include isoproterenol, isoniazid, and penicillin.[7]

Approaches based on drug modification are sensitive to in vivo conditions. An important objective of sustained release formulation is to minimize the effect of in vivo variables on drug release. An alternate approach, which has been advanced by Banker, involves preparation of drug dispersions through "molecular scale drug entrapment" in suitable carrier materials that act to retard release.[8] Compositions of this type can be prepared by induced flocculation of a polymer latex (e.g., acrylic copolymers). Control of drug release is accomplished by varying the nature of the carrier material, the loading dose of drug, and particle size of the product (i.e., surface area). These systems follow a scheme similar to that suggested for drug adsorbates. They also have the advantage of allowing formulation of different dosage forms and may, with appropriate selection of the carrier, be less influenced by in vivo variables.

Since the extended release form of the drug, whether complex, prodrug, or solid dispersion, when formulated as a liquid suspension, is in contact with a fluid medium, an equilibrium is estabhshed in the formulation with respect to "free" drug and "bound" drug. The chemical stability of these systems with respect to the conversion of "bound" to "free" drug, in addition to physical stability problems characteristic of suspensions, adds an additional dimension to their overall formulation. The development of injectable depot forms as suspensions of physicochemically modified drugs has been proven to be an effective means of achieving controlled release in antibiotic therapy.

Approaches Based On Dosage Form Modification

Most peroral sustained release products have been formulated as encapsulations or tablets. Formulations based on modification of the physicochemical properties of these dosage forms can be classed into three product types: encapsulated slow release beads (or granules), tabletted mixed or slow release granulations, and slow release (core) tablets. Fabrication of tablets allows for direct incorporation of loading doses, by preparation of either multilayered or press-coated tablets. One layer or the outer coat of the tablet is prepared from a potentially rapid disintegrating granulation, leaving the less quickly disintegrating layer or core, which contains the maintenance dose. Systems prepared as tabletted mixed released granulations may or may not be designed to disintegrate quickly, simulating the administration of an encapsulated form in the latter case.

Encapsulated sustained release dosage forms have two specific advantages over core tablet designs. (1) Undisintegrated tablets may remain in the stomach for extended periods of time, excessively delaying absorption of the maintenance dose. Disintegration of the capsule shell in the gastric fluid releases particles that can pass unimpeded through the pyloric valve. (2) There is statistical assurance of drug release with encapsulated forms, since release of drug by a significant fraction of the granules is highly probable. If a core tablet fails to release drug, all of the maintenance dose is lost.

Two general principles are involved in retarding drug release from most practical sustained release formulations involving dosage form modification. These are the embedded matrix and the barrier principle, which are schematically shown in Figures 14-8 and 14-9. In the

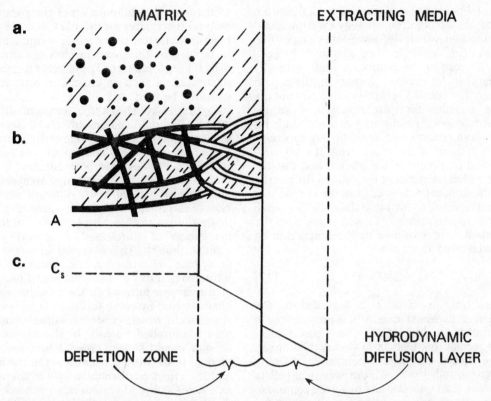

MATRIX   EXTRACTING MEDIA

a.

b.

A

c. C$_s$

DEPLETION ZONE   HYDRODYNAMIC
                                DIFFUSION LAYER

FIG. 14-8. *Embedded matrix concept as a mechanism of controlled release in sustained release dosage form design. Network model (a): drug is insoluble in the retardant material. Dispersion model (b): drug is soluble in the retardant material. Diffusion profile (c) characterizes drug release from a matrix system.*

former case, drug is dispersed (embedded) in a matrix of retardant material, which may be encapsulated in particulate form or compressed into tablets. Release is controlled by a combination of several physical processes. These include

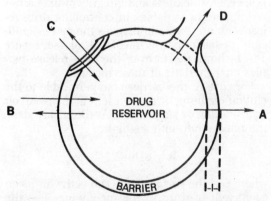

FIG. 14-9. *Barrier-mediated models of sustained release dosage form designs. A, Drug diffusion through the barrier. B, Permeation of barrier by elution media followed by drug diffusion. C, Erosion of barrier, releasing drug. D, Rupture of barrier as a result of permeation of elution media.*

permeation of the matrix by water, leaching (extraction or diffusion) of drug from the matrix, and erosion of matrix material. Alternately, drug may dissolve in the matrix material and be released by diffusion through the matrix material or partitioned between the matrix and extracting fluid. Matrices may be prepared from insoluble or erodable materials (e.g., silicone polymers or lipids).

Higuchi has provided the theoretic basis for defining drug release from inert matrices.[9] The equation describing drug release from the planar surface of an insoluble matrix is:

$$Q = [(D\epsilon Cs/\tau)(2A - \epsilon Cs)t]^{\frac{1}{2}} \qquad (16)$$

where Q is the amount of drug released per unit surface after time t, D is the diffusion coefficient of the drug in the elution medium, τ is the tortuosity of the matrix, ϵ is the porosity of the matrix, Cs is the solubility of the drug in the elution medium, and A is the initial loading dose of drug in the matrix. This expression was derived assuming a linear diffusion gradient as diagrammed in Figure 14-8c. Drug release is triggered by penetration of eluting media into the matrix, dissolving drug, thereby creating channels through which diffusion takes place (Fig. 14-8b). The depletion zone gradually extends into the core of the matrix. A high tortuosity means that the effective average diffusion path is large. The porosity term takes into account the space available for drug dissolution; an increased porosity results in increased drug release. Both porosity and tortuosity are functions of the amount of dispersed drug, the physicochemical properties of the matrix, and the dispersion characteristics of the drug in the matrix.

If the drug is freely soluble in the elution medium, i.e., $Cs \gg A$, such that the dissolution rate is rapid, then equation (17), which describes the release of drug from a solution entrapped in an insoluble matrix, applies:

$$Q = 2A(Dt/\pi\tau)^{\frac{1}{2}} \qquad (17)$$

Release rate is directly proportional to the amount of dispersed drug, A; it is proportional to $A^{\frac{1}{2}}$ for insoluble drugs if $2A = Cs$. These expressions predict that plots of Q versus $t^{\frac{1}{2}}$ be linear.

The theory has been extended to defining matrix-controlled release from spherical pellets as well as from cylindric and biconvex compacts. In Chien's description of the application of a general expression for the case of a drug dispersed in a matrix in which the drug dissolves (Fig. 14-8a), both matrix and partition control are possible.[10] The drug has low solubility in the elution media, partition control dominates, and the release is zero-order, that is:

$$Q = KDCst/h \qquad (18)$$

where K is the partition coefficient ($K = Cs/Cp$), Cp is the solubility in the matrix phase, and h is the thickness of the hydrodynamic diffusion layer. A modified form of equation (16) applies in the former case (diffusion takes place in the matrix phase), in which the drug has a high solubility in the elution media.

These expressions have been successfully applied to interpreting drug release from insoluble polymer matrices as well as from such potentially erodable materials as wax-lipid compositions and hydrophilic polymers. With the latter, hydration of the polymer forms a gel, which controls the initial stages of drug release. The variables affecting drug release, which have been studied using these models, have included the nature of retardant, drug solubility, effect of added diluents, drug loading, drug mixtures, and drug-matrix interaction.[11] The rate of drug release from embedded matrices is capable of

adjustment by manipulation of the parameters defined by equations (16), (17), and (18). The release characteristics of a base formulation can be defined by the slopes of plots of cumulative drug released versus $t_{\frac{1}{2}}$. The effect of formulation modifications such as change in drug loading can then be predicted.

Figure 14-10 shows the forms of different drug-release profiles from different dosage form planar models, including zero-order (curve A), first-order (curve B), and square root of time (curve C). Profiles have been adjusted to show 50% release at the same time. Analysis of in vitro release data of many different sustained release formulations has demonstrated a pseudo-first-order release characteristic, if the log percentage of unreleased drug was plotted against time.[12]. The observed apparent first-order rate constants, however, could not be interpreted in terms of the fundamental properties of the dosage form as in the case for systems characterized by curve C. Curve D represents a situation in which erosion is superimposed on matrix-controlled release. In the planar case, erosion should be zero-order, a function of the product of the drug concentration in the matrix and the effective dissolution rate of the retardant. Release due to erosion is, in general, more rapid than matrix-controlled release. This has been demonstrated with dispersions of chlorpheniramine maleate in methylcellulose matrices.[13]

The barrier concept of controlled release implies that a layer of retardant material is imposed between the drug and the elution medium.[14] Drug release results from diffusion of drug through the barrier, permeation of the barrier by moisture, and/or erosion of the barrier. In addition to barrier composition and physicochemical properties, thickness and integrity of the barrier are important variables in controlling drug release. Figure 14-9 summarizes the more significant models of barrier-mediated release. Figure 14-11 shows the form of the drug-release profiles characteristic of these models.

For case A, the barrier is impermeable to the elution medium; drug is present in the reservoir as a solution or suspension. At the steady state, the release rate into a sink is:

$$R = SDmC_{sm}/1 \qquad (19)$$

where S is the surface area, Dm is the diffusion coefficient of drug in the membrane, 1 is the thickness of the membrane barrier, and Cs_m is the solubility of drug in the membrane, assuming constant activity of drug in the reservoir. For the membrane-encapsulated solution, release is

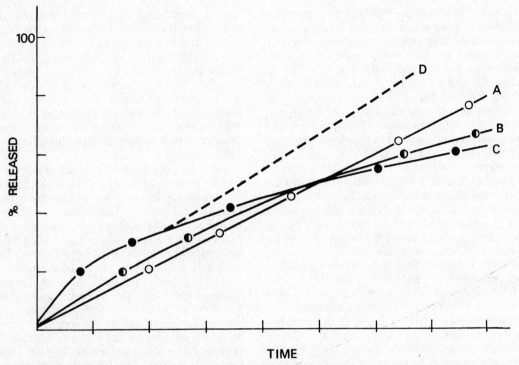

FIG. 14-10. *Drug-release profiles characteristic of different dosage form models representing embedded matrix systems. A, Zero-order model. B, First-order model. C, Diffusion model. D, Diffusion model with erosion.*

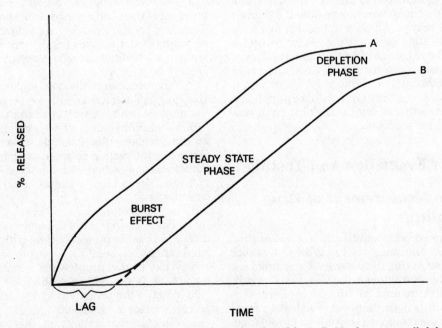

FIG. 14-11. *Drug-release profiles characteristic of barrier-mediated models. A, B, Membrane-controlled diffusion.*

first-order. If membrane diffusion is slower than dissolution, release is zero-order for membrane-encapsulated suspensions. Two forms of release profiles may be observed: a burst effect if the membrane is saturated with drug (Fig. 14-11, curve A), and a time lag if drug has not penetrated the membrane (Fig. 14-11, curve B). Drug release approximates first-order kinetics during the depletion phase. This principle has been successfully applied in the development of ophthalmic, intravaginal, and transdermal controlled release devices.

For case B (Fig. 14-9), in which the barrier is permeable to the elution media, a time lag is involved since drug is not released until moisture has penetrated the barrier, dissolving drug in the reservoir. Additional mechanisms might involve timed erosion of the barrier (case C) or rupture of the barrier after sufficient moisture has permeated the membrane (case D).

The pharmaceutical formulator can select from a variety of potential sustained release dosage form designs.[15] Those based on drug modification are limited to drugs with appropriate structural characteristics. In principle, dosage form designs may be applied to all drug types; however, the selection of a particular dosage form may be limited by the specific drug properties (e.g., solubility, dissociation constant, stability, etc.), the manufacturing technology available, and the methodology needed to establish the validity of the design. For example, water-insoluble drugs may not be suited to designs based on the embedded matrix principle using insoluble matrices, but may be suited to barrier controlled release, which is applicable to a wide variety of drug characteristics. Prior to beginning the development of a practical formulation, the formulator must have established an in vitro testing methodology to serve as an aid to formulation, and have a clear view of the requirements for in vivo testing of drug availability from sustained release products.

Product Evaluation and Testing

In Vitro Measurement of Drug Availability

It is not possible to simulate in a single in vitro test system the range of variables that affect drug release during the passage of sustained release medication through the GI tract. Properly designed in vitro tests for drug release serve two important functions, however. First, data from such tests are required as a guide to formulation during the development stage, prior to clinical testing. Second, in vitro testing is necessary to ensure batch-to-batch uniformity in the production of a proven dosage form. Different methods are usually required by these two distinctly different testing situations. Although attempts to correlate in vitro release profiles with clinical performance are useful once sufficient clinical testing has been completed, in-vitro/in-vivo correlation must not be assumed. In vitro studies are not sufficient to establish the efficacy of a new preparation.

Tests developed for the purpose of quality control are generally limited to USP dissolution testing methods, using either the rotating basket (apparatus 1), the paddle (apparatus 2), or the modified disintegration testing apparatus (apparatus 3). In many instances in which USP test procedures are followed, upper and lower limits are specified for drug release in simulated gastric and/or intestinal fluid. Measurements are made at specified time intervals appropriate to the specific product. Complete release profiles are not measured unless automated techniques are used. At present, there are no specific USP specifications for sustained release dosage forms. Procedures are determined by nature of the dosage form (e.g., tablet or capsule), the principle utilized to control drug release (e.g., disintegrating or nondisintegrating), and the maintenance period.

During formulation development, testing methods should be designed to provide answers to the following questions.

1. Does the product "dump" maintenance dose before the maintenance period is complete? Sustained release products are subject to either of two modes of failure: Insufficient dose is released, or too much drug is made available too quickly.

2. What fraction of the dose remains unavailable, i.e., what fraction will not be released in the projected time of transit in the GI tract?

3. What is the effect of physiologic variables on drug release? For example, delayed gastric emptying, interaction between drug and GI constituents, composition and volume of GI fluids, and variation in intensity of agitation should be considered.

4. Is the loading dose (if present) released immediately? Is release of the maintenance dose delayed? If so, is the delay time within the desired range?

5. What is the unit-to-unit variation? How predictable is the release profile?

6. What is the sensitivity of the drug release profile to process variables?

7. What is the stability of the formulation with respect to its drug release profile?

8. In short, does the observed release profile fit expectations?

The methods used to measure drug release profiles should have the following characteristics. The analytic technique should be automated so that the complete drug release profile can be directly recorded. Allowance should be made for changing the release media from simulated gastric to simulated intestinal fluid at variable programmed time intervals, to establish the effect of retention of the dosage form in gastric fluid as well as to approximate more closely the pH shifts that the dosage form is likely to encounter in vivo. In addition, the hydrodynamic state in the dissolution vessel should be controllable and capable of variation. The apparatus should be calibrated using a nondisintegrating dissolution standard (e.g., salicylic acid compacts).

Besides the USP dissolution testing apparatus, testing equipment used for in vitro testing of sustained action formulations have included the rotating bottle, stationary basket/rotating filter, Sartorius absorption and solubility simulator, and column-type flow-through assembly. The rotating bottle method was developed for evaluation of sustained release formulations.[16] Samples are tested in 90-ml bottles containing 60 ml of fluid, which are rotated end over end in a 37° bath at 40 rpm. The method is not adaptable to automated analysis, however, or to easy manipulation of the dissolution media. The Sartorius device includes an artificial lipid membrane, which separates the "dissolution" chamber from a simulated plasma compartment in which drug concentrations are measured. Alternately, a dialysis type membrane may be used. Systems of this type are advantageous in measuring release profiles of disintegrating dosage units, and suspension, granular, and powdered material, if the permeability of the membrane is properly defined. The column flow-through apparatus possesses similar advantages since drug release is confined to a relatively small chamber by highly permeable membrane filters. This apparatus is flexible, well-defined, and meets all the necessary requirements for measurement of drug release profiles from sustained release dosage forms. It can also be adapted to measurements under near sink conditions if the release medium is passed only once through the dissolution chamber, directly measuring the rate of release. Alternately, the dissolution fluid might be recirculated continuously from the reservoir, allowing measurement of the cumulative release profile. The composition of the release media as well as the flow rate can readily be altered.

The time of testing may vary from 6 to 12 hours, depending on the design specifications of the dosage form. If formulations contain retardants whose function depends on the action of normal constituents of the GI fluids (e.g., bile salts, pancreatin, and pepsin), then the appropriate materials must be included in the simulated release media. Apparatus of the Sartorius type would be advantageous in these circumstances if the analytic procedure for the drug would be adversely affected by the presence of these substances. Otherwise, the simulated fluids consisting of pH 1.2 and 7.2 buffers, as well as intermediate pH-values, which represent the transition between gastric and intestinal pH, would suffice at 37°. For insoluble dosage forms, flow rates should be set at the practical maximum to minimize diffusion in the hydrodynamic layer at the dosage form interface as a significant factor affecting release. For disintegrating or erodable units, measurements should be obtained at several rates of fluid flow to establish the effect of this variable, so that conditions can then be established to generate a release profile encompassing the length of time the dosage form is designed to release drug in vivo. Encapsulated products should be removed from the capsule shell for testing.

Figure 14-12 shows the observed release profile of an encapsulated slow release bead form of papaverine hydrochloride, measured in a flow-

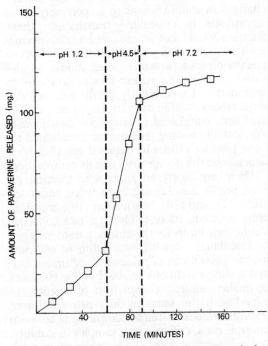

FIG. 14-12. *In vitro release profile of a papaverine hydrochloride sustained release capsule.*

through apparatus at three pH-values.[17] No significant effect of flow rate was observed for this product. The profiles show that the amount of drug released depends on the length of time the formulation is in contact with gastric fluid, and more significantly, on the length of time it is exposed to media of pH 4 to 5, i.e., the transition between gastric and intestinal pH. In effect, release is controlled by the dissolution characteristics of the drug and apparently not by the dosage form design. Papaverine has maximum solubility at pH 4.5. These data demonstrate the importance of measuring release profiles from dosage units exposed to a variety of conditions in a single test.

As with all pharmaecutical dosage forms, stability testing is an important aspect of the development stage. The same standards that apply to conventional dosage forms with respect to active ingredient stability and dosage form integrity should be used. The stability testing program includes storage of the formulation under both normal (shelf) and exaggerated temperatures so that appropriate extrapolations for long-term stability can be made. The stability of the release profile in addition to that of the active ingredient must be assessed.

Most sustained release formulations are complex. They may be formulated with ingredients that often present special problems regarding their physical stability upon storage. Furthermore, accelerated stability testing may induce changes in some systems (e.g., polymorphic or amorphous to crystalline transitions); these changes would not be observed under normal shelf storage conditions. In addition, observed release profiles measured after storage at elevated temperatures reflect loss of drug due to degradation. Consequently, predictions of long-term release profile stability based on accelerated tests could lead to erroneous conclusions. The stability testing program for a sustained release product cannot be outlined specifically. It depends on the dosage form and its composition.

There are many advantages to treating release-profile data kinetically by using equations (16), (17), and (18), or equation (19), or a first-order approximation, to obtain a rate constant. Confidence limits for the kinetic parameters can be calculated, allowing establishment of limits for the percentage of released drug under limited testing conditions established for purposes of quality control. Comparison of results obtained with the same product using different testing methods as well as comparisons between multiple runs, different lots, samples in stability, and different products can be made more readily.

In Vivo Measurement of Drug Availability

Validation of sustained release product designs can be achieved only by in vivo testing. The basic objective is to establish the bioequivalence of the product for which a controlled release claim is to be made with conventional dosage forms of the formulated drug.[18] Since no unnecessary human testing should be done, animal models, such as dogs, should be used initially during the product development stage to tune the formulation to the desired specifications. It is necessary to verify that dumping or insufficient drug availability are not observed in vivo. Tests in both animal and subsequent human trials should include periodic blood level determinations, comparison of urinary excretion patterns, serial radiophotographs (in humans) to follow the course of the dosage form in the GI tract, and sequential observations of pharmacologic activity. In some instances (e.g., with insoluble core tablets), egested dosage forms should be recovered and assayed for drug content. If drug level cannot be measured in biologic fluids, then the pharmacologic effect must be observed as a function of time, or clinical trials must be designed, to establish the effectiveness of the drug product.

The FDA has promulgated the general bioavailability and bioequivalence requirements for drug products.[19] These are made to ensure that the new drug product meets its controlled release claims, that no dose dumping occurs, that performance is consistent between individual dosage units, and that steady-state drug levels obtained with the product are equivalent to currently marketed products with approved new drug applications (NDAs). Reference materials can include the pure drug substance in solution or suspension as well as conventional dosage forms administered according to their usual dosage schedules or according to the dosage schedule of the controlled release product. Bioavailability studies are ordinarily single-dose comparisons of tested drug products in normal adults in a fasting state. A crossover design in which all subjects receive both the product and reference material on different days is preferred. Guidelines for clinical testing have been published for multiple-dose steady-state studies as well as for single-dose studies. Correlation of pharmacologic activity or clinical evidence of therapeutic effectiveness with bioavailability may be necessary to validate the clinical significance of controlled release claims.

Figure 14-13 shows one example of the type of data required in an in vivo study designed to

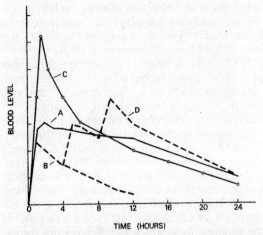

FIG. 14-13. *In vivo validation of a sustained release tablet of phendimetrazine tartrate. A, 105-mg sustained release tablet. B, 35-mg nonsustained release tablet. C, 105-mg nonsustained release tablet. D, 35-mg nonsustained release tablet administered q4h for three doses.*

demonstrate the validity of a sustained release product design.[20] Comparison is made between blood level profiles observed after administration of a single unit of the sustained release product (curve A), a conventional tablet form containing the usual single dose of active ingredient (curve B), the total dose in the sustained release form as a tablet (curve C), and the total dose administered as three divided doses at the recommended dosing interval (curve D). Samples should be taken over a period of 24 hours or three half-lives of the active ingredient at sufficient frequency to permit reasonable estimation of peak concentrations. Pharmacokinetic model-independent methods are best employed to quantitate the data. The data represented in Figure 14-13 show the equivalence between administration of the sustained release form and that of three divided doses of drug. Equivalence is demonstrated by comparison of measured blood levels and the AUC-values (area under blood level curve).

While single-dose studies are usually sufficient to establish the validity of sustained release dosage form designs, multiple-dose studies are required to establish the optimum dosing regimen. They are also required when differences may exist in the rate but not the extent of absorption, when there is excessive subject-to-subject variation, or when the observed blood levels after a single dose are too low to be measured accurately. A sufficient number of doses must be administered to attain steady-state blood levels. According to an extensive study of sustained release theophylline products, for ex-

ample, encapsulated forms showed less peaking during multiple dosing, and therefore, better control of blood level within the desired limits.[21]

Attempts to correlate in vivo performance with in vitro availability tests generally have been based on "single-point" measurements. For example, AUC-values, peak blood levels, or peak times might be correlated with the time required for 50% of drug to be released in vitro. The best that can be expected from this approach is a rank-order correlation. Significant bioavailability difference between formulations might be masked by improper in vitro methods, or drug release studies might indicate a greater difference than is actually seen in vivo.

Two general approaches to interrelating in vivo and in vitro measurements of drug release have been suggested. In one approach, an in vitro release profile is transformed into a predicted in vivo response. A weighting function characterizing a reference product is determined between the release profile and the average in vivo response, which is measured in a panel of human subjects by the mathematical operation of deconvolution. The in vivo response, predicted in vitro, of the dosage form undergoing testing is obtained by convolution of the observed release profile and the weighting function. The method has been successfully applied to prediction of plasma levels of warfarin and acetazolamide from tablet dissolution data. The technique is computationally complex, but maximizes the amount of information derived from in vitro dissolution testing.[22] Alternately, a reference blood level profile is used as the input to a feedback-controlled dissolution testing apparatus, which is subsequently forced to yield a release profile close to the standard by dynamically changing release media and flow rates. The conditions established using the reference product are used for testing other formulations. Application of these techniques to sustained release products requires a similar formulation as the reference.

In the second approach, the apparent in vivo drug release profile is computed from smoothed blood level or urinary excretion data.[23] This technique requires knowledge of the pharmacokinetic model of the drug. The in vivo data are used as input to a computer simulation of the pharmacokinetic model; the output represents the amount of drug released at the absorption site as a function of time. Beckett, in applying this method to a sustained release form of phendimetrazine, found that measured in vitro release rates were significantly faster than computed in vivo release rates.[23]

In vivo testing involves a number of simplifying assumptions regarding the uniformity of the absorption process and the suitability of using average data points to represent the population. Since the formulator has no control over physiologic variables, it is essential that clinical studies be based on sufficiently large cross-sections of the population to provide meaningful results. Both in vivo and in vitro testing methods play a major part in validating the effectiveness of sustained release formulations.

Practical Formulation

Drug Complexes

The principal advantage of preparing drug derivatives for sustained release is that such materials can be formulated into diverse dosage forms. This approach has proven effective in the development of injectable depot forms, in which release profiles are not subject to the variability characteristic of the gastrointestinal tract. Sensitivity to in vivo variables is a definite disadvantage of perorally administered forms: in vivo studies may not consistently support sustained release claims.

If an alcoholic solution of a basic drug and tannic acid are mixed in a 5:1 drug:tannic acid ratio at reduced temperature, tannate complexes containing one amine per digallyl moiety are precipitated. These complexes are split by hydrolysis in gastric and intestinal fluid. Amphetamine and antihistamine tannates were once marketed in both tablet and suspension forms with sustained release claims. Breakdown of the tannate complex depended on pH, being somewhat faster in gastric than intestinal fluid, as well as on the low solubility of the complex. Other complex acids used to prepare relatively insoluble and degradable complexes of basic drugs have included polygalacturonic acid, alginic acid, and arabogalactone sulfate. Products obtained by interaction of montmorillonite clays (e.g., bentonite) with cationic drugs or amine salts and certain nonionic drugs have also been investigated.[24] Both cation exchange and strong chemisorption contribute to the interaction. The release profiles can be varied by altering the drug:clay ratio. A 1:20 complex of amphetamine, for example, is reported to release drug effectively in intestinal fluid, with little release in gastric fluid. Since the clays are anionic, effective adsorbates cannot be prepared from anionic drugs.

Ion-exchange resin complexes, which potentially can be prepared from both acidic and basic drugs, have been more widely studied and mar-keted. Salts of cationic or anionic exchange resins are insoluble complexes in which drug release results from exchange of "bound" drug ions by ions normally present in GI fluids (Na^+, H^+, Cl^-, OH^-). Resins used are special grades of styrene/divinyl benzene copolymers that contain appropriately substituted acidic groups (carboxylic or sulfonic for cation exchangers) or basic groups (quaternary ammonium for anion exchangers) on the styrene moiety of the resin. Ion-active sites are distributed uniformly throughout the resin structure. Variables relating to the resin are the degree of cross-linking, which determines the permeability of the resin, its swelling potential, and the access of the exchange sites to the drug ion; the effective pKa of the exchanging group, which determines the exchange affinity; and the resin particle size, which controls accessibility to exchange ions.

Drug-resin salts, for example, may be prepared by percolation or equilibrium of the resin in acid form with a concentrated solution of drug hydrochloride salt. The resin is washed with ion-free water and partially dried. The resulting product can be encapsulated, tabletted, or suspended in ion-free vehicles. The following equations represent the preparation and exchange reaction affecting drug release in vivo:

$$RESIN - SO3Na + DRUGHCl$$
$$= NaCl + RESIN - SO3.DRUGH$$
$$RESIN - SO3.DRUGH + NaCl$$
$$= DRUGHCl + RESIN - SO3Na$$

A strong acid resin must be used to minimize exchange of drug by hydrogen ion, to avoid excessive drug release in the gastric fluid. The percentage of cross-linking is the most important variable affecting release profiles. Resins with minimum cross-linking show maximum swelling when converted from free acid to salt forms. Subsequent contact with acid can cause shrinkage and reduction of pore volume at the resin periphery, thus entrapping large ions. However, more drug is available for release at higher pH-values. Increased cross-linking decreases resin porosity, not only reducing drug availability but also limiting access of exchange groups to drug ions during preparation. Particle size control becomes important when pore and molecular size are important. Similar observations apply to drug resinates, which are prepared by reaction of sodium salts of acidic drugs with resin chlorides.

The amount of drug that can be incorporated in these systems is limited to a maximum of 200 to 300 mg, since larger doses require too much resin. Release profiles characteristic of resin complexes are sensitive to variation of in vivo ion concentrations. Coating of the resin beads with appropriate polymers, which act as a diffusion barrier to both exchange ions and exchanged drug and water, provides a controllable rate-limiting factor that minimizes the effect of in vivo variables.[25] In one process, the resin particles are pretreated with polyethylene glycol to provide a base for a subsequent coating of ethylcellulose plasticized with a refined vegetable oil. Release profiles can be controlled by appropriate mixing of both coated and uncoated drug-resin complexes. The complexes can be formulated in encapsulated or suspension forms. Different drugs might be readily combined as coated resin forms with independently controlled release characteristics in the same product.

Encapsulated Slow Release Granules

The first significant marketed sustained-release dosage forms were encapsulated mixed slow release beads, to which was applied the barrier principle of controlling drug release, based on model D (Fig. 14-9). For low-milligram potency formulations, nonpareil seeds (20/25-mesh sugar-starch granules) are initially coated with an adhesive followed by powdered drug, and the pellets are dried. This step is repeated until the desired amount of drug has been applied. The resultant granules are subsequently coated with a mixture of solid hydroxylated lipids such as hydrogenated castor oil or glyceryl trihydroxystearate mixed with modified celluloses. The thickness of the barrier was regulated by the number of applied coatings to obtain the desired release characteristic. The original formulations utilized glyceryl monostearate beeswax compositions, which tended to be physically unstable, showing altered release patterns on aging.

A unit of this type contains hundreds of color-coated pellets divided into 3 to 4 groups, which differ in the thickness of the time-delay coating. A typical mix consists of uncoated pellets providing the loading dose and pellets designed to release drug at 2 or 3 hours, 4 or 6 hours, and 6 or 9 hours. The key factor controlling drug release is moisture permeation of the barrier, which depends on coating thickness. Absorption of moisture by the core and subsequent swelling rupture the coating, releasing drug. Some pellets within each group release drug at intervals overlapping other pellet groups, resulting in a smooth rather than discontinuous release profile. Variables that can be manipulated to alter the release pattern include the amount of drug per pellet, the composition and thickness of the coating, and the number of pellets included in each group. Regulation of coating and maintenance of the proper mix of beads during encapsulation present specific production difficulties.

In the case of high-milligram potency formulations, individual crystals of drug or pelletized drug may be coated by pan or fluidized-bed processes with a retardant barrier. Combinations of waxes, fatty acids, alcohols, and esters can be applied using fluidized-bed technology. Such enteric materials as cellulose acetate phthalate and formalized gelatin, as well as lipid compositions, have been used to control release by erosion. Microencapsulation by spray-drying or coacervation has also been used to prepare sustained release encapsulations.[26]

Many encapsulation formulations that implement barrier controlled release have been designed to produce granules with uniform rather than mixed release characteristics, thus eliminating some of the production complexities associated with the manufacture of mixed release pellets. One group of products consists of pellets coated with a hydrolyzed sytrene maleic acid copolymer, which produces a pH-sensitive barrier. Formulations of methylprednisolone have been described as releasing 5% drug in 2 hours at pH 1.2, and 90 to 100% drug in 4 hours at pH 7.5. Delayed release ascorbic acid consisting of ascorbic acid crystals encapsulated in partially hydrogenated cottonseed oil has been marketed for the food industry. Typical formulations contain up to 50% lipid. Pseudo-latexes of ethylcellulose modified by the addition of dibutyl sebacate and plasticized by triethyl citrate have been shown to produce effective retardant barriers whose permeability can be altered by varying the additive concentration. A near zero-order release is claimed with a coating containing 24% sebacate.[27]

A unique application of the barrier concept involves the preparation of granules described as microdialysis cells (model B, Fig. 14-9). Drug-containing pellets might be coated with ethylcellulose, a water-insoluble and pH-insensitive polymer, modified by the addition of suspended sodium chloride particles or other water-soluble materials (e.g., polyethylene glycol). Leaching the salt from the film results in a dialytic membrane formed in situ. This allows permeation of water, dissolution of drug, and diffusion of drug through the essentially intact membrane. These microdialysis cells have been applied to produce a sustained release form of nitroglycerin, which is claimed to be independent of the composition of the GI fluids; however, release of acidic or basic drugs from this system is generally pH-dependent. Pellet cores containing propoxyphene in a buffer system are claimed to produce a pH-independent drug release if formulated as microdialysis cells.[28] Drug may also be microencapsulated in ethylcellulose using a thermally induced phase separation technique in which polyisobutylene is used to control particle size and release rate.[29]

Alternately, placebo pellets may be coated with polyethylene glycol modified ethylcellulose, shellac, or cellulose acetate phthalate containing suspended drug, which is leached from the coating as it is eroded by the action of intestinal fluid. This approach combines both barrier and embedded matrix models of drug release. Release profiles conform to patterns C or D in Figure 14-10, depending on the relative importance of erosion.[30]

The embedded matrix principle has also been applied to prepare sustained release encapsulations. Medicaments are dispersed in molten lipid materials to form a slurry, which may be spray-congealed, or after solidification, granulated. Preferred retardant materials include hydrogenated oils, glyceryl stearates, fatty alcohols, and microcrystalline wax. The addition of 2 to 10% wicking agents, i.e., finely divided powders of methylcellulose, alginic acid, or carboxymethylcellulose, is claimed to produce a greater uniformity of drug release, which more nearly approximates a zero-order process in in vitro testing. These agents promote the permeation of moisture into the matrix, facilitating its erosion. Time-delay matrix materials may constitute 45 to 75% by weight of the formulation. Spray-congealing is advantageous since spherical pellets varying in size from 250 to 2000 microns can be obtained. Sustained release is achieved in part by the random mix of different particle sizes and random dispersal of drug in the matrix.[31]

Suspension or emulsion polymerization has been used to produce resin beads containing drug for sustained release. For example, methyl methacrylate monomer containing drug and methacrylic acid, a water soluble monomer that is added to contribute a swelling characteristic to the final product, are dispersed in an aqueous solution containing appropriate suspending and deflocculating agents. Benzoyl peroxide is added to catalyze the polymerization. The resulting product consists of uniformly sized beads that can be encapsulated.[32] Vinyl acetate and epoxy resins have also been used successfully to pro-

duce sustained release beads. With the latter, curing agents are required, and the reaction is carried out in a silicone oil phase in which the curing agent and the drug dispersed in the liquid resin are insoluble. Drug release from such systems is controlled by both matrix diffusion and partitioning as defined by equation (19).

Tabletted Slow Release Granulations

Compression of timed-release granulations into tablets is an alternate to encapsulation. Such tablets should be designed to disintegrate in the stomach so as to simulate the administration of a capsule form having the advantages associated with sustained release encapsulations, while retaining the advantages of the tablet dosage form. Three examples, each utilizing a different process, illustrate this type of formulation. The first is a tabletted mixed release granulation in which binders with different retardant properties are used to prepare three different granulations, which are color coded for identification, blended, and tabletted. The first is a conventional nonsustained release granulation prepared using gelatin as a binder; the second uses vinyl acetate, and the third uses shellac, as binders. Drug release is controlled by erosion of the granulation in intestinal fluid—the vinyl acetate granulation disintegrates at a faster rate than the shellac granulation.

The second example is illustrated by a sustained release aspirin formulation based on the microdialysis cell principle. Aspirin crystals are microencapsulated in a retardant barrier and are compressed to form a tablet that rapidly disintegrates into sustained release granules. The barrier approach is particularly advantageous for formulation of high-milligram-potency drugs such as aspirin, since only a relatively small amount of retardant is required in the formulation. The third example is represented by a sustained release form of theophylline, which is claimed to release drug zero-order for a 12-hour dosing interval. The tablet is formulated as a matrix of loading dose of theophylline containing theophylline pellets encapsulated in a semipermeable coating. Disintegration of the matrix in the stomach releases the extended action pellets. The loading dose granulation should have physical characteristics, e.g., size, similar to the maintenance dose pellets to ensure homogeneous mixing of the two granulations during compression.

Matrix Tablets

One of the least complicated approaches to the manufacture of sustained release dosage forms involves the direct compression of blends of drug, retardant material, and additives to form a tablet in which drug is embedded in a matrix core of the retardant. Alternately, retardant-drug blends may be granulated prior to compression. Table 14-7 identifies examples of the three classes of retardant material used to formulate matrix tablets, each class demonstrating a different approach to the matrix concept. The first class consists of retardants that form insoluble or "skeleton" matrices; the second class represents water-insoluble materials that are potentially erodable; and the third class consists of polymers that form hydrophilic matrices. Loading doses are best included as the second layer of a two-layer tablet or in a coating applied to the matrix core.

Insoluble, inert polymers such as polyethylene, polyvinyl chloride, and acrylate copolymers have been used as the basis for many marketed formulations. Tablets prepared from these materials are designed to be egested intact and not break apart in the GI tract. Tablets may be directly compressed from mixtures of drug and ground polymer; however, if ethyl cellulose is used as the matrix former, a wet granulation procedure using ethanol can be employed. The rate-limiting step in controlling release from these formulations is liquid penetration into the matrix unless channeling (wetting) agents are included to promote permeation of the polymer matrix by water, which allows drug dissolution and diffusion from the channels created in the matrix. Formulations should be designed so that pore diffusion becomes rate-controlling, release is defined by equation (16) or (17), and the release profile is represented by curve C (Fig. 14-10). Drug bioavailability, which is critically dependent on the drug:polymer ratio, may be modified by inclusion of diluents such as lactose in place of polymer in low-milligram-potency formulations.[33]

Egested tablets contain unreleased drug in the core. In one study of polyvinyl chloride matrix tablets containing prednisolone disodium phosphate, egested tablets contained 72% of the maintenance dose for matrices containing 87% plastic and 2% drug, and 28% drug for matrices containing 84% plastic and 3% drug.[34] These forms of matrix tablets are not useful for high-milligram-potency formulations in which the polymer content would be insufficient to form a matrix, or for highly water-insoluble drugs in which dissolution in the matrix would become rate-limiting. Release of water-soluble drugs, however, should be unaffected by the amount of liquid, pH-value, enzyme content, and other physical properties of digestive fluids, unless the drug is in a salt form that precipitates within

TABLE 14-7. *Materials Used as Retardants in Matrix Tablet Formulations*

Matrix Characteristics	Material
Insoluble, inert	Polyethylene Polyvinyl chloride Methyl acrylate-methacrylate copolymer Ethylcellulose

Insoluble, erodable	Carnauba wax
	  Stearyl alcohol
	  Stearic acid
	  Polyethylene glycol
	Castor wax
	  Polyethylene glycol monostearate
	Triglycerides

Hydrophilic	Methylcellulose (400 cps, 4000 cps) Hydroxyethylcellulose Hydroxypropylmethylcellulose (60 HG, 90 HG, 25 cps, 4000 cps, 15,000 cps) Sodium carboxymethylcellulose Carboxypolymethylene Galactomannose Sodium alginate

the matrix pores on dissolution when penetrated by acid or basic media.

Waxes, lipids, and related materials form matrices that control release through both pore diffusion and erosion (curve D, Fig. 14-10). Release characteristics are therefore more sensitive to digestive fluid composition than to the totally insoluble polymer matrix. Total release of drug from wax-lipid matrices is not possible, since a certain fraction of the dose is coated with impermeable wax films. Release is more effectively controlled by the addition of surfactants or wicking agents in the form of hydrophilic polymers, which promote water penetration and subsequent matrix erosion.

Carnauba wax in combination with stearyl alcohol or stearic acid has been utilized as a retardant base for many sustained release matrix formulations. Mixtures of (1:1) hydrogenated castor oil and propylene glycol monostearate and of carnauba wax and stearyl alcohol or stearic acid have been extensively studied as retardants for both water-soluble and water-insoluble compounds. Materials with melting points that are too low or materials that are too soft cannot be readily processed to form tablets with good physical stability. Such retardants as carnauba wax or hydrogenated castor oil provide the necessary physical characteristics to form an easily compressible stable matrix. If used singly, these materials excessively delay drug release.

Three methods may be used to disperse drug and additive in the retardant base. A solvent evaporation technique can be used, in which a solution or dispersion of drug and additive is incorporated into the molten wax phase. The solvent is removed by evaporation. Dry blends of ingredients may be slugged and granulated. A more uniform dispersion, however, can be prepared by the fusion technique, in which drug and additive are blended into the molten wax matrix at temperatures slightly above the melting point (approximately 90° C for carnauba wax). The molten material may be spray-congealed, solidified and milled, solidified and flaked, or poured on a cold rotating drum to form sheets, which are then milled and screened to form a granulation.

In the absence of additives, drug release is prolonged and nonlinear. Apparent zero-order release can be obtained by addition of additives such as polyvinyl pyrrolidone or polyoxyethylene lauryl ethers. In a study by Dahkuri et al., 10 to 20% hydrophilic polymer effectively controlled release from carnauba-wax/stearyl-alcohol matrices of tripelennamine hydrochloride.[35] Matrices prepared from carnaubà-wax/polyethylene-glycol compositions have also been used to prepare sustained release theophylline tablets. The wax:glycol ratio could be adjusted to vary the release characteristics.

A novel approach to the development of a lipid matrix utilizes pancreatic lipase and calcium carbonate as additives, with triglycerides as retardants. The lipase is activated on contact with moisture and thus promotes erosion independent of intestinal fluid composition. The release profile is controlled by the calcium carbonate, since calcium ions function as a lipase accelerator.[36] In another technique, drug is mass-blended with stearyl alcohol at a temperature above its glass transition (approximately 60°C), and the mass is cooled and granulated with an alcoholic solution of zein. This formulation is claimed to produce tablets with stable release characteristics. Since natural waxes and lipids are complex mixtures, and a fusion process is usually required for processing, hardening with decrease in effective drug release on aging may be observed, owing to polymorphic and amorphous to crystalline transitions.

The third group of matrix formers represents nondigestible materials that form gels in situ. Drug release is controlled by penetration of water through a gel layer produced by hydration of the polymer and diffusion of drug through the swollen, hydrated matrix, in addition to erosion of the gelled layer (curve D, Fig. 14-10). The extent to which diffusion or erosion controls release depends on the polymer selected for the formulation as well as on the drug:polymer ratio. Low-molecular-weight methylcelluloses release drug largely by attrition, since a significant intact hydrated layer is not maintained. Anionic polymers such as carboxymethyl cellulose and carpolene can interact with cationic drugs and show increased dissolution in intestinal fluid. Carboxypolymethylene does not hydrate in gastric fluid. The best matrix former in this group is hydroxymethylcellulose 90 HG 15,000 cps, an inert polymer that does not adversely interact with either acidic or basic drugs, and that on contact with water slowly forms a gel that is more resistant to attrition. Release rates can be adjusted for low-milligram-potency formulations by replacing polymer with lactose. High drug:polymer ratios result in formulations from which drug release is controlled by attrition.[37]

The process used to prepare formulations for compression depends on the polymer and drug:polymer ratio. With high drug:polymer ratios, a wet granulation process is required. Low-milligram-potency formulations may be directly compressed or granulated using alcohol if the polymer is not in a form amenable to direct compression. Formulations of this type are designed to release 100% of drug in vivo, unlike the other matrix forms, which may be partially egested and consequently must be formulated to contain drug in excess of that required to attain the desired therapeutic effect.

Pseudo-latex forms of the normally water-insoluble enteric polymers, such as cellulose acetate phthalate and acrylic resin, can be used as granulating agents for high-milligram-potency drugs. Erodable matrix tablets can be prepared from these granulations. This approach has been tested with theophylline.[38]

Controlled Release Technology

Controlled release dosage forms are designed to release drug in vivo according to predictable rates that can be verified by in vitro measurements. Of the many approaches to formulation of sustained-release medication described in this chapter, those fabricated as insoluble matrix tablets come closest to realization of this objective, since release of water-soluble drug from this form should be independent of in vivo variables. Controlled release technology implies a quantitative understanding of the physicochemical mechanism of drug availability to the extent that the dosage form release rate can be specified. Potential developments and new approaches to oral controlled release drug delivery include hydrodynamic pressure controlled systems, intragastric floating tablets, transmucosal tablets, and microporous membrane coated tablets.[39]

One example of a dosage form design that illustrates the application of controlled release technology to pharmaceutical formulation is the orally administered elementary osmotic pump shown in Figure 14-14A. This device is fabricated from a tablet that contains water-soluble osmotically active drug, or that is blended with an osmotically active diluent, by coating the tablet with a cellulose triacetate barrier, which functions as a semipermeable membrane.[40] A laser is used to form a precision orifice in the barrier. Since the barrier is permeable only to water, initial penetration of water dissolves the outer part of the core, resulting in the development of an osmotic pressure difference across the membrane. The system imbibes water at a rate proportional to the water permeability and effective surface area of the membrane and to the osmotic gradient of the core formulation. The device delivers a volume of saturated solution equal to the volume of water uptake through the membrane. After an initial lag time (approximately 1 hour) during which the delivery rate

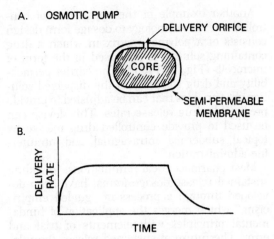

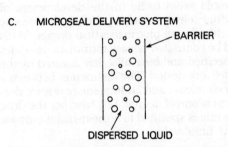

FIG. 14-14. *Controlled release dosage forms. A, Cross-section of osmotic pump. B, Release rate profile characteristic of osmotic pump. C, Micro-seal drug delivery system.*

increases to its maximum value, drug release is zero-order, as shown in Figure 14-14B, until all solid material is dissolved. Thereafter, the delivery rate decreases parabolically to zero.

The diameter of the orifice must be smaller than a maximum size to minimize drug delivery by diffusion through the orifice, and larger than a minimum size to minimize the hydrostatic pressure in the system, which acts in opposition to the osmotic pressure. For devices containing potassium chloride, orifices can range from 75 to 275 μm in diameter. The device can be used as a drug delivery system for any water-soluble drug and can be designed to deliver significant fractions of the total dose at zero-order rates unaffected by in vivo conditions. Since ions do not diffuse into the device, release of acidic and basic drugs is independent of gastrointestinal pH.

A design that provides zero-order release of potassium chloride consists of the soluble tablet core coated with a microporous membrane, which controls the diffusion rate. The membrane is produced in situ by leaching out sucrose that has been suspended in a polyvinyl chloride membrane.[41]

Another example of the application of controlled release technology to dosage form design consists of a polymer matrix in which a drug containing solution is dispersed in the form of microcells (Fig. 14-14C).[42] The barrier permeability and drug solubility in the dispersed solution are variables that can be adjusted to provide predictable drug release rates. This device can be used to provide controlled drug release by topical, subdermal, intravaginal, and intrauterine administration.[43]

Most pharmaceutical formulations, including sustained release dosage forms, have been developed through a process of "guided empiricism," which merges the application of fundamental principles with elements of trial and error. The future of sustained release formulation would seem to lie in the development of novel drug delivery systems, such as the osmotic pump. Ideally, all pharmaceutical dosage forms should be controlled release formulations—with rate specified and bioavailability assured by the drug delivery design. The distinction between a sustained release and an immediate release dosage form is one of degree, i.e., whether the drug release rate is specified to be near-instantaneous or some finite value.

References

1. Ballard, B.E.: An overview of prolonged action drug dosage forms. In Sustained and Controlled Release Drug Delivery Systems. Edited by J.R. Robinson. New York, Marcel Dekker, 1978.
2. Urquhart, J.: Controlled-Release Pharmaceuticals. Washington, DC, American Pharmaceutical Association, 1981.
3. Robinson, J.R., and Eriksen, S.P.: J. Pharm. Sci., 55:1254, 1966.
4. Manion, C.V., et al.: J. Pharm. Sci., 66:981, 1977.
5. Welling, P.G., and Dobrinska, M.R.: Multiple dosing of sustained release systems. In Sustained and Controlled Release Drug Delivery Systems. Edited by J.R. Robinson, New York, Marcel Dekker, 1978.
6. Kwan, K.C.: Pharmacokinetic considerations in the design of controlled and sustained release drug delivery systems. In Sustained and Controlled Release Drug Delivery Systems. Edited by J.R. Robinson. New York, Marcel Dekker, 1978.
7. Sinkula, A.A.: Methods to achieve sustained drug delivery—The chemical approach. In Sustained and Controlled Release Drug Delivery Systems. Edited by J.R. Robinson. New York, Marcel Dekker, 1978.
8. Banker, G.S., and Larson, A.B.: J. Pharm. Sci., 65:838, 1976.
9. Higuchi, T.: J. Pharm. Sci., 52:1145, 1963.
10. Chien, Y.W., and Lambert, H.J.: J. Pharm. Sci., 63:515, 1974.
11. Desai, J., et al.: J. Pharm. Sci., 55:1224, 1966.
12. Wagner, J.C.: Drug Standards, 27:178, 1959.
13. Lapidus, H., and Lordi, N.G.: J. Pharm. Sci., 57:129, 1968.
14. Baker, R.W., and Lonsdale, H.K.: Controlled release: Mechanisms and rates. In Advances in Experimental Medicine and Biology. Vol. 47. Edited by A.C. Tanquary and R.E. Lacey. New York, Plenum Press, 1974.
15. Williams, A.: Sustained Release Pharmaceuticals. Park Ridge, NJ, Noyes Development Corp., 1969.
16. Krueger, E.O., and Vliet, E.B.: J. Pharm. Sci., 51:181, 1962.
17. Timko, R.J., and Lordi, N.G.: J. Pharm. Sci., 67:496, 1978.
18. Lazarus, J., and Cooper, J.: J. Pharm. Sci., 50:715, 1961.
19. Federal Register, 40:26164, 1975.
20. Hadler, A.J.: J. Clin. Pharmacol., 8:113, 1968.
21. Upton, R.A., et al.: J. Pharmacokinet. Biopharm., 8:131, 1980.
22. Smolen, V.F., Ball, L., and Scheffler, M.: Pharm. Tech., 3:88, 1979.
23. Beckett, A.H., Staniforth, D.H., and Raisi, A.: Drug Dev. and Ind. Pharm., 6:121, 1980.
24. McGinity, J.W., and Lach, J.L.: J. Pharm. Sci., 66:63, 1977.
25. Raghunathan, Y., et al.: J. Pharm. Sci., 70:379, 1981.
26. Harris, M.S.: J. Pharm. Sci., 70:391, 1981.
27. Banker, G.S., and Peck, G.E.: Pharm. Tech., 5:55, 1981.
28. Bechgaard, H., and Baggesen, S.: J. Pharm. Sci., 69:1327, 1980.
29. Kawashima, Y., et al.: Drug Dev. and Ind. Pharm., 10:467, 1984.
30. Chandrasekaran, S.K., and Hillman, R.: J. Pharm. Sci., 69:1311, 1980.
31. Lantz, R.J., and Robinson, M.J.: U.S. Patent 3,146,167 (1964).
32. Khanna, S.C., and Jecklin, T.: J. Pharm. Sci., 59:614, 1970.
33. Salomon, J.L., and Doelker, E.: Pharm. Acta Helv., 55:174, 1980.
34. D'Arcy, P.F., et al.: J. Pharm. Sci., 60:1028, 1971.
35. Dahkuri, A., Butler, L.D., and DeLuca, P.P.: J. Pharm. Sci., 67:357, 1978.
36. Javaid, K.A., Fincher, J.H., and Hartman, C.W.: J. Pharm. Sci., 60:1709, 1971.
37. Salomon, J.L., and Doelker, E.: Pharm. Acta Helv., 55:189, 1980.
38. McGinity, J.W., Cameron, C.G., and Cuff, G.W.: Drug Dev. and Ind. Pharm., 9:57, 1983.
39. Chien, Y.W.: Drug Dev. and Ind. Pharm., 9:1291, 1983.
40. Theeuwes, F.: J. Pharm. Sci., 64:1987, 1975.
41. Kallstramd, G., and Ekman, B.: J. Pharm. Sci., 72:772, 1983.
42. Chien, Y.W., Rozek, L.F., and Lambert, H.J.: J. Pharm. Sci., 67:214, 1978.
43. Chien, Y.W.: Novel Drug Delivery Systems. New York, Marcel Dekker, 1982.

15

Liquids

J. C. BOYLAN

The oral use of liquid pharmaceuticals has generally been justified on the basis of ease of administration to those individuals who have difficulty swallowing solid dosage forms. A more positive argument can be made for the use of homogeneous liquids (systems in which the drug or drugs are in solution). With rare exceptions, a drug must be in solution in order to be absorbed. A drug administered in solution is immediately available for absorption, and in most cases, is more rapidly and efficiently absorbed than the same amount of drug administered in a tablet or capsule.

The formulation of solutions presents many technical problems to the industrial pharmacist. Some drugs are inherently unstable; this property is magnified when the drug is in solution. Special techniques are required to solubilize poorly soluble drugs. The final preparation must satisfy the requirements of pharmaceutical elegance with regard to taste, appearance, and viscosity. This chapter discusses those factors particularly important in the formulation and manufacture of solutions. The various dosage forms that fall under this general classification are treated as a group. No attempt is made to treat each dosage form individually. Whenever possible, however, specific examples are given to illustrate the application of the principles discussed.

Formulation Considerations

To solve the formulation problems encountered with pharmaceutical liquids, an interesting dichotomy of investigative skills is required. On the one hand, solubility and stability factors can be approached with the precision long associated with the exact sciences; on the other hand, flavoring and other organoleptic characteristics remain subjective factors for which the application of the scientific method still plays a distressingly minor role. Thus, the successful formulation of liquids, as well as other dosage forms, requires a blend of scientific acuity and pharmaceutical "art."

Solubility

Whether or not a substance dissolves in a given system and the extent to which it dissolves depend largely on the nature and intensity of the forces present in the solute, the solvent, and the resultant solute-solvent interaction. The nature of these interaction energies and the interplay of electronic and steric factors in determining the solubility of substances in various classes of solvents has been clearly presented by Martin et al.[1]

The equilibrium solubility of the drug of interest should be determined in a solvent that is similar to the one intended for use in the final product. This can readily be done by placing an excess of drug (the drug should be finely powdered to minimize the time required to attain equilibrium) in a vial along with the solvent. The tightly closed vial is then agitated at constant temperature, and the amount of drug in solution is determined periodically by assay of a filtered sample of the supernate. Equilibrium is not achieved until at least two successive samplings give the same result.

Solubility studies are generally conducted at fixed temperatures, preferably at temperatures somewhat higher than room temperature (e.g., 30°C), so that constant conditions can be maintained regardless of normal laboratory temperature variations. During the normal distribution process, however, it is possible and even likely that the product will be exposed to a wide range of temperature conditions. For this reason, information relative to the influence of temperature on solubility should be generated. As a rule, a solution should be designed in which the solubility of the solute is not exceeded even at temperatures as low as 4°C.

The approach used when the required concentration of drug exceeds the aforementioned solubility criteria depends on the chemical nature of the drug and the type of product desired.

pH. A large number of modern chemotherapeutic agents are either weak acids or weak bases. The solubility of these agents can be markedly influenced by the pH of their environment. Through application of the law of mass action, the solubility of weakly acidic or basic drugs can be predicted, as a function of pH, with a considerable degree of accuracy. Consider, for example, the reactions involved in the dissolution of a weakly acidic drug, DH:

$$DH \text{ (solid)} \rightleftharpoons DH \text{ (solution)} \qquad (1)$$

where DH (solution) is equal to the solubility of the undissociated acid in moles per liter and is a constant generally referred to as Ks.

The undissociated acid is also in equilibrium with its dissociation products:

$$DH \text{ (solution)} \rightleftharpoons D^- + H^+$$

$$Ka = \frac{[D^-][H^+]}{[DH]} \qquad (2)$$

$$[D^-] = Ka\frac{[DH]}{[H^+]} \qquad (3)$$

The total amount of drug in solution is the sum of the ionized form $[D^-]$ and the un-ionized form $[DH]$. The equation for total solubility, S_T, therefore can be written as:

$$S_T = [DH] + [D^-]$$

$$= [DH] + Ka\frac{[DH]}{[H^+]} \qquad (4)$$

since DH has previously been defined as equal to Ks:

$$S_T = Ks + Ks\frac{Ka}{[H^+]} = Ks\left(1 + \frac{Ka}{[H^+]}\right) \qquad (5)$$

This equation is a most useful one for determining the total solubility of a weak acid at a specific hydrogen ion concentration. Since the question most frequently asked is "What must the pH of the formulation be to maintain X

amount of drug in solution?" a modified form of equation (4) is frequently useful:

$$S_T - Ks = \frac{KsKa}{[H^+]} \qquad (6)$$

or

$$[H^+] = \frac{KsKa}{S_T - Ks} \qquad (7)$$

For example: What must the pH of an aqueous formulation be to maintain in solution 10 mg/ml of a weakly acidic drug, molecular weight (MW) = 200, K = 1×10^{-5}, Ks = 0.001 M/L?

The desired molar $\left(\dfrac{g/L}{MW}\right)$ concentration of

$$drug = \frac{0.010 \times 1000}{200} = 0.05M.$$

$$[H^+] = \frac{(1 \times 10^{-3})(1 \times 10^{-5})}{0.05 - 0.001} = \frac{1 \times 10^{-8}}{0.049}$$

$$[H^+] = 2.04 \times 10^{-7}$$

$$pH = 7 - \log 2.04 = 7 - 0.31$$

$$pH = 6.69$$

An equation that is useful for poorly soluble, weakly basic drugs can be similarly derived:

$$DOH \text{ (solid)} \rightleftharpoons DOH \text{ (solution)}$$
$$Ks = DOH \text{ (solution)}$$

and DOH (solution) is equal to the solubility of the undissociated base in moles/liter.

The dissociation of the weak base can be written as:

$$DOH \text{ (solution)} \rightleftharpoons D^+ + OH^-$$

$$Kb = \frac{[D^+][OH^-]}{DOH \text{ (solution)}} \qquad (8)$$

$$D^+ = \frac{Kb[DOH \text{ (solution)}]}{OH^-} \qquad (9)$$

The total solubility of the base, S_T, is the sum of the ionized form $[D^+]$ and the un-ionized form [DOH]:

$$S_T = [DOH] + [D^+]$$

$$= [DOH] + \frac{Kb[DOH]}{OH^-} \qquad (10)$$

$$S_T = Ks + \frac{KbKs}{OH^-} \qquad (11)$$

Since:

$$Kw = [H^+][OH^-]$$

$$[OH^-] = \frac{Kw}{H^+}$$

then:

$$S_T = Ks + \frac{KbKs}{\dfrac{Kw}{H^+}} = Ks + \frac{KsKb}{Kw}[H^+] \quad (12)$$

Rewriting to solve for $[H^+]$:

$$\frac{S_T}{[H^+]} - \frac{Ks}{[H^+]} = \frac{KsKb}{Kw} \quad (13)$$

or:

$$[H^+] = \frac{Kw}{KsKb}(S_T - Ks) \quad (14)$$

In practice, these equations hold reasonably well; however, there are limitations that the reader should be aware of:

1. The values for the solubility constant Ks and the dissociation constants Ka or Kb that are reported in the literature (or determined in preformulation studies) are usually for the drug in distilled water. These values may be considerably different in a pharmaceutical dosage form such as an elixir, which contains a high percentage of solids and cosolvents. In general, cosolvents such as alcohol or glycerin have the effect of increasing Ks and decreasing the dissociation constant, as shown in Figures 15-1 and 15-2.[2]

2. The equations assume little or no interactions between the solute and itself or between the solute and other formulation components. At low concentrations of solute (below several percent), this assumption is generally valid.

In selecting the pH environment for adequate solubility, several other factors should be considered. The pH that satisfies the solubility requirement must not conflict with other product requirements, such as stability and physiologic compatibility. In addition, if pH is critical to maintaining drug solubility, the system must be adequately buffered. The selection of a buffer must be consistent with the following criteria:

1. The buffer must have adequate capacity in the desired pH range.

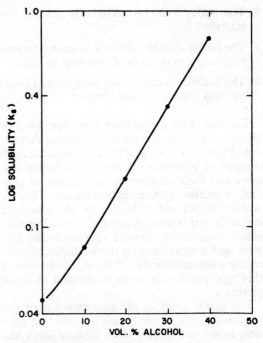

FIG. 15-1. *Effect of alcohol concentration on the solubility (Ks) of un-ionized sulfathiazole. (From Higuchi, T., Gupta, M., and Busse, L.W.: J. Am. Pharm. Assoc., Sci. Ed., 42:157, 1953.)*

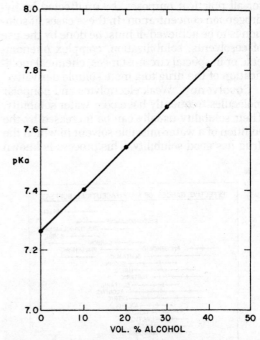

FIG. 15-2. *Effect of alcohol concentration on the dissociation constant (Ka) of sulfathiazole. (From Higuchi, T, Gupta, M., and Busse, L.W.: J. Am. Pharm. Assoc., Sci. Ed., 42:157, 1953.)*

2. The buffer must be biologically safe for the intended use.

3. The buffer should have little or no deleterious effect on the stability of the final product.

4. The buffer should permit acceptable flavoring and coloring of the product.

The first three points have been discussed by Windheuser[3]; the last needs no further elaboration. Figure 15-3 is a graphic representation of a number of pharmaceutically useful buffer systems and their effective buffer ranges. In general, a buffer system has adequate capacity within one pH unit of its pK. As an example of research in this area, Wang and Paruta have recently studied the effect of aqueous buffer systems and temperature on the solubility of commonly used barbiturates.[4,5] Basic information of this type is valuable to the formulator of liquid products.

For many drugs, a pH adjustment does not provide an appropriate means for effecting solution. In the case of very weak acids or bases, the required pH may be unacceptable in terms of physiologic considerations or owing to the effect of pH extremes on the stability of formulation adjuvants (such as sugars and flavors) or of the drug itself. The solubility of nonelectrolytes will, for all practical purposes, be unaffected by hydrogen ion concentration. In these cases, if solution is to be achieved, it must be done by the use of cosolvents, solubilization, complex phenomena, or in special circumstances, chemical modification of the drug to a more soluble derivative.

Cosolvency. Weak electrolytes and nonpolar molecules frequently have poor water solubility. Their solubility usually can be increased by the addition of a water-miscible solvent in which the drug has good solubility. This process is known as *cosolvency*, and the solvents used in combination to increase the solubility of the solute are known as *cosolvents*. The mechanism responsible for solubility enhancement through cosolvency is not clearly understood. It has been proposed that a cosolvent system works by reducing the interfacial tension between the predominately aqueous solutions and the hydrophobic solute.[6] Recent work supports the theory that amides adsorb to the solute at the interface with water, thereby diminishing the hydrophobic surface or solute/water interfacial tension.[7] As a result, the soluble hydrophilic portion of the amide cosolvent remains oriented toward the aqueous phase. Some workers have looked upon the phenomenon as a result of the independent solubility of the solute in each cosolvent. This is obviously a gross oversimplification, since the solubility of a substance in a blend of solvents is usually not equal to the value predicted on the basis of its solubility in the pure solvents. For example, undissociated phenobarbital has a solubility of approximately 1.2 g/L in water and 13 g/L in ethyl alcohol. The ratio of solvents, as well as pH, can alter solubility (Fig. 15-4).

Ethanol, sorbitol, glycerin, propylene glycol,

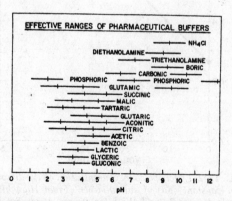

FIG. 15-3. *Commonly used pharmaceutical buffers and their effective buffer ranges. (From Windheuser, J.: Bull. Parenteral Drug Assoc., 17:1, 1963.)*

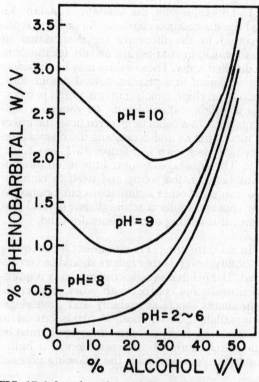

FIG. 15-4. *Interdependence of pH and alcohol concentration on the solubility of phenobarbital. (From Lin, K.S., Anschel, J., and Swartz, C.J.: Bull. Parenteral Drug Assoc., 25:44, 1971.)*

and several members of the polyethylene glycol polymer series represent the limited number of cosolvents that are both useful and generally acceptable in the formulation of aqueous liquids. Spiegel and Noseworthy, in their review of nonaqueous solvents used in parenteral products, cited a number of solvents that might also be useful in oral liquids.[8] These include glycerol dimethylketal, glycerol formal, glycofurol, dimethylacetamide, N-(β-hydroxyethyl)-lactamide, ethyl lactate, ethyl carbonate, and 1,3-butylene glycol. It should be emphasized, however, that with the possible exception of dimethylacetamide, all of these solvents are unproven with respect to their acceptability for systemic use. Dimethylacetamide has been used as a cosolvent in parenteral products, but its use in oral liquids is seriously limited, owing to the difficulty of masking its objectionable odor and taste. Thus, the spectrum of solvents from which one may make a selection is extremely narrow. Nevertheless, the frequency of their use is high, as can readily be seen by reviewing the formulas for a variety of official and proprietary oral liquids.

Cosolvents are employed not only to effect solubility of the drug, but also to improve the solubility of volatile constituents used to impart a desirable flavor and odor to the product.

Much of the early data on the solubility of pharmaceutical solutes in mixed solvents have been reported as a function of solvent composition; no attempt has been made to explain the data. In recent years, much more emphasis has been placed on cultivating a basic understanding of this phenomenon, with the objective of developing a mathematical approach to interpreting and predicting solubility behavior. Hildebrand and Scott have developed an equation that yields a thermodynamic measure of the cohesive forces that exist within a homogeneous substance.[9,10] This number is often referred to as *Hildebrand's solubility parameter.*

There are several serious limitations to the practical application of the solubility parameter concept to pharmaceutical systems. The approach is restricted to what Hildebrand terms "regular solutions." A regular solution has been defined as one in which there are no interactions between the various solvents present and between the solute and the solvents. All molecules are randomly distributed and oriented in the system. In thermodynamic language, this may be stated as "a solution involving no entropy change when a small amount of one of its components is transferred to it from an ideal solution of the same composition, the total volume remaining unchanged."[10] An additional liability

to the solubility parameter approach is the thermodynamic values that must be known to solve the Hildebrand-Scott equation for solubility:

$$\log X_2 = \frac{\Delta Hm^F}{4575}\left(\frac{Tm - T}{TmT}\right)$$
$$+ \frac{\Delta Cp}{4575}\left(\frac{Tm - T}{T}\right)$$
$$- \frac{\Delta Cp}{1.987}\log\frac{Tm}{T}$$
$$- \frac{V_2}{4.575T}(\delta_1 - \delta_2)^2\phi_1^2 \qquad (15)$$

where:

X_2 = mole fraction solubility at temperature T

ΔHm^F = heat of fusion of the solute at its melting point Tm

$\Delta Cp = Cp^l - Cp^s$ where Cp^l and Cp^s are the molal heat capacities of the liquid and solid forms

V_2 = molar volume of the solute

$\left.\begin{array}{l}\delta_1 = \text{solubility parameter of the solvent} \\ \delta_2 = \text{solubility parameter of the solute}\end{array}\right\} = \left(\dfrac{\Delta E^V}{V}\right)^{1/2}$ or $\left(\dfrac{\Delta H - RT}{V^l}\right)^{1/2}$

ϕ_1 = volume fraction of the solvent

Assuming that the solubility parameter values were known for all pharmaceutically useful solvents, the thermodynamic data for each solute of interest would still have to be determined.

Martin and co-workers attempted to use this theory in their study concerning the solubility of benzoic acid in mixed solvent systems.[11,12] The solubility of benzoic acid was found to be in general agreement with the values predicted by the Hildebrand equation, particularly when the solubility parameter of the mixed solvent was approximately equal to the solubility parameter of benzoic acid. The same general conclusions were reached when the solubility of a series of p-hydroxybenzoic acid esters were studied, and the experimental data were compared with the value predicted by the solubility parameter approach. Other authors have extended solubility studies with benzoic acid to other binary and ternary solvent systems.[13]

Dielectric Constant. A more practical, although admittedly less rigorous, approach to the solubility problem may be found in what has come to be known as the "dielectric requirement" for solubility.[14-18] According to this theory, every solute shows a maximum solubility, in any given solvent system, at one or more specific dielectric constants.*

The absolute solubility of a solute may vary considerably in two different solvents of the same dielectric constant, but the solubility profile, as a function of dielectric constant, appears to be similar for a solute in a wide variety of solvent systems.

Solubility profiles as a function of dielectric constants have been reported for numerous pharmaceuticals in a variety of liquid solvent systems. Examples of substances studied include barbiturates, parabens, xanthine derivatives, antipyrine, and aminopyrine.[19-26]

The dielectric constants of most pharmaceutical solvents are known;[27,28] values for a number of binary and tertiary blends have been reported,[15] and if not reported, can be readily estimated. Molal boiling point and dielectric constant equations may be used to estimate solubility of pure solvents and miscible solvent blends.[29] The use of each varies, depending upon the literature values and/or laboratory equipment available. To determine the dielectric requirement of the substance of interest, dioxane-water blends having known dielectric constants are used, and the dielectric constant(s) at which maximum solubility is attained is noted. Pharmaceutical formulations of comparable dielectric constant(s) can then be prepared, and the most appropriate system can be selected on the basis of the solubility requirements, stability, and organoleptic characteristics.

Solubilization. Solubilization has been defined by McBain as the spontaneous passage of poorly water-soluble solute molecules into an aqueous solution of a soap or a detergent, in which a thermodynamically stable solution is formed.[30] The mechanism for this phenomenon has been studied quite extensively and involves the property of surface-active agents to form colloidal aggregates known as micelles. When surfactants are added to a liquid at low concentra-

tions, they tend to orient at the air-liquid interface. As additional surfactant is added, the interface becomes fully occupied, and the excess molecules are forced into the bulk of the liquid. At still higher concentrations, the molecules of surfactant in the bulk of the liquid begin to form oriented aggregates or micelles; this change in orientation occurs rather abruptly, and the concentration of surfactant at which it occurs is known as the *critical micelle concentration (CMC)*. Solubilization is thought to occur by virtue of the solute dissolving in or being adsorbed onto the micelle. Thus, the ability of surfactant solutions to dissolve or solubilize water-insoluble materials starts at the critical micelle concentration and increases with the concentration of the micelles.

Solubilizing agents have been used in pharmaceutical systems for many years. As early as 1868, it was reported that cholesterol was markedly more soluble in aqueous soap solutions than in pure water.

In recent years, the application of solubilization phenomena to pharmaceutical systems has greatly increased. Table 15-1 shows the type of solubilizing agents most frequently used in pharmaceutical systems and the types of drugs for which these agents have been effective. The acceptability of these surfactants for oral use should be determined on an individual basis.

It is readily apparent from this tabulation that a wide variety of substances can be solubilized. McBain has stated, "Any material can be solubilized in any solvent by proper choice of solubilizing agent."[38] This may well be true, but the questions that must be asked and answered are: To what extent can the substance be solubilized? How is the proper solubilizing agent selected? What effect will the solubilizing agent have on the stability, efficacy, and physical characteristics of the product?

It has generally been observed that lyophilic surface active agents with hydrophilic-lipophilic balance (HLB) values higher than 15 are the best solubilizing agents. Final selection of solubilizing agents should be based on phase solubility studies in a manner similar to that employed by Guttman et al. in their studies concerning the solubilization of prednisolone, methyl prednisolone, and fluorometholone with Triton WR-1339.[39] They determined the equilibrium solubility of the steroids at 25°C as a function of surfactant concentration. Figure 15-5 is a plot showing the apparent solubility of steroid as a function of Triton WR-1339. A similar plot could be constructed in which the solubility of a specific substance is determined as a function of surfactant concentration, and several surfac-

---

*The dielectric constant is the property of a solvent relating to the amount of energy required to separate two oppositely charged bodies in the solvent as compared with the energy required to separate the same two oppositely charged bodies in a vacuum. By definition, the dielectric constant of a vacuum is unity. The dielectric constant of water at 25°C is 78.5; thus, it takes 78.5 times more energy to separate two oppositely charged bodies in a vacuum than in water. This property is closely related to the polarity of solvents, and it is therefore not surprising that a solute shows a preference for solvent systems having a specific dielectric constant.

TABLE 15-1. *Solubilizing Agents Used in Pharmaceutical Systems*

Solubilizer	Solubilizate	Reference
Polyoxyethylene sorbitan	Acetomenaphtone	31
Fatty acid esters (Tween® series)	21-Acetoxypregnenolone	31
	Barbital	32
	Caffeine	32
	Benzocaine	32
	Chloramphenicol	31
	Chloroform	31
	Chlorotrianisene	31
	Cortisone acetate	31
	Cyclocoumarol	31
	Desoxycorticosterone acetate	31
	Dicoumarol	31
	Dienestrol	31
	Diethylstilbestrol	31
	Digitoxin	31
	Volatile oils	33
	Essential oils	31
	Estrone	31
	Ethylbiscoumacetate	31
	Hexestrol	31
	Menthol	32
	Methyltestosterone	31
	Phenobarbital	32
	Progesterone	31
	Reserpine	34,35
	Salicyclic acid	32
	Testosterone	31
	Vitamin A (alcohol and esters)	31
	Vitamin D	31
	Vitamin E (alcohol and esters)	31
	Vitamin K	31
Polyoxyethylene monoalkyl ethers (BRIJ® and MYRJ® series)	Essential oils	36
	Volatile oils	36
	Benzocaine	31
	Benzoic acid derivatives	31
	Chloroxylenol	31
	Iodine	31
Sucrose monoesters	Vitamin A (alcohol and esters)	31
	Vitamin D	31
	Vitamin E (alcohol and esters)	31
Lanolin esters and ethers	Essential oils	37
	Volatile oils	37
	Hexachlorophene	37
	Vitamin A palmitate	37

®Registered trademarks of I.C.I. United States, Inc.

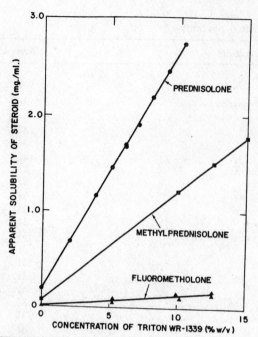

FIG. 15-5. *The effect of varying concentrations of Triton WR-1339 in water on the solubility of some anti-inflammatory steroids. (From Guttman, D.E., Hamlin, W.E., Shell, J.W., and Wagner, J.G.: J. Pharm. Sci., 50:305, 1961.*

tants of interest are included in the study. The appropriate surfactant can then be selected on the basis of its efficiency as a solubilizer and its effect on other product characteristics.

The major producers of surface active agents have carried out extensive studies on the physiologic effects of products that they recommend for pharmaceutical use. Although the agents are, in themselves, generally free of toxicity, their use must be tempered with a full understanding of the secondary effects that they may produce. While nontoxic surfactants have been shown to improve the stability of vitamin A,[40,41] other surfactants have been shown to have a deleterious effect on formulation components such as dyes.[42] Addition of surface active agents to drug systems has in some instances enhanced gastrointestinal absorption and pharmacologic activity, and in other cases inhibited the same. Of comparable importance is the effect that surfactants can have on formulation adjuvants. The activity of several preservatives, for example, has been found to be significantly decreased in the presence of a number of surface active agents.

Complexation. Organic compounds in solution generally tend to associate with each other to some extent. Frequently, this association is too weak to be detected by standard techniques. In other cases, the intermolecular association, or

complex, can be readily observed and quantitated by one or more of numerous published techniques.[1] One of the more widely used methods, and one that is highly germane to this discussion, is the solubility analysis technique. Every substance has a specific, reproducible equilibrium solubility in a given solvent at a given temperature. Any deviation from this inherent solubility must be due to the formation of a new species in solution.* In the case of weakly acidic and basic compounds, the total solubility is equal to the *inherent* solubility of the undissociated compound plus the concentration of the dissociated species. Similarly, when complex formation occurs, the total solubility is equal to the inherent solubility of the uncomplexed drug plus the concentration of drug complex in solution. Consider the interaction between a drug, D, and a complexing agent, C:

$$xD + yC \rightleftharpoons D_xC_y \qquad (16)$$

where x and y denote the stoichiometry of the interaction. For simplicity, only the case in which one species of complex is formed is considered here; it is possible for several species of complexes to coexist.

The total solubility of drug in this case is:

$$S_T = [D] + X[D_xC_y] \qquad (17)$$

where:

[D] = the solubility of uncomplexed drug
= Ks

$X[D_xC_y]$ = concentration of drug in complexed form

By use of the solubility analysis technique, the stoichiometry of this interaction, as well as its equilibrium constant, can be determined. This is carried out by placing excessive quantities of the drug, together with solutions containing various concentrations of complexing agent, in

---

*Apparent solubility can be influenced by the size and shape of solute particles when the particles are in the micron size range. The observed solubility increased with decreasing particle size in accordance with the equation:

$$\log \frac{S}{So} = \frac{2\gamma v}{2.303RTr}$$

where S is the observed solubility. So the inherent equilibrium solubility, γ the surface tension of the particles, v the molar volume, R is the gas constant (8.314×10^7 ergs/deg mole), T is the temperature absolute, and r is the radius of the particles.

well-closed containers. The containers are agitated at a constant temperature until equilibrium is achieved. Aliquot samples of the supernatant liquid are then removed and assayed for total concentration of drug. A typical solubility analysis profile is shown in Figure 15-6.

The increase in solubility of drug from points S to A is due to complex formation. At point A, the solution is saturated with respect to both the drug and the complex. The composition of the solution does not vary from point A to B because as drug in solution interacts with complexing agent, it is replaced from the excess present in the system and the additional complex-formed precipitates, since the solution is already saturated with respect to this component. At point B, all of the excess drug has been consumed, and the further addition of complexing agent results in a depletion of the uncomplexed drug in solution. If no higher complexes were formed, the curve would approach a value equal to the solubility of the complex $(R - S)$. The increase in this case indicates the formation of one or more secondary complexes.

The stoichiometry of the interaction can be determined as follows.

The excess drug remaining in the system at point A is entirely converted to complex at point B. The amount of drug entering into the complex over this range is equal to the total amount of drug added to the system (D_T) less the amount of drug in solution at point A(R). The amount of complexing agent entering into the reaction over the plateau region can be read directly from the abscissa and is equal to $b - a$. Therefore, the stoichiometry is given by:

$$\frac{D_T - R}{b - a} =$$

$$\frac{\text{moles of drug in complex}}{\text{moles of complexing agent in complex}} \quad (18)$$

If the ratio of drug to complexing agent is found to be 1, then the complexing reaction may be written as:

$$D + C \rightleftharpoons DC$$

and the stability constant is:

$$K = \frac{[DC]}{[D][C]} \quad (19)$$

where:

$[DC]$ = total drug in solution at point A less the solubility of the uncomplexed drug (S)

$[D]$ = solubility of the uncomplexed drug (S)

$[C]$ = the concentration of complexing agent added to the system at point A (a) less the amount of complexing agent in the drug complex [DC]

The extent to which the solubility of the drug can be increased in the foregoing example is limited by the solubility of the complex (Fig. 15-6). In other cases, the limitation may be imposed by the solubility of the complexing agent. To the pharmaceutical investigator, however, the major concerns are how much drug can be put into solution by a specific complexing agent and how the resultant complex affects the safety, stability, and therapeutic efficacy of the product.

The formulator must also be aware of potential detrimental interaction between ingredients. An example of such interaction is the complexation of nonionic surfactants, such as polysorbate 80, with parabens resulting in the inactivation of the preservatives. Certain polyols have been shown to inhibit this complexation, thus maintaining paraben antimicrobial activity. Unfortunately, a commonly used polyol, sorbitol, does not inhibit these complexation reactions, probably because it is too polar to partition into the surfactant micelle (Fig. 15-7).[40]

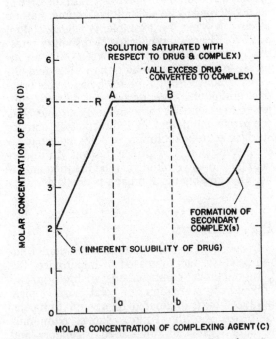

FIG. 15-6. *Phase diagram showing the effect of varying concentrations of complexing agent on the apparent solubility of drug.*

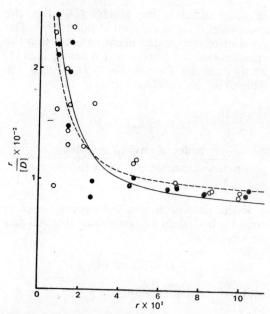

FIG. 15-7. *Influence of sorbitol on the binding of methylparaben to 10% (w/v) polysorbate 80 to 30°. Key: ○, methylparaben alone; and ●, methylparaben plus sorbitol (1:1). (From Blanchard, J., Fink, W.T., and Duffy, J.P.: J. Pharm. Sci., 66:981, 1977. Reproduced with permission of the copyright owner, the American Pharmaceutical Association.)*

Hydrotrophy. The term hydrotrophy has been used to designate the increase in solubility in water of various substances due to the presence of large amounts of additives.[43,44] The mechanism by which this effect occurs is not clear. Some workers have speculated that hydrotrophy is simply another type of solubilization, with the solute dissolved in oriented clusters of the hydrotrophic agent. Hydrotrophic solutions do not show colloidal properties, however. Others feel that this phenomenon is more closely related to complexation involving a weak interaction between the hydrotrophic agent and the solute. Still others reason that the phenomenon must be due to a change in solvent character because of the large amount of additive needed to bring about the increase in solubility.

The influence on large concentrations of sodium benzoate on the solubility of caffeine is a classic example of this phenomenon applied to a pharmaceutical system. Other examples include the solubilization of benzoic acid with sodium benzoate, and of theophylline with sodium acetate and sodium glycinate. Except for these examples, little use has been made of hydrotrophy in pharmaceutical systems, probably due to the large amount (in the range of 20 to 50%) of additive necessary to produce modest increases in solubility.

The practical application of complexation and hydrotrophy is quite limited with respect to solubility enhancement in pharmaceutical liquids. Many agents have been studied that associate with a variety of drug substances. The degree of association, however, and the extent to which the solubility can be increased are generally not adequate for practical use in formulation research. These deficiencies are further complicated by the fact that many of the known complexing agents are either physiologically active substances (i.e., the xanthines) or are of unknown biologic character.

Wolfson and Banker have reported significant increases of barbiturate solubilities as a result of complexation with poly-N-vinyl-5-methyl-2-oxazolidone.[45] Polyvinylpyrrolidone participates in complex formation with a variety of organic and inorganic pharmaceuticals, the most dramatic of which is the well known PVP-iodine complex. The principle of hydrotrophy has been effectively applied in the solubilization of adrenochrome monosemicarbazone with sodium salicylate (Adrenosem ampuls and oral liquid, Massengill).

Chemical Modification of the Drug. Many poorly soluble drugs can be chemically modified to water-soluble derivatives. This approach has been highly successful in the case of corticosteroids. The solubility of betamethasone alcohol in water, for example, is 5.8 mg/100 ml at 25°C. The solubility of its 21 disodium phosphate ester is greater than 10 g/100 ml, an increase in solubility greater than 1500-fold. In general, however, this approach has severe practical limitations. New derivatives must be subjected to essentially the same testing protocol as the parent compound, including biologic activity studies, acute and chronic toxicity, pharmaceutical evaluation, and clinical testing. An undertaking of this magnitude can be justified only if no other reasonable approach is available.

Preservation

In recent years, adequate preservation of liquid products has increased in importance. Reports of clinical complications arising from microbial contamination of oral and topical products have originated in several European countries and the United States. Numerous product recalls and tightened regulatory and compendia limits have re-emphasized the need for the formulator to carefully and thoroughly consider all aspects of the preservative system chosen for a particular formula.[46,47] In addition to presenting a health hazard to the user, microbial growth can cause marked effects on product stability.

Numerous sources of contamination exist. Including among these are raw materials, processing containers and equipment, the manufacturing environment, operators, packaging materials, and the user.

Manufacturing techniques to minimize microbial contamination are presented under the heading "Manufacturing Considerations." The remainder of this section deals with preservative systems for liquid products.

An ideal preservative can be qualitatively defined as one that meets the following three criteria:

1. It must be effective against a broad spectrum of microorganisms.

2. It must be physically, chemically, and microbiologically stable for the lifetime of the product.

3. It must be nontoxic, nonsensitizing, adequately soluble, compatible with other formulation components, and acceptable with respect to taste and odor at the concentrations used.

No single preservative exists that satisfies all of these requirements for all formulations. The selection of a preservative system must be made on an individual basis, using published information and "in house" microbiologic studies for guidance. Frequently, a combination of two or more preservatives are needed to achieve the desired antimicrobial effect.

The antimicrobial agents that have been used as preservatives can be classified into four major groupings: acidic, neutral, mercurial, and quaternary ammonium compounds. Table 15-2 lists some representative members of these groupings and the concentration ranges at which they have been used.

The phenols are probably the oldest and best known pharmaceutical preservatives, but are little used in oral pharmaceuticals, owing to their characteristic odor and instability when exposed to oxygen. The more useful members of the series, for this application, are the parahydroxybenzoic acid esters, and the salts of benzoic and sorbic acid. They are adequately soluble in aqueous systems and have been demonstrated to possess both antifungal and antibacterial properties.

Frequently, a combination of two or more esters of parahydroxybenzoic acid are used to

TABLE 15-2. *Some Pharmaceutically Useful Preservatives*

Class	Usual Concentration (%)
Acidic	
Phenol	0.2–0.5
Chlorocresol	0.05–0.1
O-phenyl phenol	0.005–0.01
Alkyl esters of parahydroxybenzoic acid	0.001–0.2
Benzoic acid and its salts	0.1–0.3
Boric acid and its salts	0.5–1.0
Sorbic acid and its salts	0.05–0.2
Neutral	
Chlorbutanol	0.5
Benzyl alcohol	1.0
β-phenylethyl alcohol	0.2–1.0
Mercurial	
Thimerosal	0.001–0.1
Phenylmercuric acetate and nitrate	0.002–0.005
Nitromersol	0.001–0.1
Quaternary Ammonium Compounds	
Benzalkonium chloride	0.004–0.02
Cetylpyridinium chloride	0.01–0.02

achieve the desired antimicrobial effect. Methyl and propyl parahydroxybenzoic acid, for example, are often used together in a ratio of 10 to 1, respectively. The use of more than one ester makes possible a higher total preservative concentration, owing to the independent solubilities of each, and according to some researchers, serves to potentiate the antimicrobial effect. The solubilities of a series of parabens have been studied at four temperatures. The solubilities were expressed in terms of ideal, actual, and excess free energies.[48]

The remaining three classes of preservatives have been widely used in ophthalmic, nasal, and parenteral products, but have been little used in oral liquids. The neutral preservatives are all volatile alcohols, and their volatility introduces odor problems as well as concern for preservative loss on aging. The mercurials and quaternary ammonium compounds are excellent preservatives. They are, however, subject to a variety of incompatibilities, with mercurials being readily reduced to free mercury and the quaternary compounds being inactivated by a variety of anionic substances. The incompatibilities common to these and other preservatives are discussed by Lachman.[49]

Syrups containing approximately 85% sugar

resist bacterial growth by virtue of their exosmotic effect on microorganisms. Syrups that contain less than 85% sucrose, but a sufficient concentration of polyol (such as sorbitol, glycerin, propylene glycol, or polyethylene glycol) to have an exosmotic effect on microorganisms, similarly resist bacterial growth. It is possible, however, for surface dilution to take place in a closed container as a result of solvent evaporation followed by condensation, with the condensate flowing back onto the liquid surface. The resulting diluted surface layer makes an excellent medium for bacterial and fungal growth. These products, therefore, should be designed so that even after dilution, they do not support microbial growth. This can be done either by incorporating a sufficient concentration of preservative, so that a diluted sample of the product resists microorganism growth, or by including approximately 5 to 10% ethanol in the formulation. The vapor pressure of ethanol is greater than that of water and normally vaporizes to the surface of the liquid and the cap area, preventing, or at least minimizing, the potential for microorganism growth as a result of surface dilution.

An effectively designed preservative system must retain its antimicrobial activity for the shelf-life of the product. To ensure compliance with this precept, the preservative characteristics of the product in its final form (including formulation and package) must be studied as a function of age. The best method of demonstrating preservative characteristics is by microbiologic evaluation.

To determine whether a specific organism is hazardous, one must consider the nature of the product and its dose, the state of health of the user, and clinical reports on the frequency and severity of infections caused by the microorganism.

The FDA distinguishes between organisms that are "always objectionable" and "usually objectionable." The former designation is based on only two factors—pathogenicity of the organism and site of use. The latter designation is based on an additional determinant, the state of health of the user. The official compendia are continually reevaluating their standards based on the latest FDA data and guidelines.

Specific organisms generally recognized as undesirable in oral liquids include Salmonella species, Escherichia coli, Enterobacter species, Pseudomonas species (commonly P. aeruginosa), proteolytic species of Clostridium, and Candida albicans. Some liquid pharmaceuticals (i.e., ophthalmic solutions) must be processed aseptically and rendered sterile.

Chemical analysis for the antimicrobial constituent frequently provides a helpful guide but can be misleading. Molecular interactions involving preservatives and commonly used pharmaceutical adjuvants, such as surfactants and cellulose derivatives, have been observed. For example, it has been shown that Tween 80 interacts to a significant extent with the methyl and propyl esters of parahydroxybenzoic acid, and that the preservative-surfactant complex is essentially devoid of antibacterial activity.[49] Chemical analysis for the parahydroxybenzoate esters would not differentiate between the unbound substance (microbiologically active) and the bound substance (microbiologically inactive).

Subjective Product Characteristics

Many product qualities, such as taste and appearance, cannot be quantitatively measured. These characteristics are often referred to under the heading of "pharmaceutical elegance." The word elegance has, however, a superficial connotation, which is not justified. The value of a pharmaceutical product is measured by both its medical significance and its commercial success. A satisfactory performance on either of these ratings can only be achieved with a product that is convenient to use and receives patient acceptance.

Sweetening Agents

Sweetening agents generally constitute a major portion of the solids content in those dosage forms requiring them. Sucrose has had a long history of use. It is soluble in aqueous media (solutions containing approximately 85% sucrose can be prepared); it is available in highly purified form at reasonable cost, and it is chemically and physically stable in the pH range of 4.0 to 8.0. It is frequently used in conjunction with sorbitol, glycerin, and other polyols, which are said to reduce the tendency of sucrose to crystallize. One of the manifestations of sucrose crystallization is cap-locking, which occurs when the product crystallizes on the threads of the bottle cap and interferes with cap removal. This phenomenon has been studied, and several vehicles containing sucrose, glucose, sorbitol, and glycerin have been reported as acceptable in terms of product characteristics and resistance to cap-locking.[50]

Liquid glucose is an extremely viscid substance that imparts both body and sweetness to liquid formulations. It is prepared by the partial hydrolysis of starch with strong acid, and contains, as its main component, dextrose with smaller amounts of dextrins and maltose. In a manner similar to that of honey and molasses, but to a lesser degree, this agent imparts a characteristic odor and flavor to the formulations in which it is used. Although liquid glucose is not a pure chemical entity, its method of manufacture can be well controlled, and batch-to-batch variability is usually not a significant problem. The same is not true for such materials as honey and molasses. The quality of these substances varies, depending on the source from which they are obtained, and if the source is held constant, depending on the time of year they are produced and on other natural factors over which there is little or no control. The use of these and other naturally occurring materials should be predicated on a rigorous quality control regimen, which gives maximum assurance of product uniformity.

Saccharin is used to supplement sugars and polyols as sweeteners. It is approximately 250 to 500 times as sweet as sugar, but it can have a bitter aftertaste if not properly used in the formula.

Numerous countries have approved a new synthetic sweetener, aspartame, for use as a food and/or drug ingredient. Aspartame is the methyl ester of aspartic acid and phenylalanine.

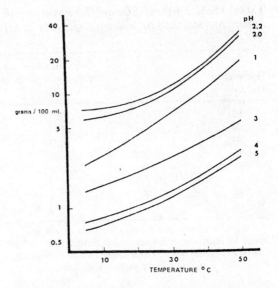

FIG. 15-8. *Effect of pH and temperature on aspartame solubility in water. (Reprinted with permission from Beck, C.I.: Application potential for aspartame in low calorie and dietetic foods. In* Low Calorie and Special Dietary Foods. *Edited by B.K. Dwivedi. CRC Press, 1978, p. 68. Copyright CRC Press, Inc., Boca Raton, FL.)*

Aspartame

It is approximately 200 times sweeter than sucrose and has none of the aftertaste of saccharin. Aspartame's aqueous solubility is quite adequate for formulation purposes (Fig. 15-8.) Although it is very stable as a dry powder, its stability in aqueous solutions is quite pH- and temperature-dependent. Aspartame's greatest stability is between pH 3.4 and 5.0 and at refrigerated temperatures (see Fig. 15-9 and Table 15-3).[51]

Sweetness enhancement by aspartame is synergistic with saccharin, sucrose, glucose, and cyclamate. In addition, its taste properties have been improved using sodium barcarbonate, gluconate salts, and lactose.[51] For further information, the pharmaceutical formulator should consult the excellent review on the food uses of aspartame by Beck.[51]

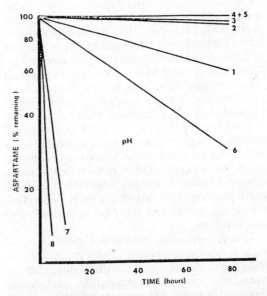

FIG. 15-9. *Effect of pH and time on aspartame stability in aqueous buffer systems at 40°C. (Reprinted with permission from Beck, C.I.: Application potential for aspartame in low calorie and dietetic foods. In* Low Calorie and Special Dietary Foods. *Edited by B.K. Dwivedi. CRC Press, 1978, p. 68. Copyright CRC Press, Inc., Boca Raton, FL.)*

TABLE 15-3. *Effect of Storage Temperature on Aspartame Stability in Aqueous Solutions at pH 4.0*

Temperature storage (°C)	Calculated time for 20% decomposition (days)
10	387
20	134
30	51
40	22
55	5
68	2
80	1
90	0.15

Reprinted with permission from Beck, C.I.: Application potential for aspartame in low calorie and dietetic foods. *In* Low Calorie and Special Dietary Foods: Edited by B.K. Dwivedi. CRC Press, 1978. Copyright CRC Press, Inc., Boca Raton, FL.

Viscosity Control

It is sometimes desirable to increase the viscosity of a liquid, either to serve as an adjunct for palatability or to improve pourability. This can be achieved by increasing the sugar concentration or by incorporating viscosity-controlling agents such as polyvinylpyrrolidone or various cellulosic derivatives (e.g., methylcellulose or sodium carboxymethylcellulose). These compounds form solutions in water that are stable over a wide pH range. Methylcellulose and carboxymethylcellulose are available in a number of different viscosity grades. Carboxymethylcellulose may be used in solutions containing high concentrations of alcohol (up to 50%) without precipitating. It is precipitated, however, as an insoluble salt of a number of multivalent metal ions such as Al^{+++}, Fe^{+++}, and Ca^{++}. Methylcellulose polymers do not form insoluble salts with metal ions, but can be salted out of solution when the concentration of electrolytes or other dissolved materials exceed certain limits. These limits may vary from about 2 to 40%, depending on the electrolyte and the type of methylcellulose involved.

Viscosity-inducing polymers should be used with a degree of caution. They are known to form molecular complexes with a variety of organic and inorganic compounds, and in so doing, influence the activity of these compounds. It is conceivable that highly viscid systems that resist dilution by gastrointestinal fluids might impede drug release and absorption.

Flavors

Flavoring can be divided into two major categories: selection and evaluation. Much has been written on both phases of pharmaceutical flavoring, but selection remains a totally empiric activity.

The four basic taste sensations are salty, bitter, sweet, and sour. Some generalizations concerning the selection of flavors to mask specific types of taste have been suggested by Janovsky,[52] and by Wesley.[53] (See Table 15-4.)

A combination of flavoring agents is usually required to mask these taste sensations effectively. Menthol, chloroform, and various salts frequently are used as flavor adjuncts. Menthol and chloroform are sometimes referred to as *desensitizing agents*. They impart a flavor and odor of their own to the product and have a mild anesthetic effect on the sensory receptor organs associated with taste. Monosodium glutamate has been widely used in the food industry, and to a lesser extent, in pharmaceuticals, for its reported ability to enhance natural flavors. A carefully selected panel reported this substance to be effective in reducing the metallic taste of iron-containing liquids, as well as the bitterness and aftertaste of a variety of other pharmaceutical preparations.[54] It cannot be used in pediatric products, however.

Chemburkar and Joslin have reported that the partitioning of parabens into flavoring oils from aqueous systems depends on the concentration of the flavoring oil, the nature and concentration of the additives, and pH.[55]

Wesley's Pharmaceutical Flavor Guide contains suggestions for flavoring over 51 types of pharmaceutical preparations.[53] It and many similar reports provide some guidance for the formulation chemist, but the final selection

TABLE 15-4. *Flavor Selection*

Taste Sensation	Recommended Flavor
Salt	Butterscotch, maple, apricot, peach, vanilla, wintergreen mint
Bitter	Wild cherry, walnut, chocolate, mint combinations, passion fruit, mint spice, anise
Sweet	Fruit and berry, vanilla
Sour	Citrus flavors, licorice, root beer, raspberry

must result from a trial and error approach. Inherent in this approach is what is referred to as taste fatigue. Repeated samplings of strong tasting substances soon result in decreased flavor acuity, and therefore, impaired ability to evaluate flavor properly. Preliminary flavoring should be carried out on diluted samples. This is done by preparing flavored vehicles and adding increments of the medicament or other formulation components responsible for the taste problem. The concentration at which the taste of the medicament is perceptible is referred to as the *minimum threshold level*. The vehicles that are most effective in masking low levels of drug are candidates for full-strength flavor evaluation.

Flavor evaluation techniques have progressed to a much greater extent than flavor selection. Taste panels can be useful in selecting one of several candidate formulations. This subject, as well as other flavor considerations, has been surveyed in an excellent book assembled by Arthur D. Little, Inc.[56]

Appearance

The overall appearance of liquid products depends primarily on their color and clarity. Color selection is usually made to be consistent with flavor, i.e., green or blue for mint, red for berry. The types of colorants available for pharmaceutical use, their relative stabilities, and areas of application have been reviewed by Swartz and Cooper.[57]

The dyes (and the maximum amounts) permitted for use in pharmaceuticals vary from country to country. Each regulatory agency also revises its approved list from time to time. Before formulating a product that may be marketed in several countries, it would be wise to check the current status of each dye. Suppliers of the dyes are usually excellent sources of information on this subject.

A purification step invariably is required to achieve maximum clarity. Particulate matter may be introduced through lint and fibers from the solvent or trace quantities of insoluble contaminants in one or more of the formulation components. It is quite common, for example, for alcoholic solutions of natural flavors to precipitate pectins and resins on addition to the bulk aqueous solution. The removal of this and other particulate matter is referred to as "polishing," and technically may be accomplished in several ways: (1) by settling and subsequent decantation, (2) by centrifugation, and (3) by filtration. Filtration is the only practical method

when large volumes of liquid are involved. A discussion of clarification and filtration procedures can be found in Chapter 7. It is in order at this point, however, to mention some of the effects that this process can have on the product. The filter pads most frequently used for oral liquids were formerly composed either entirely of asbestos or of mixtures of asbestos and cellulose. With the finding that asbestos fibers can cause cancer,[58,59] liquids are now filtered, whenever possible, through membrane filters. A number of manufacturers make available membrane filters in a variety of materials and pore sizes. Combined with filter aids and prefilters, they can be used to filter most pharmaceutical liquids.

Studies should be carried out before and after filtration to determine the extent, if any, to which actives, preservatives, flavors, colorants, and other important product components are adsorbed. Production conditions should be simulated as closely as possible, and particular attention given to filtration rate and liquid-to-filter surface area ratio.

Adsorption observed in the filtration of small batches in which the ratio of adsorptive surface to liquid volume is large may be misleading. Under production conditions, when the ratio of adsorptive surface to liquid volume is small, this effect may be insignificant. If adsorption is a significant problem and a nonadsorptive filter cannot be found, a satisfactory filtration process may require the use of an appropriate overcharge or preequilibration of the filter medium with the formulating component(s) being adsorbed.

A much less common problem is that of extraction of materials from the filter pad. This is only of concern insofar as the extracted material may affect the physical and chemical stability of the product. (Pharmaceutically acceptable filter pads and aids contain no biologically active components). For this reason, stability studies must be carried out on product made by the same process as the one to be used for ultimate production.

Stability

Chemical Stability. Techniques for predicting chemical stability of homogeneous drug systems are well defined.[60] Chemical instability of a drug invariably is magnified in solution, as opposed to solid or suspension systems. This liability, however, is to a large extent offset by the rapid and accurate stability predictions, which are possible with homogeneous systems but are extremely risky with heterogeneous dosage forms.

Studies involving evaluation of stability in liquid drug systems include the effect of amino acids on the stability of aspirin in propylene glycol solutions,[61] and a systematic study of the autoxidation of polysorbates.[62]

Physical Stability. A physically stable oral liquid retains its viscosity, color, clarity, taste, and odor throughout its shelf-life. All of these characteristics can and should be evaluated subjectively, and objectively if possible, during the course of stability assessment. A freshly made sample should serve as a reference standard for subjective evaluations.

Objective measurements should be made when such tests are practical. Color can readily be measured spectrophotometrically, and the absorbance at the appropriate wave length of aged samples can be compared with the initial value to determine the extent of color change. Clarity is best determined by shining a focused beam of light through the solution. Undissolved particles scatter the light, and under these conditions, the solution appears hazy. Light-scattering equipment is available to give a quantitative measure of turbidity. In general, however, this type of measurement is not necessary in the evaluation of oral liquids. In most cases, a liquid that becomes noticeably turbid with age is unacceptable. A quantitative measure of the turbidity is of little importance except as a tool in determining factors that influence the rate at which the liquid becomes turbid.

Taste and odor continue to be subjectively evaluated by the formulation chemist. This is done either by the pharmaceutical investigator, or preferably, by a panel of unbiased, taste-sensitive individuals. Coded aged samples are submitted to each panel member along with a similarly coded reference sample. The odor and taste of the reference sample should be known to be intact. Product that has been stored in the refrigerator frequently is used as the reference sample. Each panel member is asked to taste and compare the coded samples. If most of the panel members cannot detect a difference between samples, obviously the organoleptic character of the aged sample has not significantly changed. Some time should be allowed to pass between the preparation of a flavored sample and taste testing. Aging for about two weeks to one month is recommended to permit flavor blending.

Some attempts have been made, mainly by the perfume and flavor industry, to characterize products by vapor phase chromatography. This approach has proven useful with respect to pure flavors and perfumes, but has rarely been successfully applied to a finished pharmaceutical product.

An integral part of any stability study should include consideration of the package and the effect the package may have on the contents as well as the effect the contents may have on the package. For this reason, stability studies that are intended to support a New Drug Application and/or marketing of a drug must be carried out on the package intended for ultimate use. A well-designed stability protocol should call for a thorough evaluation of both the package and its contents at various conditions of storage, including exposure to both natural and artifical light of known amounts.

It is important to store the final product in the same container in which it was marketed until its expiration date. Flavors and colors often change with time, owing to adsorption by plastic containers or closures, or evaporation of the solvent, with a resultant concentrating of the product or chemical breakdown. One example of chemical breakdown is oxidative breakdown induced by repeated opening of a pint or gallon container to dispense prescriptions. This results in a new source of oxygen being introduced and a larger headspace with each dispensing.

Most oral liquids are packaged in either amber or flint glass containers with plastic or metal caps. Fortunately, glass is generally inert to aqueous solutions in the pH range appropriate for oral liquids. The same is not necessarily true for the cap and liner. Plastic caps may undergo stress cracking on contact with some liquids, whereas under some conditions, corrosion may be a problem with metal caps. In both cases, it is important to select a liner that on the basis of actual testing, is compatible with the package contents.

The integrity of the seal between a cap and container depends on the geometry of the cap and container, the materials used in their construction, the composition of the cap liner, and the tightness with which the cap is applied. Torque is a measure of the circular force, measured in inch-pounds, applied in closing or opening a container. The application and removal torque should be considered an integral part of any pharmaceutical development project involving a threaded package and is of particular importance with respect to liquid formulations. An inadequate cap seal may result in excessive loss of volatile components or leakage of product from the container. Extreme tightening may deform or break closures and make the cap excessively difficult to remove. Product prepared for stability evaluation should be capped with essentially the same torque as anticipated for use in production.

The optimum application torque for closures and containers varies, depending on the material used in their manufacture. The proper application torque should be determined experimentally by the use of containers and closures of the same size, neck finish, and composition as those intended for use in the final product. The recommended application torque is generally a compromise between the torque providing maximum product protection and the torque that allows for convenient cap removal.

Manufacturing Considerations

The basic principles involved in the preparation of homogeneous liquids are the same regardless of the quantity of material involved. The solubility of the solute and intramolecular and intermolecular interactions in the final solution *at equilibrium* are independent of the manner in which the solution is made. This assumes, of course, that the method of compounding does not affect the final composition of the system, as would be the case if a volatile component were charged to a heated solution. The *rate* at which equilibrium is achieved, however, is highly dependent on the details of the compounding procedure and the equipment used.

The reader is directed to an article by Carstensen and Mehta for a discussion of several factors involved in scaling-up solution dosage forms for manufacturing.[63] Areas covered include heating, agitation, and clarification. Basic equations and example calculations are provided in the article.

Liquid processing lends itself to computer-controlled automation. A few pharmaceutical firms have already instituted automated or semi-automated processes for several large-selling liquid products. Yelvigi has written a good basic review of this developing area of technology.[64]

Raw Materials

The raw materials used in manufacturing liquids should conform to well thought out specifications. These specifications should assure identity, purity, uniformity, and freedom from excessive microbial contamination. Incoming raw materials should be impounded and thoroughly tested before they are released for manufacturing. Additional processing may be necessary to obtain a desirable property, such as particle size or freedom from microorganisms. With regard to microbial contamination of raw materials, it is usually much easier to begin with low counts in the raw materials than to try to reduce these counts substantially during processing.

Aside from the active ingredient, water is usually the most important constituent in a liquid product. It should meet the USP requirements for purified water. It may be obtained by distillation or ion-exchange treatment. In recent years, manufacturers have devoted considerable effort to upgrading the microbial purity of the water supply used in oral liquids. Techniques employed include reverse osmosis purification, ultraviolet sterilization, membrane filtration, and constant circulation in piping systems that have no "dead ends" where microorganisms can thrive. In general, the most difficult microbes to remove from a purified water system are the pseudomonads. Figure 15-10 shows a purified water system designed to minimize microbial growth.

Many of the ideas incorporated in Figure 15-10 have been taken from experience gained in preparing and storing pyrogen-free water for injection and adapted to the manufacture of high-quality de-ionized water for use with liquid pharmaceutical products.

The ion-exchange resins used in the water system are important to the successful maintenance of low bacteria counts. An example of an appropriate mixed resin bed would be Ambergard XE-352 and Amberlite IR-120. Ambergard XE-352 is a large-pore, macroreticular, Type 1 quaternary ammonium anion-exchange resin. It is effective for a wide range of flow rates and for many different bacterial strains.[65] Amberlite IR-120 is a strongly acidic, cation-exchange resin that balances the chemical equilibrium of the water.

The use of ultraviolet sterilization of water has been discussed in some detail in the literature.[66,67] Two factors should be emphasized at this point: (1) The flow rate of the water should not exceed the capability of the sterilizing unit, and (2) even if sterility is achieved, a filter should still be used downstream to remove the dead microorganisms and particulate matter. Although the first point seems self-evident, it is violated surprisingly often—compromising the effectiveness of the entire system.

A number of in-line filtration units are commercially available. These filters are discussed in Chapter 7.

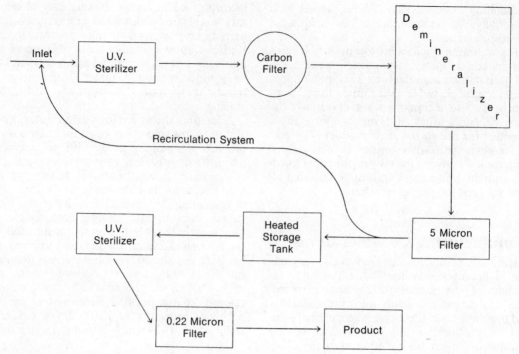

FIG. 15-10. *Schematic drawing of a deionized water system for the manufacture of liquid pharmaceutical products.*

Equipment

In the most general terms, the type of equipment used in the manufacture of oral solutions consists of mixing tanks equipped with a means of agitation, measuring devices for large and small amounts of solids and liquids, and a filtration system for the final polishing and/or sterilization of the solution. In addition, most production facilities are equipped with systems for bulk material handling, such as tote bins and tote bin discharging equipment.

FitzSimon has written a valuable and practical discussion on the design of piping, valves, mixers, pumps, and controls to produce high-quality liquid products.[68]

All equipment must be thoroughly cleaned and sanitized (sterilized if possible) before use. Appropriate disinfectants include dilute solutions of hydrogen peroxide, phenol derivatives, and peracetic acid. Equipment and lines can be sterilized by such methods as alcohol, boiling water, autoclaving, steam, or dry heat.

Tanks are usually constructed of polished stainless steel and are usually jacketed to allow for heating or cooling of the contents. They can be obtained in a number of different sizes, and are completely covered and equipped with see-through charging ports and illumination for easy observation of the contents. If tanks are used for the compounding of the bulk liquid, they have a built-in agitation system.

Water condensate that forms on the lid of mixing tanks and similar processing equipment during heating and chilling steps may provide a source of microbial contamination that is often overlooked.

The liquid is then clarified by cycling through a filtration system, and the polished solution is stored in an adjacent tank until released by the quality control department. The liquid may then be transported to the filling line, either manually by filling into portable transport tanks or by pumping (or gravity flow) through a suitable liquid delivery conduit.

The distance the product travels between the holding tank and the filling line should be held to a minimum to reduce the chance of microbial contamination. All lines should be easy to disassemble, clean, and sanitize.

A major source of microbial contamination is often the processing operators. Head covering should be worn at all times. Gloves and face masks should be worn as necessary.

An ongoing education program is recommended to maintain operator interest and concern for good work habits.

In additions, the use of portable laminar flow units can be an aid in certain operations (such as the addition of ingredients to a tank).

Compounding Procedure

Dilute solutions, prepared from rapidly dissolving materials, are simply prepared by charging the solute to the solvent and agitating until the solution is homogeneous. When more concentrated solutions are being made, or when the solute is slowly dissolving, it may be advantageous to employ heat. The syrup formula and manufacturing method presented in Table 15-5 illustrate some of the steps involved in compounding a complex liquid formulation.

The rationale for most of the steps cited in this procedure is obvious. Several steps, however, warrant some discussion. Step 1 calls for the metering of a specific amount of purified water into the compounding tank. The precise quantity of water in this case is not critical, but in spite of this, a confirmatory volumetric check is desirable, to protect against the consequences of a malfunctioning metering device. The purified water is heated in step 2 primarily to facilitate the solution of sucrose, the other solutes being rapidly soluble even in cold water. In step 5, the menthol and flavor are dissolved in an aliquot of the alcohol, and this alcohol solution is charged to the batch (step 6). As previously mentioned, the equilibrium solubility of all solutes is the same regardless of the manner in which they are charged. The rate at which solution is achieved, however, can be markedly influenced by the compounding procedure. In this case, predissolving the menthol and flavor in alcohol, in which both solutes are highly soluble, and then charging the resultant alcoholic solution to the main part of the batch effect rapid approach to equilibrium conditions.

Solutes present in small concentrations, particularly dyes and other intensely colored materials, should be predissolved prior to mixing with the main portion of the batch, as is indicated in step 8. This is done to ensure complete solution of the substance before the batch is further processed. If the solutes were charged directly to the bulk mixing tank, it would be extremely difficult to determine the presence of a small amount of undissolved material at the bottom of the tank. As a rule, complete solution should usually be confirmed at every stage in the manufacture of a homogeneous liquid.

TABLE 15-5. *Syrup Formula and Manufacturing Method*

Formula	Per ml	Per batch (5000 L)
Drug	2.00 mg.	10.0 kg.
Sodium benzoate USP	1.00 mg.	5.0 kg.
Menthol, USP	0.10 mg.	0.5 kg.
Alcohol, USP	0.05 ml. (40.8 mg.)	250.0 liters (204.0 kg.)
Flavor	0.005 ml. (4.5 mg.)	25.0 liters (22.5 kg.)
Dye FD&C Yellow No. 6	0.10 mg.	0.5 kg.
Glycerin	0.05 ml. (62.45 mg.)	250.0 liters (312.250 kg.)
Sorbitol solution, USP	0.10 ml. (128.5 mg)	500.0 liters (642.5 kg.)
Standard granulated sugar	550.00 mg.	2750.0 kg.
Purified water, USP q.s. to	1.0 ml.	5000 liters

Compounding Instructions:

1. Charge 2000 L of purified water through the water meter into the compounding tank. Check the volume against the outage chart. Heat to approximately 50°C.

2. To the water in the compounding tank, charge the following materials in the amounts specified in the batch sheet. Dissolve each one, with agitation, before adding the next: (a) drug, (b) sodium benzoate, (c) standard granulated sugar. Agitate the contents of the compounding tank until homogeneous, and then cool to 30°C.

3. Charge the specified amount of glycerin to the compounding tank. Agitate until the batch is homogeneous.

4. Charge the specified amount of sorbitol solution to the compounding tank. Agitate until the batch is homogeneous.

5. Measure 20 L of alcohol into a suitable stainless steel container. Add and dissolve the specified charge of menthol. Add and dissolve the specified charge of flavor.

6. Charge the alcoholic solution of menthol and flavor to the batch in the compounding tank. Agitate until homogeneous.

7. Charge the balance of the specified amount of alcohol to the batch. Agitate until homogeneous.

8. Charge 10 L of purified water to a clean stainless steel container. Add to the water and dissolve the specified amount of FD&C Yellow No. 6.

9. Charge the dye solution to the batch in the compounding tank, and agitate until homogeneous.

10. Add to the compounding tank sufficient purified water to bring the batch volume to 5000 L.

11. Weigh out 2.5 kg of filter aid, and charge it to the contents of the compounding tank. Agitate for 10 min. The batch is now ready to filter.

12. Cycle the batch through the filter and back to the compounding tank until the filtrate is clear. At this point, the filtrate may be discharged and collected in the designated holding tank.

13. Sample the batch, and submit for testing in accordance with standard procedure.

Step 11 calls for the addition of a specified amount of filter aid to the contents of the compounding tank. The amount and type of filter aid must be determined during the development of the product. The amount used does not usually exceed 0.5 g/L.

In the laboratory, liquids are usually measured by volume. When large quantities of liquid materials are handled, however, it is frequently more convenient and accurate to use gravimetric means of measurement. For this reason, all liquid components of the cited formula are expressed in units of both volume and weight.

Packaging

The specific method used for filling a pharmaceutical liquid varies greatly depending on the characteristics of the liquid (e.g., viscosity, surface tension, foam-producing qualities, and compatibility with the materials used in the construction of the filling machine), the type of package into which the liquid is placed, and the required production output. Three basic filling methods—gravimetric, volumetric, and constant level—are used for most liquid filling operations. The latter two methods are used most frequently in the filling of pharmaceutical liquids. Filling containers to a given weight (gravimetric filling) is generally limited to large containers or to highly viscous products. The process does not readily lend itself to high-speed, automatic equipment.

Volumetric filling is usually accomplished by positive displacement piston action.* Each filling station is equipped with a measuring piston and cylinder. The fill accuracy is controlled by the close tolerances to which the pistons and cylinders are manufactured. The fill amount is measured by the stroke of the piston, which on all machines can be varied to a limited degree. Major changes in fill amount usually necessitate changing the piston and cylinder assembly. This type of device is capable of accuracy to within fractions of a milliliter. There are, however, several significant problems associated with volume filling. Highly viscous liquids may cause the pistons to seize, resulting in either loss of fill accuracy or line breakdown. On the opposite side of the spectrum, thin liquids may flow past the pis-

ton, causing uncontrollable dripping from the filling spout and associated fill inaccuracies. These problems can be controlled to a large extent by proper engineering of the filling machine. An inherent problem with volumetric filling, however, is encountered when containers are used that are not dimensionally uniform. In this case, even though the fill amount is accurate, the fill height varies inversely with the container capacity, i.e., an oversized package appears to have a slack fill, whereas an undersized package appears to have an excessive fill.

Constant-level filling uses the container as the means for controlling the fill of each unit. The fill amount is varied by adjusting the height to which the container is filled. Any dimensional variations in the containers result in comparable variations in the net fill per unit. The oldest form of a constant-level filler involves the use of a siphon; however, this method of filling is usually slow and is rarely used when high production rates are required. The high-speed, automated, constant-level filling machines in use today are generally based on the siphon principle, with the major modification being the induced pressure differential between the liquid discharge nozzle and the constant-level overflow system. The most widely used methods can be broadly classified into three categories: vacuum filling, gravity-vacuum filling, and pressure-vacuum filling.

The principle of vacuum filling is illustrated in Figure 15-11. To fill by vacuum, a seal must be made between the filling head and the container. A vacuum is then developed within the container, which causes the liquid to flow from the bulk liquid tank to the container. The liquid level rises until it reaches the vacuum tube, which is positioned at the desired constant level. Excess liquid is drawn through the vacuum tube and can be recycled to the bulk liquid tank. In gravity-vacuum filling, the bulk liquid tanks are a level above the filling stem, so that the driving force for liquid flow results from both the negative pressure in the container and the force of gravity. Similarly, in pressure-vacuum filling, a positive pressure is applied to the bulk liquid, which in combination with the vacuum developed in the container, results in a pressure differential that allows for rapid filling of even highly viscous liquids. The latter two methods require some valve mechanism that is responsive to the presence of the container, to open and subsequently close a valve device in the filling stem assembly. Vacuum filters do not require such a mechanism, since a pressure differential to promote liquid flow can only be

---

*Volumetric filling can also be accomplished by the pumping of a liquid at a constant pressure through an orifice of constant size for a predetermined period of time. The volume can be varied by increasing or decreasing the pressure and by varying the time between opening and closing the filling nozzle.

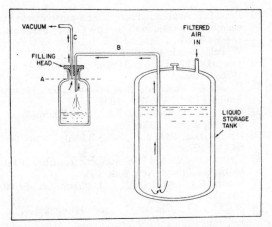

FIG. 15-11. *Schematic diagram of the principle used in* vacuum filling. *The vacuum drawn through tube C reduced pressure in the container. Pressure differential causes liquid in storage tank to flow through tube B into container. When liquid level reaches point A, excess is carried out through tube C and may be recycled to liquid storage tank. Note—In* gravity-vacuum *filling, the bottom of the liquid storage tank is at a level above the filling head. In* pressure-vacuum *filling, a positive pressure is applied to the liquid in the storage tank.*

achieved by the vacuum formed when the filling stem forms a seal with the container.

A problem that is common to all types of liquid filling machines, but that is particularly bothersome with high-speed automatic equipment, is excessive foam. Foaming during the filling operation often can be decreased by filling equipment that minimizes product turbulence, closed-system filling to limit the introduction of air or other gases that participate in the formation of foam, mechanical defoaming devices, and reduction in the speed of the filling line.

All of these methods introduce considerable engineering and production difficulties. It would be preferable to formulate the product with careful consideration of the problems that eventually might be encountered in large-scale production and high-speed filling operations.

A microbial survey should be performed on all packaging materials that come into contact with the product to ensure that microbial contamination is not introduced at this point. Attention must also be paid to details during packaging operations. For example, on small-volume orders in which bottle closures or tips for plastic squeeze-spray containers are often placed on the product by hand, this procedure can be a source of microbial contamination from the hands of operators unless gloves are used that are presterilized and periodically disinfected during use.

References

1. Martin, A.N., Swarbrick, J., and Cammarata, A.: Physical Pharmacy. 2nd Ed. Lea & Febiger, Philadelphia, 1969.
2. Higuchi, T., Gupta, M., and Busse, L.W.: J. Am. Pharm. Assoc., Sci. Ed., 42:157, 1953.
3. Windheuser, J.: Bull. Parenteral Drug Assoc., 17:1, 1963.
4. Wang, L.-H., and Paruta, A.N.: Drug Dev. and Ind. Pharm., 10:667, 1984.
5. Wang, L.-H., and Paruta, A.N.: Drug Dev. and Ind. Pharm., 10:861, 1984.
6. Yalkowsky, S.H., Amidon, G.L., Zografi, G., and Flynn, G.L.: J. Pharm. Sci., 64:48, 1975.
7. Lee, C.H., and Lindstrom, R.E.: Drug Dev. and Ind. Pharm., 7:223, 1981.
8. Spiegel, A.J., and Noseworthy, M.M.: J. Pharm. Sci., 52:917, 1963.
9. Hildebrand, J.H., and Scott, R.L.: The Solubility of Nonelectrolytes. Reinhold, New York, 1950.
10. Hildebrand, J.H., and Scott, R.L.: Regular Solutions. Prentice-Hall, Englewood Cliffs, NJ, 1962.
11. Chertkoff, M.J., and Martin, A.N.: J. Am. Pharm. Assoc., Sci. Ed., 49:444, 1960.
12. Restaino, F.A., and Martin, A.N.: J. Pharm. Sci., 53:636, 1964.
13. Acree, W.E., Jr., and Bertrand, G.L.: J. Pharm. Sci., 70:1033, 1981.
14. Paruta, A.N., Sciarrone, B.J., and Lordi, N.G.: J. Pharm. Sci., 51:704, 1962.
15. Sorby, D.L., Bitter, R.G., and Webb, J.G.: J. Pharm. Sci., 52:1149, 1963.
16. Lordi, N.G., Sciarrone, B.J., Ambrosio, T.J., and Paruta, A.N.: J. Pharm. Sci., 53:463, 1964.
17. Paruta, A.N.: J. Pharm. Sci., 53:1252, 1964.
18. Cave, G., Puisieux, F., and Carstensen, J.T.: J. Pharm. Sci., 68:424, 1979.
19. Paruta, A.N., and Sheth, B.B.: J. Pharm. Sci., 55:896, 1966.
20. Paruta, A.N., and Irani, S.A.: J. Pharm. Sci., 55:1055, 1966.
21. Sheth, B.B., Paruta, A.N., and Ninger, F.C.: J. Pharm. Sci., 55:1144, 1966.
22. Paruta, A.N., and Sheth, B.B.: J. Pharm. Sci., 55:1208, 1966.
23. Paruta, A.N.: J. Pharm. Sci., 56:1565, 1967.
24. Paruta, A.N.: J. Pharm. Sci., 58:364, 1969.
25. Breon, T.L., and Paruta, A.N.: J. Pharm. Sci., 59:1306, 1970.
26. Breon, T.L., Mauger, J.W., Osborne, G.E., et al.: Drug. Dev. Comm., 2:521, 1976.
27. The Handbook of Chemistry and Physics. 45th Ed. The Chemical Rubber Co., Cleveland, OH, 1964, p. 30.
28. Margott, A.A., and Smith, E.R.: Table of Dielectric Constants of Pure Liquids. N.B.S. Circ. 514, U.S. Govt. Printing Office, Washington, DC, 1951.
29. Breon, T.L., Mauger, J.W., and Paruta, A.N.: Drug Dev. and Ind. Pharm., 6:87, 1980.
30. McBain, J.W.: Advances in Colloid Science. Vol. I. Interscience, New York, 1942.
31. Swarbrick, J.: J. Pharm. Sci., 54:1229, 1965.
32. Kuettel, D.: Pharm. Zentralhalle, 102:116, 1963 (through Chem. Abstracts).

33. MonteBovi, A.J., Halpern, A., and Mazzola, P.: J. Am. Pharm. Assoc., Pract. Ed., 15:162, 1954.
34. Harned, H.S., and Owen, B.B.: The Physical Chemistry of Electrolyte Solutions. 3rd Ed. Reinhold, New York, 1958, p. 161.
35. Leyden, A.F., Pomerantz, E., and Bouchard, E.G.: J. Am. Pharm. Assoc., Sci. Ed., 45:773, 1956.
36. Bulletin, Atlas Chemical Industries Inc., Wilmington, DE.
37. Conrad, L.I., Kalmen, M., and Maso, H.F.: Drug and Cosmetic Industry, 83:160, 1958.
38. McBain, M.E.L., and Hutchinson, E.: Solubilization. Academic Press, New York, 1965.
39. Guttman, D.E., Hamlin, W.E., Shell, J.W., and Wagner, J.G.: J. Pharm. Sci., 50:305, 1961.
40. Kern, C.J., and Antoshkiw, T.: Ind. Eng. Chem., 42:709, 1950.
41. Coles, C.L.J., and Thomas, D.F.W.: J. Pharm. Pharmacol., 4:898, 1952.
42. Scott, M.J., Goudie, A.J., and Huetteman, A.J.: J. Am. Pharm. Assoc., Sci. Ed., 49:467, 1960.
43. Neuberg, C., et al.: Biochem. Z., 76:107, 1916.
44. Neuberg, C., et al.: Biochem. Z., 229:467, 1930.
45. Wolfson, B.B., and Banker, G.S.: J. Pharm. Sci., 54:195, 1965.
46. McGregor Scott, H.: Manuf. Chem. Aerosol News, 1972.
47. Bruch, C.W.: Drug and Cosmetic Industry, 110:32, 1972.
48. Alexander, K.S., LaPrada, B., Mauger, J.W., and Paruta, A.N.: J. Pharm. Sci., 67:624, 1978.
49. Lachman, L.: Bull. Parenteral Drug Assoc., 22:127, 1968.
50. Ward, D.R., Lathrop, L.B., and Lynch, M.J.: Drug and Cosmetic Industry, 99:48, 1966.
51. Beck, C.I.: Application potential for aspartame in low calorie and dietetic foods. In Low Calorie and Special Dietary Foods. Edited by B.K. Dwivedi. CRC Press, W. Palm Beach, FL, 1978, p. 68.
52. Janovsky, H.L.: Drug and Cosmetic Industry, 86:335, 1960.
53. Wesley, F.: Pharmaceutical Flavor Guide. Fritzsche Brothers Inc., New York, 1957.
54. Caul, J.F., and Rockwood, E.L.: J. Am. Pharm. Assoc., Sci. Ed., 42:682, 1953.
55. Chemburkar, P.G., and Joslin, R.S.: J. Pharm. Sci., 64:414, 1975.
56. Flavor Research and Food Acceptance. Arthur D. Little Inc., Reinhold, New York, 1958.
57. Swartz, C.J., and Cooper, J.: J. Pharm. Sci., 51:89, 1962.
58. Selikoff, I.J., Chung, J., and Hammond, E.C.: J.A.M.A., 188:22, 1964.
59. Selikoff, I.J., Hammond, E.C., and Chung, J.: J.A.M.A., 204:106, 1968.
60. Garrett, E.R.: Kinetics and mechanisms in stability of drugs. In Advances in Pharmaceutical Sciences. Vol. 2. Academic Press, New York, 1967.
61. Narang, P.K., and Lim, J.K.: J. Pharm. Sci., 68:645, 1979.
62. Donbrow, M., Azaz, E., and Pillersdorf, A.: J. Pharm. Sci., 67:1676, 1978.
63. Carstensen, J.T., and Mehta, A.: Pharm. Tech., 6:64, 1982.
64. Yelvigi, M.: Pharm. Tech., 8:47, 1984.
65. Scruton, S.H.: Pharm. Tech., 4:39, 1980.
66. Ellner, G.G., and Ellner, S.: Drug and Cosmetic Industry, 104:54, 1969.
67. Olson, S.W.: Amer. Perfumer. Cosmetic, 85:97, 1970.
68. FitzSimon, R.: Drug Dev. Commun., 2:1, 1976.

16

Pharmaceutical Suspensions

NAGIN K. PATEL, LLOYD KENNON,* *and* R. SAUL LEVINSON

Suspensions form an important class of pharmaceutical dosage forms. These disperse systems present many formulation, stability, manufacturing, and packaging challenges. The primary objective of this chapter is not to develop a formulary, but rather to put forth some of the basic theoretic and practical considerations that apply to suspension systems, and to relate these principles to formulation methods, evaluation procedures, and manufacturing techniques. The reader is assumed to have at least some knowledge of basic pharmaceutical technology.

For the most part, only aqueous suspensions are discussed, and little attention is paid to oils or aerosol propellants as suspension vehicles. Also, this discussion is limited to suspensions with particles having diameters greater than 0.2 micron, approximately the lower limit of resolution of optical microscopes; for purposes of comparison, a human hair has a diameter of about 75 microns (0.003 in.). Systems with particles smaller than 0.1 to 0.2 micron are generally considered to be colloidal, and they exhibit properties that lie between those of true molecular solutions and suspensions of visible particles. Thus, although suspended particles do not exhibit all the properties of colloids, such as the so-called colligative properties, they do have heightened surface properties, that is, whatever surface properties exist are magnified because of the increased surface area. In actual experience, this additional action expresses itself as an enhanced power of adsorption. The colligative properties just noted depend on the number of "particles" (molecules, ions, aggregates) rather than on their nature. They are possessed by true solutions and by many colloidal solutions and are manifested as freezing-point depression,

boiling-point elevation, and osmotic-pressure phenomena.

Suspensions are heterogeneous systems consisting of two phases. The *continuous* or *external phase* is generally a liquid or semisolid, and the *dispersed* or *internal phase* is made up of particulate matter that is essentially insoluble in, but dispersed throughout, the continuous phase; the insoluble matter may be intended for physiologic absorption or for internal or external coating functions. The dispersed phase may consist of discrete particles, or it may be a network of particles resulting from particle-particle interactions. Almost all suspension systems separate on standing. The formulator's main concern, therefore, is not necessarily to try to eliminate separation, but rather to decrease the rate of the settling and to permit easy resuspendability of any settled particulate matter. A satisfactory suspension must remain sufficiently homogeneous for at least the period of time necessary to remove and administer the required dose after shaking its container. Traditionally, certain kinds of pharmaceutical suspensions have been given separate designations, such as mucilages, magmas, gels, and sometimes aerosols; also included would be dry powders to which a vehicle is added at the time of dispensing.

Theoretic Considerations

A knowledge of the theoretic considerations pertaining to suspension technology should ultimately help the formulator to select the ingredients that are most appropriate for the suspension and to use the available mixing and milling equipment to the best advantage. Some understanding of wetting, particle interaction, electrokinetics, aggregation, and sedimentation concepts facilitates the making of good formulatory decisions.

*Deceased

Wetting

A frequently encountered difficulty that is a factor of prime importance in suspension formulation concerns the wetting of the solid phase by the suspension medium. By definition, a suspension is essentially an incompatible system, but to exist at all, it requires some degree of compatibility, and good wetting of the suspended material is important in achieving this end.

When a strong affinity exists between a liquid and a solid, the liquid easily forms a film over the surface of the solid. When this affinity is nonexistent or weak, however, the liquid has difficulty displacing the air or other substances surrounding the solid, and there exists an angle of contact between the liquid and the solid. This contact angle, θ, results from an equilibrium involving three interfacial tensions, specifically, those acting at the interfaces between the liquid and vapor phases, at the solid and liquid phases, and at the solid and vapor phases. These tensions are caused by unbalanced intermolecular forces in the various phases similar to the familiar analogous phenomenon of the convex "skin" formation over the surface of a glass of water filled to the brim. The contact angle concept is important because it affords a method of considering degrees of wettability and indicates that surface properties are important. An involved mathematical treatment of wetting is possible, but needed data usually are not available to make any equations useful. It is easier for the formulator simply to try a few surfactants to find a good wetting agent.

Certain solids are readily wet by liquid media whereas others are not. In *aqueous* suspension terminology, solids are said to be either *hydrophilic* (lyophilic or solvent-loving, rarely lyotropic) or *hydrophobic* (lyophobic). Hydrophilic substances are easily wet by water or other polar liquids; they may also greatly increase the viscosity of water suspensions. Hydrophobic substances repel water but can usually be wetted by nonpolar liquids; they usually do not alter the viscosity of aqueous dispersions. Hydrophilic solids usually can be incorporated into suspensions without the use of a wetting agent, but hydrophobic materials are extremely difficult to disperse and frequently float on the surface of the fluid owing to poor wetting of the particles or the presence of tiny air pockets.

A frequently helpful pharmaceutical technique for modifying the wetting characteristics of powders involves the use of surfactants (sometimes with shearing) to decrease the solid-liquid interfacial tension. The mechanism of surfactant action is thought to involve the preferential adsorption of the hydrocarbon chain by the hydrophobic surface, with the polar moiety of the surfactant being then directed toward the aqueous phase. Other materials that can be used to aid dispersion of hydrophobic solids are hydrophilic polymers such as sodium carboxymethylcellulose and certain water-insoluble hydrophilic materials such as bentonite, aluminum-magnesium silicates, and colloidal silica, either alone or in combination. These materials also exert viscosity-building effects, depending on the specific type and concentration used. These hydrophilic agents may, if used at too high a concentration, cause an undesirable gelling instead of just the desired degree of viscosity or thixotropy; the latter term refers to the formation of a gel-like structure that is easily broken and becomes fluid upon agitation. Rheologically, the liquid is said to have a *yield value*. Incidentally, Carless and Ocran reported that in pharmaceutical suspensions, the yield value of a vehicle having the density of water must be about 0.3 dyne cm^{-2} to support solid particles having a diameter of 0.2 micron and a density of 1.5.[1]

Various screening techniques have been devised to facilitate the comparison of possible alternatives during the selection of a wetting agent. Some examples follow. Hiestand,[2] in an excellent review of suspensions, suggested the use of a narrow lyophobic trough, one end of which holds the powder while a solution of the wetting agent is placed in the other end. The relative rates of penetration of different agents can then be directly observed, the better agents showing the faster rates. Another technique involved measuring the relative ability of solutions of different wetting agents to carry powder through a gauze as the solutions are dropped onto the gauze supporting the powder. Obviously, the better wetters are able to function more effectively as vehicles and carry more powder through the gauze than the poorer wetters.

With respect to determining wettability, it is interesting to note that there have also been developed methods of comparing the wetting of powders by nonaqueous liquid vehicles; such wetting can be enhanced by certain lanolin derivatives. Obviously, lanolin derivatives, of which many lipophilic and hydrophilic types are available, find their major use in topically applied preparations. Two techniques developed by the paint industry that could be applied pharmaceutically involve determining the so-called wet and flow points. The wet point measures the amount of vehicle needed to just wet all of the powder. Reduction of the wet point by an additive indicates initial surface wetting by that agent in that powder-vehicle combination. The flow point measures the amount of vehicle needed to produce pourability. The extent to which the flow point of a powder-vehicle system is reduced by a surface active agent measures the degree to which the agent deaggregates the system, i.e., inhibits the buildup of a network-like structure by the solid phase. A low wet point coupled with a low flow point (and a small difference between the two) indicates good deaggregation or dispersion.

The wet point method involves incorporating the additive in the powder by rubbing the mixture on a glass plate with a spatula. The vehicle is then added drop-wise and worked thoroughly through the mass after each addition. The endpoint is reached when just enough vehicle has been incorporated to form a coherent mass that does not break or separate. Good reproducibility in the determination of the endpoint can be obtained. The sharpness of the endpoint values depends on the powder, vehicle, and additive employed. The wet point is expressed as milliliters per 100 grams and may, for example, have values of 15 to 45 with a 10% additive concentration. The better the wetting agent, the lower is the wet point value.

The flow point is also measured by mixing the additive with the powder, but in a beaker rather than on a plate. The vehicle is added and incorporated by thorough mixing. The endpoint is reached when just enough vehicle has been added to permit the mixture to flow from the spatula in a uniform stream. The flow point may be expressed as milliliters per 100 grams. The sharpness of the endpoint varies, as in the wet point determination, depending on the powder, vehicle, and additive. The flow point may have values at a 10% additive level in the range of 50 to 250, with the better wetting agents producing the lower values.

Testing an additive at only one concentration may not present an accurate evaluation of its effectiveness as a dispersant because dramatic decreases in the flow or wet points may be caused by concentration changes of only a small percentage. It is wise to investigate several additive concentrations before drawing conclusions relating to the utility of any particular agent.

A similar technique could be applied to aqueous systems. In this analogous method, water is added to a mixture of the material to be wetted and the various additives to be evaluated. Some test method modifications may be required to ensure that the powder and additive are mixed well, that is, in both tests, the additive and powder must be in intimate contact. This may best

be achieved by coating the powder with the additive in alcohol, which is then evaporated from the slurry. When lanolin derivatives are used with powders such as talc, titanium dioxide, or ferric oxide, values for the flow and wet points are in the same general range as previously mentioned, although somewhat lower values tend to be observed.

Particle Interactions and Behavior

The terms lyophobic (hydrophobic) and lyophilic (hydrophilic) were mentioned in the previous section. These terms are sometimes considered synonymous with nonwetting and wetting, respectively. The primary behavioral difference between these two classes of materials is their sensitivity to the presence of electrolytes. Lyophobic materials in suspension are sensitive to the addition of salts, whereas lyophilic materials are not. A lyophilic material, such as a gum, is readily wet by water, although in this instance, large amounts of electrolyte may affect the solution by salting out effects. As distinct from lyophobic materials, dilution with the vehicle reverses the precipitation of lyophilic solids. However, one may not observe aggregation, the desired form of matrix formation during sedimentation, in the case of the lyophobic particle. The stability of lyophobic colloids is also reduced by lowering the repulsive potential of the electrochemical double layer or by decreasing the degree of hydration.

In addition to the repulsion between particles resulting from the diffuse double layer, the ionic strength and the valence and size of the ions on the surface and in the double layer influence both the total charge (range: 0 to 50 millivolts) and the thickness of the double layer; these factors also influence hydration. Some of these overall interrelationships are illustrated in Figure 16-1. Note that increasing the concentration of ions in the solution decreases the thickness of the diffuse double layer by "swamping," and therefore aggregation is encouraged. Specific adsorption of an ion by the system also neutralizes the surface charge of the particle and allows aggregation. The concentration of electrolyte needed to effect optimal aggregation depends on the balance and type of interacting ion; addition of electrolyte past this point may result in a reversal of charge, which in turn would cause deaggregation and ultimate caking of the system. These ion effects can be systematized by referring to the Schulze-Hardy rule.

The Schulze-Hardy rule states that the va-

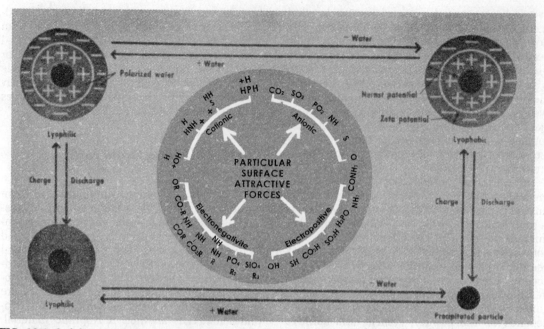

FIG. 16-1. *Stability of colloidal particles in aqueous suspension depends on hydration and electrostatic charge; these depend on the chemical composition and structure of the substrate at the liquid-solid interface. (From Industrial and Engineering Chemistry, 54:39, 1962. Reprinted by permission of the American Chemical Society.)*

lence of the ions having a charge opposite to that of the hydrophobic particle appears to determine the effectiveness of the electrolyte in aggregating the particles. The aggregating value or efficiency therefore increases with the valence of the ions. Divalent ions are ten times as effective as monovalent; trivalent are one thousand times as effective as monovalent. It is important to remember that this rule is valid only for systems in which there is no chemical interaction between the aggregating electrolyte and the ions of the double layer of the particle surface. Note also, incidentally, that aggregating forces are of sufficient magnitude to overwhelm the electrostatic repulsion between particles having net charges of the same sign. With respect to actual electrolyte concentrations used, satisfactory aggregation has been found to occur at the following approximate ion concentrations: 25 to 150 mmol/L for monovalent ions, 0.5 to 2.0 mmol/L for divalent ions, and 0.01 to 0.1 mmol/L for trivalent ions. The influence of valence and concentration on the aggregation of a lyophobic particle suspension can be determined experimentally by either measuring the change in zeta potential or by observing the degree of aggregation in terms of some measurable parameter such as sediment height.

Although it is not pharmaceutically useful to a great extent, the Hofmeister or lyotropic series

rule applies to hydrophilic particles in a manner somewhat analogous to the Schulze-Hardy rule, and takes into account not only the charge but also the ionic size and hydration capability. In order of decreasing aggregating ability, the monovalent cation and anion progressions are respectively Cs^+, Rb^+, NH_4^+, K^+, Na^+, Li^+, and F^+, IO_3^-, $H_2PO_4^-$, BrO_3^-, Cl^-, ClO_3^-, Br^-, NO_3^-, ClO_4^-, I^-, CNS^-.

Although there have been several attempts in the literature to clarify the imprecise terminology used to describe aggregation phenomena, the problem of definition is formidable.[3,4] The terms used in colloid science and pharmaceutical science do not coincide, and to make matters worse, individual workers tend to use the terms "flocculation," "coagulation," and "aggregation" interchangeably. Regardless of the mechanism of aggregation, it is convenient to classify the end result of the aggregation of suspension particulates on the basis of the morphologic characteristics of the aggregate.

Note first the open network aggregate, or *floccule*. This aggregate is characterized by a fibrous, fluffy, open network of aggregated particles,[4] as illustrated by Figure 16-2. The structure is quite rigid; hence, these aggregates settle quickly to form a high sediment height and are easily redispersible because the particles constituting individual aggregates are suffi-

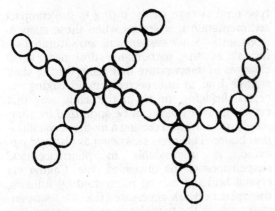

FIG. 16-2. *An artist's conception of open-network suspension aggregate.*

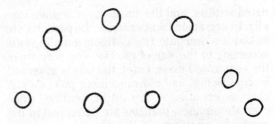

FIG. 16-4. *An artist's conception of dispersed suspension form.*

ciently far apart from one another to preclude caking.

Note second the closed aggregate, or *coagule*. This aggregate is characterized by a tight packing produced by surface film bonding,[4] as shown by Figure 16-3. These aggregates settle slowly to low sediment heights that approach the sediment density of a dispersed particulate system, which is discussed in the following paragraph. Characteristically, sediments composed of closed aggregates are not easily redispersed. The affinity of surface films to each other is responsible for the tenacity of the aggregate not only within an individual aggregate, but also to surrounding aggregates. Upon sedimentation, the aggregates tend to form a single large "film-bonded" aggregate, which is difficult, if not impossible, to redisperse. The surface films that lead to coagule formation are often surfactants, gases, immiscible liquids, and in the case of nonaqueous suspensions, water.

In addition to the two aggregation types just discussed, one should be cognizant of the deaggregated or dispersed form. In this suspension type, the individual particles are dispersed as discrete entities,[4] as illustrated by Figure 16-4. This suspension type sediments slowly (as compared with the closed and open aggregate types), attains the lowest possible sediment height, and owing to the closeness of the particle surfaces upon sedimentation, possesses a high potential for caking, because of the ease of formation of extensive crystal bridging, which is mentioned later in this chapter. Obviously, a pharmaceutical suspension must be redispersible on only mild agitation to ensure dosage uniformity.

The tendency of particles to aggregate depends on the forces of attraction and repulsion between them. If the repulsion is of sufficient strength, the particles remain dispersed; if not, they aggregate. The attractive forces between particles is thought to be due to London or van der Waals forces. The van der Waals forces of intermolecular attraction were named after a scientist who used certain constants in the gas equation he formulated as a correction to the ideal gas law. The forces are due to combinations of ionic, dipole, and induced dipole interatomic and intermolecular phenomena effected through dipole moments; the London forces terminology emphasizes the induced dipole aspects. For example, in a suspension of clay particles, as an increasing amount of sodium chloride is added, the repulsive forces decrease. As increasing amounts continue to be added, the repulsive forces can no longer counteract the van der Waals attraction, and the system aggregates.

Sedimentation and aggregation rates are properties of suspension systems governed by particle size, particle-particle interactions, densities of the particles and the medium, and the viscosity of the continuous phase. Subsidence is a term often used to describe the settling of an aggregated system and refers to the settling rate or descending of the boundary between the sediment and the clear supernatant above it. In polydispersed systems (i.e., those having many different particle sizes present), this measurement is of little value because the boundary is not well defined. In this case, the large particles settle downward more rapidly than the smaller particles, whereas in concentrated aggregated suspensions, the larger particles exhibit hin-

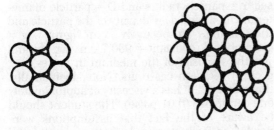

FIG. 16-3. *An artists's conception of closed suspension aggregate.*

dered settling, and the smallest settle more rapidly. In aggregated suspensions, the particles are linked together into flocs, which initially settle according to the size of the floc and porosity of the aggregated mass. Later, the rate is governed by compaction and rearrangement processes. A clear supernatant is formed on settling, since even the smallest particles are entrapped in the mesh-like network of the floc. Intermediate states are possible in which all particles are not associated with flocs.

As experimental examples, it is noted that Jones, Matthews, and Rhodes studied the stability of sulfaguanidine suspensions as they were affected by electrolyte (aluminum chloride), type and concentration of surfactant (cetyltrimethylammonium bromide, polysorbate 80), and nature of vehicle (water with various amounts of glycerol).[5] They achieved optimum stability by balancing the adjuvants to obtain a controlled aggregation. Also of interest, Carless and Ocran related, in hectorite dispersions, for example, particle shape, particle interaction mediated by added electrolytes, and some rheologic properties.[6] As reported in a patent, Storz,[7] doing research on intramuscular injectables containing steroidal and other water-insoluble medicaments, found that a pharmaceutically elegant, readily redispersible, stable, well-preserved, moderately aggregated suspension would form in an aqueous vehicle having as additives a nonionic polyether surfactant (up to 1% of, for example, polysorbate 80, PEGs, or polyoxyethylenepolyoxypropylene block polymers) and normal preservative concentrations of benzyl alcohol (0.5 to 1.5%) *and* the parabens (0.1 to 0.3%).

To determine whether a suspension is aggregated, a differential manometer can be used to compare the pressure of a suspension near its bottom and top in a container. This device has been described by Tingstad.[8] An aggregated suspension shows the same pressure at both points, as it exerts little or no pressure on the liquid because the particles essentially support each other. A deaggregated suspension, however, exerts more pressure near its bottom.

Caking is defined as the formation of a nonredispersible sediment within a suspension system. The major causes of caking are crystal bridging and closed aggregate (coagule) formation.

In crystal bridging, particle surface crystal growth occurs on two or more particles simultaneously and results in the steady formation of crystal-linked particles, ultimately leading to the formation of a highly linked sediment akin to concrete or plaster. Suspensions of the dispersed type tend to cake easily, owing to the compact sedimentation that occurs when these suspensions settle. Since suspensions are saturated solutions of the particulate substance, small changes in temperature that occur during shelf storage lead to unexpectedly rapid caking via crystal bridging, much in the same way that crystal growth yields can be optimized by alternately warming and cooling a mother crystallization liquor. This process, known as *Ostwald ripening*, is unavoidable in pharmaceutical suspensions of the dispersed type. Caking via crystal bridging can be minimized by utilizing the open network aggregate (floccule) suspension type, as the particles cannot sediment to a close proximity because of the rigidity of the aggregate. From a practical point of view, since fully aggregated suspensions are often unsightly, partial aggregation is often a desired objective, as it leads resistance to caking and imparts esthetic qualities to a suspension formulation.

Caking can also occur by extensive closed aggregate (*coagule*) formation, although the mechanism of nonredispersibility is different in that crystal bridging is not involved. A sedimented, highly coagulated suspension tends to form large coagules as the surface films present on coagulated particles cause the "filmed" particles to cling to each other. Although crystal growth may not occur upon sedimentation because of the presence of the surface films, the end result of a film-bonded sediment that cannot be redispersed is often observed for coagulated suspensions.

Sedimentation Rates

With regard to actual settling rates, the well-known Stokes relation describes the sedimentation velocity of a particle in suspension:

$$v = \frac{2r^2(d_1 - d_2)g}{9\eta} = \frac{D^2(d_1 - d_2)g}{18\eta}$$

where v = velocity of the sedimentation in cm/sec; r = particle radius and D = particle diameter in cm; d_1 and d_2 = density of the particle and the liquid, respectively, in g/ml; g = gravitational constant = 980.7 cm sec^{-2}; and η = the viscosity of the medium in poises, i.e., g cm^{-1} sec^{-1} in cgs units. Note, incidentally, that water at 20° has a viscosity of approximately one centipoise (0.01 poise). The student should be aware of the fact that assumptions were needed to facilitate the derivation of this relationship. Pharmaceutical systems containing less than 2 g of solids per 100 ml generally follow the Stokes equation. Obviously, if the two densities involved are such that a negative velocity results, this is the rate of flotation or creaming.

To illustrate by example a Stokes Law calculation, one could find the settling rate of a particle having a radius of 4 microns and a specific gravity of 4 in a medium with a viscosity of 100 cps and a specific gravity of 1.2. Using the Stokes equation (after changing the radius and viscosity to the proper units), a velocity of approximately 1×10^{-4} cm/sec is found. This means that this suspension packaged in a 10-cm high bottle would settle in 10^5 sec or in a little over one day. Similar "ideal calculations" make it clear that pharmaceutical suspensions are destined to settle, even though one can slow the process, well within the shelf-life times of pharmaceutical products. As the equation indicates, the parameter most powerful in changing the velocity of the settling is the particle diameter or radius, as it is a squared term; as technologists, the formulators are most able to control this and the viscosity of the medium.

Although the Stokes equation has been presented in the pharmaceutical literature for many years, a reader of Stokes' original publications will discover, as a point of historical interest, that pharmaceutical suspensions were not an object of his studies. George Gabriel Stokes, a professor of mathematics at the University of Cambridge more than a century ago, wrote papers on hydrostatics that dealt with the motion of fluids around spheres and with the motions of pendulums in fluids.

To handle more concentrated pharmaceutical suspensions (i.e., those containing more than 10 g of solid per 100 ml) requires the development of equations that go beyond the Stokes derivation. Obviously, the mathematics becomes even more complex if one tries to handle heterodispersed particles (i.e., not all particles are the same size), and in addition, irregularly shaped particles. One can, however, bring basic physical and chemical thinking to the kinetic settling and creaming problems; although exact and completely useful equations may not be developed, some conceptual value is gained.

T. Higuchi,[9] among others, has approached this problem of the hindered settling of relatively concentrated suspensions and has obtained an equation with somewhat fewer limitations. By recasting the problem, he considered the settling phenomenon to be equivalent to the movement of an external liquid phase through a bed of internal phase. (Note the similarity to the studies of Stokes mentioned in the second last paragraph.) Fluid flow through packed beds had been previously treated mathematically by Kozeny. Starting with the Kozeny equation, Higuchi developed an equation that somewhat resembles the Stokes equation with respect to the parameters needed to solve it. Specifically, one needs all the factors in Stokes' Law except the particle radius, and in addition, one needs an empiric constant, the volume fraction of the phases (which is a measure of the porosity of the "bed"), and the specific surface area of the particles, i.e., the area in cm^2/g.

Such an equation does not take into account the size or size distribution of the particles (an advantage over Stokes), and it is of some validity where it can be used, i.e., in more concentrated systems in which the suspended phase forms a sort of bed or where the aggregated structure is relatively firm. The equation has not been subjected to a great deal of experimental verification, but sample calculations show that the Stokes relationship (which does not take into account explicitly the concentration of the internal phase) gives too fast a rate of settling as opposed to actual observations made on more concentrated suspensions. The newer equation shows that the rate of settling decreases rapidly with the concentration of solid phase. Pharmaceutically speaking, the extension of this concept corroborates the observation that pastes do not settle in the usual sense, although small quantities of liquid components may separate. The new equation neglects, as does Stokes' Law, the contribution made to suspension stability by the various particle interactions. In summary, it is interesting to observe that suspensions are complex systems from a theoretic standpoint.

Regarding sedimentation and factors affecting it, it should be remembered that as the solids content is increased, viscosity also is increased. Hence, study of the viscosity characteristics of the vehicle alone may not always produce valid observations. Also, the discussions of particle charges, aggregation, zeta potential, and sedimentation rates dealt with aqueous systems. The vehicles used for pharmaceutical suspensions are usually aqueous, but may be oleaginous. Examples of oleaginous vehicles include peanut, sesame, cottonseed, corn, safflower, and castor oils and also fluorocarbon aerosol propellants. Particle-particle and particle-liquid interaction vary greatly depending on the vehicle. Since the electrical potential between two charges is inversely proportional to the dielectric constant of the medium between them, the distribution of ions in the double layer also depends on the dielectric constant of the vehicle. In low dielectric liquids such as oils, the double layer is many times thicker than in aqueous systems with high dielectric constants. It is therefore much more difficult to produce an aggregated particle structure in a low dielectric medium.

Crystal Habit

Crystal habit may be defined as the outward appearance of an agglomeration of crystals. Although seemingly trivial, crystal habit can be of great importance in suspension redispersibility, sedimentation, physical stability, and appearance. For example, sulfisoxazole can be produced in a single geometric crystal form having relatively similar sizes, but an agglomerate of the crystals can have physical properties vastly different from those of single crystals. Small clumps of sulfisoxazole crystals may exhibit little tendency to disperse because of the tenacity of the clump. These clumps may exhibit retarded dissolution and thus retarded bioavailability rates due to the inability of a dissolution fluid to penetrate to the interior crystal components of the clump.

A mental picture of the effect of crystal habit can be gained by considering sucrose in all of its commercial forms. Rock candy, lump sugar, granulated sugar, and powdered confectioner's sugar are all crystalline sucrose having identical crystalline geometry. Each of these forms of sucrose, however, possesses distinctly different dissolution rates in water. The effect is directly attributable to the crystal habit. Much in the same way, crystalline drugs destined for suspension formulation can exhibit different physical properties due to the influence of different crystal habits.

Traditionally, crystal habit was classified on the basis of the geometry of the agglomerate (needle, prism, plate, etc.), but in reality, most crystal habit morphology is of a nondescript form. The relatively strong, rigid crystalline structure that exists within a crystal is not responsible for the agglomeration of crystals. Rather, weak van der Waals interactions occurring at crystal surfaces hold the agglomerate of crystals in form. Mostly, this occurs as nongeometrically classifiable clumps.

For reasons delineated previously, it is important for the pharmaceutical formulator to specify the desired crystal habit for component crystalline ingredients in pharmaceutical formulations and to specify quality control procedures so that possible changes in crystal habit, which may adversely affect a finished pharmaceutical preparation, may be adequately tracked.

Crystal Structure Factors

A question of fundamental importance arises when formulations are prepared by either dispersion or precipitation techniques. It concerns the effect, if any, that the method of preparing the particles has on their initial or subsequent physical stability in the suspension. Effects on the properties of the crystals are more often produced when the precipitation procedure is used to create the particles. Closely allied in importance to the way the particles are prepared are the nature of the vehicle used and its effect on suspension properties. Smith, Buehler, and Robinson, during development of a sustained action suspension of an insoluble derivative of dextromethorphan, noted that dramatic differences in physical behavior and stability were encountered when the derivative was coated by different methods and crystallized from different solvent systems.[10]

The factors controlling crystal characteristics involve basically either the production of a change in crystal habit (physical shape such as needle, plate, prism) or the production of no change in crystal habit. When there is no change in the crystal habit, the following factors may still be considered: drug decomposition leading to salting in or out, pH changes with changes in the particle size distribution, and the effect of change in temperature. When there is a change in crystal habit, solvation and polymorphism (presence of one or more crystalline and/or amorphous forms) are of importance. It is also notable that the rate of physiologic absorption can be greatly altered, depending on which crystalline or amorphous forms are administered.

Drug breakdown may occur because the products of decomposition cause a shift in pH, which in turn, could have a marked effect on solubility. A salting in effect also may exert an autocatalytic effect on the rate of drug decomposition. These effects are particularly apparent when the chemical stability of suspensions is studied at elevated temperatures. This is a good reason for viewing data obtained from high temperature storage studies with caution because these conditions may contribute to the manifestation of greater chemical instability than may occur at room temperature.

The effect of cyclic temperature changes, as mentioned in the discussion of caking, is important in measuring suspension stability from a physical as well as chemical standpoint. The temperature effects depend on the magnitude of the change in temperature over a given period of time, the time interval, the effect of temperature on the solubility of the suspended drug, and on recrystallization phenomena. With respect to the latter point, it is known that at each crystal contact point there exists a thin layer of supersaturated solution that facilitates crystal growth. The type of inherent crystal form may be needles, plates, cubes, rods, or prisms, and production of these is determined by the factors that govern the rate of crystal growth. The rate of cooling, the extent and degree of agitation, and the size and number of nuclei are all elements that affect the degree of supersaturation of the solution in contact with the crystal. Other important factors include pH, solvent effects, and perhaps most important, the impurities present. The formation of distinct new crystalline entities during storage due to solvation and polymorphism is also a possibility. An originally anhydrous drug in suspension may rapidly or slowly form a hydrate.

Experimentally, Varney investigated the factors controlling the sensitivity of crystalline suspensions to temperature fluctuations.[11] He showed that crystal growth increases with an increase in particle solubility; thus, excipients that increase the particle solubility should be kept to a minimum. Also demonstrated was the fact that in a dilute suspension, growth increases with stirring (as compared to a quiescent formulation), since the mean free diffusion path of the solute molecules is reduced. Similarly, if sedimentation occurs—even if the sediment is easily redispersed—the local increase in particle concentration increases particle growth.

Polymorphism as applied to crystals specifically refers to the different crystal structures the same chemical compound may have. These various forms may exhibit different solubilities, melting points, and x-ray diffraction patterns. The storage temperature, the solvent chosen for crystallization, and the rate of cooling are important factors in determining which polymorph is obtained, and at what speed it is obtained. All organic substances appear to exist in several polymorphic forms. In fact, experts have remarked that the number of forms found and characterized is directly proportional to the time and money spent looking for them. It is usually economically prohibitive to prepare a large number of polymorphic forms and then proceed to test them to find the most stable ones. Quite extensive studies have been done on cortisone, however; of the four polymorphic forms of cortisone acetate known, only one is stable in aqueous media. Another example that may be cited is prednisolone; of the prednisolone polymorphs, only one is stable in aqueous media.

The rate of conversion of a metastable to a stable polymorph may be rapid or slow. When this rate of conversion is very slow, it may be feasible to use the metastable form commercially. On the other hand, if it occurs within days, as for example in the case of cocoa butter, the metastable form may not interfere with the material when used in a marketed product. Conversions of intermediate speed, i.e., those that occur gradually over a period of one to several months, could be troublesome.

Suspension Formation

Precipitation Methods

Three precipitation methods are discussed in this section: organic solvent precipitation, precipitation effected by changing the pH of the medium, and double decomposition.

Water-insoluble drugs can be precipitated by dissolving them in water-miscible organic solvents and then adding the organic phase to distilled water under standard conditions. Examples of organic solvents used include ethanol, methanol, propylene glycol, and polyethylene glycol. Several important considerations are involved when this method is used. Perhaps the most important factor next to particle size control is that the "correct" polymorphic form or hydrate of the crystal be obtained. For example, different forms are obtained when prednisolone is precipitated from aqueous methanol as opposed to aqueous acetone. The methanolic precipitate forms a sesquihydrate when dried, whereas the acetone precipitate forms a metastable, anhydrous, crystalline product; only the former is easily suspended in water. Besides the influence of the solvent on crystal characteristics, the following additional factors may need to be considered: possible preparation under sterile conditions, inherent solvent entrapment and subsequent toxicity, the volume ratios of the organic to the aqueous phase, rate and method of addition of one phase to the other, temperature control (cooling rate and drying conditions), method of drying the precipitate (forced air, vacuum, or freeze drying), and finally, the washing of the precipitate. Sometimes, the need for a narrow particle size range for parenteral or inhalation therapy is indicated. With respect to the latter point, the particles should be in the 1- to 5-micron range. If they are too small, they are exhaled; if too large, they are not able to get to and be absorbed from the lung area. The combined use of sterile precipitation, drying, micronization, ethylene oxide sterilization, and sterile resuspension may be necessary. Where pertinent, sterilant residues should not be overlooked (e.g., ethylene glycol from ethylene oxide gas sterilization procedures).

The method of changing the pH of the medium is perhaps more readily accomplished and does not present the same difficulties associated with organic solvent precipitation. The technique, however, is only applicable to those drugs in which solubility is dependent on the pH value. For example, estradiol suspensions can be prepared by changing the pH of its aqueous solution; estradiol is readily soluble in such alkali as potassium or sodium hydroxide solutions. If a concentrated solution of estradiol is thus prepared and added to a weakly acidic solution of hydrochloric, citric, or acetic acids, under proper conditions of agitation, the estradiol is precipitated in a fine state of subdivision. The type of crystal or polymorphic form depends on such factors as the concentrations of acid and base and the degree and type of fluid shear imparted to the system.

Insulin suspensions also may be prepared by a pH change method. Insulin has an isoelectric point of approximately pH 5. When it is mixed with a basic protein, such as protamine, it is readily precipitated when the pH is between the isoelectric points of the two components, i.e., pH 6.9 to 7.3. Protamine zinc insulin (PZI) contains an excessive quantity of zinc to retard absorption. According to the British Pharmacopoeia of 1958, a phosphate buffer is added to each individual vial containing the acidified solution of insulin, protamine, and zinc, so that the pH is between 6.9 and 7.3; the preparation is compounded in the final container by mixing the PZI and the buffer in the filling operation. Adrenocorticotropin (ACTH) zinc suspensions are prepared in a similar manner. The precipitate formed in the process is zinc hydroxide or zinc phosphate, on which the ACTH is adsorbed; this combination results in a long acting preparation when administered. The addition of phosphate salts and organic phosphate to prepare an even longer acting ACTH preparation is also possible.

When either the change in pH or the organic solvent precipitation method is used to prepare a suspension, a degree of supersaturation is brought about suddenly in the batch process to give rise to crystal nucleation and growth, after which the initial supersaturation subsides. Thus, the degree of supersaturation changes throughout the process, and neither the rate of nucleation nor the rate of crystal growth is constant; therefore, the particle size distribution is variable. The degree of supersaturation and the rate of nucleation are greatest at the beginning of the process, so that crystals formed initially become the largest because they are exposed to the supersaturated solution for the longest period of time. It appears, therefore, that when less concentrated solutions are used, the particle size distribution is broader than when more concentrated solutions are used.

Making suspensions by double decomposition involves only simple chemistry, although some of the aforementioned physical factors also come into play. The reader is referred to standard pharmacy texts to review the preparation of White Lotion (NF XIII), that is, forming zinc "polysulfide" by mixing zinc sulfate and sulfurated potash solutions.

Dispersion Methods

When the dispersion method is utilized for suspension preparation, the vehicle must be formulated so that the solid phase is easily wetted and dispersed. The use of surfactants is desirable to ensure uniform wetting of hydrophobic solids. The use of suspending agents, such as the synthetic polymeric polyelectrolytes, natural gums, or clay, may be indicated, depending on the specific application. The actual method of dispersing the solid is one of the more important considerations because particle size reduction may or may not result from the dispersion process. If particle-size reduction occurs, the particles obtained may have different solubilities if a metastable state is involved, and this may lead to transient supersaturation of the system. A number of dispersion methods are used to prepare suspension products. For present purposes, there is no need to describe and discuss the comminuting and shearing equipment commercially available because information on such equipment is easily obtained. The reader need only recall that much of what has been and will be discussed with respect to basic suspension technology applies regardless of how the suspension is made.

Formulation of Suspensions

As the discussion thus far implies, many factors must be considered in the course of developing a suspension dosage form. The basic concern involves the fact that suspensions settle, and it is necessary to redistribute them before using or dispensing them as products. A desirable suspension should be easily redispersed by shaking, should remain suspended long enough to withdraw an accurate dose, and should have the desired flow properties. In the early phases of formulation, a decision must be made as to the general type of suspension system desired. As noted, aggregated systems usually exhibit a minimum of serious separation, depending on the solids content and the degree of aggregation that has taken place. At times, an aggregated system may appear to be coarse because of the aggregates formed. On the other hand, in a dispersed system, the particles are well distributed and settle singly but more slowly than an aggregated system. The particles, however, have a tendency to form a sediment or cake that is difficult to redisperse.

Aggregated (Open Network Aggregate) Systems

Before aggregating the suspension particles in the open network aggregate, it is important to ensure that the particles are well dispersed in the aqueous phase or other vehicle. A proper surfactant in appropriate concentration improves the dispersion by reducing the interfacial tension. For example, if surfactants with negative charges are adsorbed on the particles, this prevents or minimizes aggregation in the presence of positive ions because of the mutual repulsion of like charges. Examples of such agents include sodium lauryl sulfate and sodium dioctyl sulfosuccinate.

The concentration of added electrolyte necessary to produce the aggregated state corresponds to the quantification expressed in the Schulze-Hardy rule previously discussed. In some cases in which incompatibility factors are absent, very small amounts of aluminum chloride or potassium biphosphate may act as aggregating agents. In practice, a nonionic surfactant is usually used to aid the dispersion of the insoluble phase. Polyoxyethylene ethers of mixed partial fatty acid esters of sorbitol anhydrides (Tweens),* the same compounds without the hydrophilic oxyethylene groups (Spans),* higher molecular weight polyethylene glycols (Carbowaxes),* and molecular combinations of polyoxyethylene and polyoxypropylene (Pluronics),* are frequently used in this manner. One

*Tween and Span are trademarks of ICI United States Inc., Concord Pike and New Murphy Road, Wilmington, DE 19897. Carbowax is a trademark of the Union Carbide Corporation, Chemicals and Plastics, 270 Park Avenue, New York, NY 10017. Pluronic is a trademark of BASF Wyandotte Corporation, 1609 Biddle Avenue, Wyandotte, MI 48192.

must be careful, especially with the nonionic surfactants, not to use too high a concentration of the agent. Over the critical micelle concentration, intact micelles are adsorbed to particle surfaces, providing a continuous film for coagule formation, as discussed previously.

Suspension systems intended for oral, parenteral, ophthalmic, or topical use may not appear elegant because they usually exhibit poor drainage in vials or bottles due to the clusters of particles. These properties may be improved by the addition of protective colloids. Protective colloids differ from surfactants in that they do not reduce interfacial tension. Their solutions differ in viscosity and are used in higher concentrations than are surfactants. Protective colloids also differ from other agents in that their effect is due not only to their ability to increase the zeta potential, but also to their formation of a mechanical barrier or sheath around the particles. An example of this approach is the use of silica gel, a form of precipitated silicic acid. It is used in concentrations up to 10% and may be gelled with surfactants; it is primarily limited to topical preparations. Another example involves the use of aluminum hydroxide gel as a vehicle; commercially, this approach was employed in a triple sulfonamide suspension. When this type of vehicle is used, it is important to consider the alkalinity present and its possible effect on the active ingredient. Hence, the use of a nonreactive type of gelling agent may be advantageous.

Dispersed Systems

As previously discussed in the section "Particle Interactions and Behavior," the individual particles in dispersed systems are generally dispersed with the aid of an agent to lower the interfacial tension. To maintain this state, however, a viscosity-imparting suspending agent is usually required as an adjunct. These agents retard settling and agglomeration of the particles by functioning as an energy barrier, which minimizes interparticle attraction and ultimate aggregation. The general choice of suspending agents includes protective colloids, viscosity-inducing agents, surfactants, and dispersing agents. Combinations of various types of suspending agents may be used to achieve the desired rheologic properties. It is particularly with dispersed suspension systems that the following factors involved in Stokes' Law become important: the particle size, the density of the vehicle and of the particle, and the viscosity of the medium. Some of the suspending agents used to a large extent in formulation include modified cellulose polymers, proteins such as gelatin, and totally synthetic polymers. Of the modified cellulose polymers, sodium carboxymethylcellulose (CMC),* methylcellulose (Methocel),* and hydroxypropylmethylcellulose (Methocel, HG)* are widely used in oral, topical, and parenteral dosage forms. Sodium carboxymethylcellulose is an anionic polymer, whereas methylcellulose and hydroxypropylmethylcellulose are nonionic. Sodium carboxymethylcellulose is used in concentrations of up to 0.5% in injectable preparations. In oral dosage forms, they are frequently used in higher concentrations because of the higher solids content of the systems. Sodium carboxymethylcellulose does have some disadvantages: it is incompatible with a number of electrolytes and quaternary ammonium compounds, and it forms complexes with certain surfactants. Methylcellulose and hydroxypropylmethylcellulose gel on heating and are affected by electrolytes. One of the more useful of the totally synthetic polymers is polyacrylic acid (Carbopol);* it is used mostly in external lotion and gel preparations. After being uniformly dispersed in water, it is neutralized with an organic amine such as triethanolamine or with inorganic alkali to achieve the desired viscosity in a range from pH 6 to 10. The material is extremely sensitive to electrolytes, but is suited for use equally in aqueous and nonaqueous systems. These polymeric agents function primarily as protective colloids and alter the viscosity of the medium.

As a group, the clays (essentially hydrated aluminum and/or magnesium silicates) are also quite useful in suspension formulating. They hydrate further in water to a high degree to form colloidal dispersions having high viscosities. The manner in which the members of the group are prepared, however, has a profound effect on the final product. The clay should always be added to the water with high shear to effect uniform dispersion and maximum hydration. The pH of aqueous clay dispersions is somewhat alkaline, in the range of pH 8.5 to 9.5; therefore, they also possess some acid neutralizing capacity. The viscosity of aqueous dispersions of these agents varies, depending on the type and amount of solids dispersed. In general 5 to 10% concentrations of the clay form firm opaque gels.

Clays can be formulated in systems in which the pH is between 6 and 11, but they are most stable between pH 9 and 11. Alkaline buffers usually are included to maintain the pH. All dispersions of the clays are drastically affected by electrolytes in accordance with the Schulze-Hardy rule; ethanol also affects these agents by dehydrating the colloid, thereby reducing the viscosity. Clay suspensions and gels are excellent media for mold and bacterial growth, and should therefore be adequately preserved with nonionic antimicrobial preservatives. The paraben esters and benzoates are useful, but cationic "quaternary" preservatives are ineffective. Heat and aging usually increase the viscosity of clay mixtures, but this may become less significant in the more concentrated systems.

As noted, another Stokes' Law factor that is especially important in deaggregated systems is the density of the medium. There are several ways to approach density adjustment when feasible. The addition to the system of nonionic substances such as sorbitol, polyvinylpyrrolidone, glycerine, sugar, or one of the polyethylene glycols (or combinations of these) may be helpful. In addition to the change in the density of the medium, a considerable effect on the viscosity also may be achieved, owing to the viscosity-building effects created by hydrogen bonding of the water molecules and the glycols. When suspensions of higher solids content are prepared, as in toothpastes, for example, the use of a combination of a clay and a gum such as sodium carboxymethylcellulose may be desirable.

Rheologic Considerations

The rheologic characteristics of a pharmaceutical suspension can be of great importance as the determining factor in the optimization of the physical stability of the suspension system. In particular, a suspension that possesses highly developed thixotropy is most desirable. Such a suspension, properly formulated, can prevent sedimentation, aggregation, and caking by virtue of a high yield-value/viscosity at rest, while sharp agitation reduces the viscosity to permit pouring and thus dispensing of the product. The high viscosity can reform rapidly when the suspension is again at rest, virtually eliminating the possibility of the physical instabilities previously discussed. The bentonite clays and some polymeric resins tend to form well-developed aqueous thixotropic media.

The pharmaceutical formulator would be well advised to expend efforts to avoid certain rheo-

---

*CMC is a trademark of Hercules Inc., 910 Market Street, Hercules Tower, Wilmington, DE 19899. Methocel is a trademark of the Dow Chemical Company, Abbott Road, Midland, MI 48640.

*Carbopol is a trademark of the B. F. Goodrich Chemical Company, 6100 Oak Tree Boulevard, Cleveland, OH 44131.

logic characteristics in a pharmaceutical product under development. In particular, the following rheologic characteristics are most undesirable because of their poor physical stability: pseudoplastic (in which there is no yield value), dilatant, and rheopexic (in which viscosity increases with shear force).

Formulation Adjuvants

Certain aspects of suspension formulation pertain to both aggregate and dispersed suspension systems and are therefore discussed together. Suspension adjuvants must be considered. These agents include the preservative, color, perfume, and flavor; they may materially affect the characteristics of the suspension system. In general, most colors are used in small quantities and are usually compatible; flavors and perfumes are similarly used and are also usually compatible with the vehicle. To illustrate that one must be on guard against adjuvant interaction, it is noted that Bean and Dempsey showed that the adsorptive power of kaolin suspensions can reduce the activity of some preservatives.[12] Kaolin hurt the quaternary benzalkonium chloride (BAK), but not the nonionic and less surface-active m-cresol. Similarly, it was shown that procaine penicillin adsorbed the quaternary and that the supernatants of the BAK systems had less activity than the suspensions; thus, the adsorbent acted as a reservoir.

Perhaps the final "adjuvant" one should consider is the package. Usually, initial laboratory screening employs conventional graduates or readily available bottles. When final packaging is considered, it should be noted that various types of glass are available. The types vary with respect to their ability to resist water attack, the degree of attack being related to the amount of alkali released from the glass. The USP should be consulted for further details, as it describes both the tests and standards that should be met by containers to be used for packaging parenteral and nonparenteral (oral or topical) products. One point of terminology may be noted: "flint" refers to clear, colorless, brilliant glass. Originally, it contained lead and was also called "lead" or "crystal" glass; today in commerce, nonlead, highly color-free, soda-lime-silica glasses, the most common general-purpose transparent glasses, are also called flint. Parenteral multiple-dose vials may be "flint" (colorless) or amber, and may be silicone-coated to improve drainage of the suspensions. (Silicone coating also minimizes the leaching of alkali from the glass.) This technique of silicone coating is used widely for suspensions of steroids and combinations of penicillin and dihydrostreptomycin. It is also used in preparations with high solids content, in which formulation modifications cannot measurably improve the drainage of the preparation.

There has been a trend to package suspension systems for oral and topical administration in polyethylene or other plastic containers. Many factors must be considered when a suspension is evaluated in such a container. These factors include loss of flavor and perfume, preservative adsorption, and leaching into the product of substances from the container. Before evaluative procedures are discussed per se, it must be stressed that after the initial stability observations are completed, the determination of the stability of the suspension in the *final package* is an important step of the product development procedure.

Preparative Techniques

The actual preparation of suspensions involves choosing the ingredients (utilizing principles already discussed) and determining the type of manufacturing equipment to be used. Needless to say, each suspension is a separate case and absolute generalization is not possible.

If the suspension is made by a dispersion process, it is best to achieve pulverization of the solid by a micronization technique. This involves subjecting the particles to a turbulent air chamber in which they collide with each other and fracture. Particles under 5 microns are readily obtained. Although it is not widely used for this purpose, spray-drying also can be considered a method of comminution to produce a finely divided solid phase.

If the suspension is made by controlled crystallization, a supersaturated solution should be formed and then quickly cooled with rapid stirring. This causes the formation of many nuclei and hence many crystals; it is just the opposite of letting crystals grow large.

At some time during suspension formation, it is likely that shearing will be desired. This homogenization can be accomplished by the conventional stator-rotor colloid mills. Ultrasonic equipment also can be used to effect high intensity mixing, but usually, this technique is not applied commercially. Of interest, however, is the work of Sheikh, Price, and Gerraughty, who studied the effect of ultrasound on polyethylene spheres in aqueous suspension.[13] The ultrasound reduced the sphere size only when surfactants were added, especially those having high HLBs. When such agents were used as additives, the particles were readily dispersed and hence completely surrounded by liquid. Since ultrasound waves and cavitation shock waves are transmitted to the particles through the liquid medium, a poor suspension would not be as susceptible to size reduction as a better dispersed one. Excessive shearing (or high temperatures) may irreversibly damage polymeric materials such as gums, so that viscosity loss is suffered. Instead of trying to hydrate gums and clays by massive shearing, it is often better, when possible, to give the material the necessary time to hydrate under conditions of mild shearing. An alternate procedure is to mix with, or preferably spray the gum with, a chlorinated hydrocarbon, acetone, or alcohol solution of a wetting agent (e.g., sodium dioctyl sulfosuccinate). About 0.4% (based on the gum weight) of the wetting agent should be added to the gum. This technique can produce a marked beneficial effect, as wetting of the gum and hence hydration is greatly accelerated.

A final comment is that processing studies in a pilot plant are needed because it is axiomatic that the scale-up operation from laboratory batches to production lots brings with it many troubles and unexpected results.

Evaluation of Suspension Stability

Since stability testing is discussed elsewhere in the pharmaceutical literature, the only emphasis here is on the most pertinent aspects of suspension stability. Techniques for the evaluation of heterogeneous systems generally are complex and are far from being completely satisfactory. Some test methods are so drastic that the stability information is obtained during an evaluation that destroys the system being evaluated. Some methods are somewhat empiric in nature, i.e., the exact basis on which they operate cannot be explicitly defined mathematically. All test procedures suffer some limitations, and the results, therefore, must be cautiously evaluated and interpreted. As the methodology involved in the pertinent stability studies is often somewhat complicated, this section of the chapter is more fully referenced so that further details can be obtained if desired. The purpose here is to point out explicitly one method, and then indicate only the general nature of some of the other approaches taken. Use of evaluation techniques permits the formulator to screen the initial preparations made and also to compare the improved formulations to competitive commercial products. The latter point should not be treated lightly even though it does not deal with absolute standards.

Sedimentation Volume

Since redispersibility is one of the major considerations in assessing the acceptability of a suspension, and since the sediment formed should be easily dispersed by moderate shaking to yield a homogeneous system, measurement of the sedimentation volume and its ease of redispersion form two of the most common basic evaluative procedures.

The concept of sedimentation volume is simple. In short, it considers the ratio of the ultimate height (H_u) of the sediment to the initial height (H_o) of the total suspension as the suspension settles in a cylinder under standard conditions. The larger this fraction, the better is the suspendability.

Methods utilizing the sedimentation volume obtained in a cylinder offer a practical approach to the determination of the physical stability of suspension systems. Particularly good is the fact that the system remains undisturbed. Specifically, it is worth knowing how to use the H_u and H_o concepts. The formulator should obtain the H_u/H_o ratios and plot them as ordinates with time as the abscissae. Note that although the conventional H_u is called the "ultimate" height of the sediment, ultimate really means the height at any particular time. The plot just described will at time zero start at 1.0, with the curve then being either horizontal or gradually sloping downward to the right as time goes on. One can compare different formulations and choose the best by observing the lines, the better formulations obviously producing lines that are more horizontal and/or less steep. Another technique that utilizes essentially the same parameters may be used to evaluate highly concentrated suspensions, which might be difficult to compare because there would be only minimum supernatant liquid. The technique involves diluting the suspension with additional vehicle, i.e., with the total formula with all ingredients except the insoluble phase. As an example, one could dilute 50 ml of a suspension to a volume of 100, 150, or 200 ml. The H_u reading then becomes the volume of sediment in the diluted sample, and H_o equals the original volume of the sample before dilution. The H_u/H_o ratio may in this case be greater than 1. Regardless, the ratio is again plotted against time, and comparisons between formulas are made as before.

One additional concept should also be considered by the formulator. In all the comparisons just mentioned, the screening technique results only in a relative ranking; this indicates which preparations are the better ones. It is also useful, however, to consider the possibility of making an absolute evaluation; this may be done as follows. The degree of settling can be related to the amount of sediment that would be produced in the ultimate dispersed state. To obtain the completely dispersed suspension form, which represents the least void space for the solid phase and hence the smallest sedimentation volume, electrolytes that promote settling may be added or the preparation may be centrifuged. The H_u/H_o ratio observed is then the lowest figure obtainable. This figure serves as a base line and gives some idea of the degree of aggregation obtained because ratios higher than this minimum represent the existence of the desired aggregated state. In reference to the plots discussed, it is clear that data that produce a line that quickly drops toward this reference point do not represent a good suspension, as any aggregation if there is any at all, is too temporary and infirm.

Another use for H_u/H_o data is possible, and particularly pertinent are the various relationships of Ward and Kammermeyer.[14] In essence, these workers attempted to quantitate settling further using H_u and H_o values. It is known that the ultimate height of the solid phase after settling depends on the concentration of solids and the particle size. These workers found that if H_o and H_u readings (taken on a series of different concentrations of the same solids having a particular average particle size range) are measured in a certain vehicle, the resulting data form a straight line plot if the logarithm of the weight percentage of solids is plotted against the ratio H_u/H_o. One can then predict H_u for any given solids concentration by multiplying H_o by the "relative concentration factor," i.e., by H_u/H_o.

As noted, the evaluation of redispersibility is also important. To help quantitate this parameter to some extent, a mechanical shaking device may be used. It simulates human arm motion during the shaking process and can give reproducible results when used under controlled conditions. It should be remembered, however, that the test conditions are not the same as those encountered under actual use, and further testing should be considered. Nevertheless, the test results are useful and provide guidance during screening procedures.

Rheologic Methods

In addition to techniques involving sedimentation and redispersibility factors, rheologic methods can also be used to help determine the settling behavior and the arrangement of the vehicle and particle structural features for purposes of comparison.

The majority of rheologic investigations of suspension systems have been done at high shear rates and on systems that must be made uniform before evaluation. For present purposes, the importance of using low shear rates and undisturbed samples cannot be overemphasized. The prime reason for this is the fact that the structure achieved on storage is what should be evaluated. A practical rheologic method involves the use of the Brookfield viscometer mounted on a helipath stand. The T-bar spindle is made to descend slowly into the suspension, and the dial reading on the viscometer is then a measure of the resistance the spindle meets at various levels in a sediment. In this technique, the T-bar is continually changing position and measures undisturbed samples as it advances down into the suspension. This technique also indicates in which level of the suspension the structure is greater, owing to particle agglomeration, because the T-bar descends as it rotates, and the bar is continually entering new and essentially undisturbed material. Data obtained on samples variously aged and stored indicate whether undesired changes are taking place. Thus, using the T-bar spindle and the helipath, the dial reading can be plotted against the number of turns of the spindle. This measurement is made on undisturbed samples of different ages. The results indicate how the particles are settling with time. In a screening study, the better suspensions show a lesser rate of increase of dial reading with spindle turns, i.e., the curve is horizontal for a longer period.

A method combining the use of both rheologic and sedimentation parameters is illustrated by the work of Foernzler, Martin, and Banker,[15] who studied the effect of thixotropy on stability. Although this method does not observe the system under equilibrium conditions and is subject to some challenge, the authors attempted to predict physical stability by a rheologic evaluation of thixotropy. Incidentally, Wood used these workers' data to develop additional correlations.[16] It is important to note that the use of most viscometers and centrifuges in stability studies is not ideal for aggregated systems because their use destroys the structure formed.

Wood, Catacalos, and Lieberman studied aging magnesium aluminum silicate suspensions and uncovered interesting, logarithmic, atypical kinetic relationships involving the time and temperature of storage and shear rate and shear stress.[17] It would not be useful to discuss this further in detail, but for practical purposes, it is noted that work such as this illustrates that clay and gum hydration is not attained instantaneously, but is part of the aging process and hence is not necessarily completed even by the stress a formulation undergoes in a manufacturing procedure.

Although the previously mentioned Brookfield instrument sees wide industrial application, many types of viscometers are available. It is worth noting that various types of rheologic equipment, together with their applications, have been discussed and reviewed in the book by Van Wazer, Lyons, Kim, and Colwell.[18]

Electrokinetic Techniques

In a discussion of the physicochemical principles involved in suspensions, Martin noted the applicability of an electrophoretic method that employed a microelectrophoresis apparatus.[19] Such instrumentation permitted measurement of the migration velocity of the particles with respect to the surface electric charge or the familiar zeta potential; the latter has units of viscosity times electrophoretic mobility, or more familiarly, volts. Stanko and DeKay also evaluated suspensions by electrokinetic methods and showed that the zeta potential changes upon the addition of additives and is related to stability.[20] Haines and Martin studied some of the formulation factors that influence the stability of suspensions.[21] They correlated the zeta potential to visually observed caking; zeta potential was again determined by microscopic electrophoresis. It was found that certain zeta potentials produced more stable suspensions because aggregation was controlled and optimized. Nash has also published an excellent review of this subject.[22,23]

Particle Size Changes

The freeze-thaw cycling technique is particularly applicable to stressing suspensions for stability testing purposes. This treatment promotes particle growth and may indicate the probable future state of affairs after long storage at room temperature. Thus, it is of prime importance to be alert for changes in absolute particle size, particle size distribution, and crystal habit. With respect to the latter point, Carless et al. investigated the various crystal forms of cortisone acetate and also noted the acceleration of sulfathiazole crystal growth in suspensions that underwent temperature cycling.[24,25] Obviously,

the physiologic availability and thus the therapeutic effect of the active ingredients may be influenced by such changes. Particle size distributions are sometimes determined by microscopic means. This method of necessity requires dilute suspensions that are counted with the aid of an ocular grid. In some instances, photomicrographs may be taken for permanent records. This method is quite tedious, especially when large numbers of samples are to be evaluated.

It is worth noting that certain suspension components, e.g., the preservative or the protective colloid, may have a profound effect on the physical performance of the suspension under freeze-thaw conditions. When a low solids content steroid injectable preparation containing sodium carboxymethylcellulose (CMC)* and benzyl alcohol, and one containing CMC,* methylparaben, and propylparaben, were subjected to freezing and thawing, the former suspension caked badly, while the latter was unaffected. Protective colloids may thus be adversely affected by freezing, thawing, or elevated temperatures; for example, gelatin is sensitive to low temperatures whereas methylcellulose is adversely affected by higher temperatures. Although freeze-thaw cycle studies are useful guides, the best stability information is still obtained from studies conducted at room temperature.

Reviews

Stability testing methods pertaining to the suspension product form have been reviewed by Kennon.[26] Additionally, Matthews and Rhodes reviewed and interpreted suspension stability, coagulation, and aggregation processes on the basis of a comparison of the forces of electrostatic repulsion and of van der Waals attraction.[27,28] Somewhat similarly, Ho, Toguchi, and Higuchi made a comparison of theoretic equations involving electrostatic repulsion.[29] Also pertinent here is the review by Hiestand of the physical properties of coarse suspensions, particularly as it helped to clarify the mechanisms of the control of floc structure.[30] Although measurement problems still exist, it appears that a study of the potential structural changes in floc may be more useful in predicting shelf life than are sedimentation-caking studies. Experimentally, Carstensen and Su studied the sedimentation kinetics of aggregated suspen-

*As noted previously, CMC is a trademark of Hercules Inc.

sions to derive equations that were consistent with both experimental data and with theory.[31] Also, Matthews and Rhodes used a Coulter counter and digital computer to evaluate the stability of aggregating monodisperse polystyrene systems,[27,32] and in another study, Matthews used microelectrophoresis (to measure zeta potential) along with other standard stability tests to monitor the stability of various griseofulvin suspensions.[28]

Illustrative Examples

This section presents certain formulas that demonstrate some of the principles discussed in this chapter. Additives exert a great influence on the stability and the drug bioavailability of formulations. The whole area of suspension product development is a study of the performance characteristics of adjuvants. Skill in finding and matching the everlasting marriage between the suspending characteristics and desired drug bioavailability determines the degree of excellence represented in the final product. It is also the purpose of this section to discuss biopharmaceutical aspects of the suspending agents in contemporary suspensions.

Illustrative formulations are discussed here in these categories: (a) suspensions with wetting and aggregating agents; (b) suspensions with low solids content; (c) suspensions with high solids content; (d) antacids; (e) biopharmaceutical considerations.

Suspensions With Wetting and Aggregating Agents. A patent by Macek describes a noncaking aqueous parenteral suspension of cortisone acetate and the wetting principle as follows.[33]

Ingredients	Percentage in Formula
Cortisone acetate, USP microfine	2.5
Polysorbate 80,* USP (wetting agent)	0.4
Carboxymethylcellulose sodium, USP (suspending agent)	0.5
Sodium chloride, USP (for isotonicity)	0.9
Benzyl alcohol, NF (preservative)	0.9
Water for injection, USP, q.s. to make	100.0

*Marketed as Tween 80 by ICI Americas, Inc., Wilmington, DE 19899.

On the industrial scale, all the ingredients except cortisone acetate can be dissolved in water for injection using suitable mixing equipment. Cortisone acetate can now be dispersed in the solution. The entire dispersion may be passed through a colloid mill (e.g., Gaulin type with an aseptic provision).*

The principles of aggregation and wetting may also be observed by making the preparations labeled A through F in the table below.

Comparison of preparations A and B demonstrates the value of a wetting agent. It is easy to disperse sulfamerazine in B, but it settles on standing and forms a cake because of its deaggregated nature. In C, the inclusion of the cati-

*Gaulin high-energy homogenizer, marketed by Gaulin Corporation, Everett, MA 02149.

| Ingredients | Percentage in Preparations | | | | | |
	A	B	C	D	E	F
Sulfamerazine, USP	2.0	2.0	2.0	2.0	2.0	2.0
Docusate sodium,* USP	—	0.2	0.2	0.15	0.2	—
Aluminum chloride hexahydrate,† USP	—	—	0.1	0.1	—	0.25
Carboxymethylcellulose sodium (7MP),‡ USP	—	—	—	0.02	—	0.15
Potassium biphosphate, NF	—	—	—	—	0.1	—
Purified water, USP q.s. to make	100	100	100	100	100	100

*Add as 0.2% solution.
†Add as 1% solution.
‡Add as 0.1% solution.

onic aluminum (which should be added last) yields an aggregated suspension. Although the aggregates settle rapidly, they form a high-volume sediment that does not cake and is easily redispersed.

Preparation D is similar to C except that it contains carboxymethylcellulose, which acts as a protective colloid and a viscosity builder. Therefore, this aggregated suspension does not cake on standing and settles more slowly than C. From a physical stability point of view, D is the best suspension in this series. Suspension E cakes on standing because the anionic biphosphate does not cause aggregation as was evident in C, in which the cationic aluminum acted as an aggregating agent. Preparation F illustrates a gross incompatibility of a negatively charged cellulose derivative with the positively charged aluminum ions.

For additional examples illustrating the phenomena of aggregation and wetting in aerosol dispersion systems, the reader is referred to Chapter 20, "Pharmaceutical Aerosols."

Suspensions With Low Solids Content. Table 16-1 illustrates the components that are required to prepare a model parenteral suspension. This route of administration limits the formulator to a rather narrow range of additives. The samples are best prepared by making a concentrate of the dispersant in a volume equal to 10% of the final volume, thoroughly mixing in the active ingredient with the help of a colloid mill or other device, and adding the remaining components to a solution of the preservative(s). The latter should be prepared using about 80% of the final total volume. This solution is then added to the portion containing the active ingredient, and sufficient purified water is added to bring it to the final volume. Note that the preservatives are added in a slightly excess amount to compensate for their binding to polysorbate 80. This binding has been shown to inactivate the preservative in direct proportion to the amount bound.[34,35]

The following observations are made with respect to Table 16-1:

A— No dispersion or very little wetting of solid; this may depend on the recrystallization solvent (acetone versus dimethylformamide).
B— Good dispersion, rapid settling, caking.
C— Good dispersion, rapid settling, severe caking, poor redispersibility, deaggregation.
D— Good dispersion, rapid settling, slight aggregation.
E— Good dispersion, slow settling, moderate aggregation.
F— Good dispersion, slow settling, fine aggregation.
G— Good dispersion, slow settling, aggregation.
H— Good dispersion, slow settling, coarse aggregation.

TABLE 16-1. *Low Solids Content Suspensions*

Sample	Concentration in mg/ml							
	A	B	C	D	E	F	G	H
Steroid*	25	25	25	25	25	25	25	25
Polysorbate 80[†] (dispersant)	—	1.0	1.0	1.0	1.0	1.0	1.0	1.0
Sodium citrate (buffer)	—	—	—	10.0	—	—	—	—
Sodium chloride (for isotonicity)	9.0	9.0	9.0	—	9.0	9.0	9.0	9.0
Benzyl alcohol (preservative)	—	—	9.0	9.0	9.0	—	9.0	—
Chlorobutanol (preservative)	—	—	—	—	5.0	5.0	—	—
Methylparaben (preservative)	—	—	—	—	—	—	1.8	1.8
Propylparaben (preservative)	—	—	—	—	—	—	0.2	0.2
Purified water q.s. to make 1.00 ml								

*Cortisone acetate or prednisolone acetate.
[†]Tween 60 or Tween 40 could also be used. These are trademarks of ICI Americas, Inc., Wilmington, DE 19899.

It is important to note that protective colloids, such as polyethylene glycol 4000, carboxymethylcellulose sodium, and methylcellulose all modify these characteristics. Sorbitol or dextrose can be included to adjust density.

Suspensions With High Solids Content. Table 16-2 illustrates a different set of sample preparations. Again, it should be recognized that additives often markedly affect the properties of the formulation.

The samples are best prepared as follows. The lecithin is added to the penicillin G, then the remaining vehicle containing the other components is added. The product is first passed through a 40-mesh screen, then through a colloid mill, so that the procaine penicillin G is uniformly coated with the lecithin. The products must be placed in silicone-treated vials or cylinders for proper study because of the poor drainage from the walls of containers that are not so treated.

The samples exhibit characteristics that are not as readily distinguishable as those seen with the low solids content suspensions. Phase separation is not the primary criterion for evaluating the physical performance of the product as it is with the low solids suspensions.

The following is observed if the products are shaken after standing for about one week at room temperature. Samples A, B, and E are diffi-cult to redisperse; samples C, D, F, and G are easily redispersed. If samples are stored for longer periods of time at room temperature, samples A to D show color formation, while E to G do not show color formation (or show it only slightly), owing to the antioxidant effect. Since the product is normally refrigerated during storage, the antioxidant is an added safeguard against deterioration. A good test of the influence of preservatives on the products involves drawing 5 ml of the preparations into a hypodermic syringe fitted with a 22-gauge needle, and trying to eject the contents of the syringe. Samples A, B, and E are difficult to eject, whereas the aggregated samples C, D, F, and G, because of their structure, are more easily emptied, and as indicated before, are generally redispersible.

Antacid Suspensions. Antacids constitute a single class of drugs available in both suspension and tablet forms; consumers prefer the suspension form. This is due to in vivo effectiveness of a well-formulated antacid suspension superior to that of its tablet counterpart. (Detailed discussion is in the next section.) Therefore, antacid formulations merit special treatment.

Aqueous aluminum hydroxide (but not magnesium hydroxide) antacid suspensions tend to thicken or gel during their shelf-life. This gelling

TABLE 16-2. *High Solids Content Suspensions*

Sample	Concentration in mg/ml						
	A	B	C	D	E	F	G
Penicillin G procaine,* USP	200,000[†]	200,000	200,000	200,000	200,000	200,000	200,000
Procaine hydrochloride, USP	20.0	20.0	20.0	20.0	20.0	20.0	20.0
Sodium citrate, USP (buffer)	20.0	20.0	20.0	20.0	20.0	20.0	20.0
Lecithin (protective) colloid)	2.0	2.0	2.0	2.0	2.0	2.0	2.0
Sodium formaldehyde sulfoxylate, USP (antioxidant)	—	—	—	—	2.5	2.5	2.5
Benzyl alcohol, NF (preservative)	—	5.0	—	—	5.0	—	—
Butylparaben, NF (preservative)	—	—	0.15	—	—	0.15	—
Methylparaben/propylparaben, NF (preservatives)	—	—	—	1.0/0.1	—	—	1.0/0.1
				Purified water q.s. to make 1.0 ml			

*Micronized, sterile.
[†]Based on 1000 units/mg.

accelerates during storage under warm conditions (30 to 40°C). Dramatic thickening is observed in the case of high-potency antacids containing large amounts of aluminum hydroxide gel. A patent by Alford teaches how to circumvent this problem by the addition of a hexitol (sorbitol or mannitol) in concentrations from 0.5 to 7%, depending on the concentration of aluminum hydroxide in the suspension.[36] This gelling can also be prevented by the addition of 0.1 to 0.5% potassium or sodium citrate, the former of which is preferred because of consumer demand for low-sodium antacids, particularly with those of higher potency. The gel-preventing action of the citrate ions may be analogous to the mechanism of action of monobasic potassium phosphate on the positively charged bismuth subnitrate suspension.[37] Aluminum hydroxide particles have an excess of positive charge because of surrounding Al^{3+} ions. With the addition of potassium citrate to the aluminum hydroxide gel-type antacids, the apparent zeta potential may be decreased to a point at which the system exhibits a maximum aggregation with a resultant thinning effect.

The following formula demonstrates a hexitol stabilized antacid system.

Ingredients	Percentage in Formula
Aluminum hydroxide gel, AHLT-LW*	36.000
Sorbitol, NF, or mannitol, USP	7.000
Methylparaben, NF	0.200
Propylparaben, NF	0.020
Saccharin, NF	0.050
Peppermint oil, NF	0.005
Alcohol, USP	1.000
Purified water, USP q.s. to make	100.000

*Supplied by Chattem Chemicals Division, Chattem Inc., 1715 West 38th Street, Chattanooga, TN 37409.

The formula can be prepared by dissolving the methylparaben, propylparaben, saccharin, and peppermint oil in the alcohol and transferring the solution, with agitation, to a vessel containing nearly one half of the volume of purified water with agitation. The aluminum hydroxide gel, AHLT-LW, is added and then dispersed using a high-speed propeller or other high-speed disperser. To demonstrate the effect of sorbitol or mannitol, the preparation should be made with and without it. Each product is then stored in bottles at ambient temperature and at 40°C. The addition of sucrose, dextrose, propylene glycol, glycerin, or polyethylene glycol 400 in place of sorbitol or mannitol does not prevent gelling.

Aluminum hydroxide has a constipating effect. Therefore, it is normally combined with the laxative effect of magnesium hydroxide in commercial antacid formulations, as shown in the table at the top of page 499. These formulas can be manufactured by dissolving the methylparaben, propylparaben, saccharin, and peppermint oil in alcohol and then transferring the mixture, with agitation, to a vessel containing nearly one third of the volume of purified water in which either the potassium citrate or the sorbitol solution has been dissolved. The aluminum hydroxide gel, AHLT-LW, is added along with the magnesium hydroxide paste, and the mixture is agitated with a high-speed disperser. Alternately, the entire product can be passed through a colloid mill. The final volume is made up with purified water. A neutral gum-type suspending agent may be included to reduce the separation.

The taste of an antacid must be considered for consumer acceptance. Potassium citrate or sorbitol solution are included to prevent gelling; however, potassium citrate has its own unpleasant taste, while the sorbitol has a cool sweet taste that is pleasant. The parabens at the concentrations given previously impart a numbing aftertaste to the tongue, especially in the presence of the peppermint flavor. The paraben concentrations may be reduced to some extent provided the following factors are considered. The pH of the antacid product is around 8, and the pKa of the parabens is approximately 8.[38] Thus, 50% of the parabens are in the inactive ionized form. The concentrations can be somewhat reduced, however. This can be accomplished by either including an oxidizing-type preservative with a decomposing half-life of about two weeks or by pasteurizing the final bottled product.

Biopharmaceutical Considerations. On a theoretic basis, one would expect the drug bioavailability from a suspension to be equal or somewhat better than that from a tablet during the first hour after administration of the dosage form. This is because the tablet must invariably undergo disintegration before drug dissolution can occur. The suspension, on the other hand, already contains discrete drug particles. Data showing that the suspension drug dosage form is either equally or more bioavailable during the first hour after administration have been documented in the literature.[39,40]

In suspension, the drug is present in the form of solid particles, which must disperse in the gastrointestinal media and dissolve in them. The rate of drug dissolution, and potentially the drug bioavailability, can be affected by such

Ingredients	Percentage in Formula	
	A	B
Aluminum hydroxide gel, AHLT-LW*	23.330	28.750
Magnesium hydroxide (Hydro-magma)[†] paste	13.110	16.400
Sorbitol solution, (70%) USP	—	10.000
Potassium citrate, USP	0.600	—
Methylparaben, NF	0.200	0.200
Propylparaben, NF	0.020	0.020
Saccharin, NF	0.100	0.050
Peppermint oil, NF (or other flavor)	0.005	0.005
Alcohol, USP	1.000	1.000
Purified water, USP q.s. to make	100.000	100.000

*Supplied by Chattem Chemicals Division, Chattem Inc., 1715 West 38th Street, Chattanooga, TN 37409.
[†]Hydro-magma is a trademark of Merck & Co. Inc., 126 East Lincoln Avenue, Rahway, NJ 07065.

physical factors as dispersibility, particle size and shape, and polymorphism.

Considering the hydrodynamic conditions generated by the mild agitation of the gastrointestinal musculature, one would expect the suspending agents to influence the efficacy of suspensions with poor dispersion characteristics in the gastric milieu. Antacid suspensions are the case in point. This class of products also demonstrates that the suspension dosage form is far better than the tablet in terms of in vivo efficacy.[41,42] Using their peristaltic assembly, Simmons and co-authors demonstrated an excellent correlation between the in vitro and in vivo neutralization capacity of a commercial alumina and magnesia oral suspension.[43] Using the in vitro method, which is claimed to simulate the mild agitation in the stomach, they showed that there were significant differences in the neutralization capacity of various commercial antacid suspensions. One product in particular failed to disperse through the reaction medium, which can be attributed to the nature of the suspending agent in this product. Similarly, Fordtran and co-authors,[41] and Drake and Hollander,[42] have shown the varying neutralization capacity of numerous commercial antacid suspensions, as illustrated in Table 16-3.

In addition to the suspending agent, the nature of the raw material and the manufacturing

TABLE 16-3. *In Vitro Neutralization Capacity of Several Commercial Antacids*

Product (Manufacturer)	Neutralization Capacity (mEq/ml)*	Antacid Content (mg/ml)[‡]	
		Aluminum hydroxide	Magnesium hydroxide
Maalox TC[†] (Rorer)	4.2	120	60
Mylanta II** (Stuart)	4.14	80	80
Delcid[†] (Merrell-Dow)	4.1	120	133
Gelusil II[†] (Parke-Davis)	3.0	80	80
Aludrox** (Wyeth)	2.81	61.4	20.6
Maalox** (Rorer)	2.58	45.4	40
Di-Gel** (Plough)	2.45	56.2	17.4
Mylanta** (Stuart)	2.38	40	40
Silain-Gel** (Robins)	2.31	56.4	56.4
Maalox Plus[†] (Rorer)	2.3	45.4	40
Gelusil[†] (Parke-Davis)	2.2	40	40
Amphogel** (Wyeth)	1.93	64	—
Kolantyl Gel** (Merrell-Dow)	1.69	15	15

*A mEq of antacid is defined as the mEq of HCl that is required to maintain the antacid suspension at pH 3 in vitro for a specific time.
**pH 3 maintained for 2 hours.[42]
[†]pH 3 maintained for 1 hour.[43]
[‡]Estimated from Facts and Comparisons, J.B. Lippincott Co., Philadelphia, 1984.

process (milling and homogenization) exert a significant effect on the neutralization capacity of antacid suspensions. For example, aluminum hydroxide gel, AHLT-LW (Chattem Chemicals Division, Chattem Inc.), showed superior neutralization capacity in comparison with other similar raw materials when tested under mild agitative conditions.[43] Because of its fluid nature, this raw material is also pumpable during large-scale production of the antacid suspension. The milling operation reduces the size of the suspended antacid particles, thereby making them more reactive with the gastric acid under mild agitation. The aforementioned factors may account for the observed differences in the neutralization capacity of various commercial antacids in Table 16-3, and of those reported elsewhere.[43]

Howard and associates illustrate a dissolution profile of a prednisolone acetate ophthalmic suspension that is relatively inferior, owing to the presence of hydroxypropyl methylcellulose in a commercial and also an experimental formulation as compared with formulations not having this suspending agent.[44]

The remainder of the chapter deals with the physicochemical factors, influence of excipients, and the drug absorption effects due to body movements, as they relate to bioavailability of parenteral suspensions.

During preparation of a physically stable and therapeutically effective parenteral suspension, the formulator should consider the effects of possible changes in the crystal form (polymorphism) and adjuvants on the absorption process. There exists a very thin layer of saturated drug solution around the suspended crystal. Depending on the conditions, e.g., shelf temperature cycles and crystallization properties of the drug from a particular vehicle, there may be a growth in the crystal. This change may be accompanied by a change in crystal habit (external shape), which thereby causes the formation of one or more polymorphic or solvate forms of the drug. This often results in a change in the particle size distribution of the parenteral formulation. Macek's work demonstrates how one crystal form of cortisone acetate in an aqueous parenteral suspension underwent conversion to a stable form when allowed to stand undisturbed for some time at room temperature.[33] It was accompanied, however, by crystal growth and caking, which made the product unacceptable.

The influence of particle size, vehicle, and additive on the absorption profile of intramuscular procaine penicillin G suspensions is discussed in the extensive work of Buckwalter and Dickinson.[45] Their study showed that larger crystals of drug suspended in water, sesame oil, and peanut oil gave delayed drug absorption with prolonged blood levels; however, when 2% aluminum monostearate was included as a gelling agent in sesame and peanut oils, the micronized drug form exhibited a more prolonged blood level in rabbits. This effect was further confirmed by a study in humans. It might have been due to the incipient depot formation brought about by the gelling agent. Frederick proposed that it was a result of the marked cementing action of the fine particles.[46]

An important factor affecting drug absorption from an intramuscular parenteral suspension is that of body movement (stirring) at the injection site. Thus, Robinson administered an intramuscular injection of procaine penicillin G suspension in which small drug particles were suspended in peanut oil with 2% aluminum monostearate.[47] She showed that active ambulatory patients had serum penicillin levels that were initially higher than those of sedentary patients. She believes this was due to increased massage of the injection site, which released penicillin into the bloodstream earlier. Other workers have confirmed that the degree of body movement influences the onset and duration of benzathine penicillin G depot preparation.[48]

As stated in the previous discussions and as demonstrated in this section, the desired form of sedimentation is a state of controlled aggregation. Complete aggregation may produce a formulation with too coarse an appearance, but just the right degree provides a truly elegant final product. In terms of bioavailability, a suspension should be easily dispersed upon shaking, allowing for removal of a precise drug dose during administration. The suspending agent should permit free and easy drug dispersion in the gastric (or other body) medium under mild agitational conditions.

References

1. Carless, J.E., and Ocran, J.: J. Pharm. Pharmacol., 24:717, 1972.
2. Hiestand, E.N.: J. Pharm. Sci., 53:1, 1964.
3. Ecanow, B., Levinson, R.S., and Takrur, H.: Am. Cosmetics, Perfumer., 84:30, 1969.
4. Ecanow, B., Gold, B., and Ecanow, C.: Am. Cosmetics, Perfumer., 84:27, 1969.
5. Jones, R.D.C., Matthews, B.A., and Rhodes, C.T.: J. Pharm. Sci., 59:518, 1970.
6. Carless, J.E., and Ocran, J.: J. Pharm. Pharmacol., 24:637, 1972.
7. Storz, G.K.: U.S. Patent No. 3,733,408 (1973).
8. Tingstad, J.E.: J. Pharm. Sci., 53:955, 1964.
9. Higuchi, T.: J. Pharm. Sci., 47:657, 1958.
10. Smith, W.E., Buehler, J.D., and Robinson, M.J.: J. Pharm. Sci., 59:776, 1970.

11. Varney, G.: J. Pharm. Pharmacol., *19 (Suppl.)*:19S, 1967.
12. Bean, H.S., and Dempsey, G.: J. Pharm. Pharmacol., 23:699, 1971.
13. Sheikh, M.A., Price, J.C., and Gerraughty, R.J.: J. Pharm. Sci., 55:1048, 1966.
14. Ward, H.T., and Kammermeyer, K.: Ind. Eng. Chem., 32:622, 1940.
15. Foernzler, E.C., Martin, A.N., and Banker, G.S.: J. Am. Pharm. Assoc., Sci. Ed., 49:249, 1960.
16. Wood, J.H.: Am. Perfumer, 76:37, 1961.
17. Wood, J.H., Catacalos, G., and Lieberman, S.V.: J. Pharm. Sci., 52:354, 1963.
18. Van Wazer, J.R., Lyons, J.W., Kim, K.Y., and Colwell, R.E.: Viscosity and Flow Measurement—A Laboratory Handbook of Rheology. Interscience, New York, 1963.
19. Martin, A.M.: J. Pharm. Sci., 50:513, 1961.
20. Stanko, G.L., and DeKay, H.G.: J. Pharm. Sci., 47:104, 1958.
21. Haines, B.A., Jr., and Martin, A.N.: J. Pharm. Sci., 50:753, 756, 1961.
22. Nash, R.A.: Drug & Cosmetic Ind., 97:843, 1965.
23. Nash, R.A.: Drug & Cosmetic Ind., 98:39, 1966.
24. Carless, J.E., Moustafa, M.A., and Rapson, H.D.C.: J. Pharm. Pharmacol., *18 (Suppl.)*:1908, 1966.
25. Carless, J.E., and Foster, A.A.: J. Pharm. Pharmacol., 18:697, 1966.
26. Kennon, L.: J. Soc. Cosmetic Chemists, 17:313, 1966.
27. Matthews, B.A., and Rhodes, C.T.: J. Pharm. Sci., 59:521, 1360, 1970.
28. Matthews, B.A.: J. Pharm. Sci., 62:172, 1973.
29. Ho, N.F.H., Toguchi, H., and Higuchi, W.I.: J. Pharm. Sci., 62:851, 1973.
30. Hiestand, E.N.: J. Pharm. Sci., 61:268, 1972.
31. Carstensen, J.T., and Su, K.S.E.: J. Pharm. Sci., 59:666, 671, 1970.
32. Matthews, B.A., and Rhodes, C.T.: J. Pharm. Sci., 57:557, 569, 1968.
33. Macek, T.J.: U.S. Patent No. 2,671,750 (1954).
34. Patel, N.K., and Kostenbauder, H.B.: J. Am. Pharm. Assoc., Sci. Ed., 47:289, 1958.
35. Patel, N.K.: Can. J. Pharm. Sci., 2:77, 1967.
36. Alford, C.E.: U.S. Patent No. 2,999,790 (1961).
37. Martin, A., Swarbrick, J., and Cammarata, A.: Physical Pharmacy. 3rd Ed. Lea & Febiger, Philadelphia, 1983, p. 549.
38. Patel, N.K.: Ph.D. Dissertation. University of Maryland, College Park, MD, 1962.
39. Bates, T.R., Lambert, D.A., and Johns, W.H.: J. Pharm. Sci., 58:1468, 1969.
40. Meyer, M.C., Straughn, A.B., Ramachander, G., et al.: J. Pharm. Sci., 67:1659, 1978.
41. Fordtran, J.R., Morawski, S.G., and Richardson, C.T.: N. Engl. J. Med., 288:923, 1973.
42. Drake, D., and Hollander, D.: Ann. Internat. Med., 94:215, 1981.
43. Simmons, D.L., Patel, N.K., Chenier, M., et al.: Drug Dev. Ind. Pharm., 7:621, 1981.
44. Howard, S.A., Mauger, J.W., and Phusanti, L.: J. Pharm. Sci., 66:557, 1977.
45. Buckwalter, F.J., and Dickinson, H.L.: J. Am. Pharm. Assoc., Sci. Ed., 47:661, 1958.
46. Frederick, K.J.: J. Pharm. Sci., 50:531, 1961.
47. Robinson, J.M.: J. Michigan State Med. Soc., 48:337, 1949.
48. Lukash, W.M., and Fraser, P.F.: Am. J. Med. Sci., 246:429, 1963.

17

Emulsions

MARTIN M. RIEGER

This chapter is divided into three parts. The first part deals with emulsions in a nonmathematical, descriptive way. The second part covers the equipment and the chemical and physical conditions for the preparation of emulsions. The last portion of the chapter is devoted to a discussion of the physical and chemical characteristics and stability of emulsions.

Overview

A precise definition of the term *emulsion* depends on the observer's point of view. The physical chemist defines an emulsion as a thermodynamically unstable mixture of two essentially immiscible liquids. For the product development technologist, it is more useful to regard an emulsion as an intimate mixture of two immiscible liquids that exhibits an acceptable shelf life near room temperature. Other definitions exist, but the two given here suffice for the purpose of this chapter.

Practical Definitions

When two immiscible liquids are mechanically agitated, both phases initially tend to form droplets. When the agitation is stopped, the droplets quickly coalesce, and the two liquids separate. The lifetime of the droplets is materially increased if an *emulsifier* is added to the two immiscible liquids. Usually, only one phase persists in droplet form for a prolonged period of time. This phase is called the *internal (disperse or discontinuous) phase,* and it is surrounded by an *external (continuous) phase.* An assembly of close-packed monodisperse* spherical droplets as the internal phase can occupy no more than

*All particles have the same size.

approximately 74% of the total volume of an emulsion. It is evident, however, that the internal phase can exceed 74% if the spherical particles are not monodisperse (as in most emulsions). A further increase in the ratio of internal:external phase can result if the internal phase is assumed to consist of polyhedra rather than spheres.[1]

An emulsifier functions and is operationally defined as a stabilizer of the droplet form (globules) of the internal phase. On the basis of their structure, emulsifiers (wetting agents or surfactants) may be described as molecules comprising both hydrophilic (oleophobic) and hydrophobic (oleophilic) portions. For this reason, this group of compounds is frequently called *amphiphilic* (i.e., water- and oil-loving).

It is almost universally accepted that the term emulsion should be limited to *liquid-in-liquid* systems. Emulsions are normally formed by "mixing" two immiscible liquids. If necessary, the two phases are heated to ensure that they are liquids during emulsification. The most common types of pharmaceutical or cosmetic emulsions include water as one of the phases and an oil or lipid as the other. If the oil droplets are dispersed in a continuous aqueous phase, the emulsion is termed *oil-in-water (o/w)*; if the oil is the continuous phase, the emulsion is of the *water-in-oil* type *(w/o)*. It has been observed that o/w emulsions occasionally change into w/o emulsions and vice versa. This change of *emulsion type* is called *inversion.*

Since approximately 1978, two additional types of emulsions, classified as *multiple emulsions,* received the attention of surface chemists. It is entirely feasible to prepare a multiple emulsion with the characteristics of *oil-in-water-in-oil (o/w/o)* or of *water-in-oil-in-water (w/o/w)* emulsions. Such emulsions also can invert; however, during inversion they usually form "simple" emulsions. Thus, a w/o/w emulsion normally yields an o/w emulsion.[2]

The particle size of the disperse phase determines the appearance of an emulsion. The radius of the emulsified droplets in an opaque, usually white, emulsion ranges from 0.25 to 10 microns. It is fairly well established that dispersed particles having a diameter of less than $1/4$ the wave length of visible light, i.e., less than approximately 120 nm, do not refract light and therefore appear transparent to the eye. Dispersions of a liquid to such small particle sizes yield *microemulsions* or *micellar emulsions*. Often, these terms are erroneously used interchangeably because such emulsions appear transparent to the human eye in daylight. In a microemulsion, disperse globules having a radius below the range of 10 to 75 nm are present.

The production of a transparent dispersion of an oil by micellization* does not result in the formation of droplets, but in the inclusion of the lipid into micelles, which may, but need not, possess spherical shapes. In terms of size, micelles have dimensions ranging from about 5 to 20 nm. To the practicing technologist, transparent emulsions, solubilized oils, micellar emulsions, and microemulsions are one and the same because they appear clear. However, solubilization in any form represents an entirely different phenomenon from that of emulsification.

Applications and Utility

Emulsions are sometimes difficult to prepare and require special processing techniques. To warrant this type of effort and to exist as useful dosage forms, emulsions must possess desirable attributes and cause a minimum of associated problems. The "mixing" of immiscible liquids for various purposes has been met by the emulsification process for centuries. Today, emulsions continue to have a variety of cosmetic and pharmaceutical applications. The latter may be further classified by route of administration, i.e., topical, oral, or parenteral. In principle, cosmetic applications and topical pharmaceutical applications are similar and together form one of the most important groups of emulsions.

Patient acceptance undoubtedly is the most

*Micelles are the result of self structuring of surface active materials in order to reach a state of minimum energy. For example, sodium stearate, in a clear aqueous solution at a concentration above the *critical micelle concentration (CMC)*, forms structures with the nonpolar ends of several molecules in contact with each other (hydrophobic bonding) and with the polar ends exposed to the surrounding water.

important reason why emulsions are popular oral and topical dosage forms. Many medicinal agents have an objectionable taste or texture, and can be made more palatable for oral administration when formulated into emulsions. As a result, mineral oil-based laxatives, oil-soluble vitamins, and high-fat nutritive preparations are commonly administered as o/w emulsions. The utility of orally administered emulsions resides in their efficacy, i.e., absorption or bioavailability of the drug. It has been demonstrated that some drugs are more readily absorbed when they are administered orally in the form of emulsions.[3] It has even been reported that normally unabsorbable macromolecules, such as insulin and heparin, are absorbed when they are incorporated into emulsions.

Patient acceptance is also important in topically applied emulsions. Emulsions possess a certain degree of elegance and are easily washed off whenever desired. In addition, the formulator can control the viscosity, appearance, and degree of greasiness of cosmetic or dermatologic emulsions.

With regard to emulsion type, o/w emulsions are most useful as water-washable drug bases and for general cosmetic purposes. W/o emulsions are employed more widely for the treatment of dry skin and emollient applications. The utility of topical emulsions depends on their ability to "penetrate." This much abused term has entirely different meanings to the layman and to the technologist. To the former, rapid "penetration" is desirable and refers to the disappearance of the product or of oiliness from the skin during inunction. It is generally believed that this process of penetration into the skin is facilitated if the emulsion is thixotropic, i.e., if it becomes less viscous during shearing. To the technologist, penetration of the vehicle is of secondary importance; instead, rapid and efficient penetration of the drug moiety to the site that needs to be treated is desired.[4]

Emulsions have been used for the intravenous administration of lipid nutrients, which is facilitated by emulsification and probably would be impossible unless the lipid were in the form of an emulsion. Such emulsions of the o/w type require the most rigorous control of the emulsifying agent and/or particle size (normally less than 100 nm).

Some other pharmaceutical and clinical applications of emulsions include the following. Radiopaque emulsions have been used as diagnostic agents in x-ray examinations. W/o emulsions have been employed to disperse water-soluble antigenic materials in mineral oil for intramuscular depot injection. The presence of emulsifiers in injectable drugs that are relatively insoluble in water (or serum) may help lower the tendency of the drug to crystallize and cause thrombophlebitis. Finally, emulsification of perfluorinated hydrocarbons is required to make them useful as oxygen carriers in blood replacements.

Emulsions also possess an important cost advantage over single-phase preparations. Most lipids and solvents for lipids that are intended for application to or into the human body are relatively costly. As a result, dilution with a safe and inexpensive diluent, such as water, is highly desirable from an economic point of view as long as efficacy or performance is not impaired.

Descriptive Theory of Emulsification

The fundamental principles of surface chemistry and of emulsification are included in Chapter 5. Therefore only a few concepts of practical importance need be discussed here to make the formulation steps better understood. When oil and water are mixed and agitated, droplets of varying sizes are produced. A tension exists at the interface because the two immiscible phases tend to have different attractive forces for a molecule at the interface. A molecule of phase A is attracted into phase A and repelled by phase B. In general, the greater the degree of immiscibility, the greater is the interfacial tension. For example, liquid hydrocarbons, such as those found in mineral oil, exhibit an interfacial tension against water of approximately 50 dynes/cm, whereas a more polar vegetable oil, such as olive oil, exhibits a value of 23 dynes/cm. The interfacial tension at a liquid interface is defined as the work required to create 1 cm^2 of new interface.

A fine dispersion of oil and water necessitates a large area of interfacial contact, and its production requires an amount of work equal to the product of interfacial tension and the area change. Thermodynamically speaking, this work is the interfacial free energy imparted to the system. A high interfacial free energy favors a reduction of interfacial area, first by causing droplets to assume a spherical shape (minimum surface area for a given volume) and then by causing them to coalesce (with a resultant decrease in the number of droplets). This is the reason for including the words "thermodynamically unstable" in the classic definition of opaque emulsions.

Droplet Stabilization. Two conceptual alternatives exist for creating opaque, i.e., milky-appearing, emulsions. Such dispersions can be formed and stabilized by lowering the interfacial tension and/or by preventing the coalescing of droplets. According to classic emulsion theory, surface active agents are capable of performing both objectives: They reduce interfacial tension, and they act as barriers to droplet coalescence since they are adsorbed at the interface, or more precisely, on the surface of the suspended droplets. Emulsifying agents assist in the formation of emulsions by three mechanisms:

1. Reduction of interfacial tension—thermodynamic stabilization.

2. Formation of a rigid interfacial film—mechanical barrier to coalescence.

3. Formation of an electrical double layer—electrical barrier to approach of particles.

Interfacial Tension. Even though reduction of interfacial tension lowers the interfacial free energy produced on dispersion, it is the role of emulsifying agents as interfacial barriers that is most important. This can be seen clearly when one considers that many polymers and finely divided solids, not efficient in reducing interfacial tension, form excellent interfacial barriers, act to prevent coalescence, and are useful as emulsifying agents.

Interfacial Film. The formation of films by an emulsifier on the surface of water or oil droplets has been studied in great detail. The concept of an oriented (monomolecular) film of the emulsifier on the surface of the internal phase of an emulsion is of fundamental importance to an understanding of most theories of emulsification.[5] Scheme 1 in Figure 17-1 illustrates how emulsifiers are believed to surround the droplets of the internal phase.

It is reasonable to expect an amphiphilic molecule to align itself at a water-oil interface in the most energetically favorable position—oleophilic portion in the oil phase and hydrophilic portion in the aqueous phase. It is also well established that the surface-active agents tend to concentrate at interfaces and that emulsifiers are adsorbed at oil-water interfaces as monomolecular films. If the concentration of the emulsifier is high enough, it forms a rigid film between the immiscible phases, which acts as a mechanical bar to both adhesion and coalescence of the emulsion droplets. Measurements of the area occupied by a single molecule of surface-active agent at the interface of emulsion

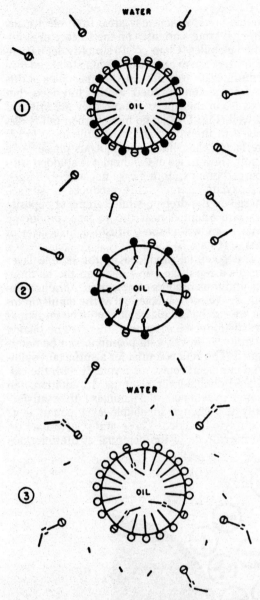

FIG. 17-1. *Schematic representation of the relationship between mixed film formation, mechanical strength, and the stability of emulsions. (From Schulman and Cockbain.*[6]*) 1, ⊖ Cetyl sulfate Na; ● cholesterol; closely packed condensed complex; excellent emulsion. 2, ⊖ Cetyl sulfate Na; ● oleyl alcohol; no closely packed condensed complex; poor emulsion. 3, ○ Cetyl alcohol; ⊖ sodium oleate; fairly closely packed monolayer; negligible complex formation: rather poor emulsion.*

droplets have shown that in stable emulsions, the molecules of surface-active agents are in fact closely packed and form a tough interfacial film.

This concept is illustrated by the classic study of Schulman and Cockbain.[6] They found that o/w emulsions stabilized by mixtures of sodium cetyl sulfate and cholesterol, which were known from other experiments to form rigid and tightly packed films, were extremely stable (scheme 1, Fig. 17-1). When oleyl alcohol was substituted for cholesterol, however, the steric effect of a double bond (which produces a kink in the carbon chain) resulted in the formation of a poor interfacial complex, and emulsion stability was proportionately low (scheme 2, Fig. 17-1). On the other hand, if this last system was changed somewhat by using sodium oleate and cetyl alcohol, it was possible to obtain a rather poor emulsion, but one that was more stable than that of the previous case (scheme 3, Fig. 17-1). Thus, a tightly packed emulsifier film contributes to the stability of the emulsion. This steric argument by Schulman and Cockbain has been used to explain the well-known fact that mixed emulsifiers are often more effective than single emulsifiers. The ability of the mixture of emulsifiers to pack more tightly contributes to the strength of the film, and hence, to the stability of the emulsion. Most emulsifiers probably form fairly dense gel structures at the interface and produce a stable interfacial film.

Recent studies have helped to clarify further the nature of these interfacial films. Stable emulsions are now believed to comprise liquid crystalline layers on the interface of emulsified droplets with the continuous phase.[7-9] In their pioneering studies, Friberg and co-workers were able to show by optical (polarized light) and electron microscopy and low-angle x-ray diffractometry that mixed emulsifiers can interact with water to form three-dimensional association structures. The classic concept of emulsions as two-phase systems with a monomolecular layer of emulsifier at the interface must be revised. Emulsions should instead be viewed as three-component systems comprising oil, water, and lamellar liquid crystals, the latter consisting of consecutive layers of water-emulsifier-oil-water (Fig. 17-2).

Interlamellar layers representing the internal and external phases of an emulsion have recently been identified by freeze fracture micrography of o/w creams.[10] In addition, it has recently been learned that emulsion droplets can be surrounded by liquid crystals of a closed lamellar type in appropriately prepared emulsions.[11]

This field of emulsion science is currently undergoing active investigation by scientists throughout the world. Efforts have been made to measure the mechanical properties of association structures by studying interfacial shear vis-

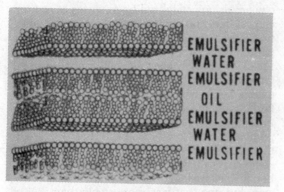

FIG. 17-2. *A lamellar liquid crystal consists of consecutive layers of water - emulsifier - oil - emulsifier - water. (From Friberg.[9])*

cosity.[12] These investigations are expected to lead to a fuller understanding of the complex droplet-droplet interactions that lead to coalescence and emulsion instability. There is little doubt that nonionic emulsifiers, proteins, and macromolecular gums stabilize emulsions by forming interfacial films.

Electrical Repulsion. It has just been described how interfacial films or lamellar liquid crystals significantly alter the rates of coalescence of droplets by acting as barriers. In addition, the same or similar film can produce repulsive electrical forces between approaching droplets. Such repulsion is due to an electrical double layer, which may arise from electrically charged groups oriented on the surface of emulsified globules (Chap. 5). To simplify, let us consider the case of an o/w emulsion stabilized by a sodium soap. Not only are the molecules of this surfactant concentrated in the interface, but because of their polar nature, they are oriented as well (Fig. 17-3). The hydrocarbon tail is dissolved in the oil droplet, while the ionic heads are facing the continuous aqueous phase. As a result, the surface of the droplet is studded with charged groups, in this case negatively charged carboxylate groups. This produces a surface charge on the droplet, while cations of opposite sign are oriented near the surface, producing what is known as the (diffuse) double layer of charge (Chap. 5).

The potential produced by the double layer creates a repulsive effect between the oil droplets and thus hinders coalescence. Although the repulsive electrical potential at the emulsion interface can be calculated, it cannot be measured directly for comparison with theory. The related quantity, however, zeta potential, can be determined. The zeta potential for a surfactant-stabilized emulsion compares favorably with the calculated double-layer potential. In addition, the change in zeta potential parallels rather satisfactorily the change in double-layer potential as electrolyte is added. These and related data on the magnitude of the potential at the interface

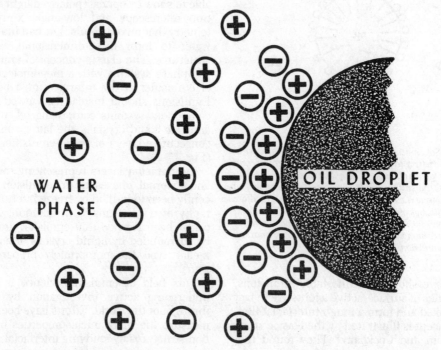

FIG. 17-3. *Idealized representation of the electrical double layer at an oil-water interface.*

can be used to calculate the total repulsion between oil droplets as a function of the distance between them.

Droplet Interaction. A plot of the total repulsive potential between two charged droplets as a function of the interparticle distance has been shown in Figure 5–20. This potential includes not only the repulsive electrical potential, but also a series of other interactions, known as van der Waals forces or London interactions. The repulsive potential at large distances is small and then rises sharply as the distance between the droplets decreases. To the left of the peak, the repulsive force drops rapidly to zero, and this corresponds, of course, to coalescence of emulsion droplets. The barrier to coalescence is high (many multiples of kT, the translational energy) and probably cannot be overcome by two approaching droplets. If, as is now believed, liquid crystal phases surround the emulsified droplets, and if these phases adhere tenaciously, their presence can be expected to cause a change in the van der Waals potential. The distance at which this change occurs depends not only on the droplet radius but also on the surrounding liquid crystalline phase, and the compressibility and rheology of this assembly.

Another important point is that the curve has two minima, and the minimum at a separation of approximately 5 to 15 nm is responsible for the initial adhesion of emulsion particles. When the droplets fall into this secondary minimum of the potential energy curve, they flocculate. The smallness of this minimum explains why emulsion flocculation is a reversible process. It is believed that flocculated droplets may remain in this minimum for a fairly long time, but that some rearrangements of the surface active compound occurs at the interface. This modifies the potential picture and allows coalescence to take place.

Emulsion Type. Only o/w and w/o emulsions have achieved commercial and practical importance. To understand the various factors that determine whether an o/w or a w/o emulsion will be produced, one must again think in terms of two critical features: (1) droplet formation and (2) formation of an interfacial barrier. The phase volume ratio, i.e., the relative amount of oil and water, determines the relative number of droplets formed initially and hence the probability of collision; the greater the number of droplets, the greater is the chance for collision. Thus, normally, the phase present in greater amount becomes the external phase.

To predict the type of emulsion formed under a given set of conditions, the interaction of various parameters must be estimated. This estima-

tion is nearly impossible, and only a few generalized and somewhat empiric rules can be given.

1. If the amphiphile is essentially water-soluble (e.g., potassium soap or polyoxyethylene alkyl ether with more than 5 ethylene oxide units), it will usually favor o/w emulsification; if the surfactant is primarily soluble in the lipid portion (calcium soap, polyoxyethylene alkyl ether with less than 5 ethylene oxide units), it may yield w/o emulsions if the other conditions are favorable.

2. The polar portions of emulsifier molecules are generally better barriers to coalescence than their hydrocarbon counterparts. It is, therefore, possible to make o/w emulsions with relatively high internal phase volumes. On the other hand, w/o emulsions (in which the barrier is of hydrocarbon nature) are limited in this regard and invert easily if the amount of water present is significant. For example, a water-mineral oil-sorbitan monooleate system, ordinarily expected to favor w/o emulsion formation because of the lack of ethylene oxide units, does so only if the amount of water present constitutes less than 40% by volume. At higher amounts of water, only o/w emulsions form.

3. Even at 20% and 30% water, w/o emulsions form only if the water is added to the oil with mixing. The addition of both phases together, followed by mixing, favors o/w emulsions at all concentrations above 10% water.

4. Finally, the type of emulsion formed is influenced to some extent by the viscosity of each phase. An increase in the viscosity of a phase aids in making that phase the external phase.

Despite these complications, one can expect a predominantly water-soluble emulsifier to form o/w emulsions, whereas the reverse is true of primarily oil-soluble surfactants. Occasionally, it is desirable to determine the type of emulsion formed. Methods for this purpose are shown in Table 17-1.

Microemulsions. Operationally, microemulsions may be defined as dispersions of insoluble liquids in a second liquid that appear clear and homogeneous to the naked eye. Microemulsions are frequently called *solubilized* systems because on a macroscopic basis they seem to behave as true solutions. Careful examination of these complex systems has shown that clear emulsions can exist in several differentiable forms. Microemulsions should not be confused, however, with solutions formed by *cosolvency*, e.g., the clear system consisting of water, benzene, and ethanol.

Blending of a small amount of oil with water results in a two-phase system because "water and oil do not mix." If the same small amount of

TABLE 17-1. *Methods for the Determination of Emulsion Type*[*]

Test	Observation	Comments
Dilution test	Emulsion can be diluted only with external phase.	Useful for liquid emulsions only.
Dye test	Water-soluble solid dye tints only o/w emulsions and reverse. Microscopic observation usually helpful.	May fail if ionic emulsifiers are present.
CoCl$_2$/filter paper	Filter paper impregnated with CoCl$_2$ and dried (blue) changes to pink when o/w emulsion is added.	May fail if emulsion is unstable or breaks in presence of electrolyte.
Fluorescence	Since oils fluoresce under UV light, o/w emulsions exhibit dot pattern, w/o emulsions fluoresce throughout.	Not always applicable.
Conductivity	Electric current is conducted by o/w emulsions, owing to presence of ionic species in water.	Fails in nonionic o/w emulsions.

[*]For details, consult Becher,[13] p. 413.

oil is added to an aqueous solution of a suitable surfactant in the micellar state, the oil may preferentially dissolve in the interior of the micelle because of its hydrophobic character. This type of micellar microemulsion, which was observed by McBain many years ago, has also been called an o/w micellar solution. Similarly, w/o solubilization—especially that by a nonionic surfactant—has recently been attributed to the existence of swollen micelles. In these systems, sometimes called reverse micellar solutions, water molecules are found in the polar central portion of a surfactant micelle, the nonpolar portion of which is in contact with the continuous lipid phase. A third type of microemulsion (usually of the w/o type) is formed by ionic surfactants (e.g., sodium stearate) in the presence of cosurfactants (e.g., pentanol or dioxyethylene dodecyl ether) with hydrocarbons (e.g., hexadecane) and water.

In general, microemulsions or solubilized systems are believed to be thermodynamically stable. Transparent or clear emulsions in which a water-insoluble oil or drug is "dissolved" in an aqueous surfactant system play an important role in drug administration. In addition, a wide variety of clear proprietary and toiletry products are in fact clear emulsions of all types of oils and lipids in water.

Formation of Emulsions

The spontaneous formation of an emulsion is a relatively rare occurrence. Instead, emulsion preparation by the commonly employed dispersion method requires a sequence of processes for breaking up the internal phase into droplets

and for stabilizing them in the external phase. The complete process must be designed in such a way that these two steps are carried out before the internal phase can coalesce. Usually, the breakup of the internal phase (by physical means) is fairly rapid; however, it is believed that the stabilization step and the rate of coalescence are time- and temperature-dependent. It is therefore a requirement in the design of any emulsification process that the variable physical and chemical parameters are selected and controlled to favor emulsion formation.

Physical Parameters

The application of energy in the form of heat, mechanical agitation, ultrasonic vibration, or electricity is required to reduce the internal phase into small droplets. The amount of work input depends on the length of time during which energy is supplied; thus, timing (scheduling of work input) becomes another important physical parameter.

Heat. Vaporization is an effective way of breaking almost all the bonds between the molecules of a liquid. It is possible, therefore, to prepare emulsions by passing the vapor of a liquid into an external phase that contains suitable emulsifying agents. This process of emulsification, called the condensation method, is relatively slow, is limited to the preparation of dilute emulsions of materials having a relatively low vapor pressure, and is therefore primarily of theoretical importance.

The more practical emulsification by dispersion is affected by heat—or better, changes in temperature—in a number of ways. The interactions are complex, and it is almost impossible to predict whether a raise in temperature will favor emulsification or coalescence. An increase in temperature decreases interfacial tension as well as viscosity. One would therefore predict— and this is usually true—that emulsification is favored by an increase in temperature. At the same time, however, an increase in temperature raises the kinetic energy of droplets and thereby facilitates their coalescence. This type of instability is normally observed when emulsions are stored at elevated temperatures for long periods of time. Changes in temperature alter the distribution coefficients of emulsifiers between the two phases and cause emulsifier migration. The distribution of the emulsifier as a function of temperature cannot be correlated directly with either emulsion formation or stability, since changes in surface tension and viscosity occur simultaneously.

Phase Inversion Temperature. The most important influence that temperature has on an emulsion is probably inversion. Almost 50 years ago it was observed that w/o emulsions of benzene in water that were stabilized with sodium stearate invert to o/w emulsions upon heating and reform w/o emulsions upon cooling. The temperature at which the inversion occurs depends on emulsifier concentration and is called *phase inversion temperature (PIT)*. This type of inversion can occur during the formation of emulsions, since they are generally prepared at relatively high temperatures and are then allowed to cool to room temperature. Emulsions formed by a phase inversion technique are generally considered quite stable and are believed to contain a finely dispersed internal phase. The PIT is generally considered to be the temperature at which the *hydrophilic* and the *lipophilic* properties of the emulsifier are in *balance* and is therefore also called the *HLB* temperature.

Shinoda's description of the processes at or near the PIT is almost universally accepted today.[14] An o/w emulsion stabilized by a nonionic polyoxyethylene-derived surfactant contains oil-swollen micelles of the surfactant as well as emulsified oil. When the temperature is raised, the water-solubility of the surfactant decreases*; as a result, the micelles are broken,

and the size of emulsified oil droplets begins to increase. A continued rise in the temperature causes separation into an oil phase, a surfactant phase, and water. It is near this temperature that the now water-insoluble surfactant begins to form a w/o emulsion containing both water-swollen micelles and emulsified water droplets in a continuous oil phase.

Timing. Timing, just like variation in temperature, exerts a profound and complex influence on the process of emulsification. During the initial period of agitation required for emulsification, droplets are formed; however, as agitation continues, the chance for collision between droplets becomes more frequent, and coalescence can occur. It is generally advisable, therefore, to avoid excessive periods of agitation during and after the formation of an emulsion. On the other hand, it is impossible to specify the time required for agitation, and the optimum period necessary for emulsification is usually determined empirically.

The criticality of the interaction between agitation and timing was demonstrated more than 50 years ago by Briggs. In the most obvious manner of preparing an emulsion, two immiscible liquids are mixed in a suitable container in the presence of an emulsifier and are then shaken until the emulsion has formed. Briggs showed that the best way of forming an emulsion by this technique is to use intermittent shaking. He found that he could emulsify 60% by volume of benzene in 1% aqueous sodium oleate by mechanically shaking 750 times during a period of four to five minutes. The same mixture, however, could be completely emulsified with merely five hand shakes in about two minutes, if the emulsion was allowed to rest for 20 to 30 seconds after each shake. The reasons for the observed time-dependent droplet stabilization may be distribution of the emulsifier between the phases, slow formation of the (double-layer) film on the surface of the benzene droplets, or interruption of droplet formation by continuous shaking.

Timing or scheduling also affects the speed with which the two immiscible liquids are blended. In the case of an o/w emulsion, for example, the rate at which the oil phase is added to the aqueous phase can materially affect particle size and ultimate stability of the finished emulsion. Finally, there is a relationship between temperature and timing, i.e., the cooling/heating cycle. It is routine to prepare emulsions at elevated temperatures. The cooling rate of the initially formed emulsion also has a profound influence on the ultimate characteristics of the emulsion. Unfortunately, it is impossible to pre-

*The water solubility of ether-type surfactants depends on the formation of hydrogen bonds between water and the O-atoms of the ether. The surfactant's solubility decreases when H-bonds are broken by heat and/or the presence of electrolytes. The cloud point, i.e., the temperature at which the solution of an emulsifier becomes cloudy, is an important analytic criterion for nonionic amphiphiles.

dict whether a slow or a rapid cooling cycle is desirable for a given emulsion.

Low-Energy Emulsification. The classic process of emulsification just described requires considerable expenditure of energy during both the heating and cooling cycles of emulsion formation. The principle of low energy emulsification has been formalized by Lin in recent years, although some of his suggestions may have been previously used by other practitioners.[15,16] In low-energy emulsification, all of the internal phase, but only a portion of the external phase, is heated. After emulsification of the heated portions, the remainder of the external phase is added to the emulsion concentrate, or the preformed concentrate is blended into the continuous phase. In those emulsions in which a phase inversion temperature exists, the emulsion concentrate is preferably prepared above the PIT, which results in emulsions having extremely small droplet size. As in the case of the classic emulsification technique, the temperature for the preparation of the emulsion concentrate is critical. It is important to effect in situ neutralization of acidic emulsifying components during the emulsion step. By careful control of the variables (emulsification temperature, mixing intensity, the amount of the external phase employed during emulsification, and the method of blending), it is reportedly possible to produce emulsions with smaller and more uniform particle size than those resulting from the conventional process.

Mechanical Equipment for Emulsification

Almost all methods used for breaking up the internal phase into droplets depend on "brute force" and require some sort of agitation. When a liquid jet of one liquid is introduced under pressure into a second liquid, the initially cylindric jet stream is broken up into droplets. The factors that enter into the breakup of a liquid jet include the diameter of the nozzle, the speed with which the liquid is injected, the density and the viscosity of the injected liquid, and of course, the interfacial tension between the two liquids. A similar breakup into droplets occurs when a liquid is allowed to flow into a second liquid that is agitated vigorously. Once the initial breakup into droplets has occurred, the droplets continue to be subject to additional forces due to turbulence, which cause deformation of the droplet and further breakdown into smaller droplets.[11]

Various types of equipment are available to effect droplet breakup and emulsification either in the laboratory or in production. Regardless of size and minor variations, such equipment can be divided into four broad categories: (1) mechanical stirrers, (2) homogenizers, (3) ultrasonifiers, and (4) colloid mills.

During the formulation of an emulsion, the mechanical requirements of preparation, and particularly the problems associated with scale-up to production-size equipment, must be considered. The most important factor involved in the preparation of an emulsion is the degree of shear and turbulence required to produce a given dispersion of liquid droplets. The amount of agitation required depends on the total volume of liquid to be mixed, the viscosity of the system, and the interfacial tension at the oil-water interface. The latter two factors are determined by the emulsion type, the phase ratio, and the type and concentration of emulsifiers. For this reason, no single method of dispersion can be used for all emulsions, and conversion from one method to another is difficult.

Mechanical Stirrers. An emulsion may be stirred by means of various impellers mounted on shafts, which are placed directly into the system to be emulsified. Simple top-entering propeller mixers are adequate for routine development work in the laboratory and for production purposes, if the viscosity of the emulsion is low. If more vigorous agitation is required, or if the preparation has moderate viscosity, turbine type mixers are employed both in the laboratory and in production. Other mixers, provided with paddle blades, counter rotating blades, or planetary action blades, are available for special requirements. The degree of agitation is controlled by the speed of impeller rotation, but the patterns of liquid flow and the resultant efficiency of mixing are controlled by the type of impeller, its position in the container, the presence of baffles, and the general shape of the container (Chaps. 5 and 15). Despite the variation in flow behavior and the efficient mixing that can be produced, the use of stirrers for the formation of emulsions is often limited when vigorous agitation of viscous systems is required, when extremely fine droplets are needed, or when foaming at high shear rates must be avoided.

Homogenizers. In a homogenizer, the dispersion of two liquids is achieved by forcing their mixture through a small inlet orifice at high pressures. A homogenizer generally consists of a pump that raises the pressure of the dispersion to a range of 500 to 5,000 psi and an orifice through which this fluid impinges upon the homogenizing valve held in place on the valve seat by a strong spring (Fig. 17-4). As the pressure builds up, the spring is compressed, and some of the dispersion escapes between the valve and the valve seat. At this point, the energy that has been stored in the liquid as pressure is released instantaneously and subjects the product to intense turbulence and hydraulic shear.

Homogenizers can also be built with more than one emulsifier stage, and it is possible to recycle the emulsion and pass it through the homogenizer more than one time. Homogenizers of varying designs are useful for handling either liquids or pastes, since the rate of throughput is little affected by viscosity. It must be remembered, however, that homogenization raises the temperature of the emulsion, and subsequent cooling may be required. The use of a homogenizer is warranted whenever a reasonably monodisperse emulsion of low particle size (1 nm) is required. Another useful piece of equipment, which combines mixing with some homogenizing action, is the rotor-stator homogenizer described in Chapter 23.

Ultrasonifiers. The use of ultrasonic energy to produce pharmaceutical emulsions has been demonstrated, and many laboratory-size models are available. These transduced piezoelectric devices have limited output and are relatively expensive. They are useful for the laboratory preparation of fluid emulsions of moderate viscosity and extremely low particle size. Commercial equipment is based on the principle of the Pohlman liquid whistle shown in Figure 17-5. The dispersion is forced through an orifice at modest pressures and is allowed to impinge upon a blade. The pressures required range from approximately 150 to 350 psi and cause the blade to vibrate rapidly to produce an ultrasonic note. When the system reaches a steady state, a cavitational field is generated at the leading edge of the blade, and pressure fluctuations of approximately 60 tons psi can be achieved in commercial equipment.

Colloid Mills. Homogenizers and ultrasonic equipment depend on sudden changes in pressure to effect the dispersion of liquids. By contrast, colloid mills operate on the principle of high shear, which is normally generated between the rotor and the stator of the mill (Chap. 23). Colloid mills are used primarily for the comminution of solids and for the dispersion of suspensions containing poorly wetted solids but are also useful for the preparation of relatively viscous emulsions.

Spontaneous Emulsification. Spontaneous emulsification occurs when an emulsion is formed without the application of any external

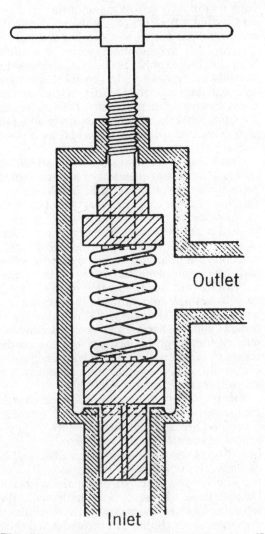

FIG. 17-4. *Schematic representation of a homogenizer.*[17]

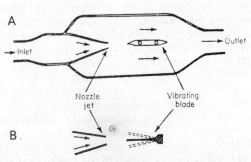

FIG. 17-5. *Principle of Pohlman whistle. A, Nodally supported blade. B, Edge-mounted blade. (From Gopal, E.S.R.: Principles of emulsion formation. In Emulsion Science. Edited by P. Sherman. Academic Press, London, 1968, p. 47.)*

agitation. Emulsifiable concentrates and micro-emulsions are typical examples. The former are blends of the internal phase with emulsifiers, which "bloom" when they are added to the external phase. Microemulsions commonly form spontaneously, but not all spontaneous emulsions are transparent. The phenomenon of spontaneous emulsification is observable when a drop of oil is placed on an aqueous solution of an emulsifier, in which case the interface becomes extremely unstable and results in the formation of fine droplets. Spontaneous emulsification evidently is not practiced commercially.

Production Aspects. In routine production, it is customary to prepare emulsions by a batch process using kettles, agitators, and related equipment. However, it is possible to design combinations of equipment that permit continuous manufacturing of emulsions. The selection of commercial equipment for the production of emulsions is based in part on the production capacity and the power requirements for various types of apparatus. Propeller-type agitators and turbine impellers require the least amount of energy and are capable of handling large quantities of product. Their greatest utility is for the slow mixing of emulsions that have been prepared by the melting of waxes followed by slow cooling. The power requirements for homogenizers are much higher than those for simple agitators; nevertheless, their output is slower. The least efficient type of mixer is the colloid mill, which has the highest power requirements and the slowest production rate of any commercially useful equipment.

Foaming during Agitation. During the agitation or transfer of an emulsion, foam may be formed. Foaming occurs because the water-soluble surfactant required for emulsification generally also reduces the surface tension at the air-water interface. To minimize foaming, emulsification may be carried out in closed systems (with a minimum of free air space) and/or under vacuum. In addition, mechanical stirring, particularly during the cooling of a freshly prepared emulsion, can be regulated to cause air to rise to the top. If these precautions should fail to eliminate or reduce foaming, it is sometimes necessary to add foam depressants (antifoams); however, their use should be avoided, if at all possible, since they represent a chemical source of incompatibility. Sometimes the use of ethyl alcohol accelerates the coalescence of foam on the surface of emulsions. On the other hand, the most effective defoamers are long-chain alcohols and commercially available silicone derivatives, both of which are generally believed to spread over the air-water interface as insoluble films.

Chemical Parameters

It is difficult to designate a general approach or a set of rules for selecting the components and their amounts to yield a desired emulsion. The ingredients of any pharmaceutical or cosmetic emulsion must conform to various requirements. There are situations in which certain oils, emulsifiers, and other ingredients must be avoided or used exclusively. Usually, however, ingredient selection is made on the basis of the experience and personal tastes of the formulator and by trial and error.

Formulators are cautioned to establish the safety and regulatory acceptance of emulsion ingredients for a particular application.

Chemical Stability. Chemical inertness is an absolute and almost obvious requirement for emulsion ingredients. For example, it would be futile to utilize a soap as an emulsifier in a system having a final pH of less than 5. Similarly, one would not use an easily hydrolyzed ester in an emulsion that is either acidic or alkaline. Some lipids are subject to chemical changes due to oxidation (rancidity); in general it is simpler to avoid their use than to depend on antioxidants to ensure their stability. It is important, therefore, that the chemical nature of all emulsion constituents be understood before a selection for a given preparation is made.

Unfortunately, predictions of hydrolytic stability made by classic chemical or pharmaceutical procedures may on occasion be unreliable, as a result of micellar catalysis. This type of catalysis can be observed whenever the reactive species is present on or near the micellar surface. Under these conditions, hydrolytic (and substitution) reactions can be accelerated. The decomposition of drugs via micellar catalysis has not been studied extensively, but the hydrolysis of alkyl sulfates is a simple and particularly important example of micellar catalysis. The hydrolysis of dodecyl sulfates has been shown to depend not only on the pH of the medium, but also on the presence of a variety of electrolytes and on the concentration of the surfactant; in addition, it is subject to micellar catalysis.[18,19]

Safety. Safety and toxicologic clearance of components of pharmaceutical and cosmetic emulsions are absolute requirements. It is essential, therefore, for the formulator to depend heavily on toxicologic information from suppliers or in the scientific literature, as well as on regulatory activities by governmental agencies. Despite these almost obvious limitations, the formulator has an enormous choice of emulsion ingredients, which differ in their cost and their ability to yield the desired product.

Choice of the Lipid Phase. The materials making up the oil portion of an emulsion and their relative amounts are determined primarily by the ultimate use of the product. For pharmaceutical and cosmetic products, the oil phase, unless it is the active ingredient, may include a wide variety of lipids of natural or synthetic origin. The consistency of these lipids may range from mobile liquids to fairly hard solids. Some of the lipids useful for pharmaceutical or cosmetic emulsions are listed in Table 17-2.

A drug in an emulsion type of dosage form distributes itself between the oil phase and the aqueous phase in accordance with its oil/water partition coefficient. The drug's absorption by the gastrointestinal tract or the skin can be expected to depend on its solubility in the oil phase, and this is an important pharmacokinetic observation (Chap. 9). In principle, the less soluble an active ingredient is in the nonvolatile portion of the vehicle, the more readily it penetrates into and through a barrier. On the other hand, a finite solubility of the active ingredient in the vehicle is necessary to ensure its presence in a fine state of subdivision. It is generally accepted that the release of a medicinal agent from a dosage form is a function of the solubilities of the agent in the base and in the body membrane. The key point is that the drug must not be so soluble preferentially in the base that it prevents penetration or transfer.

A final consideration in the selection of a lipid component for a topical preparation is its "feel." Emulsions normally leave a residue of the oily components on the skin after the water has evaporated. Therefore, the tactile characteristics of the combined oil phase are of great importance in determining consumer acceptance of an emulsion.

Phase Ratio. The ratio of the internal phase to the external phase is frequently determined by the solubility of the active ingredient, which must be present at a pharmacologically effective level. If this is not the primary consideration, the phase ratio is normally determined by the desired consistency. As a rule of thumb, it can be assumed that fluid emulsions result from low levels of the internal phase, whereas heavier emulsions are the result of higher percentages of the internal phase. Also, a high internal phase ratio normally requires a high level of emulsifying agent; this point affects the decision concerning the phase ratio.

Choice of Emulsifying Agents. It is customary to differentiate three broad classes of emulsifying agents: the surfactants, the hydrophilic colloids, and the finely divided solids. Although hydrophilic colloids and finely divided solids can be used as the only emulsifier, their greatest utility is in the form of auxiliary emulsifiers; accordingly, they are discussed under this heading.

A particular class of emulsifier is selected primarily on the basis of required "shelf-life" stability, the type of emulsion desired, and emulsifier cost.

Choice of Surfactant. The number of surfactants available for the formation of emulsions is so huge that even a cursory description is impossible. Only a general classification can be given here (Table 17-3). Important and useful sources for background material are the trade literature and the publications that originate from commercial suppliers.

Emulsion technologists have for many years selected emulsifiers from an intuitive knowledge of their hydrophilic, lipophilic behavior and of the type of emulsion produced with a given

TABLE 17-2. *Ingredients for Oil Phase of Emulsions*

Class	Identity	Consistency
Hydrocarbon	Mineral oils	Fluids of varying viscosity
Hydrocarbon	Petrolatum	Semisolid
Hydrocarbon	Polyethylene waxes	Solids
Hydrocarbon	Microcrystalline waxes	Solids
Ester	Vegetable oils	Fluids of varying viscosity
Ester	Animal fats	Fluids or solids
Ester	Lanolin	Semisolid
Ester	Synthetics (e.g., *i*-propylmyristate)	Fluids
Alcohols	Long-chain (natural & synthetic)	Fluids or solids
Fatty acids	Long-chain (natural & synthetic)	Fluids or solids
Ethers	Polyoxypropylenes	Fluids of varying viscosity
Silicones	Substituted	Fluids of varying viscosity
Mixed	Plant waxes (e.g., Candelilla)	Solid
Mixed	Animal waxes (e.g., Bees)	Solid

TABLE 17-3. *Classification of Surfactants for Pharmaceutical Emulsions*

	Typical Representatives*	Utility
Anionic Group		
Carboxylic acids	Soap	T
	Lactylates	TO
	Polypeptide condensates	T
Sulfuric acid esters	Sulfated monoglycerides	TO
	Alkyl sulfates	TO
Alkyl and alkyl-aryl sulfonates	Dodecylbenzene sulfonates	T
Phosphoric acid esters	Trioleyl phosphate	T
Substituted alkyl amides	Sarcosinates	TO
	Taurates	T
Hemiesters	Sulfosuccinates	TO
Cationic Group		
Amines	Alkoxyalkylamines	T
Quaternaries	Benzalkonium chloride	TO
Amphoteric Group		
Ammonium carboxylates	N-alkylaminoacids	TO
Ammonium phosphates	Lecithin	TOP
Nonionic Group		
Polyalkoxyethers	Polyoxyethylene alkyl/aryl ethers	T
	Polyoxyethylene polyoxypropylene block polymers	TOP
Polyalkoxyesters	Polyoxyethylene fatty acid esters	TO
	Polyoxyethylene sorbitan acid esters	TO
Polyalkoxyamides		T
Fatty acid esters of polyhydric alcohols	Sorbitan esters	TO
	Glyceryl esters	TO
	Sucrose esters	TO
Fatty alcohols	Lauryl alcohol	T

*Illustrative examples only.
T = some representatives useful in topicals.
O = some representatives useful in oral preparations or ingested drugs.
P = some representatives useful in parenterals.

lipid or aqueous phase. This approach is most readily illustrated with nonionic surfactants, but the principles involved can be extrapolated to any type of emulsifier or combination of emulsifiers. For example, a number of emulsions with surfactants of different polarities can be prepared using polyoxyethylene derivatives having the same nonpolar group but varying numbers of ethylene oxide units, and can be evaluated on their appearance and stability. It is apparent that the choice of specific emulsifiers by this method, although practical, is empiric and tedious.

To systematize the hydrophilic/lipophilic approach to emulsifier selection, Griffin in 1947 developed the (still somewhat empiric) system of the *Hydrophilic-Lipophilic Balance (HLB)* of surfactants. The HLB value of an emulsifier can be determined experimentally or can be computed as long as the structural formula of the surfactant is known. The HLB value of individual emulsifiers or their combinations is of little value unless some specific information is also available for determining the HLB value required for the formation of a particular type of emulsion. Despite some pitfalls, the HLB system continues to be used by formulators for the selection of emulsifiers or emulsifier blends. It is appropriate, therefore, to describe the practical application of this approach in some detail.

Griffin defined the HLB value of a surfactant as the mol % of the hydrophilic group divided by 5. A completely hydrophilic molecule (without any nonpolar group) has an HLB value of 20. The simple arithmetic determination of the HLB value is applicable only to polyoxyethylene ethers; as a result, the HLB for many other materials must be estimated by laborious experimental methods. A useful means of finding the HLB of an unknown emulsifier is that proposed by Davies, which permits calculation of the HLB value by algebraically adding the values assigned to a particular atomic grouping within the molecule of the emulsifier.20 Only a few HLB values are listed in Table 17-4, but a more comprehensive listing has been compiled by Fox. In general, molecules that are oil-soluble or oil-dispersible have low HLB values; those that are water-soluble have high HLB values. This simplified classification of HLB values by dispersibility in water is included in Table 17-4.

Efforts have been made to provide a theoretic basis for the HLB values of surfactants. As a result, it has been possible to establish correlations between the practical term HLB and several theoretic concepts of surface chemistry,[13,22] especially the solubility parameter.[23]

The HLB required for emulsifying a particular oil in water can be determined by trial and error, i.e., by preparing appropriate emulsions with emulsifiers having a range of HLB values and then determining that HLB value that yields the "best emulsion." Although the numbers have been derived empirically, they are useful starting points for the preparation of a variety of emulsions. A list of required HLB values for lipids that are of interest in pharmaceutical preparations is shown in Table 17-5. The knowledge of the required HLB permits selection of an emulsifier or a combination of emulsifiers that will produce the required HLB.

Occasionally, it will be found that a single

TABLE 17-4. *HLB Values of Selected Emulsifiers*

Chemical Designation	HLB	Water Dispersibility
Ethylene glycol distearate	1.5	No dispersion
Sorbitan tristearate	2.1	
Propylene glycol monostearate	3.4	
Sorbitan sesquioleate	3.7	
Glyceryl monostearate, non-self-emulsifying	3.8	Poor dispersion
Propylene glycol monolaurate	4.5	
Sorbitan monostearate	4.7	
Diethylene glycol monostearate	4.7	
Glyceryl monostearate, self-emulsifying	5.5	
Diethylene glycol monolaurate	6.1	Milky dispersion (not stable)
Sorbitan monopalmitate	6.7	
Sucrose dioleate	7.1	
Polyethylene glycol (200) monooleate	8.0	
Sorbitan monolaurate	8.6	
Polyoxyethylene (4) lauryl ether	9.5	Milky dispersion (stable)
Polyoxyethylene (4) sorbitan monostearate	9.6	
Polyoxyethylene (6) cetyl ether	10.3	
Polyoxyethylene (20) sorbitan tristearate	10.5	Translucent to clear dispersion
Polyoxyethylene glycol (400) monooleate	11.4	
Polyoxyethylene glycol (400) monostearate	11.6	
Polyoxyethylene (9) nonyl phenol	13.0	
Polyethylene glycol (400) monolaurate	13.1	
Polyoxyethylene (4) sorbitan monolaurate	13.3	
Polyoxyethylene (20) sorbitan monooleate	15.0	
Polyoxyethylene (20) oleyl ether	15.4	
Polyoxyethylene (20) sorbitan monopalmitate	15.6	
Polyoxyethylene (20) cetyl ether	15.7	
Polyoxyethylene (40) stearate	16.9	
Sodium oleate	18.0	
Polyoxyethylene (100) stearate	18.8	
Potassium oleate	20.0	
Sodium lauryl sulfate	Approx. 40	

TABLE 17-5. *HLB Values Required by Commonly Used Lipids*

	O/W Emulsion (Fluid)	W/O Emulsion (Fluid)
Cetyl alcohol	15	—
Stearyl alcohol	14	—
Stearic acid	15	—
Lanolin, anhydrous	10	8
Mineral oil, light and heavy	12	—
Cottonseed oil	10	5
Petrolatum	12	5
Beeswax	12	4
Paraffin wax	11	4

emulsifier can yield the desired type of emulsion at the desired viscosity. More often, however, especially in the case of o/w emulsions, stable emulsions can be prepared readily by utilizing a combination of a lipophilic and a hydrophilic surfactant. Such combinations appear to produce mixed interfacial phases of high surface coverage as well as of sufficient viscosity to prevent creaming and promote stability (see "Specific Formulation Considerations; Consistency"). HLB values of combinations may be determined by taking weighted averages of the individual surfactant HLB values. For example, Table 17-5 indicates that a w/o emulsion of lanolin requires an HLB of about 8. Thus, a 68:32 mixture of sorbitan monostearate (HLB 4.7) and polyoxyethylene (20) sorbitan monooleate (HLB 15.0) could be used to yield an emulsifier exhibiting an average HLB value of about 8.0.* In fact, almost any HLB can be obtained by appropriate blending of emulsifiers, with the additional advantage, in most cases, of greater efficiency at lower concentrations. However, optimal emulsion stability and desirable rheologic characteristics cannot be achieved by random blending of emulsifiers. Shinoda and co-workers point out that the blending of two emulsifiers of very high and very low HLB to achieve an intermediate HLB can result in an unstable emulsion unless an emulsifier of medium HLB is included.[24] Therefore, a 65:35 blend of sorbitan tristearate and polyoxyethylene (100) stearate, which has an HLB of about 8, could be expected to be inferior for the indicated emulsification to the blend of sorbitan monostearate and polyoxyethylene (20) monooleate.

Emulsion specialists generally agree that the HLB system is useful and that it may be used judiciously and with caution. It is a dictum of the HLB concept that the HLB value is critical, but this is not always the case. There is no assurance that a stable emulsion prepared from one chemical class of emulsifiers at a particular HLB can be duplicated by another class of emulsifiers exhibiting the same HLB. Thus, marked differences in emulsion type, viscosity, and time for phase separation were noted when polyoxyethylene ether derivatives were compared to polyoxyethylene ester-type surfactants having the same HLB and concentration. Additional complications arise from the observations that the HLB required for a particular emulsion to some extent depends on the phase ratio and the salt content.

Several improvements on the classical HLB system for the selection of emulsifiers have been proposed. The phenol index, developed by Marszall, makes it possible to determine the "effective" HLB of nonionics as a function of their concentration and in the presence of additives such as alcohols and glycols.[25] Shinoda has pointed out that the HLB-temperature (or PIT) can be determined easily on a series of test emulsions of varying HLB.[26] For optimal stability of an o/w emulsion, this temperature should be 25 to 70°C higher than the proposed storage temperature of the emulsion. The selection of the emulsifier system best suited for an emulsion thus becomes relatively easy. The PIT can be particularly critical for the high-temperature stability and appearance of clear emulsions.

It is generally believed that more hydrophilic emulsifiers favor o/w emulsions, whereas more nonpolar surfactants favor w/o emulsions. Griffin originally proposed that emulsifiers with HLB values ranging from 3.5 to 6.0 should be used for w/o emulsions, but Ford and Furmidge showed that correlation between emulsion type and HLB is far from perfect.[27] Stable mineral oil-in-water emulsions have been obtained with a combination of nonionic ethers having an HLB

*$0.68 \times 4.7 + 0.32 \times 15.0 \approx 8.0$

value as low as 1.9. HLB may be one consideration in the preparation of a stable emulsion; another is the solubility of the emulsifier's lipid chain in the oil phase.

A final complication arises from the observation that a hydrophilic surfactant placed into one of the phases of an emulsion prior to emulsification migrates to the other phase after or during emulsification until equilibrium is established.[28] The rate of surfactant migration is believed to depend on the presence of a second (hydrophobic) surfactant, which retards the establishment of this equilibrium and influences emulsion formation and stability. In a recent report, Lin and co-workers point out that the significance of surfactant location before emulsion might be related to phase inversion.[29] Their studies and those of Shinoda[26] show that an emulsion prepared by a process involving phase inversion exhibits smaller particle sizes and possesses improved emulsion stability.

The practical importance of emulsification temperature on emulsion stability has been known to formulators for many years. As a rule, maximum particle size reduction occurs at or near the PIT. At that temperature, surfactants that are normally water-soluble may actually become soluble in the oil phase. As the emulsion cools, emulsifiers migrate, e.g., by changing their location from the internal to the external phase of the emulsions. How this alters emulsion formation, particle size, and stability has not been rigorously studied; however, some of Lin's data in Table 17-6 illustrate these points.[29] In this simple system of one single emulsifier at HLB 9.9, complete placement of the surfactant into the oil phase seems most advantageous regardless of the temperature. However, the emulsification will be successful regardless of the location of the emulsifier as long as the temperature exceeds the PIT during emulsification.

This discussion of the selection of emulsifiers would be incomplete without a brief examination of how one can determine that surfactant mixture of which the least amount is required for optimal stability of an emulsion. Often, this goal can be achieved by determining the amount of water that can be solubilized in a given oil-plus-surfactant(s) mixture under carefully controlled temperature and stirring conditions.[30] For this purpose, 10 g of the lipid/surfactant mixture is weighed into a 68-ml capacity square glass vial. After equilibration at a temperature at which this (not always homogeneous) system is fluid, water is added in 0.10-ml increments. The mixture is shaken and allowed to stand at the equilibration temperature until all air bubbles have escaped. The addition of water (in 0.10-ml increments) is continued until the system remains permanently turbid. If the initial lipid/surfactant mixture is not clear, it will usually become clear upon addition of water and then become cloudy again upon continued addition of water. This second cloudpoint is the end of the titration. As a rule, the most stable o/w emulsion with the finest particle size results at that surfactant/oil ratio that can tolerate the largest quantity of water and still remain clear.

Most of our current knowledge of the selection of emulsifiers is based on the HLB concept and is applied to the commonly used nonionic surfactants. Recently, the optimization of the stability of a parenteral, ultrasonically emulsified nutrient oil preparation stabilized with various phospholipids and a nonionic has also been explained on the basis of HLB.[31] A somewhat different interpretation of the emulsifying efficacy of phospholipids, which does not involve HLB, was offered by Rydhag.[32] She reported that the best soya bean oil in water emulsions can be obtained with mixed (commercial) phospholipids containing the largest amounts of negatively charged phospholipids (i.e., phosphatidyl inositol, phosphatidic acid, and phosphatidyl serine). Pure phosphatidyl choline (or its combination with phosphatidyl ethanolamine) yields the least stable emulsion. These findings are best explained by the phase-forming ability of these emulsifiers as postulated by Friberg.[7-9]

TABLE 17-6. *Effect of Surfactant Lotion and Emulsification Temperature on Droplet Size*

	Average Droplet Size (μm) at Emulsification Temp.			
Percentage of Emulsifier in Oil Phase*	30°C	40°C	50°C	60°C
0	15.0	13.0	11.0	0.2
40	13.0	10.0	9.0	0.2
80	2.0	2.0	1.5	0.2
100	1.5	1.5	0.9	0.2

*The emulsion consists of 30% mineral oil, 5% polyoxyethylene (5) oleyl ether, and 65% water. The emulsifier was added to one or both phases before emulsification at the indicated temperatures.

Choice of Auxiliary Emulsifiers. *Solids.*

Finely divided solids have been shown to be good emulsifiers, especially in combination with surfactants and/or macromolecules that increase viscosity. Included are polar inorganic solids, such as heavy metal hydroxides, certain nonswelling clays, and pigments. Even nonpolar solids, e.g., carbon or glyceryltristearate, can be used. Polar solids tend to be wetted by water to a greater extent than by the oil phase, whereas the reverse is true for nonpolar solids. In the absence of surfactants, w/o emulsions are favored by the presence of nonpolar solids, presumably because the wetting by oil facilitates the coalescence of oil droplets during the initial steps of emulsification. An analogous interpretation may be given for the tendency of polar solids to favor water as the external phase.

In the presence of wetting agents, i.e., when such solids are used as auxiliary emulsifiers, their behavior is controlled by the so-called Young equation, which was given in Chapter 5, equation (18). For example, barium sulfate in the presence of sodium laurate (at pH 12) favors o/w emulsions, whereas barium sulfate coated with sodium dodecyl sulfate favors w/o emulsions. In view of the limited utility of such solids as primary emulsifiers, or even as auxiliary emulsifiers, they are not of major interest to the formulator.

Hydrophilic Colloids.

Polymers that are water-sensitive (swellable or soluble) have some utility as primary emulsifiers; however, their major use is as auxiliary emulsifiers and as thickening agents. Natural and synthetic clays of the smectite or amphibole groups are commonly used for building the viscosity of emulsions or for suspending solids, such as pigments, in makeup preparations. A large variety of natural and synthetic clays is available, and the selection of a useful clay is occasionally difficult. The most commonly used clays, bentonites, are derived from montmorillonite, a typical smectite clay. These swell in the presence of water but raise the viscosity of aqueous media only at pH 6 or higher. Clays derived from the amphibole group, such as attapulgite, thicken not by swelling but primarily because of particle anisotropy, which interferes with formation of a compact sediment.

The naturally occurring gums and synthetic hydrophilic polymers listed in Table 17-7 are useful as emulsifiers and as emulsion stabilizers. Most natural hydrocolloids are polysaccharides, and their chemistry is extremely complex. These gums exhibit some type of incompatibility or instability depending on the presence of various cations, on pH, or on a second hydrophilic polymer. Some of the most useful synthetic hydrocolloids are ethers derived from cellulose. Among the completely synthetic group of polymers, the carboxyl vinyl polymers deserve special mention: Their outstanding characteristic is their ability to impart a yield value to aqueous systems.* These materials are also included in Table 17-7.

The water-sensitive hydrocolloids generally favor o/w emulsions because they form excellent hydrophilic barriers. Their use is warranted whenever it is desired to increase the viscosity of an emulsion without a corresponding increase

*A system is said to possess a yield value if a minimum shear is required before the system exhibits any flow.

TABLE 17-7. *Organic Hydrocolloids Useful in Emulsion Technology*

Source	Name	Comment
Tree exudate	Gum Arabic (Acacia)	Essentially neutral polysaccharide
	Gum Ghatti	Essentially neutral polysaccharide
	Karaya	Essentially neutral polysaccharide
	Tragacanth	Essentially neutral polysaccharide
Sea weeds	Agar, Carrageenan	Sulfated polysaccharide
	Alginates	Acidic polysaccharide
Seed extracts	Locust bean	Essentially neutral polysaccharide
	Guar	Essentially neutral polysaccharide
	Quince seed	Essentially neutral polysaccharide
Synthetic (fermentation)	Xanthan gum	Essentially neutral polysaccharide
Cellulose	Methyl-, hydroxyethyl-hydroxypropyl-ether	Neutral polysaccharide
	Carboxymethyl-ether	Anionic polysaccharide
Collagen	Gelatin	Amphoteric protein
Synthetic	Polyoxethylene polymer	Neutral
	Carboxyvinyl polymer (cross-linked)	Anionic

in the lipid portion of the emulsion. Proteins, as a group, are effective not only as primary emulsifiers but also as auxiliary emulsifiers. They are particularly useful in oral dosage forms. The theoretical basis for effectiveness, i.e., amphilic characteristics, and the practical application of proteins as emulsifiers have been reviewed by Cante and co-workers.[33]

Multiple emulsions of the w/o/w type are normally prepared by first forming a w/o emulsion with the aid of a low HLB emulsifier. This w/o emulsion is then slowly incorporated into an aqueous phase that contains an emulsifier of a significantly higher HLB, i.e., approximately 12 to 14.

Specific Formulation Considerations. *Consistency.* Once the desired emulsion and emulsifiers have been chosen, a consistency that provides the desired stability and yet has the appropriate flow characteristics must be attained. It has already been mentioned that the viscosity of an emulsion can be altered by manipulating the composition of the lipid phase, by variations in the phase ratio and the surfactants and by the addition of gums. It is well known that the creaming of fluid emulsions depends on their rheologic character as well as on the surface characteristics of the interfacial film. The use of gums, clays, and synthetic polymers in the continuous phase of emulsions is a powerful tool for enhancing an emulsion's stability. As was pointed out in Chapter 16, the sedimentation or creaming rate of suspended spherical particles is inversely proportional to the viscosity in accordance with Stoke's law. When all other variables are held constant, an increase in viscosity generally minimizes creaming, rising, or sedimentation.

Since emulsions should flow or spread, and since higher viscosity favors stability, thixotropy in an emulsion is desirable.* In the case of emulsions that also contain suspended solids, the presence of a yield value assures at least reasonable stability.

It is routinely observed that the building up of viscosity in a freshly prepared emulsion requires some time. It is recommended, therefore, that a newly formulated emulsion be allowed to rest undisturbed for 24 to 48 hours before it is determined whether its rheologic properties correspond to those that are required.

The viscosity of emulsions responds to changes in composition in accordance with the following generalizations.[34-37]

*Shear thinning refers to the phenomenon in which the viscosity of a preparation is reduced by agitation but increases after agitation has been stopped.

1. There is a linear relationship between emulsion viscosity and the viscosity of the continuous phase: (The use of gums and clays for o/w emulsions has already been noted.) In the case of w/o emulsions, the addition of polyvalent metal soaps or the use of high melting waxes and resins in the oil phase can be used to increase viscosity. Emulsion viscosity is not very sensitive to viscosity changes of the internal phase.

2. The greater the volume of the internal phase, the greater is the apparent viscosity.

3. To control emulsion viscosity, three interacting effects must be balanced by the formulator: (1) The viscosity of o/w and w/o emulsions can be increased by reducing the particle size of the dispersed phase, (2) emulsion stability is improved by a reduction in particle size, and (3) flocculation, or clumping, which tends to structure the internal phase, can be a stabilizing effect, but it increases viscosity.

4. As a rule, the viscosity of emulsions increases upon aging.

Clear Emulsions. In general, the considerations applicable to opaque emulsions are also pertinent to the preparation of clear emulsions. The amount of internal phase in clear emulsions or in solubilized systems is generally lower than that in opaque emulsions. Most emulsion technologists have found that an increase in the surfactant concentration(s) reduces the opacity of all types of emulsions, and if carried further, can result in solubilization.

Cosmetic and pharmaceutical microemulsions usually do not employ the cosolvents required for the more classic microemulsions of theoretic interest. Instead, modern commercial solubilized systems are frequently based on nonionic emulsifiers, which results in the formation of micellar solutions. If the solubilizate is a drug, the drug available for absorption through the skin may not equal the total amount of drug in the product. That portion of the drug that is incorporated into the interior of micelles may not be available for absorption unless the micelles exhibit instability. The actual location of the drug is described by a micellar distribution coefficient defined as:

$$Km = \frac{Sm}{Sw}$$

where Sm is the solubility of the active ingredient in the micellar phase and Sw is its solubility in water.[38] The value for Km is established by classic solubility determinations. The value for Sm, e.g., in the case of dexamethasone, increases linearly with increasing concentrations of a nonionic surfactant, such as polyoxyethylene (20) stearyl alcohol.[39] Comparable results are obtained by equilibrium (or differential) dialysis through membranes that are impermeable to surfactant micelles but permeable to the free steroid, which also yields a slightly different distribution coefficient, $K'm$. In the case under discussion, Km is large (≈ 400) and almost identical to $K'm$.

During the processing of solubilizates, these "clear" emulsions are frequently opaque at high temperatures (in view of the PIT). Clearing of the emulsion occurs as the preparation cools, and solubilized systems (in the absence of cosolvents) usually remain clear to temperatures close to the freezing point of one of the major components. In the case of nonionic o/w solubilizates, it is sometimes helpful to include a small amount of a surfactant with a high HLB (e.g., alkyl sulfate) to raise the PIT if it is too close to the expected storage temperature.

Whenever it is desirable to "dissolve" a small amount of a flavor or fragrance in an essentially aqueous system, the formulator should be guided by some important practical rules: 1. Surfactants in the HLB range of 15 to 18 are ideal solubilizing agents for this purpose (see Tables 15-1 and 17-4). 2. It sometimes helps to add a small amount of a surfactant with an HLB in the range of 8 to 12. 3. As a rule, 3 to 5 times as much surfactant as oil is required to effect solubilization. 4. The oil should always be blended with the surfactant before addition to the (warmed) aqueous phase. This is particularly important for the oil-soluble vitamins. 5. The incorporation of a flavor or fragrance into solubilizing systems generally reduces the organoleptic impact of the oil, since as described above, part of it is entrapped into micelles. To enhance flavor or fragrance intensity, it is sometimes necessary to use a cosolvent, such as ethanol.

Choice of an Antimicrobial Preservative. Emulsions often contain a number of ingredients, such as carbohydrates, proteins, sterols, and phosphatides, all of which readily support the growth of a variety of microorganisms. Even in the absence of any of the aforementioned natural ingredients, the mere presence of a mixture of lipid and water in intimate contact frequently allows microorganisms to establish themselves. As a result, the inclusion of a preservative is a necessary part of the formulation process. Several points must be kept in mind in selecting a preservative. Microbial contamination may occur during the development or production of an emulsion or during its use. Frequently, the microbial contamination can arise from the use of impure raw materials or from poor sanitation during preparation. Alternately, contamination may be the result of invasion by an opportunistic microorganism. Finally, the consumer may actually inoculate the product during use. It is commonly believed that a preservative or a system of preservatives can protect the emulsion against all of these possibilities. The formulation of a self-sterilizing emulsion is exceedingly difficult without the use of potent antimicrobial agents, most of which have been or are in the process of being reviewed by governmental regulatory agencies. Prevention of contamination is recommended, and certain cardinal rules must be observed. The most important one is the use of uncontaminated raw materials, including the water. A second precaution is meticulous housekeeping and careful cleaning of equipment (with live steam). Once a microbiologically uncontaminated product has been prepared, a relatively mild antimicrobial agent suffices to protect the product against chance contamination by microorganisms. It is also desirable that the preservative system be effective against invasion by a variety of pathogenic organisms and be adequate to protect the product during use by the consumer.

As is true of most ingredients of a formulation, the preservative system must first meet the general criteria of low toxicity, stability to heat and storage, chemical compatibility, reasonable cost, and acceptable taste, odor, and color. Efficacy against a variety of organisms is required since fungi, yeasts, and bacteria are common contaminants. The more important groups of preservatives and some popular examples used in emulsions are shown in Table 17-8. The activity of the antimicrobial agents listed in the table varies widely and depends on the microorganism involved.

The concentration of preservative required in an emulsion depends to a large extent on its ability to interact with microorganisms. Since microorganisms can reside in the water or the lipid phase or both, the preservative, regardless of its water-oil partition coefficient, should be available at an effective level in both phases. It is almost inconceivable that a single preservative could distribute itself at effective concentrations between the phases, regardless of their compositions. It is therefore customary to include a preservative that is soluble in the water phase and one that is primarily soluble in the oil phase. The esters of p-hydroxybenzoic acid are particularly good examples because the methyl ester is water-soluble, whereas the propyl and higher esters exhibit almost no water solubility. The distribution of a preservative between the lipid

TABLE 17-8. *Some Typical Preservatives Used in Pharmaceutical and Cosmetic Emulsions*

Type	Example	Characteristics & Utility
Acids and acid derivatives	Benzoic acid	
	Sorbic acid and salts	
	Propionic acid and salts	Antifungal agent
	Dehydroacetic acid	
Alcohols	Chlorobutanol	Eye preparations
	Phenoxy-2-ethanol	Synergist
Aldehydes	Formaldehyde	
	Glutaraldehyde	Broad spectrum
Formaldehyde donors	Hexamethylenetetramine	
	Mono- (and di-) methyloldimethyl hydantoin	
Phenolics	Phenol	
	Cresol	
	Chlorothymol	
	o-Phenylphenol	
	p-Chlorometaxylenol	
	Methyl p-hydroxybenzoate	
	Propyl p-hydroxybenzoate	
	Benzyl p-hydroxybenzoate	Broad spectrum
	Butyl p-hydroxybenzoate	
Quaternaries	Chlorhexidine and salts	
	Benzethonium chloride	
	Benzalkonium chloride	
	Cetyltrimethyl ammonium bromide	
	Cetylpyridinium chloride	
Mercurials	Phenylmercuric acetate	
	Sodium ethylmercurithiosalicylate	
Miscellaneous	6-Acetoxy-2, 4-dimethyl-m-dioxane	
	2, 4, 4′Trichloro-2′-hydroxy-diphenylether	Primarily against gram positive bacteria
	(1-(3-Chloroallyl)-3,5,7-triazo-1-azoniaadamantane chloride	Broad spectrum and synergist
	Imidizolidinyl urea compound	Synergist
	Bromo-2-nitropropanediol-1,3	
	5-Bromo-5-nitrol-1,3-dioxane	
	2-Thiopyridine N-oxide (and salts)	Broad spectrum
	2-Methyl-4-isothiazolin-3-one and 5-chloro derivative	

This tabulation is not complete and may include antimicrobial agents, use of which is prohibited in some countries. Formulators must consult pertinent regulations and toxicity studies.

and the aqueous phase of emulsions can be determined by procedures commonly employed for evaluating distribution coefficients.[40,41]

Complex problems arise whenever the preservative interacts with one of the emulsion ingredients. Such interactions may inactivate the preservative. The interaction with emulsion ingredients of various alkyl hydroxybenzoates (the most widely used preservatives in emulsions) has been studied for many years and is illustrated by the data in Table 17-9.[42,43] As a rule, the so-called bound preservatives are not readily available to exert antimicrobial activity. It is apparent that the phenolic preservatives are especially susceptible to interaction with compounds containing polyoxyethylene groups.

A basic mathematical model for understanding the relationship between preservative concentration and microbiological activity was developed by Garrett. This basic concept was confirmed by Kazmi and Mitchell[41] with the aid of a dialysis method and by Shimamoto and co-workers[44] with the aid of an ultrafiltration technique. The current interpretation of preserva-

TABLE 17-9. *Interaction of Parabens with Emulsion Ingredients*

Macromolecular Compounds	Methyl-p-hydroxy benzoate		Propyl-p-hydroxy benzoate	
	free (%)	bound (%)	free (%)	bound (%)
Gelatin	92	8	89	11
Methyl cellulose	91	9	87	13
Polyethyleneglycol 4000	84	16	81	19
Polyvinylpyrrolidone	78	22	64	36
Polyoxyethylene monostearate	55	45	16	84
Polyoxyethylene sorbitan monolaurate	43	57	14	86
Polyoxyethylene sorbitan monooleate	43	57	10	90

tive inactivation by surfactants rests on the concept that part of the preservative is unavailable for activity by virtue of incorporation into surfactant micelles or other relatively stable surfactant phases.[45] This concept is no different from the rationale proposed for the unavailability of a solubilized drug, which was briefly described before.

To compensate for the loss of preservative by interactions, an amount equal to the complexed material may be added. It has also been found that the addition of various alcohols seems to activate p-hydroxybenzoate esters in the presence of nonionics; propylene glycol appears to be especially useful.

Several other factors can alter the ability of preservatives to protect a product against microbial contamination. The pH is known to exert a major influence on the ability of acidic or phenolic preservatives to interfere with microbial growth. These agents are almost completely inactivated by converting them into anions.[42,43] Other factors include the phase ratio, the degree of aeration during preparation, and especially the presence of flavors and perfumes, some of which have antimicrobial properties. Combinations of preservatives are often used, since they have been shown to increase the effectiveness of preservative action, either by an enhancement of the spectrum of activity or by some synergistic behavior.

Although much has been written on the subject of preservation and on the utility of a particular preservative or preservative combination, the selection of a preservative for actual use in a specific emulsion is somewhat empiric. Formulators are cautioned not to depend on chemically determined availability of preservatives to establish the microbiologic cleanliness of a product. Instead, rigorous microbiologic examination of the final composition is required to determine whether an emulsion is properly preserved.[46,47]

Choice of Antioxidant. Many organic compounds are subject to autoxidation upon exposure to air, and emulsified lipids are particularly sensitive to attack. Many drugs commonly incorporated into emulsions are subject to autoxidation and resulting decomposition.

Upon autoxidation, unsaturated oils, such as vegetable oils, give rise to rancidity with resultant unpleasant odor, appearance, and taste. On the other hand, mineral oil and related saturated hydrocarbons are subject to oxidative degradation only under rare circumstances.

Autoxidation is a free radical chain oxidation reaction. It can be inhibited, therefore, by the absence of oxygen, by a free radical chain breaker, or by a reducing agent. Materials that are useful as antioxidants by one or more of these three mechanisms are listed in Table 17-10. The choice of a particular antioxidant

TABLE 17-10. *List of Antioxidants*

Gallic acid	L-Tocopherol
Propyl gallate	Butylated hydroxytoluene
Ascorbic acid	Butylated hydroxyanisol
Ascorbyl palmitate	4-Hydroxymethyl-2,6-di-*tert*-butylphenol
Sulfites	

Although incomplete, this listing includes materials, use of which may be restricted by governmental regulations.

depends on its safety, acceptability for a particular use, and its efficacy. Antioxidants are commonly used at concentrations ranging from 0.001 to 0.1%.

Butylated hydroxyanisole (BHA), butylated hydroxytoluene (BHT), L-tocopherol, and the alkyl gallates are particularly popular in pharmaceuticals and cosmetics. BHT and BHA have a pronounced odor and should be used at low concentrations. Alkyl gallates have a bitter taste, whereas L-tocopherol is well suited for edible or oral preparations, such as those containing vitamin A. Almost all antioxidants are subject to discoloration in the presence of light, trace metals, and alkaline solutions. Combinations of two or more antioxidants have been shown to produce synergistic effects. In some cases, compounds completely devoid of antioxidant activity by themselves enhance the effectiveness of certain antioxidants. For example, alkyl gallates, BHT, and BHA are much more effective in the presence of citric, tartaric, or phosphoric acids. A related way of enhancing the activity of phenolic antioxidants involves the use of a small amount of a sequestrant for heavy metal, calcium, and magnesium ions.

Additional Recommendations. In the laboratory development of emulsions, it is common practice to prepare an oil phase containing all the oil-soluble ingredients and to heat it at about 5 to 10°C above the melting point of the highest melting ingredient. The aqueous phase is normally heated to the same temperature, and then the two phases are mixed. A laboratory beaker containing a hot emulsion cools fairly rapidly to room temperature, but a production tank filled with hundreds of gallons of hot material cools more slowly unless external means of cooling are employed. This is one reason that the simple transfer of a laboratory process to production requires extensive studies of the cooling and agitation schedule. It is also advisable to utilize jacketed equipment for the large-scale preparation of emulsions, so that the heating and cooling cycles can be carefully controlled.

In the preparation of anionic or cationic o/w emulsions, it is customary to add the oil phase to the water phase, although some technologists prefer the inversion technique, i.e., addition of the water phase to the oil phase. In the case of nonionic emulsions, which exhibit a PIT, the inversion technique is not required since temperature alone can be used to control this stage of emulsification. If soap is used as the emulsifier, it is usually prepared in situ by combining the alkali with the water phase and the fatty acid with the oil phase. Similarly, oil-soluble emulsifiers are commonly added to the lipid phase, whereas the water-soluble emulsifiers are dissolved in the aqueous phase. Occasionally, it may prove advantageous to include even the water-soluble emulsifier in the oil phase. In the preparation of w/o emulsions, it is almost always necessary to add the water phase slowly to the oil/emulsifier blend.

To avoid losses, volatile flavors or perfumes are preferably added at the lowest temperature at which incorporation into the emulsion is possible (usually 55 to 45°C).

If a gum is employed, it should be completely hydrated or dissolved in the aqueous phase before the emulsification step. If a heat-sensitive gum is used, it may be necessary to incorporate the gum solution after the emulsion has been formed. The use of two different organic gums can cause incompatibility. It is also noted that anionic and cationic emulsifiers in about equimolar quantities rarely yield satisfactory emulsions.

Not unexpectedly, emulsions designed for parenteral administration can be prepared with only a limited number of emulsifiers (see Table 17-3). Since the use of conventional preservatives is contraindicated, such preparations require sterilization at high temperature but must still yield acceptable emulsions after this heating/cooling cycle. It is recommended, therefore, that parenteral emulsions, especially those designed for intravenous injection, be homogenized until a satisfactory particle size is achieved.

Whenever an emulsion is formed at elevated temperatures, the loss of water due to evaporation must be made up. This is done best by adjusting to "final weight" with water when the emulsion reaches about 35°C.

Practical Examples. A few selected formulations that have been published in the literature are presented below.* They have not been prepared by the author nor have they been screened for stability or safety. They are cited here merely to illustrate the utility of various emulsifiers and to indicate some practical means for forming various emulsions. Only the first one is discussed in detail.

1. Oral Emulsion (o/w)

(A) Cottonseed oil, winterized	460.0 g
Sulfadiazine	200.0 g
Sorbitan monostearate	84.0 g

*Some additional emulsions are discussed in Chapter 18.

(B) Polyoxyethylene (20) sorbitan
   monostearate   36.0 g
   Sodium benzoate   2.0 g
   Sweetener   qs
   Water, potable   1000.0 g
(C) Flavor oil   qs

Procedure:

1. Heat (A) to 50°C and pass through colloid mill.
2. Add (A) at 50°C to (B) at 65°C and stir while cooling to 45°C.
3. Add (C) and continue to stir until room temperature is reached.

Discussion and Critique. Sulfadiazine is essentially water-insoluble. A suspension or emulsion is required to yield a fluid oral dosage form. To maintain sulfadiazine in suspension, the viscosity of the final product must be reasonably high. This could be achieved by the use of gums or by developing an emulsion high in internal phase. The choice of a cottonseed oil o/w emulsion is probably arbitrary except for the fact that o/w preparations are quite palatable.

Table 17-4 shows that an HLB of about 10 is required to yield a fluid emulsion of cottonseed oil. Although a single emulsifier, such as polyoxyethylene (4) sorbitan monostearate (HLB 9.6), might be satisfactory, the use of mixed emulsifiers is generally preferred. In view of their "safety" and availability, a blend of sorbitan monostearate (HLB 4.7) and polyoxyethylene (20) sorbitan monostearate (HLB 14.9) seems promising. The ratio required to yield an HLB of 10.0 is computed from $a \times 4.7 + b \times 14.9 = 10$, where a and b are the weight fraction of each of the two emulsifiers and where $a + b = 1$. It is found that a blend of 48% of the lipophilic and 52% of the hydrophilic emulsifier yields the desired HLB. In fact, the formula calls for 70% of the hydrophobic emulsifier, equivalent to an HLB of the blend of 8.2. This must be attributed to the presence of the sulfadiazine and the need for a high viscosity emulsion. The ratio of emulsifiers:oil (about 1:4) is high and again points toward an unpredictable effect of the sulfadiazine.

To develop a smooth product, it is necessary to reduce the particle size of the sulfadiazine. For this purpose, the blend of the drug, the oil, and the oleophilic emulsifier is warmed slightly and passed through a colloid mill. The emulsion itself is formed by adding the drug suspension to the aqueous phase, but in contrast to usual emulsion technique, the two phases are blended at different temperatures. Presumably, heating of the drug suspension to 65°C would materially lower its viscosity and cause excessive settling of the drug particles unless specialized stirring equipment were employed.

The addition of the flavoring oils at a lower temperature prevents loss due to volatility. The following additional points are pertinent: Since sulfadiazine has a broad antimicrobial spectrum, the absence of a preservative in the oil phase is not surprising. Nevertheless, the emulsion should be protected against molds and fungi; the use of sodium benzoate for this purpose is of doubtful merit. The absence of an antioxidant in this emulsion suggests the presence of additives in the cottonseed oil.

2. Medicated Ointment Base (w/o)

	% wt/wt
(A) Mineral oil, U.S.P. (125/135 Saybolt units at 100°F)	25.0
Microcrystalline wax (M.P. 170–180°F)	10.0
Cetyl alcohol	5.0
Mixed lanolin alcohols (high in cholesterol)*	10.0
Sorbitan sesquioleate	3.0
Propyl *p*-hydroxybenzoate	0.1
(B) Glycerine	3.0
Methyl *p*-hydroxybenzoate	0.1
Deionized water	43.8
(C) Medicament	q.s.

*Rita Chem. Corp.

Procedure:

1. Heat (A) and (B) separately to 75°C.
2. Add (B) to (A) and stir while cooling to 45°C.
3. Add (C), mix, and package.

Discussion and Critique. This emulsion illustrates a conventional approach (the addition of solid oil-soluble components) for increasing the viscosity of the external phase in a w/o emulsion. Lanolin and its derivatives are generally useful for formulating w/o emulsions and may assist in effecting dissolution of the medicament. The addition of preservatives to both phases is noteworthy.

3. Emollient Cream (o/w)

	% wt/wt
(A) Acetylated lanolin*	2.00
Stearic acid	2.00
Petrolatum	4.00
Lanolin absorption base*	6.00
Glyceryl monostearate, pure	12.00
Propyl *p*-hydroxybenzoate	0.15
(B) Water	62.90
Glycerol	10.00
Sodium lauryl sulfate	0.50
Methyl *p*-hydroxybenzoate	0.15
Perfume	0.30

*Amerchol Division, C.P.C. International

Procedure:

1. Heat (A) and (B) separately to 75°C.
2. Add (A) to (B) and stir until temperature reaches 45°C.
3. Add perfume and continue to stir gently until room temperature is reached.

Discussion and Critique. This cosmetic preparation illustrates the use of relatively high concentrations of glyceryl monostearate to create a viscous o/w emulsion. Lanolin absorption bases are blends of lanolin (and its derivatives) with hydrocarbons and a small amount of emulsifier. They are normally employed in the formulation of w/o emulsions. Evidently, the method of emulsification and the use of the extremely hydrophilic sodium lauryl sulfate permit formation of an o/w emulsion. Particularly striking is the use of free stearic acid as a means of bodying the lipid portion of this cream. The preparation's viscosity would be reduced significantly if the stearic acid were neutralized, e.g. with triethanolamine..

4. Makeup Cream (o/w)

	% wt/wt
(A) Magnesium aluminum silicate*	2.60
Sodium carboxymethyl cellulose[†]	0.40
Water, distilled	42.40
(B) Dispersing agent*	0.30
Propylene glycol	5.00
Water, distilled	12.30
(C) Talc	18.50
Kaolin	1.30
Titanium dioxide	3.70
Iron oxides	1.50
(D) Isopropyl myristate	5.00
Stearyl alcohol	2.00
Lanolin absorption base[‡]	2.00
Sorbitan monolaurate	0.75
Polyoxyethylene (20) sorbitan monolaurate	2.25
Preservative	q.s.
Perfume	q.s.

*R. T. Vanderbilt Co.
[†]Hercules, Inc.
[‡]Amerchol Div., C.P.C. International

Procedure:
1. Blend solids of (A) and add to water at 80°C; stir until smooth.
2. Micropulverize (C) and add to (B); pass through colloid mill to yield smooth paste.
3. Add (B) + (C) to (A) and heat to 60 to 65°C.
4. Heat (D) to 70°C and add to (A) + (B) + (C) blend; stir until temperature reaches 45°C; add perfume and mix until cool.

Discussion and Critique. This composition illustrates the use of an organic gum and an inorganic clay to achieve viscosity and a yield point in order to reduce settling of heavy pigments. The need for a pigment dispersing agent (a complex alkyl-aryl sulfonate) can generally be avoided by blending the micropulverized pigments (C) with the warm oil phase (D) and passing this blend through a colloid mill. The mixture of (C) + (D) can then be added to the aqueous phase containing the gums, humectants, and a trace of surfactant (about 0.1% sodium lauryl sulfate).

5. Fat Emulsions for Parenteral Nutrition (o/w)

	wt/vol
(A) Cottonseed oil, winterized	15.0
Polyethylene glycol	
200 monopalmitate, purified*	1.2
Tartaric acid ester of cotton seed fatty acid mono glyceride, purified*	0.3
(B) Polyoxyethylene-poly oxypropylene block polymer*	0.3
Isotonic glucose solution	83.2

Procedure:
1. Blend and heat (A) and (B) separately to 45°C.
2. Circulate (B) in a two-stage homogenizer at 3000 psi
3. Add (A) to (B) at 40 to 45°C and raise pressure to 4000 psi
4. Continue homogenization until the emulsion has been cycled five times.
5. Package and autoclave at 121°C for 17 min.

*For details consult Singleton, W. S., et al.: J. Am. Oil Chem. Soc., 39:260, 1961.

Discussion and Critique. This emulsion is unusual since it could be expected to show signs of hydrolysis of the lipid and a drop in pH upon storage. Better stability could be achieved through use of a system of Pluronic F68 and L-α-phosphatidyl choline as described by Guay and Bissailon[31]:

Soybean oil	10.0%
Dextrose	4.0%
Emulsifier (blend of L-α-phosphatidyl choline and Pluronic F-68 at HLB 10)	3.0%
Water	q.s. 100.0%

The aqueous phase (at 95°C) was added to the oil phase (also at 95°C), and the blend was mechanically stirred for 45 min. Two hundred grams of this mixture was then sonicated in a 400 ml beaker—using a model W140D (20 kHz) sonifier (Branson Sonic Power Co.)—in an ice bath at 16 kHz for 12 min. The emulsion was then autoclaved at 121°C and 15 psi for 15 min. The resulting product exhibits good pH stability and resistance to creaming and coalescence during centrifugation.

6. *High Internal Phase Emulsion (w/o)*

	% wt/wt
(A) Glyceryl monoisostearate	2.5
Isoparaffin (C_{10}-C_{12})	5.0
Mineral oil (light)	5.0
Microcrystalline wax	0.3
Acetylated lanolin	1.0
Propyl *p*-hydroxybenzoate	0.1
(B) Monosodium glutamate	3.0
Methyl *p*-hydroxybenzoate	0.2
Water	82.7
Perfume	0.2

Procedure:
1. Heat (A) and (B) separately to about 60°C.
2. Add the aqueous phase to the oil phase and homogenize.
3. Add perfume at about 40 to 45°C.

Discussion and Critique. This low viscosity skin cream illustrates the concept that exceptionally high internal phase ratio products can exhibit reasonable stability. Glyceryl monoisostearate probably has an HLB of about 3.5 to 4.0 and is a good w/o emulsifier. The key to the stability of this preparation is the use of an amino acid salt as an emulsion stabilizer. The practical feasibility of this approach is documented in European Patent #0,009,404 of 4/2/80, but no theoretic basis for this concept has been provided.

7. Mouthwash

1. Cetylpyridinium chloride	1.00 g
2. Citric acid, USP	1.00 g
3. Sweetener (sodium saccharin)	0.40 g
4. Flavor oils (peppermint, eucalyptus, and clove oils)	1.50 ml
5. Polyoxyethylene (20) sorbitan monostearate	3.00 g
6. Alcohol, USP	100.00 ml
7. Sorbitol solution (70%)	200.00 g
8. Water, potable	q.s. 1000.00 ml

Procedure:

1. Dissolve components 1, 2, and 3 in a sufficient amount of the water and add component 6.
2. Mix components 4 and 5 and add blend slowly to the hydroalcoholic solution while stirring.
3. Add the remaining ingredients (7 and 8).

Discussion and Critique. The level of surfactant in this preparation is surprisingly low, as is the level of alcohol. It would appear that the level of sorbitol (14%) in this product contributes to the solubilization efficacy of this mouthwash. Cetylpyridinium chloride, which is included primarily as an antimicrobial agent, also contributes to the solubilizing power of the system. This product illustrates the use of alcohol in the presence of a solubilizer to increase flavor impact (see under previous section "Clear Emulsions.").

Properties and Stability of Emulsions

Becher has indicated that the physical properties of an emulsion and its stability cannot be considered separately.[13] Accordingly, this section is concerned with the more important physical properties of emulsions, their changes under external influences, and their relationship to emulsion stability.

Emulsion Stability

It has already been noted that on purely thermodynamic grounds, emulsions are physically unstable. A reduction of the interfacial area by coalescence reduces the system's energy, and this process is thermodynamically favored. For this reason, Garrett defined a stable emulsion as one that "would maintain the same number of sizes of particles of the dispersed phase per unit volume of weight of the continuous phase. The total interfacial energy must be invariant with time to conform to this definition."[48]

Thermodynamic stability of emulsions differs from stability as defined by the formulator or the consumer on the basis of entirely subjective judgments. Acceptable stability in a pharmaceutical dosage form does not require thermodynamic stability. If an emulsion creams up (rises) or creams down (sediments), it may still be pharmaceutically acceptable as long as it can be reconstituted by a modest amount of shaking. Similar considerations apply to cosmetic emulsions; however, in the latter, creaming is usually unacceptable because any unsightly separation makes the product cosmetically inelegant. It is important, therefore, to remember that the standard of stability depends to a large extent on the observer, since subjective observations or opinions by themselves do not suffice to define such a parameter as acceptable stability. Stability should be defined in the sense given to it by Garrett, i.e., on a purely objective basis. Shelf life is a useful term to describe the subjective evaluation of stability.

A product's shelf life may be directly related to its "kinetic" stability. Kinetic stability means that the physicochemical properties of an emulsion do not change appreciably during a reasonably long period of time. On the other hand, "thermodynamic" stability of the type commonly postulated for solubilized systems or microemulsions is generally temperature-dependent. Thus, after the temperature of a solubilized product has been disturbed, it will *eventually* return to its original (and in this particular case clear or transparent) state when the temperature is returned to "normal." Thermodynamics does not and cannot predict how quickly the original (clear) state is restored.

Symptoms of Instability. As soon as an emulsion has been prepared, time- and temperature-dependent processes occur to effect its separation. During storage, an emulsion's instability is evidenced by creaming, reversible aggregation (flocculation), and/or irreversible aggregation (coalescence).

Creaming. Under the influence of gravity, suspended particles or droplets tend to rise or sediment depending on the differences in specific gravities between the phases. If creaming takes place without any aggregation, the emulsion can be reconstituted by shaking or mixing. The Stokes equation (see Chap. 16 under "Sedimentation Rates) is most useful in gaining an understanding of the process of creaming, even though Stokes made a number of unrealistic assumptions: The equation is based on spherical particles that have essentially the same size and are separated by a distance that makes the movement of one particle independent of that of another. In fact, creaming involves the movement of a number of heterodisperse droplets, and their movements interfere with each other and may cause droplet deformation. If flocculation takes place, the criterion of sphericity is lost, and complex corrections for these variations must be made before Stokes' law can be applied quantitatively to the behavior of emulsions.

Despite its defects, Stokes' equation is qualitatively applicable to emulsions. It shows that the rate of creaming is a function of the square of the radius of the droplet. Thus, larger particles cream much more rapidly than smaller particles. It is also apparent that the formation of larger aggregates by coalescence and/or by flocculation will accelerate creaming. The reverse is also true, i.e., the smaller the particle size of an emulsion, the less likely it is to cream. Stokes' equation predicts that no creaming is possible if the specific gravities of the two phases are equal. Adjusting the specific gravity of the dispersed phase is frequently a practical means of achieving improved emulsion stability. Finally, Stokes' law shows that the rate of creaming is inversely proportional to the viscosity; this is the reason for the well known fact that increased viscosity of the external phase is associated with improved shelf life.[34–37]

Flocculaticm. Emulsion flocculation in terms of energetics has been mentioned in this chapter, and the importance of controlled flocculation for suspensions of solids in a liquid medium is discussed in Chapter 5.

Flocculation of the dispersed phase may take place before, during, or after creaming. It is best described as reversible aggregation of droplets of the internal phase in the form of three-dimensional clusters. Flocculation is influenced by the charges on the surface of the emulsified globules. In the absence of a protective (mechanical) barrier at the interface, e.g., if an insufficient amount of emulsifier is present, emulsion droplets aggregate and coalesce rapidly. Flocculation of emulsion droplets can occur only when the mechanical or electrical barrier is sufficient to prevent droplet coalescence. In other words, flocculation differs from coalescence primarily by the fact that the interfacial film and the individual droplets remain intact. The reversibility of this type of aggregation depends on the strength of the interaction between particles, as determined by the chemical nature of the emulsifier, the phase volume ratio, and the concen-

tration of dissolved substances, especially electrolytes and ionic emulsifiers. For example, a 2% hexadecane-in-water emulsion stabilized with 0.09% Aerosol O.T., a negatively charged surfactant, remains deaggregated in the form of single droplets, presumably as a result of repulsion between negatively charged oil droplets. An increase of the ionic strength with electrolytes or an increase of the emulsifier concentration tends to promote flocculation. Although electrolytes are commonly used for demulsification, a modest level of electrolyte is frequently helpful in stabilizing emulsions. A typical example is the observation by Vold and Groot that sodium chloride reduces oil separation in a Nujol/water emulsion exposed to ultracentrifugation.[49]

A high internal phase volume, i.e., tight packing of the dispersed phase, tends to promote flocculation. However, gum acacia can produce a flocculated o/w emulsion with as little as 0.002% of orange oil. Thus, it is probably safe to say that most practical o/w and w/o emulsion systems exist in a flocculated state.

Flocculation, emulsion viscosity, and shear thinning may be closely related. The viscosity of an emulsion depends to a large extent on flocculation, which restricts the movement of particles and can produce a fairly rigid network. Agitation of an emulsion breaks the particle-particle interactions with a resulting drop of viscosity, i.e., shear thinning.

Coalescence. Coalescence is a growth process during which the emulsified particles join to form larger particles. Any evidence for the formation of larger droplets by merger of smaller droplets suggests that the emulsion will eventually separate completely. The major factor which prevents coalescence in flocculated and unflocculated emulsions is the mechanical strength of the interfacial barrier. This is particularly true in o/w systems containing nonionic surfactants and in w/o emulsion-systems in which electrical effects are negligible. Thus, it is widely recognized that good shelf life and absence of coalescence can be achieved by the formation of a thick interfacial film from macromolecules or from particulate solids.[50] This is the reason a variety of natural gums and proteins are so useful as auxiliary emulsifiers when used at low levels, but can even be used as primary emulsifiers at higher concentrations.

Assessment of Emulsion Shelf Life

The final acceptance of an emulsion depends on stability, appearance, and functionality of the packaged product. The most obvious problems facing the formulator are (1) What is acceptable emulsion shelf life? and (2) What are the predictive indicators of shelf life? The formulator requires unequivocal and quantitative answers to these questions.

As is true with most dosage forms, the container used for packaging an emulsion may be expected to be a source of incompatibility. Possible problems include interaction of ingredients with the container, extraction of material from the container, and loss of water and volatile ingredients through the container or the closure. For this reason, whatever the nature of the container, final evaluation of the product must be conducted in the container that will be used commercially.

No quick and sensitive methods for determining potential instability in an emulsion are available to the formulator. Instead, he is forced to wait for interminable periods at ambient conditions before signs of poor shelf life become clearly apparent in an emulsion. To speed up his stability program, the formulator commonly places the emulsion under some sort of stress. Alternately, he may seek a test or parameter that is more sensitive for the detection of instability than mere macroscopic observations. Both approaches may be faulty. The first one may eliminate many good emulsions because excessive artificial stress has been applied. An accelerated aging test should speed up only the processes involved in instability under "normal" storage conditions. If the stress is excessive, abnormal processes may come into play. The second one may eliminate only those emulsions that are extremely poor unless the parameter correlates well with shelf life. It is therefore essential to use sound judgment and great care in setting up a meaningful stability program for a given emulsion.

Stress Conditions. Stress conditions normally employed for evaluating the stability of emulsions include (1) aging and temperature, (2) centrifugation, and (3) agitation.

Aging and Temperature. It is routine to determine the shelf life of all types of preparations by storing them for varying periods of time at temperatures that are higher than those normally encountered. The Arrhenius equation, which predicts that a 10°C increase in the temperature doubles the rate of most *chemical* reactions, is not applicable to emulsions. The Arrhenius equation is based on the concept that the *same* chemical reactions take place at all temperatures albeit at different rates. It is generally recognized that in the case of emulsions, changes in temperature bring into play new re-

actions. It is important, therefore, for the formulator to realize that exposure to unrealistically high temperatures may produce meaningless results. It is clearly established that many emulsions may be perfectly stable at 40 or 45°C, but cannot tolerate temperatures in excess of 55 or 60° even for a few hours. The varied effects of temperature changes on emulsion parameters have been discussed before: viscosity, partitioning of emulsifiers, inversion at the phase inversion temperature, and crystallization of certain lipids. In view of these problems, shelf life cannot be predicted by studying emulsions at temperatures in excess of 50°C even for relatively short periods of time, unless there is some reason to believe that the preparation will be exposed to such a high temperature in normal handling, such as in sterilization of parenteral emulsions.

A particularly useful means of evaluating shelf life is cycling between two temperatures. Again, extremes should be avoided, and cycling should be conducted between 4 and 45°C. This type of cycling approaches realistic shelf conditions, but places the emulsion under enough stress to alter various emulsion parameters.

The normal effect of aging an emulsion at elevated temperature is acceleration of the rate of coalescence or creaming, and this is usually coupled with changes in viscosity. Most emulsions become thinner at elevated temperature and thicken when allowed to come to room temperature. This thickening can be excessive if the emulsion is not agitated during the cooling cycle; sometimes, the low viscosity can be "frozen" into the emulsion if it is chilled rapidly. In view of these variations, the formulator must evaluate each emulsion separately and on the basis of his own personal experience. Freezing can damage an emulsion more than heating, since the solubility of emulsifiers, both in the lipid and aqueous phases, is more sensitive to freezing than to modest warming. In addition, the formation of ice crystals develops pressure that can deform the spherical shape of emulsion droplets.

Centrifugation. It is commonly accepted that shelf life under normal storage conditions can be predicted rapidly by observing the separation of the dispersed phase due to either creaming or coalescence when the emulsion is exposed to centrifugation. Stokes' law shows that creaming is a function of gravity, and an increase in gravity therefore accelerates separation. Becher indicates that centrifugation at 3750 rpm in a 10-cm radius centrifuge for a period of 5 hours is equivalent to the effect of gravity for about one year.[13] The modest speed suggested by Becher is probably reasonable. On the other hand, ultracentrifugation at extremely high speeds (approximately 25,000 rpm or more) can be expected to cause effects that are not observed during normal aging of an emulsion. Ultracentrifugation of emulsions creates three layers: a top layer of coagulated oil, an intermediate layer of uncoagulated emulsion, and an essentially pure aqueous layer. Rapid formation of a clear oily layer is the first clue to "abnormal" phenomena taking place during ultracentrifugation. Groot and Void showed how the rate of oil formation in a Nujol: water: sodium dodecyi sulfate (50:50:0.2%) emulsion depends on the rate of centrifugation.[51] Separation was extremely rapid at 56,000 rpm, somewhat slower at about 40,000 rpm, and no oil was separated after 2½ hours of centrifugation at approximately 11,000 rpm. These findings suggest that the force of ultracentrifugation does not cause oil separation until it is high enough to break or rupture the absorbed layer of emulslfier that surrounds each droplet. It is concluded that centrifugation, if used judiciously, is an extremely useful tool for evaluating and predicting shelf life of emulsions.

Agitation. It is a paradigm of emulsion science that the droplets in an emulsion exhibit Brownian movement. In fact, it is believed that no coalescence of droplets takes place unless droplets impinge upon each other owing to their Brownian movement. Simple mechanical agitation can contribute to the energy with which two droplets impinge upon each other. It is rarely appreciated how useful the evaluation of an emulsion by agitation at or near room temperature can be. It was already noted that excessive shaking of an emulsion or excessive homogenization may interfere with the formation of an emulsion. As a corollary, agitation can also break emulsions. A typical case, well known to all, is the manufacture of butter from milk. Some clear microemulsions become cloudy upon short agitation in a blender due to coalescence of particles. Similarly, conventional emulsions may deteriorate from gentle rocking on a reciprocating shaker. This is related in part to impingement of droplets and in part to reduction of viscosity of a normally thixotropic system.

Chemical Parameters. The need for chemical stability of the components of emulsions has already been noted. A typical problem encountered in the presence of polyethylene glycols or derivatives of polyethylene glycol is their propensity toward autoxidation. This phenomenon can cause formation of undesirable odors, of acidic components, and of all types of oxidative byproducts.[52] The instability of nonionic esters leading to hydrolytic degradation may result in changes in the dielectric constant of the emulsion. This phenomenon parallels observations of physical instability and has been attributed to the formation of stearic acid from, for example, polysorbate 80.[53]

Physical Parameters. The most useful parameters commonly measured to assess the effect of stress conditions on emulsions include (1) phase separation, (2) viscosity, (3) electrophoretic properties, and (4) particle size analysis and particle count.

Phase Separation. The rate and extent of phase separation after aging of an emulsion may be observed visually or by measuring the volume of separated phase. It is important to differentiate between creaming and coalescence, since the means of correcting these defects are different.*

Relatively little quantitative information is available concerning oil separation in practical systems in the absence of centrifugation. A study of mineral oil-water emulsions stabilized with either polyoxyethylene sorbitan monooleate or sodium lauryl sulfate showed that the amount of coalescence observed at room temperature depends on the concentration of emulsifier.[54] At low levels, i.e., below 0.1%, visible coalescence of the oil phase occurs after only one month's storage. When the concentration of emulsifier is raised to 2 or 5%, the amount of visible coalescence is negligible even after two years' storage. Two additional points are noteworthy: The two emulsifiers perform similarly, and coalescence can be observed quite early.

A particularly simple means of determining phase separation due to creaming or coalescence is apparently so trivial that it has evidently not been described in the literature. It involves withdrawing small specimens of the emulsion from the top and the bottom of the preparation after some period of storage and comparing the composition of the two samples by appropriate analysis of water content, oil content, or any suitable constituent.

Viscosity. Although the viscosity of an emulsion is an essential performance criterion, its use for shelf life studies is not concerned with the absolute values of viscosity, but with changes in viscosity during aging. The number of instruments available for the determination of consistency/viscosity is overwhelming.[55] Since

*Creaming can usually be controlled by an increase in viscosity or by addition of an emulsifier having high solubility in the external phase; coalescence generally requires examination of alternate systems of emulsifiers.

emulsions are generally non-Newtonian and since the instrument should have universal utility, it is best to avoid capillary and falling sphere viscometers. Viscometers of the cone-plate type are particularly useful for emulsions, but instruments utilizing coaxial cylinders are the easiest to use. In the case of fairly viscous materials, the use of a penetrometer is often helpful in detecting changes of viscosity with age.

As a rule, globules in freshly prepared w/o emulsions flocculate quite rapidly. Consequently, the viscosity drops quickly and continues to drop for some time (5 to 15 days at room temperature), and then remains relatively constant.[56] O/w emulsions behave quite differently. In this case, globule flocculation causes an immediate increase in viscosity. After this initial change, almost all emulsions show changes in consistency with time, which follow a linear relationship when plotted on a log-log scale.[57] The complete absence of a slope (no change in viscosity with age) is believed to be ideal, although most acceptable systems exhibit modest increases of viscosity between 0.04 and 400 days (Fig. 17-6). Other emulsions exhibit much more drastic and sudden nonlinear increases in viscosity after two or three months' aging; such behavior is frequently followed by a drop in viscosity, which is probably associated with phase separation.

A practical approach for the detection of creaming or sedimentation, before it becomes visibly apparent, utilizes the Helipath attachment of the Brookfield viscometer.* As a result of emulsion separation, the descending rotating spindle meets varying resistance at different levels and registers fluctuations in viscosity. For example, Lotion A in Figure 17-7 contains solids suspended in an emulsion, and the high viscosity near the top is due to nonwetted solid and creamed emulsion; the high viscosity at lower levels is due to sedimented particles. The addition of polyoxyethylene sorbitan monooleate and methylcellulose (Lotion B) yields a much more uniform viscosity pattern after eight weeks' storage.

The collection of such data is certainly useful; however, it is apparent from these two examples that it is impossible to predict long-term viscosity behavior from data collected during the first few weeks of storage after an emulsion has been prepared. According to Sherman, the best way of using viscosity determinations for the prediction of shelf life is to relate them to changes in particle size.[34-37] As a rule, a decrease in viscosity with age reflects an increase of particle size due to coalescence and is indicative of poor shelf life.

*The Brookfield viscometer determines the resistance encountered by a rotating spindle or cylinder immersed in a viscous material. The Helipath attachment slowly lowers the rotating spindle into the medium so that the resistance measured is always that of previously undisturbed test substance.

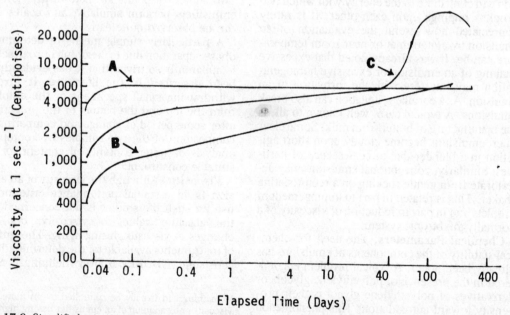

FIG. 17-6. *Simplified aging curves of emulsions. Ideal shelf life (A), typical shelf life (B), and questionable shelf life (C). (After Wood and Catacalos.[57])*

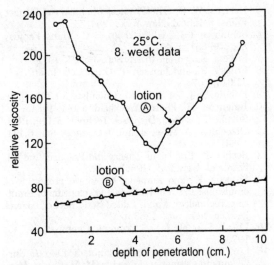

FIG. 17-7. *Use of the Helipath in the evaluation of creaming and sedimentation. Lotion B is the same as A except that 0.1% polysorbate 80 and 0.25% methyl cellulose have been added. (From unpublished results from the Upjohn Co., Kalamazoo, MI.)*

Viscosity measurements should be carried out in undisturbed containers to avoid changes due to previous stresses. To avoid artefacts, replicate samples should be prepared in advance, or special studies must be carried out to determine the time necessary for a disturbed emulsion to recover its original viscosity. It must always be remembered that the act of measuring the viscosity disturbs the system. Also, the viscosity of emulsions at several different shear rates must be determined to obtain a clear picture of the rheologic behavior of an emulsion. Measurements at low shear rates frequently reflect aspects of flocculation. High shear rates overcome the attractive forces between particles and can result in a precipitous loss of viscosity.

Electrophoretic Properties. The zeta potential of emulsions can be measured with the aid of the moving boundary method or, more quickly and directly, by observing the movement of particles under the influence of electric current. The zeta potential is especially useful for assessing flocculation since electrical charges on particles influence the rate of flocculation.[58] If the instability is due to coalescence, the determination of the surface charges of particles may not be relevant for the prediction of shelf life.

The measurement of electrical conductivity has been claimed to be a powerful tool for the evaluation of emulsion stability shortly after preparation.[59] The electrical conductivity of o/w or w/o emulsions is determined with the aid of Pt electrodes (diameter 0.4 mm; distance 4 mm) nucroamperometrically to produce a current of about 15 to 50 ;µA. Measurements are made on emulsions stored for short periods of time at room temperature or 37°C. Reportedly, the conductivity depends on the degree of dispersion. O/w preparations with fine particles exhibit low resistance; if the resistance increases, it is a sign of oil droplet aggregation and instability. A fine emulsion of water in a w/o product does not conduct current until droplet coagulation, i.e., instability occurs.

Particle Size Number Analysis. Changes of the average particle size or of the size distribution of droplets are important parameters for evaluating emulsions. Particle size analysis may be carried out by a number of methods, each giving a somewhat different average for heterodisperse systems.[60] For example, microscopic measurements of the apparent diameter give an average value dependent on the number of particles of each size.[29] On the other hand, some electronic counting devices measure particle volume, and since the volume of a sphere is $\pi d^3/6$, they give greater weight to larger particles when volume is converted to diameter. Such counting devices, e.g., the Coulter counter, also require that the emulsion be diluted, sometimes with a conducting electrolyte. The changes caused by these steps as well as changes caused by sampling, even for a microscopic assessment of particle size, often make the counted sample no longer representative of the bulk emulsion.

Light scattering and related reflectance relationships have been used for particle size determinations. Thus, the change of reflectance at wave length at which the colored internal phase partially absorbs the incident light has been found to be inversely proportional to a power of the particle diameter (see Chap. 26).

The utility of particle size for predicting or interpreting emulsion shelf life is somewhat doubtful. Two studies utilizing fairly stable emulsions have shown that the initial increase in particle size is rather rapid, but is followed by a much slower change.[54-6] Almost no change in particle size has been noted, even in the case of emulsions that show appreciable coalescence due to a low level of emulsifier.[62] One would expect that particle size, the number of particles, the droplet surface area, or the droplet volume should vary linearly with time. Hill and Knight claim good correlation with experimental data by plotting the total surface area of all droplets (Σ) in accordance with the following equation: $1/\Sigma = at + b$, where a and b are constants and t equals time.[62]

Practical Recommendations for Shelf Life Predictions. The preceding discussion has pointed out that surprisingly little evidence exists to suggest that instability under stress can be related to normal shelf life. It is most important, therefore, to set up a realistic stability program to assess the shelf life of emulsions.

A typical test program for an "acceptable" emulsion (in the temperate zone) might establish the following: The emulsion should be stable with no visible signs of separation for at least 60 to 90 days at 45 or 50°C, 5 to 6 months at 37°C, and 12 to 18 months at room temperature. Similarly, there should be no visible signs of separation after one month's storage at 4°C and preferably after two or three freeze-thaw cycles between −20 and +25°C. An emulsion should survive at least six or eight heating/cooling cycles between refrigerator temperature and 45°C with storage at each temperature of no less than 48 hours. A stable emulsion should show no serious deterioration by centrifuging at 2,000 to 3,000 rpm at room temperature. The emulsion should not be adversely affected by agitation for 24 to 48 hours on a reciprocating shaker (approximately 60 cycles per minute at room temperature and at 45°C).

During the testing period just described, the samples stored at various conditions should be observed critically for separation, and in addition, monitored at reasonable time intervals for the following characteristics:

Change in electrical conductivity

Change in light reflection

Change in viscosity

Change in particle size

Change in chemical composition

In addition to these physical measurements, a shelf life program for emulsions should include testing of the emulsion for microbiologic contamination at appropriate intervals. It should be remembered that the distribution of emulsifiers in a freshly prepared emulsion is different from distribution of one that has been aged for several months at 45°C. As a result, an emulsion's resistance to microbial contamination may be affected by redistribution or micellization of the preservative.

References

1. Lissant, K. J.: J. Soc. Cosmetic Chemists, 21:141, 1970.
2. Frenkel, M., et al.: J. Coll. Interf. Sci., 94:174, 1983.
3. Carrigan, P. J., and Bates, T. R.: J. Pharm. Sci., 62:1476, 1973.
4. Idson, B.: Drug Metab. Rev., 14:207, 1983.
5. Harkins, W. D.: The Physical Chemistry of Surface Films. Reinhold, New York, 1954.
6. Schulman, J. J., and Cockbain, E. G.: Trans. Faraday Soc., 36:651, 1940.
7. Friberg, S.: J. Coll. Interf. Sci., 37:291, 1971.
8. Friberg, S., and Jansson, P. O.: J. Coll. Interf. Sci., 55:614, 1976.
9. Friberg, S.: J. Soc. Cosmetic Chemists, 30:309, 1979.
10. Junginger, H.: Pharm. Weekblad, 6:141, 1984.
11. Suzuki, T., et al.: J. Disp. Sci. Technol., 5:119, 1984.
12. Orecchioni, A. M., et al.: Int. J. Cosmetic Sci., 6:131, 1984.
13. Becher, P.: Emulsions Theory and Practice. 2nd Ed. Reinhold, New York, 1965.
14. Shinoda, K., and Kunieda, H.: Phase properties of emulsions: PIT and HLB. In Encyclopedia of Emulsion Technology. Vol. I. Edited by P. Becher. Marcel Dekker, New York, 1983, p. 337.
15. Lin, T. J., et al.: J. Soc. Cosmetic Chemists, 29:745, 1978.
16. Lin, T. J., et al.: Low energy emulsification. In Surfactants in Cosmetics. Edited by M. M. Rieger. Marcel Dekker, New York, 1985, p. 87.
17. Griffin, W. C.: Emulsions in Kirk Othmer Encyclopedia of Chemical Technology. Vol. 8. 3rd Ed. Wiley Interscience, New York, 1979, p. 922.
18. Garnett, C. J., et al.: J. Chem. Soc., 79:953, 1983.
19. Garnett, C. J., et al.: Faraday Trans. I, 965, 1983.
20. Davies, J. T.: Proc. 2nd Int. Congress Surface Activity, London, 1:426, 1957.
21. Fox, C.: Cosmetic emulsions. In Emulsions and Emulsion Technology. Part II. Edited by K. J. Lissant. Marcel Dekker, New York, 1974, p. 701.
22. Becher, P.: J. Soc. Cosmetic Chemists, 11:325, 1960.
23. Schott, H.: J. Pharm. Sci., 73:790, 1984.
24. Shinoda, K., et al.: J. Dispersion Sci. Technol., 1:1, 1980.
25. Marszall, L.: Cosmetics Toiletries, 93:53, 1978.
26. Shinoda, K., and Saito, H.: J. Coll. Interf. Sci., 30:258, 1969.
27. Ford, R. E., and Furmidge, C. G. L.: J. Coll. Interf. Sci., 22:331, 1966.
28. Lin, T. J., and Lambrechts, J. C.: J. Soc. Cosmetic Chemists, 20:627, 1969.
29. Lin, T. J., et al.: J. Soc. Cosmetic Chemists, 26:121, 1975.
30. Lin, T. J.: J. Soc. Cosmetic Chemists, 30:167, 1979.
31. Guay, F., and Bisaillon, S.: Drug Develop. Ind. Pharm., 5:107, 1979.
32. Rydhag, L.: Fette Seifen Anstrichm., 81:168, 1979.
33. Cante, C. J., et al.: J. Am. Oil Chem. Soc., 56:71A, 1979.
34. Rogers, J. A.: Cosmetics Toiletries, 93:49, 1978.
35. Sherman, P. J.: J. Phys. Chem., 67:2531, 1964.
36. Sherman, P. J.: J. Pharm. Pharmacol., 18:589, 1966.
37. Lissant, K. J.: Basic theory. In Emulsions and Emulsion Technology. Part I. Edited by K. J. Lissant. Marcel Dekker, New York, 1974, p. 1.
38. Humphrey, K. J., and Rhodes, C. T.: J. Pharm. Sci., 57:79, 1968.
39. Moes-Henschel, V., and Jaminet, F.: Internat. J. Cosmetic Sci., 2:193, 1980.
40. Garrett, E. R.: J. Pharm. Pharmacol., 18:589, 1966.
41. Kazmi, S. J. A., and Mitchell, A. G.: J. Pharm. Sci., 60:1422, 1971.
42. Nowak, G. A.: Soap, Perfumery & Cosmetics, 36:914, 1963.

43. Pisano, F. D., and Kostenbauder, H. B.: J. Am. Pharm. Assoc., Sci. Ed., 48:310, 1959.
44. Shimamoto, T., et al.: Chem. Pharm. Bull., 21:316, 1973.
45. Rieger, M. M.: Cosmetics Toiletries, 96:39, 1981.
46. Moore, K. E.: J. Appl. Bacteriol., 44:S29, 1978.
47. Davis, J. G.: Soap Perfumery Cosmetics, 53:133, 1980.
48. Garrett, E. R.: J. Pharm. Sci., 54:1557, 1965.
49. Vold, R. D., and Groot, R. C.: J. Soc. Cosmetic Chemists, 14:233, 1963.
50. Ottewill, R. H.: J. Coll. Interf. Sci., 38:357, 1977.
51. Groot, R. C., and Vold, R. D.: Proc. 4th Int. Congress Surface Activity, 11:1233, 1967.
52. Rieger, M. M., Cosmetics Toiletries, 90:12, 1975.
53. Reddy, R. B., and Dorle, A. K., Cosmetics Toiletries, 99:67, 1984.
54. Rowe, E. L.: J. Pharm. Sci., 54:260, 1965.
55. Sherman, P.: Rheology of Emulsions. Academic Press, London, 1968.
56. Sherman, P.: Industrial Rheology. Academic Press, London, 1970.
57. Wood, J. H., and Catacalos, G.: J. Soc. Cosmetic Chemists, 14:147, 1963.
58. Sherman, P.: Soap, Perfumery & Cosmetics, 44:693, 1971.
59. Mrukot, M., and Schmidt, M.: Parfumerie Kosmetik, 57:337, 1976.
60. Groves, M. J., and Freshwater, D. C.: J. Pharm. Sci., 57:1273, 1968.
61. Rehfeld, S. J.: J. Coll. Interf. Sci., 24:358, 1967.
62. Hill, R. A. W., and Knight, J. T.: Trans. Faraday Soc., 61:170, 1965.

General References

Books

Adamson, A. W.: Physical Chemistry of Surfaces. 3rd Ed. Interscience, New York, 1976.

Becher, P.: Emulsions Theory and Practice. 2nd Ed. Reinhold, New York, 1965.

Becher, P.: Encyclopedia of Emulsion Technology. Vol. I. Marcel Dekker, New York, 1983.

Lissant, K.: Emulsions and Emulsion Technology. Marcel Dekker, New York, 1974.

Rosen, M. J.: Surfactants and Interfacial Phenomena. John Wiley and Sons, New York, 1978.

Sherman, P.: Emulsion Science. Academic Press, London, 1968.

Sherman, P.: Rheology of Emulsions. Academic Press, London, 1968.

Sherman, P.: Industrial Rheology. Academic Press, London, 1970.

Shinoda, K.: Principles of Solution and Solubility. Marcel Dekker, New York, 1978.

Recommended Reading

Becher, P.: J. Disp. Sci. Technol., 5:81, 1984. (Update on HLB)

Bornfriend, R.: Cosmetics Toiletries, 93:61, 1978. (Processing)

Florence, A. T., and Rogers, J. A.: J. Pharm. Pharmacol., 23:153, 233, 1971. (Emulsion stabilization)

Freese, E., and Levin, B.C.: Action mechanisms of preservatives and antiseptics. *In* Developments in Industrial Microbiology. Vol. 19. Edited by L. S. Underkofler. American Institute Biological Sciences, Washington, DC, 1978, p. 207 (Preservation)

Groves, M. J., and Freshwater, D.C.: J. Pharm. Sci., 57:1273, 1968. (Particle size)

Mulley, B. A.: Medicinal emulsions. *In* Emulsions and Emulsion Technology. Part I. Edited by K. J. Lissant. Marcel Dekker, New York, 1974, p. 291. (Pharmaceutical emulsions)

Quack, J. M.: Cosmetics Toiletries, 91:21, 1976. (Emulsion stability)

Reynolds, J. A.: Interactions between proteins and amphiphiles. *In* Lipid-Protein Interaction. Vol. 2. Edited by P. C. Jost and O. H. Griffith. John Wiley and Sons, New York, 1982, p. 193. (Amphilic/protein interactions in vitro and in vivo)

Rieger, M. M.: Cosmetics Toiletries, 97, VIII:27, 1982. (Prediction of stability)

Rieger, M. M.: Cosmetics Toiletries, 97, X:49, 1982. (Solubilization)

Takamura, A., et al.: J. Pharm. Sci., 73:676, 1984. (In vitro drug release methodology)

18

Semisolids

BERNARD IDSON *and* JACK LAZARUS*

Pharmaceutical semisolid preparations include ointments, pastes, cream emulsions, gels, and rigid foams. Their common property is the ability to cling to the surface of application for reasonable duration before they are washed or worn off. This adhesion is due to their plastic rheologic behavior, which allows the semisolids to retain their shape and cling as a film until acted upon by an outside force, in which case they deform and flow.[1]

Ointments, in general, are composed of fluid hydrocarbons meshed in a matrix of higher-melting solid hydrocarbons. While most ointments are based on mineral oil and petrolatum, there are alternative types. Polyethylene can be incorporated into mineral oil to yield a plastic matrix (e.g., Plastibase, manufactured by Squibb). Mixtures of polyethylene glycols can yield products of ointment consistency that are water-soluble. Most ointments are prepared by melting the components together. Drugs or other components are added in the fluidized state. If the solids are insoluble and to be suspended, the system is put through a milling process (a colloid mill, homogenizer, or ultrasonic mixer) so that the solids are fully dispersed.

Pastes are basically ointments into which a high percentage of insoluble solids has been added. They are valuable as protective barriers on the skin, such as for treating diaper rash or protecting the face and lips from the sun. Pastes are usually prepared by incorporating a solid directly into a congealed system by levigation with a portion of the base to form a paste-like mass. The remainder of the base is added with continued levigation until the solids are uniformly dispersed in the vehicle.

Creams are semisolid emulsion systems with opaque appearances, as contrasted with translucent ointments. Their consistency and rheologic character depend on whether the emulsion is a water-in-oil or oil-in-water type and on the nature of the solids in the internal phase. The subject of emulsions is treated in Chapter 17.

Gels are semisolid systems in which a liquid phase is constrained within a three-dimensional polymeric matrix (consisting of natural or synthetic gums) in which a high degree of physical (or sometimes chemical) cross-linking has been introduced. The polymers used to prepare pharmaceutical gels include the natural gums tragacanth, pectin, carrageen, agar, and alginic acid and such synthetic and semisynthetic materials as methylcellulose, hydroxyethylcellulose, carboxymethylcellulose, and the Carbopols, which are synthetic vinyl polymers with ionizable carboxyl groups. Gels are prepared by either a fusion process or a special procedure necessitated by the gelling characteristics of the gellant.

The bulk of these semisolid preparations are applied to the skin, where they usually serve as vehicles for topically applied drugs, as emollients, or as protective or occlusive dressings. A lesser portion of topical semisolid dosage forms are applied to mucous membranes, such as rectal tissue, buccal tissue, vaginal mucosa, urethral membrane, external ear lining, nasal mucosa, and cornea. The mucous membranes permit more ready access to the systemic circulation, whereas normal skin is relatively impenetrable. The emphasis of this chapter is on the skin and on dermatologicals, but the general concepts and rationale apply to all semisolid topical therapy.

*Deceased.

Skin

The skin is a large multilayered organ that in the average adult weighs about eight pounds, excluding fat. It covers a surface exceeding 20,000 cm² and has varied functions and properties. The skin serves as a barrier against physical and chemical attack. Some materials, such as nickel ions, mustard gas, and the oleoresins from Rhus toxicodendron, commonly known as poison ivy, can penetrate the barrier, but most substances cannot. The skin acts as a thermostat in maintaining body temperature, shields the body from invasion by micro-organisms, protects against ultraviolet rays, and plays a role in the regulation of blood pressure.

Anatomically, the skin has many histologic layers, but in general, it is described in terms of three tissue layers: the epidermis, the dermis, and the subcutaneous fat layer. Figure 18-1 represents an idealized section of the skin, showing the glands, hair follicles, nerves, blood vessels, and other skin accessories. The outermost layer is the stratum corneum, or horny layer, which consists of compacted, dead, keratinized cells in stratified layers with a density of 1.55. Because of the dense nature of the stratum corneum, values of diffusion coefficients in this tissue are a thousand or more times smaller than in any other skin tissue, which results in higher resistance and general impenetrability.[2]

The stratum corneum is the rate-limiting barrier that restricts the inward and outward movement of chemical substances. Structurally, the stratum corneum is a heterogeneous tissue composed of flattened keratinized cells, the outer

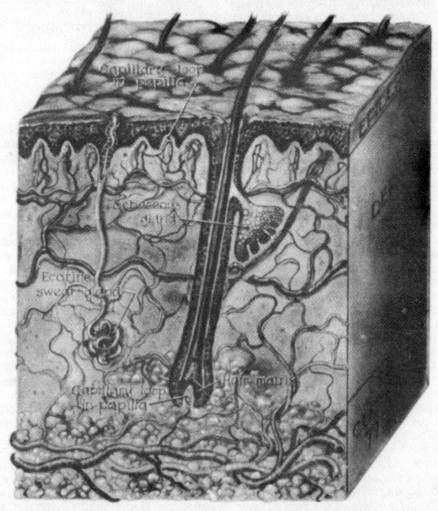

FIG. 18-1. *Stratified organization of the skin. (From Pillsbury, D. M.: A Manual of Dermatology. W. B. Saunders, Philadelphia, 1971).*

layers of which are less densely packed than those adjacent to the underlying granular layer. The stratum corneum exhibits regional differences in thickness over the body. It is as thick as several hundred micrometers on the palms of the hand and soles of the feet in an adult, but over most of the body it is about 10 μm thick when dry, increasing to about 40 to 50 μm when fully hydrated.[3]

There is limited knowledge of the chemical composition of the barrier. The main cellular components are the proteins, lipid, and water, combined into an ordered structure. The approximate composition in the dry state is 75 to 85% protein, 15 to 20% lipid, and 15% water. Although the surface lipids offer little resistance to the passage of compounds, studies of the removal of lipids from the cutaneous surface indicate that they participate in epidermal water function.[4–10] Barrier function is restored when the extracted lipids are returned to the skin, which suggests variations in biologic membrane permeability, depending largely on the specific nature or distribution of the lipid contained in the cell membrane.

Beneath the stratum corneum are the metabolically active layers of the epidermis. The basal or germinal layer lies right above the dermis. Epidermal cells start their mitotic journey upward to the surface; the cells flatten and shrink as they slowly die from lack of oxygen and nutrition.

The next distinctive histologic layer shown in Figure 18-1 is the dermis, or corium, which is approximately one eighth of an inch thick and constitutes the main mass of the skin. The dermis essentially consists of about 80% of protein in a matrix of mucopolysaccharide "ground substance."[11]

Contained and supported within the dermis are numerous blood vessels, lymphatics, and nerves, as well as the epidermal appendages such as the hair follicles, sebaceous glands, and sweat glands. Hair follicles are distributed over the entire skin surface with the exception of the soles of the feet, the palms of the hand, the red portion of the lips, and select portions of the sex organs. Each hair follicle is associated with one or more sebaceous glands, which are outgrowths of epithelial cells. The fractional area of the skin surface occupied by the hair follicles has been estimated to be roughly 1/1000 of the total surface.[12] The sweat glands are divided into the eccrine and apocrine types. They are widely distributed over the surfaces of the body. The eccrine glands are particularly concentrated in the palms and soles. The principal function of the glands is for heat control, as they secrete a dilute salt solution. The apocrine glands are found in the axillae (armpits), in anogenital regions, and around nipples. They are coiled tubular glands about ten times larger than eccrine glands and extend entirely through the dermis and well into the subcutaneous layer.[11]

Percutaneous Absorption

The usual object of dermatologic drug therapy is to produce a desired therapeutic action at specific sites on the epidermal tissue. While certain topical drugs such as emollients, antimicrobials, and deodorants act primarily on the surface of the skin, the target area for most dermatologic disorders lies in the viable epidermis or upper dermis. This requires diffusive penetration of the skin or percutaneous absorption.

Routes of Penetration

When a drug system is applied topically, the drug diffuses out of its vehicle onto the surface tissues of the skin. There are three potential portals of entry: through the follicular region, through the sweat ducts, or through the unbroken stratum corneum between these appendages. There is little convincing evidence that eccrine sweat glands play any significant role in cutaneous permeability. Material may enter the ducts, and even the glands, but there appears to be no penetration from these areas to the dermis.

For substances absorbed by the transepidermal route, penetration is fairly rapid, although slower than intestinal tract absorption, and is almost always accompanied by some degree of pilosebaceous penetration as well. For substances that are absorbed through both pathways, the transepidermal route is the principal portal of entry because of the total, relatively small, absorbing surface offered by the pilosebaceous units. The epidermis presents a surface area 100 to 1000 times greater than the other routes of absorption. The appendages, sweat glands, and hair follicles are scattered throughout the skin in varying numbers, but are comparatively sparse; their total cross-sectional area is probably between 0.1 and 1.0% of the skin area.

The particular route a substance may take and the relative importance of one in contrast with the other, depend almost entirely on the physicochemical properties of the drug and the condition of the skin. Under the appropriate conditions, each of the contending routes of permeability may change and be the overwhelmingly dominant one. In particular, the transient diffusion that occurs shortly after the application of a substance to the surface of the skin is shown to be potentially far greater through the appendages than through the matrix of the stratum corneum. After steady-state diffusion has been established, the dominant diffusion mode is probably no longer intra-appendageal, but occurs through the matrix of the stratum corneum. Flux through shunts is difficult to measure experimentally, except possibly through hair. The recognition of transient diffusion, occurring primarily via follicles and ducts, and steady-state diffusion, occurring primarily through the intact stratum corneum, results in a considerably more self-consistent and orderly treatment of the process of percutaneous absorption.

Once a substance passes through the stratum corneum, there is apparently no significant further hindrance to penetration of the remaining epidermal layers and corium; there is then a ready entry into the circulation via the capillaries. The concentration gradient essentially ends in the dermal layer at the beginning of the circulation. The systemic circulation acts as a reservoir or "sink" for the drug. Once in the general circulation, the drug is diluted and distributed rapidly with little systemic buildup.[1]

Diffusion through the horny layer is a passive process. There is little evidence to support specialized active transport systems for cells of the stratum corneum. The passive process is affected only by the substance being absorbed, by the medium in which the substance is dispersed, and by ambient conditions. On the other hand, percutaneous absorption is a more complicated process, of which epidermal diffusion is the first phase, and clearance from the dermis the second. The latter depends on effective blood flow, interstitial fluid movement, lymphatics, and perhaps other factors that combine with dermal constituents.[5]

Study Methods

In Vitro Technique. The principal in vitro technique for studying skin penetration involves use of some variety of a diffusion cell in which animal or human skin is fastened to a holder and the passage of compounds from the epidermal surface to a fluid bath is measured. The simplicity of methods and equipment ranges from just stretching human skin over the mouth of a funnel to using special glass chambers. The penetration rates can be quantitated, particularly by radioactive measurements. The area of spread of radioactive agent on the surface is detected with autoradiographs, allowing expression in terms of quantity per unit area per unit time. Radioactive agents have not taken over completely. Many chemical agents penetrate in sufficient concentration to be determined by one or the other techniques of physical or chemical analysis.

More recently, model systems have been used that do not use membranes. Solvents such as alcohol-water have been utilized as models chosen to have negligible solubility in the phase representing the skin, but in which the drug is fairly soluble.[13–17] A receptor phase or "sink" is used to receive the penetrant. Chloroform and isopropyl myristate have served as sinks. Since they are immiscible with the alcohol-water, it is not necessary to introduce an artificial membrane to separate these sinks from the vehicles. The important factors influencing the release into the receptor phase are the solubility in the vehicle and the partition coefficient of the drug between the vehicle and the receptor phase. Optimal release is obtained from vehicles containing the minimum concentration of solvent required for complete solubilization of the drug.[13]

In Vivo Technique. The major in vivo methods are histologic techniques, use of tracers, analysis of body tissues and fluids, and elicitation of a biologic response. Tissue changes in skin following the application of various substances to the cutaneous surface can yield information about the specific tissue affected, so that not only absorption, per se, is revealed, but also the route of penetration. The method is limited to dyes and to a small number of other substances that yield perceivable colored end products with specific chemical reactions. Following the movements of penetrants through dyes, fluorescence and radioactive labeling represent the most widespread tracer methods. The studies are always combined with other techniques such as histologic or chemical analysis of tissues or fluids. While radioactive methods give information on the amount of the compound that moves across the skin, they yield little or no information on the route of penetration or on the localization of the penetrant within the structure of the skin.

Urine analysis is by far the most frequently used method. Although the urinary method is extremely valuable, caution is indicated since the recovered agent will not necessarily by the original material or the amount needed to penetrate the skin. Some of the applied agent may have gone elsewhere than into the urine; some may have been metabolized and therefore may be no longer detectable. A steady state between absorption and excretion needs to be reached before measurements can be accepted. The use of topical agents that elicit a physiologic reaction when they reach the dermis makes it possible to demonstrate not only penetration, but also the time required for a reaction to occur. The method is intriguing because it is simple and has practical applications. For example, responses such as sweat secretion, vasoconstriction, vasodilation, pigmentation, and vascular permeability can be recorded with reasonable accuracy by visual observation.

Various methods have been used for studying in vitro and in vivo percutaneous absorption. There are three variables in all the methods: application of the medicament, apparatus, and measurement of the medicament. The combinations of these variables lead to numerous methods, and comparisons between investigations is difficult.[18]

Factors in Skin Penetration. The factors that influence skin penetration are essentially the same as those for gastrointestinal absorption, with the rate of diffusion depending primarily on the physicochemical properties of the drug and only secondarily on the vehicle, pH, and concentration. Differing physiologic variables involve the condition of the skin, i.e., whether it is intact or injured, the skin age, the area of skin treated, the thickness of the skin barrier phase, the species variation, and the skin moisture content.

The principal physicochemical factor in skin penetration is the hydration state of the stratum corneum, which affects the rate of passage of all substances that penetrate the skin. Hydration results from water diffusing from underlying epidermal layers or from perspiration that accumulates after application of an occlusive vehicle or covering on the surface. Under occlusive conditions, the stratum corneum is changed from a tissue that normally contains little water (5 to 15%) to one that contains as much as 50% water. The clinical importance of hydration can be found in the use of occlusive plastic film in steroid therapy. Here, the prevention of water loss from the stratum corneum and the subsequent increased water concentration in this skin layer apparently enhances the penetration of the steroid. The temperature of the skin and the concentration of drug play significant roles, but they are secondary to that of hydration.

The solubility of a drug determines the concentration presented to the absorption site, and the water/lipid partition coefficient influences the rate of transport. An inverse relationship appears to exist between the absorption rate and the molecular weight. Small molecules penetrate more rapidly than large molecules, but within a narrow range of molecular size, there is little correlation between the size and the penetration rate. Materials of higher molecular weight also show variable penetration. Very large molecules, such as proteins and polysaccharides, go through poorly, if at all.[19,20]

Vehicles and Skin Penetration. The efficiency of various types of vehicles in aiding penetration can be reasonably predicted by the way in which the vehicle alters the activity of water in the stratum corneum and influences the stratum corneum/vehicle partition coefficient. Greases and oils are the most occlusive vehicles and induce the greatest hydration through sweat accumulation at the skin-vehicle interface. This is accentuated if the skin is covered with occlusive bandages or plastic. Emulsions of the water-in-oil type are somewhat less occlusive than greases. Substances in the vehicle, such as humectants, which have a high affinity for water, may under certain circumstances dehydrate the stratum corneum and decrease penetration. Similarly, powders increase the surface area and increase the rate of evaporation of water, and so decrease the extent of hydration. Conversely, vehicles may also affect penetration by their ability to reduce loss of water vapor on the skin surface. Paraffin bases suppress transepidermal water diffusion, whereas a number of other standard vehicles cause a lesser degree of transepidermal water loss suppression.

The role of vehicles on skin penetration is often confusing and contradictory, since the emphasis has generally been placed on the compatibility, stability, and appearance of the product. Only in recent years has attention been given to the influence of components in the vehicle on the movement of the drug through the skin. The release of a substance is favored by the selection of vehicles that have a low affinity for the penetrant or in which the drug is least soluble. This is consistent with the view that the rate of release is governed by the vehicle-to-receptor phase (stratum corneum) partition coefficient. For a given concentration of drug in certain vehicles, the activity coefficient of the drug at that concentration may vary by as much as 1000-fold from one vehicle to the other. The thermodynamic activity of the drug in the vehicle is the product of the concentration of the drug and the activity coefficient of the drug in the vehicle. Solutes held firmly by the vehicle, such as those occurring when the drug forms a soluble complex with the vehicle, exhibit low activity coefficients: hence, the rate of release from such drug-vehicle combinations is slow. Solutes held "loosely" by the vehicle (with less affinity of the vehicle for the drug or solute) exhibit high activity coefficients; therefore, the rate of release from such drug-vehicle combinations is fast. Varied materials require individual formulation based on solubility characteristics, and the formulation may also need modification for different concentrations of the agent to obtain maximal release rates.

Materials have been experimentally studied in attempts to increase the rate of absorption of topically applied drugs. These agents are often called "accelerants." They appear to swell the stratum comeum and leach out essential structural material, thus reducing the diffusional resistance and increasing the permeability. The most effective is dimethylsulfoxide (DMSO) followed by dimethylformamide (DMF), dimethylacetamide (DMA), urea, propylene glycol, and surface-active agents. DMSO, DMF, and DMA are all strongly hygroscopic and it is likely that the presence of these substances in the stratum comeum increases the hydration of the tissue and therefore its permeability. These agents are currently restricted to experimental use. Surface-active agents appear to increase the permeability of the skin to water by altering the physical state of water in the skin in such a way as to permit greater freedom to the passage of charged hydrophilic substances. When penetration occurs, anionlcs penetrate best, followed by cationics and nonionic surfactants. Among anionic substances, the laurate ion is reported to have the greatest penetration and the greatest effect on the penetration of other solutes. Soaps of different fatty acids have this property in varying degrees, with penetration more significant for salts of fatty acids having a carbon length of 10 or less. The penetration of fatty acid soaps varies inversely with pH. At higher pH (approximately 11), the action of the anionic surfactant appears to be attenuated or overshadowed by the influence of the more alkaline pH itself.

Raw Materials

More raw materials are available for use on the skin than for oral use, and in turn, more are available for oral use than for parenteral use. The difference in the number of materials available for each route of administration is due to the type of absorption barrier and physicochemical environment surrounding the absorption sites. Substances such as isopropyl myristate and butyl stearate may be used topically without toxic effects, yet these esters may not be used orally, because hydrolysis of the esters by digestive enzymes yields poorly tolerated alcohols. The absence of comparable hydrolytic enzymes on the skin surface makes these compounds satisfactory for dermatologic medication.

The Federal Food and Drug Administration (FDA) approves chemical substances and states the maximum concentration that is considered to be safe for use in a particular food or cosmetic. The information is published in the "Federal Register," and a compilation of all such substances is available.[21] All raw materials should be checked against this list if there is any doubt regarding the current status of a particular substance; however, each new pharmaceutical dosage form must receive individual approval. The supplier of a chemical substance usually indicates in his brochure, or upon request, the safety tests that have been performed and whether approval from the FDA has been received for its use in a particular form. The tests should be thorough and well designed; they should include human patch tests, eye irritation studies, determination of minimum lethal dose on at least two animal species, and chronic toxicity studies.

Names of suppliers of various raw materials for semisolids, manufacturing equipment, and other pertinent information can be obtained from trade and scientific journals. Consultation with representatives of suppliers frequently reduces the development time required for a new pharmaceutical semisolid, but independent critical judgment is needed.

The suppliers of raw materials such as emollients, emulsifiers, fats, oils, waxes, cellulose derivatives, humectants, lanolin derivatives, and water absorption bases have detailed knowledge of their specific products. Many of the suppliers have well-equipped laboratories in which workers are constantly developing new uses for their materials in the pharmaceutical, cosmetic, toiletries, and chemical specialties fields. The formulator must be cautious, however, in accepting a supplier's claims about the utility of a raw material. It is necessary to ascertain the biologic properties as well as the significant physical and chemical parameters of the substance and its stability on storage at different temperatures.

It is a fundamental concept in formulating any dosage form that chemical and physical incompatibilities that affect the therapeutic efficacy of a drug must be avoided. In advance of any formulation, the physicochemical properties of the drug must be evaluated. The stability of the active substance under alkaline or acidic conditions can be established from its pH profile. The sensitivity of the drug to oxidation and reduction, moisture, and light, and its solubility in various materials, indicate the type of base most suitable for the stability of the drug and for its absorption. Compatibility with the container is of equal importance, and it is necessary to conduct stability studies of the product in the finished container.

Perfumes generally are not included in the semisolid formulations because in the past many dermatologists have objected to their use for the treatment of a skin condition in view of the danger of sensitization. Many manufacturers of fragrances have run toxicity, sensitization, and irritation tests on the various perfume materials and can supply fragrances that have successfully passed critical testing in animals. However, such animal tests do not obviate the need for testing on humans.

The industrial pharmacist who develops the dosage form must be aware of the chemical composition of the materials at his disposal and their physical properties, so that he can set or have specifications set for the raw materials. Broad specification limits may lower the cost of a raw material, but represent false economy if the quality of the product is affected. New raw materials suitable for use in semisolids are continually being introduced. Flynn has published an excellent compilation of these materials that includes their functions in formulations.[1]

Hydrocarbons

Except for water, petrolatum and mineral oil are perhaps the most widely used substances in semisolids. Petrolatum is a complex mixture of semisolid hydrocarbons, containing aliphatic, cyclic, saturated, unsaturated, branched, and unbranched substances in varying proportions. Although extensively used for more than 85 years, petrolatum still has broad physical and chemical specifications in the USP. Wide density and melting point ranges, as well as variation in chemical composition, are permitted in the official compendia throughout the world.

Petrolatum is available in the form of a short or long "fiber." The type of fiber possessed by the petrolatum is usually determined by dipping the index finger into the petrolatum sample and then withdrawing it slowly. The long fiber type tends to form a transparent continuous film or thread joining the finger and the sample. The short fiber variety ruptures easily and does not exhibit this film. The long fiber petrolatum is preferred for an occlusive dressing because of the continuous film it forms over the surface of the skin.

Mineral oil is obtained from petroleum, as is petrolatum, by collection of a particular viscosity-controlled fraction. It is produced in many viscosity and specific gravity ranges. The lower viscosity oils are preferred for semisolids, since

they are less tacky and greasy. An excellent review of the chemistry and the properties of petrolatum and mineral oil has been published.[22]

Hydrocarbon Waxes

Hydrocarbon waxes frequently are employed in the manufacture of creams and ointments to increase the viscosity of mineral oil in order to prevent its separation from an ointment. *Ozokerite* is a mined wax with a melting point range of 65 to 75°C and consists of a mixture of saturated hydrocarbons ranging in carbon content from C_{35} to C_{55}. *Paraffin wax* is obtained from petroleum and is available in a variety of melting points ranging from 35 to 75°C. Another wax that is often used is *ceresin*, which is a mixture of ozokerite and paraffin wax. Its melting point varies, depending on the paraffin wax content. Ozokerite and ceresin possess the property of retaining oils within a matrix-like structure without the sweating or oozing of the oils.

Synthetic waxes have been developed from vegetable oils and naturally occurring waxes by a process of hydrogenation and catalytic splitting that involves long C_{18}–C_{36} hydrocarbon chains. Like all true waxes, the synthetic waxes exhibit thermoplastic, crystalline properties and are not pure chemical compounds but complex mixtures of mainly long chain saturated aliphatic chemical entities. The synthetic waxes are chemically closely related to the naturally occurring waxes in that they contain long chain wax fatty acids, but are not considered to be direct replacements for them. However, they may be used in conjunction with or can replace the natural waxes in some formulations to achieve certain desired properties. Synchrowaxes,* the brand name of a series of such waxes, have unique gelling characteristics that may be used in formulating synthetic petrolatums with occlusive properties to help moisturize the skin without the inelegant properties of natural petrolatum.

Oleaginous Substances

Vegetable oils such as peanut oil, almond oil, sesame oil, and olive oil are mono-, di-, and triglycerides of mixtures of unsaturated and saturated fatty acids. Trace metal contaminants in the oils may catalyze oxidation reactions that can be prevented by the addition of antioxidants, such as butylated hydroxyanisole, butylated

*Synchrowaxes are available from Croda, Inc., New York, NY.

hydroxy toluene or propyl-gallate, and by the addition of metal chelating agents such as salts of ethylenediamine tetraacetic acid.

Antioxidants may produce problems of drug compatibility or dermal sensitivity in some patients. The exact chemical composition of a particular vegetable oil varies from lot to lot because of its natural origins. Its composition depends on the climatic conditions, the soil, the amount of rainfall during the growth of the vegetable crop, and the storage conditions of the harvested crop and the oil.

The trend toward the isolation and synthesis of pure chemical entities present in the vegetable oils is evident in the literature and supplier's catalogs. Perhaps when these chemically pure substances are available in quantity, the influence of a homologous series of compounds, either individually or in combination, on the quality of an emulsion and the release of a drug from such a base can be more rigidly controlled.

Fatty Acids and Alcohols

The commercially available fatty acids are really mixtures of related fatty acids. Stearic and palmitic acids are present in the greatest proportion in triple pressed stearic acid along with varying quantities of other fatty acids. Various fixed ratios of stearic/palmitic acids can be obtained from the suppliers. A slight change in the ratio of the saturated fatty acids changes the structure and size of the fatty acid crystal, the x-ray diffraction pattern, and the solubility. For this reason, stearic acid of rigidly controlled purity is used in many topical preparations.

Similar variations in chemical structure exist in almost all materials of natural origin, in polymeric substances having a long chain length, and in combinations of polymers with fatty acids or alcohols. The number of moles of ethylene oxide, for example, in a polyethylene reaction product such as $ROCH_2CH_2[OC_2H_4]_nOH$ merely represents an average rather than an exact amount. Rigid purchasing and quality control specifications must be established for such materials if variations in the quality and consistency of semisolid emulsions are to be avoided.

Stearic acid is used in water-removable creams as an emulsifier to develop a certain consistency in the cream and to give a matt effect on the skin. When a stearate soap is used as an emulsifier, enough potassium hydroxide or triethanolamine usually is added to react with about 8 to 20% of the stearic acid. The unreacted fatty acid increases the consistency of the cream. These creams are soft and develop a sheen or luster upon aging, owing to the forma-

tion of stearic acid crystals. Creams formed with sodium stearate are much firmer in consistency.

Stearyl alcohol and *cetyl alcohol* (palmityl alcohol) are used in creams as auxiliary emulsifiers and emollients. In sufficient quantity, stearyl alcohol produces a firm cream that may be softened with cetyl alcohol.

For a description of waxes of animals, insect, and vegetable origin such as lanolin, beeswax, carnauba wax, candelila wax, silicones, branched chain compounds, isopropylesters, polyols, cellulose ethers, and other raw materials suitable for creams and ointments, the reader is advised to check sources such as the CTFA Cosmetic Ingredient Dictionary,[23] as well as suppliers' catalogs.

A list of the various raw materials and their functions has recently been published.[1] Another listing of cosmetic raw materials appeared in the FD&C Reports ("The Rose Sheet")[24] which was reproduced from the Japan Cosmetic Ingredient Dictionary of 148 government-approved raw materials. The dictionary is the result of a collaborative effort between the Cosmetic, Toiletry and Fragrance Association (CTFA), the U.S. Commerce Department, the Japanese Government, and the Japan Cosmetic Industry Association (JCIA). The second supplement to the dictionary lists 173 raw materials and is reproduced in a later issue of the same trade periodical.[24] The dictionary will eventually list approximately 2,000 to 3,000 raw materials. According to the CTFA, inclusion of the raw materials in the dictionary is based on "(1) chemical (not brand name), (2) whether the substance is free from patent and/or 'technical know-how problems,' (3) whether it is free of safety problems, and (4) a specified alkyl group." The interest and purpose of CTFA is "to eliminate testing, certification, and standards activities that act as barriers to trade with Japan."

Emulsifiers

The water-soluble soaps were among the first emulsifiers used for semisolid oil-in-water emulsions. The viscosity of the cream or ointment prevents coalescence of the emulsified phases and helps to stabilize the emulsion. The addition of fatty polar substances, such as cetyl alcohol and glyceryl monostearate, tends to stabilize the semisolid oil-in-water emulsion. The interfacial film formed around the dispersed phase globules in such a system is generally solid, thereby making the emulsified preparation more rigid. Polyvalent ions, such as magnesium, calcium, and aluminum, tend to stabilize water-in-oil emulsions by cross-linking with the polar groups of the fatty materials. Nearly all semisolid creams and emulsified ointments require more than one emulsifier. The combination of a surface active agent with an oil-soluble auxiliary emulsifier is referred to as a *mixed emulsifier system*. Triethanolamine stearate soap combined with cetyl alcohol is an example of an oil-in-water mixed emulsifier; beeswax and divalent calcium ions or small quantities of a water-soluble surface active agent exemplify mixed emulsifiers for a water-in-oil emulsion. Maximum stability of an emulsion occurs when a complex interfacial film is formed. Such a film forms when an oil-soluble substance is added and reacts at the interface with the water-soluble surfactant. Soft water-in-oil cream bases can be made with calcium ions as an auxiliary emulsifier. The bases can be made firmer by decreasing the mineral oil content. Formula #1 is used to make a soft water-in-oil cream base employing divalent calcium ions in the form of water-soluble saccharated lime.

Formula #1

	%
A Mineral oil, 65 to 75 viscosity	30.00
Lantrol*	3.00
Microcrystalline wax†	2.00
Acidlan 20*	4.00
Propylparaben	0.20
B Borax	0.20
Methylparaben	0.20
Water	49.75
C Saccharated lime	0.65
Purified water	10.00

*Available from Emery Industries, Cincinnati, OH.

†Should have a melting point of 75 to 79°C and should be tested for safety on animal and human skin, since petroleum residues may be present in the wax.

Procedure: Heat parts A, B, C separately to 78°C. Add B to A. After the emulsion has formed, add C. Cool and pass through a homogenizer.

The clay, magnesium aluminum silicate, has been used as a thickener, suspending agent, and oil-in-water emulsion stabilizer because of the colloidal structure of its aqueous dispersions. It also contributes to the stability of water-in-oil emulsions when used with suitable emulsifiers, probably owing to its thickening action on the internal phase whereby it inhibits coalescence. The magnesium aluminum silicate may migrate to the interfacial area, resulting in a stronger film.[25]

Formula #2

	%(w/w)
A Magnesium aluminum silicate (MAS)*	2.0
Purified water	37.0
B Mineral oil, light	20.0
Petrolatum	9.0
Isopropyl myristate	5.0
Lantrol (lanolin oil)†	3.0
70% sorbitol solution	20.0
Arlacel 186 (glyceryl oleate and propylene glycol)‡	1.0
Polysorbate 80	1.0
Preservative	q.s.

*Available from Veegum, R.T. Vanderbilt Co., Norwalk, CT.
†Available from Emery Industries, Cincinnati, OH.
‡Available from ICI Americas, Inc., Wilmington, DE.

Procedure: Add the MAS to the water slowly, agitating continually until smooth. Heat A to 70 to 75°C. Heat B with stirring to 70 to 75°C. Add A to B, and mix until cooled.

The soap-type emulsion may be unstable in the presence of acidic substances. Cationic or nonionic emulsifiers are preferable for drugs requiring an acid pH. Quaternary ammonium compounds like cetyl trimethyl ammonium chloride help to stabilize these emulsions in combination with such fatty alcohols as cetyl alcohol.

The nonionic emulsifiers are employed for both oil-in-water and water-in-oil emulsified pharmaceutical semisolids because they are compatible with many drug substances. The nonionic emulsifiers are versatile and may be used with strongly acidic salts or with strong electrolytes.

Formula #3
Tripelennamine Hydrochloride Cream*

	%(w/w)
Oil Phase	
Cetyl alcohol	5.0
Glyceryl monostearate	15.0
Sorbitan monooleate	0.3
Polysorbate 80, USP	0.3
Aqueous Phase	
Tripelennamine HCl	2.0
Methylcellulose 100 cps	1.0
Purified water, q.s. ad	100.0
Preservative	q.s.

*Available from ICI Americas, Inc., Wilmington, DE.

Procedure: Disperse the methylcellulose in hot water in which the preservative has been dissolved, and then chill at 6°C until dissolved. Heat the oil phase to 70°C. Heat the methylcellulose solution to 72°C, and add to the oil phase, stirring continuously. Add the tripelennamine HCl at 35°C, and stir continuously until dissolved.

Recently, a series of emulsifiers have been marketed that contain chemically bonded lactic acid with fatty acids. These acyl lactylates are claimed to be mild and nonirritating to the skin and eyes,* to produce an emollient feel to the skin, and to serve as oil-in-water or water-in-oil emulsifiers. The sodium salts are suggested for use in oil-in-water. The particular fatty acid lactylate that is selected should be based on the desired application of the final product as well as on the most compatible fatty acid derivative. Some of the available lactylates and the calculated HLB values are as follows:

Types of Fatty Acid	Calculated HLB
1. Stearic	6.5
2. Stearic/Palmitic	8.3
3. Lauric/Myristic	14.4
4. Capric/Lauric	11.3
5. Isostearic	5.9

Items 3 and 4 are foamers. Item 4 shows good bacteriostatic properties, owing to the presence of the moderately short chain capric acid.

An example of an oil-in-water cream utilizing one of the emulsifiers that can serve as a vehicle for a compatible active substance follows:

Formula #4

	%(w/w)
A Oil Phase	
Cetearyl alcohol	5.0
Silicone oil, 200 fluid	1.0
Isopropyl myristate	2.0
Sodium stearoyl-2-lactylate	2.0
B Aqueous Phase	
Propylene glycol	5.0
Sodium citrate	0.2
Preservative	q.s.
Purified water, q.s. ad	100

Procedure: Mix A and heat to 65°C. Combine B and heat to 70°C. Add B to A with suitable agitation. Mix with moderate agitation while cooling.

To achieve adequate stability in creams in which the oil content exceeds 10%, the supplier recommends the use of a co-emulsifier to achieve adequate stability. The HLB system should be utilized to calculate the ratio between the two emulsifiers for the lipid(s) being used. Several ratios should be checked to either side of the calculated HLB value to optimize the emulsion.

Formula #5
Antiperspirant Cream

	%(w/w)
A Oil Phase	
Mineral oil	23.0
Calcium stearoyl-2-lactylate	3.2
PEG 400 dioleate	0.8
B Aqueous Phase	
Glycerine	3.0
Sodium lactate (60%)	10.0
Purified water	20.0
C Aluminum chlorohydrate (50%)	40.0

Procedure: Heat A, B, and C to 70°C in separate vessels. Add B to C immediately before adding to A. Mix with moderate agitation while cooling.

The Promulgens* are a series of nonionic emulsifiers composed of a mixture of fatty alcohols and their ethoxylates. Two types, D and G, are available and are described in the boxed area below.

The two types differ in melting point and in consistency of the emulsions that they form. According to the supplier, the emulsions formed with type D are usually thicker in consistency. Since there are no ester linkages, these emulsifiers are not subject to hydrolysis. In addition, they are compatible with anionic surfactants of the sodium lauryl sulfate type or with cationics such as quaternary ammonium compounds. Type D tends to form creams, and type G tends to form liquid emulsions. It is suggested that they be used in combination to achieve a desired viscosity level.

	Promulgen D	Promulgen G
CTFA adopted name—	Cetearyl alcohol and Ceteareth-20	Stearyl alcohol and Ceteareth-20
Chemical description—	Cetearyl alcohol and ethoxylated cetearyl alcohol	Stearyl alcohol and ethoxylated cetearyl alcohol
Melting point—	47 to 55°C	55 to 63°C

*Available from Patco Products, Kansas City, MO.

*Available from Amerchol Corporation, Edison, NJ.

Polyols

Glycerine, propylene glycol, sorbitol 70%, and the lower molecular weight polyethylene glycols are used as humectants in creams. The choice of a humectant is based not only on its rate of moisture exchange, but also on its effect on the texture and viscosity of the preparation. These materials prevent the cream from drying out and prevent the formation of a crust when the cream is packaged in a jar. They also improve the consistency and rub-out qualities of the cream when it is applied to the skin, permitting the cream to be spread without rolling. Increasing the humectant content tends to cause tackiness.

Sorbitol 70% is more hygroscopic than glycerine and is used at a lower concentration, usually 3% as compared to 10% for glycerine. Propylene glycol and the polyethylene glycols occasionally are used in combination with glycerine, since their ability to absorb moisture is less than that of glycerine.

Insoluble Powders

Insoluble drugs must be uniformly dispersed throughout the vehicle to ensure homogeneity of the product. The solid must be impalpable to the touch; otherwise, grittiness results. Particles less than 74 microns in size, equivalent to the mesh openings in a 200-mesh sieve in the U.S. Standard Sieve series, are impalpable to most people. Milling to a finely divided state provides more surface area for contact with the dermal site and increases the rate of dissolution of poorly soluble substances.

Some powders do not disperse uniformly, but tend to aggregate in the base, whereas others present no difficulties even though the particle size is the same. The difference may be due to the electrically charged surface condition of the particles after milling. Aggregation of particles becomes a problem for those that are 5 microns or smaller in size. For particles below 0.5 microns in size, the dispersion problems increase exponentially. Different powdered substances show similar problems of aggregation in the submicron size.

Many drug substances used in topical preparations (e.g., prednisolone; fluorocortisone acetate) exist in several polymorphic states. Compounds that exist in different crystalline forms at room temperature possess varying amounts of free energy or thermodynamic activity. The physiologic activity and availability of a drug substance often are directly related to its thermodynamic activity[26] and the choice of the proper crystalline form for use in the semisolid is vitally important. Following its incorporation into the semisolid, the maintenance of the selected polymorphic form in the semisolid is of equal concern. The components of the vehicle and the method of preparation of the semisolid dosage form affect the stability of the polymorphic form.

Types of Vehicles

The vehicle used for a pharmaceutical differs from that used for a cosmetic because with a cosmetic, penetration into the skin is not desired. Penetration or protection is desired in a pharmaceutical semisolid, and its cosmetic effect or appearance on the skin is less important. A well-formulated pharmaceutical semisolid should be both therapeutically effective and cosmetically appealing, with the major effort in the medical direction.

The therapeutic preparations included in the semisolids classification are products intended for application to the skin, scalp, and certain body orifices. These preparations include ophthalmic ointments, nasal jellies, gels, and sterile lubricants for surgical use. In this chapter, however, attention is given to those dosage forms that are used in the prevention or treatment of skin disease.

The solubility and stability of the drug in the base, as well as the nature of the skin lesion, determine the choice of the semisolid vehicle. The United States Pharmacopeia (USP) XX recognizes four classes of semisolids under the general classification of ointments: hydrocarbon bases, absorption bases, (anhydrous form and emulsion form), water-removable bases, and water-soluble bases.[27]

Hydrocarbon Bases

Petrolatum and white ointment, which is petrolatum with 5% beeswax, are typical of this class of lipophilic vehicles. The most commonly used raw material in ointment vehicles is petrolatum because of its consistency, its bland and neutral characteristics, and its ability to spread easily on the skin. These bases are difficult to wash off the skin and may be used as occlusive coverings to inhibit the normal evaporation of moisture from the skin. A thin film of petrolatum produces a sensation of warmth on the skin because the insensible moisture does not evaporate. Very little water can be incorporated into these greasy bases without the addition of other substances.

Absorption Bases

The absorption bases are formed by the addition of substances miscible with hydrocarbons and possessing polar groupings, such as the sulfate, sulfonate, carboxyl, hydroxyl, or an ether linkage. Lanolin, lanolin isolates, cholesterol, lanosterol and other sterols, acetylated sterols, or partial esters of polyhydric alcohols (e.g., sorbitan monosterate or monooleate) may be added to make the hydrocarbon bases hydrophilic. Such hydrophilic mixtures have been known as "absorption bases," although the term "absorption" is a misnomer. The bases do not absorb water on contact, but with sufficient agitation, they do absorb aqueous solutions and can be considered water-in-oil emulsions. (The notations o/w for oil-in-water and w/o for water-in-oil are convenient abbreviations for the respective emulsion types.)

The absorption bases are of two types: the anhydrous form and the emulsion form. Anhydrous lanolin and hydrophilic petrolatum are examples of anhydrous vehicles that absorb water to form water-in-oil emulsions.

Formula #6
Hydrophilic Petrolatum (USP XX)

	g
Cholesterol	30.0
Stearyl alcohol	30.0
White wax	80.0
White petrolatum	860.0
	1000.0

The maximum amount of water that can be added to 100 g of such a base at a given temperature is known as the water number. To determine the water number, the base is stirred continuously as the water is being added. Distilled or deionized water should be used. The end point is reached when no more water can be "absorbed" into the base, as evidenced by droplets of water remaining in the container.

In a study involving the separate addition of a series of surfactants to a semisolid base, it was found that the water-absorbing capacity of the base increased as the HLB number (hydrophilic-lipophilic number) of the surfactant decreased[28] (see Table 18-1).

Hydrous lanolin was the prototype or forerunner of the absorption bases because of its ability to absorb water. Various absorption bases were developed as various lanolin isolates and derivatives became commercially available. Many of these lanolin fractions aid in the formation of water-in-oil emulsions. A typical example of a lanolin absorption base follows:

Formula #7
Lanolin Absorption Base

	%
Lanolin alcohols	10
Lanolin	25
Mineral oil, low viscosity	30
Purified water	35

Mineral oil is added to reduce the tackiness of the base. Nonionic water-in-oil emulsifiers, such as glyceryl monostearate, cholesterol, cetyl alcohol, and the sorbitan fatty acid derivatives, may be added for improved stability and water-absorbing capacity. These vehicles have "emollient" properties and deposit an oily film upon the skin. Examples of water-in-oil emulsion vehicles that utilize the absorption base principle are given in Formulas #8 and #9.

Formulas	#8* %	#9† %
Oil Phase		
Lanolin, anhydrous USP	3.1	15.0
Petrolatum, white, USP	25.0	—
Mineral oil, heavy	25.0	8.0
Beeswax (white wax, USP)	10.0	7.0
Sorbitan sesquioleate	1.0	—
Propylparaben	0.05	0.05
Amerchol CAB	—	20.0
Aqueous Phase		
Sodium borate, USP	0.7	—
Polyethylene glycol 1500	—	5
Methylparaben	0.15	0.15
Purified water	35.0	49.8

*Available from Hans Schott, Temple University, Philadelphia, PA.

†Available from Amerchol, a Unit of CPC International, Inc., Edison, NJ.

Procedure: Heat the oil phase to 70°C, and add the aqueous solution at 72°C to the oil phase, stirring continuously.

Cold cream base, which reportedly dates back to Galen, was the forerunner of these water-in-oil emulsion vehicles.

The cold cream type of emulsion frequently utilizes a borax-beeswax combination as the emulsifier, with mineral oil or a vegetable oil as the continuous phase. A protective oil film remains on the skin following the evaporation of the water. The slow evaporation of water gives the skin a cooling effect.

TABLE 18-1. *Determination of Water Numbers Using 10-g Samples*

Surfactant	HLB	Grams Water Absorbed		Water Number
		Sample 1	Sample 2	
(Control: White petrolatum)		0.40	0.40	4.0
Sorbitan monolaurate	8.6	5.21	5.41	53.1
Sorbitan monopalmitate	6.7	8.20	8.52	83.6
Sorbitan monostearate	4.7	10.59	10.17	103.8
Sorbitan monooleate	4.3	24.75	25.25	250.0
Sorbitan sesquioleate	3.7	29.84	31.04	304.4
Sorbitan trioleate	1.8	41.95	40.31	411.3

From Mendes, R.W., et al.: Drug Cosm. Ind., 95:34, 1964.

Semisolid water-in-oil emulsions of the borax-beeswax type frequently exhibit poor long-term physical stability. The development and large-scale commercial manufacture of water-in-oil emulsifiers have made it possible to prepare stable semisolids that are oily to the touch. Also, relatively nongreasy water-in-oil emulsions may be prepared by a judicious combination of raw materials.

Synthetic substances are replacing natural raw materials as the latter become restricted in availability. As an example, the supplies of natural beeswax have declined with the steady price rises that result from both supply and inflation. A number of synthetic beeswaxes have appeared with properties quite similar to the natural. Synthetic spermaceti types have replaced the natural grade since the latter was banned as a result of endangering the whale. Formula #10 illustrates the use of synthetic beeswax in a relatively nongreasy cold cream.

Hydrophilic ointment is an example of a water-in-oil absorption base type vehicle that does not have any lanolin or its derivatives in the formula.

Formula #11
Hydrophilic Ointment (USP XX)

	%
Methylparaben	0.25
Propylparaben	0.15
Sodium lauryl sulfate	10.00
Propylene glycol	120.00
Stearyl alcohol	250.00
White petrolatum	250.00
Purified water	370.00

Formula #10
Cold Cream[29]

		%
A	Purified water	34.60
	Borax	1.00
	Methylparaben	0.25
B	Light mineral oil	50.00
	Synthetic beeswax flakes	13.00
	Glyceryl monostearate, pure	1.00
	Propylparaben	0.15

Procedure: Dissolve the methylparaben and borax in water at 75 to 80°C. Dissolve the propylparaben in a well-mixed mixture of phase B heated to 75 to 80°C. Add phase A to phase B while stirring rapidly.

This ointment can be used as a vehicle for many drug substances, but is not a cosmetically elegant preparation. The high petrolatum content leaves an unctuous residue upon the skin that may be uncomfortable. Modification of the formulation by reducing the petrolatum content, and the addition of other emollients such as cetyl alcohol, hexadecyl alcohol, and fatty acid esters (isopropyl myristate or palmitate), can add cosmetic appeal to the preparation. The effect of such modifications on the activity of a drug substance incorporated in the base must be determined.

Formulas #12 and #13 represent different types of hydrophilic ointment bases.

Formula #12
Hydrophilic Ointment Base*

	%
Oil Phase	
Amerchol CAB*	50.0
Cetyl alcohol	2.0
Stearyl alcohol	2.0
Aqueous Phase	
Sodium lauryl sulfate	2.0
Water	34.0
Methyl gluceth-20	10.0
Preservative	q.s.

*Available from Amerchol, a Unit of CPC International, Inc., Edison, NJ.

Procedure: Add the water phase at 80°C to the oil phase at 80°C. Cool while mixing to just above congealing temperature.

Variations: For greater firmness, increase ratio of stearyl to cetyl alcohol.

Formula #13
Hydrophilic Ointment Base*

	%
Oil Phase	
Acetylated lanolin*	5.0
Mineral oil 70 vis.	5.0
Amerchol L-500*	10.0
Amerchol CAB*	15.0
Microcrystalline wax, 195°C	5.0
Cetyl alcohol	5.0
Brij 52†	6.0
Brij 58†	4.0
Aqueous Phase	
Water	40.0
Methyl Gluceth-20	5.0
Preservative	q.s.

*Available from Amerchol, a Unit of CPC International, Inc., Edison, NJ.

†Available from ICI Americas, Inc., Wilmington, DE.

Procedure: Add the water phase at 80°C to the oil phase at 80°C. Cool while mixing to just above congealing temperature.

Water-Removable Bases

The water-removable bases are oil-in-water emulsions and are referred to as "creams." The vanishing cream bases fall into this category. The vanishing creams are so termed because upon application and rubbing into the skin, there is little or no visible evidence of their former presence. Formulas for some typical van-ishing cream bases in which different types of emulsifiers are used are given in Table 18-2.

Removal of these creams from skin or clothing is facilitated by the oil-in-water emulsifiers they contain. Creams may be applied to moist skin lesions, since the oil-in-water vehicle tends to absorb any serous discharge. The water removable bases form a semipermeable film on the site of application following the evaporation of water. The semisolid water-in-oil emulsions, however, tend to form a hydrophobic layer on the skin.

Semisolid emulsions are intimate, relatively stable mixtures or dispersions of a hydrophilic phase with a lipophilic phase. The phase that is dispersed in the form of fine microscopic globules is referred to as the discontinuous or internal phase; the other is the continuous or external phase. The vanishing cream type vehicles are representative of the oil-in-water emulsions, whereas the absorption bases are generally water-in-oil emulsions.

Water-Soluble Bases

Water-soluble vehicles are prepared from mixtures of high- and low-molecular-weight polyethylene glycols, which have the general formula: $HOCH_2[CH_2OCH_2]_nCH_2OH$. The low-molecular-weight glycols in this category are liquids; those with a moderately higher molecular weight are somewhat unctuous; and the higher molecular weight polyethylene glycols are solids. Suitable combinations of high- and low-molecular-weight polyethylene glycols yield products having an ointment-like consistency, which soften or melt when applied to the skin. No water is required for their preparation. They are water-soluble because of the presence of many polar groups and ether linkages.

If the polyethylene glycol ointment has a high percentage of crystalline material, the softening and melting of the ointment rubbed onto the skin will not be as gradual as with petrolatum, since the crystalline material melts sharply with an increase in temperature. The polyethylene glycol ointments are much less occlusive than in water-in-oil emulsions of the absorption base type; they mix with skin exudates and are readily washed from the skin. The polyethylene glycol vehicles are softened by the addition of water, owing to solution of the glycols. The USP states that 5% of the polyethylene glycol 4000 may be replaced with an equal amount of stearyl alcohol when 6 to 25% of aqueous solution is to be added to the vehicle.

The "water-soluble" bases are also known as greaseless ointment bases. The compatibility of these bases with drug substances and their release rate must be evaluated for each class of drugs.

Pastes, Gels, and Jellies

Pastes are dispersions of high concentrations of insoluble powdered substances (20 to 50%) in a fatty or aqueous base. The fatty bases are less greasy as well as stiffer in consistency than ointments because of the large amount of powdered material present. These pastes adhere well to the skin and are of benefit in the treatment of chronic or lichenified lesions. Zinc gelatin paste, USP XX, for example, is used when a protective film on the skin is desired following the evaporation of water. Pastes provide a protective layer, and when covered with suitable dressings, prevent excoriation of the patient's skin by scratching.

Jellies are water-soluble bases prepared from natural gums such as tragacanth, pectin, alginates, and boroglycerin, or from synthetic derivatives of natural substances such as methylcellulose and sodium carboxymethylcellulose.

Gels are usually clear transparent semisolids containing the solubilized active substance. Carbomer 940 swells when dispersed in water in the presence of such alkaline substances as triethanolamine or diisopropanolamine to form a semisolid.

Formula #18

		%
A	Carbomer 940*	0.5
	Water	42.5
	Sorbitol 70% solution	2.0
B	Ameroxol OE 20†	10.0
	Solulan 98†	3.0
	Polyvinylpyrrolidone (PVP) K-30	1.0
	Triethanolamine	1.0
	S.D. alcohol #40	40.0

*Available from B.F. Goodrich Company, Cleveland, OH.

†Available from Amerchol, a unit of CPC International, Inc., Edison, NJ.

Procedure: Phase A—Disperse Carbomer 940 thoroughly in water with good stirring. Add sorbitol solution. Phase B—Add the Ameroxol OE 20 to the alcohol, warm to 35°C, and stir until uniform. Add Solulan 98, PVP, and triethanolamine consecutively, mixing after each addition. Add phase B to phase A with gentle mechanical mixing until gel forms.

Formula #19

	%
Carbomer 940	0.75
Purified water	34.25
Solulan 98*	3.00
S.D. alcohol #40	50.00
Diisopropanolamine, 10% in water	12.00

*Available from Amerchol, a unit of CPC International, Inc., Edison, NJ.

Procedure: Prepare a Carbomer slurry in water with gentle agitation, and add mixture of SDA #40 and Solulan mixture, mixing until no particles are visible. Neutralize carefully with diisopropanolamine solution to avoid incorporating air.

For greater firmness, increase the concentration of the Carbomer and diisopropanolamine.

Gels are also formed with celluloses such as hydroxypropylcellulose and hydroxypropylmethylcellulose. A popular over-the-counter benzoyl peroxide gel contains 6% polyoxyethylene lauryl ether, 40% ethyl alcohol, colloidal magnesium aluminum silicate, hydroxypropylmethylcellulose, citric acid, and purified water.

Ophthalmic Ointments

Semisolid ophthalmic vehicles frequently contain soft petrolatum, a bland absorption base, or a water-soluble base. The water-soluble base may be prepared with polyethylene glycols or with a water-soluble gum. Mineral oil is frequently added to petrolatum to lower its fusion point, but its addition introduces a problem of separation upon storage. Such oil separation may be prevented by the addition of small quantities of natural waxes such as ozokerite, ceresin, or microcrystalline wax. The amount of wax added should not appreciably raise the melting point of the base.

All materials used in the ophthalmic ointment should be impalpable to avoid eye discomfort and possible irritation. Ophthalmic ointments, especially when used on injured eyes, should be sterile.

Numerous variations of the aforementioned basic vehicles are possible because of the availability of new raw materials, which permit the pharmacist to vary his formulation to obtain the desired therapeutic effect and to make a semisolid that is both convenient and comfortable for the patient to apply. A minimal number of materials should be used in a semisolid dosage form, since fewer constituents reduce inventory, decrease the possibility of chemical interference with the analytic procedure, and decrease the

TABLE 18-2. *Formulas for Vanishing Cream Bases*

	#14 Anionic Stearate Emulsifier % By Weight	#15 Anionic Emulsifier % By Weight	#16 Nonionic Emulsifier % By Weight	#17 Cationic Emulsifier % By Weight[30]
Stearic acid	13.0	7.0	14.0	
Stearyl alcohol	1.0	5.0		
Cetyl alcohol	1.0	2.0	1.0	
Glyceryl monostearate				10.0
Isopropyl palmitate			1.0	
Lanolin				2.0
Methylparaben	0.10	0.10	0.10	0.1
Propylparaben	0.05	0.05	0.05	
Sorbitan monostearate			2.0	
Glycerin	10.0	10.0		15.0
Sorbitol solution [70%]			3.0	
Potassium hydroxide	0.90			
Sodium lauryl sulfate		1.0		
Polysorbate 60			1.5	
Stearyl colamino formyl methyl pyridinium chloride				1.5
Purified water. q.s. ad	100	100	100	100

danger of allergic reactions in unusually sensitive patients.

Many formulas for creams and ointments can be found in the scientific literature, formularies, and catalogs of chemical suppliers of emulsifiers and other raw materials. These formulas should only serve as a guide for developmental work, because many of them have not been checked for stability, ease of application, or ability to release the drug to the absorption site. The requirements of the drug should determine what materials are used. Only by subsequent experimentation can the typical problems regarding consistency, application, and stability be overcome.

In the past, many pharmaceutical semisolids used to treat skin disease lacked the elegance and aesthetic appeal of the better cosmetics and toiletries. However, the availability of a host of new and safe raw materials suitable for use as dermatologic semisolids has made it possible for the patient to apply to his skin a preparation that is therapeutically effective and cosmetically acceptable. For cosmetic appeal, the semisolid should be easy to apply and feel comfortable on the skin. It should not feel clammy, excessively moist, or too dry. When a protective film is formed or deposited on the skin, the film should not be tacky or excessively adhesive. All these properties may be summed up under the expression "pharmaceutical elegance."

Preservation from Microbial Spoilage

Chemical preservatives for semisolids must be carefully evaluated for their stability with regard to the other components of the formulation as well as to the container. Plastic containers may absorb the preservative and thereby decrease the quantity available for inhibiting or destroying the microorganisms responsible for spoilage. Some preservatives may sting or irritate the mucous tissues of the eye or nasal passages. Methylparabens and propylparabens tend to be more irritating when applied in the nose than quaternary ammonium compounds (e.g. benzalkonium chloride) or the phenylmercuric salts. Boric acid may be used in the ophthalmic preparations, but is omitted from products to be used in the nose because of possible toxic effects if absorbed in large quantities.

The preservatives are added to semisolids to prevent contamination, deterioration, and spoilage by bacteria and fungi, since many of the components in these preparations serve as substrates for these microorganisms. Several terms are used to describe microbial organisms associated with pharmaceutical and cosmetic products: "harmful," "objectionable," and "opportunistic."

The USP XX uses the term "harmful" to refer to microbial organisms or their toxins that are responsible for human disease or infection. Examples of organisms that must not be present in a product are given, namely, Salmonella species, Escherichia coli, certain species of Pseudomonas, including P. aeruginosa, and Staphylococcus aureus. An "objectionable" organism can cause disease, or its presence may interrupt the function of the drug or lead to the deterioration of the product. Organisms are defined as "opportunistic" pathogens if they produce disease or infection under special environmental situations, as in the newborn or the debilitated person. Included in the latter group are the aged, those undergoing extensive surgical or accidental trauma, and the compromised host, defined as those who are on antibiotic, anticancer, or immunosuppressive therapy. The newborn has increased susceptibility to gram-negative infections, while the other individuals have various forms of immunologic deficiency, which increase the susceptibility to infections. Recognized opportunistic pathogens are "objectionable."[31] The following objectionable organisms should not be present in a pharmaceutical or cosmetic product: P. putida, P. multivorans, P. maltophilia, Proteus mirabilis, Serratia marcescens, Klebsiella sp., Acinetobacter anitratus (Bacterium anitratum), and Candida sp.[32]

The success or failure of a preservative in protecting a formulation against microbial spoilage depends upon many factors. The interaction of the preservative with surfactants, active substances, other components of the vehicle, sorption by polymeric packaging materials, and product storage temperature may change the concentration of the unbound or free preservative in the aqueous phase.

Perfumes, high concentrations of glycerine, and electrolytes make the environment less favorable to microbial growth, thus enhancing the effectiveness of the preservatives. Preservative action appears to depend on the concentration of the free preservative in the aqueous phase. Surfactant solubilized preservative may be bound within the micelles and there inactivated, or on the contrary, the micelles may act as reservoirs of preservative in an actively preserved system.

The minimum inhibitory concentration of preservative necessary to prevent microbial spoilage may be estimated by (1) the use of experimentally determined physicochemical parameters such as the oil/water partition coefficient, concentration of surfactant, the number of independent binding sites on the surfactant, oil/water phase ratio, and concentration of free preservative in the aqueous phase;[33] (2) an ultracentrifuge technique;[34] and (3) direct dialysis.[33] These techniques provide an approximate

value for the minimum preservative concentration required for a formulation, but to ensure quality, the product must be tested for its ability to withstand accidental and deliberate microbial contamination.[35]

Preservative efficacy in a formulation is determined by the addition of pure or mixed cultures of microbial organisms to the finished preparation. The number of microorganisms initially present in the inoculated material is determined by plating aliquots of suitable dilutions. Table 18-3 gives the USP XX procedure and the investigational FDA procedure for topicals, including the organisms used, the levels of inoculum, sampling periods, and the measure of effectiveness. Various neutralizers for the preservative are added to the culture media to recover a maximum number of organisms. A TAT broth consisting of tryptone (2%), azolectin (0.5%), and polysorbate 20 (4%) has been found to be a suitable medium for topical products. Azolectin is a neutralizing agent for quaternary ammonium compounds and polysorbate 20 inactivates parabens. The samples should be tested at intervals for both slow-growing and rapidly proliferating organisms.

The USP XX has procedures for determining the microbial content of raw materials and finished products. Suitable limits on the number

TABLE 18-3. *Preservative Efficacy (High-Level Inocula Challenge) Tests*

A. USP XX Procedure
1. Organisms used: C. albicans, A. niger, E. coli, S. aureus, P. aeruginosa.
2. Inoculum: 0.1ml/20 ml; 100,000 to 1,000,000 cells/ml.
3. Sampling at 7, 14, 21, and 28 days following inoculation.
4. Effectiveness: vegetative cells not more than of 0.1% of initial concentrations by 14th day; concentration of viable yeasts and molds at or below initial concentration after 14 days; concentration of each test organism remains at or below these levels after 28 days.

B. Investigational FDA Procedure for Topicals
1. Organisms used: same as USP XX plus P. putida, P. multivorans, Klebsiella sp., S. marcescens.
2. Inoculum: 0.2 ml/20 ml; $0.8-1.2 \times 10^6$ cells/ml.
3. Sampling: weekly observations.
4. Effectiveness: vegetative cells <0.01% survival by 28 days; C. albicans <1% survival; A. niger <10% survival.
5. Re-inoculate: vegetative cells: $1-2 \times 10^5$ cells/ml; 0.1% survival in 28 days.

Modified from Bruch: Drug and Cosm. Ind., *110*:32, 1972.

and types of microorganisms have not been officially specified, however. All materials must be free of the harmful microorganisms listed in the USP XX. Manufacturers have set up their own microbiologic specifications suitable to their raw materials and finished products. A typical manufacturer's microbiologic specification may read as follows: (1) The material must be free of viable organisms restricted by the USP XX. (2) The total aerobic count must not be more than 5000 microorganisms per gram; (3) not more than 100 molds per gram; (4) not more than 100 yeasts per gram; and (5) not more than 90 coliforms per gram.

Microbiologic quality guidelines have been established by The Cosmetic, Toiletry and Fragrance Association, Inc.[36] These have been grouped according to product type:

1. Baby products—not more than (nmt) 500 microorganisms per gram or milliliter;

2. Products used about the eye—nmt 500 microorganisms per gram or milliliter;

3. Oral products—nmt 1000 microorganisms per gram or milliliter;

4. All other products—nmt 1000 microorganisms per gram or milliliter.

There is a further specification that the products must be free from microorganisms recognized "as harmful to the user as determined by standard plate count procedures."[36]

Limits on the maximal microbial content of potable and purified water are stated in the United States Public Health Service regulations.[37] The test is made for the presence of the coliform group of bacteria, since experience has shown that this group is a significant indicator of pollution. The membrane filter technique, as well as the fermentation tube method, is used for detecting and estimating the number of coliform bacteria present.

Raw materials of botanical or animal origin

that contain high levels of microorganisms must be treated before use to remove these contaminants. The greatest source of contamination in nasal jellies, for example, are the natural gums, but treatment of the thickener with ethylene oxide vapor destroys the bacterial and fungal contaminants. Tests for ethylene oxide residues should be made before using the material. The amount of allowable ethylene oxide residues have not been established. The residues are ethylene oxide (ETO), ethylene chlorohydrin (ETC), and the various monomeric forms of ethylene glycol (ETG). Bruch has stated: "Recent studies have shown the LD_{50} (Gm./Kg.) by different routes for different animal species to approximate the following: ETC > ETO > ETG (least toxic). Acute topical irritation studies show on Gm./Kg. basis that the activity is ETO > ETC > ETG."

The FDA has proposed the following:[38] "Each drug product of a type listed in this paragraph for which ethylene oxide is used as a sterilant in the manufacture of the finished product, its components, or its market container shall not, when tested as packaged in its market container, exceed the following residue levels . . . ." (See Table 18-4.)

The manufacturer cannot depend on the preservative or a type of sterilizing process, such as radiation sterilization or a liquid chemical sterilant, to eliminate organisms introduced during the manufacturing process or by contaminated raw materials. Though the microbiologic quality of a product may be high as a result of the sterilization process, endotoxins may be present as a result of lysing of the bacterial cells. Some endotoxins have been shown to be allergens. These substances should be absent from semisolids just as sterile products should be free of pyrogens. Methods for detection of endotoxins are being investigated.[39]

A manufacturer can lessen the microbial hazards in his products by following the Good Manufacturing Practices (GMPs) recommended by

TABLE 18-4. *Residue Limits of Ethylene Oxide and Derivatives (Parts per million)*

Drug product	Ethylene oxide	Ethylene chlorohydrin	Ethylene glycol
Ophthalmics (for topical use)	10	20	60
Injectables (including veterinary intramammary infusions)	10	10	20
Intrauterine device (containing a drug)	5	10	10
Surgical scrub sponges (containing a drug)	25	250	500
Hard gelatin capsule shells	35	10	35

From Federal Register, 43(122), June 23, 1978, part 221, p. 27482.

the FDA.[40] These procedures do not spell out the specific details that a manufacturer should follow to avoid contamination with microbial or foreign matter in pharmaceutical products. An interesting sanitary guideline was developed with the food industry in mind, but it is applicable to any industry in which sanitary procedures must be followed. The Sanitary Design Principles are in the form of a checklist covering many details, such as the construction of the manufacturing plant, processing and packaging equipment, floors, walls and ceilings, plant services, and the relative ease of cleaning both equipment and the environment.[41]

If the bacterial count in the finished product is high despite precautions taken to prevent contamination in the raw materials, including the water supply, then the pipelines, filling equipment, and containers must be checked for sources of contamination or interference with the activity of the preservatives. For example, some filling equipment may still contain some of the semisolid after rinsing or flushing of the equipment during the cleaning operation. In such cases, complete disassembly and thorough cleaning are mandatory.

The container may contribute to contamination by harboring bacterial spores, or by sorption or chemical interaction with the preservative, which thereby lowers its concentration in the preparation. Plastic containers, rubber seals, and closures have been shown to react with some preservatives.[42] Reduced preservative concentration also can occur through chemical complexation with the surfactant or gum as shown in Table 18-5.

In the presence of 5% polysorbate 80, 80% of the total methylparaben present in the aqueous phase is inactive.[44] Such inactivation also occurs with benzalkonium chloride, benzoic acid, cetylpyridinium chloride, dehydroacetic acid, and sorbic acid. The partial inactivation of the

preservative can be overcome by an excess of the same preservative, by the substitution of a noncomplexing preservative, or by the substitution of a noncomplexing emulsifier system.

The antibacterial or bacteriostatic activity of the preservative depends also on its partition coefficient. The preservative may partition between the oil and the aqueous phase, and if the preservative is more soluble in one phase than another, an additional quantity of the preservative must be added so that both phases are protected from microbial spoilage. Hence, methylparaben and propylparaben are frequently used in semisolids because of their better solubility in aqueous and oil phases, respectively.

Many of the preservative studies reported in the literature are performed in simple aqueous systems. It is comforting to know that the preservatives appear to be more effective in the finished formulations than indicated in the complexation studies. The interactions occurring in a complex emulsion system in a semisolid apparently do not apply.[45] However, in view of the fact that interaction of preservatives with macromolecules does occur, the finished formulation should be tested microbiologically for preservative adequacy.

The p-hydroxybenzoate esters are used in combination with one another because of their synergistic action. In general, they are employed at a concentration level approaching their maximum solubility in water. The solubilities of some commonly used preservatives are given in Table 18-6. The propyl or butyl ester is usually dissolved in the fat phase and should be increased for vehicles with a high fat content. Satisfactory protection of the emulsion against microbial growth may possibly be attained with sorbic acid, in which the p-hydroxybenzoate esters prove to be ineffective.[45]

The paraben esters of p-hydroxybenzoic acid are still popular as preservatives because their toxicity is low, they are odorless, they do not discolor, and they are nonirritating to the skin. On the negative side, the parabens have a low solubility in water and are less effective against gram-negative bacteria than molds and yeasts. Combining the parabens with phenoxyethanol,[47] or with imidazolidinyl urea (Germall II),[48] improves their activity against bacteria, yeast, and molds. The supplier* claims that the combination system retains activity against yeast and mold even when paraben activity has been diminished by interaction with nonionics or other substances in the formulation, or has

TABLE 18-5. *Degree of Binding of p-Hydroxybenzoate Esters by Various Macromolecules*

Macromolecule 2% w/v	Unbound Methylparaben %	Unbound Propylparaben %
Gelatin	92	89
Methylcellulose	91	87
Carbowax 4000	84	81
PVP	78	64
Myrj 52	55	16
Tween 20	43	14
Tween 80	43	10

From Barkley, E. L.: Am. Perf. Aromat., 73:33, 1959.

*Sutton Laboratories, Inc., Chatham, NJ

TABLE **18-6.** Solubilities of Some Preservatives in g/100 ml Solvent at 25°C

	Water	Mineral Oil	Propylene Glycol
Bithional	0.0004	1.0	0.5
Butyl-p hydroxybenzoate	0.02	S	110
p-Chloro-m-xylenol	0.0025	SS	1.5*
Dehydroacetic acid	0.10	0.01	1.7
Ethyl paraben	0.075		
Methyl-p-hydroxybenzoate	0.25	0.03	22
Propyl-p-hydroxybenzoate	0.06		26
Sorbic acid	0.2		5.5

S = soluble; SS = slightly soluble; * = in glycerin. These descriptive terms are approximate solubilities as defined in USP XX.

migrated into the oil phase. Germall II is used in concentrations of 0.1 to 0.5% alone or in combination with the parabens. It should be added to the product below 60°C.

The solid parabens may be difficult to incorporate into some formulations because of their low water solubility. A 50% by weight oil-in-water emulsion (Liqua Par*) has been marketed. The oil phase is a mixture of p-hydroxybenzoic acid esters: n-butyl, isobutyl and isopropyl. The aqueous portion contains water with emulsion stabilizers. The solubility of the active ingredients in water at 25°C is 0.06 g/100 g and is freely miscible with propylene glycol. The preservative should be added to the aqueous phase at a temperature not exceeding 70 to 75°C and stirred until thoroughly dissolved before the preparation of the emulsion. Paraben hydrolysis may occur if the temperatures exceed 80°C. The supplier recommends the use of a concentration ranging from 0.05 to 0.3% active ingredient.

Another preservative that is available is Dowicil 200f, which is described as a broad-spectrum antimicrobial effective against bacteria, yeast, and molds at concentrations of 0.02 to 0.3% weight. It is not inactivated by nonionic, anionic, or cationic formulation ingredients. The substance is extremely soluble in water but is virtually Insoluble in oils and organic solvents. Chemically, it is the cis isomer l-(3-chloroallyl)-3,5,7-triaza-l-azoniaadamantane chloride. The preservative should not be heated above 50°C and is unstable in solution below pH 4 and above pH 10. Discoloring of this material may occur, but can be prevented by the addition of sodium sulfite. Strong oxidizing or reducing agents should be avoided since these may adversely affect the antimicrobial efficacy.

Newer preservatives are being marketed, but all of these substances must be thoroughly evaluated for their effectiveness in the product, and their effect on the physicochemical stability of the product. As with all new dermatologicals under development, patch testing must be conducted to eliminate any possibility of skin irritation or sensitivity with the products containing these substances.

Rapid determination of preservative efficacy in semisolids can be done in 48 hours for bacteria and 7 days for molds.[49] The method utilizes the so-called D-value, or decimal reduction time, which is calculated from a plot of the log number of surviving organisms per gram against time of inoculation of the product with specific organisms. The D-value is a numerical value of rate of destruction of a particular organism in a specific product. Since it is a quantitative expression, it can be used to compare the rate of inactivation of different organisms in one or more products. The D-value permits the calculation of the time required for the complete destruction of any size population of organisms.

The method consists of inoculating the product with known amounts of the test organisms. The products are then sampled periodically to record the population of each test organism, and the log of the surviving organisms at each sample time is plotted. The slope of the line is determined by linear regression, and the negative reciprocal of the slope represents the D-value. The time predicted for complete destruction of the test organism in a product is calculated by linear estimate of the x-intercept. Figure 18-2 shows the effect of different concentrations of parabens on the death rate of Staphylococcus aureus in a cream.

The D-values for the control, the cream with the lower, and the cream with the higher concentrations of parabens were 18, 4, and 0.6 hr, respectively. The times predicted for the complete destruction of S. aureus in these samples were 63, 19, and 3 hr for the control, low-paraben-content cream, and high-paraben-

*MaUinckrodt, Inc., St. Louis, MO.
†Dow Chemical, U.S.A., Midland, MI.

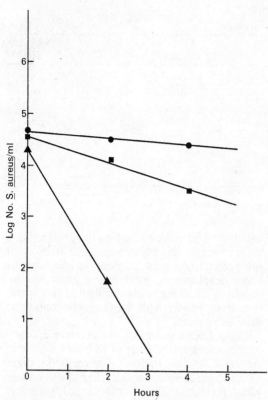

FIG. 18-2. *Survivor curves showing the effects of different concentrations of parabens on the rate of death of Staphylococcus aureus in a cream. Symbols: ●—●, cream with no parabens (control): ■—■, cream with 0.12% methyl- and 0.08% propyl-paraben; and ▲—▲, cream with 0.2% methyl- and 0.1% propyl-paraben. (From Orth, D. S.: J. Soc. Cosm. Chem., 30:321, 1979.)*

Antioxidants

Antioxidants are added to semisolids whenever oxidative deterioration is anticipated. The antioxidant system is determined by the components of the formulation, and the selection depends on several factors, such as toxicity, irritancy, potency,·compatibility, odor, discoloration, solubility, and stability. Often, two antioxidants are used, since the combination is often synergistic. Listed in Table 18-8 are some physical and chemical properties of antioxidants in common use. Acids such as citric, maleic, phosphoric, or tartaric may be added to the combination to chelate trace quantities of metals.

Industrial Processing

Pilot plant or small-scale production equipment is essential in developing a manufacturing procedure for a production-size batch. The preparation of many batches, ranging in size from 2.5 to 25.0 or more kilograms, for product evaluation and clinical testing provides opportunity to observe, correct, or improve the effects of minor but important variations in the manufacturing technique or formula. Mixing and stirring operations are critical in the preparation of emulsions, and in the laboratory these operations can be carefully controlled in 0.5- or 1.0-kg batches of finished product.

The electrically operated propeller-type mixer can be manually adjusted and positioned in the laboratory mixing vessel to achieve maximum turbulence. The angle of entry of the propeller shaft and the depth of the propeller can be easily varied in the laboratory to prevent aeration. A metal spatula can be held or positioned in the beaker during mixing to serve as a baffle to increase turbulence without entrainment of air. Similar maneuverability and control of the mixing action is more limited with larger stationary equipment used for the manufacture of semisolids. High-speed agitation may introduce air into the product, and slow mixing may not form a satisfactory emulsion.

Such problems occur in large-scale manufacture, but would not be apparent in small 1- or 2-kg batches for which a beaker and a laboratory mixer are used. Small-scale equipment similar to the production models can approximate production conditions. It may not be possible to predict the exact mixing time and rotational speed of the agitator, but the overall processing characteristics can be ascertained if identical mixers are used.

Aeration of the semisolid should be avoided,

content cream, respectively. The time required for the complete destruction of a specific organism of known population in a particular product may be predicted from the D-value. If the mean D-value for S. aureus in a product is 2.5 hr, the time for 10^6 S. aureus per milliliter to be totally inactivated is given by the product of the log number of the organisms per milliliter multiplied by the D-value, or 6×2.5 hr = 15 hr.

Table 18-7 shows the composition of the vehicles of several corticosteroid creams. It is designed to show how currently marketed semisolids utilize the principles described in the previous sections, namely, the different physiologically innocuous fatty materials used in the fat phase, the emulsifier systems, and the humectants, preservatives, antioxidants, and chelating agents.

since it may lead to emulsion instability and variation in density within a batch, resulting in weight variation of the ointment or cream in its container. Entrainment of air can occur during the mixing, homogenizing, or milling stage, during the transfer of the product to storage and/or filling equipment, and during the filling or packaging operation.

Aeration may be prevented at the primary emulsion step if one phase is introduced into the other in such a manner that splashing and streaming are avoided. The Incoming liquid should enter the mixing kettle below the surface of the other liquid. Vortexing and splashing are overcome by careful adjustment of the mixing conditions and liquid flow pattern.

Completely enclosed kettles are available for the manufacture of semisolids, which tend to aerate excessively. The sealed vessels can be operated under vacuum; mixing and emulsification can then be performed without entralnment of air. Loss of moisture and volatile substances may present problems, however, because of the vacuum.

A closed system prevents aeration of the product during homogenizatlon or milling, and when the material is transferred to the storage tanks, vessels, or hoppers of the filling machines. When an auger device or a wormdrive is used in the hopper to deliver the material to the tube or jar at the filling outlet, the hopper must be kept full of product, or the rotation of the auger will drive air into the semisolid.

Rheologic Changes. Homogenization frequently Increases the consistency of a semisolid emulsion because it increases the number of emulsified particles. It can also have the opposite effect, that of decreasing the viscosity of the product owing to an electrolyte effect. Some products retain their viscosity if they are not homogenized. Consistency also is affected by the number of passes through the homogenizer, the pressures used for homogenization with the valve-type homogenizer, or the clearance between the rotor and stator if a colloid mill is used.

Some commercial creams are sensitive to agitation and stress. The continuous rotation of an auger in the hopper of the filling machine may cause a cream to liquefy. Such creams may be made more resistant to agitation by a formula change; however, the soft and easy spreading properties of the cream on the skin may then be lost. The replacement of the auger by another, gender feeding device is of value.

Fusion Method. Anhydrous ointments are manufactured by the fusion process. The active substance is dissolved in the melted fats and waxes, or in one of the components of the vehicle, and then mixed with the base. The melted mass must be mixed while cooling because the fatty alcohols, fatty acids, and waxes do not form true solutions with petrolatum and mineral oil, but crystallize from the melt as the temperature falls.

Manufacture of Emulsions. Time, temperature, and mechanical work are the three variables in the manufacture of emulsified semisolids. The three factors are interrelated and must be carefully controlled if the same high-quality batches are to be manufactured repeatedly.

Equipment is available for automatically controlling many aspects of emulsion manufacture, such as the complete control of the temperature in the jacket and regulation of the mixing time and rate of agitation. If the volume warrants the cost, the entire operation can be automated. The kettles must be thoroughly cleaned before re-use because the presence of small quantities of foreign contaminants or the residue from a previous batch may have an adverse effect on the stability and quality of the emulsion.

Preparation of Oil and Aqueous Phases

The components of the oil or fat mixture are placed into a stainless steel steam-jacketed kettle, melted, and mixed.

Some of the solid components (e.g., stearic acid, cetyl alcohol) are available in many different forms: cakes, flakes, or powder. The flakes are preferable because of the convenience of handling. The powder may have occasional fine metal contaminants from the pulverizing equipment. Petrolatum is inconvenient to handle unless it is melted and transferred by pumping or pouring from its drum. Transfer of large quantities of petrolatum is expedited by heating the petrolatum in the steel drum in which it is received from the supplier by means of immersion heaters, or by placing the drums in a hot room (60 to 62°C) until the petrolatum is fluid. The liquefied petrolatum can then be transferred to the mixing kettle by metering pump through metal-reinforced inert plastic hoses and insulated pipes. The oil phase is then strained through several layers of cheese cloth to remove any foreign matter. Alternatively, the petrolatum can be passed through a filter medium, particularly for an ophthalmic preparation. The oil phase is transferred by gravity or pump to the emulsion mixing kettle whose walls have been

TABLE 18-7. Components of Some Typical Corticosteroid Cream Bases

	Cordram Cream	Kenalog Cream	Lidex Cream	Locorten Cream	Aristocort Cream	Oxylome Cream	Synalar Cream	Synalar Emollient Cream	Valisome Cream
Emulsifiers									
Sorbitan monostearate		X					X	X	
Sorbitan monooleate							X		
Sodium lauryl sulfate				X					
Polyoxyethylene sorbitan monostearate					X		X	X	X
Polyoxy 40 stearate	X								
Polyethylene glycol 100 monocetyl ether					X				
Polysorbate 80									
Fat Phase Components									
Glyceryl monostearate	X	X			X	X			
Cetyl alcohol	X	X		X				X	
Spermaceti		X			X	X			
Stearyl alcohol			X		X			X	
Stearic acid	X						X		
Petrolatum									X
Liquid petrolatum	X							X	X
Cetostearyl alcohol		X							X
Isopropyl palmitate					X				
Squalane									

Ingredient	1	2	3	4	5	6	7	8	9
Polyols									
Glycerin	X								
Propylene glycol		X		X			X	X	
Polyethylene glycol 400		X	X			X			
Polyethylene glycol 6000			X						
1,2,6 Hexanetriol									
Sorbitol solution					X				
Antimicrobial agents									
Methylparaben		X		X		X			
Propylparaben		X		X			X		
Ethylparaben	X								
Butylparaben						X			
4-chloro-m-cresol									X
Thimerosal								X	
Sorbic acid					X				
Potassium sorbate					X				
Buffering agents									
Citric acid			X	X			X	X	
Phosphoric acid									X
Monobasic sodium phosphate									X
Purified water	X	X			X		X	X	X

TABLE 18-8. *Commercial Antioxidants*

Common name	BHA	BHT	propyl gallate
Chemical name	(Butylated hydroxyanisole)	(Butylated hydroxytoluene)	
	3-t-butyl-4-hydroxyanisole	3,5-di-5-butyl-4-hydroxytoluene	alkyl gallate
	2-t-butyl-4-methoxyphenol	2,6-di-t-butyl-4-methylphenol	
Melting point	55°–60°C	70°C	150°C
Solubility at 25° in % [approx.]			
Propylene glycol	70	insoluble	55
Peanut oil	40	30	0.5

Modified from Rosenwald, R.H.: Am. Perf. Cos., 78:41, 1963.

heated to the temperature of the oil phase to prevent some of its higher-melting components from congealing. The components of the aqueous phase are dissolved in the purified water and filtered. A soluble drug may be added to the aqueous phase at this time, provided the high temperature does not degrade the active substance or the emulsion is not adversely affected; otherwise, the soluble drug may be added in solution after the emulsion has formed and has cooled.

Mixing of Phases. The phases are usually mixed at a temperature of 70 to 72°C, because at this temperature intimate mixing of the liquid phases can occur. The phase mixing temperature can be lowered a few degrees if the melting point of the fat phase is low enough to prevent the premature crystallization or congealing of its components. Decreasing the temperature at which the phases are mixed decreases the cooling time, which is a significant factor when the batch size is large. The properties of some emulsions (borax-beeswax type) depend on the temperature at which the phases are mixed. The initial mixing temperature must be raised above 70 to 72°C, because intimate mixing of the components at monolayer levels cannot occur, since the emulsion that forms immediately has a high viscosity. The phases can be mixed in one of three ways: (1) simultaneous blending of the phases, (2) addition of the discontinuous phase to the continuous phase, and (3) addition of the continuous phase to the discontinuous phase.

The simultaneous blending of the phases requires the use of a proportioning pump and a continuous mixer. This method of emulsification is satisfactory for continuous or large-batch operation. The second method may be used for emulsion systems that have a low volume of dispersed phase. The third process is preferred for many emulsion systems, since the emulsions undergo an inversion of the emulsion type during the addition of the continuous phase, which results in a finer dispersed phase globule. The disperse or aqueous phase in an oil-in-water emulsion is added slowly to the inner phase with agitation. The initial low concentration of water in relation to the concentration of oil results in the formation of a water-in-oil emulsion. The viscosity of the emulsion continues to increase as more water is added, and the volume of the oil phase also increases up to a point of its maximum expansion. Beyond this point, the viscosity decreases, and emulsion inversion is said to occur. The phases reverse themselves, and the inner phase is finely dispersed.

Batch sizes are on a weight basis, which is independent of variations in temperature and density. To measure the weight in a kettle, load cells are placed onto the bases of the manufacturing kettle. The kettle exerts a pressure on the cell, which is transmitted by means of a hydraulic force exerted by a layer of oil seated on a diaphragm and can be read on a dial or recorded. Figure 18-3 is a schematic presentation of a load cell. Figure 18-4 is a photograph of a manufacturing kettle resting on a load cell.

Cooling the Semisolid Emulsion. Following the addition of the phases, the rate of cooling is generally slow to allow for adequate mixing while the emulsion is still liquid. The temperature of the cooling medium in the kettle jacket should be decreased gradually and at a rate consistent with the mixing of the emulsion and scraping of the kettle walls to prevent formation of congealed masses of the ointment or cream, especially when the semisolid contains a large percentage of high-melting substances. Figure 18-5 is a photograph of a manufacturing kettle showing agitator and sweep blades. Aeration may occur if the semisolid thickens considerably upon cooling, and steps should be taken to prevent this. If perfume is to be added to an oil-in-water emulsion, it is best done while the mixture is at a temperature of 43 to 45°C to avoid chilling the emulsion and to facilitate dissolution of the perfume oil in the still incompletely congealed oil phase. The perfume may be added

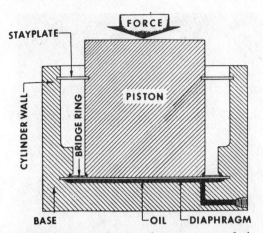

FIG. 18-3. *Schematic diagram of a cross-section of a hydraulic load cell. The hydraulic load cell is a frictionless piston and cylinder assembly with a fixed acting area. It is specifically designed for the conversion of force or weight into a proportional hydraulic pressure. This pressure may be connected to a dial indicator, a recorder, a controller, or transducers. (Courtesy of the A. H. Emery Company, New Canaan, CT.)*

near room temperature to a water-in-oil emulsion, since dissolution of the perfume oils is to occur in the outer phase of the system.

The drug is added in solution form, if not already incorporated, or as crystals, provided it is soluble in the external phase. An insoluble powder should be dispersed in the continuous phase

prior to removing the semisolid from the kettle for homogenization and/or storage. Figure 18-6 shows a Gifford-Wood homomixer after it has been withdrawn from a kettle used for dispersing solids. The cooling of the semisolid stored in a large covered vessel is not uniform, since cooling is more rapid at the surface or the walls of the container. Hence, variation in physical properties of the semisolid may occur, such as differences in the size of the fat and wax crystals and the dispersed globules.

Adjustment of the final water content of a water-in-oil emulsion is not easy once the emulsion has been formed. Several batch runs help to determine the amount of water lost on heating in the particular process, and this lost water should be added to the required amount at the start of manufacture. The oil film surrounding each emulsified water droplet in a water-in-oil emulsion tends to retard evaporation, so that water loss is not excessive following this type of emulsification.

Low-Energy Emulsification

The high cost of energy has prompted re-evaluation of manufacturing procedures in an attempt to limit the amount of thermal and mechanical energy expended in the production of emulsions. It has been shown that the use of a minimum amount of the emulsion phase in the

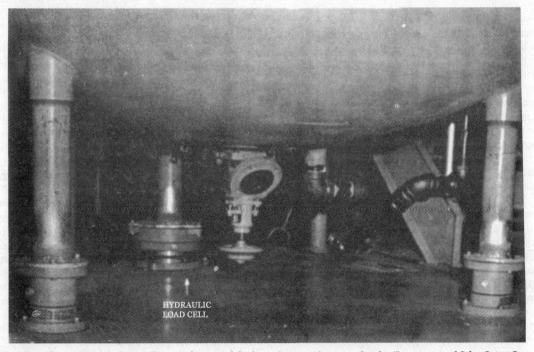

FIG. 18-4. *Photograph of a load cell set under one of the legs of a manufacturing kettle. (Permission of Ciba-Geigy Corp.)*

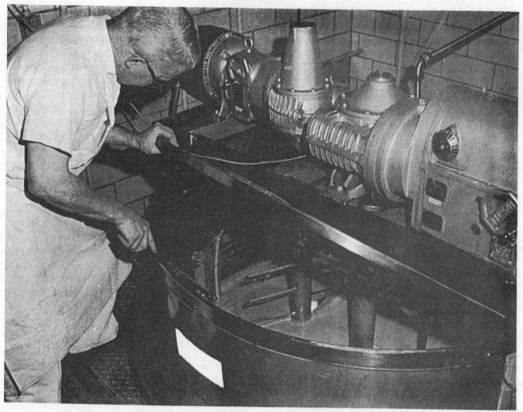

FIG. 18-5. *Stainless steel jacketed mixing kettle equipped with a slow-speed, anchor-type sweep blade agitator which takes the material from the side wall and swirls it around the secondary, bar-type mixer. The bar-type mixer rotates at a higher speed and directs the flow of material downward for thorough agitation. (Permission of Ciba-Geigy Corp.)*

emulsification stage can result in a considerable reduction in energy requirements and processing time without compromising the quality of the product. The major cost saving is achieved by heating both the oil phase and a portion of water or external phase to the required temperature to form a concentrated emulsion. The balance of the aqueous phase is added at room temperature during the cooling state. Thus, the energy used to heat the aqueous phase and the mechanical energy of mixing during the cooling stage are reduced.

Figure 18-7 illustrates the usual method of emulsion manufacture. The internal phase of an oil-in-water emulsion usually consists of fats, waxes, preservative, and perhaps an emulsifier. The external phase contains the water-soluble substances. Both are heated to a high temperature and then mixed to form an emulsion. The emulsion is then cooled. The low-energy method, illustrated in Figure 18-8, shows that a major portion of the aqueous phase, which may be as much as 70%, can be added at the cool

dilution stage. The savings in energy could be considerable.

The quality, stability, rheologic properties, and the particle size distribution of the internal phase of the finished product prepared by this process depend on several variables. These include the temperature required for forming the concentrated emulsion, the ratio of the external phase to the internal phase forming the concentrated emulsion, the phase inversion temperature, the type and intensity of mixing, and the rate of addition of the external phase.[50,51]

Homogenization. The creams or ointments that require further treatment are then transferred or pumped to the proper homogenizer, the selection of which is governed by the degree and rate of shear stress required. The choices include a low-shear gear pump, a roller mill, a colloid mill, a valve-type homogenizer, and a suitable sonic homogenizer. Uniform dispersion of an insoluble drug in a semisolid, as well as reduction of the size of the fatty aggregates can be attained by the passage of the warm (30 to 40°C)

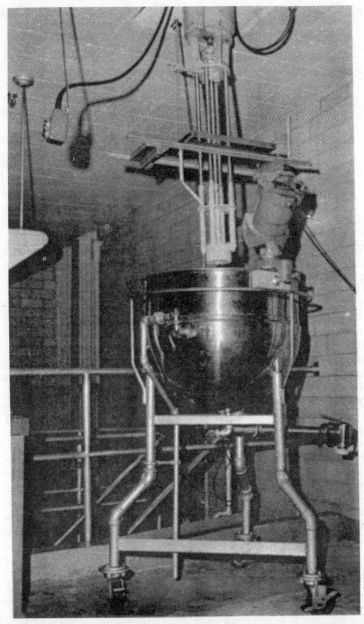

FIG. 18-6. *The high shear Homo-Mixer is attached to an electrically driven lift mechanism for raising or lowering it into the jacketed kettle used for dispersing solids in liquids. (Permission of Ciba-Geigy Corp.)*

ointment or cream through a homogenizer or mill.

Storage of Semisolids. Unless rapid in-process methods of analysis are developed, it is the usual practice to store the semisolid until the specified quality control tests have been completed before packaging into appropriate containers: tubes, jars, or single-dose packets. A product is considered to be "in-process" until it

has been packaged. These preliminary quality control tests are time-consuming and delay the packaging process; however, it is less costly to wait for the assay and to store the material until it can be scheduled for filling than to package and then perhaps be compelled to empty the containers to recover the material, should the semisolid fail to meet the established specifications for the product. Some semisolids have a

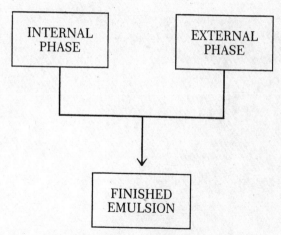

FIG. 18-7. *Conventional emulsion processing. (Modified from Lin, T.J.: J. Soc. Cosm. Chem., 29:745, 1978.)*

tendency to "set up" or exhibit an increase of viscosity on storage, and such products cannot be stored for any length of time. The industrial pharmacist must be aware of the delays caused by quality control requirements and packaging schedules, so that he can develop formulations that tolerate storage in bulk without undergoing marked changes in consistency which might cause filling problems. The active substance in the cream or ointment may react with the storage container unless a highly resistant #316, stainless steel, is used for bulk storage. Evaporation of water from a cream must be retarded; this can be effectively accomplished by placing nonreactive plastic sheeting in direct contact with the cream, as well as covering the storage container with a tight-fitting stainless steel lid.

Transfer of Material For Packaging. The semisolid may be gravity fed, if it is a two-level operation, or pumped to the filling equipment. It must be able to resist the shear stress developed in the transfer of the product, as well as that due to the mechanical action of the filling equipment.

Once a formal manufacturing procedure has been established, there should be no deviation from it. If a change is necessary, however, the problem should be carefully re-evaluated, first in the research and development laboratory and then at the pilot plant and manufacturing level.

Although the design and the evaluation of semisolids usually does not include the equipment cleaning operation following the manufacture and filling of the product, it is mandatory that the cleaning operation be thorough to avoid any contamination between batches. Cleaning of large-scale equipment is facilitated and labor costs and downtime of equipment can be reduced through the use of high-pressure (up to 1000 psi), low-volume pump systems now available. The cutting force of high-pressure hot water that may contain detergent can be applied like a knife edge to clean difficult-to-reach tight spots inside kettles and tanks and a variety of manufacturing and processing equipment, eliminating old-fashioned manual scrubbing. Homogenizers, pumps, and filling equipment that have areas wherein pockets of water or product may accumulate and that are ordinarily inaccessible must be completely disassembled, cleaned, sanitized, and dried before reassembly. Ball valves and sanitary (Ladish) type or sanitary threaded piping should be used throughout. The packing material used as lubricant for the shafts of mixers should also be replaced during the cleanup process if there is any possibility that they may harbor microorganisms. The manufac-

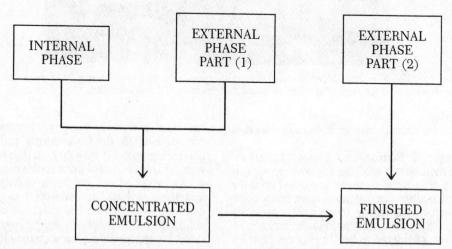

FIG. 18-8. *Low-energy emulsion processing. (Modified from Lin, T.J.: J. Soc. Cosm. Chem., 29:745, 1978).*

turing and packaging equipment should be sanitized following thorough cleaning with detergents. They should be flushed with chlorinated water, formalin, or other suitable sterilant followed by a bacteria-free water rinse. Water and swab samples should be taken to verify microbial elimination.

References

1. Flynn, G.L.: Percutaneous absorption. In Modern Pharmaceutics. Edited by G.S. Banker and C.T. Rhodes. Marcel Dekker, New York, 1979.
2. Scheuplein, R.J., and Blank, I.H.: Physiol. Rev., 51:762, 1971.
3. Scheuplein, R.J.: J. Invest. Derm., 46:334, 1965.
4. Blank, I.H.: J. Invest. Derm., 18:433, 1952.
5. Blank, I.H., Gould, E., and Theobald, A.B.: J. Invest. Derm., 42:363, 1964.
6. Wurster, D.E., and Kramer, S.F.: J. Pharm. Sci., 50:288, 1961.
7. Winsor, T., and Burch, G.E.: Arch. Intern. Med., 74:428, 1944.
8. Onken, H.D., and Moyer, C.A.: Arch. Derm., 87:584, 1963.
9. Stoughton, R.B.: Arch. Derm., 91:657, 1965.
10. Sweeney, T.M., and Downing, D.T.: J. Invest. Derm., 55:135, 1970.
11. Woodbourne, R.T.: Essentials of Human Anatomy, Oxford University Press, New York, 1965.
12. Scheuplein, R.J.: J. Invest Derm., 48:79, 1967.
13. Schutz, E.: Arch. Exp. Path. Pharmacol., 232:237, 1957.
14. Poulsen. B.J., Young, E., Coquilla, V., and Katz, M.: J. Pharm. Sci., 57:928, 1968.
15. Coldman, M.F., Poulsen, B.J., and Higuchi, T: J. Pharm. Sci., 58:1098, 1969.
16. Busse, M.J., Hunt, P., Lees, K.A., et al.: Brit. J. Derm., 81:103, Suppl. 4, 1969.
17. Poulsen, B.: Brit. J. Derm., 82:49, Suppl. 6, 1970.
18. Nugent, F.J., and Wood, J.A.: Canad. J. Pharm. Sci., 15:1, 1980.
19. Tregear, R.T.: The permeability of the skin to molecules of widely differing properties: In Progress in the Biological Sciences in Relation to Dermatology-2. Edited by A. Rook. University Press, Cambridge, 1964, p. 275.
20. Tregear, R.T.: Physical Functions of the Skin. Academic Press, New York, 1966.
21. Food and Color Additives Directory. Hazelton Laboratories, Inc., Falls Church, VA.
22. Franks, A.J.: Soap, Perf. and Cosm., 37:221, 319, 1964.
23. CTFA Cosmetic Ingredient Dictionary. 2nd Ed. The Cosmetic, Toiletry and Fragrance Association, Inc., Washington, DC.
24. The Rose Sheet. FDC Reports. Washington, DC, 2(37), Sept. 14, 1981, p. 8.
25. Ciullo, P.A.: Drug and Cosm. Ind., 126:50, 1980.
26. Shefter, E., and Higuchi, T.: J. Pharm. Sci., 52:781, 1963.
27. United States Pharmacopoeia XX, Mack Publishing Co., Easton, PA, 1980.
28. Mendes, R.W., Morris, R.N., and Brown, E.T.: Drug Cosm. Ind., 95:34, 1964.
29. Abrutyn, E.: Drug and Cosm. Ind., 126:46, 1980.
30. Strianse, S.J.: Hand creams and lotions. In Cosmetics: Science and Technology. Edited by E. Sagarin. Interscience, New York, 1957.
31. Bruch, C.W.: Drug and Cosm. Ind., 111:51, 1972.
32. Bruch, C.W.: Drug and Cosm. Ind., 110:32, 1972.
33. Kazmi, S.J.A., and Mitchell, A.G.: J. Pharm. and Pharmacol., 16:533, 1964.
34. Garrett, E.R.: J. Pharm. and Pharmacol., 18:589, 1966.
35. Kazmi, S.J.A., and Mitchell, A.G.: Soap, Perf. and Cosmetics., 45:549, 1972.
36. Microbiological Limit Guidelines for Cosmetics and Toiletries. Revised Aug. 18, 1972. The Cosmetic, Toiletry and Fragrance Association, Inc., Washington, DC.
37. Standard Methods for the Examination of Waste and Waste Water. 13th Ed. American Public Health Association, New York, 1971.
38. Federal Register, 43(122), June 23, 1978, part 221, p. 27482.
39. Evans, J.R., Gilden, M.M., and Bruch, C.W.: J. Soc. Cosm. Chem., 23:549, 1972.
40. Federal Register, 36:601, 1971.
41. Baur, F.J. (ed.): Sanitary design principles. Food Processing, January 1973.
42. Marcus, E., Kim, H.K., and Autian, J.: J. Am. Pharm. Assoc., Sci. Ed., 48:457, 1958.
43. Barkley, E.L.: Am Perf. Aromat., 73:33, 1959.
44. Patel, N.K., and Kostenbauder, H.B.: J. Am. Pharm. Assoc., Sci. Ed., 47:289, 1958.
45. Blaug, S.M., and Ahsan, S.S.: J. Pharm. Sci., 50:441, 1961.
46. Charles, R.D., and Carter, P.J.: J. Soc. Cosm. Chem., 10:383, 1959.
47. Boehm, E.E., and Maddox, D.N.: Amer. Perf. and Cosm., 85:31, 1970.
48. Berke, P.A., and Rosen, W.E.: J. Soc. Cosm. Chem., 31:37, 1980.
49. Orth, D.S.: J. Soc. Cosm. Chem., 30:321, 1979.
50. Lin, T.J.: J. Soc. Cosm. Chem., 29:117, 1978.
51. Lin, T.J.: J. Soc. Cosm. Chem., 29:745, 1978.

19

Suppositories

LARRY J. COBEN *and* HERBERT A. LIEBERMAN

A suppository is a medicated solid dosage form generally intended for use in the rectum, vagina, and to a lesser extent, the urethra. Rectal and urethral suppositories usually employ vehicles that melt or soften at body temperature, whereas vaginal suppositories, sometimes called *pessaries,* are also made as compressed tablets that disintegrate in the body fluids.

Oleum Theobromae was first recommended to American pharmacists by A. B. Taylor in 1852, and it soon grew in popularity as the suppository base of choice. Glycerinated gelatin mixtures did not appear as suppository vehicles until about 1875. In 1913, Bruno Solomon published a critical study of suppository bases, in which he classified them into three broad types: (1) cocoa butter, (2) fat and wax combinations with cocoa butter, and (3) glycerinated gelatin bases.

In the 1930s, several unwanted side effects and disadvantages inherent to oral therapy focused attention, principally in Europe, on the rectal route for administering drugs. Industrial concerns, principally in Germany and France, synthesized special lipid excipients, which were designed to replace cocoa butter. Water-soluble polyethylene glycol type bases were introduced as an improvement on glycerinated gelatin and lipid type suppository bases.

For the combined prescription and over-the-counter market, suppositories represent about 1% of all medications dispensed in the United States. The suppository is a far more popular medication in Europe and South America than in the United States.

Dose Characteristics

Opinion is mixed concerning the amount of drug that should be given rectally as compared with the oral dose. In general, for rectal administration, one-half to two or more times the oral dose is given for all but very potent drugs. The range in dose can be attributed to the availability of the drug from the particular suppository base used. The correct dose for any drug depends on the rate of release of the drug from the suppository. As a consequence, the suppository base and the amount of drug must be considered concomitantly. Since the vehicle can change the rate of drug absorption, the amount of drug to be given in suppository form depends on the vehicle and the chemical and physical form of the drug given.

Rectal suppositories for adults weigh about 2 g and are usually tapered to resemble a torpedo shape. Children's suppositories weigh about 1 g and have a corresponding reduction in size. Vaginal suppositories weigh about 3 to 5.0 g and usually are molded in the globular or oviform shape, or compressed on a tablet press into modified conical shapes. Urethral suppositories, sometimes called *bougies,* are pencil-shaped and pointed at one extremity. Urethral suppositories intended for males weigh about 4 g each and are 100 to 150 mm long; for females, they are 2 g each and usually 60 to 75 mm in length. Figure 19-1 illustrates a representative sampling of several commercially available suppositories.

Therapeutic Uses

Drugs may be administered in suppository form for either local or systemic effects. Such action depends on the nature of the drug, its concentration, and the rate of absorption. Emollients, astringents, antibacterial agents, hormones, steroids, and local anesthetics are dispensed in suppository form for treating local conditions of either the vagina, rectum, or urethra.

Many articles have been published recently

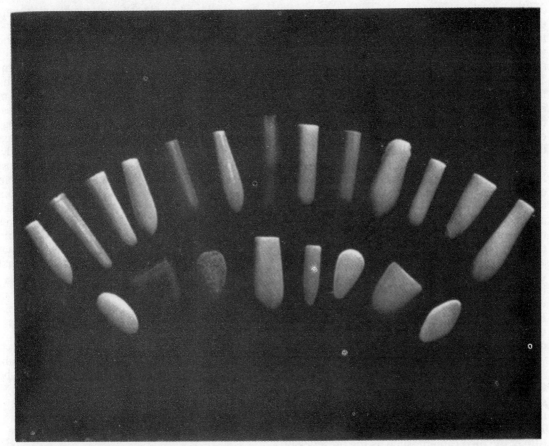

FIG. 19-1. *Types and shapes of suppositories.*

on the use of prostaglandin-containing vaginal suppositories for interruption of early pregnancy.

Rectal suppositories are primarily intended for the treatment of constipation and hemorrhoids. Suppositories are also administered rectally for systemic action. A wide variety of drugs are employed, e.g., analgesics, antispasmodics, sedatives, tranquilizers, and antibacterial agents.

Rectal suppositories are also utilized for systemic actions in conditions where oral medication would not be retained or absorbed properly, such as during severe nausea and vomiting or in paralytic ileus.

Factors Affecting Drug Absorption from Rectal Suppositories

Physiologic Factors

A number of drugs cannot be administered orally, because either the drugs are affected by the digestive juices, or their therapeutic activity is modified by the liver after absorption. After a drug is absorbed from the small intestine, the drug is carried by the hepatic portal vein to the liver. The liver modifies many drugs chemically and thereby often reduces their systemic effectiveness. On the other hand, a major portion of the same drugs can be absorbed from the anorectal area and still retain therapeutic values. The lower hemorrhoidal veins surrounding the colon and rectum enter into the inferior vena cava and thus bypass the liver. The upper hemorrhoidal vein does connect with the portal veins leading to the liver. More than half (50 to 70%) of rectally administered drugs were reported absorbed directly into the general circulation.[1] The lymphatic circulation helps also in absorbing a rectally administered drug and in diverting the absorbed drug from the liver.[2]

The pH of the rectal mucosa plays a significant rate-controlling role in drug absorption. Schanker reported that the rat colon has a pH of approximately 6.8, a pH slightly more acidic than previously believed.[3] Rectal fluids have virtually no buffer capacity, and as a consequence, the dissolving drugs determine the pH existing in the anorectal area. Schanker states that weaker acids and bases are more readily absorbed than the stronger, highly ionized ones. These findings suggest that the barrier separating the colonic lumen from the blood is preferentially permeable to the un-ionized forms of drugs. Thus, the absorption of a drug would be enhanced most likely by a change in the pH of the rectal mucosa that would increase the proportion of un-ionized drug. The effect of intraluminal pH on the absorption of several acidic and basic drugs is shown in Table 19-1.

As shown in Table 19-1, absorption of acidic drugs was markedly increased when the pH of the surrounding fluids was lowered. The absorption of salicylic acid rose from 12% at a pH of approximately 7 to 42% at pH 4. In contrast, with a basic drug like quinine, which becomes more ionized at the lower pH values, absorption was decreased from 20% at pH 7 to 9% at pH 4. Phenol is a weak acid and is almost completely un-ionized at both pH 7 and pH 4. Consequently, there was little change in absorption when the pH was lowered.

Riegelman and Crowell have demonstrated that one of the rate-limiting steps in drugs absorption is the diffusion of the drug to the site on the rectal mucosa at which absorption occurs. This diffusivity is influenced not only by the nature of the medicament, such as the presence of surfactant or the water-lipoidal solubility of the drug, but also by the physiologic state of the colon, that is, the amount and chemical nature of the fluids and solids present.

The state of the anorectal membrane also plays a role in drug absorption.[4] This membra-nous wall is covered with a relatively continuous mucous blanket, which can act as a mechanical barrier for the free passage of drug through the pore space where absorption occurs.

Drugs absorbed from the small and large intestines would most likely be absorbed from the anorectal area. The similarity in the patterns of drug absorption from the small and large intestines makes it unlikely that a drug that has passed through the small intestine would be significantly absorbed from the colon.[5] Conversely, a drug that can be absorbed from the colon most likely would have been completely absorbed in the small intestine before reaching the colon.

It should be recognized that although average body temperature is 37°C, patient temperatures may vary from 36 to 38°C, owing to daily and monthly cycles. The suppository formulator must bear in mind the lower limit as a "worst case."

Physicochemical Characteristics of the Drug

The sequence of events leading to drug absorption from the anorectal area can be diagramatically represented as follows:

Drug in vehicle $\longrightarrow$ Drug in colon fluids $\longrightarrow$ Absorption through the rectal mucosa

In order for the drug to be available for absorption, it must be released from the suppository and distributed by the surrounding fluids to sites of absorption. By dissolving in the fluids, there is wide contact of the drug with the lumen walls, thereby increasing drug contact with a large number of absorption sites. If the drug has a lipid-water coefficient favoring fat solubility, the drug is released slowly from its suppository excipient. Allawala and Riegelman report that a drug that is very soluble in cocoa butter and present in low concentration does not escape to the surrounding aqueous solution as readily as the drug that is slightly soluble in the cocoa butter vehicle and present at levels at or close to saturation.[6] Thus, water-soluble, oil-insoluble salts are preferred in fat-base suppositories. For water-soluble suppository type bases, from which the drug is released as the vehicle dissolves, the water-soluble type salt is the one of choice for quicker drug absorption. For example, to increase the absorption rate from suppositories, ephedrine sulfate and quinine hydrochloride, as well as sodium barbital and sodium salicylate, are preferred to their corresponding bases and acids.

TABLE 19-1. *Effect of Intraluminal pH on Absorption from the Rat Colon*

Drug	pKa	pH of the Perfusion Solution	
		6.8–7.2*	3.6–4.0†
Acid		% Absorbed	% Absorbed
Salicylic	3.0	12	42 ± 3
Benzoic	4.2	19	50 ± 7
Phenol	9.9	36	37 ± 1
Base			
Aniline	4.6	44	32 ± 5
Quinine	8.4	20	9 ± 1

*The solution, which entered the colon with a pH of 7.2 and left with a pH of 6.8, is a weakly buffered saline solution.

†This highly buffered solution entered the colon with a pH of 3.6 and left with a pH of 4.0.

The rate-limiting step in drug absorption from suppositories is the partitioning of the dissolved drug from the melted base and not the rate of solution of the drug in the body fluids. Riegelman and Crowell have shown that the rate at which the drug diffuses to the surface of the suppository, the particle size of the suspended drug, and the presence of surface-active agents are factors that affect drug release from suppositories.[4] Solution of the drugs in solid polyethylene glycol and oleaginous bases resulted in prolonged absorption times, because the drug is slowly eluted into the surrounding fluids. As would be expected, the larger the particle size, the slower the rate of solution, and as a consequence, the drug absorption rate is decreased with an increase in drug particle size. Surfactants can both increase and decrease drug absorption rate. For instance, in the case of sodium iodide, absorption is accelerated in the presence of surfactants and appears to be proportional to the relative surface tension lowering of the vehicle. In addition, Riegelman and Crowell state that the acceleration of sodium iodide absorption might also be attributed to the mucus-peptizing action of the vehicle.[4] The rectal membrane is covered by a continuous mucous blanket, which may be more readily washed away by colonic fluids that have reduced surface tension. The cleansing action caused by the surfactant-containing vehicle may make additional pore spaces available for drug absorption, thus facilitating drug movement across the rectal membrane barrier. In the case of phenol-type drugs, absorption rate is decreased in the presence of surfactant, probably because of the formation of a drug-surfactant complex.

Schanker showed that the absorption of several acid and base compounds in solution, as in a retention enema, was not affected over a 10-fold range of concentration. In the case of the retention enema, the absolute amount of drug absorbed was directly proportional to the initial saturation concentration present and not to any excess beyond this amount. If the luminal concentration of drug is above a particular amount, which varies with the drug, the rate of absorption does not change with further increases in drug. Thus, colonic absorption of drugs is a matter of simple diffusion across the colonic membrane. In suppositories, however, concentration does play a role in determining the rate of release of the drug from suppository bases.

Once the drug is released from the suppository base and reaches the site of absorption on the lumen wall, the lipid-soluble undissociated drug is the most readily absorbed form. Completely ionized drugs like quaternary ammonium compounds and sulfonic acid derivatives are poorly absorbed. Un-ionized substances that are lipid-insoluble also are poorly absorbed.[3]

The relation between the degree of ionization and the rate of absorption of drugs is illustrated in Table 19-1. Weak acids with a pKa below 4.3 and weak bases with a pKa below 8.5 are usually readily absorbed.[3] Highly ionized compounds are poorly absorbed. Acids having pKa values below 3.0 and pKa values for bases above 10.0 (quaternary ammonium salts) indicate negligible absorption rates. This relation suggests that the anorectal and colonic mucosae are selectively permeable to the uncharged drug molecule, whereas the ionized drugs penetrate the mucosa poorly or negligibly. Thus, drug absorption can be increased by the use of buffer solutions or salts that convert the pH of the anorectal area to a value that increases the concentration of un-ionized drug.

In summary, absorption of drugs from the anorectal area is affected by such physiologic factors as colonic contents, circulation, pH, lack of buffering capacity, physiologic state, and the mucous blanket on the lumen wall. The physicochemical characteristics of drugs affecting absorption are the lipid/water partition coefficient and the degree of ionization. When the amount of drug in the rectal fluids is above the rate-determining level, marked increases in drug concentration play no role in altering established drug absorption rates. Drug concentration is related, however, to release rates from suppository bases. The presence of surfactant may or may not aid absorption, depending on concentration and possible interaction with the drug. Drug particle size is directly related to absorption rate.

Physicochemical Characteristics of the Base and Adjuvants

Various properties of the suppository base can affect drug absorption. Heinmann et al. reported that with use of sodium phenobarbital, the absorption rate is faster from fatty bases having a lower melting range than from those with higher melting ranges.[7] It was also shown that absorption rate increases along with hydroxyl values. Pasich et al.,[8] using polyethylene glycol bases, showed a decrease in absorption time with increase in the molecular mass of the polyethylene glycols (PEGs) used.

Since fatty bases may harden for several months after molding, this rise in melting range certainly would affect absorption (see "Examples of Typical Stability Problems," presented later in this chapter).

Adjuvants in the formula can affect drug absorption through changes in the rheologic properties of the base at body temperature, or by affecting the dissolution of the drug in the media of the dosage form.

In emulsion type bases, it was shown that the amount of water-soluble drug released increased with the water content of the base, and that the rate of drug released could be prolonged by the addition of an aqueous polymer.[9]

Addition of hydrophobic colloidal silicon oxide to fat base suppositories dramatically changed the rheologic behavior of the mass.[10]

Salicylates were found to improve the rectal absorption of water-soluble antibiotics in lipophilic bases.[11]

Drug release from cylindric hydrogels of hydroxyethyl methacrylate decreased as increasing percentages of the cross-linking agent ethylene glycol dimethacrylate were used.[12] (See "Unusual Types of Suppositories," in this chapter.)

Blood Levels From Different Dosage Forms

The literature is replete with conflicting information concerning the effectiveness of drugs administered in suppository form. The information is difficult to correlate because of different or inadequate methods for determining blood levels, the nature of the drug and the suppository base, as well as the inability of many patients to retain the suppository. In some studies, blood levels from suppositories were obtained, and in some of these studies, these blood levels were considered therapeutically effective.

Rudolfo et al. reported on blood levels resulting from the oral, rectal, and intravenous administration of theophylline derivatives (Fig. 19-2).[13] Rectal retention enemas and intravenous injections showed that these two routes are similarly effective if allowance is made for the approximately 30-min delay required for drug absorption from the rectum.

The fact that the rectum or colon is a dependable site for drug absorption seems well established, but not all investigators agree that the suppository dosage form yields therapeutically adequate blood levels. Several investigators report adequate absorption of drug from suppositories. Enesco and co-workers made a comparative study on the absorption time of six drugs, namely sodium salicylate, chloral hydrate, methylene blue, atropine, morphine, and sodium iodide.[14] The first five drugs are absorbed rectally more quickly and at therapeutically more effective levels than with oral administration. Ab-

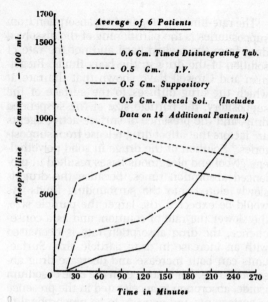

FIG. 19-2. *Plasma concentration of theophylline following single dose of theophylline monoethanolamine (gamma per 100 ml). (From Rudolfo et al.[13])*

sorption of sodium iodide is slower by the rectal route than by the oral route, but varies considerably from one individual to another. Shichiri et al. reported increased intestinal absorption of insulin from a suppository.[15] Copsidas and Ward-McQuaid found pentazocine suppositories equal in relief of moderate pain to pethidine injections and saw less side effects with the suppository.[16] Turrell, Marino, and Nerb report the same dosage requirement for sulfanilamide in glycerinated gelatin suppositories as in tablets.[17] Higher concentrations of the sulfonamide are found in the blood following its administration by enema than by suppository. Thus, in some cases, the suppository does yield effective therapeutic blood levels, although the enema yields faster and higher concentrations of drug in the blood. To maintain the therapeutic effectiveness of a drug in a suppository requires, therefore, a wise choice of both the drug salt and the suppository base.

Types of Suppository Bases

A variety of substances have been used as suppository bases throughout the history of medicine. Their uses and applications were prompted by availability rather than scientific knowledge. More exacting requirements and specifications were applied, however, to this area of pharmaceutical dosage form in the past decades. The use of chemical and physical measurements has provided the yardsticks with which to set standards for suppository bases, as well as for the finished suppositories, and some of these parameters are included with the bases given in Table 19-2.

Specifications for suppository bases usually include any number of the following.

1. Origin and Chemical Composition. A brief description of the composition of the base reveals the source of origin (i.e., either entirely natural or synthetic, or modified natural products) and chemical makeup (i.e., compound, or a well-defined or poorly elucidated mixture). Physical or chemical incompatibilities of the base with the other constituents may be predicted if the exact formula composition is known, including preservatives, antioxidants, and emulsifiers.

2. Melting Range. Since fatty suppository bases are complex mixtures of triglycerides and therefore do not have sharp melting points, their melting characteristics are expressed as a range indicating the temperature at which the fat starts to melt and the temperature at which it is completely melted. Although the "melting range" is usually determined by the USP method, manufacturers of bases occasionally use different methods for determining melting characteristics, such as "Wiley melting point," "capillary melting point," "softening point," "incipient melting (or thaw) point," and others.[18]

3. Solid-Fat Index (SFI). From this graph of the percentage of solids versus temperature, one can determine the solidification and melting ranges of fatty bases as well as the molding character, surface feel, and hardness of the bases (see Fig. 19-3).

A base with a sharp drop in solids over a short temperature span proves brittle if molded too quickly. This type of base requires a reduced differential between mold temperature and mass temperature for trouble-free molding. Suppository hardness can be determined by the solids content at room temperature. Since skin temperature is about 32°C, one can predict a product that would be dry to touch from a solids content over 30% at that temperature.

Since SFI is determined by dilatometry, which necessitates melting the base to carry out measurements, this set of data is reflective only of the base immediately after molding and not of an equilibrium or hardened state. (See "Examples of Typical Stability Problems," in this chapter.)

4. Hydroxyl Value. This is a measure of unesterified positions on glyceride molecules and reflects the monoglyceride and diglyceride content of a fatty base. The number represents

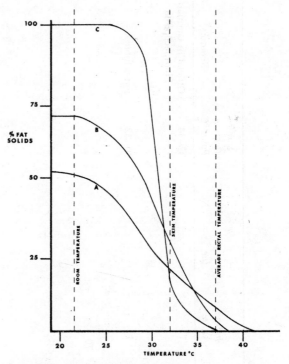

FIG. 19-3. *Typical solid-fat indices.*

the milligrams of KOH that would neutralize the acetic acid used to acetylate 1 g of fat.

5. Solidification Point. This value allows prediction of the time required for solidifying the base when it is chilled in the mold. If the interval between the melting range and solidification point is 10°C or more, the time required for solidification may have to be shortened by augmenting refrigeration to produce a more efficient manufacturing procedure.

6. Saponification Value. The number of milligrams of potassium hydroxide required to neutralize the free acids and saponify the esters contained in 1 g of a fat is an indication of the type (mono-, di-, or tri-) glyceride, as well as the amount of glyceride present.

7. Iodine Value. This value expresses the number of grams of iodine that reacts with 100 g of fat or other unsaturated material. The possibility of decomposition by moisture, acids, and oxygen (which leads to rancidity in fats) increases with high iodine values.

8. Water Number. The amount of water, in grams, that can be incorporated in 100 g of fat is expressed by this value. The "water number" can be increased by the addition of surface active agents, monoglycerides, and other emulsifiers.

9. Acid Value. The number of milligrams of potassium hydroxide required to neutralize the

TABLE 19-2. *Suppository Bases*

Name	Supplier	Composition	Melting Range °C	Saponification Value	Iodine Value	Hydroxyl Value	Water No.	Solidification Point °C	Remarks
Adeps Solidus		Triglycerides of saturated fatty acids with mono- and diglycerides	33.5–35.5	225–240	<7			32–34	Official in German Pharmacopoeia
Cebes Pharma 16	Aarhus Olifabrik, A/S, Aarhus, Denmark	Modified palm kernel oil	33–35	240–250	<1			30–32	Fat-soluble
Cotomar	Procter and Gamble, Cincinnati, OH	Partially hydrogenated cottonseed oil	37	191	70				
S-70-XX95 S-70-XXA	Best Foods/Refined Oils, Div. of CPC International, Englewood Cliffs, NJ	Rearranged hydrogenated vegetable oils	34.4 35.6 38.2 39.3						
Hydrokote 25	Capital City Products Company, Columbus, OH	Higher melting fractions of coconut and palm kernel oil; upon request, may contain 0.25% lecithin	33.6 36.3	235–245	<4			31–33	Narrow melt. range
Hydrokote 711			39.5 44.5	230–240	<4			35–37	Broad melt. range
Hydrokote SP			31.1 32.3	245–255	<6			30–32	Sharp melt. range
Idropostal (water-soluble)	Medifarma, Milan, Italy	Condensation product of polyethylene oxide	53–60	<1			Sol.	50	Water-soluble; in powder form
Kaomel	Durkee Foods, Rockville Center, NY	Fractionated Hydrogenated Triglycerides	35–38	194	59	<10			
Massa Estarinum A	Edelfett-Werke Werner Schluter, Hamburg, Germany (Kay-Fries, Inc., Montvale, NJ)	Mixture of tri-, di-, and monoglycerides of saturated fatty acids $C_{11}H_{23}COOH$ to $C_{17}H_{35}COOH$	33–35	225–240	<1	35–45	30–40	29–31	Emulsifies aqueous solution; delayed release for drugs with local effect

Name	Manufacturer	Composition							Remarks
Massa Estarinum AB			29–31	235–245	<3	25–40		26.5–28.5	Low melting mass for melting point correction
Massa Estarinum B			33.5–35.5	225–240	<3	20–30		31–33	Melts below body temperature; universal base
Massa Estarinum C			36–38	225–235	<3	20–30		33–35	For addition to drugs that lower melting-point; for tropical climates
Massa Estarinum D			40–42	220–230	<3	30–40		38–40	High melting base
Massa Estarinum E			34–36	215–230	<3	45–60		30–32	Emulsifies water, alcohol, glycerin
Massa Mf 13 (fat-soluble)	Medifarma, Milan, Italy	Mixture of di- and triglycerides of saturated fatty acids	36–37	225–235	2–3			33–35	Fat-soluble; specific weight 0.93–0.94
Massuppol 15	Croklaan, B. V., Wormerveer, Holland		34–37	230–240	<3		50–100	29.5–31.5	For compression and molding; especially suitable for mass production; fat-soluble
Neosuppostal-N (fat-soluble and water-dispersible)	Medifarma, Milan, Italy	Hydrogenated triglyceride with fatty alcohols and emulsifiers	37–38	112	9–11		unlimited	36–37	Suitable also for vegetable extracts; compatible with antibiotics and vitamins
Paramount B	Durkee Foods, Rockville Center, NY	Hydrogenated interesterified vegetable oils	34.5–35.5	235–245	<3	<10			
Satina III		Fractionated hydrogenated triglycerides	33–35	242	1	<10			
Suppocire AIML	Establissements Gattefosse, Paris, France (Gattefosse Corp.,	Eutectic mixtures of mono-, di-, and triglycerides derived from nat-	33–35	225–245	<2	20–30			
Suppocire AM			35–36.5	225–245	<2	<6			
Suppocire AP			33–35	200–220	<1	30–50			
Suppocire BS2X			36–37.5	220–240	<3	15–25			

TABLE 19-2. *Suppository Bases (Continued)*

Name	Supplier	Composition	Melting Range °C	Saponification Value	Iodine Value	Hydroxyl Value	Water No.	Solidification Point °C	Remarks
Suppocire NA$_0$	Elmsford, NY	ural vegetable oils	35.5–37.5	225–245	<2	<3			For light and voluminous additives
Novata Type AB	Henkel International Dusseldorf, Germany (Henkel, Inc. Teaneck, NJ)	Mixture of tri-, di- and monoglycerides of saturated fatty acids	29–31	235–245	<3			26.5–28.5	
Type A			33.5–35.5	225–240	<3			29–31	For extreme cooling
Type B			33.5–35.5	225–240	<3			31.5–33.5	Standard for retail pharmacy work
Type BC			33.5–35.5	225–240	<3			30.5–32.5	Good elasticity; for industrial production
Type BD			33.5–35.5	225–240	<3			32–34	Low hydroxyl value; relatively nonreactive
Type BBC			34–36	225–240	<3			30.5–32.5	For automatic processing
Type E			34–36	215–230	<3			29–31	Emulsion-type; for water pickup
Type BCF			35–37	225–240	<3			30–32	For heavy crystalline substances
Type C			36–38	225–235	<3			33–35	For drugs with lower melting point; also for tropical use
Novata Type D			40–42	220–230	<3			38–40	For increasing melting point
Type 229			33.5–35.5	240–255	<3			31.5–33.5	For groups that react with hydroxyl groups

Suppostal-N	Meditarma, Milan, Italy	Hydrogenated triglyceride with fatty alcohols and emulsifiers	37–38	98	16–18	54	36–37	Compatible with chloral hydrate and other eutectic substances; fat-soluble
Suppostal-Es			38–39	99	18–20	50	37–38	Takes up essential oils, balsams; fat-soluble
Wecobee W	PVO International, Inc., Boonton, NJ	Triglycerides	31.7–32.8	242–252	<4	30–40	30–31	Narrow melting range
Wecobee R		Higher melting fractions of coconut oil and palm kernel oil (may contain 0.25% lecithin)	33.9–35	236–246	<4	30–40	31–32	Narrow melting range
Wecobee S			38–40.5	236–246	<4	30–40	32–34	Broad melting range above body temperature
Wecobee M			33.3–36	238–248	<3	30–40	29–31	Narrow melting range; low melting point
Wecobee FS			39.4–40.5	236–248	<3	30–40	32–34	Narrow melting range above body temperature
Witepsol H12	Dynamit Nobel, Koln-Mulheim, Germany (Dynamit Nobel of America, Northvale, NJ)	Triglyceride of saturated vegetable fatty acids with monoglycerides (formerly marketed as "Imhausen bases")	32.3–33.5	240–245	<7	100	29–31	Universal base for industry
Witepsol H15			33.5–35.5	230–240	<7	100	32.5–34.5	Universal base for industry; higher melting point
Witepsol W35			33.5–35.5	225–235	<7		29–32	Suitable for quick cooling, small-scale production

TABLE 19-2. Suppository Bases (Continued)

Name	Supplier	Composition	Melting Range °C	Saponification Value	Iodine Value	Hydroxyl Value	Water No.	Solidification Point °C	Remarks
Witepsol S55			33.5–35.5	220–230	<7			29–32	Good dispersibility for vaginal suppository
Witepsol E75			37–39	220–230	<7		45	32–34	Special high melting point for eutectic mixtures and tropical suppositories
Witepsol E85			42–44	220–230	<7		45		
Polyethylene Glycols	Dow Chemical Co., Midland, MI; Union Carbide Chemicals Co., Dallas, TX	Linear polymers of ethylene oxide							
1000			38–41				Sol.	38	Soft, waxy
1450			42–47				Sol.	42	Solid
4000			40–48				Sol.		
6000			49				Sol.		
Tween 61	ICI Americas Inc., Wilmington, DE	Polyethylene glycol sorbitan mono-stearate	35–49	95–115		165–195			Used alone or in combination with fats or emulsified bases; waxy consistency

free acid in 1 g of substance is expressed by this value. Low "acid values" or complete absence of acid are important for good suppository bases. Free acids complicate formulation work, because they react with other ingredients and can also cause irritation when in contact with mucous membranes.

The Ideal Suppository Base

The ideal suppository base may be described as follows. (1) Having reached equilibrium crystallinity, the majority of components melt at rectal temperature 36°C but bases with higher melting ranges may be employed for eutectic mixtures, addition of oils, balsams, and suppositories intended for use in tropical climates. (2) The base is completely nontoxic and nonirritating to sensitive and inflamed tissues. (3) It is compatible with a broad variety of drugs. (4) It has no metastable forms. (5) It shrinks sufficiently on cooling to release itself from the mold without the need for mold lubricants. (6) It is nonsensitizing. (7) It has wetting and emulsifying properties. (8) The "water number" is high, i.e., a high percentage of water can be incorporated in it. (9) It is stable on storage, i.e., does not change color, odor, or drug release pattern. (10) It can be manufactured by molding by either hand, machine, compression, or extrusion.

If the base is fatty, it has the following additional requirements: (11) "acid value" is below 0.2; (12) "saponification value" ranges from 200 to 245; (13) "iodine value" is less than 7; (14) the interval between "melting point" and "solidification point" is small or the SFI curve is sharp.

A suppository base containing all of these properties has not been found. Indeed, some of the properties are mutually exclusive and are not ideal in all situations. Often, the addition of drugs changes the desirable characteristics of the base. Judicious formulation requires the use of the physical values described, for they help in the choice of the base for the drug.

Cocoa Butter (Theobroma Oil)

Cocoa butter is the most widely used suppository base; it is often used in compounding prescriptions when no base is specified. It satisfies many of the requirements for an ideal base, since it is innocuous, bland, and nonreactive, and melts at body temperature. Cocoa butter has several disadvantages, however. It can become rancid, melt in warm weather, liquefy when incorporated with certain drugs, and with overheating, isomerize to an undesirable lowered melting point.

Cocoa butter is primarily a triglyceride, with the predominant glyceride chains being oleopalmitostearin and oleodistearin. It is a yellowish-white, solid, brittle fat, which smells and tastes like chocolate. Its melting point lies between 30°C and 35°C (86°F to 95°F), its iodine value is between 34 and 38, and its acid value is no higher than 4. Because cocoa butter can easily melt and become rancid, it must be stored in a cool, dry place and be protected from light.

Cocoa butter exhibits marked polymorphism (the property of existing in different crystalline forms), a phenomenon probably attributable to the high proportion of unsaturated triglycerides. Each of the different forms of cocoa butter has different melting points, as well as different drug release rates. When cocoa butter is heated above its melting temperature (about 36°C) and chilled to its solidification point (below 15°C), immediately after returning to room temperature this cocoa butter has a melting point of about 24°C, approximately 12° below its original state. A knowledge of these polymorphic states is essential for an understanding of how uniform drug release patterns can be obtained from suppository bases consisting primarily of cocoa butter.

Cocoa butter is thought to be capable of existing in four crystalline states:

1. The α form, melting at 24°C, is obtained by suddenly cooling melted cocoa butter to 0°C.
2. The β' form crystallizes out of the liquefied cocoa butter with stirring at 18 to 23°C. Its melting point lies between 28 and 31°C.
3. The β' form changes slowly into the stable β form, which melts between 34 and 35°C. This change is accompanied by a volume contraction.
4. The γ form, melting at 18°C, is obtained by pouring a cool (20°C) cocoa butter, before it solidifies, into a container, which is cooled at deep-freeze temperature.

The formation of the various forms of cocoa butter depends on the degree of heating, on the cooling process, and on conditions during this process. At temperatures below 36°C, negligible amounts of the unstable forms are obtained, but prolonged heat above that critical temperature causes the formation of the unstable crystals with resulting lowered melting points. The reconversion to the stable β form takes one to four days, depending on the storage temperature—the higher the temperature, the faster the change.

The formation of the unstable forms can be avoided by various methods. (1) If the mass is not completely melted, the remaining crystals prevent the formation of the unstable form. (2) Small amounts of stable crystals added to the melted cocoa butter accelerate the change from the unstable to the stable form; this process is called "seeding." (3) The solidified melt is tempered at temperatures between 28 and 32°C for hours or days, causing a comparatively quick change from the unstable to the stable form.

All of these properties of cocoa butter may cause considerable difficulties in the manufacturing process. As a general rule, the minimal use of heating in the process of melting the fats is recommended. Prolonged heating must be avoided as much as possible. There are several additional disadvantageous characteristics inherent to cocoa butter as a suppository base. Low contractility during solidification causes the suppositories to adhere to molds and necessitates the use of mold release agents or lubricants.

The solidification point of cocoa butter lies about 12 to 13° below its melting point. This property can be utilized in working with cocoa butter in suppository formulations, in which the mass can be kept in a fluid state at comparatively low temperatures. Constant agitation maintains cocoa butter liquid at temperatures below its solidification point.

Cocoa butter does not contain emulsifiers and therefore does not take up large quantities of water (maximum 20 to 30 g of water to 100 g of cocoa butter). The addition of emulsifiers such as Tween 61 (5 to 10%) increases the water absorption considerably. Emulsifiers also help to keep insoluble substances suspended in the fat. Suspension stability is further obtained by the addition of materials (aluminum monostearate, silica) that give melted fats thixotropic properties. There is always the possibility that the suppositories containing these additives will harden on storage. Therefore, prolonged, careful stability observations are recommended.

Such drugs as volatile oils, creosote, phenol, and chloral hydrate lower the melting point of cocoa butter to a considerable extent. To correct this condition, wax and spermaceti were commonly used. Now special bases with high melting ranges are available for this purpose. Examples of these bases can be found in Table 19-2.

The quality of cocoa butter varies with the origin and treatment. Thus, it is quite possible to obtain different physical characteristics with two cocoa butters from different sources, although both are within all specifications of the USP. The selection of a reliable source of supply is imperative to eliminate broad variations in color and consistency between batches.

Cocoa Butter Substitutes

The mechanization of suppository manufacture, as well as the disadvantages inherent to cocoa butter, have prompted a search for suitable substitutes. The satisfactory ones maintain the many desirable properties of cocoa butter, and attempts are made to eliminate the objectionable ones.

Typical Treatment of Vegetable Oils to Produce Suppository Bases

Fat-type suppository bases are produced from a variety of materials, either synthetic or natural in origin. For example, such vegetable oils as coconut or palm kernel oil are modified by esterification, hydrogenation, and fractionation at different melting ranges to obtain the desired product.

An inexpensive method involves hydrogenating corn oil to reduce unsaturation and so increase the percentage of solid triglycerides at room temperature. The triglycerides with lower melting points are then removed by solvent extraction or by pressing. Manufacturers of fats and oils refer to this type of product as a "hard butter."

A common method of producing fats intended for use as suppository bases involves *interesterification*. In this process, coconut oil, palm kernel oil, and/or palm oil (all chosen for their high content of lauric acid moieties) are refined to remove free fatty acids, deodorized to remove volatiles, hydrogenated as described previously, and then interesterified. This final step, catalyzed by sodium methoxide, more equally distributes the fatty acid moieties among the glycerin molecules, creating more common triglycerides, and therefore a more narrow melting range.

A third method utilizes re-esterification. First, the oil is split into fatty acids and glycerin by treatment with high-pressure steam. The glycerin is removed from the mixture, and the remaining free fatty acids consist of C_6–C_{18} chain length compounds, namely caproic, caprylic, capric, lauric, myristic, palmitic, oleic, and stearic acids. Caproic, caprylic, and capric acids are removed by fractional vacuum distillation, because they are readily rancidified and also may cause irritation of mucous membranes. The remaining fatty acids, consisting mainly of lauric acid, are hydrogenated to harden the mixture and lower its iodine value. The catalyst used in the hydrogenation process is removed, and then the fatty acid mixture is re-esterified with an excess of glycerin to form a mixture of triglycerides, diglycerides, and monoglycerides. The manufacturer controls the re-esterification to build into the base the desired characteristics, e.g., melting range, good mold release, smoothness, and viscosity. In the final steps, the base is deodorized and purified by filtration.

The solid-fat indices of bases produced by these methods are illustrated in Figure 19-3. Index A represents a typical hard butter. Indices B and C represent interesterified and re-esterified products respectively.

Typical Suppository Bases

A number of suppository bases are available commercially, manufactured for specific purposes. These bases are listed and described in 19-2.

Certain characteristics are usually considered in the selection of a suppository base: (1) a narrow interval between the melting and the solidification points (e.g., melting point 34°C, solidification point 32°C), which is useful in prescription pharmacy and in certain small-scale hospital and industrial formulations; (2) high melting ranges (37 to 41°C) for incorporating drugs that lower melting points of bases—camphor, chloral hydrate, menthol, phenol, thymol, and several types of volatile oils—or for formulating suppositories for use in tropical climates; (3) low melting ranges (30 to 34°C) when the substances added to the suppository base or large amounts of total solids increase the viscosity of the melted suppository; (4) low acid values (below 3) and iodine values (below 7) which are essential characteristics for suppository bases intended for long shelf-life.

Hydrophilic Suppository Bases

Glycerin Suppositories

USP XX described the following formula for *glycerin suppositories* for use as a cathartic:

Glycerin	91 g
Sodium stearate	9 g
Purified water	5 g
To make approximately	100 g

The glycerin is heated in a suitable container to about 120°C. The sodium stearate is dissolved, with gentle stirring, in the heated glycerin, after which the purified water is added and mixed, and the hot mixture is immediately poured into a suitable mold.

In addition to the above official preparation, USP XX also provided an unofficial formula for *glycerated gelatin suppositories:*

Drug and purified water	10 g
Gelatin	20 g
Glycerin	70 g

This formula is most often used in vaginal suppositories, where local application of antimicrobial agents is intended. The suppository dissolves slowly to prolong the activity of the drug. Because glycerin is hygroscopic, these suppositories are packaged in materials that protect them from environmental moisture.

Glycerinated gelatin suppositories do not melt at body temperature, but rather dissolve in the secretions of the body cavity in which they are inserted. Solution time is regulated by the proportion of gelatin/glycerin/water used, the nature of the gelatin used, and the chemical reaction of the drug with gelatin.

Glycerinated gelatin suppositories support mold or bacterial growth, and as a consequence, they are stored in a cool place and often contain agents that inhibit microbial growth.

The Polyethylene Glycols

The various polyethylene glycol polymers are marketed in the United States as Carbowax and Polyglycols and are suggested for use as suppository bases. Long-chain polymers of ethylene oxide have the general formula $HOCH_2(CH_2OCH_2)_xCH_2OH$ and exist as liquids when their average molecular weight ranges from 200 to 600, and as wax-like solids when their molecular weights are above 1000. Their water solubility, hygroscopicity, and vapor pressure decrease with increasing average molecular weights. The wide range of melting points and solubilities makes possible the formulation of suppositories with various degrees of heat stability and with different dissolution rates. They do not hydrolyze or deteriorate, are physiologically inert, and do not support mold growth.

Several combinations of polyethylene glycols have been prepared for suppository bases having different physical characteristics. Examples of these formulas can be illustrated by a few suggested in the work of Collins, Hohmann, and Zopf.[19]

| Polyethylene glycol 1000 | 96% |
| Polyethylene glycol 4000 | 4% |

This base is low-melting and may require refrigeration during the summer months. It is useful when rapid disintegration is desired.

Base 2

| Polyethylene glycol 1000 | 75% |
| Polyethylene glycol 4000 | 25% |

This base, more heat stable than Base 1, may be stored at higher temperatures than the previous one. It is useful when a slow release of active ingredients is preferred.

Bases 1 and 2, which do not contain water, are usually dipped in water before insertion, so that possible irritation to mucous membranes may be eliminated. This irritation, or "sting," is caused when the water is drawn from the mucosa. Most patients do not feel discomfort from the use of these suppositories. Cheymol, Buffet, and Lechat suggested the addition of 10% water to facilitate solution of the suppository after insertion.[20]

The polyethylene glycol suppositories can be prepared by both molding and cold compression methods. A mixture of 6% hexanetriol-1,2,6 with polyethylene glycol 1540, and 12% of the polyethylene oxide polymer 4000 are especially suitable bases for the cold compression technique.[3,21] The drug is incorporated by dissolving or dispersing in the molten base. Special precautions are necessary in preparing a molded suppository with the polyethylene glycol bases. The mold must be dry because of the solubility of the base in water. The melted mass must be allowed to cool almost to the congealing point before pouring, or the resultant suppository will be fissured owing to the crystallization and contraction of the polymer. Such suppositories may be easily fractured in packaging or handling. The polyethylene glycol base suppositories cannot be prepared suitably by hand rolling. Polyethylene glycol suppositories do not require a mold lubricant and are easier to prepare than cocoa butter suppositories.[15]

Disintegration times of polyethylene glycol type suppository bases, measured in vitro by determining the rate of solution in water at body temperature, do not coincide with the human in vivo results, measured by x-ray study of suppositories containing barium sulfate. See Table 19-3 for comparative results.[19] Thus, clinical results seem the best criterion for choosing the desired polyethylene glycol base, and in vitro test methods should be used for controlling product uniformity of different production lots.

Reports of many workers on adverse reactions of these polymers indicated little difference in sensitivity to individual bases, but a diminished reaction with the 6000 polymer. In one study, the problem of safety, sensitization, and chemical inertness was attributed to impurities and not to the base itself.[22]

Water-Dispersible Bases

Several nonionic surface active materials, closely related chemically to the polyethylene glycols, have been developed as suppository vehicles. Many of these bases can be used for formulating both water-soluble and oil-soluble drugs. The water-dispersible bases offer the additional advantages of storage and handling at elevated temperatures, with claims of broad drug compatibility, nonsupport of microbial growth, nontoxicity, and nonsensitivity.

The surfactants most commonly used in suppository formulations are the polyoxyethylene sorbitan fatty acid esters (Tween*), the polyoxyethylene stearates (Myrj*), and the sorbitan fatty acid esters (Span* and Arlacel*). These surface active agents may be used alone, blended, or used in combination with other sup-

*Atlas Chemical Industries, Inc., Wilmington, DE.

TABLE 19-3. *Comparison of In Vivo Solution Time to In Vitro Disintegration Time of Three Suppository Bases*

Base	Solution Time	Disintegration Time
Polyethylene glycol 1000	13 min	15 min
Cocoa butter	3 min	3 min
A base made of:		
Polyethylene glycol 1540—94%		
Hexanetriol 1,2,6—6%	18 min	40 min

From Collins, A. P., Hohmann, J. R., and Zopf, L. E.: American Professional Pharmacist, 23:231, 1957.

pository vehicle materials to yield a wide range of melting points and consistencies.

Caution must be exercised in the use of surfactants with drugs. There are reports indicating increased rate of drug absorption,[23-26] and other reports showing interaction of these surface active agents with drugs and a consequent decrease in therapeutic activity.[4,6,23,27] Each formulation must be tested in vivo to evaluate its medicinal effectiveness, as well as its safety.

Gross and Becker recommend a water-dispersible, high-melting-point (50°C) suppository base consisting of polyoxyethylene 30 stearate (Myrj 51), water, white wax, and dioctyl sodium sulfosuccinate (Aerosol OT*).[28] The use of the Aerosol OT in the formula is claimed to lend synergism to the surfactant and thus aid in the rapid disintegration of the suppository. The drugs studied were phenobarbital, quinine hydrochloride, tannic acid, and chloramphenicol.

Whitworth and Larocca studied, by in vivo and in vitro methods, nineteen different formulas for suppository bases.[24] These suppositories contained hydrogenated cottonseed oil as the main constituent and varying amounts of surfactant to increase the release of a dye, which was intended to represent a drug. Judging from the rate of release of dye, the bases containing 35 to 40% of the emulsifying agents studied (combinations of Tweens, Tweens and Spans, and Tweens and Arlacel) gave best release.

Ward reports on several polyoxyethylene sorbitan derivatives (Tweens), which are designed to melt at body temperature into liquids that disperse readily in the body fluids.[29] A 2.5 g suppository consisting of Tween 61 (60%) and Tween 60 (40%), and one of Tween 61 (90%) and glyceryl laurate (10%), melted at 37.5°C in about 16 min. The combination of Tween 61 (85%) and glyceryl laurate (15%) melted in about 12 min.

Another type of water-dispersible suppository vehicle reported is based on the use of water-soluble cellulose derivatives, such as methylcellulose and sodium carboxymethylcellulose.[30]

Compressed Tablet Suppositories

Rectal suppositories usually are not compressed as tablets, because the amount of liquid in the rectal cavity is inadequate for tablet disintegration. Effervescent base tablets, which contain dried sodium biphosphate, sodium bicarbonate, and to further aid disintegration, starch or finely divided cellulose, have been described as carbon-dioxide-releasing laxative suppositories.[31] These effervescent base tablets require a small amount of water for rapid disintegration. This compressed rectal suppository is dipped in or sprayed with a thin coating of water-soluble polyethylene glycol to add an external film for protection of the core and for aid in insertion into the rectum.

Compressed tablets weighing about 3 g are used as vaginal suppositories. Fat base vaginal suppositories are sometimes rejected because of the discomfort resulting from the seepage obtained from suppositories with a water-insoluble base. The moisture level of the vagina is sufficient to allow ready dissolution of a tablet if it is formulated to require minimum water for disintegration.

The compressed tablet for vaginal use is usually almond-shaped to ease insertion and to provide maximum surface area, which facilitates tablet disintegration and hastens dispersion of the drug on the vaginal wall. A typical vaginal tablet contains active ingredients, with lactose and/or anhydrous dextrose as excipients, and boric and/or phosphoric acid(s) for adjusting the acidity of the vagina to approximately pH 5.

Vaginal suppositories are usually used for topical therapy, as in the treatment of vaginitis, or as a spermatocide. They also can be used for introducing drugs with systemic effects.

Unusual Types of Suppositories

There is a patent that describes a layered suppository comprising an outer shell that has a melting point of 37 to 38°C and a core that has a melting point of 34 to 35°C and that is contained within and completely surrounded by the shell.[32] Each layer contains different drugs. The layering also may be accomplished by multilayering the suppository in the horizontal plane. This is accomplished by partially filling the mold, allowing the mass to congeal, and pouring additional layers on those previously solidified. Multilayered suppositories serve the dual purpose of separating incompatible drugs in different layers and providing different melting characteristics for controlling the rate of drug absorption.

Coatings have been applied to suppositories to protect them from fast disintegration, to act as lubricants, and to prevent coalescing of adjacent suppositories during storage. Polyethylene glycol, cetyl alcohol, or a patented polyvinyl alcohol and Tween coating is applied for these purposes by dipping the suppository in the coating solution until the desired coating thickness is obtained.[33]

*American Cyanamid and Chemical Corp., New York, NY.

Soft gelatin capsules of varying shapes, filled with either liquid or solid mixtures of the drug, have been made for rectal and vaginal use.

Gstirner described a novel procedure for making suppositories.[34] Solutions of either gelatin, alginates, cellulose derivatives, polyvinylpyrrolidone, or silicates mixed with the desired active ingredients are poured into the appropriately shaped molds and lyophilized. The resultant suppositories are nonmelting, but readily dissolve in body fluids.

Rectal administration of a cylindrical hydrogel for 12-hour periods after it has been soaked in an aqueous drug solution, followed by withdrawal and replacement by a second soaked cylindrical hydrogel, was described by DeLeede, DeBoer, and Breimar.[35] Use of an osmotic delivery system was also detailed.[36]

Manufacture of Suppositories

Four methods are used in preparing suppositories, namely molding by hand, compression, pour molding, and compression on a regular tablet press.

Hand Molding

The simplest and oldest method of preparing a suppository is by hand, i.e., by rolling the well-blended suppository base containing the active ingredients into the desired shape. The base is first grated and then kneaded with the active ingredients by use of a mortar and pestle, until the resultant mass is plastic and thoroughly blended. The active ingredients are usually finely powdered, or dissolved in water, or sometimes mixed with a small amount of wool fat to help incorporation with the suppository base. The mass is then rolled into a cylindric rod of desired length and diameter, or into vaginal balls of the intended weight. Starch or talcum powder on the rolling surface and hands prevent the mass from adhering. The rod is cut into portions, and then one end is pointed. This method is practical and economical for the manufacture of small numbers of suppositories.

Compression Molding

A more uniform and pharmaceutically elegant suppository can be made by compressing the cold-grated mass into a desired shape. A hand-turned wheel pushes a piston against the suppository mass contained in a cylinder, so that the mass is extruded into molds (usually three). Hand-operated instruments and procedures for making suppositories in this manner are described in basic pharmacy texts.

The cold compression method is simple and results in a more elegant appearance than does hand molding. It avoids the possibilities of sedimentation of the insoluble solids in the suppository base, but is too slow for large-scale production. One of the major disadvantages in the use of the cold compression technique for molding fat type base suppositories is air entrapment. This unavoidable inclusion of air makes close weight control impossible and also favors the possible oxidation of both the base and active ingredients.

Pour Molding

The most commonly used method for producing suppositories on both a small and a large scale is the molding process. First, the base material is melted, preferably on a water or steam bath to avoid local overheating, and then the active ingredients are either emulsified or suspended in it. Finally, the mass is poured into cooled metal molds, which are usually chrome- or nickel-plated.

Automatic Molding Machine

The molding operations (pouring, cooling, and removal) can be performed by machine. All filling, ejecting, and mold-cleaning operations are fully automated. The output of a typical rotary machine ranges from 3500 to 6000 suppositories an hour.

In the rotary molding machine, as illustrated in Figure 19-4, chrome-plated brass molds are installed radially in the cooling turntable. First, the prepared mass is fed into a filling hopper where it is continuously mixed and maintained at constant temperature. The suppository mold is lubricated by brushing or spraying and then filled to a slight excess. After the mass solidifies, the excess material is scraped off and collected for re-use. All pumping and scraping units are heated electrically at controlled temperatures. The cooling cycle is adjusted, as required by the individual suppository mass, by adjusting the speed of the rotary cooling turntable. The solidified suppositories are moved to the ejecting station, where the mold is opened and the suppositories are pushed out by steel rods. The mold is closed, and then moved on to the spraying station for lubrication and a repeat of the cycle.

Temperatures and output speeds are regulated to create optimal conditions for continuous, automatic production. Molds must be kept

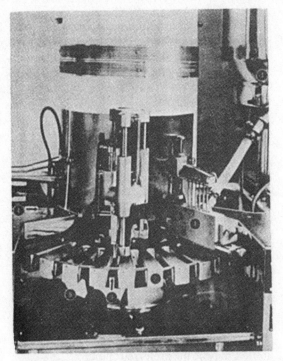

A

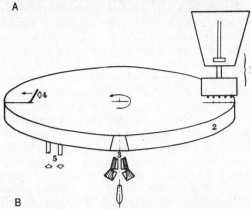

B

FIG. 19-4. A and B, *Rotary suppository molding machine: 1, feeding device and filling hopper; 2, rotating cooling turntable; 3, suppository ejection station; 4, scraping device; 5, refrigerant inlet and outlet. (Crespi, Milano, Italy.)*

clean to prevent any deposition of mass from interfering with their proper closure. Incomplete closure of the molds results in overweight suppositories with mold marks. Air jets blow loose particles out of the molds and thus help to minimize machine downtime for cleaning.

On the straight-line machine, molds are arranged for increased productivity, that is, up to about 10,000 suppositories per hour. The straight-line machine carries out the same steps as the rotary model. The individual molds are carried on a track through a cooling tunnel, where scrape-off and ejection occur.

Packaging of Molded Suppositories

Suppositories must be packaged so that each suppository is overwrapped, or they must be placed in a container in such a manner that they do not touch each other. Staining, breakage, or deformation by melting caused by jostling or adhesion can result from poorly wrapped and packaged suppositories.

Suppositories in direct contact with one another are marred by fusion resulting from changes in ambient temperature. Partially melted suppositories stain the outer package unless they are overwrapped or are packaged with some other barrier that prevents contact with the outer container. Suppositories usually are foiled in tin or aluminum; paper and plastic strips are also used.

Overwrapping of suppositories is done by hand or machine. Hand packaging is slow and yields a nonuniform and generally inelegant preparation. Modern packaging machines overcome these difficulties. They are capable of wrapping uniformly about 8000 suppositories per hour. In one type of machine, the chill-hardened suppositories are placed in a notched turntable and then fed to the packaging station, where the foil is unwound from a roll, cut to size, and finally rolled around each suppository. In other machines, the suppositories are enclosed in cellophane or heat-sealing aluminum foils. Plastic may be thermoformed into two package halves, with the suppository placed mechanically in one half and the second half sealed on afterward. The heat sealer makes contact with the plastic strips only momentarily and at a sufficient distance, so that the suppository is not affected by the heat.

Many suppositories are not individually wrapped. In such cases, they are placed into cardboard boxes or plastic containers that have been molded to provide compartments for six to 12 suppositories.

The individually wrapped suppositories are usually packaged in slide, folding, or set-up boxes. Occasionally, hygroscopicity or volatility of ingredients necessitates packaging the suppositories in glass or plastic containers. In the case of glycerinated gelatin suppositories, a well-sealed package is required. Changes in weight of suppositories depend on the types of packaging materials used.[37]

In-Package Molding

A significant advance in suppository manufacturing was the development of automated methods for molding suppositories directly in their wrapping material. This is currently accomplished with either plastic or aluminum foil. Machines utilizing plastic either thermoform the mold and fill the mold in sequence, or simply fill the mass into previously thermoformed molds. Machines using aluminum foil/polypropylene/lacquer laminates emboss two parallel strips of foil so that when they are sealed together, molds are formed.

In both plastic and aluminum approaches, the tops of the molds are left open for the entrance of filling nozzles. After the mass has been injected, usually by means of small, variable-throw piston pumps, the tops are sealed. The strips are then passed in an upright position through a cooling station. Using these techniques, one machine can make 12,000 to 20,000 suppositories per hour. The advantages of in-package molding include high production rates, no generation of scrapings, no bulk handling or storage of unwrapped suppositories, and maintenance of strict temperature controls. The disadvantages are dependence on the shape of the formed mold and seal completeness for the shape of the suppository and depression formation in the rear of the suppository since no scraping takes place.

Disposable molds have the additional advantage of being suited for suppositories intended for tropical climates. If the mass should melt at the high storage temperatures, the mold still retains it in its proper shape, so that upon cooling it can be dispensed without distortion.

An Approach to Formulating Suppositories

The first considerations of the formulator are:

1. Is the medication intended for local or systemic use?

2. Is the site of application rectal, vaginal, or urethral?

3. Is the desired effect to be quick, or slow and prolonged?

Preliminary suppository bases to be studied are first evaluated by measuring drug availability from the suppository in water at 36 to 37°C. Stability of both active ingredients and base containing drug(s) at 4°C and room temperature is the next consideration. To reduce the number of suppository bases chosen for stability studies, ease of molding and release in the manufacturing equipment are simultaneously studied. After these parameters are established, toxicity (irritancy) and drug availability are measured in animals before the medication is ready for human clinical trials.

Suppositories for Systemic Effect

A selection of possibly desirable suppository bases should be made, e.g., by choosing from those suggested in Table 19-2. Availability and cost of the suppository bases must be considered before the formulation work is begun. Whichever base is used, the drug should be homogeneously dispersible in it, but releasable at the desired rate to the aqueous body fluids surrounding the suppository. Therefore, the solubility of the active ingredient(s) in water or other solvents should be known. If the drug favors water, a fatty base with low water number may be preferred. On the other hand, if the drug is highly fat-soluble, a water-type base, perhaps with the addition of a surfactant to enhance solubility, may be the preferred choice.

The theoretically desirable suppository formulations are molded in the laboratory and stored at room temperature ($25 \pm 3°C$) for at least 48 hours before undergoing in vitro testing for release rate, to be described in the section "Testing of Suppositories." To enhance the homogeneity of drug in the desired base, either a suitable solvent is used or the drug is finely comminuted before incorporation. A drug that is soluble in a minimal quantity of water, or in another liquid miscible with the base, can be dissolved and the solution added to the molten base. If the drug is to be incorporated directly into the base, it should be finely ground so that 100% can be passed through a 100-mesh USP screen. Fragility, brittleness, and ease of handling the suppository formulations on production equipment are some of the screening tests performed before the time-consuming and costly animal and human tests begin.

The fluid content in the rectum is small. Therefore, in vitro findings of release rates, in which comparatively large amounts of water are generally used, can be regarded only as a general guideline for formulation and after the formula is in production, as a quality control procedure. In many cases, there is reasonable correlation of in vitro to in vivo release rates (see Table 19-3), but this is not necessarily so. In vivo clinical findings in man are the ultimate criteria for choosing a desired formulation, and the suppository formulation so chosen yields the in vitro release rate pattern that is to be used as the desired standard. The clinical findings may be based on blood levels of the drug and/or desired clinical effects in man. Thus, since the suppository formula is not chosen until the desired clinical effects in man are determined, screening of several prototype formulas by laboratory tests is the practiced procedure. Chemical and physical stability, consistency of in vitro drug release patterns within theoretically desired ranges, and animal toxicity are some characteristics studied before suppository formulas are chosen for human clinical trials.

Once several likely candidates are chosen for intense human clinical studies, at least two formulations, each containing different batches of acceptable-quality ingredients, are placed on prolonged stability tests. The parameters tested are described in the section "Specific Problems in Formulating Suppositories." The suppositories are stored at room temperature (25 ± 3°C) and at 4°C. They are tested at regular intervals (1- ,3-, and 6-month and 1- and 2-year periods) for changes in appearance, melting and softening range, drug stability, base stability, and in vitro drug release pattern. The minimum age of the samples to be used in clinical trials should be determined by the stability of the melting range of the formula, since nearly all shift upward initially, but the time required to reach equilibrium varies.

Suppositories for Local Effect

Drugs intended for local action are generally nonabsorbable, e.g., drugs for hemorrhoids, local anesthetics, and antiseptics. The bases used for these drugs are virtually nonabsorbable, slow in melting, and slow in drug release, as contrasted with suppository bases intended for systemic drugs. Local effects are generally delivered within a half hour and last at least 4 hours.

The base chosen is one intended for local action; several such bases are depicted in Table 19-2. The drug must be homogeneously distributed in the suppository base. This is accomplished as described previously for incorporating the drug in a systemic base. The suppository is tested 48 hours after molding by immersion in a 36 or 37°C water bath. (See the section "Testing of Suppositories.") The desired base should release an adequate amount of drug within a half hour, and completely melt with release of all drug between 4 and 6 hours. A suppository that does not melt within the 6-hour test period would probably not completely release its drug, cause discomfort to the patient, and be expelled by the patient before it is fully utilized.

Tests in animals must show no irritancy if the suppository is to be used in man. The stability testing program is as described above for suppositories intended for systemic use, the stability testing program is as described previously.

Specific Problems in Formulating Suppositories

Water in Suppositories

Use of water as a solvent for incorporating substances in suppository bases should be avoided for the following reasons.

1. Water accelerates the oxidation of fats.
2. If the water evaporates, the dissolved substances crystallize out.
3. Unless the water is present at a level significantly higher than that required for dissolving the drug, the water has little value in facilitating drug absorption. Absorption from water-containing suppositories is enhanced only if an oil-in-water emulsion exists with more than 50% of the water in the external phase.[38]
4. Reactions between ingredients contained in suppositories are more likely to occur in the presence of water. Sometimes, anhydrous chemicals are used to avoid this possibility.
5. The incorporation of water or other substances that might be contaminated with bacterial or fungal growth necessitates the addition of bacteriostatic agents such as the parabens.

Hygroscopicity

Glycerinated gelatin suppositories lose moisture by evaporation in dry climates and absorb moisture under conditions of high humidity. Polyethylene glycol bases are also hygroscopic. The rate of moisture change in polyethylene glycol bases depends not only on humidity and temperature, but also on the chain length of the molecule. As the molecular weight of these ethylene oxide polymers increases, the hygroscopicity decreases, with a significant drop for the 4000 and the 6000 series.

Incompatibilities

Polyethylene glycol bases were found to be incompatible with silver salts, tannic acid, aminopyrine, quinine, ichthammol, aspirin, benzocaine, iodochlorhydroxyquin, and sulfonamides. Many chemicals have a tendency to crystallize out of polyethylene glycol, e.g., sodium barbital, salicylic acid, and camphor. Higher concentrations of salicylic acid soften polyethylene glycol to an ointment-like consistency, and aspirin complexes with it. Penicillin G, although stable in cocoa butter and other fatty bases, was found to decompose in polyethylene glycol bases. Fatty bases with significant hydroxyl values may react with acidic ingredients.

Viscosity

The viscosity of the melted suppository mass is important in the manufacture of the suppository and to its behavior in the rectum after melting. Melted cocoa butter and some of its substitutes have low viscosities, whereas the glycerinated gelatin and polyethylene glycol type base have viscosities considerably higher than cocoa butter. In the manufacture of suppositories made with low-viscosity bases, extra care must be exercised to avoid the sedimentation of suspended particles. Poor technique can lead to nonuniform suppositories, particularly in the distribution of active ingredients. To prevent segregation of particles suspended in molten bases, the well-mixed mass should be handled at the lowest temperature necessary to maintain fluidity, constantly stirred without entrapping air, and quickly solidified in the mold.

The following approaches may be taken to overcome the problems caused by use of low viscosity bases.

1. Use a base with a more narrow melting range that is closer to body temperature.
2. The inclusion of approximately 2% aluminum monostearate not only increases the viscosity of the fat base considerably, but also aids in maintaining a homogeneous suspension of insoluble materials. Cetyl, stearyl, or myristyl alcohols or stearic acid are added to improve the consistency of suppositories.

Brittleness

Suppositories made from cocoa butter are quite elastic and do not fracture readily. Synthetic fat bases with a high degree of hydrogenation and high stearate contents, and therefore a higher solids content at room temperature, are usually more brittle. Fracturing of the suppository made with such bases is often induced by rapid chilling (shock cooling) of the melted bases in an extremely cold mold. Brittle suppositories are troublesome not only in manufacturing, but also in the subsequent handling, wrapping, and use. To overcome this difficulty, the temperature differential between melted base

and mold should be as small as possible. Addition of a small amount of Tween 80, Tween 85, fatty acid monoglycerides, castor oil, glycerin, or propylene glycol imparts plasticity to a fat and renders it less brittle.

Density

To calculate the amount of drug per suppository, the density of the base must be known. The volume of the mold cavity is fixed, and therefore, the weight of the individual suppository depends on the density of the mass. Knowledge of the suppository weight can be obtained from a given mold and density of the chosen base; the active ingredients can then be added to the bulk base in such an amount that the exact quantity of drug is present in each molded suppository. If volume contraction occurs in the mold during cooling, additional compensation must be made to obtain the proper suppository weight. Thus, density alone cannot be the sole criterion for calculating suppository weight per fixed volume mold. When volume contraction occurs, the suppository weight is determined empirically by small batch runs.

Volume Contraction

This phenomenon occurs in many melted suppository bases after cooling in the mold. The results are manifested in the following two ways.

1. Good mold release. This is caused by the mass pulling away from the sides of the mold. This contraction facilitates the removal of the suppositories from the mold, eliminating the need for mold release agents.
2. Contraction hole formation at the open end of the mold. This undesirable feature results in lowered suppository weight and imperfect appearance of the suppository. The contraction can be eliminated by pouring a mass slightly above its congealing temperature into a mold warmed to about the same temperature. In volume production using standard molds, where adequate control of temperature may not be feasible, the mold is overfilled so that the excess mass containing the contraction hole can be scraped off.

Lubricants or Mold Release Agents

Cocoa butter adheres to suppository molds because of its low volume contraction. These suppositories are difficult to remove from the molds, and various mold lubricants or release agents must be used to overcome this difficulty. Mineral oil, an aqueous solution of sodium lauryl sulfate, various silicones, alcohol, and tincture of green soap are examples of agents employed for this purpose. They are applied by wiping, brushing, or spraying. The release of suppositories from damaged molds was improved by coating the cavities with polytetrafluoroethylene (Teflon).[37]

Dosage Replacement Factor

The amount of base that is replaced by active ingredients in the suppository formulation can be calculated. The replacement factor, f, is derived from the following equation:

$$f = \frac{100(E - G)}{(G)(X)} + 1$$

where: E = weight of pure base suppositories
G = weight of suppositories with X% active ingredient

Most commonly used drugs are tabulated by replacement factor, using cocoa butter arbitrarily assigned the value 1 as the standard base:

Boric acid	0.67
Phenobarbital	0.81
Mild silver protein	0.61
Balsam Peru	0.83
Bismuth subgallate	0.37
Bismuth subnitrate	0.33
Camphor	1.49
White or yellow wax	1.0
Spermaceti	1.0
Chloral hydrate	0.67
Quinine hydrochloride	0.83
Digitalis leaves, powdered	0.61
Ichthammol	0.91
Castor oil	1.0
Phenol	0.9
Procaine hydrochloride	0.8
Resorcin	0.71
Salol	0.71
Sulfanilamide	0.6
Sulfathiazole	0.62
Theophylline sodium acetate	0.6
Zinc oxide	0.15–0.25

Others can be found in the literature.[39,40]

Weight and Volume Control

The amount of active ingredient in each suppository depends on (1) its concentration in the mass; (2) the volume of the mold cavity; (3) the specific gravity of the base; (4) the volume variation between molds—good machining of the molds should keep the volume of each cavity within 2% of a desired value; (5) weight variations between suppositories due to the inconsistencies in the manufacturing process, e.g., incomplete closing of molds, uneven scrapings. Regardless of the reason for the variation in weight, it should be within ±5%.

The German and Russian Pharamcopeias state individual weight variations of rectal suppositories at ±5% of the average weight. The Pharmacopeia Nordica allows ±10% of the average weight for 90% of the suppositories, but these deviations must not exceed ±20%.

Rancidity and Antioxidants

Many investigators confuse the acidity of fats with rancidity. The presence of free fatty acids in either small or large quantities is no indication of rancidity, or that such a product may necessarily become rancid.

Rancidity results from the autoxidation and subsequent decomposition of unsaturated fats into low- and medium-molecular-weight (C_3–C_{11}) saturated and unsaturated aldehydes, ketones, and acids, which have strong, unpleasant odors. The lower the content of unsaturated fatty acid constituents in a suppository base, the greater is its resistance to developing rancidity. Since this reaction begins with the formation of hydroperoxides, a measure of autoxidation in progress is the peroxide value. This peroxide or active oxygen value is a measure of the iodine liberated from an acidified solution of potassium iodide by the so-called "peroxide oxygen" of the fats.

Examples of effective antioxidants are phenols, such as m- or p-diphenols; α-naphthol; quinones, such as hydroquinone or β-naphthoquinone; tocopherols, particularly the β and α forms; gossypol present in cottonseed oil; sesamol present in sesame oil; propyl gallate and gallic acid; tannins and tannic acid; ascorbic acid and its esters; butylhydroxyanisole (BHA); and butylhydroxytoluene (BHT).

Testing of Suppositories

The literature is well documented with test methods to assure that each manufactured lot of suppositories consistently meets the standards established during the manufacture of early experimental lots.[41-44] Finished suppositories are routinely inspected for appearance, and after being sliced lengthwise, for uniformity of the mix. They are assayed for active ingredients to ensure that they individually conform to labeled content. Melting range tests are performed to check the physical and absorption characteristics of each manufactured batch. Fragility tests are carried out to ascertain that the suppositories can be packaged and shipped with minimal breakage.

Melting Range Test

This test is also called the *macromelting* range test and is a measure of the time it takes for the entire suppository to melt when immersed in a constant-temperature (37°C) water bath. In contrast, the *micromelting* range test is the melting range measured in capillary tubes for the fat base only. The apparatus commonly used for measuring the melting range of the entire suppository is a USP Tablet Disintegration Apparatus. The suppository is completely immersed in the constant water bath, and the time for the entire suppository to melt or disperse in the surrounding water is measured.

The in vitro drug release pattern is measured by using the same melting range apparatus. If the volume of the water surrounding the suppository is known, then by measuring aliquots of the water for drug content at various intervals within the melting period, a time-versus-drug content curve (in vitro drug release pattern) can be plotted.

Liquefaction or Softening Time Tests of Rectal Suppositories

A modification of a method developed by Krowczynski is another useful test of finished suppositories.[45,46] It consists of a U-tube partially submersed in a constant-temperature water bath. A constriction on one side holds the suppository in place in the tube. A glass rod is placed on top of the suppository, and the time for the rod to pass through to the constriction is recorded as the "softening time." This can be carried out at various temperatures from 35.5 to 37°C, as a quality control check and can also be studied as a measure of physical stability over time. A water bath with both cooling and heating elements should be used to assure control within 0.1°C.

The "softening test" measures the liquefaction time of rectal suppositories in an apparatus that simulates in vivo conditions (Fig. 19-5). A dialysis membrane, i.e., a cellophane tube, is tied to both ends of a condenser with each end of

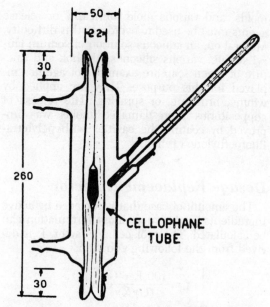

FIG. 19-5. *Apparatus for measuring the liquefaction time of rectal suppositories; the dimensions are in millimeters. The thermometer scale is divided into tenths of a degree and a scale ranging from 32 to 45° is adequate. (From Setnikar, I., and Fantelli, S.: J. Pharm. Sci., 51:566, 1962.)*

the tube open. Water at 37°C is circulated through the condenser at such a rate that the lower half of the cellophane tube collapses and the upper half gapes. The hydrostatic pressure of the water in the apparatus is approximately zero when the tube starts to collapse. When the water temperature is stabilized at 37°C, the suppository is dropped into it so that it sits at the level shown in Figure 19-5, and the time is measured for the suppository to melt completely in the tube.[44]

Breaking Test

Brittleness of suppositories is a problem for which various solutions have already been described. The breaking test is designed as a method for measuring the fragility or brittleness of suppositories. The apparatus used for the test consists of a double-wall chamber in which the test suppository is placed (Fig. 19-6). Water at 37°C is pumped through the double walls of the chamber, and the suppository, contained in the dry inner chamber, supports a disc to which a rod is attached. The other end of the rod consists of another disc to which weights are applied. The test is conducted by placing 600 g on the platform. At 1-min intervals, 200-g weights are added, and the weight at which the suppository collapses is the breaking point, or the force that

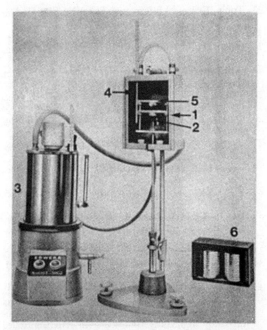

FIG. 19-6. *Breaking test apparatus: 1, double-wall chamber; 2, test suppository; 3, constant temperature water bath and pump; 4, rod; 5, disc for weights; 6, 200-g weights.*

determines the fragility or brittleness characteristics of the suppository. Differently shaped suppositories have different breaking points. The desired breaking point of each of these variously shaped suppositories is established as the level that withstands the break forces caused by various types of handling, i.e., production, packaging, shipping, and patient in-use handling.

Dissolution Testing

Testing for the rate of in vitro release of drug substances from suppositories has always posed a difficult problem, owing to melting, deformation, and dispersion in the dissolution medium. Early testing was carried out by simple placement in a beaker containing a medium.[47]

In an effort to control the variation in mass/medium interface, various means have been employed, including a wire mesh basket,[48] or a membrane,[49] to separate the sample chamber from the reservoir. Samples sealed in dialysis tubing or natural membranes have also been studied.[50] Flow cell apparati have been used, holding the sample in place with cotton,[51] wire screening,[52] and most recently with glass beads.[53]

Storage

Suppositories should be protected from heat, preferably by storing in the refrigerator. Polyethylene glycol suppositories and suppositories enclosed in a solid shell are less prone to distortion at temperatures slightly above body temperature. Glycerinated gelatin suppositories should be protected from heat, moisture, and dry air by packaging in well-sealed containers and storing in a cool place.

Examples of Typical Stability Problems

The suppository, including active ingredients and the base, must be chemically and physically stable at refrigerator temperatures as well as at room temperature storage conditions for at least two years. Storage stability studies are normally conducted at 4°C and at room temperature (25 ± 3°C).

Cocoa butter suppositories in storage sometimes "bloom," i.e., form a white powdery deposit on the surface. This is unsightly and usually can be avoided if the suppositories are wrapped in foil, and stored at uniform cool or refrigerator temperatures.

Fat base suppositories have been shown to harden for a period of time after manufacture.[54] This upward shift in melting range is due to slow crystallization to the more stable polymorphic forms of the base. Depending on the initial melting range and the formula of the suppository, this phenomenon may affect the melting of the suppository and subsequent drug absorption rates. The softening time test and differential scanning calorimetry can be used as stability-indicating test methods to predict problems of this sort. Storage immediately after manufacture at an elevated temperature below the melting range speeds up the aging process. Since the hardening phenomenon is a finite process, this tempering approach can minimize further changes in melting range, which may be worth the addition to manufacturing cycle time.

The suppository overwrap foil also can cause problems in time. For example, if the suppository contains an acid, the foil wrapping may be attacked and develop pinholes.

Stability studies of suppositories intended for tropical climates must be conducted in the final package at temperatures at which the suppositories will eventually be kept. High-melting bases, water-soluble bases, and special polyethylene shell packages must be considered. Labeling should emphasize storage in a cool place. Efforts should be made in formulating suppositories for the tropics to maintain the physical and chemical stability of these suppositories in their final package, even when they are stored at temperatures as high as 50°C (122°F).

Storage studies also should include anticipated problems resulting from shipment. To test the effects of handling the product in the field, suppositories often are shipped by the desired transport facilities to several areas in the country, and then tested physically, and occasionally chemically, for stability. Cool conditions for shipment often are required.

References

1. Bucher, K.: Helv. Physiol. et Pharmacol. Acta, 6:821, 1948.
2. Fabre, M.R., and Regnier, M.: Ann. Pharm. Franc., 9:318, 1951.
3. Schanker, L.S.: J. Pharmacol. Exptl. Therap., 126:283, 1959.
4. Riegelman, S., and Crowell, W.J.: J. Am. Pharm. Assoc., Sci. Ed., 47:115, 123, 127, 1958.
5. Schanker, L.S., Shore, P.A., and Brodie, B.B.: J. Pharm. Exptl. Therap., 120:528, 1957.
6. Allawala, N.A., and Riegelman, S.: J. Am. Pharm. Assoc., Sci. Ed., 42:267, 1953.
7. Heimann, G., Neuwald, F., and Gladtke, E.: Arzneim. Forsch., 28:1023, 1978.
8. Pasich, J., Galoch, B., and Kustra, K.: Pharmazie, 34:413, 1979.
9. Noro, S., Komatsu, Y., and Uesugi, T.: Chem. Pharm. Bull., 30:2912, 1982.
10. Tukker, J.J., Van Vught, W., and DeBlaey, C.J.: Acta Pharm. Tech., 29:187, 1983.
11. Nishihata, T., et al.: Int. J. Pharmaceutics, 21:239, 1984.
12. De Leede, L.G.J., De Boer, A.G., Pörtzgen, E., and Breimer, D.D.: Rate-controlled rectal drug delivery with a hydrogel preparation: I. Drug release in vitro. In Rate-Controlled and Site-Specific Rectal Drug Delivery. Edited by De Leede, L.G.J., Gravenhage, Drukkerij J.H. Pasmans B.V., 1983, p. 89.
13. Rudolfo, A.S., et al.: Am. J. Med. Sci., 237:585, 1959.
14. Enesco, J., Branisteanu, D., and Dangeaunu, J.: Bull. Acad. Med. Roumanie, 4:1, 1939.
15. Shichiri, M., Yamasaki, Y., Kawamori, R., et al.: J. Pharmacol., 30:806, 1978.
16. Copsidas, E., and Ward-McQuaid, J.: J. Int. Med. Res., 7:592, 1979.
17. Turrell, R., Marino, A.W.M., and Nerb, L.: Ann. Surg., 112:417, 1940.
18. Bailey, C.R.: J. Chem. Soc., 123:2579, 1923.
19. Collins, A.P., Hohmann, J.R., and Zopf, L.E.: Am. Profess. Pharmacist, 23:231, 1957.
20. Cheymol, J., Buffet, J., and Lechat, P.: Ann. Pharm. Franc., 5:59, 1947.
21. Triols. Technical Information Sheet No. 779, Carbide and Carbon Chemicals Company, New York, NY.
22. Manz, E.: Süddeut, Apoth. Ztg., 90:320, 1950.
23. Eckert, V., and Muhlemann, H.: Pharmaceutica Acta Helvetiae, 33:649, 1958.
24. Whitworth, C.W., and Larocca, J.P.: J. Am. Pharm. Assoc., Sci. Ed., 48:353, 1959.
25. Tardos, L., Ello, I., Magda, K., and Jobbagyi, L.: Acta Pharm. Hung., 29:22, 1959.
26. Tardos, L., Weisman, L.J., and Ello, I.: Pharmazie, 14:526, 1960.
27. Hennig, W.: Über die Rektale Resorption von Medicamenten. Zürich, Juris Verlag, 1959.
28. Gross, H.M., and Becker, C.H.: J. Am. Pharm. Assoc., Sci. Ed., 42:498, 1953.
29. Ward, W.C.: J. Am. Pharm. Assoc., Sci. Ed., 39:265, 1950.
30. Davies, R.E.M.: Pharm. J. 165:347, 1950.
31. U.S. Patent 3,121,663.
32. U.S. Patent 3,122,475.
33. U.S. Patent 2,477,292.
34. Gstirner, F.: Mitt. Deutsch. Pharm. Ges., 39:21, 1969.
35. De Leede, L.G.J., De Boer, A.G., and Breimer, D.D.: Rate-controlled rectal drug delivery with a hydrogel preparation: II. Drug release in vivo. An experimental study in healthy volunteers. In Rate-Controlled and Site-Specific Rectal Drug Delivery. Edited by De Leede, L.G.J., Gravenhage, Drukkerij J.H. Pasmans B.V., 1983, p. 101.
36. De Leede, L.G.J., et al.: J. Pharmacokin. Biopharm., 10:525, 1982.
37. Püffer, H.W., and Barnett, P.A.: J. Pharm. Sci., 59:848, 1970.
38. Giacomini, G., and Mascitelli, E.: Sommistrane dei Farmaci per Via rettale. Gitti Ed., Milano, 1954.
39. Büchi, J.: Pharm. Act. Helvet., 20:403, 1943.
40. V. Czetsch-Lindenwald, H.: Suppositorien. Editio Cantor. Aulendorf, Germany, 1958.
41. Mühlemann, H., and Neuenschwander, R.H.: Pharm. Act. Helvet., 31:303, 1956.
42. Büchi, J., and Oesch, P.: Pharm. Act. Helvet., 19:363, 1944.
43. Del Pozo, A., and Cemeli, J.: Galenica Acta, 6:193, 1953.
44. Setnikar, I., and Fantelli, S.: J. Pharm. Sci., 51:566, 1962.
45. Coben, L.J.: Drug Dev. and Ind. Pharm., 3:523, 1977.
46. Krowczynski, L.: Diss. Pharm., 11:269, 1959.
47. Gross, H.M., and Becker, C.H.: J. Am. Pharm. Assoc., Sci. Ed., 42:96, 1953.
48. Parrott, E.L.: J. Pharm. Sci., 64:878, 1975.
49. Krowczynski, L.: Acta Pol. Pharm., 19:127, 1962.
50. Ayres, J.W., Lorskulsint, D., Lock, A., et al.: J. Pharm. Sci., 65:832, 1976.
51. Baichwal, M.R., and Lohit, T.V.: J. Pharm. Pharmacol., 22:427, 1970.
52. Püffer, H.W., and Crowell, W.J.: J. Pharm. Sci., 62:242, 1973.
53. Roseman, T.J., Derr, G.R., Nelson, K.G., et al.: J. Pharm. Sci., 70:646, 1981.
54. Coben, L.J., and Lordi, N.G.: J. Pharm. Sci., 69:955, 1980.

20

Pharmaceutical Aerosols

JOHN J. SCIARRA *and* ANTHONY J. CUTIE

The packaging of therapeutically active ingredients in a pressurized system is not new to the pharmaceutical industry. According to present day usage, an aerosol or pressurized package is defined as "a system that depends on the power of a compressed or liquefied gas to expel the contents from the container." It is in light of this definition that the terms aerosol, pressure package, pressurized package, and other similar terms are used in this chapter.

Although pressurized packages existed during the early 1900s, it was not until 1942, when the first aerosol insecticide was developed by Goodhue and Sullivan of the United States Department of Agriculture,1 that the aerosol industry was begun. The principles of aerosol technology were applied to the development of pharmaceutical aerosols in the early 1950s. These aerosol products were intended for topical administration for the treatment of burns, minor cuts and bruises, infections, and various dermatologic conditions. Aerosol products intended for local activity in the respiratory tract appeared in 1955, when epinephrine was made available in a pressurized package. Based on their acceptability to both patient and physician, and their widespread use, pharmaceutical aerosols represent a significant dosage form and should be considered along with other dosage forms, such as tablets, capsules, solutions, etc.

An examination of the aerosol dosage form reveals the following specific advantages over other dosage forms:

1. A dose can be removed without contamination of remaining material. Stability is enhanced for those substances adversely affected by oxygen and/or moisture. When sterility is an important factor, it can be maintained while a dose is being dispensed.

2. The medication can be delivered directly to the affected area in a desired form, such as spray, stream, quick-breaking foam, or stable foam.

3. Irritation produced by the mechanical application of topical medication is reduced or eliminated.

Other advantages are ease and convenience of application and application of medication in a thin layer.

Components of Aerosol Package

An aerosol product consists of the following component parts: (1) propellant, (2) container, (3) valve and actuator, and (4) product concentrate.

Propellants

The propellant is responsible for developing the proper pressure within the container, and it expels the product when the valve is opened and aids in the atomization or foam production of the product. Various types of propellants are utilized. While the fluorinated hydrocarbons such as trichloromonofluoromethane (propellant 11), dichlorodifluoromethane (propellant 12), and dichlorotetrafluoroethane (propellant 114) find widespread use in most aerosols for oral and inhalation use, topical pharmaceutical aerosols utilize hydrocarbons (propane, butane, and isobutane) and compressed gases such as nitrogen, carbon dioxide, and nitrous oxide. The physicochemical properties of the propellants have been reviewed in other publications.[2-4] Listed in Table 20-1 are the commonly used propellants together with several of their physicochemical properties. Those properties of particular interest to the industrial pharmacist have been included. Blends of various fluorocarbon propellants are generally used for pharmaceutical

TABLE 20-1. *Physicochemical Properties of Fluorocarbon and Hydrocarbon Propellants*[5]

Chemical Name	Numerical Designation	Vapor Pressure (psia) 70°F	Vapor Pressure (psia) 130°F	Boiling Point °F	Boiling Point °C	Liquid Density (g/ml) 70°F
Trichloromonofluoromethane	11	13.4	39.0	74.7	23.7	1.49
Dichlorodifluoromethane	12	84.9	196.0	−21.6	−29.8	1.33
Dichlorotetrafluoroethane	114	27.6	63.5	38.4	3.6	1.47
Difluoroethane	152a	76.4	191.0	−11.2	−24.0	0.91
Butane	A-17	31.6	82.0	31.1	−0.6	0.58
Isobutane	A-31	45.8	111.0	10.9	−11.8	0.56
Propane	A-108	122.8	270.7	−43.7	−44.6	0.50

aerosols and are indicated in Table 20-2. By varying the proportion of each component, any desired vapor pressure can be achieved within the limits of the vapor pressure of the individual propellants.

As with the fluorocarbons, a range of pressures can be obtained by mixing the various hydrocarbons in varying proportions. Since the hydrocarbons are naturally occurring products,

however, their purity varies, and the blending is done on the basis of the desired final pressure and not on the percentage of each component present. The pressure of each individual component varies somewhat, depending on the degree of purity. Table 20-3 illustrates some of the commonly used blends that are commercially available.

The vapor pressure of a mixture of propellants

TABLE 20-2. *Blends of Fluorocarbon Propellants for Pharmaceutical Aerosols*

Propellant Blend*	Composition	Vapor Pressure (psig) 70°F	Density (g/ml) 70°F
12/11	50:50	37.4	1.412
12/11	60:40	44.1	1.396
12/114	70:30	56.1	1.368
12/114	40:60	39.8	1.412
12/114	45:55	42.8	1.405
12/114	55:45	48.4	1.390

*It is generally understood that the designation "propellant 12/114 (70:30)" indicates a composition of 70% by weight of propellant 12 and 30% by weight of propellant 114.

TABLE 20-3. *Vapor Pressure of Hydrocarbons*[6]

Designation*	Pressure (psig) 70°F	Composition (mol %) n = Butane	Propane	Isobutane	Other
A-108	108 ± 4	traces	99	1	traces of ethane
A-70	70 ± 2	1	51	48	
A-52	52 ± 2	2	28	70	
A-46	46 ± 2	2	20	78	
A-40	40 ± 2	2	12	86	
A-31	31 ± 2	3	1	96	
A-24	24 ± 2	49.2	0.6	50	0.1 each neopentane and isopentane
A-17	17 ± 2	98	traces	2	traces of isopentane

*Designations used by Phillips Chemical Company, Bartlesville, OK.

can be calculated according to Dalton's law, which states that the total pressure in any system is equal to the sum of the individual or partial pressures of the various components. Raoult's law, which regards lowering of the vapor pressure of a liquid by the addition of another substance, states that the depression of the vapor pressure of a solvent upon the addition of a solute (something added to the solvent) is proportional to the mole fraction of solute molecules in the solution. Given ideal behavior, the vapor pressure of a mixture consisting of two individual propellants is equal to the sum of the mole fraction of each component present multiplied by the vapor pressure of each pure propellant at the desired temperature. This relationship can be shown mathematically:

$$p_a = \frac{n_a}{n_a + n_b} p_A{}^0 = N_A p_A{}^0 \qquad (1)$$

where: p_a = partial vapor pressure of propellant A

$p_A{}^0$ = vapor pressure of pure propellant A

n_a = moles of propellant A

n_b = moles of propellant B

N_A = mole fraction of component A

To calculate the partial vapor pressure of propellant B:

$$p_b = \frac{n_b}{n_b + n_a} p_B{}^0 = N_B p_B{}^0 \qquad (2)$$

The total vapor pressure of the system is then obtained from:

$$P = p_a + p_b \qquad (3)$$

where P is the total vapor pressure of the system.

When one component is present in relatively low concentration, ideal behavior is approached. For practical purposes, however, the calculated pressure is sufficiently accurate for most determinations. The application of Raoult's law for calculation of vapor pressure can best be illustrated by the following example.

Calculate the vapor pressure at 70°F of a propellant blend consisting of propellant 12/11 (30:70) (see Table 20-2).

Moles of each substance:

$$\text{moles}_{11} = \frac{\text{weight}_{11}}{MW_{11}} = \frac{70}{137.38} = 0.5095$$

0.5095 moles of propellant 11

$$\text{moles}_{12} = \frac{\text{weight}_{12}}{MW_{12}} = \frac{30}{120.93} = 0.2481$$

0.2481 moles of propellant 12

From Roault's law:

$$p_{11} = \frac{n_{11}}{n_{11} + n_{12}} p_{11}0$$

$$p_{11} = \frac{0.5095}{0.5095 + 0.2481} \, 13.4 = 9.01 \text{ psia}$$

9.01 psia* partial pressure of propellant 11

$$p_{12} = \frac{n_{12}}{n_{12} + n_{11}} p_{12}0$$

$$p_{12} = \frac{0.2481}{0.2481 + 0.5095} \, 84.9 = 27.80 \text{ psia}$$

27.80 psia partial pressure of propellant 12

Vapor pressure of propellant 12/11 (30:70) then equals 27.80 + 9.01, or 36.81 psia. Gauge pressure is obtained from:

$$\text{psia} - 14.7 = \text{psig}$$

or: $\qquad 36.81 - 14.7 = 22.11 \text{ psig}$

A difference is noted in comparing the calculated value for the vapor pressure with the experimental value shown in Table 20-2. The difference is due to deviation from ideal behavior. Flanner studied the effect of various polar and semipolar solvents and prepared vapor pressure curves.[7] A curve typical of this deviation is shown in Figure 20-1.

Figure 20-2 shows the range of pressures available using various fluorinated hydrocarbons, while Figure 20-3 illustrates these ranges for hydrocarbons. Graphs that relate vapor pressure to temperature are available, and these graphs can be utilized to determine the vapor pressure at the appropriate temperature.[5]

Containers

Various materials as indicated in the following outline have been used for the manufacture of aerosol containers, which must withstand pressures as high as 140 to 180 psig at 130°F.

*The abbreviation psia is for pounds per square inch absolute, which can be converted to pounds per square inch gauge (psig) by subtracting atmospheric pressure (14.7) from psia.

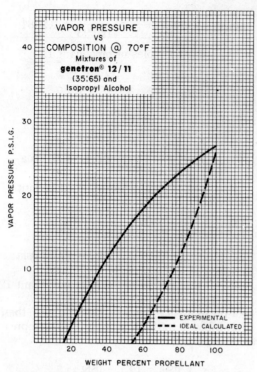

FIG. 20-1. *Deviation of vapor pressure of nonideal solutions from Roault's law. (Courtesy of Allied Chemical Corporation, Morristown, NJ.)*

A. Metal
   1. Tinplated steel
      a. Side-seam (three-piece)
      b. Two-piece or drawn
      c. Tin-free steel
   2. Aluminum
      a. Two-piece
      b. One-piece (extruded or drawn)
   3. Stainless steel
B. Glass
   1. Uncoated glass
   2. Plastic-coated glass

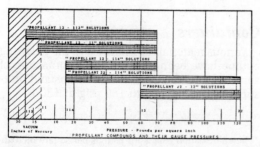

FIG. 20-2. *Range of pressures obtainable at 70° F with various fluorocarbon propellants. (Courtesy of E.I. duPont de Nemours and Co., Inc., Wilmington, DE.)*

Tinplate Containers. The tinplated steel container consists of a sheet of steel plate that has been electroplated on both sides with tin. The thickness of the tin coating is described in terms of its weight, for example, #25, #50, and #100. The size of the container is indicated by a standard system, which is a measure of the diameter and height of the container. A container said to be 202 × 214 is $2^2/16$ inches in diameter and $2^{14}/16$ inches in height.[8-13]

Brief discussion of the procedure used in the manufacture of tinplated containers might be advantageous for a better appreciation of the quality control aspects. Tinplated steel is obtained in thin sheets, and when required, it is coated with an organic material. These sheets are lithographed at this point. After the sheet is cut into sizes to make a body, a top, and a bottom, each piece is fabricated into the desired shape. The body is shaped into a cylinder and seamed via a flanging and soldering operation. The top and bottom are attached to the body, and a side seam stripe is added to the inside seam area when required. The organic coating also can be added to the finished container rather than to the flat sheets. This procedure is slower and somewhat more expensive, but a more continuous and durable coating is produced. The use of sealing compounds, types of solder, and organic coatings are discussed in this chapter under the heading "Formulation of Pharmaceutical Aerosols."

A recent development in metal tinplate containers is the welded side-seam.[14] Welding eliminates the soldering operation, saves considerable manufacturing time, and decreases the possibility of product/container interaction. In general, two processes are used: the Soudronic system (American Can Company, Crown Cork and Seal, and the Southern Can Company) and the Conoweld system (Continental Can Company). The Soudronic system is based on an electronically controlled resistance welding method that uses a copper wire as an electrode. The rounded bodies are welded and then sent to the conventional line, where the top and bottom ends are flanged as indicated previously. The Conoweld system passes the folded body through two rotating electrode rings. The rest of the container is manufactured in the usual manner.

Aluminum Containers. Aluminum is used to manufacture extruded (seamless) aerosol containers. Many existing pharmaceuticals are packaged in aluminum containers, probably because of the lessened danger of incompatibility due to its seamless nature and greater resistance to corrosion. Aluminum can be rather unpredict-

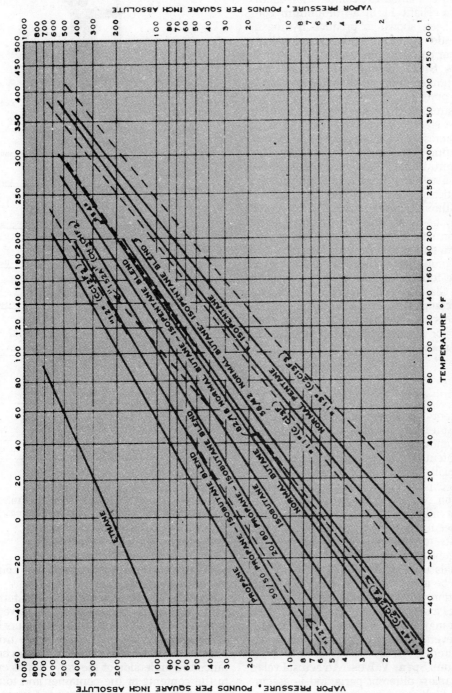

FIG. 20-3. *Vapor pressures of hydrocarbons. (Courtesy of Phillips Chemical Company, Bartlesville, OK.)*

able, however, in that it is corroded by pure water and pure ethanol. The combination of ethanol and propellant 11 in an aluminum container has been shown to produce hydrogen, acetyl chloride, aluminum chloride, propellant 21, and other corrosive products.

Stainless Steel Containers. These containers are limited to the smaller sizes, owing to production problems as well as cost. They are extremely strong and resistant to most materials. Stainless steel containers have been used for inhalation aerosols. In most cases, no internal organic coating is required.

Glass Containers. Glass aerosol containers have been used for a large number of aerosol pharmaceuticals. Glass containers are available with or without plastic coatings. The plastic coating may be totally adhered (except for the neck ring) or nonadhered and vented. By adjusting the formulation and limiting the type and quantity of propellant, satisfactory aerosol products can be formulated and packaged in glass containers. Glass aerosol containers are preferable from a compatibility viewpoint, since corrosion problems are eliminated. The use of glass also allows for a greater degree of freedom in design of the container.

Valves

The present-day aerosol valve is multifunctional in that it is capable of being easily opened and closed, and in addition, is capable of delivering the content in the desired form. Furthermore, especially in the case of pharmaceuticals, the valve is expected to deliver a given amount of medication. Valves for pharmaceuticals usually do not differ from the valves used for nonpharmaceutical aerosol products, but the requirements for pharmaceuticals are usually more stringent than for most other products.[15] The materials used in the construction of the valve must be approved by the Food and Drug Administration. Pharmaceutical aerosols may be dispensed as a spray, foam, or solid stream, and they may or may not require dosage control. The need for several different types of valves becomes apparent.

Continuous Spray Valves. An aerosol valve consists of many different parts and is assembled using high-speed production techniques. The valve manufacturers adhere to relatively close tolerances during manufacture and assembly of the valve. Various materials are used to manufacture the many components of the valve. Figures 20-4 and 20-5 illustrate typical aerosol valve assemblies for use with cans or bottles,

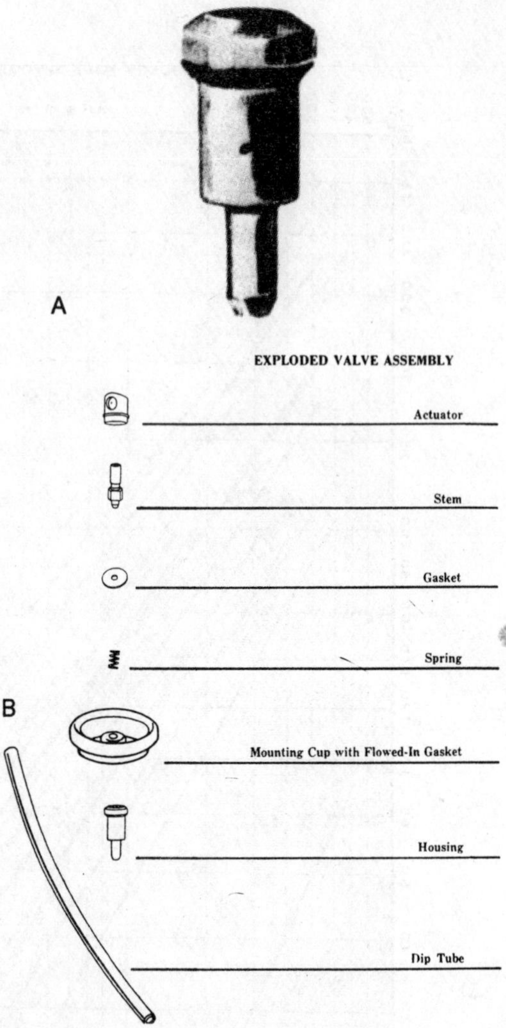

EXPLODED VALVE ASSEMBLY

Actuator

Stem

Gasket

Spring

Mounting Cup with Flowed-In Gasket

Housing

Dip Tube

FIG. 20-4. A, *Vapor tap body.* B, *Aerosol can valve assembly. (Courtesy of Precision Valve Corporation, Yonkers, NY.)*

respectively. These valve assemblies consist of the following parts.

Ferrule or Mounting Cup. The ferrule or mounting cup is used to attach the valve proper to the container. For use with containers having a one-inch opening, the cup is made from tinplate steel, although aluminum also can be used. Since the underside of the valve cup is exposed to the contents of the container and to the effects of oxygen trapped in the head space, a single or double epoxy or vinyl coating can be added to increase resistance to corrosion. Ferrules are used with glass bottles or small aluminum tubes and are usually made from a softer metal such as aluminum or brass. The ferrule is attached to the container either by rolling the end under the

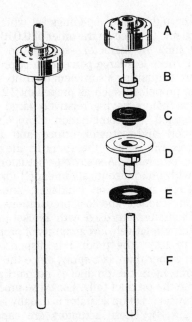

FIG. 20-5. *Aerosol bottle valve assembly: A, ferrule; B, stem; C, valve seat; D, valve body, E, mounting gasket; F, dip tube. (Courtesy of Risdon Manufacturing Co., Naugatuck, CT.)*

lip of the bottle or by clinching the metal under the lip.

Valve Body or Housing. The housing is generally manufactured from Nylon or Delrin and contains an opening at the point of the attachment of the dip tube, which ranges from about 0.013 inch to 0.080 inch.

The housing may or may not contain another opening referred to as the "vapor tap." The vapor tap allows for the escape of vaporized propellant along with the liquid product (see Fig. 20-4A). The vapor tap further produces a fine particle size, prevents valve clogging with products containing insoluble materials, allows for the product to be satisfactorily dispensed with the container in the inverted position, reduces the chilling effect of the propellant on the skin, and in the case of hydrocarbon propellants, allows for a decrease in flame extension. These vapor tap openings are available in sizes ranging from about 0.013 inch to 0.080 inch.

Stem. The stem is made from Nylon or Delrin, but metals such as brass and stainless steel can be utilized also. One or more orifices are set into the stem; they range from one orifice of about 0.013 inch to 0.030 inch, to three orifices of 0.040 inch each.

Gasket. Buna-N and Neoprene rubber are commonly used for the gasket material and are compatible with most pharmaceutical formulations.

Spring. The spring serves to hold the gasket in place, and when the actuator is depressed and released, it returns the valve to its closed position. Stainless steel can be used with most aerosols.

Dip Tube. Dip tubes are made from polyethylene or polypropylene. Both materials are acceptable for use although the polypropylene tube is usually more rigid. The inside diameter of the commonly used dip tube is about 0.120 inch to 0.125 inch, although capillary dip tubes are about 0.050 inch, and dip tubes for highly viscous products may be as large as 0.195 inch. Viscosity and the desired delivery rate play an important role in the selection of the inner diameter of the dip tube.

Metering Valves. Metering valves are applicable to the dispensing of potent medication. These operate on the principle of a chamber whose size determines the amount of medication dispensed. This is shown in Figure 20-6. Although these have been used to a great extent for aerosol products, they are limited in both size and accuracy of dosage. Approximately 50 to 150 mg ± 10% of liquid material can be dispensed at one time with the use of such valves.

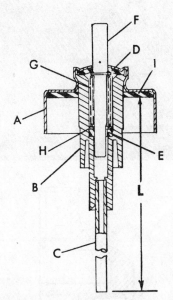

FIG. 20-6. *Metering valve for pharmaceutical aerosols: A, mounting ferrule; B, plastic housing; C, capillary dip tube; D, outlet valve seal; E, inlet valve seal; F, two-piece stainless steel stem; G, stainless steel spring; H, stainless steel washer; I, sealing gasket. (Courtesy of Emson Research, Bridgeport, CT.)*

Actuators

To ensure that the aerosol product is delivered in the proper and desired form, a specially designed button or actuator must be fitted to the valve stem.[16] The actuator allows for easy opening and closing of the valve and is an integral part of almost every aerosol package. It also serves to aid in producing the required type of product discharge.

There are many different types of actuators. Among them are those that produce (1) spray, (2) foam, (3) solid stream, and (4) special applications.

Spray Actuators. Figure 20-7 illustrates actuators that are capable of dispersing the stream of product concentrate and propellant into relatively small particles by allowing the stream to

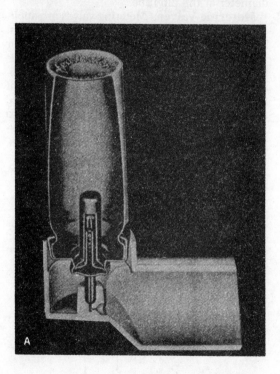

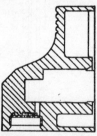

FIG. 20-7. *Actuators for pharmaceutical aerosols. A, Inhalation spray type. (Courtesy of Riker Laboratories.) B, Mechanical breakup type. (Courtesy of Risdon Manufacturing Co., Naugatuck, CT.)*

pass through various openings (of which there may be one to three on the order of 0.016 inch to 0.040 inch in diameter—see Figure 20-7A). Where there is a large percentage of propellant mixture containing a sufficient quantity of a low boiling propellant such as propellant 12 or propane, actuators having relatively large orifices can be used. The combination of propellant vaporization and actuator orifice and internal channels can deliver the spray in the desired particle size range. A spray type actuator can be used with pharmaceuticals intended for topical use, such as spray-on bandages, antiseptics, local anesthetics, and foot preparations. When these actuators are used with aerosol products containing relatively low amounts of propellants (50% or less), the product is dispensed as a stream rather than as a spray, since the propellant present in the product is not sufficient to disperse the product fully. For these products, a mechanical breakup actuator is usually required (Fig. 20-7B). These actuators are capable of "mechanically" breaking a stream into fine particles by causing the stream to "swirl" through various channels built into the actuator.

Foam Actuators. These actuators consist of relatively large orifices ranging from approximately 0.070 inch to 0.125 inch and greater (Fig. 20-8). The orifices allow for passage of the product into a relatively large chamber, where it can expand and be dispensed through the large orifice.

Solid-Stream Actuators. The dispensing of such semisolid products as ointments generally requires these actuators. Relatively large openings allow for the passage of product through the valve stem and into the actuator. These are essentially similar to foam type actuators.

Special Actuators. Many of the pharmaceutical and medicinal aerosols require a specially designed actuator to accomplish a specific purpose. They are designed to deliver the medication to the appropriate site of action—throat, nose, eye, or vaginal tract. Several are shown in Figure 20-8.

Metered-Dose Inhalers. Over the last four to five years, there has been an increased interest in modifying metered-dose inhalers (MDIs) to minimize the number of administration errors and to improve the drug delivery of aerosolized particles into the nasal passageways and respiratory airways. Some of these modifications have included the introduction of tube spacers, breath actuators, and portable plastic reservoirs with inhalation aerosols. In the case of intranasal preparations, new propellant-free metered pumps have been introduced to replace the traditional propellant delivery systems.[17]

During the late 70s and early 80s, there were a number of in vivo and in vitro studies evaluating the differences between the conventional adaptors and the expanded-chamber adaptors, referred to as "spacers," or "tube spacers."[18] At present, many conventional short-stem MDIs deliver at best only 10 to 15% of the dose actuated into the respiratory airways. The balance of the dose is either lost to the inner surface of the adaptor (approximately 10%), or is deposited through inertial impaction in the oropharynx area (80%). The latter leads to swallowing and possible systemic absorption of the therapeutic agent(s). To reduce this fraction that has been lost to the oropharynx and swallowed, a number of tube spacers of various geometric shapes and dimensions were considered, since they should, at least in theory, minimize some of the effects produced by inertial compaction, which contributes significantly to this problem.

Tobin et al., in attempting to further improve and simplify the delivery of aerosolized drug from an MDI, developed a new reservoir aerosol-type delivery system (RADS), consisting of a 700-ml collapsible plastic bag into which the aerosol can be injected.[19] This unit is designed to allow patients more time to inhale the medication after actuating than did the conventional MDI, and it eliminates some of the loss of medication associated with too rapid propulsion or inhalation of aerosolized drugs. This unit (InspirEase by Key Pharmaceuticals, Inc.) consists of a collapsible reservoir bag and a special mouthpiece that is fitted with a reed that produces a warning sound when patients are inhaling too quickly.

A new metered propellant-free intranasal pump has recently been introduced to deliver flunisolide, an effective steroidal agent in the relief of symptoms associated with seasonal or perennial rhinitus. The pump permits the administration of a metered dose of steroid without utilizing propellants, which by their cooling effects often cause smarting and irritation to the nasal mucosa. The metered aerosol pump also ensures accurate dosage and eliminates many of the administration problems associated with nose drops. The concept of propellant-free metered delivery offers a new dimension to intranasal delivery of potent therapeutic agents.

Formulation of Pharmaceutical Aerosols

An aerosol formulation consists of two essential components: product concentrate and propellant. The product concentrate consists of active ingredients, or a mixture of active ingredients, and other necessary agents such as solvents, antioxidants, and surfactants. The propellant may be a single propellant or a blend of various propellants; it can be compared with other vehicles used in a pharmaceutical formulation. Just as a blend of solvents is used to achieve desired solubility characteristics, or various surfactants are mixed to give the proper HLB value for an emulsion system, the propellant is selected to give the desired vapor pressure, solubility, and particle size.

Since one must be familiar with the physicochemical properties of surfactants, solvents, and suspending agents, it follows that the formulator of aerosol preparations must be thoroughly familiar with propellants and the effect the propellant will have upon the finished product. Propellants can be combined with active ingredients in many different ways, producing products with varying characteristics. Depending on the type of aerosol system utilized, the pharmaceutical aerosol may be dispensed as a fine mist, wet spray, quick-breaking foam, stable foam, semisolid, or solid. The type of system selected depends on many factors, including the following: (1) physical, chemical, and pharmacologic properties of active ingredients, and (2) site of application.

Types of Systems[20]

Solution System. A large number of aerosol products can be formulated in this manner. This system is also referred to as a two-phase system and consists of a vapor and liquid phase. When the active ingredients are soluble in the propellant, no other solvent is required. Depending on the type of spray required, the propellant may consist of propellant 12 or A-70 (which produce very fine particles), or a mixture of propellant 12 and other propellants as indicated in Tables 20-1, 20-2, and 20-3. As other propellants with vapor pressures lower than that of propellant 12 are added to propellant 12, the pressure of the system decreases, resulting in the production of larger particles. A lowering of the vapor pressure also is produced through the addition of less volatile solvents such as ethyl alcohol, propylene glycol, ethyl acetate, glycerin, and acetone. The amount of propellant used may vary from 5% (for foams) to 95% (for inhalation products) of the entire formulation. When a spray is produced with larger particles, a decrease is noted in the number of fine particles, decreasing the danger of inhaling these materials through formation and subsequent inhalation of airborne particles. These sprays are also useful for topical

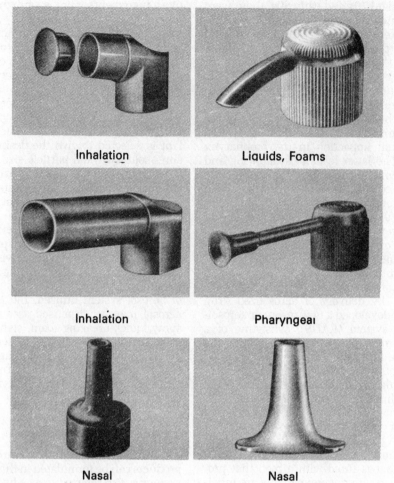

Inhalation	Liquids, Foams
Inhalation	Pharyngeal
Nasal	Nasal

FIG. 20-8. *Various actuators and applicators for pharmaceuticals. (Courtesy of Pechiney Ugine Kuhlman Development, Inc., Greenwich, CT.)*

preparations, since they tend to coat the affected area with a film of active ingredients. Depending on the boiling point of the solvent used, the rate of vaporization of the propellant is decreased, thereby increasing any chilling effect that may be present. This system can best be exemplified by the following general formulations:

	Weight %
Active ingredients	to 10–15
Propellant 12/11 (50:50)	to 100

Propellant 12/11 (30:70), propellant 12/114 (45:55), or propellant 12/114 (55:45) also can be utilized for oral inhalation aerosols or other FDA-exempted products such as contraceptive foams. As the amount of propellant 12 is increased, the pressure increases. With the exception of propellant 12/11 (30:70), the pressure of these systems necessitates packaging the contents in a metal container. If the product is to be packaged in a glass container, a mixture of propellant 12/114 (20:80) or (10:90) can be used. Table 20-4 indicates the pressure limitations in using various aerosol containers.

Aerosols intended for inhalation or for local activity in the respiratory system in the treatment of asthma may be formulated as follows:

	Weight %
Isoproterenol HCl	0.25
Ascorbic acid	0.10
Ethanol	35.75
Propellant 12	63.90

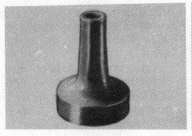

Nasal

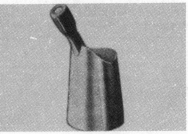

Nasal

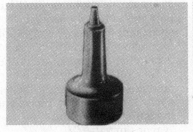

Foams

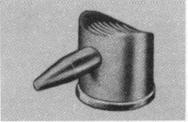

Dental Spray

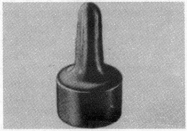

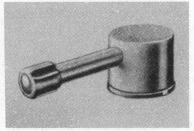

FIG. 20-8. *(Continued)* **Nasal** **Auricular**

This type of formulation is usually packaged in a 15- to 30-ml stainless steel, aluminum, or glass container. Since propellant 12 has a relatively high vapor pressure, the addition of propellant 114 is recommended in order to reduce the pressure, as illustrated by the following example:[21]

	Weight %
Octyl nitrite	0.1
Ethanol	20.0
Propellant 114	49.2
Propellant 12	30.7

Hydrocarbons in topical aerosol pharmaceutical preparations are used as follows:

	Weight %
Active ingredients	up to 10–15
Solvents such as ethanol or propylene glycol	up to 10–15
Distilled water	10–15
Hydrocarbon propellant A-46	55–70

Depending on the amount of water present, the final product may be a solution or a three-phase system. Solution aerosols produce a fine to coarse spray, depending on the concentration of the other ingredients. Hydrocarbon propellant A-70 produces a drier particle, while propellants A-17 and A-31 tend to produce a wetter spray. Hydrocarbon propellants can also be used for products packaged in plastic-coated glass bottles, provided that the amount of flammable hydrocarbon propellant present does not exceed 15% of the total product weight and that the container has a volumetric capacity not exceeding 5 fluid ounces. In addition, one of every 1000 bottles must be tested to 250 psig without failure. The manufacturer of the aerosol product must test one bottle out of each lot of 20,000

TABLE 20-4. *Pressure Limitations of Nonrefillable Aerosol Containers*

Container	Maximum Pressure (psig)	Temperature °F
Tinplated Steel		
Low pressure	up to 140*	130
2 P	from 140 to 160*	130
2 Q	from 160 to 180*	130
Uncoated glass	less than 18†	70
Coated glass	less than 25†	70
Aluminum	up to 180‡	130
Stainless steel	up to 180‡	130
Plastic	less than 25*	70

*Department of Transportation (DOT) Regulations. Consult regulations for definition of 2 P and 2 Q containers.

†Aerosol containers with a pressure less than 25 psig at 70°F and 89 psig at 130°F or a capacity of less than 4 fluid ounces are not regulated by the DOT.

‡Exemptions can be obtained for higher pressures in these containers.

bottles to the bursting point, and the bursting pressure must not be less than 300 psig. One fully charged bottle from this lot must be dropped to an unyielding surface from a height of 4 feet without producing flying glass or a shattering effect. Should either of these two bottles fail, then 10 additional bottles must be tested for each failed test. Failure of any of these 10 samples would cause the entire lot to be rejected. Finally, one fully charged bottle out of each 1000-bottle lot must be heated so that the pressure in the container is equivalent to the equilibrium pressure of the contents at 130°F, without evidence of leakage or other defect.*

Water-Based System. Relatively large amounts of water can be used to replace all or part of the nonaqueous solvents used in aerosols. These products are generally referred to as "water-based" aerosols, and depending on the formulation, are emitted as a spray or foam. To produce a spray, the formulation must consist of a dispersion of active ingredients and other solvents in an "emulsion" system in which the propellant is in the external phase. In this way, when the product is dispensed, the propellant vaporizes and disperses the active ingredients into minute particles. Since propellant and water are not miscible, a three-phase aerosol forms (propellant phase, water phase, and vapor phase). Ethanol has been used as a cosolvent to solubilize some of the propellant in the water. By virtue of its surface-tension-lowering properties, ethanol also aids in the production of small particles.

Surfactants have been used to a large extent to produce a satisfactory homogeneous dispersion. Surfactants that possess low water solubility and high solubility in nonpolar solvents have been found to be the most useful. Long-chain fatty acid esters of polyhydroxylic compounds including glycol, glycerol, and sorbitol esters of oleic, stearic, palmitic, and lauric acids exemplify this series. In general, about 0.5 to 2.0% of surfactant is used. The propellant content varies from about 25 to 60%, but can be as low as 5%, depending on the nature of the product.

To achieve the desired fine particle size with products containing large amounts of water and a low proportion of propellant, a mechanical breakup actuator must be used along with a "vapor tap valve."

A recent development that is useful for pharmaceutical aerosols is the Aquasol* Valve.[22,23] The new Aquasol system allows for the dispensing of a fine mist or spray of active ingredient dissolved in water, which is not possible with the usual three-phase system. Since only active ingredient and water are dispensed (propellant is in vapor state and present only in extremely small quantity), there is no chilling effect as occurs with the hydrocarbon propellant.

The Aquasol system is illustrated in Figures 20-9 and 20-10. It is designed to dispense pressurized products efficiently and economically using relatively small amounts of hydrocarbon propellant; however, it can also function effectively using fluorocarbon propellants. This system, which is essentially a "three-phase" aerosol, permits the use of fairly large quantities of water in the formulation.

The chief difference between the Aquasol system and the "three-phase" system is that the former dispenses a fairly dry spray with very small particles. This relative dryness and small particle size are due chiefly to the design of the valve, which dispenses vaporized propellant rather than liquefied propellant. In addition, the vaporized propellant contributes to the nonflammability of the stream of product as it is dispensed. For example, a fine, almost dry spray is obtained using six parts of water with one part of hydrocarbon propellant. Not only is the resulting spray nonflammable, but it actually extinguishes an open flame.

As can be noted from Figure 20-9, the active

*Exemption DOT-E-8008 for 4-oz. aerosol bottles—Requested and obtained by Wheaton Plasti-Cote Company.

*Precision Valve Corporation, Yonkers, NY.

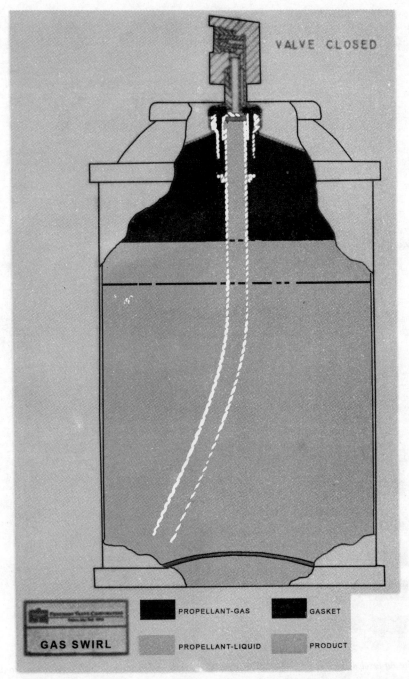

VALVE CLOSED

PROPELLANT-GAS GASKET

PROPELLANT-LIQUID PRODUCT

FIG. 20-9. *The Aquasol dispenser system—valve closed. (Courtesy of Precision Valve Corporation, Yonkers, NY.)*

ingredient is dissolved or suspended in water or in a mixture of alcohol and water. The hydrocarbon propellant floats on top of the aqueous layer and exists as both a liquid and a vapor. Depending on the amount of alcohol present in the aqueous layer, the propellant and water/alcohol layer may or may not be immiscible. As the amount of alcohol increases, the miscibility of these two layers increases. As a pure alcohol system is approached, complete miscibility occurs, at which time a two-phase system that can function satisfactorily is produced. Flammability is

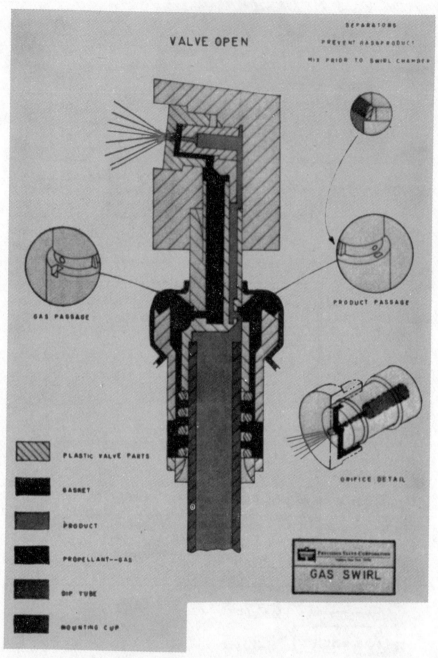

FIG. 20-10. *The Aquasol dispenser system—valve open. (Courtesy of Precision Valve Corporation, Yonkers, NY.)*

increased, however, owing to the large amount of alcohol present, as well as to the fact that liquid propellant is now also being dispensed.

In the Aquasol system, the vapor phase of the propellant and the product enter the mixing chamber of the actuator through separate ducts or channels. Moving at tremendous velocity, the vaporized propellant enters into the actuator while the product is forced into the actuator by the pressure of the propellant. At this point, product and vapor are mixed with violent force, resulting in a uniform, finely dispersed spray.

Depending on the configuration of the valve and actuator, either a *fine* dry spray or a *coarse wet spray* can be obtained. Previous studies have shown that a fine dry spray is obtained when a ratio of about 6 parts of product to 1 part of propellant is used. Up to 30 parts of product to one part of propellant has also produced a satisfactory spray, but in this case, a more coarse spray results. In the Aquasol system, it is almost impossible to dispense only the pure propellant until the package is depleted of the aqueous product.

Suspension or Dispersion Systems. Various methods have been used to overcome the difficulties encountered that are due to the use of a cosolvent. One such system involves a dispersion of active ingredients in the propellant or a mixture of propellants. To decrease the rate of settling of the dispersed particles, various surfactants or suspending agents have been added to the systems.[24,25] These systems have been developed primarily for use with oral inhalation aerosols. Several examples follow.

	Weight %
Epinephrine bitartrate (within 1 to 5 microns)	0.50
Sorbitan trioleate	0.50
Propellant 114	49.50
Propellant 12	49.50

The epinephrine bitartrate has a minimum solubility in the propellant system, but is sufficiently soluble in the fluids in the lungs to exert a therapeutic activity.

Isoproterenol sulfate	33.3 mg
Oleyl alcohol	33.3 mg
Myristyl alcohol	33.4 mg
Propellant 12	7.0 g
Propellant 114	7.0 g

The isoproterenol sulfate remains dispersed in the propellant vehicle for a sufficient length of time to allow for the dispensing of a suitable dose. The physical stability of an aerosol dispersion can be increased by (1) control of moisture content, (2) use of derivatives of active ingredients having minimum solubility in propellant system (the pharmacologic activity must also be considered), (3) reduction of initial particle size to less than 5 microns, (4) adjustment of density of propellant and/or suspensoid so that they are equalized, and (5) use of dispersing agents.

A formulation for oral inhalation that contains a steroid and is used to alleviate the symptoms of asthma would include:

Steroid compound	8.4 mg
Oleic acid	0.8 mg
Propellant 11	4.7 g
Propellant 12	12.2 g

The oleic acid is present as a dispersing agent for the steroid and is an aid in the prevention or reduction of particle growth or agglomeration. In addition, it serves as a valve lubricant and prevents the metered valve from "sticking" in the open position.

Particles of certain materials tend to agglomerate immediately following suspension or shortly thereafter, owing to solubility, moisture, or particle size growth. Caking results when the aggregates become massive. The degree of agglomeration is accelerated at elevated temperatures. This phenomenon may range in degree from flocculation, in which the particles are loosely bound, to aggregation, in which the particles are held together tightly and often fused. In severe cases, the particles may adhere to the walls of the container. Agglomeration may result in valve clogging, inaccuracy of dosage, and depending on the nature of the active ingredients, damage to the liner and possibly to the metal container.

The moisture content of both the suspensoid and the propellant affects the stability of the aerosol system and must be below 300 ppm. Higher moisture levels generally result in particle agglomeration. So that this level is not exceeded, rigid control over the conditions of manufacture must be exerted, and drying both the suspensoid and the propellant prior to manufacture becomes necessary. This can be accomplished by passing the propellant through various desiccants.

Materials suspended in a vehicle in which they are partially soluble show signs of particle size growth. To decrease this phenomenon, a chemical derivative of the drug that shows minimum solubility in the propellant vehicle must be selected. From a physiological viewpoint, the drug must show some solubility in the fluids surrounding the lung tissue. For example, a derivative such as epinephrine bitartrate is preferred when preparing a suspension of the drug in the propellant system. The hydrochloride or sulfate, however, is preferred when a solution aerosol is being formulated, since they are soluble in a hydroalcohol solution, which is miscible with the propellant.

The physical stability of a dispersed system depends primarily on the rate of agglomeration of the suspensoid. This rate is affected by the initial particle size of the drug, which must be in the range of 1 to 5 microns; the exact size depends on the nature of the active ingredient and intended use of the product. This particle size range is necessary to ensure that the particles reach the intended site of action. Suspensions containing materials intended for topical administration do not require particles of the same degree of dispersion as the inhalation aerosols, but for reasons of physical stability, the particles are seldom over 50 microns in size. The active ingredients may be reduced to required particle sizes through use of suitable grinding equipment.

Consideration must also be given to the density of the suspensoid and the propellant vehicle. By decreasing the difference between these two densities, the rate of settling of the suspensoid can be decreased. The density of both the propellant and/or suspensoid may be changed by the addition of a compound of higher or lower density, so that the density of the suspensoid may be made equal to the propellant density.

Various surfactants and lubricants have been investigated in an attempt to control the rate of agglomeration. Such agents as isopropyl myristate and mineral oil have been added to these aerosols to reduce agglomeration and to act as a lubricant for the particles in passing through the valve orifices. They have met with moderate success. The addition of surfactants to aerosol suspensions has been most successful. These surfactants exert their activity by coating each of the particles in suspension and become oriented at the solid-liquid interface. Agglomeration is reduced, thereby increasing stability by providing a physical barrier. According to investigations carried out by Young, Thiel, and Laursen,[26] nonionic surfactants were found to be most effective. Those surfactants having an HLB less than 10, such as sorbitan trioleate, could be utilized for aerosol dispersions. Other agents that were found to be useful are sorbitan monolaurate, sorbitan monooleate, and sorbitan sesquioleate. These surfactants are effective in a concentration of 0.01 to 1%, depending on the concentration of the suspensoid and the intended use of the product.

Vapor tap valves also have been used with dispersion aerosols to decrease the danger of valve clogging. The added propellant, escaping as a vapor, aids in clearing the valve of solid particles.

Foam Systems. Emulsion and foam aerosols consist of active ingredients, aqueous or nonaqueous vehicle, surfactant, and propellant, and are dispensed as a stable or quick-breaking foam, depending on the nature of the ingredients and the formulation. The liquefied propellant is emulsified and is generally found in the internal phase. Nonaerosol emulsions are usually in lotion or viscous liquid form, but aerosol emulsions are dispensed as foams, and this can be advantageous for various applications involving irritating ingredients, or when the material is applied to a limited area.

Aqueous Stable Foams. These can be formulated as follows:

	% w/w
Active ingredients ⎫	
Oil-waxes ⎪	95.0–96.5
o/w Surfactant ⎪	
Water ⎭	
Hydrocarbon propellant	3.5–5.0

While the total propellant content may be as high as 5% in certain cases, it usually is about 8 to 10% v/v or 3 or 5% w/w. As the amount of propellant A-70, A-46, etc. increases, a stiffer and dryer foam is produced. Lower propellant concentrations yield wetter foams. One type of system producing a stable foam may be illustrated by the following example:

	% w/w
Myristic acid	1.33
Stearic acid	5.33
Cetyl alcohol	0.50
Lanolin	0.20
Isopropyl myristate	1.33
Triethanolamine	3.34
Glycerin	4.70
Polyvinylpyrrolidone	0.34
Water, purified	82.93

This can be used in a pharmaceutical aerosol according to the following formula:

	% w/w
Active ingredients	2.0
Emulsion base	94.0–95.0
Hydrocarbon propellant A-46	3.0–4.0

Several different steroids, antibiotics, and other agents may be dispensed in this manner. Both hydrocarbons and compressed gas propellants may be used. Unless an exemption has been granted by the FDA, fluorocarbons are no longer used for these products. (Contraceptive foams have been exempted.)

The techniques used in preparing an aerosol emulsion are the same as those used for nonaerosol emulsions. Surfactants that showed some solubility in the propellants were most effective.

Nonaqueous Stable Foams. Nonaqueous stable foams may be formulated through the use of various glycols such as polyethylene glycol, which may be formulated according to the following:

	% w/w
Glycol	91.0–92.5
Emulsifying agent	4.0
Hydrocarbon propellant	3.5–5.0

The emulsifying agents found most effective were from the class of glycol esters, for example, propylene glycol monostearate. Various medicinal agents can be incorporated into this base.

Quick-Breaking Foams. In this system, the propellant is in the external phase. When dispensed, the product is emitted as a foam, which then collapses into a liquid. This type of system is especially applicable to topical medication, which can be applied to limited or to large areas without the use of a mechanical force to dispense the active ingredients. Quick-breaking aerosol foams may be formulated starting with the following:

	% w/w
Ethyl alcohol	46.0–66.0
Surfactant	0.5–5.0
Water	28.0–42.0
Hydrocarbon propellant	3.0–15.0

The surfactant can be of the nonionic, anionic, or cationic type. It should be soluble in both alcohol and water. If the proportion of ingredients is varied, foams may be obtained having a wide range in stability.

A specific formulation for a quick-breaking foam would consist of:

	% w/w
Polawax*	2.0
SDA 40 Anhyd.	61.0
Perfume	1.5
Menthol	0.1
Water, purified	35.4
	100.0

This is pressurized by mixing 90% concentrate and 10% propellant. The pressure should be below 25 psig, and the product can be packaged in glass aerosol containers using a valve and foam actuator.

Thermal Foams. These foams were developed several years ago and were used to produce a warm foam for shaving. They were not readily accepted by the consumer, however, and were soon discontinued, owing to inconvenience of use, expense, and lack of effectiveness. The same technology was used to dispense hair colors and dyes, but unfortunately, they were subject to some of the same problems, as well as some corrosion problems, and were therefore unsuccessful. It has been reported that these systems would be advantageous in dispensing medicated foams in which the application of heat would be desirable. The technology is available and is fully discussed in the previous edition of this book.[27]

Intranasal Aerosols. Drug delivery systems intended for the deposition of medication into the nasal passageways has long been used as a most effective means of administering drugs intended to produce either a local or systemic effect. Until recently, the modes of administering intranasal preparations have been limited to nasal drops, nonpressurized nasal sprays (mists), inhalants, and intranasal gels (jellies), creams, and ointments. A new alternative to these traditional intranasal preparations is gaining rapid popularity—the pressurized metered nasal aerosol.

The intranasal aerosol offers numerous advantages, including the delivery of a measured dose of drug, excellent depth of penetration into the nasal passageway with minimal inadvertent penetration into the lungs, reduced droplet or particle size, lower dosage than comparable systemic preparations, maintenance of sterility from dose to dose, greater patient compliance, decreased mucosal irritability, and greater flexibility in product formulation.

The following aerosol products are available for intranasal administration:

Trade Name(s)	Dosage Form	Active Ingredient	Indication
Decadron Turbinaire*	Pressurized aerosol suspension	Dexamethasone sodium phosphate	Allergic or inflammatory nasal conditions.
Beconase† Vancenase‡	Pressurized aerosol suspension	Beclomethasone dipropionate	Seasonal and perennial rhinitis.

*Merck Sharp & Dohme, West Point, PA.
†Glaxo Inc., Research Triangle Park, NC.
‡Schering Corporation, Kenilworth, NJ.

Although the dexamethasone preparation (Decadron Turbinaire) was introduced into the marketplace some 10 to 12 years ago, it was not until the introduction of beclomethasone dipro-

*Polawax is a nonionic emulsifying wax consisting of stearyl alcohol and ethylene oxide reaction products (Croda, Inc., New York, NY.)

pionate (Beconase and Vancerase) during the past two years that these nasal aerosol products have met with widespread success. This success has been responsible for the increased interest shown by pharmaceutical manufacturers in developing additional aerosols for administration by the nasal route.

The two intranasal aerosols currently marketed in the United States are suspension formulations. The basic formulation for the intranasal aerosol suspension is as follows:

Active ingredients (micronized)	up to 1.0% weight
Dispensing agent, additives, solvents, etc.	up to 1.0% weight
Propellant 12/11 (60:40)	up to 98.0% weight
	100.0% weight

In most cases, the intranasal formulation is almost identical to the comparable inhalation product (e.g., Vanceril, Vancenase; Decadron Respihaler, Decadron Turbinaire). This is not surprising since the nasal passageways, like the respiratory airways, require a fine uniform distribution of material to promote therapeutic activity and minimize irritability. Various attempts have been made to formulate these active ingredients in a nonaerosol, squeeze-bottle type of product; however, because of the relatively large particle size produced by the squeeze bottle, the product has been found to be quite irritating to the nasal mucosa, with the particles being rapidly transferred to the back of the mouth, where they are swallowed or expectorated.

Probably the major difference between the inhalation aerosol product and the intranasal aerosol product is the design of the adaptor. The nasal adaptors are considerably shorter and narrower, minimizing propellant vaporization before contacting the mucosa. This results in lower percentages of smaller particles, which is desirable because this decreases the number of particles entering the respiratory airways.

Solution and emulsion types of nasal aerosols are also regarded as vehicles for the delivery of medication through the intranasal passageways, but they have proven to be intrinsically more complex to formulate. These forms of pressurized aerosol nasal preparations introduce additional problems, such as vehicle viscosity (cilia effects), irritation from additives, and leakage from nasal passageways. Many investigators are now assessing the biopharmaceutical aspects of nasal absorption, and in the near future, one can optimistically expect to see a number of drugs administered intranasally for systemic action.[28]

Selection of Components

Propellant. Prior to 1978, fluorinated hydrocarbons were used almost exclusively as the propellants for all types of pharmaceutical aerosols. Their chemical inertness, lack of toxicity, lack of flammability and explosiveness, and their safe record of use made them ideal candidates for use. The publication of the "ozone depletion theory" in the mid-1970s, however, and the alleged implication of the fluorocarbons in depleting the ozone levels in the atmosphere, led to the phasing out and ban of the use of fluorocarbon propellants in aerosols (with few exceptions) in 1978. This ban, promulgated by the Environmental Protection Agency (EPA), Food and Drug Administration (FDA), and the Consumer Products Safety Commission, became fully effective in April 1979, when manufacturers could no longer ship aerosol products containing fluorocarbons unless the product carried a specific federal exemption.

While some propellant manufacturers indicated that there were other suitable replacements for propellants 11, 12, and 114, the only ones that have survived the necessary toxicity tests (long- and short-range) are fluorocarbons 152a, 142B, and 22, which may be of limited value. The other alternatives include hydrocarbons, compressed gases, and mechanical devices and pumps. Of these alternatives, however, hydrocarbons were restricted to use with foams and water-based aerosols, and compressed gases were of limited value in aqueous products where the propellant and water were not miscible. While compressed gases overcame the immiscibility of the components, other problems such as loss of propellant, and to a lesser degree, dispersion of the spray became apparent. Since compressed gas systems do not have a chilling effect, they are applicable to topical preparations.

With the development of newer valve technology (the vapor tap and the Aquasol valve), it was found that hydrocarbon propellants, such as butane, propane, isobutane, and their mixtures, could be safely used not only with aqueous products, but with solvent-based aerosols as well. At present, hydrocarbons can be used for all types of topical aerosols, and their flammability properties (as measured by the flame extension test) can be reduced to within safe limits as allowed by the Department of Transportation (DOT) and can meet hazard labeling requirements. As a result of this new technology, all nonexempted topical pharmaceutical aerosols have been satisfactorily reformulated using a hydrocarbon or blend of hydrocarbon as the propellant.

Inhalation aerosols for oral or nasal use have been exempted from the FDA ban, and the fluorinated hydrocarbons—namely, propellants 12, 12/114, and in some cases 12/11—are still used. Contraceptive foams are exempted and still utilize fluorocarbons as the propellant. Recently the FDA granted an exemption for a topical antibiotic aerosol. It should also be indicated that these new products will require a new drug application (NDA).

The compressed gases—nitrogen, nitrous oxide, and carbon dioxide—can be used but are of limited value. The pump system is used for liquid antiseptics, germicides, and nasal sprays.

Containers. Both glass and metal containers have been used for pharmaceutical aerosols. Glass is preferred, but its use is limited, owing to its brittleness and the danger of breakage should the container accidentally be dropped. When the total pressure of the system is below 25 psig and there is not more than 15% propellant, glass can be safely used. Pressures up to 33 psig can be utilized in conjunction with a glass container having a double plastic outer coating.

Most nonaqueous products can be placed into an unlined tinplated metal container. Depending on the degree of protection desired, ¼, ½, or 1 pound of tin per base box can be used. This type of container has been found to be satisfactory for many alcohol-based pharmaceuticals, e.g., spray-on bandages.

Products having a low pH and containing water utilize organic linings of epoxy and/or vinyl resins. Although the vinyl resin forms a tough film, it is poorly resistant to steam and cannot be used for products that must be heat sterilized or filled hot (about 200°F). For this purpose, an epoxy resin can be used since it has a greater degree of heat stability. Both materials are essentially odorless and flavorless, although less odor and flavor are found in vinyl as compared with the epoxy material. A commonly used organic coating consists of an undercoat of vinyl and a top coat of epoxy resin. This has been used to best advantage for those aqueous products of low pH.

Those products containing soaps utilize similar liners, but special attention must be given to the solder that is used for the "side-seam" of some containers. A mixture of 2% tin and 98% lead is used when the pressure is below 40 psig. When soaps are involved, lead reacts with the fatty acids present to form insoluble lead salts, which cause valve clogging. For this purpose,

pure tin or combinations of tin, silver, and other metals are used, as well as containers with a welded side-seam. It is important that specifications for containers include these considerations, and that product stability versus composition of solder be evaluated. For this reason, the welded side-seam container is now preferred for use with pharmaceuticals.

Chemical Reactions. Special attention should be given to those products containing alcohol and packaged in aluminum containers. Anhydrous ethanol is extremely corrosive to aluminum and reacts according to the following equation:

$$6Al + 6C_2H_5OH \text{ (Anhyd.)} \longrightarrow$$
$$2(C_2H_5O)_3Al + 3H_2$$

The hydrogen, which is slowly liberated, increases the pressure in the container. This increase in pressure, along with a general dissolving of some of the aluminum, may result in rupture of the container. This reaction can be reduced or prevented by anodizing the aluminum and adding water to formula. The presence of 2 to 3% water tends to inhibit the reaction. Nonpolar solvents appear to be relatively safe in aluminum containers. Polar solvents tend to be corrosive to bare aluminum, but the reaction can be controlled by the addition of water and/or other inhibitors.

Other Containers. Creams and ointments may be dispensed from a pressurized container by the use of an aluminum container that has been fitted with a piston and nitrogen or hydrocarbon as the propellant. When the valve is opened, the pressure against the piston pushes the piston, causing the product to be dispensed. The viscosity of the finished product plays an important role in the satisfactory dispensing of the product.

Many attempts have been made to separate product from the propellant. One such system utilizes an "accordion-pleated" plastic bag as shown in Figure 20-11. The product is placed inside the bag, and propellant is injected into the outer container through the rubber-plugged hole located in the bottom of the container.

Another development in barrier packs uses a laminated film made into a flexible bag. A perforated dip tube is attached to the valve and functions to prevent the bag from collapsing as the contents are used. This system, termed "Powr Flo" (American Can Company), is useful for dispensing pharamceutical ointments and creams.

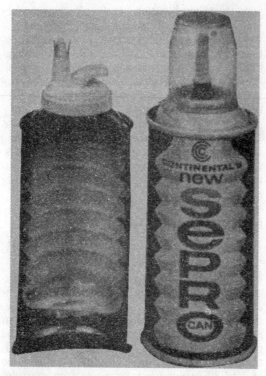

FIG. 20-11. *Sepro container. (Courtesy of Continental Can Company, Chicago, IL.)*

The Preval system not only separates the propellant from the product, but allows the product to be dispensed as a spray or powder. This system consists of an aluminum cartridge containing propellant 12 and an aerosol valve. A dip tube extends from the propellant chamber to the bottom of the container and allows for the flow of product when the valve is opened. Around the top of the valve housing, a vapor tap is placed, which extends into the propellant chamber. The product is added to the container (which need not be a pressure container), and then the valve with propellant cartridge is inserted. When the specially designed actuator is depressed, propellant vapor escapes from the propellant chamber. This creates a "venturi" effect, drawing up some of the product. At this point, mixing of propellant vapor and product takes place. The vaporized propellant then aids in carrying the product through the actuator, where it is dispersed into the desired spray. Varying ratios of propellant to product can be achieved, with results ranging from a fine to a coarse spray (Fig. 20-12).

A nonaerosol package that is self-evacuating has been developed by Plant Industries and is known as Selvac. This system utilizes a resilient bladder, which is filled with the product. As the product is filled into the bladder, the bladder stretches, thereby causing mechanical energy to squeeze out the contents as the valve is released. Since this system does not contain a gas, there is little internal pressure. Two bladders are used, assembled one inside the other. The outer bladder is usually made from natural rubber latex. The valve is inserted into the bladder, and this unit is then fitted into an outer nonpressurized container. The product is filled through the valve by means of a piston-type filler, which forces the product into the bladder.

Valves, Actuators, and Applicators. Valves are selected on the basis of materials of construction and size of various orifices. Although it is extremely difficult to indicate the proper valve for each product, suggested valve designs for specific applications are available.

Various applicators have been specially designed for use with aerosol pharmaceuticals. Inhalation actuators must have all the characteristics of spray actuators and must allow escape of propellant vapors so that the vapors are not inhaled in appreciable amounts by the user. Throat applicators must be capable of depositing the medication directly into the throat area. Elongated tubes having small internal orifices, which permit a breakup of the spray, are generally used. Nasal actuators are designed to fit into the nose and deliver the product as a fine mist.

Other applicators have been designed for specific uses, including vaginal application, ophthalmic application, and others. (See Figs. 20-7 and 20-8.)

Stability Testing of Pharmaceutical Aerosols

One of the most important considerations in the formulation of a pharmaceutical aerosol is its stability. Those aspects directly concerned with the components used to prepare the pharmaceutical aerosol must be fully studied. The effect that the container has upon the product, and conversely, the effect of product upon container, must be considered.

The same considerations apply to the valve components. Even slight changes in the various components of the valve may result in an inoperative package. The valve component of the aerosol package has several working parts made of different materials, such as natural or synthetic rubber, plastic, and stainless steel. All these materials may produce an adverse effect on the product and must be fully studied.

Since a variety of different materials are used in the make-up of the container, valve, and dip tube, it is difficult to determine whether a reac-

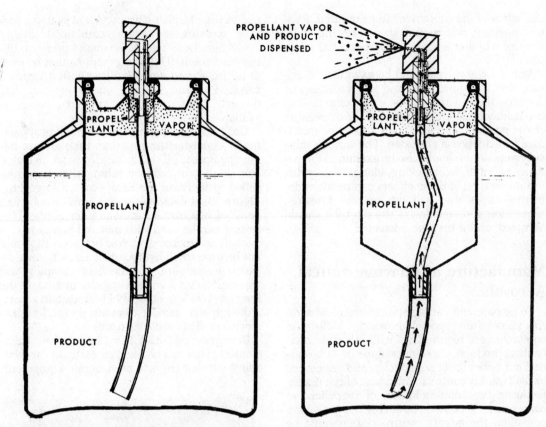

FIG. 20-12. *Schematic view of Preval. (Courtesy of Precision Valve Corporation, Yonkers, NY.)*

tion takes place between the materials and the drug. Many of the components come into intimate contact with the medicinal agent. To determine whether these reactions do occur, all materials must be studied separately and collectively. Several container coatings as well as valves with different subcomponents may be studied so that any reaction between the component and the product may be detected. Samples are prepared and packaged in glass aerosol containers as controls.

The testing of these aerosols must cover three areas: (1) concentrate and propellant, (2) container, and (3) valve. Evidence of decomposition or deterioration in any of these areas could result in an ineffective product. A more detailed discussion of the testing of aerosols can be found elsewhere in the literature.[29]

Concentrate and Propellant. Immediately after preparation, several of the important physicochemical constants of the product are determined. These vary, depending on the nature of the product, but may well include vapor pressure, spray rate of valve, pH, density or specific gravity, refractive index, viscosity, total weight, assay of active ingredients, infrared, and/or gas

chromatography curves, color, and odor. These are then used for comparison during each evaluation of the product.

These samples are usually stored on their sides so that the product comes into contact with both the valve mounting cup and the container. When three-piece metal cans are used, care should be taken to ensure that some samples have liquid as well as gaseous contact with the side-seams (soldered or welded).

Container. The contents of the container are removed by chilling the contents to a temperature of 0°F or less and opening the container. The container is then examined for signs of corrosion. These changes can be detected without much difficulty, since attack upon tinplate, tin-free steel, or aluminum is generally visible to the naked eye and under a microscope. Small pinholes can easily be detected. For those containers that have internal lacquering, the examination must ensure that the lacquer is not softened, dissolved, peeled, or blistered by the concentrate. Special attention should be paid to the side-seam and headspace, as there is a greater danger of attack upon these areas.

When glass is used for the container, an examination of the container can be omitted. Plastic containers may require special testing to determine whether leaching or sorption has taken place.

Valve. The valve should be examined to ensure that it is functional and will satisfactorily dispense the product and be easily closed. This can readily be determined during the dispensing of the product. The valve cup should be examined for evidence of corrosion. The various valve subcomponents should also be examined for evidence of softening, cracking, elongation, or distortion. Several of these effects can result in defective valves that will not operate properly. Elongation and cracking of the dip tube should be noted, and if present, corrected.

Manufacture of Pharmaceutical Aerosols

To prepare and package pharmaceutical aerosols successfully, special knowledge, skills, and equipment are required. As with other pharmaceutical products, these operations must be carried out under strict supervision and adherence to rigid quality controls. Since part of the manufacturing operation (addition of propellant to concentrate) is carried out during the packaging operation, the quality control system must be modified to account for this difference. In addition to the equipment used for the compounding of liquids, suspensions, emulsions, creams, and ointments, specialized equipment capable of handling and packaging materials at relatively low temperatures (about −40°F) or under high pressure must be available. This equipment is usually limited to aerosol or pressurized packaging, and in most instances, cannot be used for other pharmaceutical operations.

Pressure Filling Apparatus. Pressure filling apparatus consists of a pressure burette capable of metering small volumes of liquefied gas under pressure into an aerosol container. The propellant is added through the inlet valve located at the bottom or top of the burette. Trapped air is allowed to escape through the upper valve. The desired amount of propellant is allowed to flow through the aerosol valve into the container under its own vapor pressure. When the pressure is equalized between the burette and the container (this happens with low-pressure propellants), the propellant stops flowing. To aid in adding additional propellant, a hose leading to a cylinder of nitrogen or compressed air is attached to the upper valve, and the added nitrogen pressure causes the propellant to flow. Another pressure filling device makes use of a piston arrangement so that a positive pressure is always maintained. Figure 20-13 illustrates typical laboratory pressure filling equipment. This equipment cannot be used to fill inhalation aerosols fitted with a metered valve. Pressure filling equipment that fills through "pressure-fillable" metered valves is available.

Cold Filling Apparatus. Cold filling apparatus is somewhat simpler than the pressure filling apparatus. All that is needed is an insulated box fitted with copper tubing that has been coiled to increase the area exposed to cooling. Figure 20-14 illustrates such a unit, which must be filled with dry ice/acetone prior to use. This system can be used with metered valves as well as with nonmetered valves; however, it should not be used to fill hydrocarbon aerosols since an excessive amount of propellant escaping and vaporizing may form an explosive mixture at the floor level (or lowest level). Fluorocarbon vapors, although also heavier than air, do not form explosive or flammable mixtures.

Compressed Gas Filling Apparatus. Compressed gases can be handled easily in the laboratory without the use of elaborate equipment.

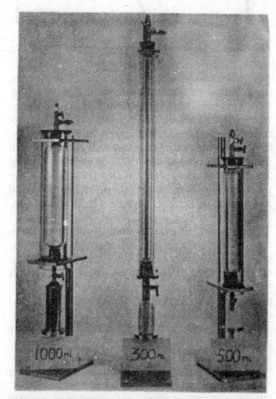

FIG. 20-13. *Pressure burets for laboratory filling of aerosols. (Courtesy of Aerosol Laboratory Equipment Corporation, Walton, NY.)*

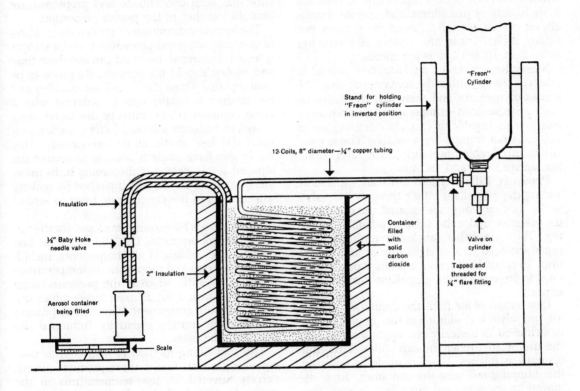

FIG. 20-14. *Apparatus for cold filling process. (Courtesy of E. I. duPont de Nemours and Co., Inc., Wilmington, DE.)*

Since the compressed gases are under high pressure, a pressure-reducing valve is required. Attached to the delivery gauge is a flexible hose capable of withstanding about 150 pounds per square inch gauge pressure and fitted with a filling head. More elaborate units utilize a flow indicator between the gauge and the flexible hose. To use this equipment for filling aerosols with compressed gases, the concentrate is placed in the container, the valve is crimped in place, and the air is evacuated by means of a vacuum pump. The filling head is inserted into the valve opening, the valve is depressed, and the gas is allowed to flow into the container. When the pressure within the container is equal to the delivery pressure, the gas stops flowing. For those products requiring an increased amount of gas, or for those in which solubility of the gas in the product is necessary, carbon dioxide and nitrous oxide can be used. To obtain maximum solubility of the gas in the product, the container is shaken manually during and after the filling operation. Mechanical shakers are also available for this purpose.

Large-Scale Equipment

Good pharmaceutical manufacturing practice requires that the filling of pharmaceutical aerosols be conducted under conditions that ensure freedom from contamination. Only equipment used specifically for aerosols is further discussed in this chapter.

Concentrate Filler. This can range from a single-stage single hopper to a large straight-line multiple-head filler or a rotary type multiple-head filler. Production schedules dictate the type of filler required. Most of these fillers deliver a constant volume of product and they can be set to give a complete fill in one or more operations. Usually, only part of the product is added at each stage, assuring a more accurate fill.

Valve Placer. The valve can be placed over the container either manually or automatically. High-speed equipment utilizes the automatic valve placer. This orients the valve and places it in position prior to the crimping operation.

Purger and Vacuum Crimper. Aerosols are packaged in both metallic and glass containers, each requiring their own style of crimper. Combination can and bottle cappers can be used for most laboratory procedures and operate manually or on air pressure (about 80 pounds per square inch). These are capable of producing more than 10 to 12 cans per minute.

Most crimpers serve a dual function, that is, to evacuate the air within the container to about 24 inches of mercury and then seal the valve in place. Single-head crimpers or multiple-head rotary units capable of vacuum crimping up to 120 cans per minute are available. These usually require both air pressure (90 to 120 pounds per square inch) and vacuum.

Pressure Filler. These units are capable of adding the propellant either through the valve stem, body, and dip tube, around the outside of the stem, or under the valve cup before crimping. They are either single- or multiple-stage units arranged in a straight line or as a rotary unit. To speed production, a positive pressure is used to force the liquid propellant into the container.

Evacuation of air from the container, crimping the valve, and addition of the propellant can be achieved in basically one operation through the use of an "under the cap" filler. This unit operates as follows. A seal is made by lowering the crimping bell onto the container, air is removed by vacuum, and propellant is then metered into the container at room temperature and high pressure. The crimping collet expands and crimps the valve into the opening. This unit can be fitted with three to nine filling heads.

Leak Test Tank. This consists of a large tank filled with water and containing heating units and a magnetized chain so that the cans or pucks for glass, aluminum, and plastic containers are carried through and submerged into the water. The length of the tank is such that the temperature of the product before it emerges from the tank is 130°F.

According to DOT regulations, "each completed container filled for shipment must have been heated until contents reached a minimum of 130°F, or attained the pressure it would exert at this temperature, without evidence of leaking, distortion, or other defects."

Manufacturing Procedure

In general, the manufacture of aerosol products takes place in two stages: manufacture of concentrate and addition of propellant. For this reason, part of the manufacturing operation takes place during the filling operation, which is quite different from nonaerosol pharmaceutical products. This necessitates special quality control measures during the filling operation to ensure that both concentrate and propellant are brought together in the proper proportion.

The aerosol concentrate is prepared according to generally accepted procedures, and a sample is tested. Testing at this point can save both time and money should the concentrate prove to be unacceptable. Once the propellant is added and the product is sealed into a container with a valve, complete rejects must be discarded, obviously a more costly solution. Early detection prevents the loss of the other components. This would also have made it possible to correct the rejected batch instead of discarding it. In many instances, this can be accomplished by making adjustments to the concentrate prior to aerosol filling.

Two methods have been developed for the filling of aerosol products. The cold filling method requires the chilling of all components, including concentrate and propellant, to temperatures of −30 or −40°F, whereas the pressure filling method is carried out at room temperature utilizing pressure equipment. The type of product and size of container usually influence the method to be used.

The cold filling method is restricted to nonaqueous products and to those products not adversely affected by low temperatures in the range of −40°F. In this method, product concentrate is chilled to −40°F and added to the chilled container. The chilled propellant is then added in one or two stages, depending on the amount. An alternating method of cold filling is to chill both concentrate and propellant in a pressure vessel to −40°F and then add their mixture to the aerosol container. A valve is then crimped in place. The container passes through a heated water bath in which the contents of the container are heated to 130°F to test for leaks and strength of container. The container is air-dried, spray-tested if necessary, capped, and labeled. (Containers may be lithographed, and as a consequence, the latter step is omitted). This filling method is no longer used to any great extent and has been replaced by the pressure filling process. Metered-dose aerosols can be filled by either process.

The pressure filling method, when first developed, was generally slower than the cold filling method. With the development of newer techniques, the speed of this method has been greatly increased to make it comparable in rate of production to the cold filling method. The concentrate is added to the container at room temperature, and the valve is crimped in place. The propellant is added through the valve or "under the cap." Since the valve contains extremely small openings (0.018 inch to 0.030 inch), this step is slow and limits production. With the development of rotary filling machines and newer filling heads, which allow propellant to be added around and through the valve stem, the speed has been increased. For those products adversely affected by the air that may be trapped within the container, the air in the headspace is evacuated prior to adding the propellant. Following the addition of the propellant, the method becomes similar to the cold filling method.

For the most part, the pressure method is also preferred because some solutions, emulsions, suspensions, and other preparations cannot be chilled. Various factors determine the method to be used. The pressure method is usually preferred to the cold method, because there is less danger of contamination of the product with moisture; high production speeds can be achieved; less propellant is lost; and the method is not limited, except for certain types of metering valves that can only be handled by the cold filling process or through use of an "under the cap" filler and valve crimper. Some metered valves that are pressure-fillable are now available.

Following the development of the aerosol product, an initial production of about 500 to 1000 units is scheduled. The initial fill is made according to the specifications of the pharmaceutical concern. These units are used for additional stability studies, and for the determination of incompatibilities with various components (containers, valves, gaskets, dip tubes). This run is also used to determine some of the problems that may become apparent in developing the product from the laboratory to full production.

A larger run of 10,000 to 25,000 units is scheduled next. At this time, all materials are identical to those utilized for the production run, and the equipment used must be the same as the production equipment. These samples can be used for clinical studies and further testing if necessary. This test run should give the following information: (1) suitability of scale-up operation, (2) number of rejects to be expected (valve, container, and other components), (3) limitations of filling process (tolerances for filling, crimping, and other operations), (4) determination of equipment to be used, and (5) check on effectiveness and acceptability of final product. Should satisfactory results be obtained at this point, arrangements for full-scale production can be made.

A typical cold filling aerosol line contains the following units arranged in the order given: un-

scrambler, air cleaner, concentrate filler (capable of being chilled), propellant filler (also capable of being chilled), valve placer, valve crimper, water bath, labeler, coder, and packing table. The comparable pressure filling line would be identical in arrangement except that (1) no refrigeration for chilling is required; (2) valve placer is located after "concentrate filler," and a purger and vacuum crimper are added; and (3) this equipment is followed by a pressure filler.

Where "under-the-cap" filling is used, the purger, vacuum crimper, and pressure filler are replaced with a single unit.

Quality Control for Pharmaceutical Aerosols

Basically, there is no difference between methods used to produce pharmaceutical aerosols and those used to produce nonpharmaceutical aerosols, but there are differences in the standards and specifications for their production.

Propellants. Propellants used in medicinal and pharmaceutical aerosols require special handling, and in many instances, special test procedures. All propellants are shipped to the user with accompanying specification sheets; however, before the propellant is used (in fact, before it is even piped into a storage tank), it is subjected to the same rigid tests necessary for all other raw materials. A sample is removed and sent to the laboratory, where its vapor pressure is determined and compared to specifications. When necessary, the density is also determined, and this is used as a further check. Gas chromatography is used to determine the identity of the propellant, and when a blend of propellants is used, to determine the composition. The purity and acceptability of the propellants is tested by moisture, halogen, and nonvolatile residue determinations. Depending on the end use of the propellants, several of these tests may be more important than others. All suppliers of propellants utilize the aforementioned tests in their own laboratories, and the tests that are run by the user are generally a check on these results, and more important, they ensure that the propellants have not become contaminated during shipment. Monographs for propellants 11, 12, and 114 are included in USP XX/NF XV (1980); monographs for the hydrocarbons are currently being written.

Valves, Actuators, and Dip Tubes. These parts are subjected to both physical and chemical inspection. The problem is more complex than with nonaerosol components since a valve is a multicomponent assembly consisting of various parts made to close tolerances. The examination at this point must determine whether the valves are fit to be used. They are sampled according to standard procedures as found in Military Standard Mil-STD-105D.[30] One manufacturer of aerosols for this purpose actually assembles valves, using component parts having similar tolerances to ensure that parts having the minimum tolerance do not engage with parts approaching maximum tolerance.

To provide the means for determining the acceptance of metered-dose aerosol valves for pharmaceutical use, a suitable test method was developed by the Aerosol Specifications Committee, Industrial Pharmaceutical Technology Section, Academy of Pharmaceutical Sciences. The object of this test is to determine the magnitude of the valve delivery and the degree of uniformity between the individual valves as related to the acceptance of any given lot of metered aerosol valves. The test is not designed to determine the suitability or the lack of suitability of the valves for a specific formulation and/or application. Detailed specifications for metered aerosol valves is a matter to be resolved between the pharmaceutical manufacturers and the aerosol valve suppliers.

The following three test solutions were proposed to rule out variations in valve delivery brought about by different formulations. These solutions were selected since they represent the range of propellants and propellant concentrations most often used in pharmaceutical aerosols. Since a metered valve delivers a specific volume of liquid with each actuation, it was proposed that metered valve delivery be designated in terms of valve delivery—volume expressed in microliters. In such a case, the test solutions recommended would apply to the control of valve delivery and uniformity for a great variety of formulations of different densities.

The test solutions may be prepared in bulk and stored in hermetically sealed containers with suitable fitments for transferring the test solution into the test units. The transfer of the test solution should be made in such a manner that no change occurs in the proportions of the ingredients of the test solution.

Test Solution A

	% w/w
Isopropyl myristate	0.10
Dichlorodifluoromethane	49.95
Dichlorotetrafluoroethane	49.95

Specific gravity at 25°C = 1.384

Test Solution B

	% w/w
Isopropyl myristate	0.10
Alcohol USP	49.9
Dichlorodifluoromethane	25.0
Dichlorotetrafluoroethane	25.0

Specific gravity at 25°C = 1.092

Test Solution C

	% w/w
Isopropyl myristate	0.10
Trichloromonofluoromethane	24.9
Dichlorodifluoromethane	50.25
Dichlorotetrafluoroethane	24.75

Specific gravity at 25°C = 1.388

Testing Procedure. A representative sampling of the valves from each shipment is made according to existing methods of sampling. Twenty-five valves are selected and placed onto suitable containers, into which has been placed the specified test solution. Where possible, the containers may be filled by the pressure process. A button-type actuator with a 0.020-inch or larger unrestricted orifice is attached. This button remains in place throughout the test procedure. The containers are placed in a suitable atmosphere at a temperature of 25 ± 1°C. When the product has attained this temperature, the valve should be actuated to the fullest extent for at least 2 sec following complete dispensing of a single delivery. This procedure is repeated for a total of ten times.

The test unit is weighed to the nearest milligram. The valve is actuated to the fullest extent for at least 2 sec following complete dispensing of a single delivery. The test unit is reweighed, and the difference between it and the previous weight represents the delivery in milligrams. The test procedure is repeated for a total of two individual deliveries from each of the twenty-five test units. The individual delivery weights in milligrams are divided by the specific gravity of the test solution to obtain the valve delivery per actuation in microliters.

Valve Acceptance. The test procedure applies to two categories of metered aerosol valves having the following limits.

For valves delivering:
  54 μL or less, the limits are ±15%.
  55 to 200 μL, the limits are ±10%.

1. Of the 50 individual deliveries, if four or more are outside the limits for the specified valve delivery, the valves are rejected.
2. If three individual deliveries are outside the limits, another twenty-five valves are sampled, and the test is repeated. The lot is rejected if more than one delivery is outside the specifications.
3. If two deliveries from one valve are beyond the limits, another twenty-five valves should be taken. The lot is accepted if not more than one delivery is outside the specifications.

Containers. Containers are sampled according to standard sampling procedures and in a manner similar to valves. Both uncoated and coated metal containers must be examined for defects in the lining. Several quality control aspects include specifications for the degree of conductivity of an electric current as a measure of the exposed metal. Glass containers must be examined for flaws. The dimensions of the neck and other parts must be checked to determine conformity to specifications. The weight of the bottle also should be determined.

Weight Checking. This is usually accomplished by periodically adding to the filling line tared empty aerosol containers, which after being filled with concentrate, are removed and then accurately weighed. The same procedure is used to check the weight of the propellant that is being added. When a propellant blend is being utilized, checks must be made to ensure a proper blend of propellants. As a further check, the finished container is weighed to check the accuracy of the filling operation.

Leak Testing. A means of checking the crimping of the valve must be available to prevent defective containers due to leakage. For metal containers, this is accomplished by measuring the "crimp" dimensions and ensuring that they meet specifications.

Final testing of the efficiency of the valve closure is accomplished by passing the filled containers through the water bath. Periodic checks are made of the temperature of the water bath, and these results are recorded.

Spray Testing. Many pharmaceutical aerosols are 100% spray tested. This serves to clear the dip tube of pure propellant (for products filled by pressure through the stem, body, and dip tube), to clear the dip tube of pure concentrate (for products filled by pressure under the cap or around the stem), and to check for defects in the valve and the spray pattern. For metered valves, it serves to prime the valve so that it is ready for use by the consumer.

Several of the basic aspects of a quality control system have been included in this section. A more detailed discussion is available.[31]

Testing of Pharmaceutical Aerosols

Aerosols are "pressurized packages," and many tests are necessary to ensure proper performance of the package and safety during use and storage. All aerosol products that are shipped in interstate commerce are subject to the regulations of the DOT. These regulations impose limitations on the pressure within the container, flash points, flame extension, and flammability. The provisions of the Hazardous Substances Labeling Act and the Food, Drug and Cosmetic Act must be applied. In addition to these federal regulations, many local officials impose further restrictions upon aerosols.

Pharmaceutical aerosols can be evaluated by a series of physical, chemical, and biologic tests, including:

A. Flammability and combustibility
1. Flash point
2. Flame extension, including flashback
B. Physicochemical characteristics
1. Vapor pressure
2. Density
3. Moisture content
4. Identification of propellant(s)
5. Concentrate-propellant ratio
C. Performance
1. Aerosol valve discharge rate
2. Spray pattern
3. Dosage with metered valves
4. Net contents
5. Foam stability
6. Particle size determination
7. Leakage
D. Biologic Characteristics

The flammability and combustibility of aerosol pharmaceuticals may be determined by the following procedures.

Flame Projection. This test indicates the effect of an aerosol formulation on the extension of an open flame. The product is sprayed for about 4 sec into a flame. Depending on the nature of the formulation, the flame is extended, the exact length being measured with a ruler.[32]

Flash Point. This is determined by use of the standard Tag Open Cup Apparatus.[32] The aerosol product is chilled to a temperature of about $-25°F$ and transferred to the test apparatus. The test liquid is allowed to increase slowly in temperature, and the temperature at which the vapors ignite is taken as the flash point. Although the test is still used, the results are of limited value because the flash point obtained is usually the flash point of the most flammable component, which in the case of topical pharmaceuticals is the hydrocarbon propellant.

Vapor Pressure. The pressure can be measured simply with a pressure gauge or elaborately through use of a water bath, test gauges, and special equipment. It is important that the pressure variation from container to container be determined, since excessive variation indicates the presence of air in the headspace. A can puncturing device is available for accurately measuring vapor pressure. Methods are available for aerosols packaged in both metal and glass containers.[32]

Density. The density of an aerosol system may be accurately determined through the use of a hydrometer or a pycnometer. These methods, which have been used for the density of nonaerosols, have been modified to accommodate liquefied gas preparations. A pressure tube is fitted with metal flanges and a Hoke valve, which allow for the introduction of liquids under pressure. The hydrometer is placed into the glass pressure tube. Sufficient sample is introduced through the valve to cause the hydrometer to rise halfway up the length of the tube. The density can be read directly.[32] Specific gravity can be determined through the use of a high-pressure cylinder of about 500-ml capacity.[32]

Moisture. Many methods have proven useful for this purpose. The Karl Fischer method has been accepted to a great extent.[32] Gas chromatography has also been used.

Identification of Propellants. Gas chromatography and infrared spectrophotometry have been used to identify the propellants and also to indicate the proportion of each component in a blend.

Aerosol Valve Discharge Rate. This is determined by taking an aerosol product of known weight and discharging the contents for a given period of time using standard apparatus. By reweighing the container after the time limit has expired, the change in weight per time dispensed is the discharge rate, which can then be expressed as grams per second.[32]

Spray Patterns. A method for comparing spray patterns obtained from different batches of material or through the use of different valves is available[32] and is shown in Figure 20-15. The

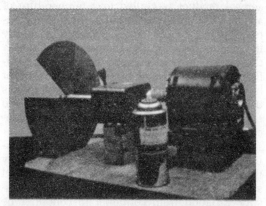

FIG. 20-15. *Apparatus for the determination of spray patterns.*

method is based on the impingement of the spray on a piece of paper that has been treated with a dye-talc mixture. Depending on the nature of the aerosol, an oil-soluble or water-soluble dye is used. The particles that strike the paper cause the dye to go into solution and to be absorbed onto the paper. This gives a record of the spray, which can then be used for comparison purposes. To control the amount of material coming into contact with the paper, the paper is attached to a rotating disk that has an adjustable slit.

Dosage With Metered Valves. Several points must be considered: (1) reproducibility of dosage each time the valve is depressed and (2) amount of medication actually received by the patient. Reproducibility of dosage may be determined by assay techniques whereby one or two doses are dispensed into a solvent or onto a material that absorbs the active ingredients. These solutions can then be assayed, and the amount of active ingredients determined.[33] Another method that can be used involves accurate weighing of filled container followed by dispensing of several doses. The container can then be reweighed, and the difference in weight divided by the number of doses dispensed gives the average dose. This must then be repeated and the results compared. Determination of the dose received by a patient is a rather difficult procedure, since all of the material dispensed is not carried to the respiratory tract. An artificial respiratory system has been developed[33] and is satisfactory for this purpose.

Net Contents. Several methods can be used to determine whether sufficient product has been placed into each container. The tared cans that have been placed onto the filling line are reweighed, and the difference in weight is equal to the net contents. The other method is a destructive method and consists of weighing a full container and then dispensing the contents. The contents are then weighed, with provision being made for the amount retained in the container. Other modifications consist of opening the container and removing as much of the product as possible. These tests are not indicated in determining the actual net weight of each container as related to the amount that can actually be dispensed. The National Bureau of Standards has issued a method that can be used for foam type, low-viscosity, high-viscosity, and food aerosols.[32] These methods standardize the manner in which the containers are to be dispensed.

Foam Stability. Various methods have been suggested for the determination of foam stability. The life of a foam can range from a few seconds (for some quickbreaking foams) to one hour or more depending on the formulation. Richman and Shangraw have indicated some of the factors involved in controlling the stability of a foam.[34] Several methods have been used, which include a visual evaluation, time for a given mass to penetrate the foam, time for a given rod that is inserted into the foam to fall, and the use of rotational viscometers.[34]

Particle Size Determination. Many methods have been advanced for the measurement of particle size aerosols.[35,36] Among those that have been used to a great extent are the Cascade impactor and "light scatter decay" methods. The Cascade impactor operates on the principle that in a stream of particles projected through a series of nozzles and glass slides at high velocity, the larger particles become impacted first on the lower velocity stages, and the smaller particles pass on and are collected at higher velocity stages. Figure 20-16 illustrates a unit suitable for the analysis of particles whose diameters range from 0.1 to 30 microns. This unit is specific for sampling aerosols comprised of particles that might be retained in the respiratory tract. Figure 20-17 shows the efficiency of this unit for determining particle size. Various modifications have been made to improve its efficiency. Porush, Thiel, and Young used the light scatter decay method for determination of particle size in epinephrine aerosols.[37] As the aerosol settles under turbulent conditions, the change in light

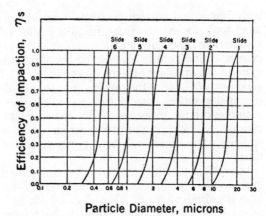

FIG. 20-17. *Impact efficiency of Cascade impactor (Model Cl-S-6).*

intensity of a Tyndall beam is measured. They noted that the mass median diameter of an epinephrine aerosol ranged from 2.7 to 3.5 microns; that 70 to 78% of the particles were less than 5 microns, that 88 to 93% were less than 7 microns, and that 98 to 100% were less than 10 microns. Sciarra and Cutie developed a method for the evaluation of different actuators based on the particle size distribution obtained.[38]

Other test methods have been covered by Johnsen, Dorland, and Dorland.[39] In addition, a test procedure for leak testing, delivery rate, and pressure testing has been included in the USP XX/NF XV. In several cases, specific test procedures are indicated in the monographs for the aerosol preparation.[40]

Biologic Testing. The final phase involved in a comprehensive research and development program for pharmaceutical aerosols must involve biologic testing. A limited number of these tests have been used to evaluate the efficiency of many products, including various antibacterial agents. These tests are similar to tests performed on nonaerosol pharmaceuticals. Biologic testing of aerosol products should include a consideration of therapeutic efficacy and toxicity.

Therapeutic Activity. Various testing procedures are available to determine the therapeutic activity of aerosols. With the exception of consideration given to the aerosol feature of the package, these procedures are similar to existing tests used for nonaerosols. The dosage of the product has to be determined for inhalation aerosols, and this must be related to particle size distribution. Topical preparations are applied to the test areas in the usual manner, and adsorption of therapeutic ingredients can be determined.

Toxicity. Toxicity testing should include

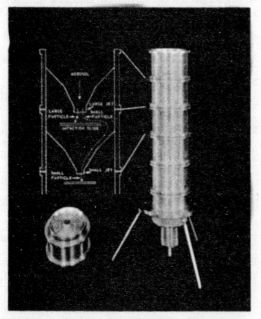

FIG. 20-16. *The Cascade impactor for determining the particle size distribution of aerosols. (Courtesy of Battelle Laboratories, Inc., Columbus, OH.)*

both topical and inhalation effects. Aerosols applied topically may be irritating to the affected area and/or may cause a chilling effect. The degree of chilling effect depends on the type and amount of propellant present. There is really no good test available at the present time, although thermistor probes attached to recording thermometers have been used to indicate the change in skin temperature when skin is sprayed with an aerosol for a given period of time.

Inhalation toxicity must also be considered even though the product may be intended for topical administration. This can be accomplished by exposing test animals to vapors sprayed from an aerosol container.

References

1. Goodhue, L.D., and Sullivan, W.M.: U.S. Pat. No. 2,321,023 (1943).
2. Sciarra, J.J.: Aerosols. In Prescription Pharmacy. 2nd Ed. Edited by J.B. Sprowls. J.B. Lippincott, Philadelphia, 1970, p. 280.
3. Sanders, P.A.: Handbook of Aerosol Technology. 2nd Ed. Van Nostrand Reinhold, New York, 1979, p. 19.
4. Root, M.J.: Aerosols. In Advances in Cosmetic Technology. Vol. 1. Edited by R. Goldemberg. Drug and Cosmetic Industry, New York, 1978, p. 97.
5. Aerosol Propellant Data Book. E.I. duPont de Nemours and Company, Wilmington, DE, 1967.
6. Sciarra, J.J.: Aerosols. In Remington's Pharmaceutical Sciences. 16th Ed. Mack Publishing, Easton, PA, 1980, p. 1614.
7. Flanner, L.: Vapor Pressures of Solvents and Propellant Mixtures. Allied Chemical Corp., General Chemical Division, Morristown, NJ, 1959.
8. Obarski, H.: Steel aerosol containers. In The Science and Technology of Aerosol Packaging. Edited by J.J. Sciarra and L. Stoller. John Wiley and Sons, New York, 1974, p. 151.
9. Industry Specifications for Fabricated Aerosol Cans. In CSMA Aerosol Guide. 6th Ed. Chemical Specialties Manufacturers Association, Washington, DC, March 1971, p. 37.
10. Johnsen, M.A.: Aerosol Age, 7:20, June 1962.
11. Johnsen, M.A.: Aerosol Age, 7:29, July 1962.
12. Johnsen, M.A.: Aerosol Age, 8:39, August 1962.
13. Johnsen, M.A.: Aerosol Age, 9:39, September 1962.
14. Mesrobian, R.B.: Aerosol Age, 19:19, July, 1974.
15. Sciarra, J.J.: Aerosol Age, 9:74, December 1964.
16. Sciarra, J.J.: Aerosol Age, 10:39, January 1965.
17. Cutie, A.J., Ertefaie, S., and Sciarra, J.J.: Aerosol Age, 29:24, March 1984.
18. Sackner, M.A., Brown, L.K., and Kim, C.S.: Chest, 805:195, 1981.
19. Tobin, M.J., Jenouri, G., Danta, I., et al.: Am. Rev. Respir. Dis., 126:670, 1982.
20. Sciarra, J.J.: Types of aerosol systems. In The Science and Technology of Aerosol Packaging. Edited by J.J. Sciarra and L. Stoller. John Wiley and Sons, New York, 1974, p. 37.
21. Porush, I., and Maison, G.: U.S. Pat. No. 2,868,691 (1959).
22. Sciarra, J.J.: Food and Drug Packaging, 37:16, December 1, 1977.
23. San Giovanni, M.L.: Aerosol Age, 22:18, July 1977.
24. Theil, C.G., Porush, I., and Law, R.D.: U.S. Pat. No. 3,014,844 (1961).
25. Abramson, B., Greif, N.I., and Silson, J.E.: U.S. Pat. No. 3,095,355 (1963).
26. Young, J.G., Thiel, C.G., and Laursen, G.A.: Nonaqueous Aerosol Dispersions. Midwestern Regional Meeting, Industrial Pharmacy Section, American Pharmaceutical Association, Chicago, IL, October 1962.
27. Sciarra, J.J.: Pharmaceutical aerosols. In The Theory and Practice of Industrial Pharmacy. 2nd Ed. Edited by L. Lachman et al. Lea & Febiger, Philadelphia, 1976, p. 281.
28. Cutie, A.J., and Sciarra, J.J.: Aerosol Age, 27:26, October 1982.
29. Sciarra, J.J.: Testing of aerosols. In The Science and Technology of Aerosol Packaging. Edited by J.J. Sciarra and L. Stoller. John Wiley and Sons, New York, 1974, p. 301.
30. Sampling Procedures and Tables for Inspection by Attributes, Mil-Std-105D, U.S. Dept. of Defense, Washington, DC, April 29, 1963.
31. Sciarra, J.J.: Quality control for pharmaceutical and cosmetic aerosol products. In Quality Control in the Pharmaceutical Industry. Vol. 2. Edited by M.S. Cooper. Academic Press, New York, 1973, p. 1.
32. CSMA Aerosol Guide. 6th Ed. Chemical Specialties Manufacturers Association, Washington, DC, March 1971.
33. Young, J., Porush, I., Thiel, C., et al.: J. Am. Pharm. Assoc., Sci. Ed., 49:72, 1960.
34. Richman, M., and Shangraw, R.: Aerosol Age, 11:45, September 1966.
35. Tollin, B.: The Determination of Particle Size of Aerosols—A Review. Selected Pharmaceutical Research References. Vol. I. Smith Kline & French Laboratories, PA, 1960.
36. Kanig, J., and Mintzer, H.: Measurement of Particulate Solid in Aerosol Systems. Aerosol Technicomment. Vol. III, No. 2. Aerosol Techniques, Inc., Milford, CT, 1960, p. 1.
37. Porush, I., Thiel, C., and Young, J.: J. Am. Pharm. Associ., Sci. Ed., 49:70, 1960.
38. Sciarra, J.J., and Cutie, A.: J. Pharm. Sci., 67:1428, 1978.
39. Johnsen, M.A., Dorland, W.E., and Dorland, E.K.: The Aerosol Handbook. Wayne E. Dorland, Caldwell, NJ, 1972, p. 377.
40. The USP XX/NF XV, The United States Pharmacopeial Convention, Inc., Rockville, MD, 1980, p. 936, 1023.

21

Sterilization

KENNETH E. AVIS *and* MICHAEL J. AKERS

Sterilization is the process designed to produce a sterile state. The traditional concept of the sterile state is the absolute condition of total destruction or elimination of all living microorganisms. This concept has given way to the reality that sterile is a term that must be given relative connotation and that the probability of having achieved the absolute can only be predicted on the basis of kinetic projection of microbial death rates. Therefore, sterility in the absolute sense cannot be shown to have been achieved, but rather, can be approached with an increasing probability of success as a sterilization process is improved. With terminal methods of sterilization of a parenteral product, particularly steam under pressure, a probability of no more than one nonsterile unit in a million (10^{-6}) is readily achievable. Even greater levels of assurance can be achieved with current technology. In this chapter, *sterile* indicates a probable condition of complete freedom from viable microorganisms with the limitations just expressed; these limitations are developed more fully later in the chapter. The term *aseptic* indicates a controlled process or condition in which the level of microbial contamination is reduced to the degree that microorganisms can be excluded from a product during processing. It describes an "apparently" sterile state.

Persons responsible for carrying out sterilization procedures must be acutely aware of the degree of effectiveness as well as the limitations of each sterilization process. They must also understand that these processes may have a deleterious effect on the material to be sterilized. In the processing of pharmaceuticals, it is often necessary to reach a compromise between the most effective sterilization procedure and one that will not have a significant adverse effect upon the material to be sterilized. For example, it may be necessary to add an antibacterial agent

to a thermally sensitive product to enhance the effectiveness of a low-temperature sterilization process; thereby decomposition is prevented while the combined effect of the antibacterial and the heat provide reasonable assurance that the product will be sterilized.

Microorganisms exhibit varying resistance to sterilization procedures. The degree of resistance varies with the specific organism. In addition, spores, the form that preserves certain organisms during adverse conditions, are more resistant than vegetative forms of the organism. The data given in Table 21-1 illustrate the varying resistance of different spores to moist and dry heat. Therefore, the conditions required for a sterilization process must be planned to be lethal to the most resistant spores of microorganisms normally encountered, with additional treatment designed to provide a margin of safety against a sterilization failure.

After consideration of the principles of microbial death and their relationship to validation of sterilization processes, the processes of interest in industrial pharmacy are studied in this chapter under the two main divisions of physical processes and chemical processes. Particular emphasis is placed on the principles involved and on applications of the processes to pharmaceuticals. For further details of sterilization processes, reference should be made to one or more of the standard textbooks on this subject.[1-4]

Validation of Sterilization Processes

All sterilization processes (thermal, chemical, radiation, and filtration) are designed to destroy or eliminate microbiologic contaminants present in a product. The official test for sterility of the product is a destructive test on a selected sam-

TABLE 21-1. *Times Required for Lethal Effect on Bacterial Spores by Thermal Exposure*

	Time (min.)					
	Moist Heat				Dry Heat	
Organisms	100°C	110°C	121°C	120°C	140°C	170°C
B. anthracis	5–15	—	—	—	180	—
Cl. botulinum	330	90	10	120	60	15
Cl. welchii	5–10	—	—	50	5	7
Cl. tetani	5–15	—	—	—	15	—
Soil bacilli	>1020	120	6	—	—	15

ple; thus, the task of proving that all units of a product are sterile must involve the employment of probability statistics. The statistics of probability depend on such parameters as the length or degree of exposure to the sterilant, the type and number of microorganisms present, the desired level of microbial destruction or elimination, and the resistance of the microorganism(s) presented to the sterilization process.

In recent years, the pharmaceutical industry has intensified its efforts to quantitate the rate and extent of microbial destruction or elimination. The Food and Drug Administration has stated in its current good manufacturing practice regulations that sterilization procedures must be validated pertaining to (1) the design of the equipment and the process used to produce batch sterilization and (2) the confirmation with reproducible data of a given probability level of residual microbial contamination upon completion of the sterilization process. Validation of sterilization processes can be facilitated by using quantitative, theoretically sound principles such as microbial death kinetic expressions.

Microbial Death Kinetic Terms

An important term in expressing microbial death kinetics for heat, chemical, and radiation sterilization is the *D value*. The D value is the time (for heat or chemical exposure) or the dose (for radiation exposure) required for the microbial population to decline by one decimal point (a 90%, or one logarithmic unit, reduction). The D value may be estimated graphically, as shown in Figure 21-1, or mathematically, as shown by equation (1):

$$D = \frac{U}{\log N_0 - \log N_u} \quad (1)$$

where U is the exposure time or exposure dose, under specific conditions, N_0 is the initial microbial population (product bioburden) and N_u is the microbial population after receiving U time

or dose units of sterilant exposure. For example, after 5 min of product exposure to a temperature of 121°C, the microbial population was reduced from 2×10^5 to 6×10^3. Then, the D value at 121°C is:

$$D_{121} = \frac{5 \text{ min}}{\log(2 \times 10^5) - \log(6 \times 10^3)} = 3.28 \text{ min}$$

Thus, at 121°C, the microbial population is decreased by 90% every 3.28 min.

D values have been defined precisely for various microorganisms contained in certain environments (liquids and solid surfaces) at specific temperatures for heat sterilization,[5] and at direct exposure to cobalt-60 irradiation.[6] D values can-

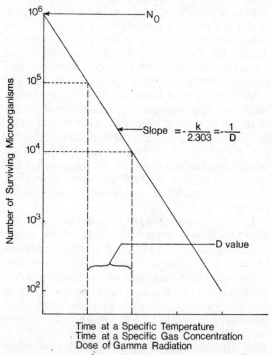

Time at a Specific Temperature
Time at a Specific Gas Concentration
Dose of Gamma Radiation

FIG. 21-1. *Graphic representation of the semilogarithmic microbial death rate.*

not be defined precisely for microorganisms exposed to such gases as ethylene oxide because of the complex interaction of heat, concentration of gas, and relative humidity.[7] D values are estimated for gas sterilization when it is possible to keep heat and humidity values constant, varying only the concentration of gas.

Other key terms used in the determination of microbial death rates include *microbial load,* or *bioburden;* the Z *value;* the F *value;* the F_0 value; and the probability of nonsterility. These terms are defined in Table 21-2, and Z value plots are shown in Figure 21-2.

The F_0 value is a term widely used in sterilization cycle design and validation. Its current application is limited to steam sterilization although an F value can be computed for any thermal method of sterilization. The F_0 value can be defined by the following two equations:

$$F_0 = \Delta t \ \Sigma \ 10^{\frac{T-121}{10}} \qquad (2)$$

where Δt is the time interval between product temperature measurements T.

$$F_0 = D_{121} (\log N_0 - \log N_u) \qquad (3)$$

where N_0 and N_u are those terms defined previously.

The F_0 value of equation (2) is obtained by physical measurement of product temperature and substitution of that temperature for T in the exponent. For example, if the product temperature was measured every 5 min from 0 to 30 min

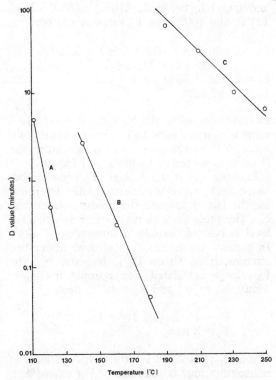

FIG. 21-2. Z *value plots of log D versus temperature.*
Key—A: Z = *10°C for* B. stearothermophilus *spores exposed to steam sterilization.*
B: Z = *22°C for* B. subtilis *var niger spores exposed to dry heat sterilization.*
C: Z = *54°C for* E. coli *endotoxin exposed to dry heat sterilization.*

TABLE 21-2. *Definition of Key Terms Employed in Microbial Death Kinetics*

Symbol	Term	Definition
N_0	Bioburden	The population or number of living microorganisms per defined unit, surface, or system.
Z	Resistance value	The number of degrees (C or F) required for a 1 log reduction in the D value. $$Z = \frac{T_1 - T_2}{\log D_2 - \log D_1}$$
F (T,z) or F_T^z	Sterilization process equivalent time	The equivalent time at temperature T delivered to a unit of product calculated using a specified value of z.
F_0	Sterilization process equivalent time	The equivalent time at a temperature of 121°C delivered to a unit of product calculated using a z value of 10°C.
N_u	Probability of nonsterility	The number of nonsterile units per batch or the theoretic or extrapolated number of living microorganisms per defined unit after a given equivalent heating time U at a specific temperature T.
$N_u = \text{antilog} \left(\log N_0 - \dfrac{U_T}{D} \right)$		

and found to be 25°C, 110°C, 118°C, 120°C, 121°C, and 100°C, the F_0 value would be:

$$F_0 = 5 \text{ min } (0 + 0.079 + 0.501 + 0.794 + 5.000 + 0.0079)$$
$$F_0 = 5 \text{ min } (6.382)$$
$$F_0 = 31.91 \text{ min}$$

By definition, when the F_0 value is used, the Z value is assumed to be 10°C. This means that for every 10°C increase in product temperature, the D value is decreased by 90%, or 1 log unit.

Equation (3) is the biologic F_0 equation because the F_0 value is calculated after determining the D_{121} value and the product bioburden, N_0. The probability of nonsterility is whatever level is desired, usually a minimum of 10^{-6}. In general, equation (3) is applied under two circumstances. Given D_{121}, N_0, and N_u, the F_0 value is calculated. For example, if $D_{121} = 1$ min, $N_0 = 10^2$, and $N_u = 10^{-6}$, then:

$$F_0 = 1 \text{ min } (\log 10^2 - \log 10^{-6})$$
$$F_0 = 8 \text{ min}$$

Given D_{121}, N_0, and F_0, the achieved level of nonsterility may be calculated. For example, if $D_{121} = 2$ min, $N_0 = 10^2$, and $F_0 = 8$ min, then:

$$N_u = \text{antilog} \left(\log N_0 - \frac{F_0}{D_{121}} \right)$$
$$N_u = \text{antilog} \left(\log 10^2 - \frac{8}{2} \right)$$
$$N_u = 10^{-2}$$

F Value Applications

The importance of F_0 values in steam sterilization cycle validation may be summarized as follows:

1. F_0 relates the killing efficiency of the process at any temperature to the killing effect produced at the desired sterilization temperature of 121°C.

2. F_0 provides a single quantitative value describing the thermal exposure time of the cycle to which the product was exposed equivalent to 121°C.

3. F_0 incorporates the contribution of the heating and cooling portions of the temperature-time profile during a cycle with the overall lethal effect of heat upon microorganisms.

4. F_0, if used to describe the lethal effect upon microorganisms at the coolest location in the sterilizer, represents the most conservative

estimate of the degree of destruction of microorganisms, and thus the safest conditions for determining cycle time.

At least three factors affect the F_0 value. They are (1) the container characteristics: size, geometry, and heat transfer coefficient, (2) the product volume and viscosity, and (3) the size and configuration of the batch load in the sterilizer.

F value equations can be applied to dry heat sterilization although most materials sterilized by dry heat can be subjected to overkill temperature-time cycles. The reference temperature T_0 would not be 121°C, of course, but it probably would be 170°C, since this temperature is specified in the USP/NF XXI. The Z value would not be 10°C, but would be in the range of 22°C for the destruction of B. subtilis var niger spores on glass to 54°C for the destruction of endotoxin.[8,9] (See Fig. 21-2.)

Aseptic processing also requires validation to assure batch to batch consistency in producing a given probability of product sterility. While D and F_0 values cannot be applied, a probability of nonsterility levels can be obtained by process simulation testing using microbiologic growth medium, a suitable type and number of challenge microorganisms, and a relevant number of containers. The percent contamination level (% C) is calculated as follows:

$$\% C = \frac{N_G}{N_T - N_D} \times 100 \tag{5}$$

where N_G is the number of undamaged containers with microbial growth, N_T is the total number of containers filled, and N_D is the number of damaged contaminated containers. Procedures for validation of aseptic fill for solution drug products have been presented in a recent publication by the Parenteral Drug Association.[10]

Validation Steps

The actual validation of a sterilization process must follow a logical, systematic series of steps and procedures. The validation procedure for a steam sterilization process may involve the following design:

1. Certify that the sterilizer has been mechanically checked and qualified.[11]

2. Select the most appropriate biologic indicator microorganism possessing the desired resistance to steam heat, while realizing the advantages and hazards of bioindicators.[12]

3. Experimentally determine the D value and Z value of the selected bioindicator.

4. Determine the distribution of heat in the empty sterilizer, and identify the coolest location.

5. Determine the distribution of heat of a defined loading size and configuration and identify the coolest location.

6. Determine the penetration of heat into the product units at the coolest location and at suspected locations where heat penetration will be slowest.

7. Evaluate the effect of such cycle parameters as time, temperature, and load configuration on the destruction of the bioindicator and the magnitude of the F_o value.

8. Determine the sterilization process time required to achieve the desired F_o value and/or the desired probability level of bioindicator destruction.

9. Repeat the process until satisfactory and reliable replication is obtained.

10. Establish a monitoring program for periodic requalification of the sterilization cycle.

11. Finalize standard operating procedures and action levels should changes or problems develop in the future.

The validation procedure for an aseptic filtration process may involve the following design:

1. Properly evaluate the facility and critical areas for proper equipment function, air quality, and other engineering criteria.

2. Perform air and surface microbial tests in the filling area to know reliably the background microbial contamination level.

3. Select a sensitive microbial growth medium.

4. Select the most appropriate challenge microorganism for aseptic filtration validation.

5. Sterilize growth medium and all filtration equipment by sterilization methods previously validated.

6. Conduct a process simulation test by filtering a desired volume of microbial growth medium containing a known concentration of challenge microorganism into an appropriate number of previously sterilized containers.

7. Incubate the filled containers at the proper conditions with proper controls.

8. Determine the percent contamination level according to equation (5).

9. Repeat the process.

10. If percent contamination level is unacceptable, for example, >0.1%, review all environmental test results, sterilization records, and other data to determine what action needs to be taken to attain a percent contamination level of less than 0.1%.

Physical Processes of Sterilization

Thermal Methods

The lethal effectiveness of heat on microorganisms depends upon the degree of heat, the exposure period, and the moisture present. Within the range of sterilizing temperatures, the time required to produce a lethal effect is inversely proportional to the temperature employed. For example, sterilization may be accomplished in 1 hour with dry heat at a temperature of 170°C, but may require as much as 3 hours at a temperature of 140°C. While it is common practice to identify cycle times in terms of the maximum temperature hold time, total heat input may be computed in terms of F values, as explained previously; however, the lethal effect must be computed in terms of the time during which the entire mass of the material is heated. The mechanism by which microorganisms are killed by heat is thought to be the coagulation of the protein of the living cell. The data given in Table 21-3 illustrate this principle, using the effect of varying amounts of water on the temperature required to coagulate egg albumin.[13] The temperature required is inversely related to the moisture present. Further, experience in the laboratory has confirmed that sterilization by thermal methods may be effected at lower temperatures in the presence of moisture.

Thermal methods of sterilization may conveniently be divided into those accomplished by dry heat and those by moist heat.

TABLE 21-3. *Effect of Moisture and Heat on Egg Albumin*

Water (%)	Temperature (°C)	Effect
50	56	coagulation
25	80	coagulation
6	145	coagulation
0	170	coagulation and oxidation

Dry Heat. Substances that resist degradation at temperatures above approximately 140°C (284°F) may be rendered sterile by means of dry heat. Two hours exposure to a temperature of 180°C (356°F) or 45 min at 260°C (500°F) normally can be expected to kill spores as well as vegetative forms of all microorganisms. This total sterilizing cycle time normally includes a reasonable *lag time* for the substance to reach the sterilizing temperature of the oven chamber, an appropriate hold period to achieve sterilization, and a cooling period for the material to return to room temperature.

Factors in Determining Cycle Time. The cycle time is composed of three parts: (1) the thermal increment time of both the chamber and the load of material to be sterilized, assuming both start at room temperature, (2) the hold period at the maximum temperature, and (3) the cooling time. The material lags behind the increasing temperature of the chamber. The time required for all of the material to "catch up" with the temperature of the chamber is longer with larger quantites of material, poorer thermal conductance properties of the material, and lower heat capacity. The relationship of these factors must be carefully determined during validation studies so that effective cycle times can be planned.

The cycle time is most commonly prescribed in terms of the hold time, for example, 2 hours at 180°C dry heat. The hold time may be shown by sensors detecting the temperature of the chamber at its coolest spot; however, a better indication of the actual thermal condition is obtained by sensing, usually with a thermocouple, the coolest spot in the load of the material to be sterilized. When such a location is used, and when this coolest spot is known from previous validation studies, the timing required for sterilization is correctly programmable. It should be remembered that other parts of the load of material may be heated for a longer period, and if it is thermally unstable, degradation could occur. Therefore, the thermal stability of the material to be sterilized must be known and the optimum method of sterilization selected to achieve effective sterilization throughout the entire mass of material while maintaining its stability and integrity.

Sterilizer Types. The ovens used to achieve hot air sterilization are of two types, natural convection and forced convection. Circulation within natural convection ovens depends upon the currents produced by the rise of hot air and fall of cool air. This circulation can be easily blocked with containers, resulting in poor heat distribution efficiency. Differences in tempera-

ture of 20°C or more may be found in different shelf areas of even small laboratory ovens of the natural convection type.[14]

Forced convection ovens provide a blower to circulate the heated air around the objects in the chamber. Efficiency is greatly improved over natural convection. Temperature differences at various locations on the shelves may be reduced to as low as ±1°C. The lag times of the load material therein also are greatly reduced because fresh hot air is circulated rapidly around the objects. The curves shown in Figure 21-3 illustrate the difference in lag time for some of the same containers of corn oil when heated in a natural convection oven as compared with the same oven equipped for forced circulation.[14]

Another type of sterilizer is the tunnel unit with a moving belt, designed to thermally sterilize glass bottles and similar items as they move through the tunnel. The items are cooled with clean air before they exit the tunnel, usually directly into an aseptic room and linked in a continuous line with a filling machine. Such units require careful validation.[15]

Effect on Materials. The elevated temperatures required for effective hot air sterilization in a reasonable length of time have an adverse effect on many substances. Cellulose materials, such as paper and cloth, begin to char at a temperature of about 160°C (320°F). At these temperatures, many chemicals are decomposed, rubber is rapidly oxidized, and thermoplastic materials melt. Therefore, this method of sterilization is reserved largely for glassware, metalware, and anhydrous oils and chemicals that can

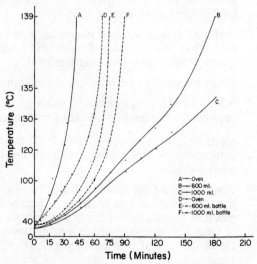

FIG. 21-3. *Rate of heating corn oil in Pyrex liter bottles in the same hot air oven with natural convection (———●———) and forced circulation (––●––).*

withstand the elevated temperature ranges without degradation. Expansion of materials is also appreciable, as they are heated from room to sterilizing temperatures. Therefore, glassware must not be wedged tightly in the oven chamber, containers for oils must be large enough to permit expansion of the oil, and provision must be made for the expansion of other substances.

Advantage may be taken of the anhydrous state achieved with this method of sterilization to provide dry glassware and metalware at the end of an adequate heating cycle. Dry equipment and containers are essential in the manufacture of an anhydrous product, but they are also desirable to prevent dilution of an aqueous product. Also, dry equipment can be kept sterile during storage more easily than wet equipment. Further, dry heat effectively destroys pyrogens, usually requiring about twice the hold time for sterilization.

To maintain a sterile condition after sterilization, environmental contamination must be excluded. The openings of equipment must be covered with a barrier material such as aluminum foil. As an alternative, items to be sterilized may be placed in a covered stainless steel box or similar protective container.

Moist Heat. Moist heat is more effective than dry heat for thermal sterilization. It should be remembered, however, that normal moist heat cycles do not destroy pyrogens.

As previously noted, moist heat causes the coagulation of cell protein at a much lower temperature than dry heat. In addition, the thermal capacity of steam is much greater than that of hot air. At the point of condensation (*dew point*), steam liberates thermal energy equal to its heat of vaporization. This amounts to approximately 540 calories per gram at 100°C (212°F) and 524 calories per gram at 121°C (250°F). In contrast, the heat energy liberated by hot dry air is equivalent to approximately only 1 calorie per gram of air for each degree centrigrade of cooling. Therefore, when saturated steam strikes a cool object and is condensed, it liberates approximately 500 times the amount of heat energy liberated by an equal weight of hot air. Consequently, the object is heated much more rapidly by steam. In addition, when steam under pressure is employed, a rapidly changing fresh supply of heat-laden vapor is applied to the object being heated. This is due both to the pressure under which steam is applied and to the partial vacuum produced at the site where steam is condensed, for it shrinks in volume by about 99% as it condenses.

Air Displacement. The density of steam is lower than that of air. Therefore, steam enters an autoclave chamber and rises to the top, displacing air downward, as illustrated by the gravity displacement autoclave shown in Figure 21-4. Objects must be placed in the chamber with adequate circulation space around each object, and so arranged that air can be displaced downward and out of the exhaust line from the chamber. Any trapped air, e.g., air in containers with continuous sides and bottoms or in tightly wrapped packs, prevents penetration of the steam to these areas and thus prevents sterilization. The air trapped in this manner is heated to the temperature of the steam, but hot air at a temperature of 120°C (248°F) requires a cycle time of 60 hours to ensure a lethal effect on spores.[16] A 20-min exposure at this temperature with hot dry air, therefore, would be entirely inadequate.

Factors Determining Cycle Time. Spores and vegetative forms of bacteria may be effectively destroyed in an autoclave employing steam under pressure during an exposure time of 20 min at 15 pounds pressure (121°C [250°F]) or as little as 3 min at 27 pounds pressure (132°C [270°F]). These time intervals are based on the assumption that the steam has reached the innermost recess of the material to be steri-

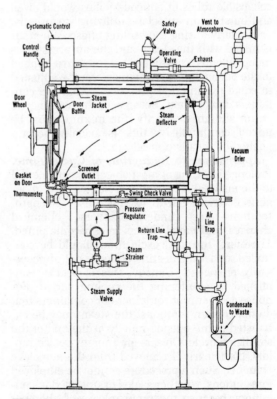

FIG. 21-4. *Cross-sectional diagram of the functional parts of an autoclave. (Courtesy of American Sterilizer Co.)*

lized, and that the temperature of the material is held for at least one half of that time interval. In the case of bottles of solution, the heat must be conducted through the wall of the container, raise the temperature of the solution to that of its environment, and generate steam within the container from the water therein. Therefore, a significant lag time is involved before the solution reaches the sterilizing temperature.

The determination of lag time and its inclusion in the planned total cycle time is no less important for moist heat sterilization than for hot air sterilization, discussed previously. By way of illustration, it has been found that 1200 ampuls, each containing 5 ml of a solution, can be effectively sterilized in an autoclave at 121°C (250°F) during an exposure time of 20 min. A single bottle containing the same total volume of solution (6 L) required an exposure of 60 min at 121°C (250°F).[17]

Air-Steam Mixtures. While air-steam mixtures have a lower temperature and lower thermal capacity than pure steam, the presence of air may be utilized to control the pressure in the chamber when flexible-walled containers of products are being sterilized. For example, plastic bags of large-volume parenterals (LVPs) or collapsible tubes of aqueous jellies would swell and burst in an autoclave utilizing steam only, particularly during the cooling phase. When air is mixed with the steam and the air pressure is independently controlled, the pressure applied to the outside of the containers can be adjusted to equal the internal pressure so that the containers do not burst. Because of the tendency of steam and air to stratify, the mixture must be mixed continuously; this is usually accomplished by means of a blower.

Approaches to Reduction of Cycle Time. Prolonged heating of most objects is detrimental to the material. For example, fabrics and rubber parts deteriorate with loss of tensile strength, solutions may undergo adverse chemical changes, and metal objects may become pitted. Therefore, the total cycle time should be controlled so that the heating period is not unnecessarily prolonged. Usually, this is best accomplished by shortening the cooling period. For nonsealed items of equipment or containers that do not contain solutions, the steam may be exhausted to the outside rapidly at the end of the sterilizing cycle. Objects are thereby cooled rapidly, particularly if removed from the autoclave chamber. Such a procedure cannot be employed for solutions, whether sealed or unsealed in containers, because the rapid release of chamber pressure would cause violent ebullition of the hot solution, with spattering of the contents of

unsealed containers and explosion of sealed containers.

One method for rapid extraction of heat from sealed containers of solutions is to spray the containers with gradually cooling water while the pressure in the chamber is concurrently reduced. Another accelerated cooling method employs short pulses of high pressure steam introduced into the loaded chamber. As the steam expands in the chamber it extracts heat from the containers of solution. The steam is exhausted from the chamber at a rate that provides for a gradual reduction of the pressure concurrent with the temperature reduction. By these methods, it is sometimes necessary to introduce pulses of air into the chamber to replace all or part of the steam so that the pressure around the containers is not reduced too rapidly. By the spray cooling method, it has been reported that the cooling time for a load of 200 one-liter bottles of solution may be reduced from about 20 hours to about 20 min.[18]

A relatively new approach to a reduction in the total heating cycle time has been the introduction of a precycle vacuum. In a specially designed autoclave, a precycle vacuum of at least 20 mm Hg is drawn. More recent studies have shown that a double vacuum drawn in sequence prior to the heating cycle removes air more effectively from porous materials.[19] The subsequent introduction of steam permits rapid penetration and load heating with complete elimination of air pockets. Since the total heating period is markedly reduced owing to the reduction in the temperature increment time, a higher temperature (usually 135°C [275°F]) may be employed with less deleterious effects on materials. This method is particularly suited to operating room packs in hospitals, where the total cycle time for large packs has been reduced from about 78 min by the conventional method to about 14 min. Such a method cannot be used for solutions or other objects that cannot withstand the high vacuum employed.

Lower Temperature Sterilization. Moist heat also is used for lower temperature sterilization procedures. Temperatures of 100°C (212°F) or lower are used for these so-called *marginal*, or *fractional*, methods. The term marginal originates from the questionable reliability of the processes. The term fractional is derived from the fact that these processes are normally performed by two or three exposures to moist heat, alternated with intervals during which the material is held at room or incubator temperatures.

Fractional methods of sterilization such as tyndallization, employing a temperature of 100°C (212°F), and inspissation, employing temperatures as low as 60°C (140°F), are relatively effective in reducing the number of vegetative forms of microorganisms, but are unreliable against spores. For certain preparations, the effectiveness of these processes may be improved by the inclusion of a bacteriostatic agent. These marginal methods of sterilization should be reserved for substances that must be processed by a thermal method but that cannot withstand higher temperatures without degradation. The assurance of sterility is comparatively low, however.

Wrapping Materials. Wrappings for equipment and supplies subjected to moist heat sterilization must permit easy penetration of steam and escape of air. They must also possess sufficient wet strength so that they will not tear or burst during the process. After sterilization, the wrapping must provide an efficient bacterial barrier so that equipment remains sterile for a reasonable time until used. In addition, maintenance of sterility depends upon complete coverage of the contents of the pack, drying of the wrapping after the process, and a static air state within. Acceptable disposable process wrapping materials include 20-lb weight Kraft paper, special parchment paper, and Tyvek. Reusable types include close-weave nylon and Dacron. Except for Kraft paper, all are low-lint materials.

Indicators for Evaluating the Sterilization Process. The duplication of proven thermal methods of sterilization cannot be taken for granted. Mechanical equipment as well as personnel are subject to failure. Therefore, indicators should be used as a check on the duplication of the conditions of a proven (validated) process, locating the indicator where there is the greatest impediment to the penetration of the heat.

Among the indicators available, the most widely used is the thermocouple. These indicators are often connected to recorders so that a continuous record of the actual temperature at the location of the thermocouple can be obtained.

For autoclave sterilization, a variety of other indicators also are used. These include wax or chemical pellets that melt at 121°C and paper strips that are impregnated with chemicals that change color under the influence of moisture and heat. All of these have limited reliability for indicating the length of time that a temperature of 121°C has been maintained.

Resistant bacterial spores in sealed ampuls or impregnated in dry paper strips are used as biologic indicators. Their destruction is evidence of the intended effect of a sterilization process. Their use to prove the effectiveness of new sterilizing equipment or processes is widely accepted,[12] but their use as indicators for routine process control is questioned by some. Among the concerns are (1) lot to lot variability of the resistance of the spores, (2) lot to lot variability in the number of viable spores, (3) difficulty in obtaining pure cultures, and (4) the inherent danger of placing viable spores in a sterilizer load of materials for human use.

Application of Thermal Methods of Sterilization. It is generally accepted that the most reliable thermal method of sterilization is the use of moist heat under pressure. Therefore, this method of sterilization should be employed whenever possible. Aqueous pharmaceutical preparations in hermetically sealed containers that can withstand the temperature of autoclaving can be rendered sterile and remain so indefinitely unless tampering with the seal occurs. Nonaqueous preparations in sealed containers cannot be sterilized in this manner during a normal cycle because no water is present within the container to generate steam and thereby effect sterilization.

Moist heat sterilization is also applicable to equipment and supplies such as rubber closures, glassware, and other equipment with rubber attachments; filters of various types; and uniforms. To be effective, however, air pockets must be eliminated. This normally requires that the items be wet when placed in the autoclave. They also will be wet at the end of the sterilizing cycle. When moisture can escape without damage to the package, part of the moisture can be removed by employing an evacuation step at the end of the cycle. Even this process does not usually completely dry the equipment. Therefore, when such equipment is used in processing, allowance must be made for the diluting effect of this water, or preferably, a small portion of the product may be used to rinse or flush the water out of the equipment. In some instances, when dry equipment is required and it must be sterilized by autoclaving, the equipment may be dried in a vacuum oven before use.

Dry heat sterilization is used for containers and equipment whenever possible because an adequate cycle results in sterile and dry equipment. High-speed processing lines recently developed have included a hot-air tunnel for the continuous sterilization of glass containers, which are heated by infrared lamps or by electrically heated, filtered, circulating air. Glass and metal equipment usually withstand dry heat sterilization without difficulty, although uneven thermal expansion may cause breakage or distortion. Rubber and cellulosic materials undergo degradation, however. Certain ingredients, such as chemicals and oleaginous vehicles, to be used in sterile pharmaceutical preparations are sometimes sterilized with dry heat at lower (usually 140°C or less) temperatures. In such cases, it must be established that the heating cycle has no deleterious effects on the ingredients and that the cycle time is adequate to achieve sterilization. They also must be carefully protected after sterilization until incorporated aseptically in the product to prevent contamination from the environment.

Nonthermal Methods

Ultraviolet Light. Ultraviolet light is commonly employed to aid in the reduction of contamination in the air and on surfaces within the processing environment. The germicidal light produced by mercury vapor lamps is emitted almost exclusively at a wave length of 2537 Angstrom units (253.7 millimicrons). It is subject to the laws for visible light, i.e., it travels in a straight line, its intensity is reduced in proportion to the square of the relative distance it travels, and it penetrates materials poorly or selectively. Ultraviolet light penetrates clean air and pure water well, but an increase in the salt content and/or the suspended matter in water or air causes a rapid decrease in the degree of penetration. For most other applications, penetration is negligible, and any germicidal action is confined to the exposed surface.

Lethal Action. When ultraviolet light passes through matter, energy is liberated to the orbital electrons within constituent atoms. This absorbed energy causes a highly energized state of the atoms and alters their reactivity. When such excitation and alteration of activity of essential atoms occurs within the molecules of microorganisms or of their essential metabolites, the organism dies or is unable to reproduce. The principal effect may be on cellular nucleic acids, which have been shown to exhibit strong absorption bands within the ultraviolet wavelength range.

The lethality of ultraviolet radiations has been well established; however, it also has been shown that organisms exposed to ultraviolet radiations can sometimes recover, a fact not surprising if the previously described theroy of lethality is correct. Recovery has been increased by the addition of certain essential metabolites to the culture, adjustment of the pH of the medium, or exposure to visible light shortly after exposure to the ultraviolet radiations. Therefore, adequate exposure to the radiations must occur before reliance can be placed upon obtaining a sterilizing effect.

The germicidal effectiveness of ultraviolet light is a function of the intensity of radiation and time of exposure. It also varies with the susceptibility of the organism. The data in Table 21-4 show some of this range of susceptibility.[20] From these data, it can be seen that if the intensity of radiation on a surface was 20 microwatts per cm^2, the minimum intensity usually recommended, it would require approximately 1100 seconds exposure to kill B. subtilis spores, but only approximately 275 seconds to kill S. hemolyticus. The intensity of ultraviolet radiation can be measured by means of a special light meter having a phototube sensitive to the 2537 Å wavelength.

Maintenance and Use. To maintain maximum effectiveness, ultraviolet lamps must be kept free from dust, grease, and scratches because of the large reduction in emission intensity that will occur. Also, they must be replaced when emission levels decrease substantially (about 30 to 50%) owing to energy-induced changes in the glass that inhibits the emission.

Personnel present in areas where ultraviolet lights are on should be protected from the direct and reflected rays. These rays cause reddening of the skin and intensely painful irritation of the eyes. The American Medical Association has recommended that the maximum safe human exposure for 1 hour be limited to 2.4 mw/cm.[2]

Ultraviolet lamps are used primarily for their germicidal effect on surfaces or for their penetrating effect through clean air and water. Therefore, they are frequently installed in rooms, air ducts, and large equipment in which the radiation can pass through and irradiate the air, and also reach exposed surfaces. Water sup-

TABLE 21-4. *Intensity of Radiation at 2537 Å Necessary to Completely Destroy Certain Microorganisms*

Organism	Energy (mw.-sec./cm.²)
Bacillus subtilis	11,000
B. subtilis spores	22,000
Eberthella typhosa	4,100
Escherichia coli	6,600
Pseudomonas aeruginosa	10,500
Sarcina lutea	26,400
Staphylococcus aureus	6,600
Streptococcus hemolyticus	5,500
Saccharomyces cerevisiae	13,200
Penicillium roqueforti	26,400
Aspergillus niger	330,000
Rhizopus nigricans	220,000

plies also have been sterilized when the limit of penetration has been carefully determined and controlled so that adequate irradiation throughout has been achieved.

Ionizing Radiations. Ionizing radiations are high-energy radiations emitted from radioactive isotopes such as cobalt-60 (*gamma rays*) or produced by mechanical acceleration of electrons to very high velocities and energies (*cathode rays, beta rays*). Gamma rays have the advantage of being absolutely reliable, for there can be no mechanical breakdown; however, they have the disadvantages that their source (radioactive material) is relatively expensive and the emission cannot be shut off as it can from the mechanical source of accelerated electrons. Accelerated electrons also have the advantage of providing a higher and more uniform dose rate output.

Electron Accelerators. Electron accelerators are of two general types, the linear and the Van de Graaff accelerators. The principle of the linear accelerator may be followed from Figure 21-5. Very high-frequency microwaves (radar) collect electrons from a cathode and accelerate them as they travel through the vacuum tube, reaching almost the speed of light. The electrons are emitted and directed to the target at an energy range of 3 to 15 million electron volts (meV). Since energy potentials of 10 meV or higher may produce radioactive materials, linear accelerators of more than 9 meV are not normally used for sterilizing.

The Van de Graaff accelerators are capable of energy potentials up to 3 meV. They utilize the force exerted on a charged particle by a high voltage potential in an electric field as a means of direct particle acceleration.

Determination of Dosage. The dosage is determined by the energy released by the gamma rays or by the number of electrons that impinge on each square centimeter of absorbing substance (the target). The *rad* is the unit of absorbed radiation, the unit of dosage now most frequently employed. It is arbitrarily defined as the absorption of 100 ergs of energy per gram of substance. The depth of penetration within a target of a given dose is directly related to the electron voltage of the source, and indirectly related to the density of the material to be irradiated.

Lethal Action and Dosage. Ionizing radiations destroy microorganisms by stopping reproduction as a result of lethal mutations. These mutations are brought about by a transfer of radiation beam energies to receptive molecules in their path, the direct-hit theory. Mutations also may be brought about by indirect action in

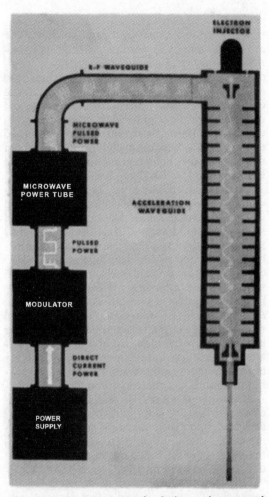

FIG. 21-5. *Operating principle of a linear electron accelerator. (Courtesy of High Voltage Engineering Corp.)*

which water molecules are transformed into highly energized entities such as hydrogen and hydroxyl ions. These, in turn, bring about energy changes in nucleic acids and other molecules, thus eliminating their availability for the metabolism of the bacterial cell. Ionizing radiations differ from ultraviolet rays in their effects on matter primarily in that the former are of a higher energy level, actually producing ionization of constituent atoms. Bacterial spores and viruses are generally four to five times more resistant than vegetating bacteria and molds. A dose of 2 to 2.5 megarads, however, is considered adequate to ensure sterility.[21] Currently, there is no evidence of reactivation of microorganisms as has been found with ultraviolet light.

Applications for Sterilization. Accelerated electrons or gamma rays may be used to sterilize select products by a continuous process. Most other product sterilization procedures must be performed in batches. Continuous-process sterilization requires exacting control so that there are no momentary lapses in sterilizing effectiveness. Assurance of adequate dose delivery, complete and uniform coverage of the product, and adequate penetration have been achieved in the effective and routine sterilization of sutures,[22] using a linear accelerator. Adequate dosage is usually determined by the effect of the absorbed energy, at the maximum determined depth of penetration, on photographic film, and/or on the biologic indicator Bacillus pumilus.

The use of radiation is increasing in frequency and extent as experience is gained with this method, particularly for the sterilization of medical plastic devices. It has been given new impetus by the question raised by the Occupational Safety and Health Administration (OSHA) on the safety of ethylene oxide and the low environmental level now being permitted. Availability of facilities for this method, using both energy sources, is increasing. An individual medical device or pharmaceutical manufacturer may not justify the high cost of a facility for radiation sterilization, but the increasing availability of centers performing contract services is making this method a more viable option.

A number of vitamins, antibiotics, and hormones in the dry state have been successfully sterilized by radiation. Liquid pharmaceuticals are more difficult to sterilize because of the potential effect of the radiations on the vehicle system as well as the drug.

Filtration. Filtration may be used for the removal of particles, including microorganisms, from solutions and gases without the application of heat. Ideally, filters should not alter the solution or gas in any way, neither removing desired constituents nor imparting undesired components. This requirement essentially limits the types of filters currently employed to the polymeric types listed in Table 21-5A, B. Furthermore, almost all of those currently in use with parenteral solutions and gases are of the membrane type, that is, tissue-thin material removing particles primarily by sieving. When a filter does remove constituents from a solution such removal is usually due to the phenomenon of adsorption, which being a surface phenomenon, occurs during only the first portion of the filtration, that is, until the surface of the filter is saturated with the adsorbed molecule or ion. The most common attack on the filter itself is due to the solvent properties of the vehicle of certain parenteral products. Since the most common solvent for parenteral solutions is water, and the use of other types of solvents is limited, this usually is not a problem. Moreover, the development of membrane filters composed of materials having high resistance to most pharmaceutical solvents has further reduced this problem.

As noted in Table 21-5A, B, membrane filters are usually composed of plastic polymers, including cellulose acetate and nitrate, nylon, polyvinyl chloride, polycarbonate, polysulfone and Teflon. Occasionally, sintered metals such as stainless steel and silver are used when highly durable characteristics are required.

Since most of the membrane filters are disposable, the problem of cleaning after use is limited to the reusable filter housing and support screen. These are usually made of stainless steel or tough plastic polymers that are cleaned rather easily. Careful attention must be given, however, to disassembly of the housing and scrubbing to remove any residues that might introduce contamination in subsequent use.

The membranes are usually rendered hydrophilic by treatment with a surface active agent at the time of manufacture. If this is not done, particularly at the lower porosities, an aqueous solution cannot be forced through the filter except under very high pressure. When nonwetting with water is desired, however, as with such nonaqueous solvents as ethanol and inert gases, the polymer is left in its hydrophobic form.

Function of Filters. Membrane filters function primarily by sieving, or by screening particles from a solution or gas, thus retaining them on the filter surface. Because of the nature of membrane filters and their limited thickness, there is little entrapment within the filter medium, this being a mechanism applicable to the function of depth filters, such as those made of glass and paper. Membrane filters also function in some instances by electrostatic attraction. This would apply particularly to the filtration of dry gases, in which electrostatic charges tend to increase because of the frictional effect of the flowing gas.

The pores, or holes, through any filter medium consist of a range of sizes. For example, if a filter is designated as 0.2 micron porosity, the porosity most commonly used to effect sterilization, the maximum mean pore diameter is 0.2 micron, with many pores much smaller than this and a few larger. The latter may have diameters as large as 0.5 micron, but they are so few in number that the probability of a microbial spore (commonly rated as being 0.5 micron in diameter) finding those few pores is highly remote. However, it must be recognized that there is a probability of this happening, even though remote. Therefore, it is no longer acceptable to consider such filters an absolute means of sterilizing a solution. To increase the probabil-

TABLE **21-5A.** *Comparative Characteristics of the Membrane Filters (0.2 µm porosity) Used for Sterilization*

Filter Type	Particular Uses	Pharmaceutical Solvents to Be Avoided	Trade Name	Company*
HYDROPHILIC				
Acrylic copolymer with nylon substrate	Aqueous solutions, alcohols, and glycols	Dimethylformamide	Versapor AN Hydrophilic Acropor	Gelman Gelman
Cellulose acetate/nitrate	Aqueous solutions	Benzyl alcohol, ethanol, propylene glycol, dimethylformamide	MF-Millipore SM 11307 Membra-Fil BA83	Millipore Sartorius Nuclepore S & S
Cellulose acetate	Aqueous solutions with selective alcohol resistance	Benzyl alcohol, ethanol, (selective), propylene glycol, dimethylformamide	GA Metricel Celotate OE66 SM 11107 SM 11607	Gelman Millipore S & S Sartorius Sartorius
Cellulose, regenerated	Aqueous solutions and pharmaceutical solvents	Solvent resistant	RC 58	S & S
Nylon 66 (polyamide)	Aqueous solutions and pharmaceutical solvents	Solvent resistant	Ultipor N_{66}	Pall
Polycarbonate	Aqueous solutions	Benzyl alcohol, dimethylformamide	Nuclepore Uni-Pore	Nuclepore Bio-Rad
Polysulfone	Aqueous solutions	Benzyl alcohol, dimethylformamide	HT Tuffryn	Gelman
Polyvinylidene difluoride	Aqueous solutions with up to 35% solvents	Acetone, dimethyl formamide	Durapore Hydrophilic	Millipore
HYDROPHOBIC				
Polytetrafluorethylene with polyethylene or polypropylene substrate	Air and nonaqueous solvents, aqueous solutions if pre-wet with ethanol	Solvent resistant	TF Teflon Fluoropore TE 35 Filinert Emflon	Gelman Millipore S & S Nuclepore Pall
Polyvinylidene difluoride	Air and aqueous solutions if pre-wet with ethanol	Acetone, dimethylformamide	Durapore	Millipore

*Bio-Rad Labs.—Richmond, CA 94804, Gelman Sciences—Ann Arbor, MI 48106; Millipore—Bedford, MA 01730; Nuclepore—Pleasanton, CA 94566; Pall Trinity Micro Corp.—Cortland, NY 13045; Sartorius—Hayward, CA 94545; Schleicher & Schuell—Keene, NH 03431

TABLE 21-5B. *Comparative Characteristics of the Membrane Filters (0.2μm porosity) Used for Sterilization*

Trade Name	Extractables	Approx. H₂O Flow Rate (ml/min./cm² at 520mm Hg)	Bubble Point (psig)	Sterilization— Autoclavable
HYDROPHILIC				
Versapor	< 3%	37	—	No, ETO
AN Hydrophilic Acropor	< 3%	20	11*	No, ETO
MF-Millipore	< 5%	15.6	55	No, ETO
SM 11307	< 0.3%	25‡	55	Yes
Membra-Fil	< 2%	18	50	Yes
BA83	1.5%	20	54	No, ETO
GA Metricel	< 3%	20	45	Yes
Celotate	—	15.6	55	No, ETO
OE66	1.5%	20	54	No, ETO
SM 11107	< 0.7%	20‡	50	Yes, and dry heat
SM 11607	negligible	25‡	50	Yes, and dry heat
RC 58	< 1.5%	25‡	54	Yes
Ultipor N₆₆	negligible	—	46	Yes
Nuclepore	negligible	15	60	Yes
Uni-Pore	negligible	26‡	—	Yes
HT Tuffryn	< 3.5%	12	36	Yes, or limited dry heat
Durapore Hydrophilic	negligible	15	45	Yes
HYDROPHOBIC				
TF Teflon	trace	15†	13†	Yes, and dry heat
Fluoropore	trace	15†	13†	Yes, and dry heat
TE 35	trace	15†	13†	Yes, and dry heat
Filinert	trace	20†	11.5†	Yes, and dry heat
Emflon	trace	4.65§	Forward flow testing	Yes, and dry heat
Durapore	negligible	15	18†	Yes

*With kerosene.
†With methyl alcohol.
‡At 700 mm Hg Δ P.
§At 207 mm Hg Δ P.

ity of achieving a sterile filtrate, some researchers are proposing that the solution be passed through a series of two 0.2-micron porosity filters. Others have suggested that a 0.1-micron porosity filter be used, but this would greatly reduce the flow rate.

Since membrane filters function primarily by sieving, particles of any kind in a solution are retained on the surface. If the content is relatively high, particles may accumulate on the surface and plug the filter so that the flow of solution decreases and perhaps stops. To avoid this problem, when solutions have a high content of solids, particularly when the solids are deformable macromolecules, the solution can best be processed by passing it through one or more prefilters, the first usually being a relatively porous depth filter. With depth filters, particles may gradually migrate through the filter if filtration time is prolonged, if there is a high pressure differential, or if there is frequent fluctuation of the pressure.

Liquid Flow Through a Filter. The flow rate of a liquid through a filter is affected by the size of the pores through the filter, the pore volume (the proportion of open space to solid matrix), the surface area of the filter, the pressure differential across the filter, and the viscosity of the liquid. Of these factors, the two most practical ways to increase flow rate is to increase the surface area of the filter or the pressure differential across the filter. There is a practical limit to increasing the diameter of a disc filter; thus, if larger surface areas are required, a pleated filter in a cartridge form is often used. In this way, a large increase in surface area may be achieved within a relatively small overall dimension of the filter unit. Within the limits of the physical strength of the filter and its housing, the pressure differential can be increased to several hundred pounds per square inch. In pharmaceutical practice, however, the pressure differential used is rarely more than 25 to 30 pounds per square inch. Usually, positive pressure is applied on the liquid upstream of the filter, but a vacuum may be drawn downstream of the filter. In the case of a vacuum, the maximum differential achievable is one atmosphere, or approximately 15 pounds per square inch. Furthermore, the negative pressure in the filtrate chamber makes it difficult to prevent the ingress of contamination from the environment. Therefore, for filtrations designed to render solutions sterile, it is preferable to apply pressure upstream of the filter using a gas filtered to be free from microorganisms. Any leakage that may occur in such a system causes loss to the outside without contamination of the sterile filtrate.

Solutions having a high viscosity normally have a slow flow rate. In most instances, the rate can be increased by warming the solution, thereby reducing its viscosity provided the warming does not have an adverse affect on the solution.

As previously mentioned, the flow rate through a filter also depends on the relative pore volume of the filter. All filters must have a solid matrix that forms the framework for the pores. The lower the amount of solid matrix is in proportion to the pore spaces, the higher are the pore volume and the flow rate.

Types of Filters. Since the filter membranes are designed to be used once and then discarded, they are disposable; further, filter housings composed of plastic polymers, which are also intended to be disposable, are becoming increasingly available. Thus, all after-use cleaning is eliminated. In addition, the membrane filter is sealed into the housing by the manufacturer, so that the risk of leakage is minimal.

Membrane filters are usually in the form of discs or pleated cylinders (cartridges). They range from 13-mm discs (approximately 0.8 cm^2) to 20-in. or longer cartridges (approximately 0.84 M^2). The housings are usually of stainless steel or of various plastic polymers.

A few years ago, it was rather common practice to use filters that were reusable, such as diatomaceous earth, sintered glass, and unglazed porcelain. Because of the problems of adequate cleaning between uses and of testing, current applications of these filters are limited.

Testing of Filters. Although membrane filters are tested and labeled by the manufacturer, the pore size and integrity of the filter should be checked before use. The least complicated method for doing this is the bubble point test. This test is performed by applying air pressure, or other gas pressure, to the upstream side of a hydrophilic filter in which the pores are filled with water. The pressure is gradually increased until bubbles pass through the filter and are detected in a liquid downstream. This bubble point pressure is inversely proportional to the diameter of the pores, and thus is a measure of the largest pores. The filter manufacturer identifies the appropriate test pressure for each pore size, for example, 55 pounds per square inch gauge for a hydrophilic membrane filter of 0.2 μm porosity as given in Table 21-5. If there is even a pinhole or similar defect in the filter, bubbling occurs at a much lower pressure than expected. For hydrophobic membranes, the filter is usually wet with ethanol or methanol prior to application of the air pressure.

For cartridge-type filters, it is practical to measure the diffusion of air, or other gas, through the water-filled pores of the filter medium because of the large surface area. Pressure is applied to the upstream side of the filter as specified by the manufacturer, at approximately 10% of the bubble test pressure. The air dissolves in the water in the pores of the membrane and is released from the downstream side of the membrane at a rate that is directly related to the pore size. This rate is measured by the volume of the air collected downstream or by the loss of pressure from the upstream side as the air diffuses.

A more direct test with respect to the ability of a filter to retain microorganisms is the microbial challenge test. A standardized culture containing a large number of small microorganisms, such as Pseudomonas diminuta, is filtered. The objective is to provide a high probability of finding oversized pores in the filter by the challenge of a large number of small microorganisms. Therefore, after filtration, the presence of bacteria in the filtrate constitutes a failure of the filter to sterilize the liquid. This type of test is normally a part of the quality control program of the filter manufacturer for each lot of sterilizing porosity membrane from which filters are made; however, it is rarely used in the pharmaceutical plant for individual filters.

Aseptic Processing. Sterilization of a solution by filtration provides an extremely clean solution, removing dirt particles as well as microorganisms in the micron size range. After sterilization, however, the filtrate must be transferred from the receiver and subdivided into the individual final containers. The objective of this process, known as *aseptic processing,* is to exclude every microorganism from all steps of the process subsequent to filtration. Accomplishing this requires a rigidly controlled aseptic environment and technique. The difficulty of maintaining such an aseptic condition is the greatest problem associated with sterilization by filtration; however, for solutions that are adversely affected by heat, this may be the only way in which sterilization can be accomplished.

Aseptic processing is technically not a sterilization process, but is mentioned here because of its close involvement with sterilization by filtration. It is used for products that cannot be *terminally sterilized*, that is, sterilized after they have been sealed in the final container. (See also Chapter 22.)

Chemical Processes of Sterilization

Gas Sterilization

Gas sterilization is not new. Such gases as formaldehyde and sulfur dioxide have been used for sterilization for many years. These gases are highly reactive chemicals, however, and are difficult to remove from many materials after exposure. Therefore, their usefulness is limited. Two newer gases, ethylene oxide and beta-propiolactone, have fewer disadvantages than the older agents and therefore have assumed importance in sterilization.[23] Undoubtedly, the advent of plastic materials and the need for a practical method of sterilizing them have spurred the development of the newer gaseous sterilizing agents, particularly ethylene oxide.

Ethylene Oxide. Ethylene oxide (EtO) is a cyclic ether ($[CH_2]_2O$) and is a gas at room temperature. Alone, it is highly flammable, and when mixed with air, explosive. Admixed with inert gases such as carbon dioxide or one or more of the fluorinated hydrocarbons (Freons) in certain proportions, ethylene oxide is rendered nonflammable and safe to handle. As a gas, it penetrates readily such materials as plastic, paperboard, and powder. Ethylene oxide dissipates from the materials simply by exposure to the air. It is chemically inert toward most solid materials. On the other hand, in the liquid state, as compressed in cylinders, ethylene oxide dissolves certain plastic and rubber materials and requires particular care in handling.

Sterilizing Process. Sterilization with ethylene oxide involves a carefully validated procedure using a pressure chamber.[24] The material to be sterilized is placed in a room or chamber and exposed to a relative humidity of up to 98% for a period of 60 min or longer. It is then placed in the chamber, previously heated to about 55°C (131°F), and an initial vacuum of approximately 27 in. Hg is drawn. The ethylene oxide is then introduced, along with moisture, to achieve a relative humidity of 50 to 60%, to the pressure required to give the desired concentration of ethylene oxide (see Table 21-6), which is maintained throughout the exposure period. Following the exposure period of 6 to 24 hours, depending on the degree of contamination, the penetrability of the material, and the concentra-

TABLE 21-6. *Exposure Conditions Used with Ethylene Oxide Mixtures at a Temperature of 55°C (131°F)**

Commercial Name	Mixture Content (%)	Ethylene Oxide Concentration (mg/L)	Chamber Pressures (Psig)	Minimum Exposure Periods (hours)
Carboxide†	10 Ethylene oxide 90 Carbon dioxide	450	28	6
Oxyfume-20†	20 Ethylene oxide 80 Carbon dioxide	670 920	18 30	4 3
Cry-Oxcide‡ (Benvicide)	11 Ethylene oxide 54 Trichlorofluoromethane 35 Dichlorodifluoromethane	450 850	5 18	5 3
Pennoxide§	12 Ethylene oxide 88 Dichlorodifluoromethane	650	7	4

*Following a humidifying (60% relative humidity) dwell period of 60 min.
†Union Carbide Chemicals Co., Niagara Falls, NY.
‡The Matheson Company, East Rutherford, NJ.
§Pennsylvania Engineering Company, Philadelphia, PA.

tion of EtO, the gas is exhausted, and a vacuum of approximately 25 inches Hg is drawn. Filtered air is then introduced into the chamber until atmospheric pressure is attained.

A heated chamber is used to decrease the time required for this sterilization process. A temperature of 55°C (131°F) has no adverse effect on most substances. It has been suggested that a rise in temperature of 17°C permits the shortening of the exposure period by about one half.[25]

Moisture also has been found to exert a significant effect on the sterilization process, although reports have varied greatly with respect to the conditions and the amount of moisture that are essential. It appears that a relative humidity (RH) of 30% or more is essential for effective antibacterial activity. Studies have shown that microorganisms must be hydrated if they are to be killed by ethylene oxide within the usual cycle time. If significantly dehydrated previously, their rehydration may require several days' exposure to relative humidities of 75% or more.[26] Moisture introduced into the sterilizing chamber along with the gas may not adequately hydrate the microorganism; the moisture must be absorbed by the surrounding material and penetrate the microorganism. Therefore, a moisturizing dwell period at up to 95% RH should be the first step in every sterilizing cycle as an aid in the distribution and absorption of moisture by the material to be sterilized. The dwell period also aids in establishing a moisture equilibrium within the chamber load, particularly for materials that preferentially absorb moisture.

The exposure conditions most frequently used with ethylene oxide are shown in Table 21-6. Note that concentrations higher than the minimum effective concentration of 450 mg per liter of chamber volume reduce the exposure period. The concentrations employed are directly related to the pressure of the various mixtures required to attain that concentration. Available equipment may limit the pressure and thereby the concentration attainable.

In addition, note that liquid ethylene oxide is frequently used instead of the mixtures with inert gases, thereby eliminating the necessity for high-pressure handling equipment. The liquid is usually vaporized into the sterilizing chamber previously evacuated to at least 720 mm (28 in.) Hg. In the absence of oxygen (in a vacuum) and a spark, there is no danger of explosion with ethylene oxide.

Normally, the dissipation of ethylene oxide from materials is accomplished readily at the end of a sterilizing cycle by the evacuation followed by a short period of aeration, that is, exposure to the normal atmosphere. It has been found, however, that certain materials—notably rubber, certain plastics, and leather—have a strong affinity for ethylene oxide and may require prolonged aeration, as long as 12 to 24 hours, before items made from these materials may safely be used. Tissue irritation may result if the ethylene oxide is not entirely dissipated. Concern also exists for the carcinogenic and mutagenic properties of EtO and residues in materials for human use. Both the Occupational Safety and Health Administration (OSHA) and the FDA have been studying this matter. As a consequence, OSHA has recently established an occupational exposure standard of 1 ppm of EtO as an 8-hour time-weighted average concentration.

Mechanism of Action. Ethylene oxide is believed to exert its lethal effect upon microorganisms by alkylating essential metabolites, affecting particularly the reproductive process.[23] The alkylation probably occurs by replacing an active hydrogen on sulfhydryl, amino, carboxyl, or hydroxyl groups with a hydroxyethyl radical. The altered metabolites are not available to the microorganism, and so it dies without reproducing.

Application. Alkylation may also occur with drug molecules in pharmaceutical preparations, particularly in the liquid state. Therefore, ethylene oxide sterilization of pharmaceuticals is limited essentially to dry powders of substances shown to be unaffected. It has extensive application, however, to plastic materials, rubber goods, and delicate optical instruments. It has also been found that stainless steel equipment has a longer useful life when sterilized with ethylene oxide instead of steam. The effective penetrability of ethylene oxide makes it possible to sterilize parenteral administration sets, hypodermic needles, plastic syringes, and numerous other related materials enclosed in distribution packages of paperboard or plastic.

Although the cycle time for sterilization with ethylene oxide is quite long and certain problems contributing to sterilization failures have yet to be elucidated, this method of sterilization has made it possible to sterilize many materials that would be virtually impossible to sterilize with other known methods.

Beta-propiolactone. Beta-propiolactone ($[CH_2]_2OCO$) is a cyclic lactone and is a nonflammable liquid at room temperature. It has a low vapor pressure, but since it is bactericidal against a wide variety of microorganisms at relatively low concentrations, no difficulty is experienced in obtaining bactericidal concentrations of the vapor. It is an alkylating agent and therefore has a mode of action against microorganisms similar to that of ethylene oxide. Studies have indicated that vapor concentrations of approximately 2 to 4 mg per liter of space are effective at a temperature not below 24°C (75°F) and a relative humidity of at least 70%, with an exposure period of at least 2 hours.[27]

The penetrability of beta-propiolactone vapor has been found to be poor. Therefore, its principal use appears to be the sterilization of surfaces in large spaces, such as entire rooms.

Surface Disinfection

The use of chemical disinfectants in the pharmaceutical industry is designed primarily to reduce the microbial population so that asepsis can be maintained in a limited, controlled environment. Most disinfectants do not destroy spores during any reasonable contact period; therefore, they do not sterilize a surface. However, as adjuncts to thorough cleaning of surfaces, disinfectants properly used may be expected to provide an aseptic condition of the surfaces involved.

The effectiveness of a disinfectant depends on the nature of the surface, the nature and degree of contamination, and the microbicidal activity of the agent employed. Hard smooth surfaces are much easier to disinfect than rough porous ones. Since most disinfectants are not effective against spores, only vegetative forms of microorganisms can be expected to be killed. The effectiveness of the agent will depend on the number of organisms present and their sensitivity to the agent. Therefore, it is essential to select an agent that has been proven effective against the common contaminants.

Hundreds of disinfectants have been made available commercially. Methods of evaluation differ significantly; therefore, comparisons of effectiveness are often quite difficult. In one comparison of 16 commercial disinfectants (identified by active constituents only) at least five were found to be ineffective by the screening method proposed. The two most effective contained a combination of four phenolic compounds.

Spaulding has provided a valuable summary of disinfectants.[29] He recommends a 2% solution of one of the phenolic germicide cleaners for floors and walls, and 1:1000 concentrations of quaternary ammonium solutions or 1 to 2% solutions of phenolic germicides for smooth hard surfaces. If the object is metallic, he recommends that 0.2% sodium nitrite be added to the quaternary ammonium solutions and 0.5%

sodium bicarbonate to the phenolic germicides to prevent rusting. Higher concentrations of disinfectants normally would be expected to be more effectively bactericidal; however, concentrations are limited by the detrimental effect that most of these solutions have on the surfaces to which they are applied. Chemical attack may be evidenced by such effects as pitting and rusting of metal surfaces and cracking and discoloration of painted surfaces.

Select disinfectants, particularly glutaraldehyde and beta-propiolactone have been found to improve the effectiveness of such physical methods of sterilization as ultraviolet light and ultrasonics. Other select combinations of chemical and physical sterilizing agents have shown increased reliability as compared with either agent alone.

Further details about the properties of the many germicides available may be found in standard textbooks.[1]

Evaluation

The effectiveness of each sterilization process must be demonstrated prior to its use under processing conditions. A thorough evaluation must be carried out, both of the functional capabilities of the equipment and of the process methods under the most demanding conditions of operation. This aspect has been discussed at the beginning of the chapter under the heading "Validation of Sterilization Processes."

Only when proved to be consistently effective can a particular procedure be considered a valid sterilization process. In addition, at frequent intervals during use, the equipment and methods should be re-evaluated to ensure that they are continuing to function properly.

Sterility Tests

Sterility tests are performed on products and materials subjected to a previously validated sterilization procedure. The results give evidence that the sterilization procedure has been repeated effectively; however, it is generally agreed that the controls exercised over an entire validated process give superior assurance of effective sterilization. These tests are performed on a sample selected to represent the entire lot of material. The sample may be taken from among final packages or containers of a product, or as a portion from a bulk tank of liquid or from other bulk material.

Details of the official test tube inoculation and filtration procedures, including modifications for certain special situations, are found in the USP.

Test Interpretations and Modifications. The principal operative factor in the test is that a portion of the material to be tested is placed in an environment designed so that any microorganisms present and viable will grow. It is well known, however, that microorganisms do not always reproduce or vegetate (spores) simply by being placed in what is thought to be a favorable environment. Attenuation resulting from ultraviolet radiation or nonlethal exposure to heat, lack of stimulation often necessary to make spores vegetate, and previous contact with a bacteriostatic agent are among the effects that may interfere with the growth of the organisms. In such cases, a false negative result would be obtained.

False negative results of a direct inoculation test also may occur as a result of antibacterial activity inherent in the product. In addition to those products in which a bacteriostatic agent has been purposely included, such an effect may arise from an excessively low pH, a high salt content, or antibacterial activity of the medicinal agent itself. Such antimicrobial effect may be determined by the introduction of viable microorganisms into tubes of culture medium with and without a serial dilution of an inoculum of the product. If comparable growth occurs in all tubes, the product is not antimicrobial (at least, against the specific organism used). If less growth occurs in some of the tubes containing an inoculum of the product, a specific inactivating agent must be used in subsequent testing, or a dilution ratio must be determined that will permit the microorganisms that are present to grow. Preferably, the filtration procedure would be used so that the product can be filtered away from any viable microorganisms retained on the filter.

A false negative result also may be obtained if the microbial population is so small that the inoculum taken from the product does not contain a microorganism. Since the product had been exposed to a sterilization process, it is conceivable that the microbial population may have been greatly reduced, but not totally so. This reduction would be more likely to occur with a marginal method of sterilization or with an aseptic procedure, although ideally, it should not occur at all. Such false results are best overcome by improving the reliability of the sterilization procedure, but in testing, they may be remedied by increasing the number or size of the sample.

A false positive test result could be caused by inadvertent contamination during the test. Such false results can be eliminated by the use of carefully and adequately trained personnel working in a properly controlled environment. In general, such results are expected to occur less than 1% of the time.

Although these limitations exist, the test is normally valid for detecting sterilization failures. The limitations of the test should be recognized, however, and the test should not be expected to yield more information than its design permits. The USP recommends that more exhaustive testing be performed at planned intervals to confirm the continued reliability of the sterilization procedures and of the testing methods. More exhaustive treatment of this subject may be found in the literature.[30]

Filtration Test Methods. The membrane filtration technique now has been accepted by the USP for large and small volume parenterals. Although a filtration technique is subject to a substantial risk from environmental contamination, it has certain distinct advantages, including the filtering away of inhibiting substances and the use of larger samples.

Essentially, this method permits the use of a sample of the liquid being tested of almost any desired volume. The liquid is filtered through a sterile membrane filter of microbial retentive porosity under strict aseptic environmental conditions. The microorganisms are retained on the filter, and the liquid under test passes into the filtrate, thereby carrying away potentially inhibitory substances. In addition, the filter may be rinsed with a sterile liquid, if necessary, to remove potentially inhibiting substances that may have adhered to the microorganisms. The filter is then placed in culture medium and incubated for growth.

Personnel conducting sterility tests must be thoroughly trained in the techniques employed. This requirement is even more stringent for persons conducting membrane filter tests because of the more complex manipulative steps involved. Likewise, persons interpreting the results from such tests must be thoroughly familiar with the limitations as well as the effectiveness of the tests.

The sterilization procedure is the vital step in achieving a sterile product, yet all other procedures and conditions required for the manufacture of the product must be designed to complement this step. Good housekeeping, an effectively controlled aseptic environment, a controlled and identified bioburden of the product, a well-planned and controlled production process, and well-trained and dedicated personnel for both production and testing are essential for the production of a sterile product. Only when all of these factors complement the findings from the sterility test can it be concluded with confidence that the product is sterile.

References

1. Block, S. S. (Ed.): Disinfection, Sterilization, and Preservation. 3rd Ed. Lea and Febiger, Philadelphia, 1983.
2. Gaughran, E. R. L., and Kereluk, K. (Eds.): Sterilization of Medical Products. Johnson & Johnson, New Brunswick, 1977.
3. Perkins, J. J.: Principles and Methods of Sterilization in Health Sciences. 2nd Ed. Charles C Thomas, Springfield, IL, 1969.
4. Phillips, G. B., and Miller, W. S. (Eds.): Industrial Sterilization. Duke Univ. Press, Durham, 1973.
5. Pflug, I. J., and Smith, G. M.: Survivor curves of bacterial spores heated in parenteral solutions. In Spore Research. Edited by A. N. Barker et al. Academic Press, London, 1976.
6. Pope, D. G., Tsuji, K., Robertson, J. H., and DeGeeter, M. J.: Pharm. Tech., 2:31, 1978.
7. Robertson, J. H., Townsend, M. W., Allen, P. M., et al.: Bull. Parenter. Drug Assoc., 31: 265, 1977.
8. Molin, G., and Östlund, K.: Can. J. Microbiol., 22:359, 1976.
9. Tsuji, K., and Harrison, S. J.: Appl. Environ. Microbiol., 36:710, 1978.
10. Technical Monograph No. 2, Parenteral Drug Association, Philadelphia, 1980.
11. Simmons, P. L.: Pharm. Tech., 3:69, 1979.
12. Myers, T., and Chrai, S.: J. Parenter. Drug Assoc., 34:234, 1980.
13. Lewith, S.: Arch. exper. Path. u. Pharmakol., 26:341, 1890.
14. Avis, K. E.: Am. J. Pharm., 129:11, 1957.
15. Akers, M. J., Avis, K. E., and Thompson, B.: J. Parenter. Drug Assoc., 34:330, 1980.
16. Bruch, C. W., Koesterer, M. G., and Bruch, M. K.: Develop. in Indus. Microbiol., 4:334, 1963.
17. Brewer, J. H.: The Becton, Dickinson Lectures on Sterilization. Seton Hall College of Medicine and Dentistry, Jersey City, NJ, April 10, 1959.
18. Wilkinson, G. R., Peacock, F. G., and Robins, E. L.: J. Pharm. Pharmacol., 12:197T, 1960.
19. Wilkinson, G. R., and Peacock, F. G.: J. Pharm. Pharmacol., 13:67T, 1961.
20. Nagy, R.: Research Paper BL-P-8-0089-6G6-3, Oct. 9, 1958, Westinghouse Electric Corp., Bloomfield, NJ
21. Ley, F. J., and Tallentire, A.: Pharm. J. 195:216, 1965.
22. Artandi, C., and Van Winkle, W., Jr.: Nucleonics, 17:86, 1959.
23. Bruch, C. W.: Ann. Rev. Microbiol., 15:245, 1961.
24. Halleck, F. E.: Med. Dev. & Diagn. Ind., 2:27, April 1980.
25. Ernst, R. R., and Shull, J. J.: Appl. Microbiol., 10:337, 1962.
26. Gilbert, G. L., Gambill, V. M., Spiner, D. R., et al.: Appl. Microbiol., 12:496, 1964.
27. Spiner, D. R., and Hoffman, R. K.: Appl. Microbiol., 8:152, 1960.
28. Ostrander, W. E., and Griffith, L. J.: Appl. Microbiol., 12:460, 1964.
29. Spaulding, E. H.: The Becton, Dickinson Lectures on Sterilization. Seton Hall College of Medicine and Dentistry, Jersey City, NJ April 1, 1958.
30. Bryce, D. M.: J. Pharm. Pharmacol., 8:561, 1956.

22

Sterile Products

KENNETH E. AVIS

Sterile products are dosage forms of therapeutic agents that are free of viable microorganisms. Principally, these include parenteral, ophthalmic, and irrigating preparations. Of these, parenteral products are unique among dosage forms of drugs because they are injected through the skin or mucous membranes into internal body compartments. Thus, because they have circumvented the highly efficient first line of body defense, the skin and mucous membranes, they must be free from microbial contamination and from toxic components as well as possess an exceptionally high level of purity. All components and processes involved in the preparation of these products must be selected and designed to eliminate, as much as possible, contamination of all types, whether of physical, chemical, or microbiologic origin.

Preparations for the eye, though not introduced into internal body cavities, are placed in contact with tissues that are very sensitive to contamination. Therefore, similar standards are required for ophthalmic preparations.

Irrigating solutions are now also required to meet the same standards as parenteral solutions because during an irrigation procedure, substantial amounts of these solutions can enter the bloodstream directly through open blood vessels of wounds or abraded mucous membranes. Therefore, the characteristics and standards presented in this chapter for the production of large-volume parenteral solutions apply equally to irrigating solutions.

Sterile products are most frequently solutions or suspensions, but may even be solid pellets for tissue implantation. The control of a process to minimize contamination for a small quantity of such a product can be achieved with relative ease. As the quantity of product increases, the problems of controlling the process to prevent contamination multiply. Therefore, the preparation of sterile products has become a highly specialized area in pharmaceutical processing. The standards established, the attitude of personnel, and the process control must be of a superior level.

The organizational divisions normally responsible for the preparation of sterile products in the pharmaceutical industry are product development, production, control, and packaging. The treatment of the subject matter in this chapter is in accordance with these four divisions of responsibility, with emphasis on the distinctive aspects of sterile product manufacturing. Particular emphasis is placed on the production division, for it is in this division that the distinctiveness of sterile product processing is particularly evident.

Requirements for components related to the product formula and its stability are considered in the product development section. Many of the principles of product development, control, and packaging are identical for sterile and nonsterile products. Since some of these principles are treated elsewhere in this text, only those that are distinctive for sterile products are covered in this chapter.

The student may wish to consult other general references for corollary reading.[1-3]

Product Development

The final objective in the development of a sterile product is the elicitation of a therapeutic effect in a patient. Concentration on the details of physical or chemical factors must not be allowed to take precedence over the prime consideration, the use of the product in a patient.

Parenteral preparations may be given by various routes: intravenous, intraspinal, intramuscular, subcutaneous, and intradermal. When injection occurs via an intravascular route, complete drug availability occurs immediately; no absorption is necessary. For all other routes, at least a blood vessel wall, and usually one or more tissue cell walls, must be permeated before the drug can enter the circulation. Most often, this occurs by passive diffusion and is most favorable when the drug has both lipophilic and hydrophilic properties, with the former being predominant. With nonvascular injections, absorption is also affected by such factors as the size and number of blood vessels supplying the tissue, the movement (exercise) of the tissue following injection, the physical and chemical properties of the drug, and such characteristics of the dosage form as whether it is a solution, suspension, or emulsion, the nature of the vehicle, and its pH. Once in the circulating blood, the physiologic effect of a therapeutic agent is affected by the extent to which it distributes throughout the body, by the degree of binding to plasma proteins, and by its rate of elimination by hepatic metabolism and/or renal excretion.[4,5]

Intravenous and intraspinal preparations rarely are given in a form other than aqueous solutions. The danger of blockage of fine capillaries, particularly in the brain, precludes the use of forms other than solutions for intravenous administration, although emulsions have been given in which the particle size of the dispersed phase is carefully controlled. The sensitivity of nerve tissues generally precludes the use of anything but the purest of solutions for intraspinal medication. Preparations given intramuscularly, subcutaneously, or intradermally can be administered as solutions, suspensions, or emulsions. Even solid pellets may be implanted subcutaneously or intramuscularly. The vehicles can range from Water for Injection, to glycols, to fixed oils. Although care must be exercised to avoid undue tissue irritation, mild local irritation is permissible at these injection sites.

The nature of a preparation can influence significantly the rapidity of onset of a therapeutic effect from a drug, the duration of the effect, and the form of the absorption pattern achieved. Therefore, the development of the formulation for a parenteral product must be integrated carefully with its intended administration in a patient.

The chemical and physical properties of a drug must be determined, its interaction with any desired excipients must be studied, and the effect of each step of the process on its stability must be studied and understood.

Solvent systems suitable for sterile products are limited to those that produce little or no tissue irritation; water is the most common. All components must be of exceptional quality. Pu-

rification beyond that obtainable in many commercial products or by normal production procedures is often necessary. Not only may chemical or physical contaminants cause irritation to body tissues, but extremely small quantities may cause degradation of the product as a result of chemical changes, particularly during the heating period when thermal sterilization is employed. For example, minute traces of copper greatly accelerate the rate of oxidation of ascorbic acid in solution. These traces of copper may come from the water vehicle, the chemical components, or even the container. Rigid specifications must therefore be developed for all ingredients.

Vehicles

By far the most frequently employed vehicle for sterile products is water, since it is the vehicle for all natural body fluids. The superior quality required for such use is described in the monograph on Water for Injection in the USP. Requirements may be even more stringent for some products, however.

One of the most inclusive tests for the quality of water is the total solids content, a gravimetric evaluation of the dissociated and undissociated organic and inorganic substances present in the water. However, a less time-consuming test, the electrolytic measurement of conductivity* of the water, is the one most frequently used. Instantaneous measurements can be obtained by immersing electrodes in the water and measuring the specific conductance, a measurement that depends on the ionic content of the water. The conductance may be expressed by the meter scale as conductivity in micromhos, resistance in megohms, or ionic content as parts per million (ppm) of sodium chloride. The validity of this measurement as an indication of the purity of the water is inferential in that methods of producing high-purity water, such as distillation and reverse osmosis, can be expected to remove undissociated substances along with those that are dissociated. Undissociated substances such as pyrogens, however, could be present in the absence of ions and not be disclosed by the test. Therefore, for contaminants other than ions, additional tests should be performed.

Additional tests for quality of Water for Injec-

*Barnstead Co., Div. of Sybron Corp., Boston, MA 02132; Beckman Instruments, Inc., Cedar Grove, NJ 07009; Corning Glass Works, Corning, NY 14830; Foxboro Analytical, Div. Foxboro Co., Burlington, MA 01803; Vaponics, Inc., Plymouth, MA 02360.

tion with permitted limits are described in the USP monographs. When comparing the total solids permitted for Water for Injection with that for Sterile Water for Injection, one will note that considerably higher values are permitted for Sterile Water for Injection. This is necessary because the latter product has been sterilized, usually by a thermal method, in a container that has dissolved to some extent in the water. Therefore, the solids content will be greater than for the nonsterilized product. On the other hand, the 10 ppm total solids officially permitted for Water for Injection may be much too high when used as the vehicle for many products. In practice, Water for Injection normally should not have a conductivity of more than 1 micromho (1 megohm, approximately 0.1 ppm NaCl).

Pyrogens. Water used in parenteral and irrigating solutions should be free of pyrogens. To achieve this, proper controls must be maintained in the preparation and storage of the water.

Pyrogens are products of metabolism of microorganisms. Most bacteria and many molds and viruses have been reported as producing pyrogens. The gram-negative bacteria produce the most potent pyrogenic substances as endotoxins. Chemically, pyrogens are lipid substances associated with a carrier molecule, which is usually a polysaccharide but may be a peptide. About 1 hour after injection into man, pyrogens produce a marked rise in body temperature, chills, body aches, cutaneous vasoconstriction, and a rise in arterial blood pressure. Antipyretics eliminate the fever, but not the other systemic effects of pyrogens.

The fever response to pyrogens in rabbits is the basis for the official pyrogen test, which is described later in this chapter. For further information, the reader is referred to the extensive reviews on the nature and significance of pyrogens that have appeared in the literature.[6,7]

Source and Elimination of Pyrogen Contamination. Pyrogens may enter a product by any means that may introduce microorganisms or the products of their growth. The most likely sources are water, contaminated solutes, and containers. Water is free from pyrogens if it has been distilled so that the condensed molecules have gone through the vapor state protected from inadvertent contamination, and if the distillate has been collected and stored in a sterile condition. To be pyrogen-free, solutes must be prepared from vehicles free from pyrogens, and must be stored in a manner designed to prevent subsequent contamination. Opened containers of solutes, capable of supporting the growth of microorganisms, invite such contamination.

Containers may be rendered free from pyrogens by adequate cleaning and heating, usually at 210°C for 3 to 4 hours. Studies also have shown that heating at 650°C for 60 sec destroys pyrogens; however, autoclaving temperatures do not destroy pyrogens during a normal cycle.

Pyrogens sometimes can be removed from solutions by adsorption on the surface of select adsorbants, but the often concurrent phenomenon of the adsorption of solute ions or molecules may prevent the use of such a method. Selective solvent extraction methods are useful in the production of antibiotics where heavy pyrogen contamination results from the fermentation process. New developments in ultrafiltration show promise of moving this process from limited research applications in molecular separations to practical production processes, which may include pyrogen separation and elimination.[8,9] For most pharmaceutical preparations, however, it is better to *prevent* pyrogenic contamination than to attempt to remove pyrogens, a task that is difficult to accomplish without adversely affecting the product.

The product development department therefore must develop purity requirements for Water for Injection which are sufficiently stringent for its use as a vehicle in the product most sensitive to contaminants. Tests other than those for solids and pyrogenic content might be required, e.g., qualitative and quantitative tests for the presence of ions such as copper and iron.

Nonaqueous Solvents. In the formulation of sterile pharmaceutical products, it is sometimes necessary to eliminate water entirely or in part from the vehicle, primarily because of solubility factors or hydrolytic reactions. A nonaqueous solvent must be selected with great care for it must not be irritating, toxic, or sensitizing, and it must not exert an adverse effect on the ingredients of the formulation. The screening of such a solvent must therefore include an evaluation of its physical properties, such as density, viscosity, miscibility and polarity, as well as its stability, solvent activity, and toxicity.[10]

Solvents that are miscible with water, and that are usually used in combination with water as the vehicle, include dioxolanes, dimethylacetamide, N-(β-hydroxyethyl)-lactamide, butylene glycol, polyethylene glycol 400 and 600, propylene glycol, glycerin, and ethyl alcohol. Water-immiscible solvents include fixed oils, ethyl oleate, isopropyl myristate, and benzyl benzoate. The most frequently used nonaqueous solvents are polyethylene glycol, propylene glycol, and fixed oils. These solvents have been reviewed elsewhere,[11,12] and the reader is referred to this review for further details.

Solutes

The physical and chemical purity of solutes used for sterile preparations must also be exceptional. Obviously, contaminants entering a product with a solute have the same effect as if they entered via the vehicle. Even small traces of contaminants may be detrimental to products, necessitating purification of the solute. For a few substances (for example, ascorbic acid and calcium gluconate), special parenteral grades are commercially available.

In addition, solutes should be free from microbial and pyrogenic contamination. This entails not only proper quality of the chemical as procured but storage conditions designed to prevent contamination, particularly after a container has been opened. Preferably, production lots should be designed to use the entire contents of packages of chemicals whenever possible.

Added Substances. Substances added to a product to enhance its stability are essential for almost every product.[13] Such substances include solubilizers, antioxidants, chelating agents, buffers, tonicity contributors, antibacterial agents, antifungal agents, hydrolysis inhibitors, antifoaming agents, and numerous other substances for specialized purposes. At the same time, these agents must be prevented from adversely affecting the product. In general, added substances must be nontoxic in the quantity administered to the patient. They should not interfere with the therapeutic efficacy nor with the assay of the active therapeutic compound. They must also be present and active when needed throughout the useful life of the product. Therefore, these agents must be selected with great care, and they must be evaluated as to their effect upon the entire formulation. An extensive review of excipients used in parenteral products and the means for adjusting pH of these products has recently been published and should be referred to for more detailed information.[14] Table 22-1 provides a list, adapted from that review, of excipients commonly used in commercial parenteral products.

Antibacterial Agents. Antibacterial agents in bacteriostatic concentration must be included in the formulation of products packaged in multiple dose vials, and are often included in formulations to be sterilized by marginal processes or made by aseptic manipulation. The requirements of activity, stability, and effectiveness of antibacterial agents in parenterals have been reviewed in published papers.[15-17]

Antioxidants. Antioxidants, included in many formulations to protect a therapeutic agent susceptible to oxidation, particularly under the accelerated conditions of thermal sterilization, may function in at least two ways., i.e., (1) by being preferentially oxidized (reducing agents) and thereby gradually used up, or (2) by blocking an oxidative chain reaction in which they are not usually consumed. In addition, certain compounds have been found to act as synergists, increasing the effectiveness of antioxidants, particularly those blocking oxidative reactions. A fourth group of compounds are useful in this connection in that they complex with catalysts that otherwise would accelerate the

TABLE 22-1. *Excipients Used for Commercial Parenteral Products*

Excipients	Concentration Range (%)
Antimicrobial Preservatives	
Benzyl alcohol	0.5–10.0
Benzethonium chloride	0.01
Butylparaben	0.015
Chlorobutanol	0.25–0.5
Metacresol	0.1–0.25
Methylparaben	0.01–0.18
Myristylgamma picolinium chloride	0.17
Phenol	0.065–0.5
Phenylmercuric nitrate	0.001
Propylparaben	0.005–0.035
Thimerosal	0.001–0.02
Solubilizers, Wetting Agents, or Emulsifiers	
Dimethylacetamide	0.01
Dioctyl sodium sulfosuccinate	0.015
Egg yolk phospholipid	1.2
Ethyl alcohol	0.61–49.0
Ethyl lactate	0.1
Glycerin	14.6–25.0

Excipients	Concentration Range (%)
Solubilizers, Wetting Agents, or Emulsifiers—continued	
Lecithin	0.5–2.3
PEG-40 castor oil	7.0–11.5
Polyethylene glycol 300	0.01–50.0
Polysorbate 20	0.01
Polysorbate 40	0.05
Polysorbate 80	0.04–4.0
Povidone	0.2–1.0
Propylene glycol	0.2–50.0
Sodium desoxycholate	0.21
Sorbitan monopalmitate	0.05
Theophylline	5.0
Buffers	
Acetic acid	0.22
Adipic acid	1.0
Benzoic acid and sodium benzoate	5.0
Citric acid	0.5
Lactic acid	0.1
Maleic acid	1.6
Potassium phosphate	0.1
Sodium phosphate monobasic	1.7
Sodium phosphate dibasic	0.71
Sodium acetate	0.8
Sodium bicarbonate	0.005
Sodium carbonate	0.06
Sodium citrate	4.0
Sodium tartrate	1.2
Tartaric acid	0.65
Bulking Substances or Tonicity Modifiers	
Glycerin	1.6–2.25
Lactose	0.14–5.0
Mannitol	0.4–2.5
Dextrose	3.75–5.0
Sodium chloride	varies
Sodium sulfate	1.1
Sorbitol	2.0
Suspending Agents	
Gelatin	2.0
Methylcellulose	0.03–1.05
Pectin	0.2
Polyethylene glycol 4000	2.7–3.0
Sodium carboxymethylcellulose	0.05–0.75
Sorbitol solution	50.0
Chelating Agents	
Edetate disodium	0.00368–0.05
Edetate calcium disodium	0.04
Edetate tetrasodium	0.01
Local Anesthetics	
Procaine HCl	1.0
Benzyl alcohol	5
Stabilizers	
Creatinine	0.5–0.8
Glycine	1.5–2.25
Niacinamide	1.25–2.5
Sodium acetyltryptophanate	0.53
Sodium caprylate	0.4
Sodium saccharin	0.03

Adapted from Wang, Y.J., and Kowal, R.R.: J. Parent. Drug Assoc., 34:452, 1980.

oxidative reaction. Because of the differences in action, combinations of these agents are sometimes used. In Table 22-2, the more commonly employed antioxidants are listed according to the above four groupings. The reader is referred to the literature for more details concerning antioxidants and their activities.[18-20]

It should also be mentioned that for those products in which oxygen enters into a degradative reaction, an antioxidant effect can be achieved by displacing oxygen (air) from contact with the product. Usually, this is accomplished by saturating the liquid with either nitrogen or carbon dioxide and sealing the final container after displacing the air above the product with the gas.

Higuchi and Schroeter have warned of the reactivity of bisulfites with drug molecules,[21] and Halaby and Mattocks have warned of the potential toxicity of sodium bisulfite absorbed from peritoneal dialysis solutions.[22]

Buffers. Buffers are added to maintain a required pH for many products; a change in pH may cause significant alterations in the rate of degradative reactions. Changes in pH may occur during storage as a result of the dissolving of glass constituents in the product, release of constituents from rubber closures or plastic components in contact with the product, dissolving of gases and vapors from the airspace in the container and diffusion through the rubber or plastic component, or reactions within the product. Buffers must have the capacity to maintain the pH of the product against these influences, but not enough to prevent the body fluids from overwhelming the buffer following administration. In most cases, the biologic effectiveness of the drug is maximum at or near the biologic fluid pH rather than at the stabilizing pH of the injected product.

Acetates, citrates, and phosphates are the principal buffer systems used, but buffer systems making use of other ingredients in the formulation are often used to reduce the total number of ingredients in the product. Buffer systems must be selected with consideration of their effective range, concentration, and chemical effect on the total product. These factors have been reviewed by Windheuser.[23]

Tonicity Contributors. Compounds contributing to the isotonicity of a product reduce the pain of injection in areas with nerve endings. Buffers may serve as tonicity contributors as well as stabilizers for the pH. Other added substances also contribute to the colligative properties of the preparation. Whenever possible such dual activity is desirable.

Although the freezing point depression of the solution is most frequently used to determine whether a solution is isotonic, isotonicity actually depends on the permeability of a living semipermeable membrane that separates the solution from a biologic cell system. Most frequently, for sterile pharmaceutical preparations, the membrane concerned is the one enclosing the red blood cells. Therefore, a preparation cannot be considered to be isotonic until it has been tested in a biologic system. A hemolytic method, using red blood cells, has been described.[24,25] Isotonicity values for various drugs have been recorded.[26-29] Testing by such a method becomes even more important when all or part of the water is replaced with another solvent, since dissociation is different when water is displaced by another solvent.

TABLE 22-2. *Antioxidants Used in Sterile Products*

Compound	Usual Concentration (%)
Antioxidants (reducing agents)	
Ascorbic acid	0.02–0.1
Sodium bisulfite	0.1–0.15
Sodium metabisulfite	0.1–0.15
Sodium formaldehyde sulfoxylate	0.1–0.15
Thiourea	0.005
Antioxidants (blocking agents)	
Ascorbic acid esters	0.01–0.015
Butyl hydroxytoluene (BHT)	0.005–0.02
Tocopherols	0.05–0.075
Synergists	
Ascorbic acid	0.01–0.05
Citric acid	0.005–0.01
Citraconic acid	0.03–0.45
Phosphoric acid	0.005–0.01
Tartaric acid	0.01–0.02
Chelating agents	
Ethylenediaminetetraacetic acid salts	0.01–0.075

Containers

Containers are in intimate contact with the product. No container presently available is totally nonreactive, particularly with aqueous solutions. Both the chemical and physical characteristics affect the stability of the product, but the physical characteristics are given primary consideration in the selection of a protective container.

Glass containers traditionally have been used for sterile products, many of which are closed with rubber stoppers. Interest in plastic containers for parenterals is increasing, and such containers are being used for commercial ophthalmic preparations and intravenous solutions.[30]

Plastic Containers. The principal ingredient of the various plastic materials used for containers is the thermoplastic polymer; the basic organic structural unit for each type commonly encountered in the medical field is given in Table 22-3. Although most of the plastic materials used in the medical field have a relatively low amount of added ingredients, some contain a substantial amount of plasticizers, fillers, antistatic agents, antioxidants, and other ingredients added for special purposes. These ingredients are not usually chemically bound in the formulation and, therefore, may migrate out of the plastic and into the product under the conditions of production and storage. Considerable variability also has been encountered in the purity of the commercially available polymers.

As the name indicates, thermoplastic polymers melt at elevated temperatures. All of the polymeric materials listed in Table 22-3 except low-density polyethylene and polystyrene can be autoclaved if they have been formulated with a low amount of plasticizers, although most of them soften at autoclaving temperatures, and care must be exercised to avoid fusing adjacent surfaces or otherwise deforming them. Also listed in Table 22-3 are certain properties of the plastic materials most commonly used for containers and components in drug packaging. These properties vary considerably with the type and amount of additive combined with the polymer.

Plastic containers are used mainly because they are light in weight, are nonbreakable, and, when low in additives, have low toxicity and low reactivity with products. Tissue toxicity can occur from certain polymers, but additives are a more common cause.[31] Reactivity due to sorption (absorption and/or adsorption) has been found to occur most frequently with the polyamide polymers, but additives leached from any of the plastic materials may interact with ingredients of the product.

Most polymers are adversely affected by the elevated temperatures required for thermal sterilization and have a relatively high permeability for water vapor (Table 22-3). Significant permeation of gases, including oxygen, may occur with some materials, polystyrene having by far the highest level of permeation of those listed.

A relatively new group of plastics, the polyolefins, deserve special mention. The two of interest today in the parenteral field are polypropylene and the copolymer polyethylene-polypropylene. Polypropylene is most widely used. It is a linear polymer that can be produced to be highly crystalline. Because of its crystallinity, it has high tensile strength, a high melting point of 165°C, and a relatively low permeability to gases and water vapor. It is translucent, abrasion-resistant, and has a high surface gloss. It will withstand normal autoclaving temperatures. It must be stabilized with an antioxidant, however, the type and concentration of which must be carefully controlled to avoid leaching on one hand or degradation of the plastic on the other.

Autian has reviewed the characteristics and use of plastic materials for parenterals.[32] Interest in the use of such materials for containers for sterile products is increasing, but careful evaluation of their potential interaction with products with which they are in contact is essential.[33] Flexible polyethylene containers are used for ophthalmic solutions to be administered in drops, and flexible polyvinyl chloride bags for intravenous solutions.[34] The latter have a particular advantage over glass bottles in that no air from the patient's bedside need enter the container as the liquid flows out; the bag simply collapses. The new group of polymers, the polyolefins, have made possible the development of bottles that are rigid enough to hold their shape during processing but can collapse under atmospheric pressure as outflow of a solution occurs during intravenous administration to a patient. Thus, the characteristics of a rigid container are utilized during processing and handling, but the advantage of collapsibility of a flexible container is achieved for aseptic administration.

The USP has provided test procedures for evaluating the toxicity of plastic materials. Essentially the tests consist of three phases: (1) implanting small pieces of the plastic material intramuscularly in rabbits, (2) injecting eluates using sodium chloride injection, with and without alcohol, intravenously in mice, and injecting eluates using polyethylene glycol 400 and sesame oil intraperitoneally in mice, and (3) injecting all four eluates subcutaneously in rabbits. The reaction from the test samples must not be significantly greater than nonreactive control samples. Guess and Autian have discussed these tests in detail.[35]

Glass Containers. Glass is still the preferred material for containers for injectable products. Glass is composed principally of the silicon dioxide tetrahedron, modified physicochemically by such oxides as those of sodium, potassium, calcium, magnesium, aluminum, boron, and iron. The two general types of glass are soda-lime and borosilicate (see Table 22-3).

TABLE 22-3. *Comparative Properties* of Container Materials*

Material	Structural Unit	Average Density	Autoclavable (Physical Stability)
Thermoplastic polymers			
Polyethylene			
Low density	$(-CH_2-CH_2-)_n$	0.92	No
High Density	$(-CH_2-CH_2-)_n$	0.96	Yes
Polypropylene	$(-CHCH_3-CH_2-)_n$	0.90	Yes
Polyvinyl chloride			
Flexible	$(-CHCl-CH_2-)_n$	1.2	Yes (cautiously)
Rigid	$(-CHCl-CH_2-)_n$	1.4	Yes (cautiously)
Polycarbonate	$(-O-C_6H_5-C(CH_3)_2-C_6H_5-CO_2-)_n$	1.2	Yes
Polyamide (nylon)	$(-CH_2-(CH_2)_4-NHCO-)_n$	1.1	Yes (repeatedly)
Polystyrene	$(-CH(C_6H_5)-CH_2-)_n$	1.05	No
Polytetrafluoroethylene (Teflon)	$(-CF_2-CF_2-)_n$	2.25	Yes (repeatedly)
Glass			
Soda-lime	$\begin{pmatrix} & O & & O & \\ & \mid & & \mid & \\ -O-&Si&-O-&Si&-O- \\ & \mid & & \mid & \\ & O & & O & \end{pmatrix}_n$	2.48	Yes
Borosilicate	$\begin{pmatrix} & O & & O & \\ & \mid & & \mid & \\ -O-&Si&-O-&Si&-O- \\ & \mid & & \mid & \\ & O & & O & \end{pmatrix}_n$	2.23	Yes
Rubber compounds			
Butyl	$(-CH_2-C(CH_3)=CH-(CH_2)_2-C(CH_3)_2-)_n$	1.3	Yes
Natural	$(-CH_2-C(CH_3)=CH-CH_2-)_n$	1.5	Yes
Neoprene	$(-CH_2-CH=CCL-CH_2-)_n$	1.4	Yes
Polyisoprene	$(-CH_2-C(CH_3)=CH-CH_2-)_n$	1.3	Yes
Silicone	$(-Si(CH_3)_2-O-Si(CH_3)_2-O-)_n$	1.4	Yes

*General relationships that vary substantially with factors such as container material formulation, thickness of wall, and temperature.

Additives† Present	Leachable Constituents‡	Water Vapor Permeation	Gas Permeation (O_2)	Potential Reaction With Product‡	Physical Properties
Low	Additives§ (Low)	High	Low	Low	Translucent, flexible
Low	Additives§ (Low)	Low	Low	Low	Translucent, semi-rigid
Low	Additives§ (Low)	Moderate	Low	Low	Translucent, semi-rigid
High	Additives§ (High)	High	Low	Moderate	Transparent, flexible
Low	Additives§ (Low)	High	Low	Low	Transparent, rigid
Low	Additives§ (Low)	High	Low	Low	Transparent, rigid
Low	Additives§ (Low)	High	Low	High	Translucent, rigid, tough
Low	Additives§ (Low)	High	High	Moderate	Transparent, rigid
Low	Additives§ (Nil)	Low	Low	Nil	Translucent, tough, rigid, temperature-resistant
High	K_2O, Na_2O, MgO, CaO (High)	None	None	High	Optically clear, rigid
Low	B_2O_3, Na_2O, CaO, (Low)	None	None	Low	Optically clear, rigid
Moderate	Additives‖ (Moderate)	Low	Moderate	Moderate	Opaque, flexible
High	Additives‖ (High)	Moderate	Moderate	High	Opaque, flexible
High	Additives‖ (High)	Moderate	Moderate	High	Opaque, flexible
High	Additives‖ (High)	Moderate	Moderate	Moderate	Opaque, flexible
Moderate	Additives‖ (Moderate)	Very high	Very high	Low	Translucent, flexible

†Substances added to modify the properties of the basic ingredient.

‡General relationships are based upon an aqueous system but may be markedly affected by other solvent systems of the product.

§May include residues of plasticizers, antistatic agents, antioxidants and other ingredients added for special purposes.

‖May include residues of vulcanizers, accelerators, lubricants, inorganic fillers, and other ingredients added for special purposes.

The glass that is most resistant chemically is composed almost entirely of silicon dioxide, but it is relatively brittle and can only be melted and molded at high temperatures. Boric oxide somewhat modifies the above characteristics as it enters the structural configuration, but most of the other oxides apparently enter the spaces within the structure and reduce the strength of the interatomic forces between the silicon and oxygen. Therefore, the latter oxides lower the melting point of the glass and are comparatively free to migrate. Consequently, they also lower the chemical resistance of the glass; that is, they may migrate into a product over a prolonged period of contact, particularly with aqueous solutions. In solution, the oxides may hydrolyze to raise the pH, catalyze reactions, or otherwise enter into chemical reactions. Glass flakes are also sometimes produced as a result of the action of the solution. These interactions are markedly accelerated during the elevated temperature required for autoclaving.

Chemical Resistance. The USP provides the Powdered Glass and the Water Attack tests for evaluating chemical resistance of glass. The test results are measures of the amount of alkaline constituents leached from the glass by purified water under controlled elevated temperature conditions; the Powdered Glass test is performed on ground, sized glass particles, and the Water Attack test is performed on whole containers. The conditions of the test must be rigidly controlled to obtain reproducible results since the quantity of alkaline constituents leached is small. The Water Attack test is used only with containers that have been exposed to sulfur dioxide fumes under controlled humidity conditions. Such treatment neutralizes the surface alkaline oxides, thereby rendering the glass more resistant chemically. This increased resistance is lost, however, if the container is subjected to repeated autoclaving, hot air sterilization, or hot detergent treatment.

On the basis of the results from the official tests, glass compounds are classified into four types, as shown in Table 22-4. The greatest chemical resistance is provided by Type I, and the least by NP (nonparenteral) glass. It should be noted, however, that within these types, as well as Types II and III, a range of compositions are available. The chemical resistance of the glass influences the selection of the type to be used for various products. Table 22-4 provides a brief summary of the general classes of products used with the four glass types. Type I glass is preferred for most sterile products, but Types II and III may be used when the product has a nonaqueous vehicle or the period of contact with the aqueous vehicle is brief, as with dry powders reconstituted just prior to use, or if the nonreactivity of the glass and product has been established. For further consideration of the interrelationships of glass with products, the reader is referred to the published literature.[36,37]

Physical Characteristics. The protection of light-sensitive products from the degradative

TABLE 22-4. *USP Glass Types, Test Limits, and Selection Guide*

Type	General Description*	Type of Test	Size† (ml)	Test Limits ml of 0.02N H_2SO_4	General Use
I	Highly resistant borosilicate glass	Powdered Glass	All	1.0	Buffered and unbuffered aqueous solutions. All other uses.
II	Treated soda-lime glass	Water Attack	100 or less Over 100	0.7 0.2	Buffered aqueous solutions with pH below 7.0 Dry powders, oleaginous solutions.
III	Soda-lime glass	Powdered Glass	All	8.5	Dry powders, oleaginous solutions.
NP	General-purpose soda-lime glass	Powdered Glass	All	15.0	Not for parenterals. For tablets, oral solutions and suspensions, ointments, and external liquids.

*The description applies to containers of this type of glass usually available.
†Size indicates the overflow capacity of the container.

effect of ultraviolet rays may be one of the important physical characteristics of a glass container. Ultraviolet rays can be completely filtered out by the use of amber glass; however, the color of amber glass is produced largely by the presence of iron oxide, traces of which may subsequently be leached into the product. If the product contains ingredients subject to iron catalyzed chemical reactions, amber glass cannot be used. The product must then be protected from ultraviolet rays by means of an opaque carton surrounding a flint (colorless) glass container.

In addition to other physical characteristics, glass containers should have sufficient physical strength to withstand the high pressure differentials that develop during autoclaving and the abuse that occurs during processing, shipping, and storage; a low coefficient of thermal expansion to withstand the thermal shocks that occur during washing and sterilization procedures; transparency to facilitate inspection of the contents; and uniform physical dimensions to facilitate handling by the mechanical machinery used for automatic production operations.

Glass containers may be manufactured by drawing from glass tubing or by blow molding. Ampuls, cartridges, and vials drawn from tubing have a thinner, more uniform wall thickness with less distortion than containers made by blow molding. The greater strength of blown vials and bottles, however, may be essential for handling by mechanical processing equipment. Large vials and bottles are made only by blow molding.

The physical dimensions of glass containers can readily be varied to meet design needs, especially those made by blow molding. An example is the double-chambered vial designed to contain a freeze-dried product in the lower chamber and the solvent in the upper chamber, separated by a rubber disc. The modifications in cartridge shapes for use with various disposable dosage units, and the wide-mouth ampuls with flat or rounded bottoms to facilitate filling dry materials or viscous liquids, also illustrate the variations in physical dimensions possible with glass containers. The development of the easy-open ampul several years ago, permitting opening without a file, was an important modification in the physical structure of these containers, marketed under the name "Color-Break"* and "Score-Break"† ampuls.

Glass containers are sometimes coated inter-nally with silicone fluid to produce a hydrophobic surface. To achieve permanency, the silicone must be baked at a temperature of approximately 150°C (300°F). This additional operation is justified for such applications as to reduce the adherence of heavy, costly suspensions or emulsions or to increase slippage of a plunger in a syringe barrel.

Container Use Considerations. The size of single-dose containers is limited to 1000 ml by the USP and multiple-dose containers to 30 ml, unless permitted otherwise in a particular monograph. The size limitation for multiple-dose vials is intended to limit the number of entries for withdrawing a portion of the contents of the vial with the accompanying risk of microbial contamination of the remaining contents. The particular advantage of these containers is flexibility of dosage offered the physician. Single-dose containers are intended to provide sufficient drug for just one dose, the integrity of the container being destroyed when opened so that it cannot be reclosed and used again. Single-dose containers may range from liter bottles of intravenous solutions to 1-ml, or smaller, cartridges. The desire for further reduction in the risk of contamination, both bacterial and viral, and an increased control over the administration of drugs, paricularly in a hospital, have led to the recent development of single-dose, disposable administration units. For most of these units, the product container is a glass cartridge with plastic and metal fitments separated from immediate contact with the product.

Rubber Closures. Rubber closures are used to seal the openings of cartridges, vials, and bottles, providing a material soft and elastic enough to permit entry and withdrawal of a hypodermic needle without loss of the integrity of the sealed container. Figure 22-1 illustrates some of the styles of rubber closures and their relationship to typical containers.

Composition and Reactivity. Rubber closures* are compounded of several ingredients,[38,39] principally, natural rubber (latex) and/or a synthetic polymer; a vulcanizing agent, usually sulfur; an accelerator, one of several active organic compounds such as 2-mercaptobenzothiazole; an activator, usually zinc oxide; fillers, such as carbon black or limestone; and a variety of other ingredients such as antioxidants and lubricants. These ingredients are combined by kneading them into a homogeneous plastic mass on a roller mill. The homogeneous com-

---

*Kimble, Division of Owens-Illinois, Toledo, OH 43601.
†Wheaton Scientific, Millville, NJ 08332.

*Faultless Rubber Co., Ashland, OH 44805; Tompkins Rubber Co., Plymouth Meeting, PA 19462; The West Company, Phoenixville, PA 19460.

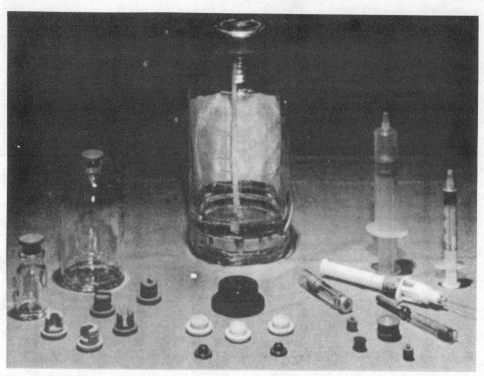

FIG. 22-1. *Rubber closures associated with vials, bottles, and cartridges. Slotted vial closures on left, flanged vial closures in center foreground, permanent hole bottle closure in center rear, and cartridge and disposable syringe closures on right.*

pound is rendered fluid and then vulcanized in the desired shape by means of molds under high pressure and temperature.

In Table 22-3 are listed the elastomeric polymers most commonly used in compounding rubber closures, as well as some of their comparative properties.

Ideally, closures should be completely nonreactive with the product with which they are in contact. No such ideal compound exists; therefore, each rubber compound should be tested for compatibility with each preparation with which it is to be used. Two general compatibility problems exist, namely, the leaching of ingredients from the rubber compound with subsequent reaction with ingredients of the product, and the removal of ingredients from the product by sorption by the rubber compound or by vapor transfer through the closure.[40,41]

Although compatibility problems are encountered with relative frequency, it should not be construed that rubber compounds invariably introduce such problems. Preliminary compatibility usually is assessed by placing the rubber closure in intimate contact with the product and maintaining the samples at elevated temperature levels for planned periods of time. At pre-

scribed intervals, samples are examined for qualitative and quantitative evidence of chemical or physical change either in the closure or in the product.

Physical Characteristics. Several properties of rubber closures are significant, particularly elasticity, hardness, and porosity. Rubber closures must be sufficiently elastic to provide a snug fit between the closure and the neck and lip of the glass container. They must also spring back to close the hole made by the needle immediately after withdrawal. Rubber closures must not be so hard that they require an excessive pressure to insert the hypodermic needle, and in doing so, must not produce a large number of fragments as the hollow needle cuts through the closure (coring). Although porous, they should not permit the easy transfer of water vapor and gases in either direction. See Table 22-3 for general comparisons. Minimal water vapor transfer is important, for example, to prevent the absorption of water by freeze-dried products.

Plastic or lacquer coatings are sometimes applied to the surfaces that will be in contact with the product. These coatings sometimes reduce vapor transfer, sorption, and leaching, but they do not usually provide the complete barrier desired. Teflon liners have been shown to provide an effective barrier against sorption and leaching.[42]

The physical shapes of closures vary with their intended use. Several common shapes are shown in Figure 22-1: the common flanged closure (center), slotted for freeze-dried products (left) or punctured for attachment of adapters for infusion sets (center, rear), and the plunger type for use with cartridges (right). Disc closures preassembled with aluminum caps are being used to increase the speed of the operation in the high-speed packaging of antibiotics and other drugs. Other designs are used as needed for particular application.

Testing. Methods of testing for lot to lot uniformity of rubber closures have been studied for many years, but because of the nature of rubber compounds, consistent test results have been difficult to obtain. Progress has been made, however, and the USP now describes physicochemical and biologic tests, but without test limits. The physicochemical tests on aqueous extracts include pH, turbidity (nephelos), residue on drying, iodine number, and heavy metals content. The biologic tests on saline, polyethylene glycol 400, and cottonseed oil extracts include acute and chronic toxicity in mice and rabbits. Further discussion of the purpose of these tests may be found in the literature.[43,44]

Devices

Devices, as considered here, are the various items of equipment used to convey the product from its container into the body of the patient or from one container to another; or the term may refer to the containers themselves. Devices associated with sterile products include the following:

Administration sets for large volume
    parenterals (LVPs)

Filter needles

Hypodermic needles

Hypodermic syringes

In-line filters

Plastic irrigating solution bottles

Plastic LVPs containers

Plastic ophthalmic dropping bottles

Transfer needles

Transfer sets

Although the contact time of the product with the device is usually brief, it is intimate; therefore, compatibility between the device and the product must be evaluated. For example, it has been shown that insulin can be adsorbed by PVC tubing during the time of contact for administrative of an i.v. solution, approximately 6 hours.[45]

The materials used for devices are mostly the same as those used for containers, but may include others if short term contact has been shown to be acceptable. For example, nylon and silicone rubber are used for i.v. catheters, and stainless steel is used for hypodermic needles. Even aluminum is sometimes used for the hub and cannula of needles, but aluminum is much more reactive with some products than stainless steel. Parts of a device that do not come into contact with the product, such as the clamp on an i.v. administration set, need not pass product stability evaluation.

All device components must be visibly clean, but the fluid path through the device should meet the same rigid standards for cleanliness as the product. Usually, this must be achieved during manufacture and assembly of the device since final wet rinse or cleaning may be difficult or impossible, owing to configuration of the device. Further, moisture residues may be detrimental to stability, causing leaching or interference with sterilization. Plastic particles from molding or metal dust from the sharpening of needles are examples of particulate matter that must be eliminated. If solvents are used to assemble components of the device, care must be taken to eliminate any excess, especially in the fluid path.

Tests performed by representative sampling of a lot of a finished device include those for toxicity as specified by the USP and functional tests appropriate for the specific device. The latter must be adequate to assure that a given lot performs as intended in use, although the criticality of a particular defect differs. Defects are usually expressed in terms of Acceptable Quality Levels (AQLs); the more critical AQLs are less than 1.0. For example, split hubs of needles would be more critical than slight discoloration of tubing, and may have AQLs of 0.065% and 2.5%, respectively. Therefore, great care must be exercised by quality control to prevent critical defects from being passed along to the user. For example, the integrity of the seal of the permeation section within a kidney dialysis unit is so critical to its use that every unit must be tested before it is released.

Formulation

The formulation of a parenteral product involves the combination of one or more ingredients with a medicinal agent to enhance the convenience, acceptability, or effectiveness of the product. Rarely is it preferable to dispense a drug singly as a sterile dry powder unless the formulation of a stable liquid preparation is not possible.

On the other hand, a therapeutic agent is a chemical compound subject to the physical and chemical reactions characteristic of the class of compounds to which it belongs. Therefore, a careful evaluation must be made of every combination of two or more ingredients to ascertain whether or not adverse interactions occur, and if they do, of ways to modify the formulation so that the reactions are eliminated or minimized. The formulation of sterile products is challenging, therefore, to the knowledge and ingenuity of the persons responsible.[46-48]

The amount of information available to the formulator concerning the physical and chemical properties of a therapeutic agent, particularly if it is a new compound, is often quite meager. Information concerning basic properties must be obtained, including molecular weight, solubility, purity, colligative properties, and chemical reactivity, before an intelligent approach to formulation can begin. Improvements in formulation are a continuing process, since important properties of a drug or of the total formulation may not become evident until the product has been stored or used for a prolonged time. However, because of the extensive test documentation required by the U.S. Food and Drug Administration (FDA), only outstanding formulations can be justified for continuance to the state of a marketed product.

The Solvent System. A parenteral therapeutic agent is given by preference as a solution. If aqueous, the solution is physiologically compatible with body tissues, and the biologic response elicited should be reasonably predictable.

The high dielectric constant of water makes it possible to dissolve ionizable electrolytes, and its hydrogen bonding potential brings about the solution of such organic substances as alcohols, aldehydes, ketones, and amines. Conversely, water is a poor solvent for nonpolar compounds, such as alkaloidal bases, which require nonpolar solvents. Since therapeutically active compounds given by injection range in property from highly polar to nonpolar, solvents having complementary properties must be employed if a solution is to be achieved. For further basic information, the reader is referred to the technical literature.[49-51]

Adding to the complexity of solvent selection is the requirement that solvents to be injected must be of low toxicity to body tissue. Ether is a solvent for testosterone, but is highly irritating to body tissue and cannot be used alone as a solvent for an injectable preparation. Frequently, the desired solubility can be achieved with mixed solvents, e.g., the use of approximately 40% ethanol in water to solubilize the digitalis glycosides.

Compounds that are dissolved in water are often subject to degradative reactions, such as hydrolysis, oxidation, decarboxylation, and racemization. Formulation must be designed, in such cases, to minimize the degradative effects. Often, these reactions are markedly affected by the pH of the solution. Epinephrine in solution undergoes racemization and oxidation, but if the pH is maintained at 3.0 or lower, little reaction occurs.[52] The oxidation reaction can be further reduced by displacing atmospheric oxygen with an inert gas and adding 0.1% sodium metabisulfite as an antioxidant. Atropine sulfate rapidly hydrolyzes in solution, but if the pH is maintained with a buffer system at about 3.5 to 4.0, hydrolysis does not occur at a significant rate.[53]

The use of a mixed solvent system often reduces degradative reactions. Barbituric acid derivatives hydrolyze readily in water, particularly at a low pH. It has been shown, however, that pentobarbital sodium is soluble and stable in a vehicle containing 60% polyethylene glycol 400 and 10% ethanol in water at a pH of 8.[54]

The aforementioned reactions do not occur in an anhydrous, nonpolar vehicle, such as fixed oil, although the presence of a small amount of water may permit slight reactions. Oleaginous injections are subjected, however, to the disadvantages of being viscous (thus difficult to administer, particularly in cold weather) and of involving frequent incidence of pain upon injection.

Additives. A variety of ingredients may be added to a formulation to provide the required stability and therapeutic efficacy. Several classes of additives have been mentioned: antibacterial agents, antioxidants, buffers, and tonicity contributors.

Additives may be included in formulations for purposes other than those already mentioned. Chelating agents may be added to bind, in nonionizable form, trace amounts of heavy metals, which if free, would catalyze degradative changes. The chelating agent most commonly used is the trisodium or calcium disodium salt of ethylenediamine tetraacetic acid in a concentration of about 0.05%. An interesting example of the use of this chelating agent is the stabilization of thimerosal in poliomyelitis vaccine. Thimerosal is present as a bacteriostatic agent, but it is unstable in the presence of cupric ions, the breakdown products of which destroy the antigenicity of the vaccine. The chelating agent stabilizes the thimerosal, and thereby stabilizes the vaccine.[55] The heavy metals extracted from rubber closures also may be bound by the presence of a chelating agent, reducing the possibility of reactions with ingredients in the formulation.

Occasionally, with slightly soluble salts it may be desirable to reduce the solubility of the compound. For example, procaine hydrochloride reduces the solubility of procaine benzylpenicillin by the common ion effect, thereby helping to stabilize the crystal size in aqueous suspensions of the antibiotic.

Inert gases have been used to displace oxygen from a solution and reduce the possibility of oxidative changes in the formulation. Inert gases may be used to stabilize solutions in other ways. For example, sodium bicarbonate injection decomposes, particularly during autoclaving, to produce sodium carbonate, carbon dioxide, and water. Saturation of the solution with carbon dioxide inhibits this reaction and stabilizes the solution.

Complexation sometimes occurs between an added ingredient and a macromolecule in the formulation. The methyl and propyl esters of p-hydroxybenzoic acid have been found to complex with polysorbate 80 with a corresponding decrease in antibacterial activity.[56] Their effectiveness can be regained, however, if the amount of the esters present is increased to offset the quantity bound by the nonionic surfactant.

Ophthalmic Preparations. Products to be instilled into the eye, while not parenterals by definition, have many similar, and often identical, characteristics. The formulation of stable, therapeutically active ophthalmic preparations requires high purity of ingredients as well as freedom from chemical, physical (particles), and microbial contaminants. These preparations usually require buffers to stabilize the pH of the product, additives to render it isotonic or nearly so, and stabilizers such as antioxidants when appropriate for the particular ingredients. Those ophthalmics used in larger quantities, such as eye irrigants, or in the care of devices such as contact lenses are usually relatively uncomplicated solutions similar to large-volume parenterals.

One characteristic not as critical for ophthalmics is freedom from pyrogens since pyrogens are not absorbed systemically from the eye; however, insofar as pyrogens are indicative of a microbiologically clean process, they should not be present.

Freeze-Dried Products. Solutions intended to be freeze-dried must be aqueous, for the drying process involves removal of water by sublimation. Since the solution is in existence for only a brief period during processing, stability problems related to the aqueous system are practically nonexistent. However, the formulation must reflect the characteristics to be imparted to the solid residue (cake) after drying,[57,58] and those required of the solution after reconstitution at the time of use. Often, the drug alone does not give sufficient solid residue or the characteristics appropriate for the product; therefore, substances often must be added to provide the characteristics desired. Among the characteristics required of a good cake are (1) a uniform color and texture, (2) a supporting matrix of solids sufficient to maintain essentially the original volume after drying, and (3) sufficient strength to prevent crumbling during storage. In addition, the nature and amount of solids in the solution largely determine (1) the eutectic temperature of the frozen solution, the subzero temperature at which the frozen material will melt, which determines the temperature below which the product must be held during freeze-drying,[59] (2) the rate of thermal and vapor transfer through the product during the process of drying, and (3) the rate of solution of the product during reconstitution.

The percentage of solids in the frozen plug should be between approximately 2 and 25%. Among the best salts for providing uniform crystal size, uniform color and texture, physical strength, and rapid reconstitution are the monobasic and dibasic sodium phosphates. Sodium chloride is often used, but when used alone, the cake tends to shrink markedly in volume and to appear crusty and crumbly. When organic substances such as mannitol, sorbitol, sucrose, and gelatin are used to provide solids for the cake, care must be taken during the heating, particularly during the terminal stages of drying, to avoid discoloration of the cake by charring. Added substances required in the formulation must not be volatile under the conditions of drying; therefore antibacterial agents such as phenol, chlorobutanol, and benzyl alcohol should not be used.

Long-Acting Formulations. Long-acting parenteral drug formulations are designed, ideally, to provide slow, constant, and sustained release of a drug over a prolonged period of time, essentially to simulate and replace the more hazardous, continuous intravenous infusion of a drug. Rarely, if ever, is the ideal achieved, but extensive research has resulted in depot dosage forms that approach the desired goal.

In one type of depot formulation, which is referred to as "dissolution-controlled," the rate of drug absorption is controlled by the slow dissolution of drug particles, with subsequent release to tissue fluid surrounding the bolus of product in the tissue. The formation of drug salts with very low aqueous solubility is one of the most common approaches to this type of formulation. Control of the particle size also can contribute to slow dissolution in that larger particles or crystals dissolve more slowly than small crystals with proportionately more surface area. Further, the suspension of the drug particles in vegetable oils, and especially if gelled with substances such as aluminum monostearate, produces prolonged absorption rates.

Another type of depot formulation is produced by the binding of drug molecules to adsorbents. Only the free portion, in equilibrium with that which is bound, can be absorbed. As drug is absorbed, a shift in equilibrium is established, and the drug is slowly released from the bound state to the free state. This is particularly exemplified by the binding of vaccines to aluminum hydroxide gel to provide a sustained release. A third type of depot preparation is the encapsulation type, in which biodegradable or bioabsorbable macromolecules such as gelatin, phospholipids, and long-chain fatty acids become a diffusion matrix for the drug. The drug is encapsulated within the matrix, and release of drug molecules is controlled by the rate of permeation out of the diffusion barrier and by the rate of biodegradation of the barrier macromolecules. A fourth type is the esterification type depot preparation, in which esters of a drug that are bioerodible are synthesized. The esterified drug is deposited in tissue at the site of injection to form a reservoir of drug. The rate of drug absorption is controlled by the partitioning of the drug esters from the reservoir to tissue fluid and by the rate at which the drug ester regenerates the active drug molecule. Often, these esters are dissolved or suspended in oleaginous vehicles, which further slow the release.

Long-acting parenteral drug formulations have been extensively reviewed in an article by Chien,[60] which should be consulted for more details of this important type of dosage form.

Suspensions. The solids content of parenteral suspensions usually ranges between 0.5 and 5%, but may go as high as 30% in some antibiotic preparations. The amount of solids and the nature of the vehicle determine the viscosity of the product, an important factor because of syringeability, the facility with which the product is passed in and out of a syringe. The property of thixotropy is sometimes utilized, particularly with oleaginous suspensions, to provide the sedimentation stability of a gelled preparation during storage and the syringeability of a fluid at the time of administration.

Probably the most important requirement for parenteral suspensions is a small and uniform particle size.[61] Various techniques are available for the reduction of particles, including dry or wet ball milling, micropulverization, fluid energy grinding, ultrasonic insonation of shock-cooled saturated solutions, and spray drying. Small, uniform particles are required to give slow, uniform rates of sedimentation and predictable rates of dissolution and drug release. Also, uniform particle size reduces the tendency for larger crystal growth during storage, since it has been found that relatively small crystals often tend to disappear and large crystals grow larger in a mixture. Such a change can cause caking of a suspension, difficult syringeability because of the large particles and changes in the dissolution and drug release rate following injection.

The stabilization of a suspension for the period between manufacture and use presents a number of problems. As indicated, solids gradually settle and may cake, causing difficulty in redispersion prior to use. Surface active agents may aid in the preparation and stabilization of a suspension by reducing the interfacial tension between the particles and the vehicle. Polysorbate 80, lecithin, Emulphor EL-620* and Pluronic F-68† are among the surface active agents that have been used in parenteral suspensions. The concurrent addition of a hydrocolloid, such as sodium carboxymethylcellulose, may enhance the effect of the surfactant and cause loss of surface charge of the dispersed particles, water repellency, and the tendency to agglomerate.[62] The following is an example of such a formulation:

Cortisone acetate, microfine	25 mg
Polysorbate 80 (surface active agent)	4 mg
Sodium CMC (protective colloid)	5 mg
Sodium chloride (for tonicity effect)	9 mg
Benzyl alcohol (antibacterial)	9 mg
Water for Injection, to make	1 ml

*GAF Corp., New York, NY 10020.
†Wyandotte Chemicals Corp., Wyandotte, MI 48192.

Among other protective colloids that have been employed are acacia, gelatin, methylcellulose, and polyvinylpyrrolidone.

Occasionally, parenteral suspensions may be improved by a slight increase in viscosity, either by increasing the amount of protective colloid or by adding a compound such as sorbitol. In other formulations, it has been found that flocculation of the suspended particles has been necessary to prevent packing to a dense cake. The addition of selected ions that increase the surface charge of the solid particles may cause them to form fluffy aggregates. These settle rapidly, but to a large sedimentation volume, which can easily be redispersed. Monosodium citrate has been used effectively for such a purpose.

Emulsions. The principal problem in the formulation of parenteral emulsions is the attainment and maintenance of uniform oil droplets of 1 to 5 microns in size as the internal phase. With emulsions, separation of the phase does not occur as readily as with suspensions because the difference in density between the oil and water is relatively small. One such product, an emulsion of a natural vitamin K_1, has been stabilized with lecithin.

Intravenous nutrient emulsions that have been made contain, for example, 15% cottonseed oil, 4% dextrose, 1.2% lecithin, and 0.3% of an oxyethyleneoxypropylene polymer, the latter two ingredients being the emulsifiers. The dispersed phase should have droplet sizes of less than 1 micron. The emulsion must be stable to autoclaving. Elevated temperatures, however, tend to produce coalescence of the dispersed phase, and excessive shaking has caused acceleration of the rate of creaming. Small amounts of gelatin, dextran, and methylcellulose have been found to aid in stabilizing the emulsions, but they are also adversely affected by elevated temperatures.

The preparation of a parenteral emulsion is troublesome. It is made more difficult by the rigid requirement for particle size control to prevent emboli in blood vessels, by the limited choice of emulsifiers and stabilizers of low toxicity, and by the preservation of the oil phase against the development of rancidity.

Effect of Route of Administration. Parenteral preparations may be given by several routes.[63] The five most common are intravenous, intramuscular, subcutaneous, intracutaneous, and intraspinal.

The intended route of administration has a marked effect on the formulation of a parenteral product. The volume in which a dose of the drug must be encompassed is one factor to consider. For intracutaneous injections a volume of more than 0.2 ml rarely is used because tissue volume is small and compact; also, absorption is quite slow owing to the lack of blood vessels. Volumes of 1 ml or less may be injected subcutaneously, and only occasionally are volumes of more than 2 ml given intramuscularly. Volumes of 10 ml or less may be given intraspinally, but only by the intravenous route may large volumes be given safely, provided careful control of the rate of administration is undertaken. It is not convenient to administer a volume of more than 20 ml by a syringe, and usually it is not practical to set up an infusion unit for less than 250 ml.

Isotonicity is a characteristic that is probably of greatest importance for intraspinal injections because the circulation of the cerebrospinal fluid is slow, and disturbances of osmotic pressure quickly cause headache and vomiting. Since intracutaneous injections are given mostly for diagnostic purposes, nonisotonic solutions may cause false signs of irritation. Isotonicity is preferable for the comfort of the patient, but is not essential for subcutaneous and intramuscular injections. For the rapid absorption of drugs given intramuscularly, a slightly hypertonic solution may increase the rate by causing local effusion of tissue fluids. Usually, intravenous fluids should be isotonic, although slow administration of a paratonic solution may be performed safely if rapid dilution with the blood occurs.

In general, only solutions of drugs in water may be given intravenously. Suspensions may not be given because of the danger of blockage of the small blood vessels. Aqueous or oleaginous suspensions and oleaginous solutions cannot normally be given subcutaneously because of the pain and irritation caused. Muscle tissue tolerates oils and suspended particles fairly well and is therefore the only route normally suitable for their administration.

The administration of a drug deep into the muscle tissue results in a pool of the product at the site of injection. From this depot, the drug is released at a rate determined to a large extent by the characteristics of the formulation. Whether the solvent is aqueous or oleaginous affects the rate of absorption; oleaginous solutions are usually more slowly absorbed. Increasing the viscosity of solutions slows the absorption, as do gelatin or polyvinylpyrrolidone in water and aluminum monostearate in oils. Utilizing modifications of the drug molecule to render it less soluble (for instance, the formation of various esters or salts) permits the production of stable suspensions, causing a marked reduction in the rate of absorption of the drug from the depot. Thus, utilizing various modifications in formulation of the product makes it possible to retard the rate at which a drug is released from a depot.

Ophthalmic preparations are formulated in much the same way as parenteral solutions. The eye is particularly sensitive to irritation; therefore formulation should be directed toward minimizing irritation. Normally, clean aqueous solutions are preferable for ophthalmic use. Suspensions of solids have been used in the eye when the therapeutic need superseded the need to avoid irritating effects, as for the suspensions of corticosteroids sometimes used. It has been found that a foreign body sensation increases as the concentration of suspended particles, regardless of size, approaches 5%.

This brief discussion of some of the factors involved in the formulation of parenteral dosage forms has been intended simply to introduce the student to this important area. This area is changing steadily as the ingenuity of research pharmacists spurs the development of new and improved formulation aids and techniques.

Stability

General principles of evaluation for stability are discussed in Chapter 26. In this chapter, it is sufficient to mention that the previous consideration of ingredients and packaging components in intimate contact with the product, and some of the problems associated with formulation, draw attention to the necessity of evaluating the effect of all the components on the stability of the product, particularly when the product is subjected to the accelerating reactivity of thermal sterilization.

Production

The production process includes all of the steps from the accumulation and combining of the ingredients of the formula to the enclosing of the product in the individual container for distribution. Intimately associated with these processes are the personnel who carry them out and the facilities in which they are performed. The most ideally planned processes can be rendered ineffective by personnel who do not have the right attitude or training, or by facilities that do not provide an efficiently controlled environment.

To enhance the assurance of successful manufacturing operations, all process steps must be carefully reduced to writing after being shown to be effective. These written process steps are often called standard operating procedures (SOPs). No extemporaneous changes are permitted to be made in these procedures; any change must go through the same approval steps as the original written SOP. Further, extensive records must be kept to give assurance at the end of the production process that all steps have been performed as prescribed, an aspect emphasized in the FDA's Good Manufacturing Practices.[64] Such in-process control is essential to assuring the quality of the product, since these assurances are even more significant than those from product release testing. The production of a quality product is a result of the continuous, dedicated effort of the quality assurance, production, and quality control personnel within the plant in developing, performing, and confirming effective SOPs.

To differentiate quality assurance from quality control, the former function is usually one of preplanning those factors that bear upon the quality of a product and is thus a preventative development process. Quality control may include this aspect, particularly if there is only one organizational group directly responsible for quality in a plant, but it more likely concentrates on those operations and tests that have been designed to evaluate the quality actually achieved in a product.

To enhance the visualization of the passage of materials through the various steps of the production process, a flow diagram is provided in Figure 22-2. In the initial step, the formula ingredients, container components, and processing equipment that have been released for use are drawn from their respective storage areas. The ingredients are compounded according to the master formula in an environment designed to maintain a high level of cleanliness. If the product is a solution, it is filtered during transfer to the aseptic filling room.

Process equipment and container components are cleaned thoroughly according to required specifications, are assembled in a clean environment, and preferably, are sterilized and depyrogenated prior to use.

All equipment and supplies introduced into the aseptic filling area should be sterile (Fig. 22-2), having come directly from the sterilization process, preferably through double-ended sterilizers (Fig. 22-3). When this is not possible, packages, hose lines from equipment, and supplies should be passed through openings (ports) of minimal size that can be reclosed promptly, under aseptic conditions. Outer wrappings of packages should be loosened and the contents received, that is, the inner wrapping grasped, by personnel already in the aseptic filling room. When double wrappings are not feasible, the outer surfaces of boxes, packages, or equipment should be wiped with a disinfectant solution as

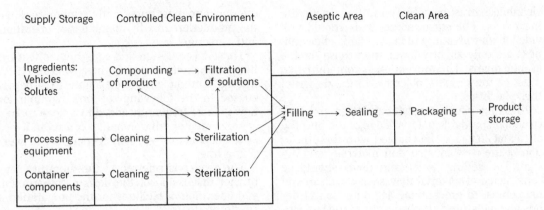

FIG. 22-2. *Diagram of flow of materials through the production department.*

they are transferred into the aseptic room. All supplies must be introduced into the aseptic filling rooms in such a manner that the aseptic state of these rooms is maintained, thereby preventing the introduction of environmental contamination into the product while it is being subdivided into individual containers. After these containers are sealed, contamination cannot enter the container and product.

As shown in Figure 22-2, the product is sealed in its final container within the aseptic room. It is them transferred to the packaging area. This area is maintained clean but need not meet the standards imposed for the aseptic rooms or for the compounding room. Packaged products are placed in quarantine storage until all tests have been completed and in-process control records have been evaluated; then the product may be released for distribution.

Facilities

The facilities for the manufacture of sterile products should be designed for control of cleanliness appropriate for each step. Near perfect

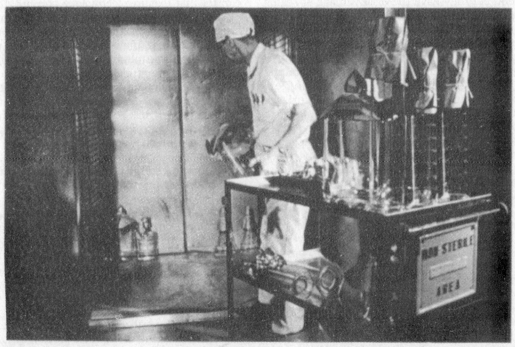

FIG. 22-3. *Double-door sterilizing oven being loaded with clean equipment. The equipment will be removed sterile from the other door in the aseptic area after the sterilization cycle. (Courtesy of Schering Corp.)*

cleanliness must be achieved in the aseptic filling rooms. The surrounding areas should provide a buffer area in which standards of cleanliness are only slightly lower than those for the aseptic rooms. The prevention of contamination must be the primary objective in the design of these facilities.

To achieve such exceptional design and construction standards, a knowledge of the purpose of the facility must be coupled with the utilization of the best construction materials and design. The ceiling, walls, and floors should be constructed of material that is easy to clean and nonporous, to prevent the accumulation of debris and moisture.[65] Probably one of the best finishes for rigid surfaces is the "spray-on-tile." This is a ceramic epoxy finish applied by spraying or painting to form a continuous, smooth, seal coating on the ceiling and walls.[66] The rigorous effects from continuous washing with detergents and disinfectants, however, can cause even this epoxy finish to degrade and wear or peal. One of the best materials for floors is a ceramic-plastic cement applied as a thick coat over existing rigid flooring to form a continuous, sealed surface. Another flooring material used increasingly in areas of less heavy traffic is sheet vinyl with heat-welded seams, coved to the side walls and applied by adhesives on underlying surfaces. Movable metal partitions are sometimes used to provide flexibility of room arrangement, but they have the disadvantage of seams and joints, which are very difficult to seal.

Glass is often used in partitions to permit supervisory view of the operation, but more importantly, to provide more pleasant, better lighted, less confining surroundings for the operators. Lighting fixtures should be recessed, and exposed piping or other dirt-collecting surfaces should not be tolerated. Furniture should be of nonporous, hard-surfaced materials, preferably stainless steel. Counters should be suspended from the wall.

Items of equipment that are difficult or impossible to sterilize should be kept out of the aseptic areas, if possible. If they must be used in the aseptic area, they should remain there and be continuously exposed to disinfecting processes. Whenever possible, operating machinery parts should be enclosed in stainless steel housing.
• The mechanical servicing of electrical, gas, water, air ventilation, and other utility lines into these areas requires careful planning. One of the most effective plans for this is to provide a floor above, space beneath, or a corridor alongside of the production area where all service connections can be accessible and properly maintained. This prevents interruption of production, and most importantly, contamination of the production area by maintenance operations and personnel.

These basic design and construction features have been continued with the advent of HEPA-filtered laminar airflow capabilities (to be discussed in the following section). Laminar airflow is most frequently added to a clean room to achieve greater environmental control in a local area, such as in a workbench enclosure or over a filling line.

The reader is referred to the literature for a further discussion of the design, construction, and operation of facilities for the preparation of sterile products.[67-69]

Environmental Control. Effective environmental control, both physical and biologic, is essential, but the level achievable is related to the characteristics of the facility, as discussed previously. Further, rigid standards from plant to plant and from one geographic location to another are not appropriate. Allowance also must be made for variations in control associated with seasonal conditions.

The standards of environmental control vary, depending on the area involved (clean-up, packaging, compounding, or filling) and the type of product being prepared. Unquestionably, the entire area used for the preparation of a product prepared aseptically (without terminal sterilization) must be maintained under the most rigid control that existing technology permits. If the product is to be terminally sterilized, somewhat less rigid biologic control of the compounding and filling areas may be acceptable, but rigid standards of cleanliness must be maintained. High standards of cleanliness, excluding daily use of the disinfecting procedures, are usually acceptable for the clean-up and packaging areas.

Traffic Control. Excellence in environmental control would be relatively easy to achieve were it not for the necessity for personnel and supplies to move from one area to another. Therefore, a carefully designed arrangement to control and minimize traffic, particularly in and out of the aseptic areas, is essential. A floor plan for a sterile products facility is shown in Figure 22-4. Note that the only access directly from the outside is to the personnel wash rooms, the equipment wash rooms, the nonsterile manufacturing area, and the capping (packaging) area. Access by personnel to the aseptic corridor and aseptic compounding and filling rooms is only through an airlock. Pass-through openings and double-ended sterilizers are provided to permit controlled passage of supplies from nonaseptic to aseptic areas.

Personnel should be permitted to enter asep-

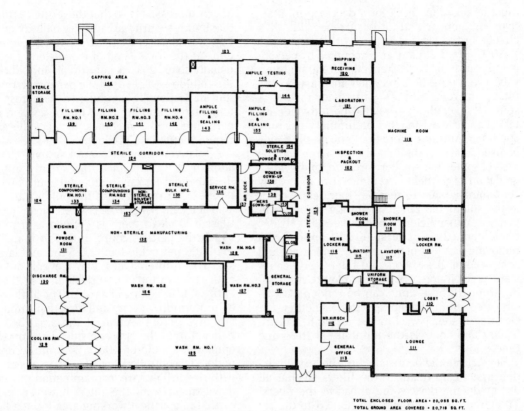

FIG. 22-4. *Floor plans for industrial sterile products production area. (Courtesy of Schering Corp.)*

tic areas only after following rigidly prescribed procedures for removing their street clothing, washing their hands, and donning gowns, hats, shoes, facemasks, gloves, and other prescribed attire. Once they have entered the aseptic area, they should not be permitted to move in and out of the area without regowning. Personnel assigned to cleaning and packaging should be restricted to these areas. Unauthorized personnel should never be permitted to enter the aseptic area.

Housekeeping. Cleaning personnel must be imbued with the philosophy that not one remaining particle of debris is acceptable. Only with such an approach will the conditions be provided for achieving and maintaining proper environmental control. It must also be recognized that many, if not most, critical contaminating particles are subvisual in size.

All equipment and surrounding work area must be cleaned thoroughly at the end of the working day. No contaminating residues from the concluded process may remain. The ceiling, walls, and other structural surfaces must be cleaned with a frequency commensurate with the design of the facility, that is, less frequently

in a laminar airflow facility than in one that is not bathed with a constant clean airflow. All cleaning equipment should be selected for its effectiveness and freedom from lint-producing tendencies. It should be reserved for use in the aseptic areas only.

Surface Disinfection. After thorough cleaning, all surfaces should be disinfected, at least in the aseptic areas. An effective liquid disinfectant should be sprayed or wiped on all surfaces (see Chap. 21, "Sterilization").

Irradiation from ultraviolet lamps that are located to provide adequate radiation intensity on the maximum extent of surfaces in a room and that are maintained free from dust and films further reduces the viable microorganisms present on surfaces and in the air. Ultraviolet rays may be particularly useful to irradiate the inside, exposed surfaces of processing tanks, surfaces under hoods, the surface of conveyor belts, and similar confined surfaces that are otherwise difficult to render aseptic; however, they cannot reach unexposed surfaces such as pipe connections to tanks, the underside of conveyors, and the inside of containers.

Ultraviolet lamps must be kept clean, and care

must be taken to check for a decrease in effective emission, a natural occurrence due to a change in the glass structure with aging.

Air Control. In any area occupied by personnel, the air must be exchanged at frequent intervals. Fresh outside or recycled air must first be filtered to remove gross particulate matter. A spun glass, cloth, or shredded polyethylene filter* may be used for this preliminary cleaning operation. At times, more than one prefilter may be used in series, the first of quite large and the next of somewhat smaller pore size, to provide a gradation of particle size removal from heavily contaminated air. To remove finer debris down to the submicron range, including microorganisms, a high efficiency particulate air (HEPA) filter, defined as at least 99.97% efficient in removing particles of 0.3 μm size and larger and composed of glass fibers and fillers† or electrostatic precipitators,‡ may be employed. Air passing through these units can be rendered virtually free from foreign matter. Another air cleaning system§ washes the air with a disinfectant and controls the humidity at the same time.

Blowers should be installed in the air ventilation system upstream to the filters so that all dirt-producing devices are ahead of the filters. The clean air is normally distributed to the required areas by means of metal (preferably stainless steel) ducts. Since it is practically impossible to keep these ducts as clean as required, it is normally preferable to install HEPA filters at the point where the clean air enters the controlled room. Alternatively, the ducts may be replaced with a room (a plenum), usually above the production area, into which clean air is blown and then distributed through openings into each of the process rooms. The entire plenum can be kept clean and aseptic.

The clean, aseptic air is distributed in such a manner that it flows into the maximum security rooms at the greatest volume flow rate, thereby producing a positive pressure in these areas. This prevents unclean air from rushing into the aseptic area through cracks, temporarily opened doors, or other openings. The pressure is re-

duced successively so that the air flows from the maximum security area to the hallway or other less critical areas for return to the filtration system. At the intake end of the system, fresh air, usually about 25%, is continually introduced for the comfort and needs of the personnel. Further, the air is usually conditioned with respect to temperature and humidity for the comfort of the personnel, and sometimes, to meet the special requirements of a product.

A relatively new air control system, based on laminar flow principles, has greatly improved the potential for environmental control of aseptic areas. Currently, it is the only means available for achieving a Class 100 clean room. A Class 100 clean room is defined as a room in which the particle count in the air is not more than 100 per cubic foot of 0.5 μm and larger in size. HEPA-filtered air is blown evenly out of the entire back or top of a workbench (Fig. 22-5), or entire side or ceiling of a room. The airflow must be uniform in velocity and direction throughout any given cross-section of the area, being exhausted from the opposite side. The air velocity employed should be 100 ± 20 ft/min. Contamination is controlled because it is swept away with the airflow. Any contamination introduced downstream from the filter, however, may be carried to a critical working area located farther downstream. This may be caused by the improper placement of supplies, the manipulation of personnel, or discharge from operating equipment. Because the risk of introducing contamination in such a manner is generally considered to be less with vertical flow from ceiling-mounted HEPA filter units, vertical flow is most frequently utilized to protect critical sections of processing lines and similar activities.[69,70] Hori-

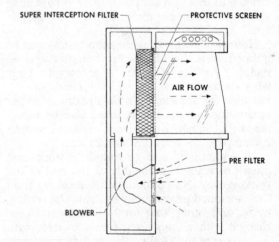

FIG. 22-5. *Horizontal laminar airflow clean bench.*

*Pliotron Corp., Niagara Falls, NY 14302.
†American Air Filter Co., Inc., Louisville, KY 40277; Cambridge Filter Corp., Syracuse, NY 13221; Flanders Filters, Washington, NC 27889; Weber Technical Products, Lawrence, MA 01842.
‡American Air Filter Co., Inc., Louisville, KY 40277; Electro-Air Div., Emerson Electric Co., McKees Rocks, PA 15136; Westinghouse Electric Corp., Sturtevant Div., Hyde Park, MA 02136.
§Midland Ross Corp., Ross Air Systems Div., New Brunswick, NJ 08903.

zontal flow, on the other hand, is used to protect processing lines and is used most frequently for workbenches.* Numerous reports have shown the marked benefit of laminar airflow for controlling working environments, from small workbenches to entire rooms.[71-75]

Although Class 100 work environments are normally specified for the most critical aseptic and/or clean operations, achieving such levels of cleanliness is expensive and requires effective maintenance and monitoring. It should be recognized that not all operations associated with parenteral medications require such an environment. To such an end, other classes are defined.[76] For example, a Class 10,000 room is one in which the particle count is no more than 10,000 per cubic foot of 0.5 μm and larger in size. Such a cleanliness level is usually considered suitable for buffer areas around Class 100 worksites in which operations such as handling precleaned containers, process filtration, and aseptic gowning of personnel may be performed. Still less stringent requirements would be applied to laboratories, stock staging areas, and finish packaging, where a Class 100,000 or similar cleanliness level would usually be considered suitable.

The effectiveness of the environmental control system is normally monitored on the basis of deviation, usually upward, from baseline counts determined from extensive testing by the environmental control procedures utilized. Biologic evaluation methods most frequently utilized are summarized in Table 22-5 and include settling and surface contact nutrient agar plates, air impingement on nutrient media, and membrane filtration.†[77-79] Particulate matter evaluation methods, also summarized in Table 22-5, include membrane filtration‡ and electronic particle counters.§[80,81] A combination of methods is

usually utilized, involving two or more that best identify the control achieved of the particular circumstances of a given environment.

Personnel. The people who produce sterile products usually are nonprofessional persons, supervised by those with professional training. To be effective operators, they must be inherently neat, orderly, reliable, and alert, and have good manual dexterity. They should be appreciative of the vital role that every movement has in determining the quality of final product, i.e., its freedom from contaminants.

All employees should be in good health and should be subjected to periodic physical examinations. They should understand their responsibility to report the developing symptoms of a head cold, a sore throat, or other infectious diseases so that they can be assigned to a less critical area until they have fully recovered.

The attire worn by personnel in the aseptic areas usually consists of sterile coveralls, hoods, face masks, and shoe covers. Sterile rubber gloves also may be required.

Personnel entering the aseptic areas should be required to follow a definite preparatory procedure.[81] This should include removing at least outside street clothing, scrubbing the hands and arms thoroughly with a disinfectant soap, and donning the prescribed uniform. A full body water and soap shower would be essential in most biologic product processing plants—usually, both when entering and leaving the area to control contamination in both directions between personnel and the product. It must be recognized, however, that removing natural oils from the skin temporarily increases particle shedding. An air shower for the fully attired worker may be used at times to blow away loose lint, although the disruptive air currents generated may be detrimental to overall air control. A vibrating foot mat or a disinfectant foot bath also may reduce the transfer of contamination.

Because people are continually shedding viable and nonviable particulate matter from body surfaces,[82] uniforms are worn to help control this emission. Preferably, they are of the coverall type and made of synthetic fibers such as Dacron. Dacron cloth is made of a continuous fiber, which makes it essentially lint-free and in air conditioned rooms, is acceptably comfortable. Hats and masks are sometimes made of special parchment paper and are discarded after use. Spun polyethylene* has recently found favor as a material for uniforms.

*Air Control, Inc., Norristown, PA 19401; The Baker Co., Inc., Sanford, ME 04005; Clean Room Products, Inc., Bay Shore, NY 11706; Envirco, Albuquerque, NM 87107; Flanders Filters, Inc., Washington, NC 27889; Laminaire Corp., Rahway, NJ 07065; Liberty Industries, Inc., Berlin, CT 06037; Vecco International, Livonia, MI 48150.
†Andersen Samplers, Inc., Atlanta, GA 30336; Flow Sensor, McLean, VA 22102; Folex-Biotest-Schleussner, Inc., Moonachie, NJ 07074; Mattson-Garvin Co., Maitland, FL 32751; New Brunswick Scientific, Edison, NJ 08817.
‡AMF-CUNO, Meridec, CT 06450; Gelman Sciences, Inc., Ann Arbor, MI 48106; Millipore Corp., Bedford, MA 01730; Nuclepore Corp., Pleasanton, CA 94566; Sartorius Filters, Inc., Hayward, CA 94545.
§Air Techniques, Inc., Baltimore, MD 21207; Bausch & Lomb, Rochester, NY 14625; Climet Instruments Co., Redlands, CA 92373; HIAC/Royco Instruments Div., Menlo Park, CA 94025; Phoenix Precision Instrument, Gardiner, NY 12525.

*Tyvek, E. I. duPont de Nemours & Co., Wilmington, DE 19898.

TABLE 22-5. *Environmental Monitoring Methods*

Method	Principle of Operation	Advantages	Disadvantages
Biologic evaluation			
Settling plates	Gravitational fallout in a given time on a given area.	Uncomplicated. Low cost.	Only heavier particles settle and are collected. Irregularities in counts due to wild air currents, physical movements of personnel, etc.
Slit sampler	Measured volume of air drawn through slit and impacted on nutrient agar as plate turns.	Measured volume of air sampled. Sampling related to time as plate turns.	Velocity of impaction likely to have lethal effect on vegetative forms. Drying effect may be lethal to vegetative cells. Must be used with access to electricity and vacuum.
Centrifugal sampler	Measured volume of air centrifugally blown on nutrient agar strip.	Measured volume of air sampled. Unit can be easily carried by hand and is battery-operated. Unit head is sterilizable and body sanitizable.	Velocity of impaction likely to have lethal effect on vegetative forms. Drying effect may be lethal to vegetative cells.
Cascade sieve sampler	Measured volume of air cascaded through up to six plates of decreasing pore size and impacted on nutrient agar plates, with the smallest particles collected on the last plate.	Measured volume of air sampled. Permits gradation of particles by size.	Velocity of impaction likely to have lethal effect on vegetative forms. Must be used with access to vacuum. Affected by high RH; best used with dry conditions.
Liquid impinger	Measured volume of air bubbled through liquid nutrient medium with impingement in liquid.	Measured volume of air sampled. Less lethal action on vegetative forms since impingement is in "soft" liquid. Accepted as reference method.	Liquid must be filtered or plated to isolate microorganisms. More complicated procedure. Time-consuming procedure.
Membrane filter sampler	Measured volume of air drawn through membrane filter with particles retained on surface and filter then incubated on nutrient agar plate.	Measured volume of air sampled. May be used also for microscopic particle counting.	Additional step of membrane being placed on nutrient agar in plate. Air pockets under membrane prevent growth. Drying effect of microorganisms on membrane is lethal to most vegetative forms. Vacuum source required.

Method	Principle of Operation	Advantages	Disadvantages
Particulate matter evaluation			
Membrane filter	Measured volume of air drawn through membrane filter with particles retained on surface.	Measured volume of air sampled. Particles microscopically visible and identifiable. Particles can be sized and dimensionally described.	Counting and sizing require experienced and trained microscopist. Identification of particles requires experienced and trained microscopist. Time-consuming procedure.
Right angle light-scattering instrumental counter	Particle in viewing cell scatters light at right angles from incident light to photodetector tube.	Quantitative count of particles in measured volume of air obtained. Instant results given. Range of sizes of particles measured.	Sizing affected by light-scattering characteristics of particle surface. No differentiation between viable and non-viable particles. Costly.
Near forward light-scattering instrumental counter	Particle in viewing cell scatters light forward from incident light to photodetector tube.	Quantitative count of particles in measured volume of air obtained. Instant results given. Range of sizes of particles measured. Greater intensity than other methods; therefore, smaller particles can be counted.	Sizing affected by light-scattering characteristics of particle surface. No differentiation between viable and non-viable particles. More costly than other methods.

Personnel working in equipment wash rooms, sterilizing rooms, and packaging areas are normally required to don clean uniforms daily and to be conscious of cleanliness, but are not required to meet the special requirements for personnel entering the aseptic areas.

Processing

The initial processing step is the procurement of acceptable components (see Fig. 22-2). In a plant, the majority of components are requisitioned from tested and approved stock, and are then subjected to whatever processing steps are required to prepare them for use. A few components, such as Water for Injection, are manufactured to specifications as needed.

Water for Injection. Water for Injection (WFI) usually is prepared by distillation in a still specifically designed to produce the high-quality water required.[83,84] Reverse osmosis, however, is a method that is now approved by the USP, and it is receiving increasing attention and use.*

The specifications for the quality of the water required have been discussed under the heading "Vehicles," earlier in this chapter.

The specifications for a still should include (1) prepurification of feed water by chemical softening, deionization, or filtration to improve the quality of the distillate and reduce the frequency of required cleaning due to insoluble scale in the boiler, (2) removal of entrained contaminants from the vapor before it is condensed by passage through an efficient baffle system, (3) ejection of volatile constituents from the top of the system before the vapor is cooled so that they will not redissolve and appear in the condensate, (4) construction of all surfaces that will come in contact with the vapor and condensate of a material that will not dissolve in even trace amounts, preferably pure tin, 304 stainless steel, or borosilicate glass.

In addition to conventional stills,* two types of stills frequently used for the production of large volumes of water are the vapor compression

*AMSCO, Erie, PA 16512; Barnstead Co., Div. of Sybron Corp., Boston, MA 02132; Culligan International Co., Northbrook, IL 60062; Millipore Corp., Bedford, MA 01730; Vaponics, Inc., Plymouth, MA 02360.

*AMSCO, Erie, PA 16512; Barnstead Co., Div. of Sybron Corp., Boston, MA 02132; Consolidated Machine Corp., Boston, MA 02134; Corning Glass Works, Corning, NY 14830; Vaponics, Inc., Plymouth, MA 02360.

stills* and the multiple effect stills.†While they operate on somewhat different principles, both utilize initially heated feed water and steam to conserve on energy consumption and cooling water. Both types are capable of producing high-purity water at rates of 50 to 1000 or more gallons per hour.

A reverse osmosis system functions by applying pressure (usually 200 to 400 psi) to raw water sufficient to force the permeation of water through a select semipermeable membrane in the opposite direction from natural osmosis. The membranes most commonly used are composed of cellulose esters or polyamides (nylon) and are effective in retaining all macromolecules and 85% or more of small ions such as Na^+ and Cl^-. Since pyrogens are macromolecules, they should be retained as well as such viable particles as microorganisms. Greater efficiency and reliability are achieved by passing the water through two membranes in series. The acceptance of reverse osmosis for the preparation of Water For Injection is increasing as experience is gained with the system and its characteristics are understood more fully.[85]

Storage and Distribution.

The storage and distribution of WFI are as important as its production.[86] A closed system is desirable, with air exchange through a filter that removes microorganisms, dirt, and vapors from the air as the tank is filled and emptied. Should microorganisms gain entrance to the tank, they may be prevented from multiplying by holding the temperature of the water at 80°C by means of a steam coil in the bottom of the tank. Normally, WFI should not be held for more than 24 hours at room temperature before it is used, but if held at 80°C, continuous addition of fresh WFI as usage occurs is common practice. The constant danger of microbial contamination, in spite of precautions, and subsequent development of pyrogenic substances in the water demand careful storage requirements.

The distribution of WFI from the storage tank to the point of use may be by direct withdrawal from the tank, or in large plants, through a pipe system. When a pipe system is used, special precautions must be followed to prevent contamination, including construction with welded stainless steel pipe, a closed system preferably with

continuous circulation to avoid stagnation, maintenance at elevated temperature, complete isolation from all other piping systems, elimination of elbows or other pockets in which water can stagnate for long periods, and a means of thorough cleaning and sanitation at frequent intervals, as with clean steam or hot alkali.

Cleaning Equipment and Containers. Equipment and containers to be used in the processing of a sterile product must be scrupulously clean.[87] New, unused containers and equipment are contaminated principally with dust, fibers, and chemical films, which usually are relatively easy to remove, often by rinsing only. Debris that is more dangerous and more difficult to remove may be present as a residue from a previous use. Such debris usually must be removed by vigorous treatment with hot detergents.

In general, equipment used previously should be scrubbed by hand immediately after use with an effective detergent that does not leave a residue of its own. Whenever possible, equipment should be disassembled so that each part can be thoroughly scrubbed and cleaned, with particular attention given to screw threads, joints, and other dirt-collecting structures. Live steam can sometimes be used to loosen debris effectively, particularly in areas that are not easily accessible. After cleaning, the equipment should be rinsed several times, with a final rinse with WFI. Just prior to reuse, large clean tanks and similar equipment should be rinsed thoroughly with WFI. Reserving equipment for use with only one type of product reduces cleaning problems.

A new method for large tanks, pipe lines, and associated equipment that can be isolated and contained within a process unit has been developed and identified as a CIP (Clean in Place) system.[88] Cleaning is accomplished primarily with high-pressure rinsing treatments delivered automatically within the equipment. This is usually followed by steam sanitization through the same system, although actual sterilization of the entire system with attached components, such as filters, is being investigated.[89]

For glass or metal equipment small enough to be transported by hand, machine washing is possible. The glassware or metalware is automatically conveyed, usually in an inverted position, through a series of rigorous, high-pressure treatments, including hot detergent, hot tap water, and final rinses with distilled water. Because many containers have restricted openings, it is essential that the treatments in any washer be introduced through tubes *into* each container, with a smooth flow out. All parts of

*Aqua-Chem. Inc., Milwaukee, WI 53201; Barnstead Co., Div. of Sybron Corp., Boston, MA 02132; Mechanical Equipment Co., Inc., New Orleans, LA 70130.
†AMSCO, Erie, PA 16512; Barnstead Co., Div. of Sybron Corp., Boston, MA 02132; Finn-Aqua America, Inc., Bellevue, WA 98007; Vaponics, Inc., Plymouth, MA 02360.

the machine coming in contact with the treatments must be noncorrosive so that metallic contaminants from the machine are not deposited on the glassware.

When high processing rates are not required, a cabinet type washer* embodying these principles may be used. In such a machine, the ware to be washed is held on a rack within a cabinet while the machine automatically goes through the sequence of treatments of the cycle.

Rinsing New Containers. In cleaning new glassware, the detergent treatment is usually eliminated, and with it, the risk of a detergent residue. Without the detergent treatment, the cycle is essentially a rinsing process. To loosen debris by rinsing, alternating hot (preferably clean steam) and cold treatments should be used. Final rinses should be done with filtered WFI. This sequence of treatments may be performed on the machines described above or on a rotary rinser.† The containers are inverted on spindles in the front of the machine and carried through a series of rinses in one rotation. For ampuls or containers with a markedly constricted opening that makes water drainage incomplete, the final treatment is usually a blast of clean air to blow out remaining water.

After cleaning, it is essential that the clean containers be protected from dust and other particulates that might be present in the environment. Therefore, the clean containers are often removed from the rinser and placed in clean stainless steel boxes for sterilization under the protection of HEPA-filtered laminar airflow (Fig. 22-6).

Conveyor type rinsers,‡ as shown in Figure 22-7, have relatively high production rates. They have an advantage over the above rinsers in that they deliver the clean container at the opposite end from that at which the unrinsed containers are loaded. The delivery end can, therefore, be in an adjoining room (Fig. 22-7), away from the dust and dirt associated with packing cartons.

To eliminate the tedious handling of each individual container, rack loading rinsers‡§ have been designed with rack sizes adapted to container packing cartons. Such a rinser is shown in Figure 22-6.

Minute quantities of oils, proteinaceous materials, or other debris retained in the rinser from a previously used container could be carried

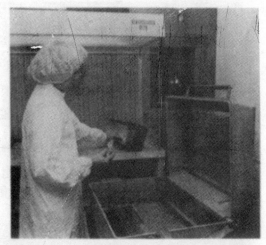

FIG. 22-6. *Rinser designed to clean vials by racks sized to shipping cartons or by individual handling. Note laminar airflow to protect clean, wet vials. (Courtesy of University of Tennessee.)*

through many rinsing operations and be deposited on glassware subsequently being processed.

High-speed processing lines often are designed to clean containers by rinsing with clean water, or sometimes simply with clean air, under high pressure. The containers are shipped from the manufacturer on a support tray enclosed within a shrunken, tightly-fitted, polyethylene sheet to minimize the accumulation of dirt during shipment. The cleaned containers are usually then fed by conveyor to hot-air sterilizing tunnels, thereby minimizing handling of the containers, increasing speed of processing, and allowing the clean sterile containers to be delivered through-the-wall into the aseptic filling room.

Cleaning Rubber and Plastic Components. Rubber closures are usually washed by mechanical agitation in a tank of hot detergent solution (such as 0.5% sodium pyrophosphate) followed by a series of thorough water rinses, the final rinse being WFI.[90] The objective is to remove surface debris accumulated from the molding operation and from handling, and leachable constituents at or near the surface. Part of the debris is attracted and held on the surface by electrostatic forces. Similarly, plastic materials accumulate surface debris.

Abrasion may occur during agitation, resulting in small, loose pieces of the rubber or plastic material. This problem is more acute with two-component closures, i.e., a rubber disc inserted in an aluminum cap, because agitation usually causes more abrasion of the aluminum and produces small aluminum fragments, which adhere

*Vernitron/Better Built, Carlstadt, NJ 07072.

†Cozzoli Machine Co., Plainfield, NJ 07060; U.S. Bottlers Machinery Co., Chicago, IL 60618; Vernitron/Better Built, Carlstadt, NJ 07072.

‡Cozzoli Machine Co., Plainfield, NJ 07060.

§Metromatic Products Corp., Oyster Bay, NY 11771.

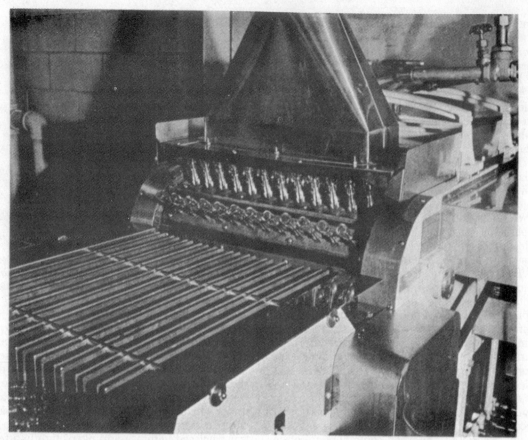

FIG. 22-7. *Conveyor rinser delivering clean vials to an adjoining clean room. (Courtesy of Schering Corp. and Cozzoli Machine Co.)*

tenaciously to the rubber disc or wedge between the disc and the cap.

Therefore, the multiple objectives for washing closures and other parts include loosening debris, minimizing abrasion, and sweeping away the loosened debris. Household clothes washers of the horizontal rotating basket type or the center post agitator type have been used, but neither meets the requirements for an ideal washer for closures. More commonly today, the closures are subjected to gentle agitation with air bubbles,* basket rotation accompanied by spray rinsing,† or simple water movement followed by extensive rinsing with WFI. Handling after cleaning must be done carefully to prevent particle generation from abrasion and to prevent pickup of dust and other particulate matter from the environment. Therefore, the clean closures are often handled under the protection of HEPA-filtered laminar airflow.

*Production Equipment, Inc., Rochelle Park, NJ 07662.
†Industrial Washing Machine Corp., Matawan, NJ 07747.

Sometimes, the closures are subjected to an autoclave cycle as a part of the cleaning process. Such treatment aids in loosening surface debris and also leaches from the closure some of the extractives, thus reducing the subsequent contamination of the product. It should be remembered, however, that excessive heating is detrimental to the life of rubber and thermoplastic materials.

Particular attention should be given to the cleaning of rubber and plastic tubing. When tubing is reused, adequate cleaning of the lumen, which is not readily accessible, may be virtually impossible. When cleaning is necessary, special brushes may be helpful in reaching the lumen. The safest approach is to retain the tubing for reuse with the same product or to discard after one use.

Sterilization of Equipment. In general, equipment, containers, closures, and all other components should be sterilized after cleaning and prior to use. The principles and practices of sterilization are discussed in Chapter 21.

Compounding the Product. The product should be compounded under clean environmental conditions (see Fig. 22-2). Aseptic conditions usually are not required since it may not be possible or feasible to sterilize some of the ingredients or the equipment, e.g., large tanks. Whenever possible, however, equipment and ingredients should be sterile to reduce the microbial load.

The accuracy of compounding should meet the rigid standards accepted in pharmaceutical procedures, regardless of the batch size, recognizing that small multiple errors may be additive. In large batches, particular attention must be given to achieving and maintaining homogeneity of solutions, suspensions, and mixtures, maintaining a given temperature, and accelerating cooling. The order of mixing ingredients may become highly significant, for example, owing to the physical problem of distributing a pH-adjusting ingredient throughout a large tank of liquid. Compounding problems for large batches of product often are different from those for small batches.

Good planning requires anticipation of reasonable stock needs for products so that a single large lot, instead of several small lots, may be prepared. If made in divided portions, each portion is "a lot" requiring separate testing, thus multiplying the time and cost required.

Filtration of Solutions. Solutions must be filtered. The primary objectives of filtration are clarification or sterilization of a solution. The two objectives differ principally in degree. Clarification is termed "polishing," and a highly polished solution requires the removal of particulate matter down to at least 3 microns in size. Further reduction in the size of the particulate matter removed, to approximately 0.3 micron, results in sterilization, the removal of viable microorganisms and spores. Where the objective of filtration is sterilization, a highly polished solution is concurrently produced. A solution having a high polish conveys the impression of exceptional quality and purity, a highly desirable characteristic for a sterile solution.

The various types of filters employed for sterile products, their selection, and use have been discussed in Chapter 7.

After filtration, the solution must be protected from environmental contamination until it is sealed in the final container. Normally, this is best accomplished by collecting the filtrate in a container that is a part of a closed system, with air exchange through a bacteria retentive filter. The filtrate is fed directly from the collecting vessel to the filling machine through sterile hose connections. A secondary "in-line" filter is often included as near the outlet from the filler as possible to collect any lint or other particulate matter picked up from the lines or equipment. It is at the moment of filtration that a solution must pass from a clean environment to an aseptic environment (see Fig. 22-2), particularly if it has been sterilized by the filtration process.

Filling Procedures. A liquid may be subdivided from a bulk container to individual dose containers more easily and uniformly than a solid. Mechanical subdivision of a mobile, low-density liquid can be achieved with light-duty machinery, but viscous, sticky, or high-density liquids require much more rugged machines to withstand the pressure required to dispense them.

Filling Equipment for Liquids. Certain fundamental features are found on all machines used for filling containers with liquids. A means is provided for repetitively forcing a measured volume of the liquid through the orifice of a delivery tube designed to enter the constricted opening of a container. The size of the delivery tube is governed by the opening in the container to be used, the viscosity and density of the liquid, and the speed of delivery desired. The tube must freely enter the neck of the container and deliver the liquid deep enough to permit air to escape without sweeping the entering liquid into the neck or out of the container. To reduce the resistance to the flow of the liquid, the tube should have the maximum possible diameter. Excessive delivery force causes splashing of the liquid and troublesome foaming, if the liquid has a low surface tension.

The delivery of relatively small volumes of liquids is usually obtained from the stroke of the plunger of a syringe. The stroke of the syringe forces the liquid through a two-way valve that provides for an alternate filling of the syringe from a reservoir and delivery to a container. For heavy, viscous liquids a sliding piston valve provides more positive action.

A drop of liquid normally hangs at the tip of the tube after a delivery. When the container to be filled is an ampul, withdrawal of the tube without wetting the long restricted neck is almost impossible, unless the hanging drop of liquid is retracted. Thus, a retraction device is designed as a part of most filling machines.

Filling machines* should be designed so that the parts through which the liquid flows can be

*Cozzoli Machine Co., Plainfield, NJ 07060; Mateer-Burt Co., Wayne, PA 19087; National Instrument Co., Inc., Baltimore, MD 21215; Perry Industries, Inc., Hicksville, NY 11802; Scientific Equipment Products Co., Baltimore, MD 21218.

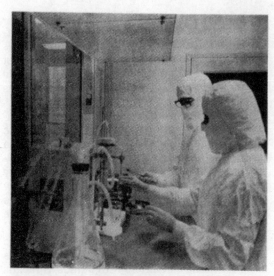

FIG. 22-8. *Aseptic filling of vials with liquid under vertical laminar airflow, followed by stoppering with forceps by hand. (Courtesy of University of Tennessee.)*

easily demounted for cleaning and for sterilization. These parts also should be constructed of nonreactive materials such as borosilicate glass or stainless steel. Syringes are usually made of stainless steel when the pressures required for delivery of viscous liquids or large volumes would be unsafe for glass syringes.

Filling machines such as the one shown in operation in Figure 22-8 can be designed to provide high delivery volume precision. The stroke of the syringe can be repeated precisely; therefore, once a particular setting has been calibrated for a delivery, high precision is possible. The precision can be affected by certain operating factors, however, such as the speed of delivery, the uniformity of speed, the expansion of rubber tubing connecting the valve with the delivery tube, and the rapidity of action of the valves.

Sterile solutions of relatively low potency dispensed in large volume (up to one liter) do not normally require the precision of filling that is required for small volumes of potent injectables. Therefore, bottles of solution are usually filled by gravity, pressure, or vacuum filling devices. Gravity filling is relatively slow, but is accomplished in a simple manner. The liquid reservoir is positioned above the filling line with a hose connection from the reservoir to a shut-off device at the filling line. The shut-off device is usually hand operated, and the bottles are filled to graduations on the bottles.

The pressure pump filler often is operated semiautomatically and differs from the gravity filler principally in that the liquid is under pressure. It is usually equipped with an overflow tube connected to a receiver to prevent excess filling of the container.

Vacuum filling* is commonly used in faster filling lines for large liquid volumes because it is more adaptable to automation. A vacuum is produced in a bottle when a nozzle gasket makes a seal against the lip of the bottle to be filled. The vacuum draws the liquid from a reservoir through the delivery tube into the bottle. When the liquid level reaches the level of an adjustable overflow tube, the seal is mechanically loosened and the vacuum released. Any liquid that had been drawn into the vacuum line is collected in a trap receiver and then returned to the reservoir.

It is obvious that the accuracy and precision of machine filling of sterile liquids vary with the method. Therefore, a method is selected to provide the degree of accuracy and precision required by the nature of the product. A slight excess is required in each container to provide for the loss that occurs at the time of administration due to adherence to the wall of the container and retention in the syringe and hypodermic needle lumen. A table of suggested excess volumes is found in the USP.

The danger of overdosage as well as economic factors limit the amount of excess desirable in a given container. A reduction of only 0.01 ml of unnecessary excess in each 1-ml ampul of a lot of 10,000 would yield approximately 100 more containers of product.

Emulsions and suspensions often require specially designed filling equipment because of their high viscosity. To obtain a reasonable flow rate, high pressures must be applied, or containers with large openings must be used, to permit the entry of large delivery tubes. Sometimes jacketed reservoir tanks can be used to raise the temperature of the product and thereby lower its viscosity. It is normally necessary to keep suspensions, and sometimes emulsions, constantly agitated in the reservoir during filling, so that the product remains homogeneous and each subdivided unit contains the required amount of drug.

Filling Equipment for Solids. Sterile solids, such as antibiotics, are more difficult to subdivide accurately and precisely into individual dose containers than are liquids. The rate of flow of solid material tends to be slow and irregular, particularly if finely powdered. Small, granular particles flow most evenly. Containers with a relatively large opening must be used; even so,

---

*Perl Machine Manufacturing Co., Inc., Brooklyn, NY 11201; U.S. Bottlers Machinery Co., Chicago, IL 60618.

the filling rate is slow, and the risk of spillage is ever present. For these reasons, the tolerances permitted for the content of such containers must be relatively large. Suggested tolerances may be found tabulated in the USP.

Sterile solids can be subdivided into containers by individual weighing. The operator can use a scoop that holds a volume approximately equal to the weight required, but the quantity filled into the container is finally weighed on a balance. This is a slow process.

When the solid is obtainable in a relatively free-flowing form, machine methods of filling may be employed. In general, these methods involve the measurement and delivery of a volume of the solid material, which has been calibrated in terms of the weight desired. Among the major problems in the use of such machines are stratification of particles due to varying particle sizes, the development of electrostatic charge within the mass of dry solid particles, the formation of air pockets, and uneven flow due to clumping of the particles. These all result in uneven filling of the container. The problems

usually can be minimized if uniform particle size of the solid is achieved and a small electric current is used to neutralize the developing charge.

One type of machine* for delivering measured quantities of free-flowing material employs an auger in the stem of the funnel-shaped hopper (see Fig. 22-9). The size and rotation of the auger can be adjusted to deliver a regulated volume of granular material from the funnel stem into the container.

In another filling machine† (Fig. 22-10), an adjustable cavity in the rim of the filling wheel is filled by vacuum as the wheel passes under the hopper. The contents are held by vacuum until the cavity is inverted over the container, when a jet of sterile air discharges the dry solids. This machine dispenses dry solids that flow less freely than those of other machines presently available.

*Chase-Logeman Corp., Hicksville, NY 11501; Mateer-Burt Co., Wayne, PA 19087.
†Perry Industries Inc., Hicksville, NY 11802.

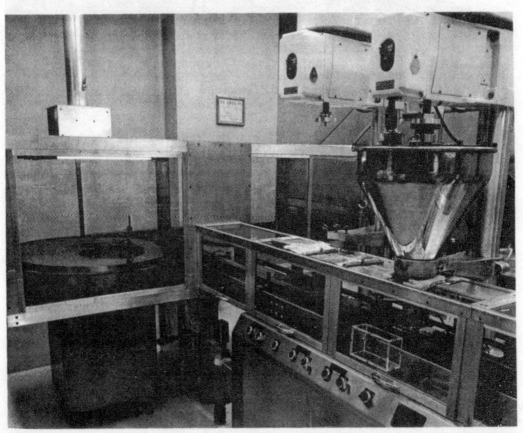

FIG. 22-9. *High-speed automated aseptic processing line protected by a hood showing unscrambler turntable at left and powder filler at right. (Courtesy of Lederle Laboratories Div., American Cyanamid Co.)*

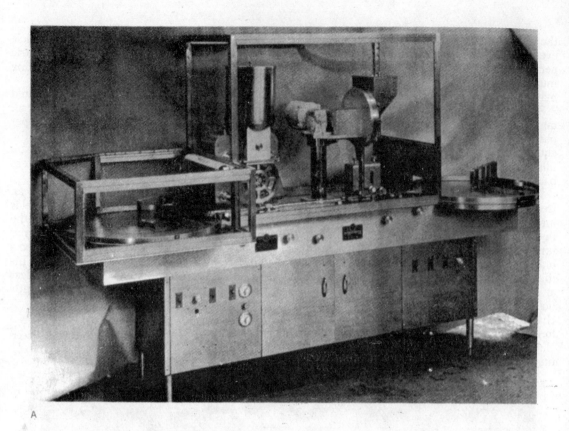

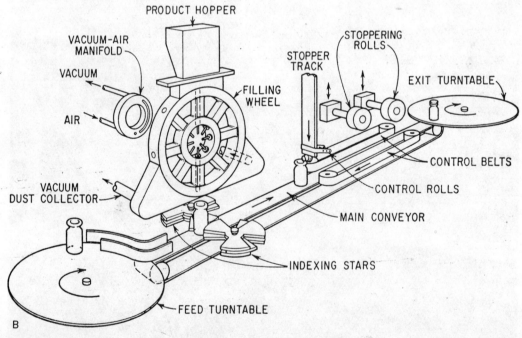

FIG. 22-10. A, *Automated filling unit for dry solids. The operation is protected by hoods to maintain an aseptic environment.* B, *The diagram represents the functioning parts with the unscrambler turntable at left, the filling machine, the rubber closure inserting device, and the collecting turntable for the filled and stoppered vials at right. (Courtesy of Perry Industries, Inc.)*

Sealing. Containers should be sealed in the aseptic area immediately adjacent to the filling machine. In addition to retaining the contents of a sterile product, sealing of containers assures the user that it has not been opened. It is obvious that a sterile container that has been opened can no longer be considered to be sterile. Therefore, tamperproof sealing is essential.

Sealing Ampuls. Ampuls may be closed by melting a portion of the glass of the neck to form either bead-seals (tip-seals) or pull-seals. Tip-seals are made by melting sufficient glass at the tip of the ampul neck to form a bead of glass and close the opening. Pull-seals are made by heating the neck of a rotating ampul below the tip, then pulling the tip away to form a small, twisted capillary just prior to being melted closed.

The heating with a high-temperature gas-oxygen flame must be even and carefully controlled to avoid distortion of the seal. Excessive heating of air and gases in the neck causes expansion against the soft glass with the formation of fragile bubbles at the point of seal. Open capillaries at the point of seal or cracks result in "leakers." Pull-sealing is a slower process, but the seals are more reliable than those from tip-sealing. Powder ampuls or other types having a wide opening must be sealed by pull-sealing.

Fracture of the neck of ampuls often occurs during sealing if wetting had occurred at the time of filling. Also, wet glass at the neck increases the frequency of bubble formation and of unsightly and contaminating deposits of carbon or oxides as a result of the effect of the heat of sealing on the droplets of product.

With some sensitive products, it may be necessary to close the ampuls with pull-seals to prevent combustion products of the flame from entering the ampul at the time of sealing, as might occur with tip-sealing. In addition, it is sometimes necessary to displace the air in the space within the ampul above the product to prevent decomposition. This may be done by introducing a stream of inert gas, such as nitrogen or carbon dioxide, during or after filling with the product. Immediately thereafter, the ampul is sealed before the gas can diffuse to the outside.

Sealing Bottles, Cartridges, and Vials. Rubber closures must fit the opening of the container snugly enough to produce a seal, but not so snugly that it is difficult to position them in or on the container. They may be inserted by hand, using sterile forceps (see Fig. 22-8). A faster hand method involves picking up the closure and inserting it into a vial by means of a tool connected to a vacuum line.

When closures are to be inserted by machines, the surface of the closure is usually halo-genated or coated with silicone to reduce the friction. This makes it possible for a closure to slide from a rotating or vibrating drum to the bottom of a chute, where it is positioned over a container, ready for insertion by a plunger or some other pressure device (Fig. 22-10). Stoppering can be done at production line speeds with such a machine.

Aluminum caps are used to hold rubber closures in place. Single caps may have a permanent center hole or a center that is torn away at the time of use to expose the rubber closure. Double aluminum caps usually have an inner cap with a permanent center hole, which in use is exposed when the entire outer cap is torn off. The triple aluminum caps are used for large bottles with rubber closures having permanent holes for attachment to administration sets. The inner cap with a permanent center hole remains in place during use to secure the rubber closure. The thin disc is used in conjunction with a thin rubber disc to seal the holes through the closure. The outer cap holds the disc in place and is torn away at the time of use.

When applied, the bottom edge of an aluminum cap is bent (crimped) around and under the lip of the glass container. It cannot be removed without destroying the cap, but perforations permit tearing away the portions of the cap to be discarded preparatory to use. Single aluminum caps may be applied by hand crimping devices,* but double or triple caps or large production lots require the use of heavy-duty motorized crimping machines.†

Automation of Processing. The need for increased production rates for sterile products eventually justifies the cost of developing and operating automatic machinery. Unquestionably, machines can be designed to carry out certain operations more rapidly and with more reliable repetition than can be performed by people. A further advantage of mechanization in processing sterile products is the elimination of the human body as a source of biologic contamination; however, the contaminating effects of abraded particles, lubricants, and dirt from the moving parts of even the cleanest aseptic machine must not be forgotten.

When machines are designed or used so that the constant attention of a human operator is required, the operation is identified as being

*The West Company, Phoenixville, PA 19460; Wheaton Scientific, Millville, NJ 08332; Production Equipment Inc., Rochelle Park, NJ 07662.
†Aluminum Co. of America, Pittsburgh, PA 15219; The West Company, Phoenixville, PA 19460; Wheaton Scientific, Millville, NJ 08332.

semiautomatic. For automatic operation, machines are usually linked together by conveyor belts in an arrangement that requires little attention from an operator (Fig. 22-10). The unscrambler or feed turntable lines up a large number of vials and feeds them one at a time to the conveyor belt. The belt carries each vial in sequence to the filling wheel, to the stoppering machine, and then out to the collecting turntable. A crimping machine could be inserted after the stoppering machine. This processing line has been permanently linked together. For greater flexibility, each machine may remain a separate unit, linked together in use by conveyor belt units in an arrangement suitable for a particular process.

Automation of the entire process would convey an empty dose container from its supply carton through the entire process until it is filled with a product, labeled, and placed in the shipping carton. A portion of such a processing line is illustrated in Figure 22-9. In this line, the vials are removed by operators from their protective cartons or "shrink-packs" and given an air rinse. A covered conveyor carries them at high speed through a sterilizing tunnel. They emerge, cooled, on the unscrambler turntable (left, Fig. 22-9) and are conveyed in sequence to the dry solids filler (right, Fig. 22-9), the stoppering and capping machines, and then into the next room for packaging, all without contact with human hands. A compact line of similar concept for processing small ampuls and vials has been developed.* Such lines are usually located in an aseptic room with the critical portions further protected with covers and bathed with HEPA-filtered air. An automated processing line such as this can be justified when high production rates are required.

Sterilization of Product. A product must be sterilized by the most reliable method possible. The methods of sterilization, their application, and the bases for their selection have been discussed in Chapter 21.

Freeze-Drying. Freeze drying (lyophilization) is a drying process applicable to the manufacture of certain pharmaceuticals and biologicals that are thermolabile or otherwise unstable in aqueous solution for prolonged storage periods, but that are stable in the dry state.

A product to be freeze-dried is prepared and handled as an aqueous solution or suspension in the same manner as discussed previously for an aseptic fill. The aqueous preparation is frozen

rapidly and cooled to an experimentally determined temperature below its eutectic point. Most commonly, it would be frozen by a mechanical refrigeration device, often the refrigerated shelves in the freeze-drying chamber, at a temperature of $-50°C$ or lower.

When the product is completely frozen and properly cooled, the chamber is sealed and evacuated. The ice in the frozen product gradually sublimes from the frozen surface and is collected in a refrigerated condenser chamber or on plates within the chamber containing the product. As the ice leaves the product, the drying residue maintains essentially its original volume and becomes porous, owing to the loss of the ice molecules. This porous structure usually increases the subsequent rate of solution of the product as compared with the original material. The rate of drying depends largely on the thermal conductance of the frozen product, the rate at which the vapor can diffuse through the progressively thicker layer of dried porous material, and the rate of transfer of the vapor through the system to the condenser surface. It has been said that the drying rate can be estimated as approximately one hour for each millimeter of depth of the product. The theory of freeze drying is more fully discussed in Chapter 3 and in the literature.[91-95]

In production, large freeze driers* are usually operated by an automatic control system. By means of a thermocouple frozen in a sample of the product, the temperature curve of the sample is duplicated in comparison with a curve experimentally found to produce a satisfactory product. During processing, the shape of the sample curve is adjusted primarily by the heat input, which provides the energy for sublimation.

The product is usually processed until there is less than 1% moisture in the dried material. After completion of the drying cycle, reabsorption of moisture must be prevented. The product must, therefore, be removed from the chamber and sealed as rapidly as possible under controlled low-humidity conditions.

Freeze driers also may be equipped for stoppering vials within the drying chamber. Special slotted rubber closures (see Fig. 22-1) are partially inserted into the neck of vials prior to freezing the product. The slots permit the escape of water vapor from the vials during the

---

*Hodes Lange Division, The West Co., Phoenixville, PA 19460.

*Hull Corp., Hatboro, PA 19040; Industrial Dynamics, Div. American Sterilizer Co., Erie, PA 16512; NRC Equipment Corp., Newton, MA 02161; Stokes Division, Pennwalt Corp., Philadelphia, PA 19120; The Virtis Co., Inc., Gardiner, NY 12525; USIFROID, Norristown, PA 19401.

drying cycle. At the end of the drying cycle a hydraulically operated plate or an expandable rubber diaphragm presses the closures firmly into the neck of the vials and seals them under vacuum. A butyl rubber compound is usually used for these closures because of its low water vapor permeability.

Numerous biologic preparations, tissue sections, and viable microorganisms are being preserved in the freeze-dried state. Multiple vitamin combinations, antibiotics, and hormone preparations are examples of pharmaceutical products preserved by this method.

Quality Control

The responsibilities of the quality control department have been discussed elsewhere in this text (Chap. 27). The discussion here is limited to those aspects of this important function that are peculiar to sterile products.

The three general areas of quality control are incoming stock, manufacturing (processing), and the finished product. For sterile products, incoming stock control encompasses routine tests on all ingredients as well as special evaluations such as pyrogen tests on WFI, glass tests on containers, and identity tests on rubber closures. It also may be necessary to perform microbial load (bioburden) tests to determine the number and types of microorganisms present. Process control in the manufacture of sterile products involves all of the innumerable tests, readings, and observations made throughout the manufacturing process of a product, including conductivity measurements during the distillation of WFI, confirmation of volume of fill in product containers, recording of cycle time and temperature for thermal sterilization of the product, and confirming the count and identity of labels for the product. The production control includes all of the final assays and tests to which the product is subjected. In addition to the usual chemical and biologic tests, a sterile product is subjected to a leaker test (when applicable), a clarity test, a pyrogen test (when applicable), and a sterility test.

Leaker Test. Ampuls are intended to provide a hermetically sealed container for a single dose of a product, thereby completely barring any interchange between the contents of the sealed ampul and its environment. Should capillary pores or tiny cracks be present, microorganisms or other dangerous contaminants may enter the ampul, or the contents may leak to the outside and spoil the appearance of the package. Changes in temperature during storage cause expansion and contraction of the ampul and contents, thereby accentuating interchange if an opening exists.

The leaker test is intended to detect incompletely sealed ampuls so that they may be discarded. Tip-sealed ampuls are more likely to be incompletely sealed than are those that have been pull-sealed. In addition, small cracks may occur around the seal or at the base of the ampul as a result of improper handling.

Leakers usually are detected by producing a negative pressure within an incompletely sealed ampul, usually in a vacuum chamber, while the ampul is entirely submerged in a deeply colored dye solution (usually 0.5 to 1.0% methylene blue). Subsequent atmospheric pressure then causes the dye to penetrate an opening, being visible after the ampul has been washed externally to clear it of dye. The vacuum (27 inches Hg or more) should be sharply released after 30 min. Only a tiny drop of dye may penetrate a small opening.

A reported study has shown that detection of leakers is more effective when the ampuls are immersed in a bath of dye* during the autoclaving cycle.[96] This has the added advantage of accomplishing both leaker detection and sterilization in one operation. Capillaries of about 15 microns in diameter or smaller may or may not be detected by these test methods.

Vials and bottles are not subjected to such a leaker test because the rubber closure is not rigid; however, bottles are often sealed while a vacuum is being pulled so that the bottle remains evacuated during its shelf-life. The presence of a vacuum may be detected by striking the base of the bottle sharply with the heel of the hand to produce the typical "water hammer" sound. Another test is to apply a spark tester probe to the outside of the bottle, moving from the liquid layer into the air space. A blue spark discharge occurs if the airspace is evacuated.

Clarity Test. Clarity is a relative term, the meaning of which is markedly affected by the subjective evaluation of the observer. Unquestionably, a clean solution having a high polish conveys to the observer that the product is of exceptional quality and purity. It is practically impossible, however, to prepare a lot of a sterile product so that every unit of that lot is perfectly free from visible particulate matter, that is, from particles that are 30 to 40 μm and larger in size. Consequently, it is the responsibility of the quality control department to detect and discard individual containers of a product that the ulti-

---

*Dye formula: F.D.&C. Red No. 1, 0.5%; F.D.&C. Red No. 2, 0.1%; and sodium lauryl sulfate, 0.25% in water.

mate user would consider to be unclean. Further, the USP states that good pharmaceutical practice requires that all containers be visually inspected and that any with visible particles be discarded. In addition, for large-volume infusions, the USP has established a limit of 50 particles of 10 μm and larger and 5 particles of 25 μm and larger per milliliter.

Normally, manufacturers of parenteral solutions can meet the above standard with the technology currently available. Further, product development, raw material quality control, and process control have eliminated any potential for widespread particulate development. In any lot of product, however, there may be a few containers having visible particles. These must be detected by visual inspection and discarded.

Although particulate matter is of primary concern in products given intravenously, all parenteral products should be free from insoluble particles. Several years ago, it was shown that the formation of pathologic granulomas in vital organs of the body can be traced to fibers, rubber fragments, and other solids present in intravenous solutions.[97] More recently, a double blind study has shown that the use of a final filter for the administration of intravenous solutions reduced the incidence of thrombophlebitis, a result believed to be due to the elimination of subvisual particles from the administered solution.[98] While there are unanswered questions relative to these toxic effects, these findings have highlighted the importance of the preparation of exceptionally clean parenteral products.

Suspensions, emulsions, or dry solids, in addition to solutions, should be compounded and processed under clean conditions to minimize the presence of foreign particles.

The visual inspection of a product container is usually done by individual human inspection of each externally clean container under a good light, baffled against reflection into the eyes, and viewed against a black and white background, with the contents set in motion with a swirling action. A moving particle is much easier to see than one that is stationary, but care must be exercised to avoid introducing air bubbles, which are difficult to distinguish from dust particles. To see heavy particles, it may be necessary to invert the container as the final step in inspection. Although a human inspector is subject to reduction in efficiency by eye strain, fatigue, distractions, and emotional disturbances, visual inspection can be done on 100% of the product units and can be done at a level of discrimination at least equal to that of the user.[99]

Instrumental methods of evaluation for particulate matter in liquids utilizing the principles of light scattering,* light absorption,† and electrical resistance‡ have been used to obtain particle counts and size distribution.[100–103] All of them, however, require destruction of the product unit to obtain the test sample, making them useful only for quality control testing. A method utilizing video image projection coupled with electronic circuitry detects moving particles without destruction of the product unit.[104] Therefore, it can be used for in-line detection of particles in product units, but at present, its use is limited to 1- to 5-ml containers.

Pyrogen Test. The presence of pyrogenic substances in parenteral preparations is determined by a qualitative biologic test based on the fever response of rabbits. Rabbits are used as the test animal because they show a physiologic response to pyrogens similar to that of human beings. If a pyrogenic substance is injected into the vein of a rabbit, an elevation of temperature occurs within a period of 3 hours. The specification limits and procedural details are given in the official test in the USP.

The housing conditions and handling are critical to obtaining consistent results with rabbits in the test. Because of this, the use of rectal thermometers has largely been replaced by rectal thermocouples, which remain in place throughout the test, eliminating the handling of the rabbits for individual temperature readings (Fig. 22-11). By this method, one person can handle 100 or more animals a day as compared with about 15 by the individual thermometer method. Critical evaluations of pyrogen testing with rabbits may be found in the literature.[105,106]

Many medical agents, if present, interfere with the test results because of their antipyretic or other interfering effects. Therefore, the pyrogen test is performed on all vehicles used for injections, but only on those finished products that do not interfere with the test, that have a high propensity for contamination with pyrogens, or that are given in large quantities. Considerably greater danger exists from the injection of large volume solutions containing pyrogens than from small volumes. Also, the pyrogenic effect is less with intramuscular injection than with intravenous injection.

Recently, an in vitro test method for pyrogens has been developed utilizing the gelling property of the lysate of the amebocytes of Limulus poly-

---

* Climet Instruments Co., Redlands, CA 92373; HIAC/Royco, Menlo Park, CA 94025; Particle Technology, Inc., Sunnyvale, CA 94086.
†HIAC/Royco, Menlo Park, CA 94025.
‡Coulter Electronics, Inc., Hialeah, FL 33010.

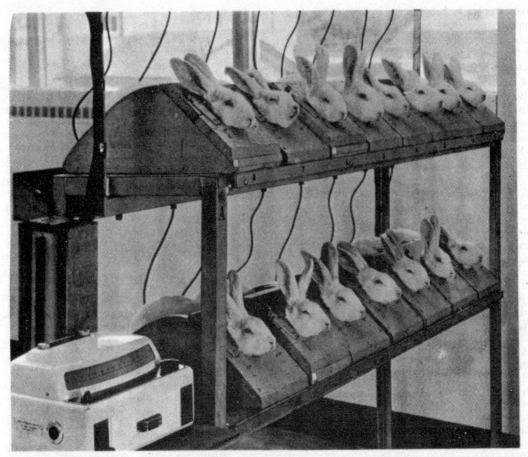

FIG. 22-11. *Rabbits being subjected to a pyrogen test with temperatures being taken by rectal thermocouples connected to an electric thermometer. (Courtesy of Wyeth Laboratories.)*

phemus (the horseshoe crab).[107] In the presence of pyrogenic endotoxins from gram-negative bacteria, a firm gel is formed within 60 min when incubated at 37° C. Although only endotoxins from gram-negative bacteria react in this way, they constitute the majority and the most potent of contaminating pyrogens. The limulus amebocyte lysate (LAL) test has been found to be 5 to 10 times more sensitive than the rabbit test and by the use of serial dilutions has been shown to be semiquantitative. There do not seem to be large numbers of substances, other than proteins, that interfere with the reaction.[108] The favorable results from many studies have brought increasing acceptance of the LAL test for in-process testing and for selective product release testing.[109] The USP now contains the specifications for a Bacterial Endotoxins Test designed to provide a means for estimating the concentration of bacterial endotoxins present in samples or on devices being tested. Debate is continuing on certain aspects of the test specifications, however, i.e., what the limits should be and how the tests are to be utilized.[110]

Sterility Test All products labeled "sterile" must pass the sterility test, having been subjected to an effective process of sterilization. The principles underlying this important test and the test procedure are discussed in Chapter 21.

Packaging

A thorough discussion of the packaging of sterile products is beyond the scope of this chapter. A few pertinent facts are presented, however. The package is an extremely important part of the product, for it presents the product to the user. It must be particularly dignified, neat, and attractive in appearance if it is to convey to the user the quality, purity, and reliability that conformance to the aforementioned principles and procedures causes to be an inherent part of the product. The package also must accurately and completely provide the user with the information necessary for its use. The labeling should be legible and the identity and strength of the drug clearly distinguishable. This is particularly difficult with the small containers used for many sterile products. Furthermore, the package should protect the product against physical damage during shipping, handling, and storage and should protect light-sensitive substances from ultraviolet radiation.

Further packaging requirements for injections are given by the USP essentially as follows:

1. The volume of an injection in single-dose containers should provide the amount specified for administration at one time and in no case is more than one liter. This requirement is intended to minimize the likelihood of someone attempting to use at a later time a residue in a container after exposure to contamination from the environment.

2. Preparations intended for intraspinal, intracisternal, or peridural administration should be packaged only in single-dose containers because of the sensitivity of nerve tissue to irritation from added substances such as antibacterial agents.

3. Normally, no multiple-dose container shall contain a volume of injection more than is sufficient to permit the withdrawal of 30 ml, because larger volumes would provide for the withdrawal of more doses, thereby increasing the potential for contamination.

4. Injections labeled for veterinary use are exempt from the above limitation to single-dose containers, and to the volume of multiple-dose containers because large animals require larger doses than man.

Details of labeling content requirements for injections can be found in the USP. When a label is applied to a container, it must be so arranged that a sufficient area of the container remains uncovered to permit inspection of the contents. While these packaging and labeling stipulations apply specifically to official injections, the Food and Drug Administration looks upon these as providing basic guidelines for all products.

The operation of the packaging department for sterile products is essentially the same as for other pharmaceutical packaging departments. The overriding objective must be that *every* unit is properly labeled and packaged, with adequate controls to be assured that this is accomplished.

Throughout the entire manufacturing process for a sterile product, the prevailing philosophy must be that no effort is too great to make the finished product as nearly perfect as possible.

References

1. Avis, K. E.: Parenteral preparations. *In* Remington's Pharmaceutical Sciences. 17th Ed. Edited by A. R. Gennaro. Mack Publishing Co., Easton, PA, 1985, p. 1518.
2. Avis, K. E., and Levchuk, J. W.: Parenteral medications. *In* Dispensing of Medication, 9th Ed. Edited by R. E. King. Mack Publishing Co., Easton, PA, 1984, p. 165.
3. Turco, S., and King, R. E.: Sterile Dosage Forms. 2nd Ed. Lea & Febiger, Philadelphia, 1979.
4. Tse, F. L. S., and Welling, P. G.: J. Parent. Drug Assoc., 34:409, 1980.
5. Tse, F. L. S., and Welling, P. G.: J. Parent. Drug Assoc., 34:484, 1980.
6. Symposium on Pyrogens. J. Pharm. Pharmacol., 6:302, 1954.
7. Hahn, H. H., Chenk, S. F., Elfenbein, C. D. S., and Wood, W. B., Jr.: J. Exp. Med., 131:710, 1970.
8. Abramson, D., Butler, L. D., and Chrai, S.: J. Parent. Sci. and Technol., 35:3, 1981.
9. Rechen, H.C.: Pharm. Manuf., 1:29, 1984.
10. Reese, D. R.: Bull, Parent. Drug Assoc., 16(5):11, 1962.
11. Spiegel, A. J., and Noseworthy, M. M.: J. Pharm. Sci. 52:917, 1963.
12. Carleton, F. J.: Bull. Parent. Drug Assoc., 21:142, 1967.
13. Scheindlin, S.: Bull. Parent. Drug Assoc., 20:61, 1966.
14. Wang, Y. J., and Kowal, R. R.: J. Parent. Drug Assoc., 34:452, 1980.
15. Akers, M. J.: Pharm. Technol., 8:36, 1984.
16. Lachman, L., Urbanyi, T., and Weinstein, S.: J. Pharm. Sci., 52:244, 1963.
17. Kohn, S. R., Gershenfeld, L., and Barr, M.: J. Pharm. Sci., 52:967, 1963.
18. Schroeter, L. C.: J. Pharm. Sci., 50:891, 1961.
19. Schou, S. A.: Am. J. Hosp. Pharm. 17:153, 1960.
20. Chipault, J. R.: Antioxidants in foods. *In* Autoxidation and Antioxidants. Vol. II, Edited by W. O. Lundberg. Interscience, New York, 1962.
21. Higuchi, T., and Schroeter, L.: J. Am. Pharm. Assoc., Sci. Ed., 48:535, 1959.
22. Halaby, S. F., and Mattocks, A. M.: J. Pharm. Sci., 54:52, 1965.
23. Windheuser, J. J.: Bull. Parent. Drug Assoc., 17(5):1, 1963.
24. Husa, W. J., and Adams, J.R.: J. Am. Pharm. Assoc., Sci. Ed., 33:329, 1944.
25. Grosicki, T. S., and Husa, W. J.: J. Am. Pharm. Assoc., Sci. Ed., 43:632, 1954.
26. Hammarlund, E. R., and Pedersen-Bjergaard, K.: J. Pharm. Sci., 50:24, 1961.
27. Ansel, H. C.: Am. J. Hosp. Pharm., 21:25, 1964.
28. Hammarlund, E. R., and Van Pevenage, G. L.: J. Pharm. Sci., 55:1448, 1966.
29. Fassett, W. E., Fuller, T. S., and Hammarlund, E. R.: J. Pharm. Sci., 58:1540, 1969.
30. Mullins, J. D.: Bull. Parent. Drug Assoc., 22:38, 1968.
31. Autian, J.; J. Pharm. Sci., 53:1289, 1964.
32. Autian, J.: Bull. Parent. Drug Assoc., 22:276, 1968.
33. Eubanks, R., and Autian, J.: Am. J. Hosp. Pharm. 28:172, 1971.
34. Petrick, R. J., Loucas, S. P., Cohl, J. K., and Mehl, B.: Am. J. Hosp. Pharm., 34:357, 1977.

35. Guess, W. L., and Autian, J.: Am. J. Hosp. Pharm. 21:260, 1964.
36. Majeske, J. P.: Bull. Parent. Drug Assoc., 16(4):1, 1962.
37. Sanga, S. V.: J. Parent. Drug Assoc., 33:61, 1979.
38. Hopkins, G. H.: J. Pharm. Sci., 54:138, 1965.
39. Keim, F.: Bull. Parent. Drug Assoc., 29:46, 1975.
40. Lachman, L., Urbanyi, T., and Weinstein, S.: J. Pharm. Sci., 52:244, 1963.
41. Hopkins, G.H.: Bull. Parent. Drug Assoc., 29:278, 1975.
42. Lachman, L., Pauli, W. A., Sheth, P. B., and Pagliery, M.: J. Pharm. Sci., 55:962, 1966.
43. Hartop, W. L.: Parent. Drug Assoc. Convention, Nov. 2, 1966.
44. Hopkins, G. H.: Bull. Parent. Drug Assoc., 23:105, 1969.
45. Whalen, F. J., LeCain, W. K., and Latiolais, C.J.: Am. J. Hosp. Pharm., 36:330, 1979.
46. Parrott, E. L.: Drug & Cosm. Ind., 96:320, 1965.
47. Macek, T. J.: Amer. J. Pharm., 137:217, 1965; 138:22, 1966.
48. Scheindlin, S.: Bull. Parent. Drug Assoc., 24:31, 1970.
49. Flynn, G. L.: J. Parenter. Sci. and Technol., 38:202, 1984.
50. Gorman, W. G., and Hall, G. D.: J. Pharm. Sci., 53:1017, 1964.
51. Lin, K. S., Anschel, J., and Swartz, C. J.: Bull. Parent. Drug Assoc., 25:40, 1971.
52. Hoevenaars, P. C. M.: Pharm. Weekblad., 100:1151, 1965.
53. Struhar, M.: Acta Fac. Bohemoslov., 9:99, 1964.
54. Bodin, J. I., and Taub, A.: J. Am. Pharm. Assoc., Sci. Ed., 44:296, 1955.
55. Davisson, E. O., et al.: J. Lab. Clin. Med., 47:8, 1956.
56. Patel, N. K., and Kostenbauder, H. B.: J. Am. Pharm. Assoc., Sci. Ed., 47:289, 1958.
57. Gross, H. M.: Drug & Cosm. Ind., 75:468, 1954.
58. Damaskus, C. W.: Bull. Parent. Drug Assoc., 11(3):25, 1957.
59. DeLuca, P., and Lachman, L.: J. Pharm. Sci., 54:1411, 1965.
60. Chien, Y. W.: J. Parent. Sci. and Technol., 35:106, 1981.
61. Nash, R. A.: Bull. Parent. Drug Assoc., 26:91. 1972.
62. Macek, T. J.: J. Pharm. Sci., 52:694, 1963.
63. Martin, E. W. (ed.): Techniques of Medication. J. B. Lippincott, Philadelphia, 1969, p. 108.
64. U.S. Food and Drug Administration, Federal Register 43:45077, Sept. 29, 1978.
65. Meckler, M.: Contam. Control, 6(3):9, 1967.
66. Leuchten, W. E.: Bull. Parent. Drug Assoc., 17(2):6, 1963.
67. Anisfeld, M. H., and Lovejoy, C. K.: J. Parent. Drug Assoc., 32:285, 1978.
68. McQuillen, D. F.: Pharm. Technol., 5:44, 1981.
69. Hertzon, L.: Med. Device & Diagn. Ind., 4(1):29, 1982.
70. Loughhead, H., and Vellutato, A.: Bull Parent. Drug Assoc., 23:17, 1969.
71. Whitfield, W. J., Mashburn, J. C., Neitzel, W. E., and Trujillo, L. C.: Basic Design Requirements for Laminar Air Flow Dust Control Devices. SC-R-64-145A, Sandia Corp., Albuquerque, NM, 1964.
72. Lamy, P. P., Davies, W. L., and Kitler, M.: Hosp. Pharm., 3:12, 1968.
73. Bowman, F. W.: Bull. Parent. Drug Assoc., 22:57, 1968.
74. Hortig, H. P.: Bull. Parent. Drug. Assoc., 27:38, 1973.
75. Gross, R. I.: Bull. Parent. Drug Assoc., 30:143, 1976.
76. Fed. Stand. No. 209B: Clean Room and Work Station Requirements, Controlled Environment. General Services Adm., Washington, DC, April 24, 1973.
77. Whitfield, W. J.: Bull. Parent. Drug Assoc., 21:37, 1967.
78. Loughhead, H. O., and Moffett, J. A.: Bull. Parent. Drug Assoc., 25:261, 1971.
79. Delmore, R. P., Jr., and Thompson, W. N.: Med. Device & Diagn. Ind., 3(2):45, 1981.
80. Lieberman, A.: Med. Device & Diagn. Ind., 4(1):43, 1982.
81. Useller, J. W.: Clean Room Technology. NASA SP-5074, Supt. of Documents U.S. Government Printing Off., Wash., DC.
82. Heuring, H.: Contam. Control. 9(7):18, 1970.
83. Klink, A. E., and Artiss, D. H.: J. Parent. Drug Assoc., 32:226, 1978.
84 DiSessa, P.: Pharm. Tech., 4:103, 1980.
85. Klumb, G. H.: Bull. Parent. Drug Assoc., 29:261, 1975.
86. Artiss D. H.: J. Parent. Drug Assoc., 32:89, 1978.
87. Anschel, J.: Bull. Parent. Drug Assoc., 31:47, 1977.
88. Grimes, T. L., Fonner, D. E., Griffin, J. C., et al.: Bull. Parent. Drug Assoc., 31:179, 1977.
89. Kovary, S. J., Agalloco, J. P., and Gordon, B. M.: J. Parenter. Sci. and Technol., 37:55, 1983.
90. Anschel, J.: Bull. Parent. Drug Assoc., 31:302, 1977.
91. Meryman, H. T.: Ann. N.Y. Acad. Sci., 85:630, 1960.
92. MacKenzie, A. P.: Bull. Parent. Drug Assoc., 20:101, 1966.
93. DeLuca, P., and Lachman, L.: J. Pharm. Sci., 54:617, 1965.
94. Couriel, B.: J. Parent. Drug Assoc., 34:352, 1980.
95. Jenning, T. A.: J. Parent. Drug Assoc., 34:109, 1980.
96. Artz, W. J. Gloor, W. T., Jr., and Reese, D. R.: J. Pharm. Sci., 50:258, 1961.
97. Garvan, J. M. and Gunner, B. W.: Med. J. Austral., 2:1, July 4, 1964.
98. DeLuca, P. P., Rapp, R. P., and Bivins, B.: Am. J. Hosp. Pharm., 32:1001, 1975.
99. Hamlin, W. E.: J. Parent. Drug Assoc., 32:63, 1978.
100. Vessey, I., and Kendall, C. E.: Analyst, 91:273, 1966.
101. Groves, M. J.: J. Pharm. Pharmacol., 18:161, 1966.
102. Hopkins, G. H., and Young, R. W.: Bull. Parent. Drug Assoc., 28:15, 1974.
103. Rebagay, T., Schroeder, H. G., Im, S., and DeLuca, P. P.: Bull. Parent. Drug Assoc., 31:57, 1977.
104. Louer, R. C., Jr., Russoman, J. A., and Rasanen, P. R.: Bull. Parent. Drug Assoc., 25:54, 1971.
105. Martin, W. J., and Marcus, S.: Appl. Microbiol., 12:483, 1964.
106. Personeus, G. R.: Pyrogen testing of parenteral pharmaceuticals. In Quality Control in the Pharmaceutical Industry. Vol. 2. Edited by M. S. Cooper. Academic Press, New York, 1973, p. 239.
107. Cooper, J. R., Hochstein, H. D., and Seligmann, E. B., Jr.: Bull. Parent. Drug Assoc., 26:153, 1972.
108. Twohy, C. W., Duran, A. P., and Munson, T. E.: J. Parent. Sci. and Technol., 38:190, 1984.
109. Mascoli, C. C., and Weary, M. E.: J. Parent. Drug Assoc., 33:81, 1979.
110. Weary, M.: J. Parenter. Sci. and Technol., 38:20, 1984.

Product Processing, Packaging, Evaluation, and Regulations

23

Pilot Plant Scale-Up Techniques

SAMUEL HARDER *and* GLENN VAN BUSKIRK

Research and development personnel expend a considerable amount of effort developing drug dosage forms with exacting specifications that guarantee adequate physical and chemical stability. These products, designed to deliver and release a drug according to specific criteria, have, up to this stage, been manufactured on a laboratory scale, or in intermediate-sized pilot plant equipment. Such equipment is usually fairly standard and available in most laboratories. In addition to the obvious requirements of clinical efficacy and safety, the ability of the experimental formulation to be reproducibly manufactured on high-speed production equipment in a cost-effective manner is often the differentiating factor between a successful product and one that is regarded as a research curiosity. To be successful, the product must be capable of being processed and packaged on a large scale, often with equipment that only remotely resembles that used in the development laboratory. In the pilot plant, a formula is transformed into a viable, robust product by the development of a reliable and practical method of manufacture that effects the orderly transition from laboratory to routine processing in a full-scale production facility.

Pilot plant studies must include a close examination of the formula to determine its ability to withstand batch-scale and process modification; it must also include a review of a range of relevant processing equipment to determine which would be the most compatible with the formulation as well as the most economical, simple, and reliable in producing the product. During this process, the availability of raw materials that consistently meet the specifications required to produce the product must be determined. Production rates and their relationship to immediate and future market requirements must be considered. The physical space required and the layout of related functions should be taken into account during the pilot plant phase with the intent to provide short-term and long-term efficiencies. The requirements, training, reporting relationships, and responsibilities of personnel are also factors in successful product scale-up.[1] During the scale-up efforts in the pilot plant, production and process controls are evaluated, validated, and finalized. In addition, appropriate records and reports are issued to support Good Manufacturing Practices (GMPs) and to provide the historical development of the production formulation, process, equipment train, and specifications.

Often, meaningful product reprocessing procedures can only be developed and validated at pilot plant scale. All critical features of a process must be identified so that as the process is scaled-up, it can be adequately monitored to provide assurance that the process is under control, and that the product produced at each level of the scale-up maintains the specified attributes originally intended.

Each of the foregoing items is discussed in more detail in the succeeding sections.

General Considerations

Reporting Responsibilities

The question of who should be responsible for pilot plant studies has been debated at great length with no clear resolution, as can be seen from the various reporting relationships in use within major pharmaceutical companies.[2-4] Pilot plant functions can be part of a research and development group with separate staffing. This arrangement is designed to provide a hierarchy of responsibility to scale-up formulations that have been developed by other formulators within research and development, thereby providing an opportunity for critique of formula/process that is independent of the initial formulation function. Alternatively, the formulators who developed the product can take it into production and continue to provide support even after the transition into production has been completed. Proponents of this system cite the advantage of historical continuity that comes from this approach. Both of these first two structures stem from the premise that if the pilot plant is a research responsibility, greater consideration is given to the preformulation and formulation experiences obtained in the initial development of a particular drug and its dosage form.

Some companies prefer to have the pilot plant and technical service group organizationally separate from research and reporting instead to the operations side of the business. The advantage here may be that such a group would be more operations-oriented, more pragmatic, and more receptive to operations priorities. Management philosophy, the nature of a company's products, and the background experience of the personnel involved in pilot plant studies help determine which arrangement is best for any one particular organization at any point in time. A few companies have adopted a composite of both approaches in hopes of achieving the best attributes of both the research and development and the operations-oriented systems.

Whatever the reporting arrangement, the goal of a pilot plant is to facilitate the transfer of a product from the laboratory into production. The effectiveness of the pilot plant is determined by the ease with which new products or processes are brought into routine production. This can best be achieved if a good relationship exists between the pilot plant group and the other groups with which they interact, namely, research and development, processing, packaging, engineering, quality assurance/control (QA/QC), regulatory, and marketing.

Personnel Requirements

The qualifications required for a position in a pilot plant organization are a blend of good theoretic knowledge of pharmaceutics and some practical experience in the pharmaceutical industry. In addition, the ability to communicate well, both in speaking and in writing, and the ability to develop good relationships with other people are important since experience and knowledge are most useful when adequately and effectively communicated. Practical experience in pilot plant operations is invaluable. Experience within the group should encompass both formulation experience and process and equipment experience in the actual production environment. Personnel in the pilot plant must recognize the intent of the formulator, and at the same time, understand the perspective of production personnel. For these reasons, successful pilot plant organizations frequently include scientists with experience in both areas.

The type and level of education within the group is important. Pharmaceutically trained scientists contribute fundamental strength to the function in their ability to assimilate the complex interrelationship between pharmaceutical processes and the potential impact on chemical, physical, biochemical, and medical attributes of dosage forms. It is also important, however, that the group possess some engineering capability since the scale-up of many of the processes involves engineering principles, which are usually not well covered in the normal pharmaceutical training. In addition, it is becoming increasingly important for the group to contain individuals who are knowledgeable in both electronics and computers.[5]

The number of people in a pilot plant group depends on the number of products being supported and on the level of support required. An experienced scientist with a knowledgeable technician should be able to handle one major project, or two major projects simultaneously depending on their complexity, while at the same time providing technical support for an additional group of marketed products.

Many established companies have production operators who have had many years of experience with particular dosage forms and equipment, and supervisors who have had considerable research experience. In such cases, the support effort required of a pilot plant group would be much reduced. In such a company, the introduction of new products involving existing technologies would require less support than the introduction of a process involving new technology. On the other hand, companies who operate their production facilities without the support of extensively trained technical personnel, and in which the supervisory function is mainly administrative, can be expected to require considerably more support during introduction and scale-up of new products or processes and also to require substantially more continuing technical support.

Space Requirements

A pilot plant has the following four types of space requirements.

Administration and Information Processing. Documentation is important. Adequate office and desk space must be provided for both the scientists and technicians. This should be adjacent to the work area but sufficiently isolated to permit people to work without undue distractions.

Since the group is the link between research, operations, and other disciplines, members of the group frequently meet with people from other departments and should have an area available where three to four people can meet and discuss subjects of mutual concern. There should also be space for a computer terminal for convenient data entry and retrieval as well as archives for stability data protocols and historical files.

Physical Testing Area. The second required area is an adequate working area in which samples can be laid out and examined and where physical tests on these samples can be performed. This area should provide permanent bench-top space for routinely used physical testing equipment (e.g., balance, pH meter, and viscometer).

Standard Pilot Plant Equipment Floor Space. The third area is discrete plant space where equipment needed for manufacturing all types of pharmaceutical dosage forms is located. The equipment should be available in a variety of sizes known to be representative of production capability. This arrangement helps assure the quality of the scale-up data collected, while meeting the concern to be prudent with expensive materials. Intermediate-sized and full-scale production equipment is essential in evaluating the effects of scale-up of research formulations and processes. Utilization of the area is most efficient when it is subdivided into areas for solid dosage forms, semisolid products, liquid preparations, and sterile products. Further subdivision of the areas should allow multiple operations to be conducted simultaneously without raising GMP concerns.

Because the utilization of pilot plant equipment is sporadic and dependent on project assignments, equipment should be made portable, where possible. The equipment can then be stored in a relatively small area and brought out into suitable work areas for use. This system helps relieve some of the congestion often found in pilot plant operations and provides more working space around equipment that is in use. Such a system also provides more space if equipment is brought in for evaluation on a loan or rental basis. An essential requirement that is frequently neglected but that is important to all pilot plant operations is the provision of adequate space for cleaning of pilot plant equipment. While some equipment can be cleaned in place, most equipment is better handled in a dedicated cleaning area.

Storage Area. The fourth area and the one most often described as inadequate is storage space. Separate provision should be made for the storage of active ingredients and excipients. These should be further segregated into approved and unapproved areas according to GMPs. There should be generous storage areas for in-process materials, finished bulk products from the pilot plant, and material from experimental scale-up batches made in production, which for GMP reasons cannot be stored in operations storage areas. Space should be provided for the storage of retained samples from pilot plant and experimental production batches. All of these space requirements are in addition to the controlled environment space allocated for storage of stability samples.

Finally, there should be storage for packaging materials. These materials tend to be bulky, but since a common requirement of the scale-up function is to evaluate alternate suppliers of packaging materials, it is essential to provide the space required to store bottles, closures, tubes, vials, ampuls, etc. Here too, it would be preferable if the material could be segregated into approved and unapproved categories.

Review of the Formula

A thorough review of each aspect of the formulation is important and should be carried out early in the scale-up process. The purpose of each ingredient and its contribution to the final product manufactured on small-scale laboratory equipment should be understood. Then, the effects of scale-up using equipment that may subject the product to stresses of different types and degrees can be more readily predicted, or recognized when they actually occur. The need to modify the formulation during scale-up is not unusual. This should be done as early as possible in phase III trials to allow time to generate meaningful long-term stability in support of a proposed new drug application (NDA). If these studies are not completed until after the application is made, long and costly delays in approval may result.

Raw Materials

One responsibility of the pilot plant function is the approval and validation of the active and excipient raw materials used in pharmaceutical products. This is necessary because the raw materials used during small-scale formulation trials may not be representative of the large-volume shipments of materials used in large-scale production, or because active ingredients, which may only have been prepared on a laboratory scale, are also being subjected to scale-up to meet the rising needs of the product. Even though all analytic specifications are met, these larger lots of active ingredient may change in particle size, shape, or morphology, resulting in different handling properties or differences in bulk density, static charges, rate of solubility, flow properties, color, etc. The quality of active ingredients needs to be verified because having alternate suppliers is usually desirable. This is an important consideration for companies who purchase their active ingredients, because a single supplier leaves the company vulnerable with respect to both supply and acquisition price. The evaluation of alternate suppliers requires that several batches of product be manufactured with these alternate materials and that their performance in the formulation and the stability of finished products be evaluated relative to the standard product.

Relevant Processing Equipment

It is almost certain that most formulation development work has been carried out on small, relatively simple laboratory equipment. During subsequent scale-up, alternative manufacturing equipment should be considered. Based on the known processing characteristics of the product, the equipment that promises to be the most economical, the simplest, the most efficient, and the most capable of consistently producing product within the proposed specifications should be evaluated. For feasibility studies, if a particular technology is not available in-house, small-scale trials can be carried out at the various equipment vendors' facilities. Then, when a decision has been made to use a particular process, the selected pilot plant equipment needs to be acquired. The size of this equipment should be such that experimental trials can be run that are meaningful and relevant to the production-sized batches that will eventually be made. If the pilot plant equipment is too small, the process developed will not scale up well. If the equipment is too large, excessive costs will be incurred, especially if the product involves the use of a large quantity of a new and expensive active ingredient.

When a reasonable process has been developed on the pilot plant equipment, intermediate-sized experimental batches should be run. Once

again, these can be made in the facilities of the equipment vendor if the equipment is not available in-house, providing some indication of the reliability of the extrapolation from the pilot plant to larger production equipment. When the decision involves equipment available from several vendors (e.g., fluid bed dryers), the next step is to determine from the various vendors the advantages of their particular equipment. Ease of cleaning should be considered, especially if multiple products are destined to be manufactured in the equipment. The time required to tear down the equipment to clean and change from one product to another should be determined. In some instances, this can be longer than the actual time required to manufacture a batch, and if frequent changeovers are anticipated, this becomes an important consideration. To evaluate these and other parameters accurately, trials should be run at the vendor's facilities. Such experiences help determine the true capability of the equipment and the quality of technical support available from the proposed vendors.

Production Rates

The immediate and future market requirements must be considered when determining the production rates and the type and size of production equipment needed. The size of the equipment should be such that it is properly utilized. The equipment and process should be chosen so as to produce batches at a frequency that takes into consideration product loss in the equipment during manufacture, the time required to clean the equipment between batches, and the number of batches that will need to be tested for release. To accommodate future growth, increased production capacity may be realized more economically through more efficient utilization of smaller equipment than through purchase of oversized equipment. For example, several smaller lots produced serially (without major clean-up) may be combined in a final blend to make a single large batch.

Process Evaluation

The previous sections have developed the product scale-up program to the point at which the manufacturing process has been proposed and the equipment for production has been evaluated, selected, installed, and debugged. The next step is to evaluate the process critically and to optimize its performance based on that evaluation.[6-9] Items that should be examined include the following:

Order of addition of components, including adjustment of their amounts

Mixing speed

Mixing time

Rate of addition of granulating agents, solvents, solutions of drugs, slurries, etc.

Heating and cooling rates

Filter sizes (liquids)

Screen sizes (solids)

Drying temperatures

Drying time

Knowledge of the effect of these important process parameters on in-process and finished product quality is the basis for process optimization and validation.[10] The purpose of process validation is to confirm that the selected manufacturing procedure assures the quality of the product at various critical stages in the process and in the finished form.[11] This is accomplished by monitoring the within-batch variation of measurable parameters, such as content uniformity, moisture content, and compressibility. These data indicate where the process is performing as intended and where problem areas may be found.

Parts of the process such as milling, mixing, heating, cooling, drying, sterilizing, compacting, and filling, which cause some measurable change in the state of the material being processed, need to be evaluated. Such process data should be accumulated for a series of batches using a particular equipment configuration and a well-documented process. If the data show that the process performs consistently at the critical steps to produce a product that falls within release specifications, then that process has been validated. The process remains validated only if there are no changes in the formula, the quality of the ingredients, or the equipment configuration.[12] Changes in any of these areas would have to be carefully evaluated and a determination would have to be made as to the need and extent of revalidation required. The personnel responsible for the process should be adequately trained to be capable of understanding the directions and to carry out the process as intended.

The manufacturing process and quality control information should be reviewed on an annual basis, and if deemed necessary, some revalidation studies should be carried out to ensure that changes have not occurred.[13] A validated process establishes a data base of cause-and-effect relationships between critical steps and in-process or end product specifications. Therefore, documentation obtained during process validation can often be used predictively to shorten the time required to identify the factor(s) in a process that has "drifted" from normal.

Preparation of Master Manufacturing Procedures

The manner in which the manufacturing directions, the chemical weigh sheet, the sampling directions, and the in-process and finished product specifications are presented is of utmost importance, as is the degree to which the processing technician understands and complies with them. The weigh sheet should clearly identify the chemicals required in a batch. Further, the weigh sheet should present these in the quantities and the order in which they will be used. To prevent confusion and possible errors, both names and identifying numbers for the ingredients should be used on batch records, and these should correspond with those on the bulk raw material containers.

The processing directions should be precise and explicit. They should be written in a style that uses language and terms with which the operators are familiar. In writing the manufacturing procedures, considerable input should come from the actual operators or from someone with current knowledge and experience in the weighing and processing areas. In accord with GMPs, the batch records need to provide space to show the weighing and addition of each ingredient with appropriate countersignatures for each. A manufacturing procedure that becomes a multipage document and takes the place of good operator training and a library of standard operating procedures (SOPs) invites problems. Too detailed or wordy directions are cumbersome, and too many sign-offs are as bad as too few. There are numerous examples in the industry of problems arising because the operators will not read or follow highly detailed procedures. Experience has shown that when too many signatures are required in a batch record, they may not be signed off in the intended sequence during the manufacturing, but instead are completed all at one time at the completion of the process. When this occurs, the intention of verifying that each step was performed correctly is lost.

The batch record directions should include specifications for addition rates, mixing times, mixing speeds, heating and cooling rates, and temperature, and appropriate ranges should be given. The actual times, temperatures, and speeds used should be documented. These can best be monitored and recorded by appropriate controller recorders, which free the operator to pay attention to the actual process and verify that all equipment is functioning properly and that the process is performing in a normal and acceptable manner. Strip charts from the controllers are used to verify the compliance with the batch directions.

The time and manner in which in-process and finished product samples are to be taken from a batch, and the way in which they are handled and stored, should be clearly specified within the batch record. Samples improperly taken or handled give rise to unreliable data that can result in lost time or can jeopardize the quality or acceptability of a batch. When this occurs, batch reassay, special stability studies, reprocessing, or extensive investigations are necessary to assure the quality of the batch before its release.

In-process specifications included in the processing directions should be realistic but slightly narrower than the finished product specification. If a specification is too broad, it cannot provide the alert desired when something goes wrong with the process. Too tight a specification results in the needless rejection of batches of acceptable quality.

Finished product specifications set the standards by which a product is evaluated and help ensure that each batch manufactured delivers the drug in the dose specified throughout the designated shelf-life of that product. Therefore, when finished product specifications and release specifications are set, they should take into consideration the capability of the process, the reliability of the test methods, and the stability kinetics of the product.

It is obvious but often forgotten that the quality of a batch cannot be determined by the analysis of the small number of samples usually required to meet compendial specifications (e.g., content uniformity). These results are only a valid estimate of the quality of a batch when process validation studies have been conducted to establish the statistical integrity of the sample. Periodic revalidation, good manufacturing procedures, and monitoring of finished product test results via control charts are essential to maintaining consistent product quality.

GMP Considerations

The term Good Manufacturing Practices means different things to different people. There are FDA guidelines describing GMP, but even these can and are interpreted differently by people in the FDA and in industry. Common sense exercised by people who have a good theoretic knowledge of pharmaceutical principles, and who are technically competent and have adequate relevant experience in manufacturing, guarantees compliance to GMP.

A checklist of GMP items that should be part of scale-up or new product or process introduction includes the following:

Equipment qualification

Process validation

Regularly scheduled preventative maintenance

Regular process review and revalidation

Relevant written standard operating procedures

The use of competent, technically qualified personnel

Adequate provision for training of personnel

A well-defined technology transfer system

Validated cleaning procedures

An orderly arrangement of equipment so as to ease material flow and prevent cross-contamination

Transfer of Analytic Methods to Quality Assurance

During the scale-up of a new product, the analytic test methods developed in research must be transferred to the quality assurance department. Early in the transfer process, the quality assurance staff should review the process to make sure that the proper analytic instrumentation is available and that personnel are trained to perform the tests. Recovery studies on the product and on spiked placebo samples should be carried out by different operators over a period of several weeks to verify that the tests perform reliably and yield results with precision and accuracy comparable to that obtained in research. If required, the assay method can be reformatted and rewritten using terminology and procedures consistent with current quality assurance laboratory practice. To complete the transfer, research personnel should review the assay procedure and the data obtained during the validation studies, to verify that the analytic methods have not been altered in a way that might affect the reliability, precision, or accuracy of the tests.

Product Considerations

Solid Dosage Forms

In scaling up the manufacture of tablets and capsules from experimental laboratory batch sizes to intermediate- and large-scale production, each stage of the operation must be carefully considered. A process using the same type of equipment performs quite differently when the size of the equipment and the amount of material involved is increased significantly. Even such simple operations as loading a mixer can become a complicated operation utilizing sophisticated equipment when large volumes are involved. In some instances, scale-up may involve a major process change that utilizes techniques and equipment that were either unsuitable or unavailable on a laboratory scale.

The following are the typical unit operations involved in production of solid dosage forms.

Material Handling

In the laboratory, materials are simply scooped, dumped, or poured by hand. This may also work well in some small- or intermediate-sized production operations, but in other intermediate- or large-scale operations, mechanical means of handling these materials often become necessary. These mechanisms range from simple post hoists or other mechanical devices for lifting, and tilting drums, to more sophisticated methods of handling materials, such as vacuum loading systems, screw feed systems, and metering pumps. The type of system selected also depends on the characteristics of the materials, e.g., density or static charge.

Any material handling system must deliver the accurate amount of the ingredient to the intended destination. Lengthy transfer lines may result in material loss, for which there must be accountability and compensation. If the system is used to transfer materials for more than one product, steps must be taken to prevent cross-contamination. This can be accomplished by the use of validated cleaning procedures for the equipment.

Dry Blending

Powders to be used for encapsulation, or to be granulated prior to tabletting or encapsulation, must be well blended to ensure good drug distribution. Inadequate blending at this stage could result in discrete portions of the batch being either high or low in potency. This could result in drug content uniformity variation, especially if

the tablet or capsule is small and the drug concentration is relatively low in the blend. Ideally, the dry blend should take place in the vessel in which any subsequent processing such as granulation occurs. Not every manufacturing facility, however, has equipment with sufficient capacity to accommodate such a process. Consequently, a larger batch may be dry blended and then subdivided into multiple sections for the granulation operation. Steps should also be taken to ensure that all the ingredients (excipient and active) are free of lumps and agglomerates prior to the dry blend. Failure to remove or break up all agglomerates could cause flow problems through the equipment, creating non-reproducible compression and encapsulation processes with a detrimental effect on the content uniformity of the product. For these reasons, screening and/or milling of the ingredients prior to blending usually makes the process more reliable and reproducible.

Granulation

To scale up a granulation process in the most efficient manner, the purposes for granulating must be clearly understood. The most common reasons given to justify granulating are (1) to impart good flow properties to the material so that the tablet presses and encapsulators can be properly fed and a uniform tablet or capsule weight maintained, (2) to increase the apparent density of the powders, and (3) to change the particle size distribution so that the binding properties on compaction can be improved. A small amount of a potent active ingredient can be dispersed most effectively in a carrier granulation when the drug is dissolved in the granulating solution and incorporated into the batch during granulation. Use of the granulation process to disperse an active ingredient is also commonly cited as a reason to granulate.

Some pieces of equipment are more suitable than others for helping to develop the desired characteristics of a finished granulation. Traditionally, wet granulation has been carried out using sigma blade or heavy-duty planetary mixers (Figs. 23-1 and 23-2). Production equipment of this type equipped with large motors of 7 to 10 horsepower can process 100 to 200 kg of material. The weight of the material and the large shear forces generated by these powerful units affect not only the granulating time but also the amount of granulating fluid required relative to that used in experimental laboratory trials.

Wet granulations can also be prepared using tumble blenders equipped with high-speed

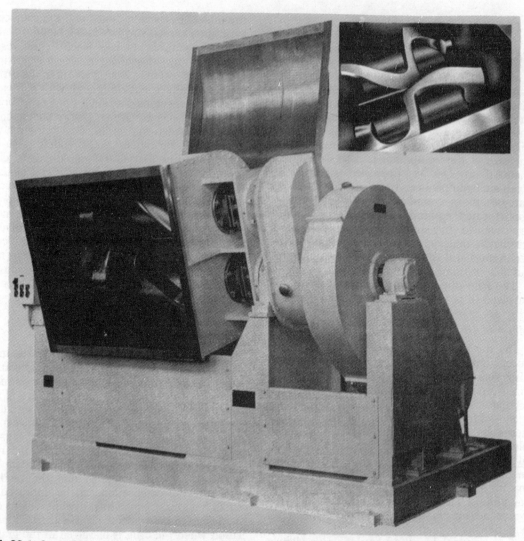

FIG. 23-1. *Sigma blade mixer. Inset shows the overlapping blades, which exert a folding and kneading action on the granulation. The blades effectively move material from the sides of the chamber to the center. (Courtesy of Day Mixing Co., Div. of Littleford Bros., Inc.)*

chopper blades (Figs. 23-3 and 23-4). High-shear mixers are often more effective in densifying light powders, but require large amounts of energy and have limited load size. There are pieces of equipment available that combine the high-shear mixing action often required for good densification with the advantages of high-speed choppers, which break up agglomerates and ensure uniform distribution of the granulating fluid and more controlled granule size (Figs. 23-5 and 23-6).

More recently, there has been a trend toward the use of multifunctional "processors." These are units that are capable of performing all the functions required to prepare a finished granulation, such as dry blending, wet granulation, dry-

ing, sizing, and lubrication in a continuous process in a single piece of equipment (Fig. 23-7). The advantages to using such equipment during scale-up of a product can be significant in terms of space and manpower requirements. Closed continuous systems have the added advantage of less handling of materials, thereby reducing the danger of personnel exposure to potent materials. This is especially important when potent and potentially hazardous compounds are involved.

Binders are used in tablet formulations to make powders more compressible and to produce tablets that are more resistant to breakage during handling. Some of these are added in the dry state and impart their binding properties

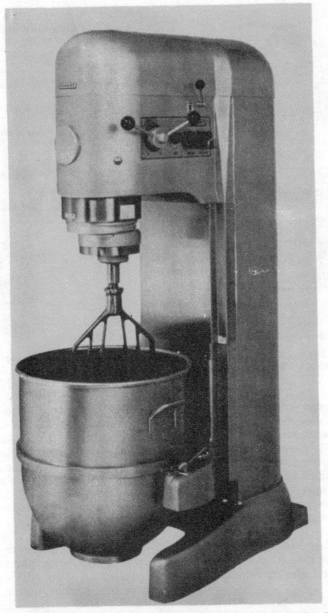

FIG. 23-2. *Planetary mixer. The beater revolves two to four times for each revolution of the head, providing double mixing action. Each revolution of the head causes the beater to complete one revolution around the bowl. (Courtesy of Hobart Corp.)*

when exposed to the granulating fluid. Others are dissolved or dispersed in the granulating fluid. In some instances, the binding agent imparts considerable viscosity to the granulating solution, so that transfer of the fluid by either pumping or pouring becomes difficult. During the scale-up of such a process, problems could be encountered during the addition of the granulating agent to the powders being processed in enclosed equipment. If the problem is anticipated during the formulation stage, the viscosity of the granulating solution can be adjusted so that scale-up problems of this type can be avoided. One way of avoiding this problem is to disperse some or all of the binding agent in the dry powder prior to granulating. The granulating liquid containing any remaining binder can then be easily pumped and metered into the batch during granulation.

Occasionally, nonaqueous solvents or solu-

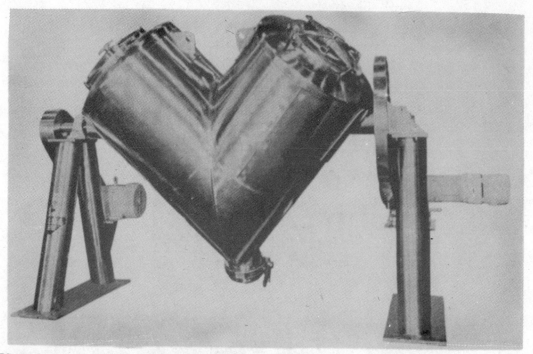

FIG. 23-3. *Twin Shell blender. Material splits and refolds as the blender rotates, producing uniform blends. Various intensifier bars can be added to handle specific applications. (Courtesy of Patterson-Kelley, Co., Division of Harsco Corp.)*

tions that are composed of water and water-miscible solvents are used to improve the granulating properties of a formulation or to disperse poorly soluble drugs. While a reduced amount of energy is required to remove the more volatile solvent(s) from the granulation, proper ventilation and additional safety precautions (against fire, toxicity, explosion) must be considered in the selection and design of the equipment and manufacturing area.[14] In addition, solvent recovery systems may be necessary to comply with Environmental Protection Agency (EPA) or Occupational Safety and Health Administration (OSHA) regulations.

Some granulations, when prepared in production-sized equipment, take on a dough-like consistency and may have to be subdivided to a more granular and porous mass to facilitate drying. This can be accomplished by passing the wet mass through an oscillating type granulator with a suitably large screen, (Fig. 23-8), or a hammer mill with either a suitably large screen or no screen at all (Fig. 23-9).

Drying

The most common conventional method of drying a granulation continues to be the circulating hot air oven, which is heated by either steam or electricity, and in which the granulation is spread on paper-lined trays on a rack truck, which is then wheeled into the oven

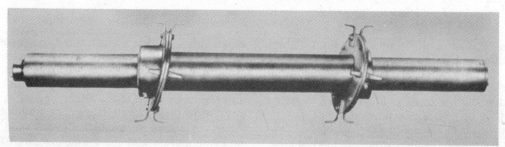

FIG. 23-4. *Liquid-dispersion bar increases or "intensifies" speed and thoroughness of liquid-solid blends. (Courtesy of Patterson-Kelley, Co., Division of Harsco Corp.)*

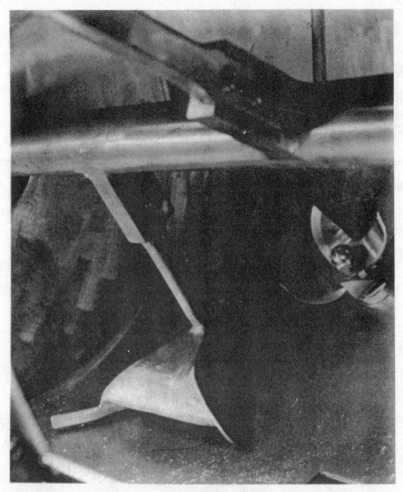

FIG. 23-5. *Large triangular-shaped plow blades and smaller high-speed choppers combine to provide intense mixing action in the Littleford mixer. (Courtesy of Littleford Bros., Inc.)*

where evaporative drying occurs. The important factors to consider as part of scale-up of an oven drying operation are airflow, air temperature, and the depth of the granulation on the trays. If the granulation bed is too deep or too dense, the drying process will be inefficient, and if soluble dyes are involved, migration of the dye to the surface of the granule may occur. During scale-up of this operation, the granulation bed depth should be carefully controlled and the drying process monitored by the use of moisture and/or temperature probes in the granulation, or by frequent multipoint sampling of the granulation for moisture content throughout the drying phase. Drying times at specified temperatures and airflow rates must be established for each product, and for each particular oven load.

Fluidized-bed dryers are an attractive alternative to the circulating hot air ovens. Their main

advantage is a reduction in drying time. Fluidized-bed drying times are usually less than 1 hour, compared with 8 hours or more in the conventional ovens. Many products can also be dry blended and granulated in a fluidized-bed granulator/dryer, further reducing the handling, and consequently the time, required to process a batch. Scale-up of a fluidized bed drying operation is more involved than scale-up of a circulating hot air oven process.[15,16] First, optimum loads must be established. Then, rate of airflow and inlet air temperature as well as the humidity of the incoming air must be established, since these all affect the drying time. If the air is drawn from outside the plant without being conditioned, the large seasonal variations in temperature and humidity that may exist can alter the drying process. Scale-up is further complicated in that it has been shown that data from

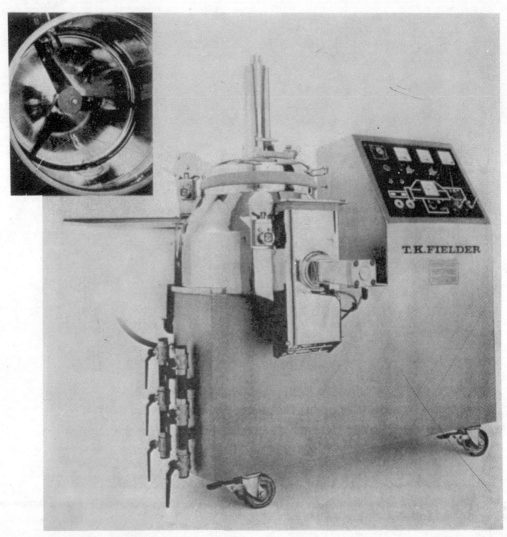

FIG. 23-6. *High-shear pharmaceutical grade mixer/granulator. Inset shows detail of mixing bowl and blades.* (*Courtesy of T.K. Fielder and Raymond Automation Company, Inc.*)

small-scale batches (1 to 5 kg) cannot be used to extrapolate processing conditions for intermediate-scale (100 kg) or larger batches. To obtain a granulation comparable to that obtained on a smaller scale, considerable experimentation and adjustments to the process are required.[17]

Reduction of Particle Size

Particle size, and especially particle size distribution, are important to the compression characteristics of a granulation. In the laboratory, hand screening or short-duration handling with small-scale milling equipment is used to obtain the desired particle size distribution prior to compression or encapsulation. When such a

process must be increased in capacity to accommodate large, high-speed presses with more elaborate feed systems, it becomes important that the equipment chosen can yield the desired throughput while controlling the particle size and size distribution of a granulation.

Compression factors that may be affected by the particle size distribution are flowability, compressibility, uniformity of tablet weight, content uniformity, tablet hardness, and tablet color uniformity. A granulation with too large a particle size and insufficient fines is unable to fill the die cavities uniformly during compression, and the weight of the tablets fluctuates considerably. For colored granulations, the coarser the granulation, the more mottled the final tablet appear-

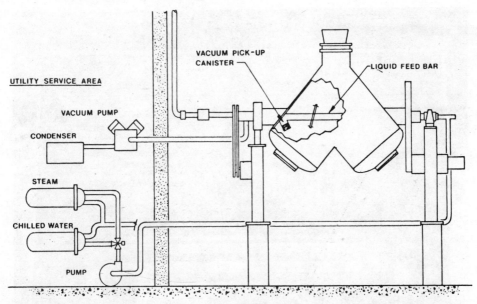

FIG. 23-7. *Schematic of a multifunction pharmaceutical processor. The system contains a solids mixing shell, which includes a liquid dispersion bar. This unit is jacketed to allow heating and cooling. Material can be dried within the unit by use of the vacuum canister and condenser. (Courtesy of Ortho Pharmaceutical Corporation.)*

ance is. If too many fines are present, tablet weight variation occurs because of flow problems. Also, the tendency toward capping increases and is further exaggerated as the speed of the press is increased. Both oversized and undersized granulations can adversely affect tablet content uniformity. Particle size reduction of the dried granulation of producdon-size batches can be carried out by passing all the material through an oscillating granulator, a hammer mill, a mechanical sieving device, or in some cases, a screening device. When a screening device is used, the retained oversized portion must be milled and then returned to the batch. Screening-off procedures that mill only the oversized granulation require a final blending to ensure uniformity throughout the batch.

The most suitable piece of milling equipment to reduce granule particle size can only be chosen by first determining the characteristics of the unmilled granulation and then selecting that piece of equipment that will produce the particle size distribution necessary for the best performance during the compression or encapsulation stages.[14] Therefore, the first step in this process is to determine the particle size distribution of the granulation using a series of "stacked" sieves of decreasing mesh openings. The percentage of a preweighed sample, which is retained on a screen, gives a distribution profile that can be compared with milled samples produced by several mill conditions (e.g., speed,

screen size, and mill type). Compressibility or encapsulation efficiency of the milled samples is used to ascertain the milling conditions and target mesh pattern for subsequent batches.

Oscillating granulators of the type shown in Figure 23-8 have long been used in the industry to screen dried granulations. They work well if the oversized portion of the granulation including lumps or agglomerates is not too hard. Unless care is exercised not to overfeed this type of equipment, an excessive number of fines is produced. Because the rub bars come in contact with the screen, the wearing action may introduce a small amount of fine metallic material into the batch. If a screen should break because of excessive wear, larger particles of potentially hazardous metal could be introduced into the granulation. The stainless steel screens commonly used today can be fabricated using special ferrous metals, so that if a break should occur, the fragments can be removed by passing the granulation through special magnetic devices or the compressed tablets through a metal checking device.

Hammer mills of the type shown in Figure 23-9 are also frequently used to mill dried granulations to a specified size distribution. They have a fairly rapid throughput, and the particle size distribution can be controlled by varying the screen size, the speed of the mill, the type and number of hammer blades used, and the rate of material feed. Usually, these mills are operated

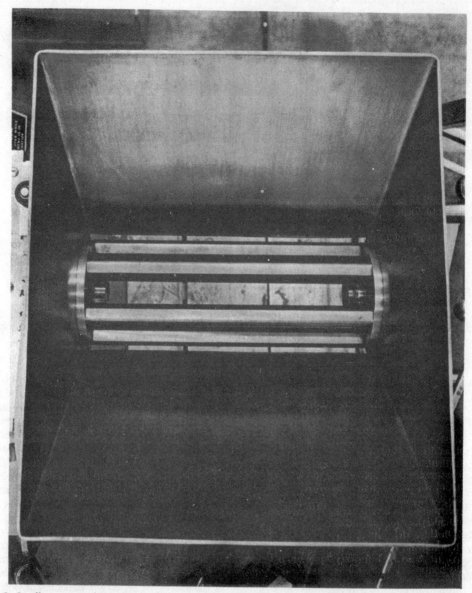

FIG. 23-8. *Oscillating granulator. Oscillating motion of horizontal bars forces granulation through a screen, resulting in uniform granules that are more easily dried. (Courtesy of Stokes Division-Pennwalt Corp.)*

at a medium to slow speed with the knives forward during sizing to prevent overmilling of the granulation. To prevent a variable particle size distribution, a uniform feed rate must be maintained. This can best be achieved by a mechanically controlled feed mechanism. Although the hammers do not come in contact with the screen, normal wear or the passage of a hard piece of granulation could cause the screen to break. Therefore, the screens should be carefully examined before and after use to ascertain whether any metal contamination has occurred.

The use of perforated plates instead of wire mesh screens also helps to reduce the chance of metal contamination (Fig. 23-10).

Many of the newer granulation operations produce material with particle size distributions already quite close to the desired range. Then, the sizing operation only requires that a small amount of agglomerates be broken down. For this type of operation, the material can either be subjected to a screening operation as described or be passed through a mechanical sieving operation, using equipment of the type shown in Fig-

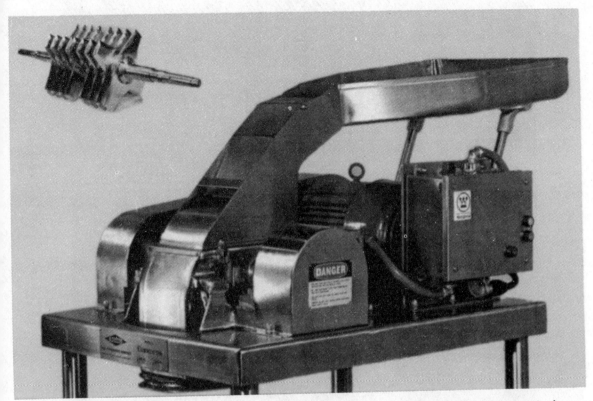

FIG. 23-9. *Hammer mill (comminuting machine). The comminuting action occurs inside the mill head (see inset), where the high-speed centrifugal force of the blades hurls the granulation through the screen, which is held in place at the discharge port. (Courtesy of Fitzpatrick Co.)*

ure 23-11. The advantage of using this type of equipment is that there is no metal-to-metal contact during the screening process, so that the possibility of metal contamination is reduced. Since there is also little milling action, the initial particle size range is not significantly reduced. In addition, the throughput is rapid, and be-

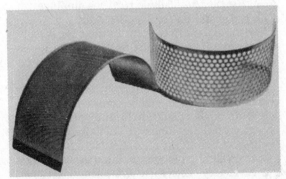

FIG. 23-10. *Perforated plate screens for hammer mills (comminuting machines). Coarse screens (right) are used for wet milling operations and finer screens (left) for dry milling. (Courtesy of Fitzpatrick Co.)*

cause of the enclosed nature of the equipment, little dust is created; consequently, material losses are low, and exposure of personnel to dust is minimized.

As part of the scale-up of a milling or sieving operation, the lubricants and glidants, which in the laboratory are usually added directly to the final blend, are usually added to the dried granulation during the sizing operation. This is done because some of these additives, especially magnesium stearate, tend to agglomerate when added in large quantities to the granulation in a blender. To assure adequate distribution of these dry additives, a preliminary dispersion of these materials is often made during the sizing operation. This part of the process must be carefully optimized so that the lubricants are not overmixed or undermixed during the screening and subsequent blending operations.[18,19]

Blending

The type of blending equipment used in production operations often differs considerably from that used in the product development laboratories, and certainly differs greatly in size.

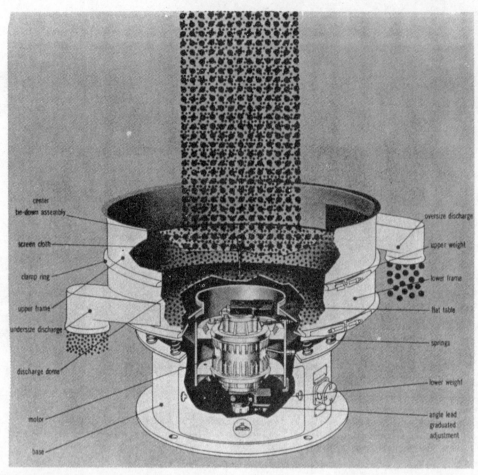

FIG. 23-11. *Mechanical Sieving Equipment. A series of stacked screens inside the vibrating body of the classifier separates the granulation. Material is collected and discharged at the take-off spouts. (Courtesy of SWECO, Inc.)*

Consequently, attention should be paid to the scale-up of this operation so that equipment of the right design is used and blender loads, mixing speeds, and mixing times are properly established.[20,21] In any blending operation, both segregation and mixing occur simultaneously.[22] Both processes are a function of particle size, shape, hardness, and density, and of the dynamics of the mixing action. Therefore, the characteristics of the different particles in the blend must be known, and the cause of segregation understood, so that the blending operation can be optimized and a uniform blend obtained.[23]

A thorough understanding of the characteristics of the material to be blended helps to make a full-scale production processing operation successful and more efficient. A product with fragile particles or agglomerates is more readily abraided, resulting in an excessive amount of fines. These fines may mix improperly and cause flow problems, and/or fill weight and content uniformity problems. Particle abrasion is more likely to occur when high-shear mixers with spiral screws or blades are used; however, even tumble blenders used for prolonged mixing times can result in an excessive particle breakdown as the free-falling particles impinge on each other and on the blender walls.

Variations that may occur in the bulk density of the raw materials must be considered in selecting a blender and in determining optimum blender load. There is an economic incentive to maximize a batch size, but the maximum batch size to be blended should be conservatively chosen so as to allow latitude for the normal variation in granulation density. The failure to do so eventually results in a low-density granulation that overfills the blender and in a loss of blending efficiency. Excessive granulation volumes have been documented as being responsible for poor content uniformity, poor lubrication of the granulation, and improper color dispersion.

Specialized Granulation Procedures

DRY BLENDING AND DIRECT COMPRESSION

Since the preferred manufacturing procedure uses the simplest, least complicated equipment and requires a minimum amount of handling and operator time, any modification in a process that simplifies it is highly desirable. Processes that yield free-flowing granulations without the aid of granulating solutions are desirable in that they do not require the time and energy necessary to volatilize the solvent used in conventional wet granulation procedures. With many of the common excipients and even active drugs now available in a form that makes them directly compressible, the possibility of dry blending and direct compression should be considered.[24] Therefore, the simplest answer to granulation problems with some formulations could be to avoid a granulation procedure by using a direct compression type of formula.

When exploring this option, a careful analysis of particle characteristics that influence mixing and segregation, such as size, size distribution, shape, and static charge should be evaluated.[25] Scaling up a dry blending operation for a directly compressible formulation requires that special attention be paid to blender loads, optimum mixing speeds, and the blending time required to assure that the drug distribution within a batch is acceptable and consistent from batch to batch. When a wet granulation is prepared, complete distribution of the active ingredients is achieved through a series of operations: dry blending, granulation, milling, and lubrication, and if any one step in this operation is inadequate to achieve content uniformity, the other processing steps often compensate. This is not the case for a single dry blend of a directly compressible formula. Consequently, optimization of the process and validation of its performance are important.

The following are aspects of the dry blending operation of directly compressible materials that can be adjusted to optimize the process.

The order of addition of components to the blender. As an example, a low-dose active ingredient may be "sandwiched" between two portions of directly compressible excipient in the blender to improve dispersion and/or to avoid loss to the surface of the blender.

The mixing speed. Examples are blade rotation speed for a planetary type mixer, and mixer tumbling or rotational speed for a twin-shell, cone-type, or similar type of mixer.

The mixing time. The mixing time can be decreased if available data show the materials to be consistently and uniformly mixed in less time than originally directed. Alternatively, the time may need to be increased if the mixing time is shown to produce material with borderline uniformity. Mixing time may also be important to compressibility of the finished blend. Excessive mixing time may fracture fragile excipients and ruin their compressibility.

The use of auxiliary dispersion equipment within the mixer. An example is an intensifier bar or chopper blade in a twin-shell mixer. These increase the efficiency of dispersion of solid and liquid ingredients added to the mixture. They also reduce agglomerates that may be present in a material, thereby aiding the efficiency of dispersion.

The mixing action. Mixing action is determined by the mechanics of the mixer and can only be changed by converting from one blender to another or by modifying the blender through addition of baffles or plates, which would alter the mixing characteristics.

The blender load. The amount of material volume to total mixer volume affects the efficiency of the blender. Each blender has an optimum working volume and a normal working range. Overloading a blender retards the free flow of the granulation and reduces the efficiency of the blender. Localized concentrations of the drug remain, causing content uniformity problems in the finished dosage form. Conversely, if the load is too small, the powders slide rather than roll in a blender, and proper mixing does not occur, or the time needed for uniform mixing of the powders increases.

SLUGGING (DRY GRANULATION)

A dry powder blend that cannot be directly compressed because of poor flow or compression properties may in some instances be processed using a slugging operation. This is done on a tablet press designed for slugging, which operates at pressures of about 15 tons, compared with a normal tablet press, which operates at pressures of 4 tons or less. Usually, extra-large tablet punches are used to form compressed slugs of the powdered material. This procedure is usually slow because the inherently poor compressibility of the powders requires slower press speeds to provide the extended compression dwell time under load needed to hold the compacted material together. Slugs range in diameter from 1 inch, for the more easily slugged material, to ¾ inch in diameter for materials that are more difficult to compress and require more pressure per unit area to yield satisfactory compacts. After compression, the slugs are broken down using either a hammer mill or an oscillating granulator to obtain a granulation with a suitable particle size distribution. If an excessive amount of fine powder is generated during the milling operation, the material must be screened and the "fines" recycled through the slugging operation. During scale-up of such an operation, the pilot plant scientist should pay particular attention to the forces used for the slugging operation, the diameter of the punches, and the subsequent sizing and screening operations. The optimization of these variables affects the particle size and particle size distribution.

Granulation by dry compaction can also be achieved by passing powders between two rollers that compact the material at pressures of up to 10 tons per linear inch. Because of the similarity in application, processes developed in the laboratory using a slugging operation might be adapted to the roller compaction process involving a Chilsonator, such as that shown in Figure 23-12. Materials of very low density require roller compaction to achieve a bulk density sufficient to allow encapsulation or compression. One of the best known examples of this process is the densification of aluminum hydroxide. Pilot plant personnel should determine whether the final drug blend or the active ingredient could be more efficiently processed in this manner than by conventional processing in order to produce a granulation with the required tabletting or encapsulation properties.

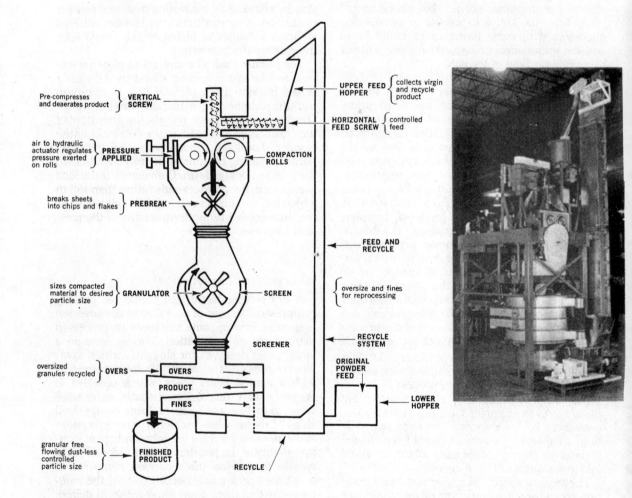

Patents Pending
©The Fitzpatrick Company, Elmhurst, Illinois 1968

FIG. 23-12. *Schematic of dry compaction operation. Dry material is fed to and compacted by a Chilsonator, then sized to remove fines, which are recycled. The finished dry compacted granulation is ready for subsequent encapsulation or compression. Inset shows actual size of a production unit. (Courtesy of Fitzpatrick Co. © The Fitzpatrick Company, Elmhurst, IL, 1968.)*

Granulation Handling and Feed Systems

The handling of the finished granulation in the compression area can be a simple operation such as hand scooping the material from a drum into the press hopper, or for larger operations, a sophisticated automated handling system using vacuum or mechanical systems to convey the granulation. For the latter system, studies should be undertaken to determine the effect that this additional handling has on the content uniformity of the drug and on the particle size distribution. Segregation due to static charges built up during vacuum and/or the mechanical handling of the granulation can lead to problems with material flow through tablet press hoppers and feed frames. This in turn makes it difficult to control tablet weight, thickness, and hardness. Poor content uniformity may be the final result.

More sophisticated material handling systems cause the added concern of cleanability. Long lengths of transfer tubes, valves, pneumatic pumps, vacuum canisters, cyclone traps, and other components of these systems must be engineered for efficient and total cleaning. Well-written, documented, and validated cleaning procedures are essential for such a system.

Compression

The ultimate test of a tablet formulation and granulation process is whether the granulation can be compressed on a high-speed tablet press.

During compression, the tablet press performs the following functions:

1. Filling of empty die cavity with granulation.

2. Precompression of granulation (optional).

3. Compression of granulation.

4. Ejection of the tablet from the die cavity and take-off of compressed tablet.

The means by which these functions are accomplished varies, depending on the design of the press. Machine design also determines the usable range of compression forces at which the machine can safely operate, and the press speed at which output can be optimized without negative impact on tablet quality.

Sometimes, because of raw material characteristics or formulation constraints, a particular product cannot be successfully compressed at the upper speed range of a press. When this occurs, the press speed is reduced, or a slower press is used, to allow more time for the dies to fill and to extend the dwell time of compression,

both of which help to facilitate the compaction process. With advances in tablet press technology, which provide better control of feeder mechanisms, precompression, and compression forces, many granulation problems or inadequacies can be overcome by making appropriate adjustments to the press. The handling and compression characteristics are important factors that must be considered in the selection of a tablet press. Output alone is not reason enough to select a press. Table 23-1 contains a partial list of presses available and their capabilities and features.

When evaluating the compression characteristics of a particular formulation, prolonged trial runs at press speeds equal to that to be used in normal production should be tried. Only then are potential problems such as sticking to the punch surfaces, tablet hardness, capping, and weight variation detected. Such preproduction trials in the pilot plant are important for identifying these problems early in the scale-up process, when changes are more easily made than during later production runs, when marketing requirements may make it difficult to interrupt production schedules to modify the formulation.

High-speed tablet compression depends on the ability of the press to interact with granulation so that a certain series of operations is successfully performed. The granulation must be delivered to the die feed system at an adequate rate. The granulation delivery must not be interrupted, nor should the flow rate vary. The delivery system must not change the particle size distribution. The system must not cause segregation of coarse and fine particles, nor should it induce static charges, which would retard the flow of the granulation and could cause the active ingredient to become segregated.[26] The die feed system must be able to fill the die cavities adequately in the short period of time that the die is passing under the feed frame. The smaller the tablet, the more difficult it is to get a uniform fill at high press speeds. The granulation must have good flow properties, a good particle size distribution, and a relatively small mean particle size to facilitate rapid but uniform fill of the die cavities. For high-speed machines, induced die feed systems are necessary. These are available with a variety of feed paddles and with variable speed capabilities, so that the optimum feed for every type of granulation can be obtained.

After the die cavities have been filled with granulation, the excess is removed by the feed frame to the center of the die table. If the feed frame has been overfilled and not all of the excess granulation is moved to the center of the die table, this excess may be thrown from the table

TABLE 23-1. *Compression Rates of Typical Production Presses*

Model	Max. Tablet Diameter (in.)	Number of Stations	Tablets per Min
Colton 216	1/2	16	600–800
Colton 233	5/8	33	2500–4000
Colton 241	7/16	41	3000–5000
Stokes B-2	7/16	22	450–900
Stokes BB-2	5/8	27	800–1400
Stokes BB-2	7/16	33	1000–1700
Stokes 540	5/8	35	800–2400
Stokes 541	7/16	41	1000–2700
Stokes 551	7/16	51	1200–3700
Stokes 552 TriPact	7/16	51	3000–5000
Stokes UltraPress 565-1	7/16	65	3500–10,000
Stokes UltraPress 565-2	5/8	53	2900–8100
Stokes Eagle-3	5/16	41	2150–6150
Stokes Eagle-2	5/8	53	2800–8000
Stokes Eagle-1	7/16	65	3500–10,000
Manesty Betapress	5/8	16	700–1500
Manesty Betapress	13/32	23	100–2000
Manesty ExPress ×20	1	20	800–2000
Manesty ExPress ×25	5/8	25	1000–2500
Manesty ExPress ×30	7/16	30	1200–3000
Manesty Rotapress	7/16	55	1300–5000
Manesty Rotapress	5/8	45	1100–4300
Manesty Rotapress Mark III	7/16	69	3300–10,000
Manesty Unipress	15/16	20	970–2420
Manesty Unipress	5/8	27	1300–3270
Manesty Unipress	7/16	34	1640–4120
Fette Perfecta 3000	15/16	37	2200–4400
Fette Perfecta 3000	5/8	45	2700–6750
Fette Perfecta 3000	1/2	55	3300–8250
Fette Perfecta 1000	5/8	28	560–2100
Courtoy R100	15/16	24	288–2300
Courtoy R100	5/8	30	360–2880
Courtoy R100	1/2	36	1260–4400
Kilian LX	15/16	15	270–1350
Kilian LX	5/8	21	400–2260
Kilian TX	5/8	30	330–3150
Kilian TX	1/2	40	440–4200
Kilian RX	15/16	41	660–5500
Kilian RX	5/8	51	830–7660
Kilian RX	1/2	67	1080–10,000
Kikusui Gemini	5/8	55	2200–7700
Kikusui Gemini	7/16	67	2680–9380
Kikusui Hercules	1 1/2	18	450–1080
Kikusui Hercules	15/16	29	725–1740
Korsch PH230	5/8	17	up to 1850
Korsch PH230	1/2	20	up to 2200
Korsch PH336	5/8	36	up to 3600
Korsch PH343	1/2	43	up to 4300
Korsch PH423	1 1/2	23	368–2300
Korsch PH431	15/16	31	500–3100
Korsch PH447	9/16	47	750–4700

by the centrifugal force of the rotating die table. For this reason, the clearance between the scraper blade and the die table must be carefully set. Too large a gap results in large granulation losses, especially if the granulation contains a lot of fines. Too close a setting causes scoring of the die table and metal contamination of the product.

Compression of the granulation usually occurs as a single event as the heads of the punches pass over the lower and under the upper pressure rollers. This causes the punches to penetrate the die to a preset depth, compacting the granulation to the thickness of the gap set between the punch surfaces. The rapidity and dwell time in which this event occurs is determined by the speed at which the press is rotating and by the size of the compression rollers. The larger the compression roller, the more gradually the compression force is applied and released. The tendency toward capping in a formulation can often be reduced by slowing down the press speed or using presses with larger compression rollers. Granulations that are difficult to compress and that have a tendency to cap can often be more effectively compressed on a press with a series of pressure rollers that impart a stepwise increase in pressure, thus allowing entrapped air to escape gradually rather than as an abrupt event at the end of a single-step compression.

Courtoy has developed a tablet press that is capable of minimizing capping by a unique compression system whereby pressure is applied to the punch heads by pressure rollers that are pneumatically loaded. Instead of the pressure profile being the customary sine wave (⌒⌒⌒) it becomes more of a square wave (⎍⎍). Thus, the dwell time at the point of maximum pressure is prolonged considerably. Subjecting the tablet to the maximum compression force for an extended time period reduces the tendency of the tablet to cap and permits running a problem granulation at higher than normal press speeds.[27]

The final event in the compression process is the ejection of the compressed tablet from the die cavity. This involves the separation of the upper punch from the upper surface of the tablet and withdrawal from the die cavity. The lower punch face then moves up through the die cavity, breaking the tablet free from the die wall and forcing it out of the die cavity. As the die table rotates, a take-off bar positioned just above the table forces the tablet to separate from the lower punch face and sweeps the tablet off the press table into a collection chute.

During compression, the granulation is compacted, and in order for a tablet to form, bonds within the compressible material must be formed.[28] The forces that give rise to strong cohesive bonds within the material also exist at the tablet interfaces and may result in adhesive bonds between the punch and die surfaces and the tablet. Embossing on the punches tends to accentuate sticking. A good internal lubricant system is necessary to prevent sticking of the tablet to the metal surface of the punches or die. If the granulation is adequately and properly lubricated, the tendency for sticking and binding of the tablet to the punch face can be eliminated. Magnesium stearate and calcium stearate are the most commonly used tablet lubricants. The level at which they should be employed and the degree to which they need to be blended with the granulation must be determined experimentally. Too high a level of lubricant or overblending can result in a soft tablet, a decrease in the wettability of the powder, and an extension of the dissolution time.[18,19]

The design and condition of the punches can also be the cause for sticking. Embossing on the punch faces often causes sticking if the embossed letters, numbers, or symbols are too high, if the angle of the embossing is too steep, or if the corners are too sharp. New punches often have to be "run in" over a 4- to 8-hour period before they can run cleanly. Microscopic nicks or pits in the punch faces can also cause sticking.

Binding at the die walls can sometimes be overcome by designing the die to be 0.001 to 0.005 inch wider at the upper portion than at the center in order to relieve pressure during ejection.

Tablet Coating

Tablet coating, which at one time consisted of sugar coating in conventional coating pans, has undergone many changes because of new developments in coating technology and changes in safety and environmental regulations. The conventional sugar coating pan has given way to perforated pans or fluidized-bed coating columns. The development of new polymeric materials has resulted in a change from aqueous sugar coating to solvent film coating, and more recently, to aqueous film coating.

Film coating is a specialized operation, and although film coating systems can be developed in a laboratory, the final coating process needs to be defined on production scale equipment.[29] A properly designed core tablet greatly facilitates the success of scale-up. The tablets must be sufficiently hard to withstand the tumbling to which they are subjected in either the coating pan or the coating column. Tablet designs with sharp edges or flat surfaces should be avoided because they are difficult to coat. Engraved surfaces also make coating more difficult. This problem can be minimized, however, if the engravings are kept shallow and the cuts are angled to avoid sharp edges. Some tablet core materials are naturally hydrophobic, and in these cases, film coating with an aqueous system may require special formulation of the tablet core and/or the coating solution.

A film coating solution may have been found to work well with a particular core tablet in a small laboratory coating pan or column, but may be totally unacceptable on a production scale. This difference in performance is due to the increased pressure and abrasion to which the tablets are subjected when the batch size is large, and to differences in the temperature and humidity environment to which the individual tablets are exposed during the coating and drying cycles. These differences are predictable from basic engineering equations that describe temperature and humidity gradients and transfer within the coating system. Operating conditions that must be established for either a pan or column operation are optimum tablet load, operating tablet bed temperature, drying airflow rate and temperature, and the solution application rate. The atomizing nozzles for typical pharmaceutical applications can be high-pressure airless or air-atomizing. For airless sprayers, the size and shape of the nozzle aperture is important. For air-atomized sprayers, the atomizing air pressure and the liquid flow rate are critical factors in establishing proper spraying characteristics. A high airflow yields a fine spray, but it also creates more turbulence and causes a spray drying effect. The coating solution can be sprayed continuously or intermittently. If it is sprayed intermittently, the cycles must be timed to prevent the rotation of dry uncoated or partially coated tablets, which would result in abrasion and edge chipping of the tablets and a poor quality coating.

Not only do chipping and abrasion affect those tablets damaged, but the debris formed adheres to the other tablets in the batch, thus ruining the whole pan or column load. In addition to increasing tablet hardness, the use of appropriate baffles in the coating pans can further reduce chipping and abrasion. These baffles prevent the tablet bed from sliding instead of rolling, and they also redistribute the weight of the tablet load, and spread the weight more uniformly over the entire tablet bed. In a column operation, the abrasion can be minimized by controlling the length and diameter of the center spouting column and controlling the force of the air fluidizing the tablets.

With the advent of computers and microprocessors, automated processing systems are available to make tablet coating a more controlled and reproducible process than it was several decades ago, when tablet coating was considered an art rather than a science.

Encapsulation for Hard Gelatin Capsules

The manufacturing process for encapsulated products often parallels that for tablets. Both tablets and capsules are produced from ingredients that may be either dry blended or wet granulated to produce a dry powder or granule mix with a uniformly dispersed active ingredient. To produce capsules on today's high-speed equipment, the processed powder blend must have the particle size distribution, bulk density, and compressibility required to promote good flow characteristics and to result in the formation of compacts of the right size and of sufficient cohesiveness to be filled into capsule shells.

Equipment used in capsule filling operations involves one of two types of filling systems. Encapsulators manufactured by Zanasi or Martelli form slugs in a *dosator* (a hollow tube with a plunger to eject the capsule plug), while the operating system of the Höfliger-Karg machines is based on formation of compacts in a die plate using tamping pins to form a compact. With both systems, the most common problems encountered in scale-up involve bulk density, powder flow, compressibility, and lubricant distribution. The common problem of weight variation can be caused by the poor flow characteristics of the granules, which may in turn be due to the bulk density and particle size distribution of the granules. Weight variation may also be caused by plugs sticking to the dosator plunger surfaces or die walls because of inadequate lubrication. Overlubrication of the granules may result in weight variation problems because the softer plugs that are formed may not be completely transferred to the capsule body.

Overly lubricated capsule granules are also responsible for delaying capsule disintegration and dissolution, which may result in reduced bioavailability. As in tablet operations, prolonged trials of many hours using multiple batches are required before a process can be judged as acceptable for routine production. The size and type of equipment used in blending, granulating, drying, sizing, and lubrication of capsule granulations or mixtures can greatly influence the characteristics of the granulation and the finished product.

Because of the differences previously noted, the type of encapsulating equipment chosen for routine production should dictate the properties required of a powder blend. During testing designed to determine the optimum process conditions, the need for controlled environmental conditions must be considered. Many encapsulation processes are less reliable than anticipated because the humidity in the processing and encapsulation rooms is not adequately controlled. Left as an unknown variable, humidity often has a significant effect on the moisture content of the granulation and on the empty gelatin capsules. Granulation moisture content can be important to chemical or physical stability of the finished product, and uncontrolled moisture leads to machine problems of flow and sticking during material transfer and filling. Empty gelatin capsules have a recommended storage condition of 15 to 25°C and a relative humidity of between 35 and 65%. This condition is designed to minimize moisture absorption or loss, and the resultant changes in physical dimensions, during the encapsulation operation. During encapsulation, the processing room humidity should be controlled to within 45 and 55%. At higher humidities, the capsules may swell because of the moisture absorbed. This may make separation of the capsule parts more difficult and interfere with the transport of the capsule throughout the encapsulation process. Low humidity conditions make the capsules brittle and increase their static charge, thereby seriously interfering with the encapsulation operation.

Liquid Dosage Forms

In the discussion that follows, liquid pharmaceuticals encountered in the pilot plant are defined as nonsterile solutions, suspensions, or emulsions. Scale-up of each of these presents a different set of processing concerns that must be considered. Sterile liquids represent an additional, unique class of pharmaceutical products; these are covered elsewhere within this book.

Simple solutions are the most straightforward to scale up, but then require tanks of adequate size and suitable mixing capability.[30] Most equipment has heating/cooling capabilities to effect rapid dissolution of components of the system. Adequate transfer systems and filtration equipment are required, but they must be monitored to assure that they can clarify the product without selectively removing active or adjuvant ingredients. All equipment must be made of suitable, nonreactive, sanitary materials and be designed and constructed to facilitate easy cleaning. Liquid pharmaceutical processing tanks, kettles, pipes, mills, filter housing, and so forth are most frequently fabricated from stainless steel. Of the two types of stainless steel used in the industry (type 308 and 316), type 316 is most often used because of its less reactive nature. Stainless steel is not nonreactive, however, it does react with some acidic pharmaceutical liquids.[31] When this situation is a concern, the problem can be minimized by prereacting the stainless steel with an acetic acid or nitric acid solution to remove the surface alkalinity of the stainless steel. This procedure, known as *passivation,* may need to be repeated at periodic intervals. For example, if an alkaline cleaning agent is being used between batches of a reactive product, passivation may need to be repeated before the subsequent batch can be prepared.

Interaction with metallic surfaces can be minimized by use of glass or polytetrafluoroethylene (Teflon) liners. Although these are highly inert surface materials, they have the obvious disadvantages of cracking, breaking, flaking, and peeling, with resultant product contamination.

Suspensions

Suspensions require more attention during scale-up than do simple solutions because of additional processing needs. The addition and dispersion of suspending agents, which on a laboratory scale may merely involve sprinkling the material into the liquid vortex, may require use of a vibrating feed system or other novel approach when production scale batches are involved.[32] A powder eductor may facilitate the addition of a material that tends to clump during the process or that is difficult to disperse. In some instance, suspending agents that are difficult to disperse can be successfully incorporated by making a slurry with a portion of the vehicle. The suspending agent in a concentrated slurry is easier to wet and can be more completely dispersed using a high-shear mixer in a smaller volume of the vehicle. Such a slurry facilitates rapid and complete hydration of the suspending agent when added to the larger portion of the vehicle. The time and temperature required to hydrate suspending agents is often critical, and unless the hydration process is complete before other ingredients are added, the quality of the suspension is adversely affected.

Active ingredients in a suspension must be uniformly dispersed throughout the batch. The best dispersion procedure to use in the production process depends on the physical characteristics of the active ingredients. If they wet easily, disperse readily, and tend not to agglomerate, a simple addition of the chemicals at a convenient stage in the manufacturing process is appropriate. If the active ingredients are difficult to wet or tend to agglomerate, however, other methods for adding these ingredients must be sought. One is to prepare a slurry with a wetting agent and with the aid of high-shear mixing equipment. Another method is to pretreat the hard-to-wet material by blending it in a high-shear powder blender with one or some of the liquid ingredients, possibly with a surfactant included. This converts a bulky material, which is difficult to handle because of static charges, to a dense, readily wettable powder, which is much easier to handle. Such approaches minimize wetting difficulties and eliminate the formation of dry agglomerates in the finished product. If these agglomerates should occur, the air trapped in this dry material may cause the product to "cream" (separate), thereby causing physical instability or poor content uniformity.

In preparing pharmaceutical suspensions, the type of mixers, pumps, and mills, and the horsepower of the motors, should be carefully selected based on scale-up performance.[33] The equipment must be selected according to the size of the batch and the maximum viscosity of the product during the manufacturing process. As an example, the use of an appropriate type of mixer is important because if the mixer is undersized, the obvious problems of inadequate distribution or excessive production time result. Mixing at too high a speed can result in the incorporation of an excessive amount of air into the product. Air that is entrapped in the product as very small bubbles is difficult and time-consuming to remove, and if not removed, can affect the physical and chemical stability of the product and/or the reproducibility of the filling operation. If air entrapment is a problem that cannot be rectified with process or equipment modifications, the air can be removed using a vacuum unit such as the Versator (Fig. 23-13). During operation of a Versator, product is drawn into a vacuum chamber through an inlet line, where it is spread onto the center of a high-speed rotating disc. The centrifugal force produced by the rotation of the disc causes the product to form a thin film on the disc surface. As the film thins and moves toward the outer edge of the vacuum chamber, the entrapped air is drawn off, and the deaerated product is collected from the outer edge of the vacuum chamber.

Unwanted and discolored particulate material in a batch can come from the raw materials or be introduced from the bags, cases, and drums in which the raw materials were supplied. Even when all precautions are taken, some unwanted material may find its way into the product during manufacturing, so that filtration of the finished suspension through an appropriate size screen is a normal batch processing step. The mesh size chosen must be capable of removing the unwanted foreign particulates but should not filter out any of the active ingredients. Such a sieve can only be selected based on production batch size trials. Most active ingredients have particle sizes less than 10 microns with almost none over 25 microns. Therefore, when dealing with particulates, screens of 150 mesh, having openings of around 100 microns, remove unwanted suspended materials that are below the easily visible range without retaining the suspended active ingredient(s).

At the completion of the batch, the transfer and filling of a finished suspension should be carefully monitored. If suspensions are not constantly mixed or recirculated during transfer processes, they may "settle out" and thereby adversely affect the uniform distribution of the active ingredient.

Emulsions

Emulsions are disperse systems similar to suspensions except that the dispersed phase is a finely divided immiscible liquid instead of a solid. The dispersed phase is usually made up of oils or waxes that may be in either a liquid or solid state. Manufacturing of liquid emulsion products entails specialized procedures, and as a result, scale-up into production equipment involves extensive process development and validation. Processing parameters and procedures that must be adjusted and controlled for the various types of emulsions include temperature, mixing equipment, homogenizing equipment, in-process or final product filters, screens, pumps and filling equipment. The degree to which the emulsion is refined by the reduction of the globule size of the internal phase affects the physical properties of the emulsion, such as appearance and viscosity, as well as the physical stability of the product. Manufacturing systems that utilize high-shear mixers are more likely to lead to air entrapment and may adversely affect the physical and chemical stability. Conversely, the use of vessels that can be operated with the

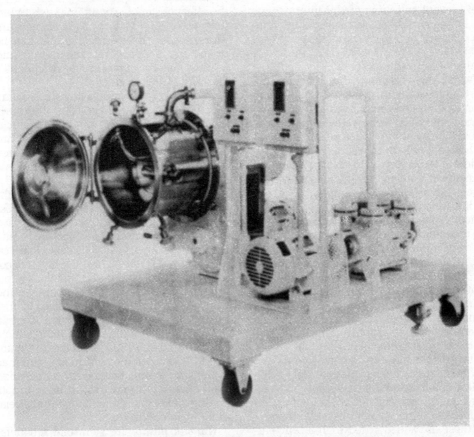

FIG. 23-13. *The Versator consists of a vacuum chamber and a high-speed revolving disc. During operation, material is spread into a thin film by the centrifugal force of the disc, and deaeration is achieved under vacuum. If desired, the unit can be pressurized to create entrainment of gas. (Courtesy of the Cornell Machine Co.)*

contents under a controlled vacuum avoids the problem of unwanted aeration. The filtration of an emulsion to remove particulates originating from the raw materials or introduced during processing can affect the quality of the emulsion. The unwanted particulates are most efficiently removed by filtering the separate oil and water phases before emulsification.

Semisolid Products

Pastes, gels, ointments, and creams are closely related to suspensions, liquids, and emulsions except that they are products with higher viscosities. The scale-up of these products involves many of the same factors that must be considered in the scale-up of the comparable lower viscosity products already discussed, but the high viscosity renders certain aspects of the scale-up of semisolid products more critical. As an example, the natural turbulence created by the mixers used to make liquid suspensions or emulsions is not adequate to produce a homogeneous ointment or cream. For these products, the mixing equipment must be capable of effectively and continuously moving the semisolid mass from the outside walls of the mixing kettle to the center and from the bottom to the top of the kettle. This action is required both to distribute the ingredients and to bring about a rapid and efficient heat transfer to and from the product during the heating and cooling steps.

The power required to carry out the mixing operation varies greatly during the manufacturing sequence and is directly related to changes in the viscosity of the product. Motors used to drive the mixing system of semisolid manufacturing equipment must be sized to handle the product at its most viscous stage. Motors that drive the mixers used to disperse or dissolve components that have been added early in the manufacturing sequence, when product viscosity is low, may be required to operate at a slower speed to prevent splashing of the intermediate phases. For this reason, most semisolid equipment is designed to provide variable speed mixing.

Many processing steps such as the mixing of oil and water phases during emulsification processing, component homogenization, addition of active ingredient, and product transfer are usually carried out at carefully predetermined temperatures. The working temperature range at which these operations are carried out are usually critical to the quality of the final product. In the formation of a cream, the aqueous phase and oil phase must be heated to a temperature above the solidification point of the oil phase, and then emulsified. Failure to have both phases at the correct temperature results in a poor-quality product with improperly dispersed wax. Consequently, an accurate understanding of the heat transfer characteristics of the system and the temperature gradient throughout the batch is important.

Reliance on the temperature recorded by a single sensor at a fixed point in the mixing vessel is often misleading. Unacceptably wide ranges in product viscosity are frequently the result of inadequate temperature control during the critical emulsification steps. Improper temperature control can have an adverse effect on the particle size of poorly soluble active ingredients. If these are added at too high a temperature, the solubility may be artificially increased, creating a metastable product. On subsequent cooling, crystal growth or recrystallization may occur from the saturated solution. This recrystallized material may be a different polymorphic form or a different crystal type or size. The result may be a change of particle size distribution, yielding a gritty, less elegant product, or one with altered stability or biologic activity.

Many cream formulations and some gel products are shear-sensitive. Handling such products during transfer from the manufacturing kettle to holding tanks or to the filling lines requires that attention be given to the amount of shear that such products will encounter. Changes in measured viscosity are frequently seen when viscous products are pumped through long transfer lines or are filtered to remove unwanted particulates. Because of this, the relationship between shear stress and the measured viscosity values of the product must be understood. When carrying out such evaluations, the pilot plant scientist needs to remember that most viscometers determine relative viscosity rather than an absolute viscosity. Therefore, the accurate evaluation of the effect of a process change on viscosity must recognize the effect of sample conditions such as temperature, processing history of the sample, and age. The more of these variables that can be controlled, the more accurate the interpretation will be of the effects of processing conditions on the viscosity of the product.[34]

The most critical processing steps that need to be carefully evaluated and controlled during the manufacture of a cream are the emulsification of the two phases and the dispersion of any suspended active ingredients. Pharmaceutical equipment used in the homogenization of the emulsion and dispersion of suspended active ingredients includes various types of high-shear mixers, homogenizers, and colloid mills, supplied by a number of different manufacturers. One of the most common pieces of equipment used for these purposes is a colloid mill consisting of a fixed stator plate and a high-speed rotating rotor plate. Material drawn or pumped through an adjustable gap set between the rotor and stator is milled or homogenized by the physical action, and centrifugal force is created by the high-speed rotation of the rotor, which operates within 0.005 to 0.010 inch of the stator (Fig. 23-14). Sonic homogenization equipment accomplishes emulsification by imparting sufficient energy to the material through rapidly vibrating vanes that break up a liquid stream into small, discrete droplets.

Transfer pumps for semisolid products must be able to move viscous material without applying excessive shear and without incorporating air. Pumps designed to meet these criteria are known as *positive displacement pumps* (Fig. 23-15). They are available from many sources with subtle differences in design, but they all operate using a rotating member inside of a close fitting stationary housing. They are self-priming and can create adequate head pressure to force product through long transfer lines and filtration equipment. In choosing the size and type of pump for a particular operation, product viscosity, desired pumping rate, product compatibility with the pump surfaces, and the pumping pressure required should be considered.

Suppositories

The manufacture of suppositories on a laboratory scale usually involves the preparation of a molten mass, the dispersion of drug in the molten base, and the casting of the suppositories in a suitable mold. When the mold has been adequately cooled, it is opened, and the suppositories are removed. Such an operation provides lit-

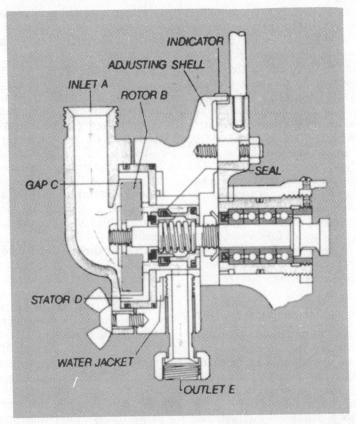

FIG. 23-14. *Operational flow pattern of rotor-stator homogenizer. Product flows by gravity or may be pumped through inlet connection (A) coming in contact with rotor (B) and is forced through first-stage processing gap (C) by high-shear impellers on front face of rotor (B). These impellers, in addition to providing intense shearing action, furnish a pumping force to move product across the periphery of the rotor (B). After traversing the periphery of the rotor (B), the product flow direction is reversed so that it is countercurrent to centrifugal force. The product then flows inward across the second-stage area between rotor (B) and stator (D) and is discharged through outlet opening (E). (Courtesy of APV Gaulin, Inc.)*

tle experience that is relevant to new processes used in large-scale production of a suppository product. However, many commercial suppositories are still produced by a fusion method in which (1) a molten mass is prepared, (2) the suppository is molded, cooled in a refrigeration tunnel, and removed from the mold, and (3) the product is packaged in an off-line wrapping or blistering operation. A detailed discussion of this operation and processing equipment can be found in Chapter 19, "Suppositories."

The manufacturing and packaging processes

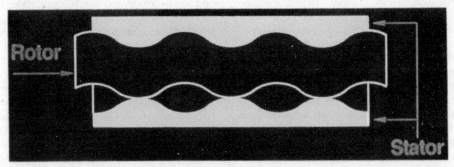

FIG. 23-15. *Schematic representation of a positive displacement pump. The helical rotor moves inside the double helical stationary housing, creating a progressing cavity, which moves the material. (MOYNO Quick Displacement Progressing Cavity Pump, courtesy of Fluids Handling Division of Robbins & Myers, Inc.)*

for suppositories have recently been simplified to a one-stage operation. This new technology eliminates many of the troublesome molding, cooling, and unmolding steps of the older technology. The basic improvement of the newer processing equipment is that the molten suppository mass is filled into formed PVC or foil shells, which serve both as the mold and finished package. Such a process eliminates many of the problems encountered during the removal of the suppository from the two-piece molds in which they were formed on the older equipment. The extra work and equipment required to complete the off-line packaging operation of wrapping or blistering are also eliminated.

The manufacture of suppositories using modern equipment can be divided into several operations involving first the manufacture of the molten suppository mass and then the molding and packaging of the suppository.

Preparation of the Molten Suppository Mass

The preparation of the suppository mass on a production scale involves heating various wax-like components of the suppository base to a temperature at which they become molten. The higher melting components should be placed in the manufacturing kettle first and the lower melting ingredients added when the first components are almost completely in the molten state. To avoid overheating the waxes and altering their melting points, this operation should be carried out in jacketed vessels in which the jacket temperature can be controlled. The best systems allow monitoring of both the temperature of the vessel jacket and the molten contents of the vessel. Systems in which only live steam or cold water are available to regulate the temperature of the molten suppository mass are almost impossible to control within the fairly narrow temperature ranges required to produce a continuous source of well-controlled heating and cooling water. The normal operating range is 35 to 65°C, with temperatures of 45 to 65°C used for melting and mixing of the suppository base material and temperatures of 35 to 45°C used during addition of active ingredients and during molding (filling). Since the viscosity of suppository masses is normally temperature-dependent, the filling operation should be conducted at a temperature just above the solidification point. Settling of suspended material during cooling is prevented through both the increased viscosity and the reduced time required to solidify the mass. Because this is the most critical step, the working range of temperature is often no larger than ±3°C around the set point.

The precise temperature control required affects the design and type of mixing system used in the melting and holding tank. The vessel in which the mass is prepared may require high-shear mixing capability to break up agglomerates of the active ingredient and to disperse the active ingredient effectively throughout the molten base. The equipment should also be capable of providing gentle stirring action that will effectively keep the active ingredients well dispersed.

Transfer of the molten mass to the filling heads of the suppository machine must be done through heated lines. When a separate holding tank is used, this must be jacketed and should be part of a recirculating loop designed to prevent settling of the active ingredient and congealing of the mass.

Any extraneous particulate material that may be present in the molten mass can be removed using an in-line filter of an appropriate mesh size. Most active ingredients in suppositories are less than 10 microns in size, so 100-mesh filters with openings of approximately 70 microns provide filtration without retention of the active ingredients. The filter's ability to remove extraneous material but not hold back any of the drug should be validated by a series of carefully monitored pilot plant trials. Extensive sampling and analysis of suppositories over an extended time period designed to mimic production conditions of filtration, holding, recirculation, and filling are required to show that the active ingredient is not retained. In addition, extensive visual inspection of filtered suppository mass is required to show that the filter is efficient in removing unwanted material.

Molding and Packaging

Current suppository manufacturing technology utilizes equipment that forms, fills, and seals the suppositories in a continuous process. The mold for the suppositories is formed from special thermoplastics sheets of PVC, polyethylene, and aluminum foil laminates. A variety of problems can occur during the forming of the shells. These can be minimized by careful attention to the temperature and dwell times used during the formation of the molded cavities. Inappropriate temperatures or dwell times that are either too short or too long produce inadequate mold shells that may leak because of improper seals. The temperature of the mass during filling is also important. If the molten mass is filled at a temperature more than a few degrees above the congealing point, a hole forms in the center of the suppository upon cooling, owing to excessive contraction. Filling at too low a temperature causes clogging of the transfer lines and filling nozzles and results in erratic fill weights. Therefore, the temperature of the molten mass in the hopper and lines must be carefully controlled, and the mass constantly stirred or recirculated, to maintain the mass within a narrow temperature range.

After filling, the shells pass through a cooling tower where the suppositories are allowed to solidify before the ends of the PVC or aluminum shell are sealed. Then the strips of suppositories are trimmed and cut into the specified length. The temperature in the cooling tower determines the cooling rate of the suppositories. If the temperature is too low and the cooling rate too fast, the suppositories can become brittle. Sufficient scale-up trials should be run to optimize the process so that the temperature of the product throughout the process is maintained at the level required for the particular formulation.

Contract Manufacture

On occasion, scale-up or manufacture of a product may need to be done at an outside contract manufacturer. The reasons for considering contract manufacture include the needs for additional manufacturing capacity, highly specialized technology, or specialized equipment. When choosing a contractor, consideration should be given to the experience, capability, and reputation of the contractor within the industry.[35] In addition, the technical competence of the contractor's personnel and compliance to good manufacturing practices are important factors in the choice of a vendor. Before pilot-size batches or larger are prepared at an outside facility, a team of personnel who are knowledgeable and experienced in production, QA, QC, and GMP should visit the potential contract manufacturer. The site visit should include an indepth assessment of facilities, equipment, personnel, and policy. The following checklist of items to be reviewed originates from the Good Manufacturing Practices regulations as set forth in the Code of Federal Regulations (21 CFR211):

Review of procedures, facilities, and personnel (training and documentation) involved in acquisition, storage, testing, and handling of raw materials (excipients and actives).

Equipment availability, utilization, and maintenance; documentation of equipment operator training, equipment cleaning procedures, and equipment calibration.

Adequacy of manufacturing facilities (size, spatial separation, cleanliness, design, cleanability; dust, temperature, and humidity control)

Adequacy of storage space for in-process, quarantine, and approved bulk finished goods storage.

Controls for preventing product mixup and cross-contamination.

Label storage, approval, dispensing, and accountability procedures and controls.

Packaging equipment utilization, maintenance, cleaning, and use controls.

Packaging component control procedures.

Structure and function of the quality control unit, including personnel, training, SOPs, and responsibilities.

Warehouse space, separation of products, control procedures, and environmental controls.

Record control policies.

After all of these checklist items have been discussed to everyone's mutual satisfaction, the visiting team can complete discussions of division of responsibilities between the originating company and the contract vendor. These discussions should be finalized in a comprehensive document that outlines all areas of responsibility and that can serve as the basis for followup investigations by the pilot plant scientist and/or the quality control department.

Technical fact-finding missions of this type can underscore the unique characteristics of the pilot plant scientist, whose scientific expertise, knowledge of production equipment and processes, awareness of GMPs and SOPs, and ability to critically evaluate facilities, personnel, and procedures are key components to the direction of subsequent negotiations.

References

1. Rhodes, C.T.: Pharm. Tech., 5:30, 1981.
2. Cooper, J.: Drug Dev. Commun., 1:1, 1974–1975.
3. Nash, R.A.: Chemtech, 6:240, 1976.
4. Wray, P.E.: Management Science Conference for the Pharmaceutical Industry, Purdue University, Lafayette, IN, September 1974.
5. Lloyd, K.A.: Chem. Ind., 3:108, 1977.
6. Estes, G.K., and Luttrell, G.H.: Pharm. Tech., 7:74, 1983.
7. Loftus, B.T.: Pharm. Ind., 42:1202, 1980.
8. Ridgway, K.: Pharm. J., 205:265, 1970.
9. Harder, S.W.: Pharm. Tech. 8:29, 1984.
10. Jeffries, J.: Interphex 82, Conference Papers, Brighton, England, May 1982.
11. Melliger, G.W.: Pharm. Ind., 42:1199, 1980.
12. Berry, I.R.: Pharm. Tech., 5:38, 1981.

13. Feature article. Drug Cosmet. Ind., *127*:44, 1980.
14. Fowler, H.W.: Manuf. Chem., Aerosol News, *40*:29, 1969.
15. Campy, D., et al.: J. Pharm. Pharmacol., *26*:76P, 1974.
16. Ceschel, G.C., et al.: Farmaco Ed. Prat., *36*:281, 1981.
17. Leuenberger, H.: Acta Pharm. Technol., *29*:274, 1983.
18. Shab, A.C., and Mlodozeniec, A.R.: J. Pharm. Sci., *66*:1377, 1977.
19. Proost, J.H., et al.: Int. J. Pharm., *13*:287, 1983.
20. Rees, J.E.: Manuf. Chem. Aerosol News, *46*:23, 1975.
21. Staniforth, J.N., et al.: J. Pharm. Pharmacol., *33*:175, 1980.
22. Lloyd, P.J., et al.: J. Soc. Cosmet. Chem., *21*:205, 1970.
23. Egermann, H.: Int. J. Pharm., Tech. Prod. Mfr., *3*:59, 1982.
24. Gioia, A.: Pharm. Tech., *4*:65, 1980.
25. Greco, G.T.: Drug Dev. Indus. Pharm., *8*:565, 1982.
26. Gold, G., and Palermo, B.T.: J. Pharm. Sci., *54*:310, 1965.
27. Ritter, A., and Sucker, H.B.: Pharm. Tech., *4*:59, 1980.
28. Jetzer, W., et al.: Pharm. Tech., *7*:33, 1983.
29. Stetsko, G., et al.: Pharm. Tech., *7*:50, 1983.
30. Carstensen, J.T., and Mehta, A.: Pharm. Tech., *6*:64, 1982.
31. List, P.H.: Dtsch. Apoth. Ztg., *117*:451, 1977.
32. Hansford, D.T., et al.: Powder Technol., *26*:119, 1980.
33. Garrison, C.M.: Chem Eng., *90*:63, 1983.
34. Fujiyama, Y., et al.: J. Soc. Cosmet. Chem., *21*:625, 1970.
35. Wasserman, M.D.: Drug Cosmet. Ind., *119*:43, 1976.

24

Packaging Materials Science

CARLO P. CROCE, ARTHUR FISCHER, *and* RALPH H. THOMAS

In the pharmaceutical industry, it is vital that the package selected adequately preserve the integrity of the product. The selection of a package therefore begins with a determination of the product's physical and chemical characteristics, its protective needs, and its marketing requirements. The materials selected must have the following characteristics: (1) they must protect the preparation from environmental conditions, (2) they must not be reactive with the product, (3) they must not impart to the product tastes or odors, (4) they must be nontoxic, (5) they must be FDA approved, (6) they must meet applicable tamper-resistance requirements, and (7) they must be adaptable to commonly employed high-speed packaging equipment.

Owing to the broad scope of the subject, a detailed treatment of the science of packaging as related to pharmaceuticals cannot be adequately covered in this chapter. To give the reader a general understanding of this subject, however, basic topics have been selected for discussion. These are limited to the protective function of commonly used packaging materials, their limitations, and their possible interaction with various drugs.

Glass Containers

Glass is commonly used in pharmaceutical packaging because it possesses superior protective qualities, it is economical, and containers are readily available in a variety of sizes and shapes. It is essentially chemically inert, impermeable, strong, and rigid, and has FDA clearance. Glass does not deteriorate with age, and with a proper closure system, it provides an excellent barrier against practically every element except light. Colored glass, especially amber, can give protection against light when it is required. The major disadvantages of glass as a packaging material are its fragility and its weight.

Composition of Glass. Glass is composed principally of sand, soda-ash, limestone, and cullet.[1] The sand is almost pure silica, the soda-ash is sodium carbonate, and the limestone, calcium carbonate. Cullet is broken glass that is mixed with the batch and acts as a fusion agent for the entire mixture. The composition of glass varies and is usually adjusted for specific purposes. The most common cations found in pharmaceutical glassware are silicon, aluminum, boron, sodium, potassium, calcium, magnesium, zinc, and barium. The only anion of consequence is oxygen. Many useful properties of glass are affected by the kind of elements it contains. Reduction in the proportion of sodium ions makes glass chemically resistant; however, without sodium or other alkalies, glass is difficult and expensive to melt. Boron oxide is incorporated mainly to aid in the melting process through reduction of the temperature required.[2] Lead in small traces gives clarity and brilliance, but produces a relatively soft grade of glass. Alumina (aluminum oxide), however, is often used to increase the hardness and durability and to increase resistance to chemical action.

Manufacture of Glass

Four basic processes are used in the production of glass: blowing, drawing, pressing, and casting.[3] *Blowing* uses compressed air to form the molten glass in the cavity of a metal mold. Most commercial bottles and jars are produced on automatic equipment by this method. In *drawing*, molten glass is pulled through dies or rollers that shape the soft glass. Rods, tubes, sheet glass, and other items of uniform diameter are usually produced commercially by drawing. Ampuls, cartridges, and vials drawn from tubing have a thinner, more uniform wall thickness, with less distortion than blow-molded containers. In *pressing,* mechanical force is used to press the molten glass against the side of a mold. *Casting* uses gravity or centrifugal force to cause molten glass to form in the cavity of the mold.

Colored Glass—Light Protection. Glass containers for drugs are generally available in clear flint or amber color. For decorative purposes, special colors such as blue, emerald green, and opal may be obtained from the glass manufacturer. Only amber glass and red glass are effective in protecting the contents of a bottle from the effects of sunlight by screening out harmful ultraviolet rays. The USP specifications for light-resistant containers require the glass to provide protection against 2900 to 4500 angstroms of light.[4] Amber glass meets these specifications, but the iron oxide added to produce this color could leach into the product. Therefore, if the product contains ingredients subject to iron-catalyzed chemical reactions, amber glass should not be used.

Glass for Drugs. The USP and NF describe the various types of glass and provide the *powdered glass* and *water attack* tests for evaluating the chemical resistance of glass. The test results are measures of the amount of alkalinity leached from the glass by purified water under controlled elevated temperature conditions. The powdered glass test is performed on crushed grains of a specific size, and the water attack test is conducted on whole containers. The water attack test is used only with type II glass that has been exposed to sulfur dioxide fumes under controlled conditions.

Type I—Borosilicate Glass. In this highly resistant glass, a substantial part of the alkali and earth cations are replaced by boron and/or aluminum and zinc.[5] It is more chemically inert than the soda-lime glass, which contains either none or an insignificant amount of these cations. Although glass is considered to be a virtually inert material and is used to contain strong acids and alkalies as well as all types of solvents, it has a definite and measurable chemical reaction with some substances, notably water. The sodium is loosely combined with the silicon and is leached from the surface of the glass by water. Distilled water stored for one year in flint type III glass (to be described) picks up 10 to 15 parts per million (ppm) of sodium hydroxide along with traces of other ingredients of the glass. The addition of approximately 6% boron to form type I borosilicate glass reduces the leaching action, so that only 0.5 ppm is dissolved in a year.

Type II—Treated Soda-Lime Glass. When glassware is stored for several months, especially in a damp atmosphere or with extreme temperature variations, the wetting of the surface by condensed moisture (condensation) results in salts being dissolved out of the glass. This is called "blooming" or "weathering," and in its early stages, it gives the appearance of fine crystals on the glass. At this stage, these salts can be washed off with water or acid. Type II containers are made of commercial soda-lime glass that has been de-alkalized, or treated to remove surface alkali. The de-alkalizing process is known as "sulfur treatment" and virtually prevents "weathering" of empty bottles. The treatment offered by several glass manufacturers exposes the glass to an atmosphere containing water vapor and acidic gases, particularly sulfur dioxide at an elevated temperature. This results in a reaction between the gases and some of the surface alkali, rendering the surface fairly resistant, for a period of time, to attack by water. The alkali removed from the glass appears on the surface as a sulfate bloom, which is removed when the containers are washed before filling. Sulfur treatment neutralizes the alkaline oxides on the surface, thereby rendering the glass more chemically resistant.

Type III—Regular Soda-Lime Glass. Containers are untreated and made of commercial soda-lime glass of average or better-than-average chemical resistance.

Type NP—General-Purpose Soda-Lime Glass. Containers made of soda-lime glass are supplied for nonparenteral products, those intended for oral or topical use.

Plastic Containers

Plastics in packaging have proved useful for a number of reasons, including the ease with which they can be formed, their high quality, and the freedom of design to which they lend themselves. Plastic containers are extremely resistant to breakage and thus offer safety to consumers along with reduction of breakage losses at all levels of distribution and use.

Plastic containers for pharmaceutical products are primarily made from the following polymers: polyethylene, polypropylene, polyvinyl chloride, polystyrene, and to a lesser extent, polymethyl methacrylate, polyethylene terephthalate, polytrifluoroethylene, the amino formaldehydes, and polyamides.[6]

Plastic containers consist of one or more polymers together with certain additives. Those manufactured for pharmaceutical purposes must be free of substances that can be extracted in significant quantities by the product contained therein. Thus, the hazards of toxicity or physical and chemical instability are avoided. The amount and nature of the additives are determined by the nature of the polymer, the process used to convert the plastic into the containers, and the service expected from the container. For plastic containers in general, additives may consist of antioxidants, antistatic agents, colors, impact modifiers, lubricants, plasticizers, and stabilizers. Mold release agents are not usually used unless they are required for a specific purpose.

Materials

At present, a great number of plastic resins are available for the packaging of drug products. A general description of the more popular ones are presented here.[1,3,7–9]

Polyethylene. High-density polyethylene is the material most widely used for containers by the pharmaceutical industry and will probably continue to be for the next several years.[10,11] It is a good barrier against moisture, but a relatively poor one against oxygen and other gases. Most solvents do not attack polyethylene, and it is unaffected by strong acids and alkalies.

Lack of clarity and a relatively high rate of permeation of essential odors, flavors, and oxygen militate against the use of polyethylene as a container material for certain pharmaceutical preparations. Despite these problems, polyethylene in all its variations offers the best all-around protection to the greatest number of products at the lowest cost.

The density of polyethylene, which ranges from 0.91 to 0.96, directly determines the four basic physical characteristics of the blow-molded container: (1) stiffness, (2) moisture-vapor transmission, (3) stress cracking, and (4) clarity or translucency. As the density increases, the material becomes stiffer, has a higher distortion and melting temperature, becomes less permeable to gases and vapors, and becomes less resistant to stress cracking. The molecular structure of high-density material is essentially the same as that of low-density material, the main difference being fewer side branches.

Since these polymers are generally susceptible to oxidative degradation during processing and subsequent exposure, the addition of some antioxidant is necessary. Usually levels of hundreds of parts per million are used. Antioxidants generally used are butylated hydroxy toluene or dilauryl thiodipropionate.

Antistatic additives are often used in bottle grade polyethylenes. Their purpose is to minimize airborne dust accumulation at the surface bottle during handling, filling, and storage. These antistatic additives are usually polyethylene glycols or long chain fatty amides and are often used at 0.1 to 0.2% concentration in high-density polyethylene.

Polypropylene. Polypropylene has recently become popular because it has many of the good features of polyethylene, with one major disadvantage either eliminated or minimized. Polypropylene does not stress-crack under any conditions. Except for hot aromatic or halogenated solvents, which soften it, this polymer has good resistance to almost all types of chemicals, including strong acids, alkalies, and most organic materials. Its high melting point makes it suitable for boilable packages and for sterilizable products. Lack of clarity is still a drawback, but improvement is possible with the construction of thinner walls.

Polypropylene is an excellent gas and vapor barrier. Its resistance to permeation is equivalent to or slightly better than that of high-density or linear polyethylene, and it is superior to low-density or branched polyethylene. One of the biggest disadvantages of polypropylene is its brittleness at low temperatures. In its purest form, it is quite fragile at 0°F and must be blended with polyethylene or other material to give it the impact resistance required for packaging.

Polyvinyl Chloride (PVC). Clear rigid polyvinyl chloride bottles overcome some of the deficiencies of polyethylene. They can be produced with crystal clarity, provide a fairly good oxygen barrier, and have greater stiffness. In its natural state, polyvinyl chloride is crystal clear and stiff, but has poor impact resistance. It can be softened with plasticizers. Various stabilizers, antioxidants, lubricants, or colorants may be incorporated. Polyvinyl chloride is seldom used in its purest form. It is an inexpensive, tough, clear material that is relatively easily processed. It must not be overheated because it starts to degrade at 280°F, and the degradation products are extremely corrosive. Polyvinyl chloride yellows when exposed to heat or ultraviolet light, unless a stabilizer is included by the resin supplier. It is virtually impossible to process vinyls at elevated temperatures without a stabilizing agent. From the standpoint of clarity, the best stabilizers are the tin compounds, but the majority cannot be used for food or drug products. Dioctyl-tin mercaptoacetate and maleate compounds have been approved by the FDA, but these have a slight odor, which is noticeable in freshly blown bottles. Other acceptable stabilizers (sulfur, calcium, and zinc salts) have a yellowish cast, which makes the plastic hazy and undesirable. In the formulation of PVC compounds with calcium-zinc stabilization materials, all ingredients are used in concentrations below their maximum extractable concentrations.

Polyvinyl chloride is an excellent barrier for oil, both volatile and fixed alcohols, and petroleum solvents. It retains odor and flavors quite well and is a good barrier for oxygen. Rigid polyvinyl chloride is a fairly good barrier for moisture and gases in general, but plasticizers reduce these properties. Polyvinyl chloride is not affected by acids or alkalies except for some oxidizing acids. Its impact resistance is poor, especially at low temperatures.

Much of the concern about the safety of plastic products has focused on polyvinyl chloride plastics and on compounds that are derived from vinyl chloride monomer. Its possible incrimination in the development of cancer of the liver (angiosarcoma) in some persons exposed to vinyl chloride monomer and polyvinyl chloride during manufacture has received widespread interest. Thus far, it seems that the only suspect is vinyl chloride, and the disease is not associated with polyvinyl chloride itself. Major reductions in the amount of residual vinyl chloride monomer have been achieved by PVC producers; the use of PVC for the fabrication of plastic bottles now represents the fastest growing application use of PVC in the United States.[12] PVC may also be used as a skin coating on glass bottles. This is accomplished by dipping the bottle in a PVC plastisol and curing the coating, which produces a shatter-resistant coating over the glass bottle.[12]

Polystyrene. General-purpose polystyrene is a rigid, crystal clear plastic. It has been used by dispensing pharmacists for years for containers for solid dosage forms because it is relatively low in cost. At present, polystyrene is not useful for liquid products. The plastic has a high water vapor transmission (in comparison to high-density polyethylene) as well as high oxygen permeability. Depending on the methods of manufacture and other factors, polystyrene containers are easily scratched and often crack when dropped. Polystyrene also easily builds up a static charge; it has a low melting point (190°F) and therefore cannot be used for hot items or other high-temperature applications. Polystyrene is resistant to acids, except strong oxidizing acids, and to alkalies. It is attacked by many chemicals, which cause it to craze and crack, and so it is generally used for packaging dry products only.

To improve impact strength and brittleness (both of which are sometimes referred to as practical toughness), general-purpose polystyrene may be combined with various concentrations of rubber and acrylic compounds. Certain desired properties diminish with impact polystyrene, e.g., clarity and hardness. The shock resistance or toughness of impact polystyrene may be varied by increasing the content of rubber in the material, and often these materials are further classified as intermediate-impact, high-impact, and super-impact polystyrene.

Nylon (Polyamide). Nylon is made from a dibasic acid combined with a diamine. Since there are many dibasic acids and many different amines, there is a great variety of nylons. The type of acid and amine that is used is indicated by an identifying number; thus, nylon 6/10 has six carbon atoms in the diamine and ten in the acid. Nylon and similar polyamide materials can be fabricated into thin-wall containers. Nylon can be autoclaved and is extremely strong and quite difficult to destroy by mechanical means. Important to the widespread acceptance of nylon is its resistance to a wide range of organic and inorganic chemicals. As a barrier material, nylon is highly impermeable to oxygen. It is not a good barrier to water vapor, but when this characteristic is required, nylon film can be laminated to polyethylene or to various other materials.

Its relative high-water transmission rate and the possibility of drug-plastic interaction have reduced the potential of nylon for long-term storage of drugs. Nylon 6, Nylon 6/6, Nylon 6/10, Nylon 11, and certain copolymers are cleared by FDA, subject to limitations or extractables.

Polycarbonate. Polycarbonate can be made into a clear transparent container. This relatively expensive material has many advantages, one being its ability to be sterilized repeatedly. The container is rigid, as is glass, and thus has been considered a possible replacement for glass vials and syringes. It is FDA-approved, although its drug-plastic problems have not been investigated adequately. It is only moderately chemically resistant and only a fair moisture barrier. The plastic is known for its dimensional stability, high impact strength, resistance to strain, low water absorption, transparency, and resistance to heat and flame.

Polycarbonate is resistant to dilute acids, oxidizing or reducing agents, salts, oils (fixed and volatile), greases, and aliphatic hydrocarbons. It is attacked by alkalies, amines, ketones, esters, aromatic hydrocarbons, and some alcohols.

Polycarbonate resins are expensive and consequently are used in specialty containers. Since the impact strength of polycarbonate is almost five times greater than other common packaging plastics, components can be designed with thinner walls to help reduce cost. Polycarbonate articles can be subjected to repeated sterilization in steam or water without undergoing significant degradation.

Acrylic Multipolymers (Nitrile Polymers). These polymers represent the acrylonitrile or methacrylonitrile monomer. Their unique properties of high gas barrier, good chemical resistance, excellent strength properties, and safe disposability by incineration make them effective containers for products that are difficult to package in other polymers. Their oil and grease resistance and minimal taste transfer effects are particularly advantageous in food packaging. This medium cost material produces a fairly clear container (not as brilliant as styrene). The use of nitrile polymers for food and pharmaceutical packaging is regulated to standards set by the Food and Drug Administration. The present safety standard is less than 11 ppm residual acrylonitrile monomer, with allowable migration at less than 0.3 ppm for all food products.

Polyethylene terephthalate (PET). Polyethylene terephthalate, generally called PET, is a condensation polymer typically formed by the reaction of terephthalic acid or dimethyl terephthalate with ethylene glycol in the presence of a catalyst. Although used as a packaging film since the late 1950s, its growth has recently escalated with its use in the fabrication of plastic bottles for the carbonated beverage industry. The development of the biaxially oriented PET bottle has had a major impact on the bottling of carbonated beverages, accounting for an estimated annual resin usage of approximately 350 million pounds. Its excellent impact strength and gas and aroma barrier make it attractive for use in cosmetics and mouth washes as well as in other products in which strength, toughness, and barrier are important considerations. Furthermore, the resin has been sanctioned for over 25 years by the FDA for food contact applications and has been the recipient of a favorable environmental impact statement.[13]

Other Plastics. Coextruded resins are being used to fabricate bottles and thermoformed blisters with barrier characteristics not previously attainable with single resins, resin blends, or copolymers. Coextrusion technology permits the use of high-barrier resins, such as ethylene vinyl alcohol, which could not be used alone because of either cost or physical or dimensional instability. The resins used in the coextrusion can be selected to provide optimum performance characteristics for the particular product needs. A coextrusion such as polypropylene/ethylene-vinyl-alcohol/polypropylene provides the mois-ture barrier of polypropylene coupled with the enhanced gas barrier of ethylene vinyl alcohol. Coextruded resins are providing packaging alternatives for products that previously were packaged only in glass.

High-barrier plastics that may compete with glass and metal containers may be available through a new processing technology developed by Du Pont Co. This technology involves dispersing nylon in a polyolefin resin so that the final polymer matrix contains a unique laminar arrangement of nylon platelets, which provide a series of overlapping barrier walls. Reportedly, this technique produces a plastic, which, when compared with the polyolefins, demonstrates a 140-fold increase as a barrier against certain hydrocarbons and an eightfold increase as a barrier for oxygen.

Drug-Plastic Considerations

A packaging system must protect the drug without in any way altering the composition of the product until the last dose is removed. The selection of a suitable package for a drug is not an easy task, inasmuch as an error can lead to serious consequences.

Drug-plastic considerations have been divided into five separate categories: (1) permeation, (2) leaching, (3) sorption, (4) chemical reaction, and (5) alteration in the physical properties of plastics or products.[6–8,14–17]

Permeation. The transmission of gases, vapors, or liquids through plastic packaging materials can have an adverse effect on the shelf-life of a drug. Permeation of water vapor and oxygen through the plastic wall into the drug can present a problem if the dosage form is sensitive to hydrolysis and oxidation. Temperature and humidity are important factors influencing the permeability of oxygen and water through plastic. An increase in temperature reflects an increase in the permeability of the gas.

Great differences in permeability are possible, depending on the gas and the plastic used. Molecules do not permeate through crystalline zones; thus, an increase in crystallinity of the material should decrease permeability. Two polyethylene materials may therefore give different permeability values at various temperatures.

Materials such as nylon, which are hydrophilic in nature, are poor barriers to water vapor, while such hydrophobic materials as polyethylene provide much better barriers.

Studies have also revealed that formulations containing volatile ingredients might change when stored in plastic containers because one or more of the ingredients are passing through the walls of the containers. Often, the aroma of cosmetic products becomes objectionable, owing to transmission of one of the ingredients, and the taste of medicinal products changes for the same reason.

The plastic container also may have an influence on the physical system making up the product. For example, certain water-in-oil emulsions cannot be stored in a hydrophobic plastic bottle, since there is a tendency for the oil phase to migrate and diffuse into the plastic.

A clearance of a plastic material from one manufacturer does not necessarily mean that the same type plastic from another blow-molder is equally satisfactory. Each bottle manufacturer has combined his own additives with the basic plastic, and each method of processing can be sufficiently different to seriously affect the stability of a product. Thus, after ascertaining that a plastic from one bottle manufacturer is satisfactory for the product, the drug or toiletry manufacturer should insist that the bottle manufacturer does not alter the components of the plastic bottle formulation or in any way alter the blow-molding process for fabricating the container.

Leaching. Since most plastic containers have one or more ingredients added in small quantities to stabilize or impart a specific property to the plastic, the prospect of leaching, or migration from the container to the drug product, is present. Problems may arise with plastics when coloring agents in relatively small quantities are added to the formula. Particular dyes may migrate into a parenteral solution and cause a toxic effect. Release of a constituent from the plastic container to the drug product may lead to drug contamination 'and necessitate removal of the product from the market.

Sorption. This process involves the removal of constituents from the drug product by the packaging material. Sorption may lead to serious consequences for drug preparations in which important ingredients are in solution. Since drug substances of high potency are administered in small doses, losses due to sorption may significantly affect the therapeutic efficacy of the preparation. A problem commonly encountered in practice is the loss of preservatives. These agents exert their activity at low concentration, and their loss through sorption may be great enough to leave a product unprotected against microbial growth.

Factors that influence characteristics of sorption from product are chemical structure, pH, solvent system, concentration of active ingredients, temperature, length of contact, and area of contact.

Chemical Reactivity. Certain ingredients that are used in plastic formulations may react chemically with one or more components of a drug product. At times, ingredients in the formulation may react with the plastic. Even micro-quantities of chemically incompatible substances can alter the appearance of the plastic or the drug product.

Modification. The physical and chemical alteration of the packaging material by the drug product is called *modification*. Such phenomena as permeation, sorption, and leaching play a role in altering the properties of the plastic and may also lead to its degradation. Deformation in polyethylene containers is often caused by permeation of gases and vapors from the environment or by loss of content through the container walls. Some solvent systems have been found to be responsible for considerable changes in the mechanical properties of plastics. Oils, for example, have a softening effect on polyethylene; fluorinated hydrocarbons attack polyethylene and polyvinyl chloride. Changes in polyethylene caused by some surface-active agents have been noted. In other cases, the content may extract the plasticizer, antioxidant, or stabilizer, thus changing the flexibility of the package. Polyvinyl chloride is an excellent barrier for petroleum solvents, but the plasticizer in polyvinyl chloride is extracted by solvents. This action usually leaves the plastic hard and stiff. Sometimes, this effect is not immediately perceptible because the solvent either softens the plastic or replaces the plasticizer; later, when the solvent evaporates, the full stiffening effect becomes apparent.

Selection of Proper Material

Some of the items to be considered in choosing the plastic material are listed in Tables 24-1, 24-2, and 24-3.

Also to be taken into consideration is the potential effect of wall thickness, which relates to barrier requirements of the package for its intended shelf-life.

Collapsible Tubes

Metal

The collapsible metal tube is an attractive container that permits controlled amounts to be dispensed easily, with good reclosure, and adequate protection of the product. The risk of contamination of the portion remaining in the tube is minimal, because the tube does not "suck back." It is light weight and unbreakable, and it lends itself to high-speed automatic filling operations.

Any ductile metal that can be worked cold is suitable for collapsible tubes, but the most common ones in use are tin (15%), aluminum (60%), and lead (25%). Tin is the most expensive, and lead is the cheapest. Since tin is the most ductile of these metals, small tubes are often made more cheaply of tin even though the metal cost is higher. Laminates of tin-coated lead provide the appearance and oxidation resistance of straight tin at lower prices.

The tin that is used for this purpose is alloyed with about 0.5% copper for stiffening. When lead is used, about 3% antimony is added to increase hardness. Aluminum work hardens when it is formed into a tube, and must be annealed to give it the necessary pliability. Aluminum also hardens in use, sometimes causing tubes to develop leaks.[1]

Tin. Tin containers are preferred for foods, pharmaceuticals, or any product for which purity is a paramount consideration. Tin is the most chemically inert of all collapsible tube metals. It offers a good appearance and compatibility with a wide range of products.

Aluminum. Aluminum tubes offer significant savings in product shipping costs because of their light weight. They provide the attractiveness of tin at somewhat lower cost.

Lead. Lead has the lowest cost of all tube metals and is widely used for nonfood products such as adhesives, inks, paints, and lubricants. Lead should never be used alone for anything taken internally because of the risk of lead poisoning. With internal linings, lead tubes are used for such products as fluoride toothpaste.

Linings. If the product is not compatible with bare metal, the interior can be flushed with wax-type formulations or with resin solutions, although the resins or lacquers are usually sprayed on. A tube with an epoxy lining costs about 25% more than the same tube uncoated.

Wax linings are most often used with water-base products in tin tubes, and phenolics, epoxides, and vinyls are used with aluminum tubes, giving better protection than wax, but at a higher cost. Phenolics are most effective with acid products; epoxides protect better against alkaline materials.

Plastic

This distinctive style of package, like its counterpart, the metal collapsible tube, excels in functional characteristics. Plastic tubes have a number of inherent practical advantages over other containers or dispensers. They are (1) low in cost, (2) light in weight, (3) durable, (4) pleasant to touch, (5) flexible, facilitating product dispensing, (6) odorless and inert to most chemicals, (7) unbreakable, (8) leakproof, and (9) able to retain their shape throughout their use. In addition, (10) they have a unique "suck-back" feature, which prevents product ooze. If too much product is dispensed with one squeeze, relaxation of hand pressure permits the product to be sucked back into the tube. If this feature is undesirable for fear of contamination, plastic tubes designed to avoid suck-back are available. Thus, the suck-back feature of plastic tubes can be an advantage or a disadvantage. When the tube is partly empty, however, this feature is a nuisance, because the air must be expelled before the product can be dispensed.

The sidewall of a plastic tube is extruded under heat and pressure as a continuous hose-like tubing and then is cut to length. The neck and shoulder are molded and joined to the tube in a separate automatic process. The tube is then decorated, mostly by offset printing. The tubes are capped with the bottoms remaining open for filling, after which they are heat-sealed to become as strong as any other part of the tube.

The most common types of material currently employed in plastic tubes are low- and high-density polyethylene. The former is less expensive and used more extensively. High-density polyethylene offers more protection than the uncoated low-density type. Coated high-density polyethylene is only slightly more protective than the coated low-density type, because in both instances, the coatings serve as a prime barrier.

Other materials include polypropylene and vinyl, but relatively high costs and various technical problems have limited their use.

Laminations

Permeation problems associated with plastic tubes, and corrosion and breakage problems experienced with metal tubes, have led to the emergence of a third type of collapsible tube, the *laminated* tube. This tube, constructed of a lamination containing several layers of plastic, paper, and foil, is fabricated from flat, printed stock. This lamination, which is specifically tailored to the product requirements, is welded into a continuous tube by heat sealing the edges of the lamination together in a machine called a "sideseamer." The tube is cut to length, and the

TABLE 24-1. *Plastic Bottle Chart*

Properties	Acrylic Multipolymer	Nitrile Polymers	Polyethylene		Polypropylene	Polystyrene	SAN (styrene acrylonitrile)	Vinyl (PVC)
			Low Density	High Density				
Resin density	1.09–1.14	1.10–1.17	0.91–0.925	0.95–0.96	0.89–0.91	1.0–1.1	1.07–1.08	1.2–1.4
Clarity[1]	Clear	Clear	Hazy transparent	Hazy translucent	Clear	Clear	Clear	Clear
Water absorption	Moderate	Moderate to low	Low	Low	Low	Moderate to high	High	Low
Permeability to: Water vapor	High	Moderate	Low	Very low	Very low	High	High	Moderate to low
Oxygen	Low	Very low	High	Moderate to high	Moderate to high	High	High	Low
CO_2	Moderate	Very low	High	Moderate to high	Moderate to high	High	High	Low
Resistance to: Acids	Poor to good	Poor to good	Fair to very good	Fair to very good	Fair to very good	Fair to good	Fair to good	Very good
Alcohol	Fair	Fair	Good	Good	Good	Poor	Poor	Very good
Alkalies	Poor to good	Good	Good	Good	Very good	Good	Good	Good
Mineral oil	Good	Very good	Poor	Fair	Fair	Fair	Fair	Good

Property							
Solvents	Poor	Fair	Good	Good	Good	Poor	Poor	Fair
Heat	Good	Fair	Poor	Fair	Good	Fair	Fair	Fair to poor
Cold	Poor	Poor	Excellent	Excellent	Poor to fair	Poor	Poor	Very poor
Sunlight	Good	Good	Fair	Fair	Fair	Fair to poor	Fair to poor	Good
High humidity	Fair	Excellent	Excellent	Excellent	Excellent	Excellent	Excellent	Excellent
Stiffness	Moderate to high	Moderate to high	Low	Moderate	Moderate to high	Moderate to high	Moderate to high	Moderate to high
Resistance to impact	Poor to good	Good	Excellent	Good	Fair to good	Poor to good	Poor to good	Fair to excellent
Unit cost	Moderate	High[2]	Low	Low	Low	Low	Moderate	Moderate
Typical uses	Foods, drugs, cosmetics	Foods, drugs, carbonated beverages, cosmetics, household chemicals, aerosols	Cosmetics, personal products, foods	Detergents, bleaches; milk, other foods; industrial cleansing powders; drugs, cosmetics	Drugs, cosmetics; syrups, juices	Dry drugs, petroleum jellies	Dry drugs	Shampoos, bath oils, detergents; whiskey, wine; floor waxes; vinegar, salad oil

[1]Bottles made from any of these resins are available in opaque colors.
[2]In production quantities, cost is expected to come down.
From Modern Packaging Encyclopedia. Volume 46, No. 12, McGraw-Hill, Inc., New York, 1973, Page 204.

TABLE 24-2. *Plastics Used for Drug Bottle Packaging*

Material (Density)	Inertness	Water Vapor Rate g/100 Sq in/24 hr @ 100°F, 95° RH	Oxygen Perm. cc/100 sq. in. @ 73°F/mil	Bottle Cost Relative to HDPE	FDA Acceptability for Foods
HIGH-DENSITY PE (0.955)	Outstanding	0.5	120	1	Yes
LOW-DENSITY PE (0.920)	Excellent	1.1	450	1.5	Yes
POLYSTYRENE (1.05)	Very poor	10.0	380	1.1	Yes
RIGID PVC (1.35)	Poor	2.7	15	2	Yes (some formulations)
POLYPROPYLENE (0.90)	Good to excellent	0.4	230	1.3	Yes
NYLON 6, 10 (1.10)	Good	2.9	3	3.0	Yes
POLYCARBONATE (1.20)	Poor	14.0	230	3.5	Yes
ACRYLIC MULTI-POLYMERS (1.10)	Fair	11.5	30	2.1	Yes

From Pinsky, J.: High-density polyethylene gets nod in Army Drug Packaging Study. Package Engineering, November, 1967.

head is injection-molded onto the tube. The head is typically molded of low-density polyethylene. Since some permeation through this molded head is possible, a head insert, made of urea formaldehyde, can be molded into the head to reduce product permeation.

Although not as impermeable as metal tubes, the laminated tube does provide a satisfactory level of barrier protection for a number of products. Laminated tubes initially served the dentifrice market but today are also found in pharmaceuticals, depilatories, hand creams, hair care products, and denture adhesives.[12]

TABLE 24-3. *Factors in Selecting a Liner*

1. Compatibility (chemical resistance)
2. Appearance, caliper, etc.
3. Gas- and vapor-transmission rates—WVTR, oxygen, CO_2, etc.
4. Removal torque
5. Heat resistance
6. Shelf-life
7. Economics

From Tang, T.: Liners and seals for closures. Modern Packaging Encyclopedia. Volume 46, No. 12, McGraw-Hill, Inc., New York, 1973, page 225.

Closures

The closure is normally the most vulnerable and critical component of a container insofar as stability and compatibility with the product are concerned. An effective closure must prevent the contents from escaping and allow no substance to enter the container. The adequacy of the seal depends on a number of things, such as the resiliency of the liner, the flatness of the sealing surface on the container, and most important, the tightness or torque with which it is applied. In evaluating an effective closure system, the major considerations are the type of container, the physical and chemical properties of the product, and the stability-compatibility requirements for a given period under certain conditions.

Closures are available in five basic designs: (1) screw-on, threaded, or lug, (2) crimp-on (crowns), (3) press-on (snap), (4) roll-on, and (5) friction. Many variations of these basic types exist, including vacuum, tamperproof, safety, child-resistant, and linerless types, and dispenser applicators.[18]

Threaded Screw Cap. When the screw cap is applied, its threads engage with the corresponding threads molded on the neck of the bot-

Color Clarity	Toughness/ Impact	Outstanding Advantages	Outstanding Disadvantages
Colorless, translucent	Excellent	Inertness, low cost, low WVT, toughness	Semi-opaque, transfer of taste ingredients, high dilute solution absorption
Colorless, hazy	Excellent	Squeeze property, inertness, low cost	Flexibility, relatively poor barrier to nonpolars, high WVT
Colorless, clear	Poor	Clarity, stiffness, low cost	High WVT, susceptibility to cracking, poor impact
Colorless, clear	Fair	Clarity, stiffness, O_2 barrier, retention of nonpolar materials	10–12 ingredients are possible; difficult processability, solvent susceptibility
Colorless, clear	Good (poor at 40°F and below)	Inertness, low cost, ESCR resistance	Low-temperature brittleness, tendency to unzip, highly stabilized content
Colorless, hazy	Excellent	Good barrier for nonpolars, tough, good O_2 barrier	Cost, water absorption, borderline for water-based materials
Colorless, clear	Outstanding	Very tough, clear, good oxygen barrier	Cost, susceptibility to solvent cracking, poor WVT, poor barrier
Colorless, clear-hazy	Good	Clarity, fair oxygen barrier, good for oils	Poor WVT, blushes, poor barrier

tle. A liner in the cap, pressed against the opening of the container, seals the product in the container by overcoming sealing surface irregularities, and provides resistance to chemical and physical reaction with the product being sealed.

The screw cap is commonly made of metal or plastics. The metal is usually tinplate or aluminum, and in plastics, both thermoplastic and thermosetting materials are used. Metal caps are usually coated on the inside with an enamel or lacquer for resistance against corrosion.

Almost all metal crowns and closures are made from electrolytic tinplate, a tin-coated steel on which the tin is applied by electrolytic deposition.

Lug Cap. The lug cap is similar to the threaded screw cap and operates on the same principle. It is simply an interrupted thread on the glass finish, instead of a continuous thread. It is used to engage a lug on the cap sidewall and draw the cap down to the sealing surface of the container. Unlike the threaded closure, it requires only a quarter turn.

The lug cap is used for both normal atmospheric-pressure and vacuum-pressure closing. The cap is widely used in the food industry because it offers a hermetic seal and handles well in sterilization equipment and on production lines.

Crown Caps. This style of cap is commonly used as a crimped closure for beverage bottles and has remained essentially unchanged for more than 50 years.

Roll-On Closures. The aluminum roll-on cap can be sealed securely, opened easily, and resealed effectively. It finds wide application in the packaging of food, beverages, chemicals, and pharmaceuticals. The roll-on closure requires a material that is easy to form, such as aluminum or other light-gauge metal.

Resealable, nonresealable, and pilferproof types of the roll-on closure are available for use on glass or plastic bottles and jars. The packager purchases these closures as a straight-sided, threadless shell and forms the threads on the packaging line as an integral part of the filling operation.

The roll-on technique allows for dimensional variation in the glass containers; each roll-on closure precisely fits a specific container.

Pilferproof Closures. The pilferproof closure is similar to the standard roll-on closure except that it has a greater skirt length. This additional length extends below the threaded portion to form a bank, which is fastened to the basic cap by a series of narrow metal "bridges."

When the pilferproof closure is removed, the bridges break, and the bank remains in place on the neck of the container. The user can reseal the closure, but the detached band indicates that the package has been opened. The torque necessary to break the bridges and remove the cap is nominal.

Non-Reusable Roll-On Closures. In some packaging applications a reusable cap is not desired. Non-reusable caps require unthreaded glass finishes. The skirts of these closures are rolled under retaining rings on the glass container and maintain liner compression. Closures of this type have tear-off tabs that make them tamperproof and pilferproof.

Closure Liners

A liner may be defined as any material that is inserted in a cap to effect a seal between the closure and the container.

Liners are usually made of a resilient backing and a facing material. The backing material must be soft enough to take up any irregularities in the sealing surface and elastic enough to recover some of its original shape when removed and replaced. It is usually glued into the cap with an adhesive, or the cap can be made with an undercut, so that the liner snaps into place and is free to rotate.

Factors in Selecting a Liner. Many factors have to be considered before an effective liner can be selected (Table 24-4). The most important consideration is that the liner be chemically inert with its product, so that the latter is protected against any possible change in purity or potency.

Gas and vapor transmission rates are usually relative and depend chiefly on the shelf-life required for the product. If the period between packing and consumer use is expected to be long, low transmission rates are necessary. Representative permeation rates are presented in Table 24-4.

Homogeneous Liner. These one-piece liners are available either as a disk or as a ring of rubber or plastic. Although they are more expensive and more complicated to apply, they are widely used for pharmaceuticals because their properties are uniform and they can withstand high-temperature sterilization.

Heterogeneous or Composite Liners. These are composed of layers of different materials chosen for specific requirements. In general, the composite liner consists of two parts: a facing and a backing. Usually, the facing is in contact with the product, and the backing provides the cushioning and sealing properties required.

TABLE 24-4. *Permeation Rate of Liner Facings**

Facing	Water	Alcohol
Polyethylene, 2-mil	0.07	0.06
Saran, 75-gauge	0.07	0.08
Aluminum foil, 1-mil	0.04	0.12
Tinfoil, 1-mil	0.09	0.20
Polyester, 50-gauge	0.12	0.10
Vinylite	0.20	0.03
Solvent-resistant	0.23	0.61
Yellow oil	0.28	0.85

*Loss in grams from a 2-oz bottle with 22-mm cap with cork-backed liner, 13 weeks at room temperature.

From Hanlon, J. F.: Handbook of Packaging Engineering. McGraw-Hill, Inc. New York, 1971.

Torque Testing

Controlling cap tightness on a packaging line with a torque tester can prevent evaporation or leakage of the product, breakage of a plastic molded closure, and application of a cap too tight to be removed. The Owens-Illinois torque tester is an instrument commonly used for this purpose.

Rubber Stoppers

Rubber is used in the pharmaceutical industry to make stoppers, cap liners, and bulbs for dropper assemblies. The rubber stopper is used primarily for multiple-dose vials and disposable syringes. The rubber polymers most commonly used are natural, neoprene, and butyl rubber.

In the manufacture of rubber closures, certain performance expectations require certain ingredients. The types of ingredients commonly found in a rubber closure are:

Rubber

Vulcanizing agent

Accelerator/activator

Extended filler

Reinforced filler

Softener/plasticizer

Antioxidant

Pigment

Special components, waxes

Since the composition of rubber stoppers is complex and the manufacturing process complicated, it is common to encounter problems with certain rubber formulas. For example, when the rubber stopper comes in contact with parenteral solution, it may absorb active ingredient, antibacterial preservative, or other materials, and one or more ingredients of the rubber may be extracted into the liquid. These extractives could (1) interfere with the chemical analysis of the active ingredient, (2) affect the toxicity or pyrogenicity of the injectable product, (3) interact with the drug preservative to cause inactivation, and (4) affect the chemical and physical stability of the preparation so that particulate matter appears in the solution.

Plastic Closures

The two basic types of plastics generally used for closures are thermosetting and thermoplastic materials. They differ greatly in physical and chemical properties, and fundamentally different manufacturing methods are used for each type.[3]

Thermosetting Resins. Phenolic and urea thermosetting plastic resins are widely used in threaded closures. The thermosetting plastic first softens under heat and then cures and hardens to a final state. Shaping must occur in the first stage of softening, because after curing there is no further mobility, even upon reapplication of heat and pressure. During the molding process, thermosets undergo a permanent chemical change, and unlike thermoplastic materials, they cannot be reprocessed. Since parts that are improperly molded must therefore be discarded, thermosetting materials are usually fabricated by compression molding. The manufacturing process is relatively slow, but allows better control and quick response to change in temperature and material flow.

Phenolics. Phenolic molding compounds are available in different grades and in dark colors, usually black or brown. Phenolics are used when a hard sturdy piece is needed, and when dark colors can be tolerated.

Rigidity, heat, chemical resistance, and strength are the outstanding properties of the phenolics. Color limitation is the main drawback, although coatings are available at a premium price. As a closure, the phenolic can withstand the torquing forces of the capping machines and maintains a tight seal over a long period of time.

The phenolics are resistant to some dilute acids and alkalies and are attacked by other, especially oxidizing, acids. Organic acids and reducing acids usually do not have any effect. Strong alkalies decompose phenolics.

Urea. This thermosetting resin is a hard translucent material that takes coloring well. It is more expensive than the phenolics, but the heat resistance and other properties of urea make it suitable for premium items. Elegant colors are obtainable with urea because the translucency gives brightness and color depth. Urea plastic is available in an unlimited range of colors and is a hard, brittle material that is odorless and tasteless. Being a thermosetting plastic, urea can withstand high temperatures without softening, but it chars at about 390°F. It absorbs water under wet conditions, but such absorption has no serious effect on the plastic.

Urea is not affected by any organic solvents, but it is affected by alkalies and strong acids. It has good resistance to all types of oils and greases. Although urea can withstand elevated temperature, it cannot be steam-sterilized. Parts may shrink as much as 0.003 inch after molding.

Thermoplastic Resins. Since their introduction, thermoplastics have become widely used in the manufacture of closures. Polystyrene, polyethylene, and polypropylenes are the materials used in 90% or more of all thermoplastic closures. Each material has specific performance advantages, and the particular resin used depends on the physical and chemical properties desired for the application and on the particular product being packaged.

Tamper-Resistant Packaging

In 1982, the vulnerability of over-the-counter (OTC) or nonprescription drug products to malicious adulteration was dramatically and tragically demonstrated with the tainting of Tylenol capsules with cyanide, which led to the deaths of several people. Public concerns about the safety of drug packaging led to various proposals by local municipalities for legislation regarding tamper-resistant packaging. To respond as quickly as possible to the safety concerns raised regarding OTC pharmaceutical packaging, and to assist the FDA in providing a consistent national standard governing tamper-resistant packaging, the Proprietary Association, a trade association for the Proprietary Pharmaceutical Industry, provided recommendations to the FDA, which were subsequently incorporated into FDA regulation 21 C.F.R. Parts 211, 314, and 700, which covers tamper-resistant packaging of OTC drugs.

The legislation enacted has had one of the greatest impacts on the packaging of pharmaceuticals in recent history. The requirement for tamper-resistant packaging is now one of the major considerations in the development of packaging for pharmaceutical products. As defined by the FDA, "a tamper-resistant package is one having an indicator or barrier to entry which, if breached or missing, can reasonably be expected to provide visible evidence to consumers that tampering has occurred. Tamper-resistant packaging may involve immediate-container/closure systems or secondary-container/carton systems or any combination thereof intended to provide a visual indication of package integrity when handled in a reasonable manner during manufacture, distribution, and retail display."

The visual indication is required to be accompanied by appropriate illustrations or precautionary statements to describe the safeguarding mechanism to the consumer. To reduce the possibility that the security mechanism can be restored after tampering, the FDA also requires either that the tamper-resistant feature be designed from materials that are generally not readily available (e.g., an aerosol system), or that barriers made from readily obtainable materials carry a distinctive design or logo that cannot be readily reproduced by an individual attempting to restore the package.

The following package configurations have been identified by the FDA as examples of packaging systems that are capable of meeting the requirements of tamper-resistant packaging as defined by FDA regulation 21 C.F.R. Parts 211, 314, and 700:

1. Film wrappers
2. Blister package
3. Strip package
4. Bubble pack
5. Shrink seals and bands
6. Foil, paper, or plastic pouches
7. Bottle seals
8. Tape seals
9. Breakable caps
10. Sealed tubes
11. Aerosol containers
12. Sealed cartons

The use of any of these concepts does not necessarily constitute compliance with the FDA ruling. The manufacturer must determine that the particular package concept provides tamper resistance for the manufacturer's specific product. By the same token, manufactures are not limited to the packaging concepts listed here, but have the flexibility of pursuing new packaging technologies that meet the objectives of the FDA ruling.

Film Wrapper

Film wrapping has been used extensively over the years for products requiring package integrity or environmental protection. Although film wrapping can be accomplished in several ways and varies in configuration from packaging equipment to packaging equipment, it can be generally categorized into the following types:

End-folded wrapper

Fin seal wrapper

Shrink wrapper

End-Folded Wrapper

The End-Folded Wrapper is formed by pushing the product into a sheet of overwrapping film, which forms the film around the product and folds the edges in a gift-wrap fashion as indicated in Fig. 24-1A. The folded areas are sealed by pressing against a heated bar. Because of the overlapping folding sequence of the seals, the film used must be heat-sealable on both surfaces. Materials commonly used for this application are cellophane and polypropylene. Cellophane, which is regenerated cellulose, is not inherently heat-sealable but requires a heat-seal coating to impart heat-sealing characteristics to the film. This is usually accomplished by coating the cellophane with either polyvinylidene chloride (PVDC) or nitrocellulose. Since PVDC also provides a durable moisture barrier, PVDC coated cellophane is often used for the overwrapping of products that are sensitive to moisture. Cellophane offers excellent machinability and crystal clarity, and for many years was the only clear film available for this type wrapping. In the early 1970s, polypropylene came onto the scene and represented a lower-cost alternative to cellophane. Because of the different handling characteristics of polypropylene, initial problems were experienced in obtaining satisfactory machinability. Machine modifications and the redesign of equipment led to the gradual replacement of cellophane by polypropylene, so that polypropylene now dominates the marketplace for this application. Heat-sealing characteristics are imparted to polypropylene by the use of heat-sealable acrylic coatings or by the addition of heat-sealable modifiers to the resin itself.

To be tamper-resistant, the overwrap must be

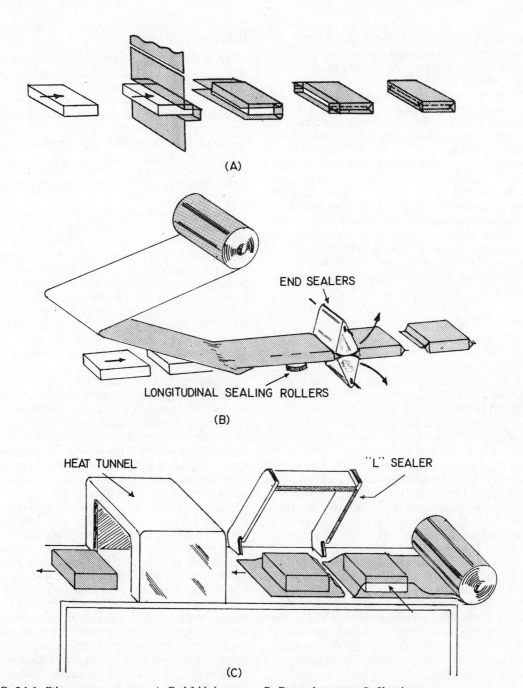

(A)

END SEALERS

LONGITUDINAL SEALING ROLLERS

(B)

HEAT TUNNEL

"L" SEALER

(C)

FIG. 24-1. *Film wrapper systems. A, End-folded wrapper. B, Fin seal wrapper. C, Shrink wrapper.*

well sealed and must be printed or uniquely decorated to exclude the possibility of having an alternate overwrap substituted in its place. The printed surface of the carton being overwrapped may also be coated with a heat-sensitive varnish, which causes the overwrap to bond permanently to the paperboard carton during the sealing of the overwrap. The removal of the overwrap would accordingly deface the carton, making the carton unsuitable for re-use.

Fin Seal Wrapper

Unlike the end-folded wrapper configuration, fin seal packaging does not require the product to act as a bearing surface against which the overwrap is sealed. The seals are formed by crimping the film together and sealing together the two inside surfaces of the film, producing a "fin" seal (Fig. 24-1B). Since the seals are formed by compressing the material between two heater bars (or nipping the film between pressure rollers) rather than sealing against the package, much greater and more consistent sealing pressure can be applied, and consequently, better seal integrity can be accomplished. For this reason, fin sealing has primarily been used when protective packaging is critical. Since the surface of the heat seal does not come in contact with the heated sealing bars on the packaging equipment, much more tenacious heat sealants, such as polyethylene or Surlyn,* can be used. With good seal integrity, the overwrap can be removed or opened only by tearing the wrapper.

Shrink Wrapper

Film overwrapping can also be accomplished with the use of a shrink wrapper. The shrink wrap concept involves the packaging of a product in a thermoplastic film that has been stretched and oriented during its manufacture and that has the property of reverting back to its unstretched dimensions once the molecular structure is "unfrozen" by the application of heat. The shrink wrap concept has a diversity of uses in packaging, one of which is its use as an overwrap. In this case, the shrink film is usually used in roll form, with the center folded in the direction of winding (Fig. 24-1C). As the film unwinds on the overwrapping machine, a pocket is formed in the center fold of the sheet, into which the product is inserted. An L-shaped sealer seals the remainder of the overwrap and trims off the excess film. The loosely wrapped product is then moved through a heated tunnel, which shrinks the overwrap into a tightly wrapped unit. The materials commonly used for this application are heat-shrinkable grades of polypropylene, polyethylene, and polyvinyl chloride. Since the various heat-shrinkable grades of film have different physical characteristics such as tear and tensile strength, puncture resistance, and shrinking forces, selection of the particular material used must be based upon specific product considerations so that the shrink wrap provides suitable integrity without crushing or damaging the product. The major advantages of this type of wrapper are the flexibility and low cost of the packaging equipment required.

*Du Pont's Ionomer Resin.

Blister Package

When one thinks of unit dose in pharmaceutical packaging, the package that invariably comes to mind is the blister package. This packaging mode has been used extensively for pharmaceutical packaging for several good reasons. It is a packaging configuration capable of providing excellent environmental protection, coupled with an esthetically pleasing and efficacious appearance. It also provides user functionality in terms of convenience, child resistance, and now, tamper resistance.

The blister package is formed by heat-softening a sheet of thermoplastic resin and vacuum-drawing the softened sheet of plastic into a contoured mold. After cooling, the sheet is released from the mold and proceeds to the filling station of the packaging machine. The semi-rigid blister previously formed is filled with product and lidded with a heat-sealable backing material. (Fig. 24-2). The backing material, or lidding, can be of either a push-through or peelable type. For a push-through type of blister, the backing material is usually heat-seal-coated aluminum foil. The coating on the foil must be compatible with the blister material to ensure satisfactory sealing, both for product protection and for tamper resistance. Peelable backing materials have been used to meet the requirements of child-resistant packaging. This type of backing must have a degree of puncture resistance to prevent a child from pushing the product through the lidding and must also have sufficient tensile strength to allow the lidding to be pulled away from the blister even when the lidding is strongly adhered to it. To accomplish this, a material such as polyester or paper is used as a component of the backing lamination. Foil is generally used as a component of the backing lamination if barrier protection is a critical requirement; however, metallized polyester is replacing foil for some barrier applications. A peelable sealant compatible with the heat-seal coating on the blister is also required since the degree of difficulty of opening is a critical parameter for child-resistant packaging. The use of peelable backing materials for blister packaging must be carefully evaluated to ensure that peel

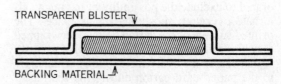

TRANSPARENT BLISTER

BACKING MATERIAL

FIG. 24-2. *Blister pack.*

TABLE 24-5. *Barrier Properties of Laminations*

Material	Oxygen Transmission*	Water-vapor Transmission†
0.002 saran/0.006 PVC	0.6	0.092
0.0015 Aclar/0.002 PE/0.0075 PVC	1.0	0.034
0.0015 Aclar/0.0075 PVC	1.1	0.035
0.002 PE/0.0075 PVC	1.3	0.170
0.0075 PVC	1.9	0.330
0.002 PE/0.005 PVC	2.6	0.200
0.005 PVC	2.7	0.520
0.001 nylon	25.0	19.000

*cc/24 hr/100 sq in. at 77°F, 50% RH.
†g/24 hr/100 sq in. at 95°F, 90% RH.
From Hanlon, J. F.: Handbook of Packaging Engineering. New York, McGraw-Hill, Inc., 1971.

strengths are sufficient to meet tamper-resistance objectives.

Materials commonly used for the thermoformable blister are polyvinyl chloride (PVC), PVC/polyethylene combinations, polystyrene, and polypropylene. For commercial reasons and because of certain machine performance characteristics, the blisters on most unit dose packages are made of polyvinyl chloride. For added moisture protection, polyvinylidene chloride (saran) or polychlorotrifluoroethylene (Aclar) films may be laminated to PVC. The moisture barrier of PVC/Aclar is superior to that of saran-coated PVC, especially under prolonged and extremely humid storage conditions. Listed in Tables 24-5 and 24-6 are several commonly used thermoformable blister materials and a comparison of their protective qualities.

Strip Package

A strip package is a form of unit dose packaging that is commonly used for the packaging of tablets and capsules. A strip package is formed by feeding two webs of a heat-sealable flexible film through either a heated crimping roller or a heated reciprocating platen. The product is dropped into the pocket formed prior to forming the final set of seals. A continuous strip of packets is formed, generally several packets wide depending on the packaging machine's limitations. The strip of packets is cut to the desired number of packets in length (Fig. 24-3). The strips formed are usually collated and packaged into a folding carton. The product sealed between the two sheets of film usually has a seal around each tablet, with perforations usually separating adjacent packets. The seals can be in a simple rectangular or "picture-frame" format or can be contoured to the shape of the product.

Since the sealing is usually accomplished between pressure rollers, a high degree of seal integrity is possible. The use of high-barrier materials such as foil laminations or saran-coated films, in conjunction with the excellent seal for-

TABLE 24-6. *Moisture Barrier Properties of Flexible Materials*

Material	Water-Vapor Transmission*
Aclar (fluorohalocarbon):	
22A, 1 mil	0.055
22A, 1½ mil	0.046
22C, 1 mil	0.045
22C, 2 mil	0.028
33C ½ mil	0.040
33C, 1 mil	0.025
33C, 2 mil	0.015
Cellulose acetate, 1 mil	80.000
Cellophane:	
140K	0.400
195K	0.450
195M	0.650
Polyester, 1 mil	2.000
Polyethylene:	
Low-density, 1 mil	1.300
High-density, 1 mil	0.300
Polypropylene, 1 mil	0.700
Polyvinyl chloride, 1 mil	4.000
Rubber hydrochloride, 1.2 mil	1.000
Saran (PVDC), 1 mil	0.200
Two-ply waxed glassine paper	0.500
Waxed glassine paper	3.000
Waxed sulfite paper	4.000

*g loss/24 hr/100 sq in./mil at 95°F, 90% RH.
From Hanlon, J. F.: Handbook of Packaging Engineering. McGraw-Hill, Inc., New York, 1971.

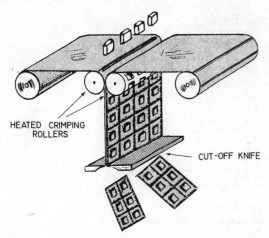

HEATED CRIMPING ROLLERS

CUT-OFF KNIFE

FIG. 24-3. *Strip packaging system.*

mation, makes this packaging mode appropriate for the packaging of moisture-sensitive products.

A number of different packaging materials are used for strip packaging. For high-barrier applications, a paper/polyethylene/foil/polyethylene lamination is commonly used. When product visibility is important, a heat-sealable cellophane or a heat-sealable polyester can be used. Also, the front and back of the package may use dissimilar materials. The choice of material used depends on both product and equipment requirements.

Bubble Pack

The bubble pack can be made in several ways but is usually formed by sandwiching the product between a thermoformable, extensible, or heat-shrinkable plastic film and a rigid backing material. This is generally accomplished by heat-softening the plastic film and vacuum-drawing a pocket into the film in a manner similar to the formation of a blister in a blister package. The product is dropped into the pocket, which is then sealed to a rigid material such as heat-seal-coated paperboard. If a heat-shrinkable material is used, the package is passed through a heated tunnel, which shrinks the film into a bubble or skin over the product, firmly attaching it to the backing card.

Shrink Banding

The shrink band concept makes use of the heat-shrinking characteristics of a stretch-oriented polymer, usually PVC. The heat-shrinkable polymer is manufactured as an extruded,

oriented tube in a diameter slightly larger than the cap and neck ring of the bottle to be sealed. The heat-shrinkable material is supplied to the bottler as a printed, collapsed tube, either pre-cut to a specified length or in roll form for an automated operation. The proper length of PVC tubing is slid over the capped bottle far enough to engage both the cap and neck ring of the bottle (Fig. 24-4). The bottle is then moved through a heat tunnel, which shrinks the tubing tightly around the cap and bottle, preventing the disengagement of the cap without destroying the shrink band. For ease of opening, the shrink bands can be supplied with tear perforations.

Foil, Paper, or Plastic Pouches

The flexible pouch is a packaging concept capable of providing not only a package that is tamper-resistant, but also, by the proper selection of material, a package with a high degree of environmental protection. A flexible pouch is usually formed during the product filling operation by either vertical or horizontal forming, filling, and sealing (f/f/s) equipment.

In the vertical f/f/s operation, a web of film is drawn over a metal collar and around a vertical filling tube, through which the product is dropped into the formed package (Fig. 24-5). The metal filling tube also acts as a mandrel, which controls the circumference of the pouch and against which the longitudinal seal is made. The formation of this seal, which can be either a fin seal or an overlap seal, converts the packaging film into a continuous tube of film. Reciprocating sealers, orthogonal to the logitudinal seal, crimp off the bottom of the tube, creating the bottom seal of the package. The product drops through the forming tube into the formed package. The reciprocation sealer moves up the film tube a distance equal to the length of the package and forms the top and final seal of the pack-

SHRINK TUBING

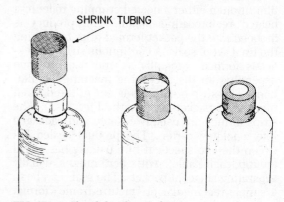

FIG. 24-4. *Shrink banding (tubing).*

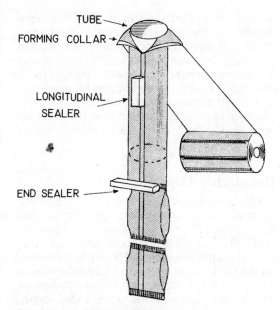

FIG. 24-5. *Vertical form/fill/seal system.*

age. This top seal of the package becomes the bottom seal of the next package and the process repeats itself. Since vertical f/f/s machines are gravity-fed, they are primarily used for liquid, powder, and granular products.

The horizontal f/f/s system is generally used for products of smaller volume, which are more amenable to the flatter format of the packages produced by this type of equipment. In this system, the web of film is folded upon itself rather than around a tube. As the folded film is fed horizontally through the equipment, a reciprocating platen creates pockets in the film by making vertical separation seals. The product is then placed into each pocket and the final top seal is made (Fig. 24-6). Packages formed on horizontal f/f/s equipment typically have a three-sided perimeter seal, but other variations are possible, depending on the type equipment used. The fin

seal wrapper illustrated in Figure 24-1B can be considered a type of horizontal f/f/s packaging system.

To provide the degree of package integrity required for tamper-resistant packaging on both horizontal and vertical equipment, inner-surface-to-inner-surface sealing should be used. This permits the use of such effective sealants as polyethylene, ethylene vinyl acetate (EVA), and Surlyn, which when properly sealed must be torn apart to access the product. These sealants must be used as part of a lamination constructed to provide the necessary characteristics for the proper performance of the packaging material. The outside surface of the lamination should provide a good printing surface and should be thermally stable since it comes into direct contact with the heater bars. The outside surface material is also used as the substrate carrier, which gives the lamination the mechanical characteristics necessary for the machining and handling of the package. The most commonly used film for a substrate carrier is paper. Polyester, nylon, and cellophane are also used if transparency, puncture resistance, or gloss are desired.

For moisture- and oxygen-sensitive products, foil is commonly used as part of the film lamination, with the foil sandwiched between the outer ply and the heat seal layer. Such laminations as paper/polyethylene/foil/polyethylene and polyester/polyethylene/foil/polyethylene are commonly used for high-barrier applications. Metallized polyester is replacing foil for some high-barrier packaging applications because of its lower cost, excellent appearance, and flexural endurance.

Bottle Seals

A bottle may be made tamper-resistant by bonding an inner seal to the rim of the bottle in such a way that access to the product can only

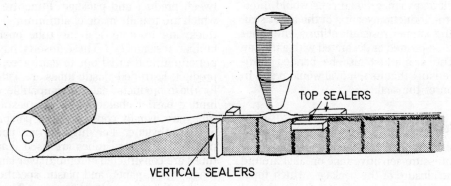

FIG. 24-6. *Horizontal form/fill/seal system.*

be attained by irreparably destroying the seal. Various inner seal compositions may be used, but the structures most frequently encountered are glassine and foil laminations.

Typically, glassine liners are two-ply laminations using two sheets of glassine paper bonded together with wax or adhesive. The inner seals are usually supplied inserted in the bottle cap and held in place over the permanent cap liner by either a friction fit into the cap or a slight application of wax, which temporarily adheres the seal to the permanent cap liner. If glue-mounted inner seals are to be used, glue is applied to the rim of the bottle prior to the capping operation. The application of the cap forces the inner seal into contact with the glued bottle rim and maintains pressure during glue curing and until the cap is removed. When the bottle cap is removed, the inner seal is left securely anchored to the bottle rim.

Pressure-sensitive inner seals can also be used. The pressure-sensitive adhesive is coated on the surface of the inner seal as an encapsulated adhesive. During the capping operation, the torque pressure ruptures the encapsulated adhesive, which then bonds the inner seal to the rim of the bottle. One type of pressure-sensitive inner seal is constructed of thin-gauge styrene foam innerseal material coated on one side with a specially formulated torque-activated adhesive. The adhesive has minimal surface tack, but when applied with a properly torqued cap, it provides excellent adhesion to both glass and plastic bottles.

A third method of application uses a heat-sensitive adhesive that is activated by high-frequency induction. This type of application requires the use of aluminum foil as part of the inner seal composition. Once the cap is applied, the bottle is passed under an induction coil, which induces high-frequency resonation in the foil. The frictional heat that is generated activates the heat-seal coating and bonds the liner to the bottle. This type of seal can only be used with plastic caps since metal caps would interfere with the induction sealing of the inner seal. To meet the tamper-resistant criteria, the inner seals must be printed or decorated with a unique design. The seal must also be bonded sufficiently to ensure that its removal would result in destruction of the seal.

Tape Seals

Tape sealing involves the application of a glued or pressure-sensitive tape or label around or over the closure of the package, which must be destroyed to gain access to the packaged product. The paper used most often is a high-density lightweight paper with poor tear strength. Labels made of self-destructing paper are available; these cannot survive any attempt at removal once they have been applied. To reduce further the possibility of removing the label intact, perforation or partial slitting of the paper can be made prior to application so that the label tears readily along those weak points if any attempt is made to remove it.

Breakable Caps

Breakable closures come in many different designs. The roll-on cap design used in the past for carbonated beverages uses an aluminum shell, which is placed over the bottle neck during the capping operation. The cap blank is held on the bottle under pressure while rollers crimp and contour the bottle tread into the cap blank. The bottom portion of the cap is rolled around and under the locking ring on the bottle neck finish. This lower portion of the cap blank is usually perforated so that it breaks away when the cap is unscrewed, which serves as a visible sign of prior opening. A ratchet-style plastic cap is also commonly used for a number of different products. In this design, the bottom portion of the closure has a tear-away strip, which engages a ratchet on the bottle neck. To remove the closure, the bottom portion of the closure must be torn away to disengage the ratchet and allow the removal of the cap.

Sealed Tubes

Collapsible tubes used for packaging are constructed of metal, plastic, or a lamination of foil, paper, and plastic. Metal tubes are still used for those products that require the high degree of barrier protection afforded by metal. Most of these are made of aluminum and are usually coated to eliminate compatibility problems between product and package. Puncture inserts, which are usually made of aluminum 3 to 5 mil thick, are used to seal the tube opening for tamper resistance.[19] These inserts have to be punctured and pried out to gain access to the product. Extruded plastic tubes are widely used for those products that are compatible with the limited barrier characteristics of plastic. These tubes are usually constructed of polypropylene or polyethylene. For high-barrier packaging, metal or laminated tubes are used. Laminated tubes are constructed of a multilayer lamination made of foil, paper, and plastic specifically tailored to the product requirements. The lamination is used for the body of the tube with the head injection molded onto the tube. Since the head is injection-molded, any number of designs are available that must be cut or broken to gain access to the product. These seal end designs are usually molded of low-density polyethylene. The tubes are filled from the other end and are sealed either by crimping the end in the case of metal tubes, or by induction sealing in the case of plastic or laminated tubes. Additional information can be found under the heading "Collapsible Tubes," a previous section in this chapter.

Aerosol Containers

The aerosol container used for pharmaceutical products is usually made of drawn aluminum. The inside of the container can be specially coated if product compatibility is a problem. A hydrocarbon propellant in its cooled liquid phase is added to the container along with the product, and a spray nozzle contained in a gasketed metal ferrule is crimped over the opening of the aerosol container. A length of polyethylene tubing, called a dip tube, is attached to the inside of the spray nozzle and dips into the product, drawing product into the spray nozzle when the sprayer is activated. The spray nozzles are usually metered to allow a specific dose to be dispensed with each spray. The design of the aerosol package makes it inherently tamper-resistant. See Chapter 20 for a further discussion on aerosol containers.

Sealed Cartons

Folding paperboard cartons have been used as a secondary package for OTC products for many years. The popularity of this packaging mode is based on both functional and marketing considerations. With the advent of mass marketing of OTC products in the self-service sections of larger stores, shelf presence and product stackability became a dominant consideration in the package design. The mass distribution of fragile products also placed a requirement on the secondary package for the prevention of breakage during distribution. Labeling requirements in many cases exceeded the limited copy area provided by the label on the primary container and consequently required additional copy area to be provided as either inserts or carton panels. All of these considerations were addressed with the use of a folding carton to contain the primary package.

The closure of folding cartons can be accom-plished in a number of ways. The most prevalent method has been the use of the "tuck end" design. The tuck end design feature allowed the ends of the carton to be held closed by the physical engagement of the side tabs at the open end of the carton, with the slits placed in the carton tuck or lid. This design feature, which has been prevalent in the folding carton industry because of its functionality and compatibility with high-speed packaging equipment, is no longer considered an acceptable closure mechanism for OTC products. If tuck end cartons are to be used, they must be augmented with some other form of tamper-resistant packaging such as film over-wrapping, tape sealing or glue sealing the carton. Seal end cartons differ from tuck end cartons in that rather than using the mechanical interlocking design of the tuck end to close the carton, externally applied glue or hot melt is used to provide carton sealing.

FDA Regulations

When the FDA evaluates a drug, the agency must be firmly convinced that the package for a specific drug will preserve the drug's efficacy as well as its purity, identity, strength, and quality for its entire shelf life. Under the provisions of the Federal Food, Drug and Cosmetic Act, however, no specifications or standards for containers or container closures are provided. Under the Act, it is the responsibility of the manufacturer to prove the safety of a packaging material and to get approval before using it for any food or drug product.

The FDA does not approve containers as such, but only the materials used in the container. A list of substances considered "Generally Recognized As Safe" (GRAS) has been published by the FDA. In the opinion of qualified experts they are safe under specified conditions, assuming they are of good commercial quality.

A material that is not included under GRAS or prior sanction, and is intended to be used with food, must be tested by the manufacturer, and the data must be submitted to the FDA.

The FDA has published regulations (part 133) that implement the Current Good Manufacturing Practice requirements of section 501 (a) of the Act.

Part 133.9 of these regulations sets forth criteria with respect to product containers, which manufacturers, processors, packers, or holders of drugs use as guidelines. The specific FDA regulation relative to drugs states that "containers, closures and other component parts of drug packages, to be suitable for their intended use, must not be reactive, additive or absorptive to an extent that the identity, strength, quality or purity of the drug will be affected."

Any drug container must be approved for such use, along with the drug, before going on the market. The drug manufacturer must include data on the container and package components in contact with the pharmaceutical product in its New Drug Application (NDA). If the FDA can determine that the drug is safe and effective, and that the package is suitable, it approves the drug and package. Once approved, however, the package may not be altered in any manner without prior FDA approval.

In the case of plastics, most resin manufacturers maintain Master Files on their resins with the FDA. Upon request from the resin manufacturer, the FDA uses this file as a reference to support a New Drug Application that which a drug manufacturer files.[20]

More detailed presentations on FDA regulations are included in Chapter 27, "Quality Control and Assurance," and Chapter 28, "Drug Regulatory Affairs."

References

1. Hanlon, J. F.: Handbook of Packaging Engineering. McGraw-Hill, New York, 1971.
2. Bacon, F. R.: Specifications of Glass Containers for Pharmaceutical Use. Owens-Illinois Co., 1970.
3. Modern Packaging Encyclopedia and Planning Guide. Vol. 46. McGraw-Hill, New York, 1973.
4. United States Pharmacopoeia XIX. Mack Publishing, Easton, PA. 1975.
5. Bacon, F. R.: The Chemical Durability of Silicate Glass. The Glass Industry. Vol. 49. 1968.
6. Cooper, J.: Plastic Containers for Pharmaceuticals Testing and Control. World Health Organization Publication, No. 4, 1974.
7. Autian, J.: J. Pharm. Sci., 52:1, 1963.
8. Autian, J.: J. Pharm. Sci., 52:105, 1963.
9. Modern Plastics Encyclopedia. Vol. 49. McGraw-Hill, New York, 1972–1973.
10. Athalye, A. S.: Popular Plastics, 16:28, 1971.
11. Pinsky, J.: Package Engineering, 12:74, 1967.
12. Package Engineering Encylcopedia. Cahners, Boston, 1982.
13. Modern Plastics Encyclopedia. Vol. 61. No. 10A. McGraw-Hill, New York, 1984–1985.
14. Autian, J.: Drug and Cosmetic Industry, 102:47, 54, 79, 1968.
15. Autian, J.: Bull. Par. Drug Assn., 19:142, 1965.
16. Griffin, R. C., and Saccharow, S.: Principles of Package Development. Ari Publishing, Westport, CT, 1972.
17. Varsano, J., and Gilbert, S. G.: Packaging of Pharmaceuticals in Plastic Containers and Films. Packaging Institute Report, October, 1968.
18. Source Book for Closures. Packaging Institute, New York, 1969.
19. A Look at 11 Solutions to O-T-C Tamper Packages. Package Engineering. Cahners, Volume 27, No. 13., December 1982.
20. Plastics Packaging for Drug Products—The Regulatory Story. The Society of the Plastics Industry Manual, New York, 1967.

25

Production Management

J. V. BATTISTA

Pharmaceutical manufacturing has long been recognized as a major industry in the United States. Its contribution to our economy is illustrated by the fact that it employs 158,000 people,* has a combined annual sales in human products of $12.9 billion, and has the second highest return on sales. When compared with all industries in the U.S. with regard to profit, most pharmaceutical corporations rank within the first 100 companies in profitability and invest proportionally more than others in research and development. In this regard, recent advances in biogenetics and gene modifications are ushering in a new era in disease treatment and the manufacture of pharmaceuticals. Clearly, then, the combination of marketing, research, manufacturing, finance, and sales reflects a high degree of professional management within the industry.

Production in a pharmaceutical company consists of the creation and maintenance of a clearly defined organization and makes effective and coordinated use of personnel, land, buildings, and equipment, including the management of inventory assets. All of these activities are performed in accordance with the highest standards and at the lowest total cost.

Before a new product can be marketed or an existing product significantly improved, the production department together with research, product development, sales, and marketing departments must define and agree upon costs, profits, marketing dates, and product quality.

All manufacturing in the pharmaceutical industry must be done in compliance with the FDA Good Manufacturing Practices Regulations (GMP); hence, all production personnel should understand GMP, at least as it applies to their

*This refers to those in the field of ethical products only.

particular area of responsibility. The deliberate contamination of drugs recently experienced in the distribution chain has added a new dimension to the responsibilities of production and has further emphasized the necessity of close and continuous cooperation between industry, FDA, and others in the protection of the public.

Good Manufacturing Practices (GMP)

To deliver to the public lifesaving drugs of the highest quality and purity, the pharmaceutical industry traditionally has cooperated with the Food and Drug Administration (FDA), even in recent years, when the regulatory agencies have become increasingly restrictive. The combined efforts of industry and government are reflected in the Good Manufacturing Practices Regulation (GMP) of 1971.[1] More recently, the FDA has increased surveillance by introducing the Intensified Drug Inspection Program (IDIP) and the Drug Enforcement Administration (DEA). In addition, the definition of drugs has been expanded to include devices and diagnostic products.

Personnel

The time-worn phrase, "Quality must be built into a product and cannot be inspected in," has a serious and particular application in pharmaceutical production. The quality control department can monitor production and indicate when a process is deviating from control standards, supply statisical data and constructive comments, and help in producing a quality product, but the production department bears the ultimate responsibility for quality. If a product fails, the production department is required to find and correct the problem.

Production is further supported by the engineering department, which must participate in such matters as the selection of equipment to ascertain that contact surfaces are not reactive or additive. Its services are basic in the matter of location of equipment and adequacy of dust pickup to prevent cross-contamination. Those in the engineering department should also be concerned with the air quality in sterile operations, the design and configuration of buildings to permit adequate storage and cleaning, proper sewage disposal, adequacy of potable water, and the like.

The GMP Regulations, although quite specific in some areas, can generally be regarded as broad and subject to wide interpretation by both the regulatory agencies and management in industry, as well as by operating personnel. In addition to adequate training and experience, the Regulations state that personnel should have "adequate information concerning the reason for the application of pertinent provisions of the GMP . . . to their respective functions." Comprehensive on-the-job training of both hourly and supervisory personnel should include interpretation of the Regulations as they apply to job responsibilities.

In most cases, the quality of production in one department has an important effect on the operations of another, and employees should be trained to understand such interrelationships. For example, if the tablet department is producing a product at the low end of the tablet hardness range, in turn causing excessive tablet breakage during packaging, then one department is transferring problems to another department, thereby making the problem more difficult and expensive to correct.

Training

It would be difficult to exaggerate the importance of personnel training. Since GMP touches on all areas of manufacturing, participation by engineering, quality control, materials handling, warehousing and distribution, purchasing, and other departments is a necessary step in ensuring compliance.

The training of hourly personnel in the manufacturing area is particularly important, since new employees may find themselves in a relatively technical environment, dealing with potent or dangerous chemicals, and working with a system of weights and measures that is unfamiliar to them. GMP clearly states that all materials going into a batch must be properly identified

and checked, and that during all steps in the manufacturing process, all containers, drying racks, and other equipment should clearly state the product name and lot number as well as the process stage. In packaging operations, a well-conceived line purgation system should ensure that all materials from a previous batch have been removed and that the new package order is properly identified with respect to the correct labeling as well as the batch number.

Shipping and distribution departments should ship only approved materials and should deal effectively with problems related to recording lot numbers on invoices, which is so critical in the development of a product recall system. Proper stock rotation and all other controls exercised at the producing location must also be provided and monitored at every warehouse and branch location. Warehousing personnel should understand the importance of any quarantine system for supplies and should never deliver unapproved materials to a processing department. In large operations, it may be difficult to place approval labels on every bag, drum, or container, and any substitute system must be clearly understood, be foolproof, and be acceptable to FDA. For these and other reasons, each employee must clearly understand why accuracy, cleanliness of operations, and strict adherence to instructions are necessary.

Written operating procedures are required under the Regulations, and they are considered helpful in an employee training program. A well-documented system and standardized procedures not only help personnel training, but also provide a basis for the development of a self-inspection program that will permit auditing of operations by production management from time to time to ensure continuing compliance. A typical self-inspection program for a packaging operation can be found in Eastern Regional Proceedings of PMA-FDA Seminar on "Quality Assurance in Drug Manufacturing."[2]

General Facilities

Sections 133.3 and 133.4 of the GMP Regulations indicate the far-reaching effect GMP has on buildings and equipment in terms of cross-contamination, sanitation, construction materials, environmental impact, equipment selection, and other factors. The value of land, buildings, and equipment represents one of the highest investments in assets by a pharmaceutical company. Improvements to avoid cross-contamination and other important problems, combined with higher costs of construction materials and labor, have caused building costs to escalate to a general average of $100 per square foot, with some specific departments running over $200 per square foot in 1982.

Cost

As an illustration of the importance of facilities, the depreciated asset values of land, buildings, and equipment of a few companies have been tabulated from 1984 annual reports (Table 25-1).

Such high expenditures in new facilities or in the refurbishment of existing ones makes it imperative that investments provide the best operations consistent with company policy and GMP requirements. Creating the best facilities and selecting the best equipment, therefore, require a continuing cooperative effort between production people who know the process parameters and engineering people who can provide the necessary designs. Such a cooperative effort avoids design and contraction mistakes, which may be expensive and difficult to correct at a later date. For example, it is best to invest in the right type of flooring for a particular area rather than incur high annual maintenance costs in cleaning or patching floors not properly specified for that area. Manufacturing areas have literally miles of service piping and ductwork overhead and along walls, and such exposed services result in high cleaning costs to avoid contaminating both the products and work areas below. Concealment of such construction errors is expensive.

In view of continuing escalation of construction costs and high cost of borrowing, companies with old or underutilized facilities have developed rationalization strategies in which operations have been consolidated into one or more plants and some facilities have been sold.

Construction materials, dust collection, and other facilities are discussed in greater detail later in this chapter.

TABLE 25-1. *Facilities Cost as Percentage of Total Assets*

	Land, Buildings, Equipment (In Millions of Dollars)	% of Total Assets
American Home Products	770	25
Warner-Lambert Co.	843	30
Merck	1913	42
Lilly	1280	35
G. D. Searle	496	30
Schering Plough	912	36

Space Allocation

As important as the provision of adequate space for production is the proper space allocation for each operation. A departmental analysis of space allocation is beyond the scope of this section, but a comparison of some major areas is of interest.

The data in Table 25-2 represent the facilities of a major pharmaceutical company whose operations extend to more than 45 countries and over 140 plants. Included in the tabulation are some domestic and international operations representing prescription products (Items 1, 5, 6, 7, & 8); proprietary products (Item 4); and for general comparative purposes, Items 2 and 3, which represent a combination of proprietaries and/or mints and chewing gum operations.

It is obvious that the production department and the warehouse occupy most of the space. One might also observe that plants 6, 7, and 8, whose total size is less than 500,000 square feet, require 21 to 39.3% of the total area for production. In plants occupying more than 500,000 square feet (1, 3, and 5), however, a significantly larger percentage of the plant (i.e., over 40%) is devoted to production.

The same table shows little percentage differ-

TABLE 25-2. *Space Allocation (Thousand Square Feet)*

	Total	Office	Production (%)		Warehouse (%)		Other
1.	1652.6	159.7	756.5	(45.7)	367.7	(22.2)	368.7
2.	615.8	7.5	163.3	(26.5)	196.3	(31.8)	248.7
3.	595.8	23.1	270.5	(45.4)	172.1	(28.8)	130.1
4.	502.7	23.4	128.3	(25.5)	300.7	(59.8)	50.3
5.	502.6	24.5	207.3	(41.2)	215.5	(42.8)	55.3
6.	304.5	40.9	84.4	(27.7)	70.5	(23.1)	108.7
7.	286.2	16.7	57.3	(21.0)	77.1	(26.9)	135.1
8.	77.7	3.2	30.6	(39.3)	16.0	(20.5)	27.9

ence in the space occupied by the warehouse, regardless of plant size. The only exceptions are plant 5, which includes a significantly larger biologic operation, and plant 4, which is a proprietary operation and has the highest warehousing occupancy of plants over 500,000 square feet and the smallest production area— just a reversal of the space allocations in pharmaceutical manufacturing. This operation is dominated by a few high-volume proprietaries that require large continuous manufacturing operations, thus minimizing space needs for production while increasing the size of warehousing areas.

Plant 2 is a combination of high-volume proprietaries and gum operations, a substantial number of which require large-batch and continuous operations. The result is a production area that is slightly smaller than the warehouse. Plant 3, a pressed mints and gum operation, is largely automated, but the massive equipment occupies considerable space. On the other hand, although there is a high volume of case goods, the product is small and compact, and less space is needed for the warehouse.

In addition to space allocation by these broad categories, GMP Section 133.3 (Buildings) states that adequate space must also be provided for the following: (1) orderly placement of equipment and materials to minimize mixups or cross-contamination; (2) receipt and storage of all material in a quarantine area prior to use; (3) holding of rejected materials; and (4) manufacturing and processing operations and others.

Environmental Factors

Materials, Lighting, and Air-Conditioning Specifications

Section 133.3 and subsection (b) of GMP refer to adequate cleaning, construction, lighting, ventilating, and other important factors in a production operation. Since the word "adequate" is used throughout GMP, one cannot be specific with respect to the amount of lighting in each department, the type of ventilation, or the materials of construction for floors and walls.

Based on personal preference and on the experiences of other companies, a choice can be made from an enormous array of available materials. These decisions are important when a new building is being designed, but become extremely difficult in the redesigning of an old facility, in which case ceiling heights, wooden floors, and other outmoded features must be taken into consideration.

One of the most significant steps taken to provide industry-wide information in these areas was a survey made by the Production and Engineering Section of the Pharmaceutical Manufacturing Association (PMA) in 1967 and updated in 1973. This publication is entitled "Survey of Current Manufacturing Practices in the Drug Industry," and it is divided into three chapters— Personnel, Buildings, and Equipment. In response to questionnaires sent out to both large and small members of PMA, a detailed summary of information has been compiled that represents a cross section of practices and materials utilized in the industry.

Table 25-3 provides a departmental checklist with a selection of materials that have proven durable over the years for walls, floors, and ceilings. Levels of lighting and general air-conditioning requirements are also listed. In the selection of construction materials, initial costs are only a partial consideration, since maintenance enters into the total cost.

The selection of decorating colors in the manufacturing and office areas is important, especially in plants with few or no windows. The sectional use of different colored paints in long corridors avoids a tunnel-like impression; and the hanging of washable wallpaper in such areas as the packaging room provides both pleasant surroundings and low maintenance costs.

Dust Collection and Cross-Contamination

Cross-contamination constitutes an ever-present danger in pharmaceutical manufacturing. Identification and removal of its causes have had a profound effect on plant layout as well as on the design and construction of production areas. In many cases, a reassessment of dust collection requirements and specifications has been necessary. For example, the development of increasingly sensitive test methods for penicillin, coupled with the awareness that some individuals are extremely sensitive to this antibiotic, necessitated a complete relocation of penicillin production into a separate facility away from all other operations to avoid possible cross-contamination.

Types of Dust-Collecting Systems. Although many types of dust collectors are available, the selection of equipment should be based primarily on its intended application. Cyclone collectors, for example, have limited application in pharmaceutical production except for their use in a spray-drying operation in which large volumes of powder are processed on a continu-

TABLE 25-3. *Facilities Guide for GMP*

	Chemical Weighing	Granulating	Tabletting	Coating	Liquid Manufacturing	Packaging	Warehousing
Floors							
High-density concrete	X	X	X	X	X	X	X
Troweled epoxy finish	X	X	X		X		
Terrazzo epoxy finish	X	X	X				
Concrete w/metal chips	X	X	X	X	X	X	X
Drains	X		X	X		X	X
Vinyl asbestos tile							
Walls							
Smooth	X	X	X	X	X	X	X
Epoxy paint	X	X	X	X	X	X	X
Washable	X	X	X	X	X	X	X
Glazed tile	X	X	X	X	X	X	
Wallpaper (washable)							
Ceilings							
Hung	X	X	X	X	X	X	
Acoustical	X		X	X	X	X	
Smooth waterproof		X					X
Open							
Lighting							
Footcandles	75	100	100	75	75	75	50
Flush mounted	X	X	X	X	X	X	
Air Conditioning							
Optional		X	X		X		
Comfort control	X	X	X		X	X	
45% RH/72°F				X			
<20% RH/72°F							

ous basis. On the other hand, replaceable filters, cloth bags, wet scrubbers, and high-efficiency particulate air filters (HEPA), or a combination of some of these, are commonly used.

Wet Collectors. A *wet scrubber* operates by mixing the dust-laden air stream with water in an enclosed chamber, which discharges the effluent into the sewer or treatment plant. A *Rotoclone* operates by spraying the air in the collector and mixing it by means of high-speed paddles. This type of scrubber is efficient and uses a minimal amount of water. Both systems are particularly effective when a dye is used as the component of a dosage form, and it is therefore necessary to prevent trace quantities from contaminating nearby operations. Either process can be used when water-soluble, volatile solvents are used in pharmaceutical manufacturing, since the entrained vapors are diluted with water to a safe level of concentration.

Filters, Bags, and High-Efficiency Particulate Air Filter. The most commonly used dust collectors are the *replaceable filter, cloth bag,* and *HEPA* types. In large operations, the collectors are placed on the roof or on a mezzanine. These air filters are rated on an efficiency basis as defined by the National Bureau of Standards (NBS) and the American Filter Institute (AFI), utilizing the Dioctyl-phthalate (DOP) test method. Figure 25-1 illustrates a DOP efficiency table for particles in the 0.3-micron range. For example: Astrocel would be rated at 99.97% efficiency, but selection of Varicel 50 lowers efficiency to 35%. Other tables are available for various particle sizes.

HEPA filters are effective at 100% in particle ranges of a few microns, and at one time, these were used exclusively in sterile operations to reduce particulate matter. The current emphasis on reducing cross-contamination, however, has resulted in their use in many dry-product operations, such as granulating, tableting, and capsule filling.

The handling of products containing at-

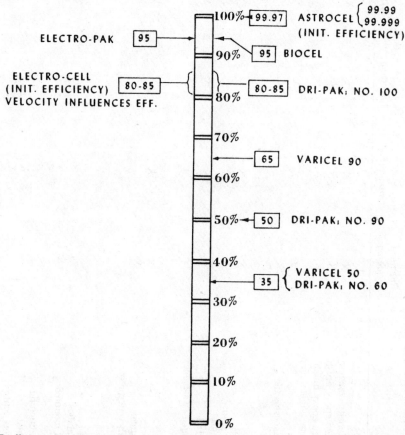

FIG. 25-1. *DOP efficiency. Dioctyl-phthalate aerosol averaging 0.3 microns. Determinations made by light-scattering method. Average value over life of media unless otherwise noted.*

tentuated viruses requires the use of HEPA filters with no return air circulation as a minimum precaution. When viable pathogenic viruses or other dangerous organisms are being processed, it is best to incinerate all exhaust air at a temperature above 800°F.

Departmental Specifications. In addition to selecting the correct type of dust collector for each department, it is desirable to provide the air volume and velocity required for the collector to do its job effectively. One of the most common failures in dust collection is an insufficient air velocity to carry all particles from the pickup location to the collector, and the most sophisticated unit can become ineffective, especially if it is located some distance away from the pickup location. For example, the dust pickup stations on a tablet press should handle not only the fine and coarse granulation, but also broken tablet pieces that may have been picked up on the turntable or placed there by the press operator.

Chemical Weighing. Figure 25-2 shows a typical weighing operation, with units located in booths, each equipped with a dust collection hood. Although a point-of-use collector may be used, a central unit gives better results when a large room is required or when several weighing booths are used. In such cases, HEPA filtration should be used. The hood for each 14 × 15 foot booth should have a capacity of 4500 cfm with a face velocity in excess of 150 feet per minute.

Tablet Granulating and Compressing. Since granulating operations use several different pieces of equipment, each with its own unique problems, dust collection can best be described in general terms. If the area is air-conditioned, it is possible to minimize cost by reusing 85% of the air, provided an HEPA filter is used. Flexible 3- or 4-inch hoses should have an air capacity of 200 to 300 cfm and a linear velocity of more than 2500 feet per minute for best results. When applied to tablet presses, however, at least 450 cfm and a velocity of over 3000 feet per minute are needed.

Coating and Tablet Packaging. A typical 42-inch coating pan should have a supply inlet of 200 cfm and an exhaust of 300 cfm when standard ducts are used. Absolute filters are preferable if 85% of the air is to be recirculated.

If solvent-type film coating is performed in a conventional Accela Cota or Pellegrini pan, not only does air volume have to be increased substantially, but the discharged air must be treated to conform to local and government environmental standards.

Flexible hoses used at tablet counters, powder fillers, and cottoning machines should handle about 200 to 300 cfm at a minimum velocity of 2000 feet per minute.

A Guide to Pharmaceutical Manufacturing Facilities

The following information on manufacturing facilities provides a guide to good manufacturing practices for a number of pharmaceutical operations.

Chemical Weighing

This first important step in the manufacturing process has been receiving an increasing amount of attention because of possibilities for cross-contamination and misbranded products due to incorrect ingredients or quantities. Many companies have adopted a central weighing department to service all of the processing areas. The advantages of this system are the centralization of responsibility, the avoidance of duplicating weighing facilities, and lower labor costs. After an item is weighed and properly initialed on the batch sheet by the weigher, check-weighed and initialed by a checker, and properly packaged and identified, additional weighing at the point of use is usually unnecessary. A chemical weighing department should be designed to provide supervision, checkers, proper weighing equipment, lighting, dust collection, and adequate sanitation.

High-potency drugs such as steroids and alkaloids should be weighed in a separate room equipped with absolute filters to avoid even minimal cross-contamination. This room could also be used for weighing dyes (see Fig. 25-2).

Sinks and drain boards should be conveniently located to facilitate frequent cleaning of measuring equipment. Cabinets should be provided for the storage of utensils.

Vacuum hoses should be available in the weighing area immediately adjacent to the weighing booths so that the tops of drums and other containers can be cleaned free of dust before they are opened for removal of contents.

Balances and scales having the proper capacity and sensitivity needed for weighing operations should be specified, and arrangements made for frequent calibration. Printing scales that record weights on formula sheets and container labels should also be provided.

Meters should be used when liquid materials are transferred from storage tanks directly to manufacturing tanks. Each quantity should be recorded on batch sheets, either manually or by

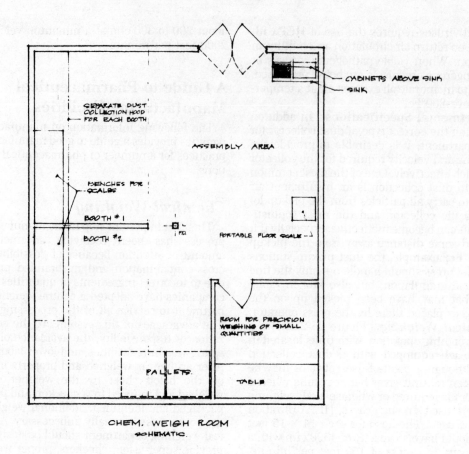

CADINETS ABOVE SINK

SINK

SEPARATE DUST
COLLECTION HOOD
FOR EACH BOOTH

ASSEMBLY AREA

BENCHES FOR
SCALES

BOOTH #1

BOOTH #2

PORTABLE FLOOR SCALE

ROOM FOR PRECISION
WEIGHING OF SMALL
QUANTITIES

PALLETS

TABLE

CHEM. WEIGH ROOM
SCHEMATIC

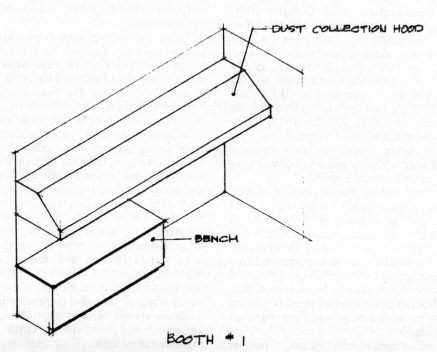

DUST COLLECTION HOOD

BENCH

BOOTH #1

FIG. 25-2. *Top, Two weighing booths together with enclosed room for weighing steroids and the like. Bottom, Work bench and hood, which should be connected to dust collector.*

means of a printing system. The meters should be calibrated and checked periodically.

Tablet Granulating

In general, several different products are in production at any given time. The numerous steps in the granulating procedure increase the possibilities of cross-contamination, incorrect product identification, and/or mixups. To eliminate these possibilities, a separate room or booth is recommended for each step. Thus, more space is required and maintenance costs are higher because the equipment and each room must be thoroughly cleaned between operations. In many cases, the cleaning costs are buried in the indirect labor category, when truly it represents changeover costs as in a packaging operation.

Compartmentalizing the granulating process has, unfortunately, fragmented the operation and increased space, capital, and labor costs. Granulating should be considered a unit operation composed of closely integrated manufacturing steps, and process development work should be directed to this area for cost reduction and process improvement. Such effects help reduce granulating costs, which are invariably higher than tabletting costs when compared on a cost-per-thousand-tablet basis.

A washing facility (Fig. 25-3) should be available for cleaning portable equipment such as granulators and mills. To facilitate cleaning of nonportable equipment, such as fluid-bed driers, mixers, etc., each room should be provided with floor drains and a pitched floor ($\frac{1}{8}$ inch per foot) as well as hot and cold water and steam for special cleaning jobs. Particular attention should be devoted to the cleaning of drying racks and trays, which should be designed for easy cleaning and made of stainless steel or other nonrusting material.

If the department is not air-conditioned, all windows should be screened against the entrance of insects.

The aforementioned precautions are equally applicable to the manufacturing of powders and bulk materials for capsule filling.

Tablet Compressing

Booths or Rooms. Separate rooms for tablet machines have now become a necessary design feature to avoid cross-contamination. When special low-humidity conditions are necessary to ensure product stability, a chemical unit employ-

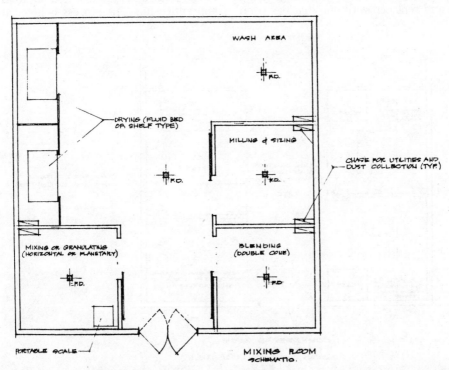

FIG. 25-3. *Typical granulating room showing separation of milling, blending, and granulating areas. Note drain in each area.*

ing lithium or silica gel is satisfactory for relative humidity levels below 20%. Such rooms should have special low vapor transmission treatment of walls and should be equipped with air locks.

Since it is now common practice to place each tablet press in its own separate location when in operation, the rooms can all be the same size or vary in size to accommodate the smallest and largest presses. When large volumes are being produced, for instance, it is practical to have a booth or room large enough to accommodate two or more tablet machines for the same batch (Fig. 25-4). The booth walls should extend from floor to ceiling and may be made of tile up to the four- or five-foot level, with a glass or transparent partition extending it to the ceiling. Tile or other hard surfaces in these booths should be used sparingly, since they contribute to the noise level. Space should also be provided for in-process testing equipment such as balances and tablet hardness testers.

Tablet Presses. Each press should be mounted on metal frames so that it can be moved by lift trucks into a cleaning area. The number of booths or rooms needed in the compressing department usually does not equal the number of tablet presses on hand, since all presses are not likely to be in operation at the same time. Once a batch has been completed, the machine should be removed promptly from the booth and replaced with one that has been cleaned and prepared for the next product. A room should be made available nearby for the cleaning of presses and replacement of punches and dies for the next product.

The exact number of tablets produced is compared to the expected yield by a process called *reconciliation*. A major discrepancy between theoretic and actual yeilds signifies that an error may have been introduced at some stage of the procedure. To discover the discrepancy, rotary presses should be equipped with automatic counters, which can be set to place the same number of tablets in each bulk drum, thereby facilitating accountability calculations and taking physical inventory. A schematic drawing of a simple mechanical counter for a double rotary press is represented in Figure 25-5. The double rotary press is equipped with a gate that is activated by a signal after a container is filled with a preset number of tablets to divert subsequent tablets into a second container placed nearby.

In this regard, commercial equipment is available that not only will count tablets but also will monitor and adjust presses to conform to weight standards.

Tablet Coating

Traditionally, tablet coating has been considered an art and has required a rather lengthy apprenticeship. The process is noisy and dusty,

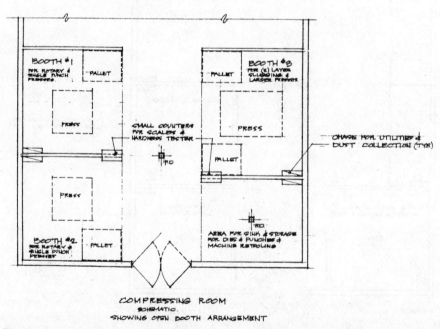

FIG. 25-4. *Two booth sizes designed to accommodate single or small rotary presses or larger slugging or multi-layer presses.*

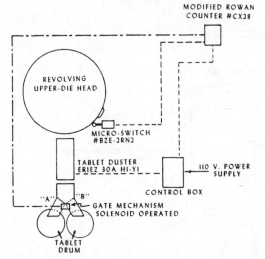

FIG. 25-5. *Mechanical tablet counter for a double rotary press.*

The figure labels read:
MODIFIED ROWAN COUNTER #CX28
REVOLVING UPPER-DIE HEAD
MICRO-SWITCH #BZE-2RN2
TABLET DUSTER ERIEZ 30A HI-YI
110 V. POWER SUPPLY
CONTROL BOX
"A" "B"
GATE MECHANISM SOLENOID OPERATED
TABLET DRUM

and since one person operates about five pans, it is a labor-consuming and somewhat inefficient procedure. In recent years, a number of technologic developments have removed some of the "art" and substituted automated techniques that have increased pan sizes and improved the drying cycles. Automated spray coating is now available, and new products as well as old ones are being given a film coating or an abbreviated thin sugar coating applied by mechanical rather than manual methods.

These technologic changes have necessitated a new approach to the design and layout of a coating department, but some of the fundamental considerations still apply. For example, regardless of coating pan size or of whether coatings are applied manually or by spraying, the pans are placed in line and may be freestanding or enclosed (Fig. 25-6). Dust collection considerations as previously described are still important even though some new designs in pans vent the dust through the back of the pan.

Enclosing pans in groups of five or more offers some advantages. The enclosure muffles the noise level to acceptable limits. This is particularly helpful in a large coating operation when the noise level approaches the maximum permitted under the OSHA (Occupational Safety and Health Administration) maximum average (80 decibels). The noise level can also be reduced in open pans by the use of insulating material or foam around the outside of the coating pan, but product temperature control is thus rendered more difficult. As indicated in Figure 25-6, each pan can be equipped with a window that can be closed during dusty operations,

thereby improving dust collection and reducing cross-contamination hazards.

Polishing cans of either the metal or cloth type should be isolated from the general coating operation, and any solvent-laden exhaust should be sufficiently diluted with air to meet fire and environmental standards of safety.

Adequate cleaning of floors and equipment can be a problem in coating operations because of dust and the frequent use of dyes. Sufficient floor drains should be provided for this purpose, and pumps should be used for the transfer of wash water from coating pans to either floor drains or nearby sinks. For large operations in which coating solutions made with dyes are formulated, it is desirable to have a small adjacent room equipped with a sink and mixing equipment for this purpose.

If coated tablets are imprinted with a monogram or a product identification number, each printing machine should be in a separate booth to avoid cross-contamination. If an in-line, one-at-a-time printing machine is used, each machine should be equipped with an electric eye or other counting device to count tablets as they move down the discharge chute. Such devices give the official yield and can be used for product reconciliation. In addition, if it is necessary to inspect coated tablets, the inspection equipment should be placed in separate booths.

Manufacturing of Liquids

In locations where oral, external, or cosmetic preparations are made, it is necessary to have separate facilities for each group. If this is not possible, a separating wall should be constructed to isolate one group from another, thereby preventing cross-contamination and the transference of odors.

Special attention should be given to the design and installation of equipment and washing facilities, especially those used for products that are susceptible to microbiologic contamination. Sanitary pumps and fittings should be used, together with stainless steel tubing with snap-on connections, to facilitate easy removal and cleaning. Troughs should also be available to permit the cleaning and soaking of piping and transfer lines on an overnight basis. They should be made of materials that withstand commercially available detergents and germicidal solutions, e.g., stainless steel.

Although the use of potable water is necessary in all operations, it is particularly important in liquid manufacturing. If deionizers and other water treatment equipment are used, special at-

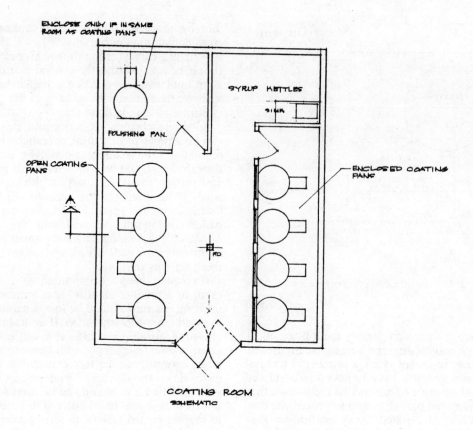

ENCLOSE ONLY IF IN SAME
ROOM AS COATING PANS

SYRUP KETTLES

SINK

POLISHING PAN

OPEN COATING
PANS

ENCLOSED COATING
PANS

FD

COATING ROOM
SCHEMATIC

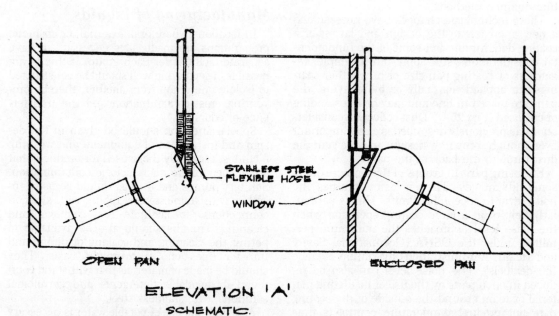

STAINLESS STEEL
FLEXIBLE HOSE

WINDOW

OPEN PAN

ENCLOSED PAN

ELEVATION 'A'
SCHEMATIC.

FIG. 25-6. Top, *An enclosed bank of coating pans. Polishing pans should be in a different location from coating pans.* Bottom, *Differences between open and enclosed pans.*

tention must be given to routine microbiologic and chemical testing. Storage tanks and piping used for bulk storage of such liquids as glycerin and mineral oil should be constructed to facilitate examination as well as cleaning.

Good Manufacturing Practices requires accurate yields for liquid preparations and reconciliation of yields as in solid dosage forms. If the same tanks are used to manufacture more than one product, liquid meters and tank calibrations are important to product reconciliation. In many cases, it is practical to install on each tank load cells that provide readout of its contents.

Manufacturing tanks located on either side or around a work platform or gantry should be sufficiently far away from each other to avoid cross-contamination, especially when dry powders are an ingredient. The elevated platforms should be sufficiently large to permit the positioning of pallets or raw materials around the tanks and still provide sufficient room for the separation of adjoining tanks.

Packaging

Packaging lines should be far enough apart to prevent cross-contamination, product mixup, or other serious problems. Normally, a separation of 15 to 20 feet is adequate, and in some opera-

tions, a wall or movable partition between packaging lines has been used.

The choice of straight lines or U-shaped lines can be made only on the basis of department layout or line speeds. If U-shaped lines are selected, essential materials-handling activities that are not related to actual filling or labeling, for both the input and output sides of the U, should be performed outside the department (Fig. 25-7). This arrangement not only eliminates noise, heavy traffic, and paper dust, but also helps to reduce air-conditioning loads in the packaging department.

Straight packaging lines, on the other hand, do not lend themselves to such an arrangement, since the output end of the line must be provided with shipping cases and case-sealing machinery, and all finished products must be carried out of the room with lift trucks.

For operations in which there are considerable numbers of labels of the same size or color, the concept of roll labeling equipment versus cut labels should be explored carefully. Roll labels have many advantages over cut labels in avoiding mislabeling or label mixups in either the label-printing operations or the storage and handling of labels in packaging. As the name implies, when the continuously printed sheet of labels comes off the printing press, it is slit, and

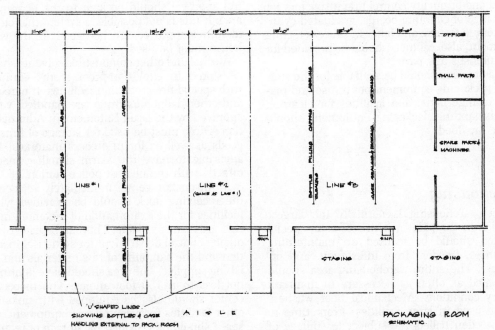

FIG. 25-7. *U-shaped lines with bottle filling and case sealing external to department. Distance between lines is 15 ft, and a divider can be used for separation when needed.*

each row of labels is wound into a roll around a center spool. Each label also has an identifying mark on it that not only provides correct label identification, but also allows electronic counting, thereby permitting good label reconciliation.

If cut labels must be used, label-scanning equipment should be provided for label identification either before the labeling operation, at the labeling machine, or at both times.

Labels should be stored in an air-conditioned room, and in winter, the air should be humidified to maintain a relative humidity of about 50% to avoid overdrying of labels. The room should have sufficient space for storage of inserts and be subdivided to separate approved from unapproved labels and inserts in accordance with GMP (see Fig. 25-7).

The department should be equipped with an adequate number of sinks to permit washing of measuring utensils such as graduates and packaging line equipment parts. Usually, one sink is sufficient for two lines.

The cleaning of dry products filling equipment by vacuum or compressed air should be conducted during shutdown hours when the danger of cross-contamination is minimized. Whenever compressed air is used for cleaning, the equipment should be removed from the line if possible or completely enshrouded during the cleaning operation.

Space should be available for use by departmental and/or quality control line inspectors for the storage of counting boards, graduated cylinders, torque testers, and other in-process testing equipment; also, cabinets should be provided for clean utensils and parts.

A staging area should be available for the storage of packaging equipment not in use and machine change parts, and facilities for cleaning and dismantling packaging equipment should also be provided.

Warehousing

Since warehousing is normally the largest operation in the plant in terms of area, special attention should be focused on maintaining cleanliness, freedom from infestation, and orderliness. The entire warehousing area should be cleaned as often as necessary to maintain sanitary conditions. Mechanical floor washers may be used in large facilities. From time to time, wooden pallets are subject to spillage of materials, and an area in which to clean pallets should be provided. Occasional pesticide treatment of pallets is also advisable to minimize insect infestation.

A quarantine area for incoming raw materials and packaging components is necessary, and an enclosed quarantine area must be provided for raw materials, packaging components, bulk products, and finished goods that have been rejected for failure to meet various standards.

Shipping and Receiving

Constant movement of materials in and out of the building subjects this area to the greatest possibility of insect and rodent infestation. This is particularly troublesome in tropical areas and when night operations are in progress. Air curtains have been used to prevent flying insects from coming into the building, but their effectiveness is somewhat limited.

When an inside dock is provided, it should be large enough to permit both the trailer and the tractor to park inside the building. Overhead doors can be used to close off the dock area. Each opening at the loading platform where trucks back into an outside wall should be equipped with compressible receptacles that effectively seal the truck's opening with the entry port into the building.

Only approved finished goods should be kept in the shipping area. Items awaiting quality control approval should be kept in the quarantine area. If this is not possible, a system that clearly identifies approved finished goods in the warehouse must be used.

Alcohol and other combustible solvents should be stored in explosion-proof rooms equipped with special fire protection facilities. If narcotics and other dangerous drugs are handled, vaults approved by the Drug Enforcement Administration (DEA) must be used for storage of finished goods as well as for in-process materials. It is advisable to have the alarm signal connected directly with the nearest police station.

An inspection center immediately adjacent to the receiving dock should be provided where facilities for the examination of incoming materials are made available. This can be used by the quality control department for statistical inspection and the sampling of raw materials and finishing supplies. The area should have lighting of not less than 150 footcandles. The inspection center should also be equipped with sinks and other facilities for washing test equipment, and space should be provided for storage of retained samples for quality control as well as permanent production records.

Dust collection hoses should be provided to clean the tops of containers prior to placement in the general warehouse.

Materials Management

The role of materials management is to convert the sales forecast into a production forecast and then into raw materials, finishing supplies, intermediates, equipment loading, and labor hours. It is then necessary to see that all of these are available at the right time and place to maximize the use of company assets and provide the best customer service with the lowest inventory investment. To do this effectively, there must be control over purchasing, receiving, shipping, warehousing, and distribution as well as production planning and scheduling, and continuous liaison is needed with production, marketing, sales, and quality control departments.

Materials management has the dual responsibility of determining the amount of inventory as well as its accountability. Inventories are an important part of a company's working capital and are reported to stockholders in the annual report.

Activities most identified with materials management are production planning and inventory control. Production and inventory control principles were developed from statistical or mathematical approaches. More recently, the evolution of operations research has permitted many production and inventory control problems to be expressed mathematically, and statistical probability theories have provided new methods for solving complex business problems by means of a computer. In this regard, the selection of computer hardware and the development or purchase of software systems are important responsibilities of the materials management department to ensure that any management information system provides timely and accurate data on thousands of daily transactions occurring in manufacturing and related operations.

Inventories

Basically, inventories are needed to satisfy future demands, and the pharmaceutical industry has relatively long process cycle times and procurement lead times. The inventories may be described as a combination of fluctuations in anticipation, lot size inventories, and inventories to cover movement of materials from one location to another. All of these are affected by fluctuations in demand and manufacturing lead times, which are covered by reserve stock or safety stock (see "Concepts of the Order Point System," later in this chapter).

Inventories are classified as follows:

1. *Materials.* These are such chemicals as active ingredients, diluents, and excipients needed to manufacture intermediates or components of the finished product. Included in this category and best shown separately are finishing supplies such as containers, labels, caps, and shippers needed in the packaging operation.
2. *Components.* These are parts or sub-assemblies needed for the final assembly of the end product (e.g., bulk tablets awaiting packaging).
3. *Work-In-Process.* As the name implies, these are materials and components on which work is being done.
4. *Finished Goods.* These are the salable items, samples, or other promotional items held in inventory awaiting customer orders or made for specific customers.

Inventory Management

It is customary in any production operation to consider return on investment in buying capital equipment, and many appropriation requests are turned down if the rate of return is too low. Commitments for inventories must be considered in the same way, and obviously, the purchase and holding of a one-month supply of an item gives a better return on investment and inventory turnover than a two-months supply. This is an oversimplification since there are many costs associated with inventory decisions, for example, ordering costs, out-of-stock costs, clerical costs, computer costs, and quality control costs; others are too numerous to list here. Examination of the annual reports of several top pharmaceutical companies that have the greatest return on equity shows that inventories can represent anywhere from 35 to 80% of working capital, and some of these have worldwide inventories approaching $700 million! Not only does it cost money to acquire inventory, it also costs money to hold it until used.

A generally accepted method of quantifying inventory costs is as follows:

Inventory Carrying Cost Breakdown (%)

Cost of money	11.0*
Storage and handling	8.5
Obsolescence	4.4
Taxes	1.0
Insurance	0.1
	25.0

*Currently about 15.0%.

A practical illustration of the importance of this quantification is as follows:

Average Worldwide Inventories
$280,000,000
Inventory Carrying Cost at 25%
$ 70,000,000/yr
A 10% reduction in investment would save
$ 7,000,000.
Inventory reduction would release in cash
$ 28,000,000.

Obviously, a well-managed inventory can exert considerable financial leverage, and inventory reduction can release much needed cash which the corporation can invest in more profitable ventures and reduce borrowing.

The inventory investment, however, must always take into consideration its effect on out-of-stock situations as well as the desired customer service level. Table 25-5 (p. 754) demonstrates the relationship between safety stocks and various customer service levels.

The ABC Concept

One of the most important and simplest tools used for inventory management is the ABC classification of inventories. This classification is based on a principle first outlined in the late 1800s by V. Pareto, an Italian engineer and mathematician. In its simplest terms, it states that in a large population in which many items are involved, relatively few items account for the major part of activity. For example, 15% of the highest-value items in inventory amounts to 70% or more of the total inventory value. Another 25% of medium-value items accounts for an additional 20% of inventory value. Therefore, the combined A and B values, which amount to only 40% of the total items, nevertheless represent a combined value of 90% of the total inventory. The remaining 60% of items represents a small value. These are classified as A, B, and C, respectively. This means that when there are a substantial number of items to be controlled, emphasis should be given to A and B items, since on the average, they constitute the major portion of total inventory value. By concentrating attention on the management of A & B items, one is in effect covering about 90% of the inventory value. Inventory levels of C items should be given little attention and can even be kept at a high level since they contribute only a small percentage to the raising or lowering of inventories.

Figure 25-8 shows that 40% of all inventory

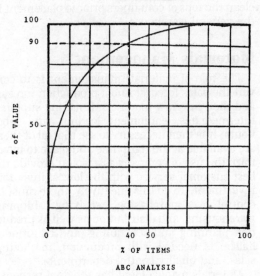

FIG. 25-8. *Pareto curve. Graph shows that 40% of items can account for 90% of total value.*

items fall on the curve at 90% of the total inventory value, and other relationships can easily be calculated from the curve.

Each item, such as raw materials, can be expressed as the total annual procurement value in descending order for easy classification.

Items	Combined Annual Value	% of Total Annual Value	Cumulative (%)
1–4	$1,800,000	36	36
5–6	600,000	12	48
7–30	500,000	10	58
31–40	1,600,000	32	90
41–200	500,000	10	100
	$5,000,000		

This table shows that the first 30 items (15% of 200) represent 58% of the total annual value. The next group of 31 through 40 items represents an additional 32%. This means that in this particular illustration, by closely following 30 raw materials that could be classified as A items, 58% of the total annual value would be covered. By examining 10 items that can be given a B classification, an additional 32% would be covered. Therefore, by closely watching 40 items out of 200, there would be a coverage of 90% of the total annual value. Obviously, little attention needs to be given to items 41 through 200, since they represent only $500,000 and 10% of total annual purchases.

Inventory Reporting and Analysis

Since inventories are reported in dollars, the figures are of little value unless they are related to something, such as the ratio to cost of goods. A commonly used expression is "Turnover" (TO), or "Stock Turn Rate" (STR), which shows the relationship of inventories to the amount of goods that could be produced from those figures when related to factory door cost on an annual basis:

$$\text{TO or STR} = \frac{\text{COST OF GOODS IN PERIOD}}{\text{COST OF INVENTORY ON HAND}}$$

If the annual cost of goods is $20,000,000 and the inventory is $10,000,000, the STR is 2.0, meaning that the inventory "turns over" twice a year. Such information is generally given to the top people in management to provide a general inventory view, but at best, it shows an incomplete picture.

In addition, a STR of 2.0 for one division of a company or one group of products may be completely unacceptable to another division or group, which may be producing large-volume consumer products and may expect inventories to be turned over more often. What the STR of 2.0 is really showing is that there is a 6-months total inventory on hand.

Inasmuch as inventories are on hand to take care of future sales demands, it is not accurate to relate today's inventories to a previous cost of goods. An expression of inventory dollars as they relate to forecasted sales would be more realistic.

To control and analyze inventories properly, it is best to develop a relationship to inventory dollars as well as to the length of time such inventory will last, expressed in number of months' supply. If it is established that a 10 million dollar inventory is too high, this figure by itself does not permit proper inventory analysis to determine in which categories the high inventory occurs. This can be done as follows.

Conversion of General Inventory Dollars to Months of Supply

The cumulative monthly forecasted cost of goods sold, which equals the inventory dollars, gives the equivalency in months of supply:

Example: If the total inventory is $10 million and finished goods total $6 million, what are the equivalents in a month's supply?

Forecasted Cost of Goods Sold (millions)
		Cumulative
January	2	2
February	2	4
March	3	7
April	2	9
May	2.5	11.5
June	3.1	14.6

By subtracting finished goods from the total inventory, the remaining balance must be supplies and work-in-process. Since the $10 million inventory falls between April and May, by interpolation, this works out to be 4.4 months.

Total Inventory	Finished Goods	Supplies and Work-in-Process
$10 million	$6 million	$4 million
4.4 mo	2.64 mo	1.76 mo
	6/10 × 4.4	4/10 × 4.4

Carried to its logical conclusion, such a report should be broken down further into individual products or product groups representing A or B items to ensure that inventories that are not in line or are above inventory policy limits will clearly show, so that investigation and further action can be taken (Table 25-4). Such a report issued monthly provides meaningful information to all managerial personnel in materials management, production, sales, and accounting, since it covers A and B items and therefore most of the inventory investment.

TABLE 25-4. *Inventory and Months of Supply by Product Classification*

Description by Classification	Raw Materials M$*	Mos	Fin Supplies M$	Mos	In Process M$	Mos	Bulk M$	Mos	Finished Goods M$	Mos
Product-A	73.0	2.2	81.4	2.7	11.5	.2	48.7	1.1	239.8	2.3
Product-B	10.8	1.6	6.2	1.8	14.2	1.3	24.0	2.1	40.0	2.9
Product-B	12.4	.9	4.8	3.2	25.6	2.4	19.3	1.5	31.0	2.2

*$ in thousands.

Sales Forecasting

The importance of a well-planned, well-executed sales forecast deserves emphasis, because therein lies the basis for many business decisions. A sales forecast dictates future personnel, equipment, and warehousing requirements. It also generates the inventory investment plan and determines the amount of cash needed to operate the business. At the same time, purchasing personnel are apprised of the amounts needed, so that they can arrive at the best prices and delivery dates.

Responsibility for Sales Forecasts. With few exceptions, sales forecasts are made by the marketing staff, and this perhaps is as it should be. They should know the conditions in the marketplace and be able to assess the effects of competition, advertising and promotion, changes in prices, and the size of the sales force in view of fluctuating demands. Poor forecasting can have serious ill effects on production operations. The production staff, on the other hand, continually calls attention to violent changes in sales demands as they affect operations. Sometimes forecast inaccuracies are offered as an excuse for problems in production management. When inventories are too high, the forecast often is blamed for not meeting the plan, and people are either laid off, or worse, kept on and underutilized, thereby increasing costs and reducing labor efficiency. Sometimes the problems are due to forecast inaccuracies and sometimes to errors in production planning. Both groups should get together to resolve significant differences.

Since sales forecasts have an effect on so many other operations, those operations most affected should be represented in the forecasting procedure. The materials management staff holds a pivotal position in this regard, inasmuch as it must be alert to significant variations between forecasted demands and actual sales.

Techniques. Basically it is more accurate to forecast for a large group of items than for any one item. It is easier, for example, to forecast the total sales of all the thyroid products in the line than to predict how many bottles of 65-mg 100s will be sold. Obviously, a forecast of tomorrow's sales can be more accurate than a prediction of sales two years hence. Additionally, forecasting should not be thought of in absolute terms, and every forecast should include an estimate of error. Before the forecast system is used, the method should be tested, especially in statistical forecasting, in which trends, seasonality, and randomness must be taken into consideration.

Averaging. *Simple Averaging.* The simplest approach is to assume that demand is steady and that sales for any new period will be the same as for the current period. Simple averaging, then, is not realistic; it treats all data equally, since there is no way of emphasizing or "weighting" some portion of the data.

Weighted Averaging. Arithmetic averages "weight" all data in terms of previous sales, which can be called the old forecast, and since inventories are for future sales, no means is provided for "weighting" future requirements. If the average weekly sales for last year were 100 pieces and the first week's sales for the new year were 70, it would be unreasonable to "weight" these numbers equally in forecasting future sales. If a "weighting factor" of 1 was used (same as 100%), it would be logical to recognize more "weight" in the 52 weeks of last year's data than in one week of the new data in computing the new forecast. For instance, consider the following:

The Weighted Average

First Week

	Simple Average	Weighted Average
"Old forecast" = (Avg/52 wks)	$100 \times 0.5 = 50$	$\times 0.9 = 90$
Sales (Latest wk)	$\underline{70} \times 0.5 = \underline{35}$	$\times 0.1 = \underline{7}$
	170 Avg 85	Avg 97

Second Week

(Using Weighted Average)

Old forecast = $97 \times 0.9 = 87$

Sales (2nd wk) = $105 \times 0.1 = \underline{11}$

New forecast = 98

In the foregoing example, the average weekly sales for the past 52 weeks (old forecast) plus the latest sales total 170, the average being 85. When an equal weight of 0.5 (50%) is given to each number, the result is an average of 85. Why should the average of 52 weeks of data be given the same weighting as data for one week? This is not a good method.

In the same illustration, one may wish to give the 52 weeks (old forecast) a value of 0.9 (90%) and the new one a value of 0.1 (10%): the results would produce a new forecast of 97 instead of 85. This in turn can be developed into forecasts for the ensuing weeks, a system well suited to computer application.

Exponential Smoothing—First-Order Equation. From the foregoing, it can be seen that it is possible to assign different weighting values to averages, and this is particularly useful on moving averages when dealing with averages of 3 months, 6 months, 39 months, and so on. In exponential smoothing, such values range from 0 to 1 using α, which is called a *smoothing constant*. Thus, to produce a new forecast, the old forecast, the current demand, and a selected value of α are needed. This can be expressed as follows and is commonly referred to as the first-order equation.

New forecast = $(1 - \alpha)$ old forecast + α new demand. Accordingly, if the old forecast is 100, current demand 120, and an assigned α 0.2, then:

(1) New forecast = $(1 - 0.2)$ 100 + 0.2 (120)
  = 80 + 24
  = 104
(2) If α is changed to 0.5
  New forecast = $(1 - 0.5)$ 100 + 0.5 (120)
  = 50 + 60
  = 110

In (1), the α of the old forecast has a value of 80, and in (2), when α is changed to 0.5, the value drops to 50. Thus, it can be seen that as the α value increases, the old average of 100 is progressively discounted and has less weighting, whereas the new data give more weighting since it moves from 24 to 60.

Forecast accuracy is best when data of 2 or 3 years are available; however, exponential smoothing can be used to advantage in forecasting for new products for which little prior sales history exists. As was seen before, the higher the α value, the less weighting there is on the old forecast, so that on new products high α values can be used to limited advantage. The following table shows the equivalency of assigned α values to months of data.

Alpha Values vs.
Equivalent Moving Average[3]

Alpha	Equivalent Months
0.500	3
0.400	4
0.333	5
0.250	7
0.200	9
0.100	19
0.050	39
0.010	199

As stated before, in any forecasting system the forecast error should always be measured by plus or minus differences between actual versus forecasted sales.

Mean Absolute Deviation (MAD). As a measure of forecast error, the monthly differences between actual and forecasted sales

should be noted and expressed as a plus or minus value from the actual. These monthly deviations are then added without regard to the sign and divided by the time period being measured. This is called mean absolute deviation (MAD).

For example—Forecast 1500

Time period (Wk or Mo)	Sales	Deviation
1	1200	−300
2	1500	—
3	1900	+400
4	1700	+200
5	1600	+100

$$\text{MAD} = \frac{1000}{5} = 200 \, Units$$

The error can also be expressed statistically by calculating the standard deviation, but this is time-consuming and requires much computation. There is an approximate relationship that is expressed, however:

$$\text{Sigma} = 1.25 \times \text{MAD}$$

which would give 250 units in the example given above.

If the MAD is watched, the forecast error is monitored frequently. This monitoring prevents overproduction or underproduction and can be used as a "tracking signal" to report significant variations, which in turn would result in production or forecast changes.

Trends and Seasonality in Forecasts. In the event of a definite sales trend, the use of the first-order equation produces forecast error differences, which on a cumulative basis gets larger and larger. In such cases, the method of "least squares" can be used; however, it is sometimes easier to use second-order smoothing. For those readers interested in statistical forecasting, the book by R. G. Brown is recommended.[4]

Economic Lot Size or Order Quantity (EOQ)

It is not uncommon to have tens of thousands of items in inventory, so that materials management personnel must decide how much to buy and when each item should be delivered, as well as when intermediates and finished products should be made. With excessively high inventories, too much cash is tied up, investment opportunities are lost, and obsolescence may be increased. Production and marketing staffs tend to favor high inventories to get longer production runs, avoid back orders, and provide the best customer service levels.

Fixed costs such as set-up and clean-up times are the same no matter how large or small the batch size or the packaging run is. Obviously, the more frequently an item is bought, the lower the carrying cost is, but such costs as quality control increases if something is purchased every month, as opposed to every third month.

Using simple figures for ease in calculation, the following trial and error method shows the EOQ.

Total Annual Cost for Various Order Quantities
Assume:

1. Annual usage of 12,000 units
2. Unit cost of $3.00
3. Cost of carrying inventory 10% per year
4. Ordering costs per order $50.

I. *Assume a delivery of 500 kg.*	Cost
Annual fixed costs (24 orders/yr × $50)	$1,200
Annual cost of carrying inventory $\left(\dfrac{500^*}{2} \times 3 \times 10\%\right)$	75
Total annual costs	1,275

II. *Assume a delivery quantity of 1,000 kg.*	
Annual fixed costs	600
Annual cost of carrying inventory	150
Total annual costs	750

III. *Assume a delivery quantity of 2,000 kg.*	
Annual fixed costs	300
Annual cost of carrying inventory	300
Total annual costs	600

IV. *Assume a delivery quantity of 3,000 kg.*	
Annual fixed costs	200
Annual cost of carrying inventory	450
Total annual costs	650

V. *Assume a delivery quantity of 4,000 kg.*	
Annual fixed costs	150
Annual cost of carrying inventory	600
Total annual costs	750

*Average inventory is half the lot size.

Therefore, when a 2,000-kg delivery quantity is ordered, the annual fixed costs and the annual carrying costs are equal, resulting in the lowest total annual costs. The interrelationship of the costs are illustrated in Figure 25-9, which shows

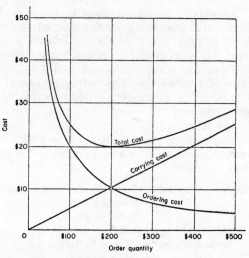

FIG. 25-9. *Graph shows relationship of changes in ordering costs and inventory carrying cost to total costs. (Data from Plossl and Wight.[5])*

that as order quantities go up, so do carrying costs, but ordering costs go down. The total cost curve shows that total costs decrease with increasing ordering quantities to a minimum of a $200 ordering quantity, after which total costs increase with larger lot sizes because of the increasing effect of inventory carrying costs. In this case, a $200 order quantity has a total cost of $20, but if a $50 order quantity were used, the total cost would be twice as much or $40.

The EOQ Formula. Considering the thousands of inventory items, a trial and error method would be impractical; in its place, the EOQ equation can be used.

$$\text{EOQ} = \sqrt{\frac{2\,\text{AS}}{\text{I}}}$$

where A is the annual usage in dollars, S is the ordering costs in dollars, and I is the inventory carrying costs expressed as a decimal.

Since the foregoing equation shows the least cost expressed in dollars, the least cost can be calculated directly as follows by substituting the figures used in the trial and error illustration.

$$\text{EOQ} = \sqrt{\frac{2(12000 \times 3) \times 50}{0.10}} = \$600$$

However, using the same example, if the number of units that give the lowest cost is required, the equation is expressed as follows:

$$EOQ = \sqrt{\frac{2\,AS}{IU}}$$

where A is the annual usage in units, S is the order cost in dollars, I is the inventory carrying costs expressed as a decimal, and U is the cost of one unit.

$$EOQ = \sqrt{\frac{2 \times 12000 \times 50}{0.1 \times 3}}$$
$$= \sqrt{4,000,000} = 2000 \text{ Units}$$

The EOQ equation shows that the most economical lot size is a function of the square root of the annual usages of items expressed in dollars.

The square root relationship also shows in a general way how much inventories should increase if the sales of a product increases by 20%. Obviously, the inventory should not be increased by 20%, and the maximum would be the square root of 20.

Generally speaking, the application of the EOQ formula for ordering and lot sizing result in good materials management. At times, however, its inappropriate use may lead to increased inventories and costs, since EOQ quantities may not balance with quantities needed for lot sizes. Set-up costs are also an important factor, and a technique called LIMIT (Lot-size Inventory Management Interpolation Techniques) can be used.[6]

For additional information on lot-size inventory and EOQ, the reader is referred to Plossl,[7] and to Plossl and Wight.[5]

Inventory Management Systems

In managing inventories, two sets of techniques can be used in a manufacturing operation: (1) statistical inventory control or order point, (2) material requirements planning (MRP).

Statistical Inventory Control vs. Material Requirements Planning. As indicated earlier in this chapter, the concepts of mathematical probability, operations research, the Pareto curve, exponential smoothing, and EOQ all indicate that mathematical expressions can be applied in the field of inventory and production control. When properly used, all constitute statistical inventory control, or the order point system which most companies are using today. Before examining its three basic concepts, a closer inspection of the system is necessary.

The order point system represents an attempt to predict on the basis of past data. It is best used when there is an independent demand. For example, one only produces finished goods in response to depletion of inventories resulting from sales demands, and therefore a sales forecast is required. However, the components in finished goods, such as raw materials and finishing supplies, need to be purchased only when supplies needed to produce the finished goods need to be replaced. These requirements can be calculated. Even so, the purchasing department should be given adequate notice. The order point system calculates the quantity and delivery date for each item separately and independently of the other items that must also be used as part of the production.

In addition to the fact that the square root approach does not balance with lot size or the other items needed simultaneously, it is not time-phased and assumes that some inventory should be replenished as soon as it is depleted. If 1,000 kg of a raw material is consumed in February and no further material is needed until June, the order point system dictates immediate replenishment, and a large inventory may result.

Concepts of the Order Point System. The following are three basic concepts of the order point system.

1. SAFETY STOCK. The function of safety stock is to ensure the best level of customer service and to keep back orders to a minimum. Such stock is necessary because all forecasting techniques have errors, which are generally expressed as MAD or in standard deviations, and safety stock compensates for such errors. The calculation of safety stock is based on the normal distribution curve and its relationship to the desired customer service level. If the MAD or standard deviation of forecast error is known, the order quantity is multiplied by either of these figures, and the result equals the reserve or safety stock. For example, if the weekly forecast is 500, the MAD is 200 units, and a 98% service is desired, the reserve stock should be 512 units (Table 25-5). This is derived by multiplying the 200 units of MAD by 2.56. The use of standard deviation results in a smaller number. Either of these figures added to the 500 units of weekly forecast results in 1,012 units or 910 units, which in turn defines the order point. Obviously, this should be applied only when there is a random demand.

Additionally, the MAD column in the table shows the enormous increase in safety stocks needed when moving from a 90% to a 99.9% service level.

TABLE 25-5. *Safety Factors for Normal Distribution*

Service Level (% Order cycles w/o stockout)	Safety Factor Using:	
	Standard deviation	Mean absolute deviation
50.00	0.00	0.00
75.00	0.67	0.84
80.00	0.84	1.05
84.13	1.00	1.25
85.00	1.04	1.30
89.44	1.25	1.56
90.00	1.28	1.60
93.32	1.50	1.88
94.00	1.56	1.95
94.52	1.60	2.00
95.00	1.65	2.06
96.00	1.75	2.19
97.00	1.88	2.35
97.72	2.00	2.50
98.00	2.05	2.56
98.61	2.20	2.75
99.00	2.33	2.91
99.18	2.40	3.00
99.38	2.50	3.13
99.50	2.57	3.20
99.60	2.65	3.31
99.70	2.75	3.44
99.80	2.88	3.60
99.86	3.00	3.75
99.90	3.09	3.85
99.93	3.20	4.00
99.99	4.00	5.00

Adapted from Plossl and Wight.[5]

2. ORDER POINT. Figure 25-10 shows that at some point in time, 25,000 items are in inventory, and as the weeks pass, the inventory is consumed as shown on the downward sloping line. This consumption continues until the inventory reaches a predetermined level or ordering point, at which time a replenishment quantity is ordered. This system assumes that usage is uniform; thus, the average inventory is equal to one-half the order quantity. The lead time, of course, is that time lapse between placement of an order and the time it is received and approved by quality control. Since both demand and lead time vary, the reserve stock is really established to take care of both. Accordingly, the order point is equal to the sum of the anticipated demand during lead time plus the reserve stock. In Figure 25-10, during the five weeks of lead time, about 5,000 units will be depleted from stock, and this amount plus the reserve of 10,000 units indicate an order point of 15,000. It must be remembered that randomness of demand during lead time and gradual inventory depletion are the underlying assumptions.

3. ORDER QUANTITY. The EOQ formula previously described assumes gradual inventory depletion, so that the lot size inventory is equal to half the order quantity.

Material Requirements Planning (MRP). As stated previously, the order point system is best applied when the demand is independent, as for finished goods. A more sophisticated and mature approach to production and inventory control is the recognition of the principles of independent versus dependent demand, first expressed by Dr. Orliky of IBM in 1965. When the demand is for all components that "go into" an item, material requirements planning is a far more satisfactory technique.

If an item such as a bulk tablet is made infrequently, or at least not on a continuous basis, and is made in a large batch, the demand is occasional, and immediate replenishment of the raw materials may not be necessary, or in fact, may be undesirable. An order point system would immediately replenish any or all of the raw materials, but in requirements planning, ordering would be postponed until the next

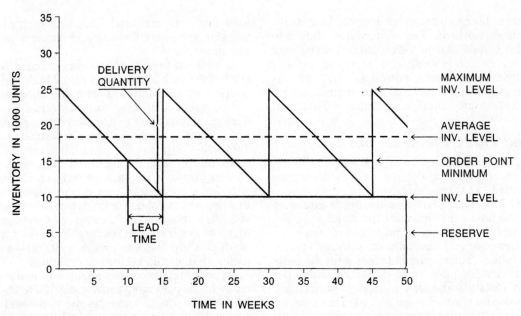

FIG. 25-10. *Graphic representation of order point.*

scheduled production day, in consideration of the lead time. In other words, in addition to holding orders until needed, this method also establishes the next requirement date and is said to be time-phased. Under these conditions, if there is a sudden change in quantity or date, the frequent updating in an MRP system permits changing in sufficient time to avoid problems.

There are three general principles to remember for an effective MRP:

1. The materials plan must be revised frequently to react to changes in requirements.

2. The smaller the time period used, the more effective the materials plan wiill be.

3. The materials plan must extend over a long enough period to cover the longest lead time of any component.

The following example illustrates the difference in order point versus MRP:

On hand	50
Plus on order	150
	200
Less gross requirement	300
Net requirement	−100

In an order point system, 100 units are needed immediately, and no one knows when the 150 on order are needed, but presumably, they are needed immediately also.

In an MRP system, the gross requirements are broken down by quantity and required date as follows:

Required	Date Needed
50	1/3
30	2/14
70	3/4
100	3/27
50	4/25
300	

It is assumed that it is now January 2, and that the lead time is four weeks. Actually, the 100 ordered for immediate delivery in the order point system do not need to be ordered until the last week in February. The 50 needed on January 3 are already on hand, whereas the 150 on order will cover 2/14, 3/4, and half of 3/27. By time-phasing the order, the material was brought in only when needed, thereby contributing to reduction of inventory and inventory carrying costs.

Cost Controls

From the sales forecast, the materials management group generates a production forecast that takes into account seasonality, deals and promotions, introduction of new products or product sizes, and other factors that create a demand on inventory, equipment, and personnel. This information in turn permits the development of the operating or expense budgets for each department. The information thus provided is applicable to a standard cost accounting system, which in its simplest terms, means that individual item costs, as well as labor and burden rates, have been fixed or standardized for a period of time, usually a calendar or fiscal year.

The Three Elements of Cost

The basic elements of cost are materials, labor, and burden; the last item is sometimes referred to as "overhead."

1. Materials. Based on the needs expressed in the production forecast, the purchasing department negotiates contracts and price arrangements, and ascertains the standard cost for each item. These standard costs form the basis of a monthly price variance report, which not only measures the effectiveness of purchasing, but also monitors changes in cost. This monitoring is paticularly important in the pharmaceutical industry, in which materials represent the largest part of the cost of goods.

The purchase price variance report shown in Table 25-6 is for the month of April and shows a favorable ($74,800) cumulative total variance through the four-month period for three operating divisions of the company as well as for advertising. For Division B, for example, there is a favorable variance of $10,200 for the month of April and $33,200 total of all divisions. Since each division shows a favorable purchase price variance, their purchases are generally within the standard cost predicted. However, to permit better analysis of price variances, the figures are broken down into major categories, such as raw materials, certain classes of finishing supplies, and others, to help pick out favorable and unfavorable price variances.

By categories, for example, the report shows that raw materials were purchased below standard costs, showing a savings of $30,100 for the month of April and a total savings of $43,300 over a four-month period. This would indicate that the purchasing division is doing a good job, and if the savings turn out to be substantial at year's end, perhaps selected raw materials cost standards could be revised downward next year. In general, it is desirable to have a favorable price variance, but on the other hand, a variance that is too high might indicate poor estimation on the part of the purchasing division; it would overstate or understate the cost of goods.

Another control occurs in the usage of materials during production. From the production forecast, production planning determines the number of batches of each product needed to meet

sales forecasts, and batch sheets for each product give the exact formula and quantity of all raw materials.

In addition to this, and in conformance with GMP, the batch sheet shows actual bulk yields, which can be compared with the theoretical yields, adjusted to take care of normal losses during manfuacturing. A materials usage variance report is issued for each department and Table 25-7 explains the cumulative results for tabletting through the month of May. This report expresses a favorable or unfavorable variance for each product, and it can be seen that this department shows a net favorable variance of $7,018. The value of this report, however, is that it shows the variances for each product, two of which show losses in excess of $2,000—a situation that should be further examined.

A similar report covers variances in materials usage in the packaging department (Table 25-7). In this case, these variances are expressed by packaging line, with respect to both variations in bulk such as tablets and liquid products, and variations in finishing supplies. For example, the May report shows that there was a total unfavorable bulk variance of $15,399 in the packaging department and an unfavorable variance of $27,796 in finishing supplies.

In all cases, the accounting, production, and quality control departments have agreed on a standard yield as compared with theory, and it probably has been derived on the basis of statistical analysis with losses built into the cost system. Variances in finishing supplies are derived by comparing the finished goods produced in packaging with the amount that should have been consumed on the packaging order and with losses on the packaging line. Both reports show that product losses on bulk can be quite expensive, and differences in yields between processing and packaging point to the need for precision in the yielding of bulk tablets, liquids, and ointments by using counters on tablet presses or meters and load cells in other areas, a practice that will help in GMP reconciliation of bulk.

As stated previously, the biggest item in pharmaceutical cost-of-goods is materials. Reports such as those illustrated are furnished to each operating department for the department head to analyze quickly and decide which products should be studied further so that problems can be corrected.

In the control of materials costs, the variances are budgeted as a hedge against unforeseeable price changes. The report described in this section is helpful to both purchasing and production departments, as it points to problems and permits their correction. Of course, the informa-

TABLE 25-6. *Purchase Price Variance Report* (In M Dollars)

| | Month of April | | | Year to Date | | | |
	Actual Purchase Price	Standard Cost	Variance	Actual Purchase Price	Standard Cost	Variance	Budget
By Division	($)	($)	($)	($)	($)	($)	($)
Division A	2.1	2.8	(.7)	27.6	30.8	(3.2)	
Division B	1,867.6	1,877.8	(10.2)	6,923.4	6,956.6	(33.2)	
Division C	671.0	684.9	(13.9)	1,526.1	1,549.2	(23.1)	
Advertising and promotion	28.6	37.0	(8.4)	78.8	94.1	(15.3)	20.0
Total	2,569.3	2,602.5	(33.2)	8,555.9	8,630.7	(74.8)	20.0
By Category							
Raw material	579.8	609.9	(30.1)	2,251.8	2,295.1	(43.3)	20.0
Bulk	213.7	184.1	29.6	501.5	463.3	38.2	
Set-up box	23.6	23.8	(.2)	56.2	58.3	(2.1)	
Folding carton	69.7	64.6	5.1	328.0	330.9	(2.9)	
Labels and inserts	74.1	73.3	.8	221.2	231.8	(10.6)	
Bottles	264.0	287.4	(23.4)	755.8	780.5	(24.7)	
Caps	44.2	47.7	(3.5)	116.9	126.0	(9.1)	
Corrugated	24.0	24.1	(.1)	59.8	56.8	3.0	
Cans, drums	32.6	34.2	(1.6)	73.5	75.7	(2.2)	
Cotton, cello	60.5	64.2	(3.7)	172.1	183.1	(11.0)	
Advertising and promotion	28.6	37.0	(8.4)	78.8	94.1	(15.3)	
Vendor charges	14.9	18.9	(4.0)	125.2	126.9	(1.7)	
Finished goods, Div. A	613.5	613.4	.1	1,437.5	1,438.9	(1.4)	
Finished goods, Div. B	493.7	487.9	5.8	1,608.9	1,603.1	5.8	
Finished goods, Other	32.4	32.0	.4	768.7	766.2	2.5	
Total	2,569.3	2,602.5	(33.2)	8,555.9	8,630.7	(74.8)	20.0

( ) Denotes favorable variance.

TABLE 25-7. *Summary—Tabletting, Granulating, and Packaging Cost Performance (Year to Date)*

Tabletting and Granulating Cost Performance

Product Name	Material Usage Variance	Std. Hrs. Delivered To Invty.	Labor Performance	Lost Time	Total Cost Over Std.
	$		$	$	$
"A"	116	615	912		1028
"B"	(1493)	948	147		(1346)
"C"	1392	648	(79)		1313
"D"	866	877	579		1445
Etc.	2211	546	1025		3236
	2568	375	1574		4142
	(896)	401	166		(730)
	(4869)	187	436		(4433)
				1992	1992
Totals	$(7018)	9042	10130	1992	5104

Packaging Cost Performance

Line No.	Packaging Line Descrip.	Mat'l Usage Var. Bulk	Mat'l Usage Var. Fin. Supply	Std. Hrs. Delivered To Invtry.	Lab. Perf.	Lost Time	Total Cost Over std.
		$	$		$	$	$
1	Tablet	1 345	3406	3767	468	1185	5404
2		2 4446	1574	3257	1234	1404	8658
3		3 (56)	1668	3559	2350	1774	5736
4		4 2553	(2498)	15190	(3561)	1277	(2229)
5		5 (976)	927	1668	3827	1468	6249
6		6 (380)	(1864)	4569	1152	1370	(725)
7		7 (432)	732	5713	3497	2459	6256
24		(141)	42	832	133	191	225
25		8531	1738	14649	12877	6612	29758
26		233	727	3567	3092	2300	6402
Totals		15399	27796		31512	36272	110979

tion is important to the accounting department and to management as well.

2. Labor. *Direct Labor.* In any manufacturing operation, the management and careful use of the labor force are important for cost control as well as for the stability and happiness of the work force. In most companies, the number of hours required in each department for production of most items is known either by virtue of historical information or as a result of time studies by industrial engineers. The latter standard is more practical, of course, since the historical data do not necessarily reflect the most efficient method of production. In either case, the production of any bulk or finished goods item is expressed as the number of direct labor hours needed to produce 1,000 bulk tablets or 1,000 bottles of 100's for every product made, including promotional samples. This information is important to several groups, e.g., the accounting department, production planning, and, of course, the operating managers.

Indirect Labor. It is easy to identify the direct labor needed for an item, but to arrive at the true cost, indirect labor hours are needed. They are difficult to measure, however. In some plants, the indirect labor has not been adequately identified, and in some departments, it represents a high percentage of the total requirements. Without indirect labor hours, it would be difficult to analyze and control available hours of work and to use the labor force efficiently. If a serviceman is bringing caps and bottles to three packaging lines, his function represents some indirect labor to each of the lines. Whenever possible, it would be best to allocate such time to the products on each line rather than completely lose its identity and cost by putting it into the indirect labor class, thereby spreading the cost over the rest of the products.

The indirect labor costs that cannot be put into a work standard should be attributed to a specific purpose, so that they can be identified and controlled. Some examples are the costs of mechanics, servicemen, equipment cleaning, line changeover, quality control inspectors, and operation of the label room in a packaging department. In a department such as packaging, which may employ 200 to 300 people, the indirect labor could amount to several hundred thousand dollars a year; therefore, each category should be budgeted and compared against actual costs on a monthly basis.

Another cost to watch is the use of direct labor for an indirect labor job. The use of direct labor people for such work should be minimized, since they have a labor rate higher than indirect labor people and would contribute to increasing the labor cost.

Every effort should be made to lower the percentage of indirect labor to total labor for good cost control. Each labor category should be examined periodically to see if it can be placed into a time standard.

It is in the interest of efficiency to break the work standard down into job skills, e.g., machine operators, table workers, and mechanics, since in the scheduling of production these services must be available when required.

3. Burden. There are two types of burden, direct and fixed.

Direct Burden. Categorized as direct burden are such expenditures as supervision and clerical help; lost time; premium on overtime; vacation, holiday, and sick pay; and such employee benefits as hospitalization, insurance, and retirement benefits.

Additional items falling into direct burden are controllable expenses incurred in the operation of each department and commonly called operating expenses.

These expenses would include such items as laundry for uniforms, maintenance department charges, travel, membership dues and seminars, and the like. An important item in each departmental budget is operating supplies. In the parenteral department, for example, would be included the cost of ethylene oxide used in sterilization and the replacement of HEPA filters. Repairs and maintenance, as well as supplies used for production equipment such as punches and dies, must be estimated since these can add substantially to the budget.

Fixed Burden. In addition to the operating departments, others such as engineering, quality control, materials management, and all departments reporting to each of them also prepare operations budgets, and the expenses and labor costs form the overhead to be charged in the manufacturing costs. In addition, the costs of fuel, electricity, land and real estate taxes, and depreciation on the building and equipment. In the case of quality control, efforts have been made by some companies to allocate as much cost as possible directly into production departments to get as close as possible to true costs. With a little effort, it is practical in some quality control services to assign reasonably accurate labor cost and expenses to some production areas. As a simplified illustration of this, if someone is keeping a facility and requires rabbits to test for the presence of pyrogens, the cost of this can be allocated to the parenteral department, which requires this service. This principle is not unlike identifying indirect labor into the direct category, and in the example used, it avoids spreading the cost of pyrogen testing over the other cost centers, which do not use this service.

References

1. *Federal Register, 36:*133, 1971.
2. Quality Assurance in Drug Manufacturing. Eastern Regional Proceedings of PMA-FDA Seminar, Rutgers University, March 1969, Workshop No. E., p. 55.
3. Pecham, H. H.: Effective Materials Management. Prentice Hall, Englewood Cliffs, NJ, 1972, p. 30.
4. Brown, R. G.: Statistical Forecasting for Inventory Control. McGraw-Hill, New York, 1959.
5. Plossl, G. W., and Wight, O. W.: Production and Inventory Control, Principles and Techniques. Prentice Hall, Englewood Cliffs, NJ, 1967.
6. Management of Lot-Size Inventories. American Production and Inventory Control Society, Chicago, 1963.
7. Plossl, G. W.: Manufacturing Control. The Last Frontier for Profits. Reston Publishing, Reston, VA, 1973.

26

Kinetic Principles and Stability Testing

LEON LACHMAN, PATRICK DELUCA, *and* MICHAEL J. AKERS

The importance of stability testing in the development of pharmaceutical dosage forms is well recognized in the pharmaceutical industry. Increased filings of Abbreviated New Drug Applications (ANDA) and Paper New Drug Applications (PNDA) by generic and nongeneric drug manufacturers have resulted in an increase in submissions of stability data to the Food and Drug Administration (FDA). With the coming of the biotechnologic age, and as bioengineered products become ready for testing in humans, stability test data for these compounds are required as part of the submissions of Investigational New Drug Applications (INDs) to the FDA to assure their quality and safety. This increase in stability testing has come at a time in which the empiric methods have, for the most part, been replaced by a more scientific approach to stability evaluation using various appropriate physical and chemical principles.

From a regulatory consideration, there are several sections of the Federal Food and Drug and Cosmetic Act that relate to the stability of pharmaceutical products. Section 505(b)(4) concerns itself with preservation of the characteristics of the new drug and is the basis for requiring stability data in the new drug application. Section 501(a)(2)(B) concerns itself with drug adulteration. A drug is considered adulterated if it does not meet the quality and purity characteristics that it is represented to possess. Section 505(h) states that a drug shall be deemed to be misbranded if found by the Health Education and Welfare Agency to be liable to deterioration unless it is packaged in such form and manner, with its label bearing a statement of such precautions, as are necessary for the protection of the public health.

Of the three sections mentioned, the one that pertains most directly to stability testing of drugs is Section 505(b)(4). The FDA Regulation dealing with this Section is 314.1(8)(p) under New Drug Applications, and requires "a complete description of and data derived from studies of the stability of the drug, including information showing the suitability of the analytical method used." It further states that stability data should be submitted for the new substance, for the finished dosage form in the container in which it is to be marketed, and, if it is reconstituted at the time of dispensing, for the solution so prepared. It requires that an expiration date appear on the label to preserve the identity, strength, quality, and purity of the drug until it is used. In fact it states, "if no expiration date is proposed, the applicant must justify its absence."

Further, the FDA current Good Manufacturing Practices (GMP) regulations under sections 211.166 and 211.167 set forth basic guidelines for stability for all drugs, and the requirement for expiration dates on pharmaceutical products. No drug product in a container-closure system is indefinitely stable, and the manufacturer or packer of a drug product is responsible for determining the stability characteristics for each of the products. In the preamble to the Good Manufacturing Guidelines published in the Federal Register of September 29, 1978,[1] the Commissioner of the FDA indicated that valid expiration dates must be established for all drug products.

In a 1983 FDA survey of regulatory actions, it was reported that 22% of GMP violations involved problems with laboratory controls, and that the most common deficiencies involved stability testing requirements of section 211.166.[2] Deficiencies included failures to have written stability testing protocols, inability to support product expiration dates, inadequate number of stability test batches, and use of assays that were not stability-indicating.

The application of certain physicochemical principles in the performance of stability studies has proved to be of considerable advantage in the development of stable dosage forms. Only through this approach is it possible to accurately and adequately make use of data obtained from exaggerated storage conditions for the purposes of predicting the stability at normal shelf storage for extended periods of time. It is extremely important that the pharmaceutical manufacturer accurately predict the shelf stability of a new product from accelerated storage data, because of the considerable economic advantage gained in marketing a new product as soon as possible after formulation. A sound stability testing program is possible only if personnel are skilled in employing these principles and if appropriate equipment is available.

Theoretic Considerations

Degradative reactions in pharmaceutical formulations take place at definite rates and are chemical in nature. They depend on such conditions as concentration of reactants, temperature, pH, radiation, and catalysts. An effective and efficient study of these reactions requires the application of chemical kinetic principles.

Order of Reaction

In many cases, by stating the order of the reaction, the manner in which the rate of a reaction varies with the concentration of the reactants can be defined. For the most part, the degradation of pharmaceuticals can be treated as zero-order, first-order, or pseudo-first-order reactions, even though many of the pharmaceutical compounds degrade by complicated mechanisms. Consequently, the lower-order reaction types are treated in detail here, and only minor consideration is given to higher-order reactions.

Zero-Order Reaction. When the reaction rate is independent of the concentration of the reacting substance, it depends on the zero power of the reactant (Rate = $k^\circ C$) and therefore is considered to be of the zero-order reaction. In this type of reaction, the limiting factor is something other than concentration, for example, solubility or absorption of light in certain photochemical reactions. When solubility is the factor, only that amount of drug that is in solution undergoes degradation. This can be depicted as follows:

$$A\,(solid) \leftrightarrows A\,(sol) \longrightarrow B \qquad (1)$$

As drug is consumed in the degradative reaction, more drug goes into solution until all solid

A has reacted. Until this occurs, the degradative reaction does not depend on the total concentration of drug, but only on the portion that is in solution, resulting in a zero-order reaction.

The rate of decomposition of the drug can be described mathematically as follows:

Rate of concentration decrease =

$$\frac{-dC_a}{dt} = k \qquad (2)$$

where: C_a = concentration of reacting material A
k = proportionality factor = reaction rate
t = time

Since C_a is a constant, x, the amount of A reacting, is identified as:

$$\frac{dx}{dt} = k \qquad (3)$$

Integration of equation (3) yields:

$$x = kt + constant \qquad (4)$$

If the data from a stability study followed a zero-order reaction, a plot of x versus t, as shown in Figure 26-1, results in straight line plots with the slope equal to k. The value k would indicate the amount of drug that is degrading per unit time, and the intercept of the line at time zero is equal to the constant in equation (4).

In the solid state, many drugs decompose according to pseudo-zero-order rates as reactions occur between the drug and moisture in the solid dosage form. The system behaves as a suspension, and because of the presence of excess solid drug, the first-order reaction rate actually becomes a pseudo-zero-order rate, and the drug loss rate is linear with time. The rate expression

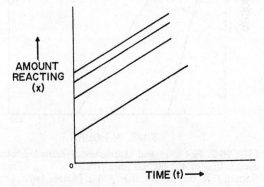

FIG. 26-1. *A representative zero-order plot of the amount of drug reacting vs. time.*

becomes similar to that in equation (3) except that k is K', which indicates the pseudo-zero-order reaction rate. Pseudo-zero-order rates of reaction frequently occur with drugs formulated as pharmaceutical suspensions.

Garrett and Carper,[3] in their study of the color stability of a liquid multisulfa preparation, showed that the color loss at 500 mμ followed zero-order kinetics. The graph in Figure 26-2 presents their data at several elevated temperatures. The straight line plots show that the degradation is behaving according to zero-order kinetics, and the slopes of their lines represent the rate of degradation at the particular temperatures.

First-Order Reaction. When the reaction rate depends on the first power of concentration of a single reactant (rate = kC_a), it is considered to be first-order. In this type of reaction, a substance decomposes directly into one or more products (A → products). The rate of reaction is directly proportional to the concentration of the reacting substance and can be expressed mathematically in the following form:

Rate of concentration decrease =

$$-\frac{dC_a}{dt} = kC_a \qquad (5)$$

Integrating equation (5) in the following form:

$$-\frac{dC_a}{C_a} = k\,dt \qquad (6)$$

we obtain:

$$-\ln C_a = kt + i, \qquad (7)$$

where i is the constant of integration. Converting from the natural logarithm (ln) yields:

$$-\log C_a = \frac{k}{2.303}t + \text{constant} \qquad (8)$$

Using the above equation for a first-order reaction, a straight line is produced when the logarithm of the concentration C_a is plotted against time, as shown in Figure 26-3. The velocity or reaction rate constant, k, can be calculated by multiplying the slope of the line by 2.303. The higher the temperature, the greater is the k value, as evidenced by the steepness of the slopes.

Integration of equation (5) between the limits C_1 and C_2 and t_1 and t_2 results in the following:

$$-\int_{C_1}^{C_2} \frac{dC}{C} = k \int_{t_1}^{t_2} dt \qquad (9)$$

$$-(\ln C_2 - \ln C_1) = k(t_2 - t_1) \qquad (10)$$

$$k = \frac{1}{t_2 - t_1} \ln \frac{C_1}{C_2} = \frac{2.303}{t_2 - t_1} \log \frac{C_1}{C_2} \qquad (11)$$

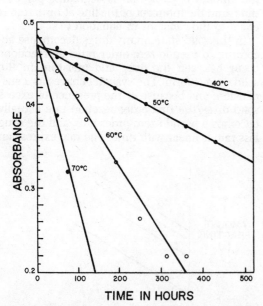

FIG. 26-2. *Plot of optical absorbance of extracted color against time at 40°, 50°, 60°, and 70°C at 500 mμ. (From Garrett, E. R., and Carper, R. F.: J. Am. Pharm. Assoc., Sci. Ed., 44:515, 1955.)*

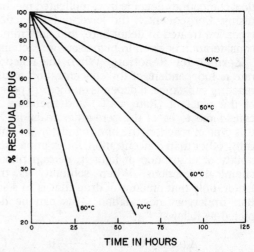

FIG. 26-3. *Representative degradation curves for a material deteriorating according to first-order kinetics.*

These equations permit the calculation of the rate of decomposition of a substance between any time interval $(t_2 - t_1)$ if the concentration of drug at these two times is known.

Where t_1 is the time at beginning of the reaction, t_0 is the time at concentration C_0, and t_2 is any time t at concentration C, then equation (11) can be expressed as follows:

$$k = \frac{2.303}{t} \log \frac{C_0}{C} \qquad (12)$$

Use of this expression permits the calculation of the rate of reaction k, by determining the concentration of drug remaining at any time t. Equation (11) or (12) can be used to ascertain whether the reaction is following first-order kinetics by determining k at several time intervals and noticing whether the values are essentially constant. Equation (12) is also written as follows:

$$k = \frac{2.303}{t} \log \frac{a}{(a - x)} \qquad (13)$$

Where $a = C_0$, x = amount reacting in time t, and $(a - x)$ the amount remaining after time t.

The constant k is called the reaction velocity constant, or more frequently, the specific reaction rate. For a first-order reaction, it is a number that expresses the fraction of the material reacting in a unit of time and may be expressed in reciprocal seconds, minutes, or hours. For example, when k has a value of 0.001 sec^{-1}, the material is decomposing at a rate of 0.1% per second.

The time necessary for a fraction of the material to degrade can be readily calculated. The half-life, $t_{1/2}$, of a drug is the time required for 50% of the drug to degrade and can be calculated as follows:

$$t_{1/2} = \frac{2.303}{k} \log \frac{C_0}{C} = \frac{2.303}{k} \log \frac{100}{50}$$

$$= \frac{2.303}{k} \log 2 = \frac{0.693}{k} \qquad (14)$$

$$\text{therefore } t_{1/2} = \frac{0.693}{k} \qquad (15)$$

In the pharmaceutical field, the time required for 10% of the drug to degrade is an important value to know, since it represents a reasonable limit of degradation of active ingredients. The $t_{10\%}$ value can be calculated as follows.

$$t_{10\%} = \frac{2.303}{k} \log \frac{100}{90} = \frac{0.104}{k}$$

$$t_{10\%} = \frac{0.104}{k} \qquad (16)$$

$$\text{or} \quad t_{10\%} = 0.152\, t_{1/2} \qquad (17)$$

It is important to note here that the $t_{1/2}$ or $t_{10\%}$ is concentration independent. In other words, it takes the same time to reduce the concentration of drug from 0.1 moles to 0.05 moles as it would to go from 0.001 moles to 0.0005 moles.

As a result of the foregoing discussion, it is obvious that knowledge of the specific rate constant, k, permits an estimation of the amount of drug that degrades within a given time. The graph in Figure 26-4 indicates the approximate interrelationship between k and the time elapsing until 10 or 50% of the drug is decomposed.

Pseudo-First-Order Reaction. If a reaction rate depends on the concentration of two reactant species (rate = $k\,C_a\,C_b$ or $k = C_a\,C_a$ or $k\,C_a^2$), it would be of a second order. A pseudo-first-order reaction can be defined as a second-order or bimolecular reaction that is made to behave like a first-order reaction. This is found in the case in which one reacting material is present in great excess or is maintained at a constant concentration as compared with the other

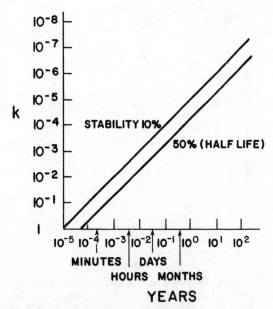

FIG. 26-4. *Approximate interrelationship between rate constant, k, and the time elapsing until 10% or 50% decomposition. (Redrawn from Schou, S. A.: Pharm. Acta Helv., 34:309, 1959.)*

substance. Under such circumstances, the reaction rate is determined by one reactant even though two are present, since the second reactant does not exhibit a significant change in concentration during the degradative reaction. An example of such a situation is the hydrolysis of an ester catalyzed by hydroxyl ion. If the hydroxyl ion concentration is high as compared with the concentration of the ester, the reaction behaves as a first-order reaction and can easily be followed by assay for residual ester. A similar approach, and one more frequently employed, is to keep the pH constant through the use of appropriate buffers.

An example of a drug that obeys pseudo-first-order kinetics is cefotaxime sodium.[4] As shown in Figure 26-5, semilogarithmic plots of cefotaxime sodium concentration versus time result in linear relationships at various pH levels demonstrating first-order rate of hydration (log k_1 vs. t). Acid catalysis occurs at ≤ pH 4, and base catalysis occurs at ≥ pH 8, in which the concentrations of H^+ and OH^- respectively are high compared with the concentration of cefotaxime sodium.

Influence of pH on Degradation

The magnitude of the rate of hydrolytic reactions catalyzed by hydrogen and hydroxyl ions can vary considerably with pH. Hydrogen ion catalysis predominates at the lower pH range, whereas hydroxyl ion catalysis operates at the higher pH range. At the intermediate pH range, the rate can be independent of pH or catalyzed by both hydrogen and hydroxyl ions. The rate constants in this pH range are usually less, however, than those at higher or lower pH values. To determine the influence of pH on the degradative reaction, the decomposition is measured at several hydrogen ion concentrations. The pH of optimum stability can be determined by the plotting of the logarithm of the rate constant versus pH, as illustrated by the pH profile in Figure 26-6. The point of inflection of such a plot represents the pH of optimum stability. Knowledge of this point is extremely useful in the development of a stable dosage form, provided the pH is within safe physiologic limits. Studies of this type can be performed at elevated temperatures so that data can be obtained in as short a time as possible. The shift of this point of inflection caused by temperature elevation is usually not of sufficient magnitude to affect seriously the conclusions drawn from such data. The plot in Figure 26-7 gives an actual example in which the point of inflection for methyl-DL-α-phenyl-2-piperidylacetate served as a guide in the development of a stable injectable solution.

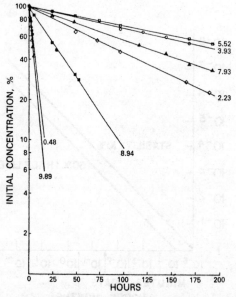

FIG. 26-5. *Observed pseudo-first-order plots for the degradation of I at various pH values, 25°, and μ = 0.5. Key: □, pH 5.52; ○, pH 3.93; ▲, pH 7.93; ◇, pH 2.23; ■, pH 8.94; ●, pH 0.48; △, pH 9.89. (From Berge, S. M., et al.: J. Pharm. Sci., 72:59, 1983. Reproduced with permission of the copyright owner, the American Pharmaceutical Association.)*

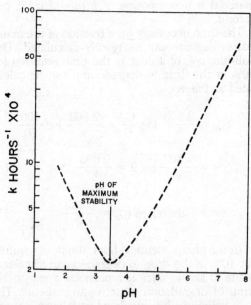

FIG. 26-6. *pH Inflection plot of maximum stability.*

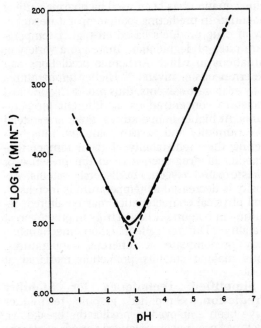

FIG. 26-7. *pH Dependency of the hydrolysis of methyl DL-α-phenyl-2-piperidylacetate at 80°. (From Siegel, S., et al.: J. Am. Pharm. Assoc., Sci. Ed., 48:431, 1959.)*

Influence of Temperature on Degradation

In order for the rate constants or velocity of degradation to be of use in the formulation of pharmaceutical products, it is necessary to evaluate the temperature dependency of the reaction. This permits the prediction of the stability of the product at ordinary shelf temperature from data obtained under exaggerated conditions of testing. According to rule-of-thumb methods, the rate of reaction is said to double for each 10° rise in temperature. Although this rule may serve as a fairly accurate estimate for certain preparations, it is not generally applicable. Therefore, to assign an overall factor for the influence of temperature on the acceleration of reactions is foolhardy. Some deterioration reactions are not measurably influenced over a 10° temperature range, while others undergo rapid degradative changes. The recommended procedure is to set up a planned schedule of accelerated tests for each formulation in order to ascertain the temperature dependency of the chemical changes in the product undergoing evaluation.

The most satisfactory method for expressing the influence of temperature on reaction velocity is the quantitative relation proposed by Arrhenius:

$$k = Se^{-Ha/RT} \qquad (18)$$

where: k = specific rate of degradation
R = gas constant (1.987 calories degree^{-1} mole^{-1})
T = absolute temperature
S = frequency factor

The constant of integration in the Arrhenius equation has been designated as the frequency factor. This value is a measure of the frequency of collisions that can be expected between the reacting molecules for a given reaction. Logarithmically, it may be expressed as follows:

$$\ln k = -\frac{\Delta Ha}{RT} + \ln S \qquad (19)$$

Converting to $\log_{10}$:

$$\log k = -\frac{\Delta Ha}{2.303\,R} \cdot \frac{1}{T} + \log S \qquad (20)$$

where log S can be considered a constant.

From equation (20), a plot of log k versus $\frac{1}{T}$ yields a slope equal to $-\dfrac{\Delta Ha}{2.303R}$ from which the value for the heat of activation can be calculated. The heat of activation (ΔHa) represents the energy the reacting molecules must acquire to undergo reaction. The higher the value for the heat of activation, the more the stability is temperature-dependent. The graph in Figure 26-8 represents a plot of k values obtained at several elevated temperatures. Since the plot is linear, the prediction of stability at shelf temperature is possible by extrapolating the curve to the lower temperatures and reading off the k value for the lower temperature. Once the k value is obtained, it can be used to estimate the time for $t_{10\%}$ degradation with the aid of equation (16).

In the event that the data available are more limited, for example, if the rate constants at two elevated temperatures or at one temperature and the heat of activation are known, it is still possible to obtain an estimate of the rate constant at a lower temperature by treating equation (19) to yield equation (22).

Using the differential form of equation (19):

$$\frac{d \ln k}{dt} = \frac{\Delta Ha}{RT^2} \qquad (21)$$

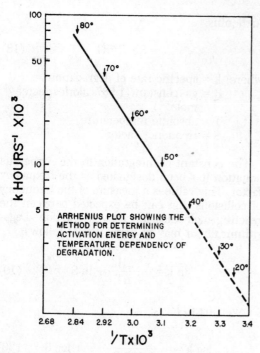

FIG. 26-8. *Temperature dependency of degradation rates.*

Upon integration between the limits k_1 and k_2 and T_1 and T_2, the following equation results:

$$\log \frac{k_2}{k_1} = \frac{\Delta Ha}{2.303 \, R} \left(\frac{T_2 - T_1}{T_2 \cdot T_1} \right) \qquad (22)$$

The utility of the temperature dependency relationship depends on the controlling mechanisms of degradation. Preparations that degrade through solvolytic processes, e.g., reactions in solution, usually have heats of activation in the range of 10 to 30 kcal/mole. Here, considerable advantage may be taken of the significant increases in rate of reaction that result with temperature elevation. On the other hand, if diffusion or photolysis are the rate determining steps of the reaction, the heat of activation is only of the magnitude of 2 to 3 Kcal/mole, and little advantage is gained by accelerated temperature studies in prediction, since the temperature effect on rate is small. For reactions such as pyrolysis of polyhydroxylic materials, in which the heat of activation can be of the magnitude of 50 to 70 kcal/mole, the rate of degradation, which may be great at elevated temperatures, may not be of any practical significance at the temperatures of marketing and storage of the pharmaceutical preparation.

Limitations of Arrhenius Relationship for Stability Prediction. Although the Arrhe-

nius equation has been used by pharmaceutical scientists in predicting room temperature stability of drug products based on higher temperature rates of degradation, there are a variety of situations in which Arrhenius predictions can be erroneous or invalid.[5,6] Higher temperatures may evaporate solvents, thus producing unequal moisture concentrations at different temperatures. At higher temperatures, there is less relative humidity and oxygen solubility, thus hindering the predictability of room temperature stability of drugs sensitive to the presence of moisture and oxygen. For disperse systems, viscosity is decreased as temperature is increased, and physical characteristics may be altered, resulting in potentially large errors in prediction of stability. Different degradation mechanisms may predominate at different temperatures, thus making stability prediction marginal at best.

Simplified Techniques for Stability Prediction. Simplified graphic techniques have been employed to predict the breakdown that may occur over prolonged periods of storage at normal shelf conditions. Free and Blythe describe such a technique for liquid products where the decomposition behaves according to the general kinetic laws.[7,8] For example, the plots in Figure 26-9 show that the degradation is following a first-order reaction. The time for the loss lines at the several temperatures to reach 90% of the theoretic potency is noted by arrows on the curve. These time values at different temperatures are plotted in Figure 26-10, and the time for 10% loss of potency at room temperature can be obtained from the resulting straight line by extrapolation to 25°C. If the extrapolated data in Figure 26-10 show that the time to reach

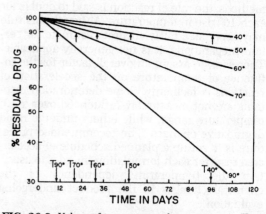

FIG. 26-9. *Values of $t_{10\%}$ at several temperatures. (From Blythe, R. H.: Product Formulation and Stability Prediction. Presented at the Production Section of the Canadian Pharm. Mfgrs. Assoc., April 1957.)*

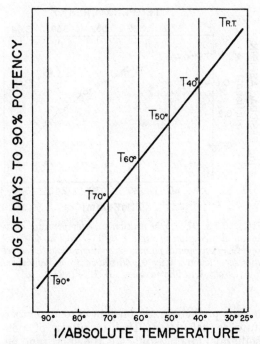

FIG. 26-10. *Plot of $t_{10\%}$ values vs. absolute temperature^{-1} (From Blythe, R. H.: Product Formulation and Stability Prediction. Presented at the Production Section of the Canadian Pharm. Mfgrs. Assoc., April 1957.)*

90% potency at room temperature is too rapid to provide an adequate shelf life for the product, it is possible to determine the overage required for the product to maintain at least 90% potency for a prescribed time. This is accomplished by drawing the loss line representative of the 90% potency value at room temperature, as shown in Figure 26-11. Then a line is drawn parallel to this from the desired shelf life back to "0" days. The example shown in Figure 26-11 indicates that by the use of a 10% overage, the product

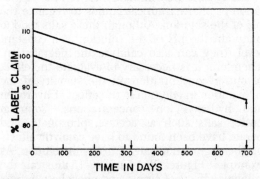

FIG. 26-11. *Plot of average and normal loss curves. (From Blythe, R. H.: Product Formulation and Stability Prediction. Presented at the Production Section of the Canadian Pharm. Mfgrs. Assoc., April 1957.)*

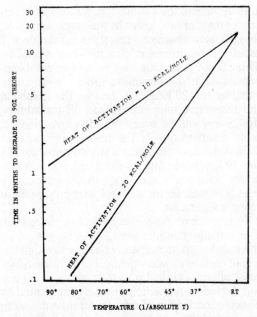

FIG. 26-12. *Two-year shelf-life goal reference decomposition. (From Kennon, L.: J. Pharm. Sci., 53:815, 1964. Reproduced with permission of the copyright owner.)*

now takes about twice as long to fall below 90% of labeled claim during shelf storage.

Kennon describes the construction of certain kinetic paths, which can be used for purposes of comparison during formulation development work.[9] Using standard kinetic equations, he calculated the paths that reactions would follow if a 10% potency loss in two years at room temperatures were permitted. By choosing activation energies of 10 and 20 kcal/mole, both of which are conservatively low, and by plotting the time in months that a formulation would take to drop to 90% potency versus 1/T, one arrives at Figure 26-12. Table 26-1 presents the data used in Figure 26-12.

If the potency of the formulation is found to remain above 90% of its original concentration

TABLE 26-1. *Maximum and Minimum Time at Which Potency Must Be at Least 90% of Label Claim at the Temperature Indicated in Order to Predict a Shelf-Life of Two Years at Room Temperature.*

Temperature	Maximum	Minimum
37°	12 months	6.4 months
45°	8.3 months	2.9 months
60°	4.1 months	3 weeks
85°	6 weeks	2.5 days

after storage at the various temperatures for certain periods of time given in the graph and table, there is good assurance that the formulation will meet the requirement of a two-year shelf-life. Thus, if the assays are over 90% of original concentration at the minimum times shown (indicated by the 20 Kcal/mole line on the graph) at the respective temperatures, in all probability, the assays will be over 90% after two years at room temperature. If the assays remain over 90% at the maximum times shown (indicated by the 10 Kcal/mole line on the graph), it is a certainty (kinetically speaking) that a potency of over 90% will be maintained after two years at room temperature.

It is evident from the foregoing discussion that considerable information can be gained on the stability characteristics of a drug through the use of certain physicochemical principles. Since most pharmaceutical preparations are complex, the degradation reaction may be complicated by possible interaction of the several ingredients in the formulation. It becomes impractical and is usually unnecessary to perform thorough basic kinetic studies on the final formulation to obtain an estimate of the shelf-life of the product. It usually is sufficient to follow the degradation or some property of the degradation as a function of time at several elevated temperatures, using the kinetic expressions presented, and then to extrapolate the data to ambient conditions to obtain an estimate of the shelf-life of the product. This is demonstrated with practical examples in the section of this chapter entitled "Chemical and Physical Stability Testing of Pharmaceutical Dosage Forms."

Thermal stability of pharmaceutical solutions and suspensions can be estimated by applying an accelerated nonisothermal kinetic method.[10,11] At suitable intervals, time and temperature are recorded, and samples of drug product are placed in a thermostated water bath whose temperature is increased at programmed intervals. The drug samples are assayed and plotted at log concentration versus time at a particular temperature. The points of the nonisothermal degradation curve, shown in Figure 26-13, are fitted according to a polynomial regression equation:

$$f(t) = a + bt + ct^2 + dt^3$$

where $f(t)$ is the concentration function, and a, b, c, and d are coefficients. The rate constants at each temperature are then calculated from the first derivative of this equation, which represents the slope of the tangent line at each point of the curve. Arrhenius plots are then generated,

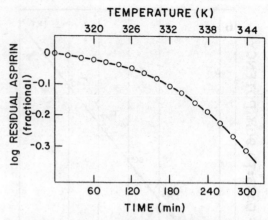

FIG. 26-13. *The concentration-time-temperature curve for the degradation of aspirin in 0.1N HCl at 40–70°C. Key: O, experimental points; —, mathematical fit (correlation coefficient = 0.9999). (Redrawn from Waltersson, J. O., et al.: Acta Pharm. Suec., 19:127, 1982.)*

and the predicted rate constant at room temperature is calculated. The advantage of nonisothermal kinetic studies is the short time period required to generate the data for estimating stability. Disadvantages include the need for programmable and sophisticated temperature control equipment and the decrease in experimental accuracy in predicting product shelf-life.

Discussions of kinetic expressions pertaining to complex mechanisms, general acid-base reactions, and the influence of ionic strength are not treated in detail but are briefly presented in a general manner to provide the reader with an awareness of the additional factors that can contribute to the stability of a drug.

General Acid-Base Catalysis of Degradation

Buffer salts are commonly used in the formulation of pharmaceutical liquids to regulate the pH of the solution. Although these salts tend to maintain the pH of the solution at a constant level, they can also catalyze the degradation. Therefore, it is necessary to evaluate the effect of buffer concentration on the stability of the preparation in addition to the effect of hydrogen and hydroxyl ion concentrations. Common buffer salts such as acetate, phosphate, and borate have been found to have catalytic effects on the degradation rate of drugs in solution. As examples, Figures 26-14 and 26-15 illustrate the catalytic effects of citrate and phosphate buffers on cefadroxil degradation at various pH.

To determine whether a particular formulation is catalyzed by the buffer system employed,

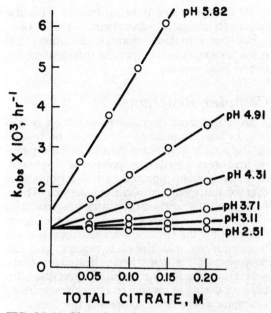

FIG. 26-14. *Plots of pseudo-first-order rate constant vs. total citrate buffer concentration for cefadroxil degradation at various pH values, 35°, and ionic strength 0.5. (Redrawn from Tsuji, K., et al.: J. Pharm. Sci., 70:1120, 1981. Reproduced with permission of the copyright owner, the American Pharmaceutical Association.)*

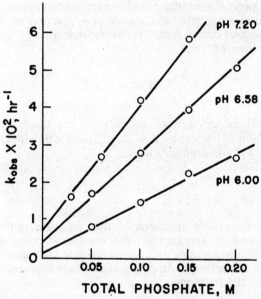

FIG. 26-15. *Plots of pseudo-first-order rate constant vs. total phsophate buffer concentration for cefadroxil degradation at various pH values, 35°, and ionic strength 0.5. (From Tsuji, K., et al.: J. Pharm. Sci., 70:1120, 1981. Reproduced with permission of the copyright owner, the American Pharmaceutical Association.)*

the ionic strength is kept constant, and the concentration of buffer is altered, while the ratio of the buffer salts is kept constant to maintain the pH. If the degradation reaction is found to be influenced by the different concentrations of buffer, then the reaction is considered to be general acid and base catalyzed. In such a case, the concentration of the buffer ratio should be kept as low as possible to diminish this catalytic effect.

Influence of Ionic Strength on Degradation

The rate of reaction can be influenced by the ionic strength of the solution in accordance with the following equation:

$$\log k = \log k_0 + 1.02\, Z_A Z_B \sqrt{u} \qquad (23)$$

where $Z_A + Z_B$ are the charges carried by the reacting species in solution, u, the ionic strength, k, the rate constant of degradation, and k_0, the rate constant at infinite dilution. The ionic strength ($u = \frac{1}{2}\Sigma c_i z_i^2$) is defined as half the sum of the terms obtained by multiplying the concentration of each of the ionic species present in the solution by the square of its valence. Plotting the logarithm of the reaction rates versus the square root of the ionic strength, as illustrated in Figure 26-16, can determine whether an increase in ionic strength increases, reduces, or has no effect on the degradation rate.

The concentration of salt employed in a liquid pharmaceutical formulation can increase or de-

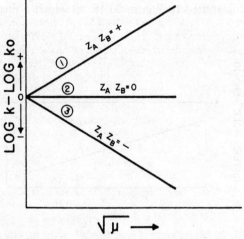

FIG. 26-16. *Dependence of reaction rates on ionic strength.*

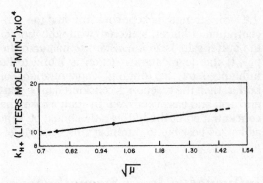

FIG. 26-17. *Influence of ionic strength on the velocity of hydronium-ion-catalyzed reaction. (From Siegel, S., et al.: J. Am. Pharm. Assoc., Sci. Ed., 48:431, 1959.)*

crease the degradation rate of the drug in solution or have no effect. When the drug is positively charged and is undergoing hydrogen ion catalysis, an increase in ionic strength caused by the addition of a salt, such as sodium chloride, causes an increase in the rate of degradation, as shown in curve 1, Figure 26-16. A decrease in the rate of degradation results if the positively charged drug is undergoing hydroxyl ion catalysis, and the ionic strength is increased by addition of a salt as shown in curve 3, Figure 26-16. If the drug undergoing degradation is a neutral molecule, changes in ionic strength by the addition of a salt would have no effect on the rate of gradation, as shown in curve 2, Figure 26-16.

The graph in Figure 26-17 shows the influence of increasing the ionic strength on the degradation rate of a positively charged drug; namely, methyl-DL-α-phenyl-2-piperidylacetate undergoing hydronium-ion-catalyzed degradation.

A negative salt effect on the degradation rate is illustrated in Figure 26-18, in which a positively charged ester is being reacted with the negatively charged hydroxyl ion.

For concentrated solutions, equation (23) must be expanded to include interactions between ionic species.

Complex Reactions

Although most degradative reactions occurring in pharmaceutical systems can be treated by the simple zero-order, first-order, and pseudo-first-order kinetics, as previously discussed, there are certain pharmaceutical formulations that exhibit more complicated reactions. These have opposing, consecutive, and side reactions along with the main reaction. In most instances, the extent of the simultaneous reactions is small in comparison with the main reaction and can be neglected. These more complicated reactions, several of which are now briefly described, include opposing or reverse reactions, consecutive reactions, and side or competing reactions.

Opposing Reactions. The simplest case of a reversible reaction is that in which both reactions are of the first order, as illustrated by the following:

$$A \underset{k^1}{\overset{k}{\rightleftharpoons}} B \qquad (24)$$

A somewhat more complicated reversible reaction is one in which the forward reaction is of a first-order type and the reverse reaction of a second-order type, as demonstrated by the following:

$$A \underset{k^1}{\overset{k}{\rightleftharpoons}} B + C \qquad (25)$$

When the forward and reverse reactions are both of the second-order type, the reaction takes on the following form:

$$A + B \underset{k^1}{\overset{k}{\rightleftharpoons}} C + D \qquad (26)$$

Reversible reactions of this type are quite common, but usually, the reverse reaction is ignored because the concentration is not significantly affected. An example of this is expressed by the following:

$$CH_3COOH + C_2H_5OH$$
$$\leftrightarrows CH_3COOC_2H_5 + H_2O$$

Initially, the reverse reaction can be ignored, but as the reaction proceeds, and the concentration

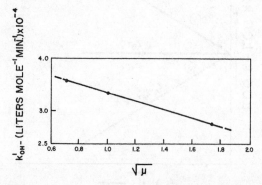

FIG. 26-18. *Influence of ionic strength on the velocity of the hydroxyl-ion-catalyzed reaction. (From Siegel, S., et al.: J. Am. Pharm. Assoc., Sci. Ed., 48:431, 1959.)*

of water and ethyl acetate increases, both reactions influence equation (26).

Since this has been given as a first example of a second-order reaction, a brief discussion of this type of reaction is presented. For equation (26), the rate of reaction is proportional to the concentration of the two reacting substances A and B for the forward reaction and C and D for the reverse reaction. For the forward reaction, if a and b represent the initial concentration of the two reacting substances, and if x denotes the moles of A and B in each liter reacting in the interval of time t, then the velocity of the reaction is expressed by the equation:

$$\frac{dx}{dt} = k(a - x)(b - x) \qquad (27)$$

When A and B are present in equal concentrations, a = b:

$$\frac{dx}{dt} = k(a - x)^2 \qquad (28)$$

Integrating equation (28) yields:

$$\frac{1}{k}\frac{dx}{(a - x)^2} = dt$$

$$\frac{1}{k}\frac{1}{(a - x)} = t + constant$$

For t = 0, constant = $\frac{1}{ka}$ (since x = 0 at t = 0).

$$k = \frac{1}{t} \cdot \frac{x}{a(a - x)} \qquad (29)$$

The half-life or time for 50% degradation ($t_{1/2}$) can be calculated by substitution.

Since x = ½a at the half-life, substituting into equation (29) results in the following equation:

$$t_{1/2} = \frac{1}{ka} \qquad (30)$$

Integrating equation (27), in which concentrations of A and B are not equal, the following equation results:

$$kt = \frac{1}{a - b} \cdot \ln\frac{b(a - x)}{a(b - x)}$$

or

$$k = \frac{2.303}{t(a - b)} \cdot \log\frac{b(a - x)}{a(b - x)} \qquad (31)$$

In such a reaction, plotting the log $\frac{b(a - x)}{a(b - x)}$

versus time (t), a straight line is obtained, and k is then obtained by multiplying the slope of the line by 2.303/(a − b).

Consecutive Reactions. When the stages of a consecutive reaction occur at rates of about the same magnitude, each stage must be considered in the kinetics of the overall reaction. The simplest case is one in which both consecutive processes are of the first order, as illustrated by the following equation:

$$A \xrightarrow{k_1} B \xrightarrow{k_2} C \qquad (32)$$

In the consecutive reaction, if k_2 is considerably greater than k_1, B can be considered an unstable intermediate, and the rate determining step for the overall reaction would be the conversion of A to B. The overall reaction could then be treated by first-order kinetics.

Side Reactions. In some processes, the reacting substance can be removed by two or more reactions occurring simultaneously, as depicted by the following equation:

$$A \begin{cases} \xrightarrow{k_1} B \\ - \\ \xrightarrow{k_2} C \end{cases} \qquad (33)$$

In general, side or competing reactions are more common to organic chemistry. The organic chemist routinely deals with the production of several compounds from two reactants; however, through the proper manipulation of conditions (e.g., pressure, temperature, concentration) the desired product predominates. An example of a competing reaction is the nitration of bromobenzene to produce ortho, meta, and para nitrobenzene as follows:

KINETIC PRINCIPLES AND STABILITY TESTING • 771

Purified insulin degrades by two mechanisms—deamidation and polymerization.[12] These degradation reactions may occur as consecutive and side reactions according to the following scheme:[13]

$$A \left\{ \begin{array}{l} \xrightarrow{k_1} B \xrightarrow{k_4} \\ \xrightarrow{k_2} C \xrightarrow{k_3} \end{array} \right\} D \qquad (34)$$

where: A = insulin
       B = desamido insulin
       C = polymerized insulin
       D = polymerized desamido insulin

The relative rates of deamidation and polymerization are pH- and temperature-dependent. This example of a complex reaction is probably representative of the complexity of degradation mechanisms that are seen with polypeptides produced by genetic engineering and developed as pharmaceutical dosage forms.

Degradative Pathways

Although the decomposition of active ingredients in pharmaceutical dosage forms occurs through several pathways, i.e., hydrolysis, oxidation-reduction, racemization, decarboxylation, ring cleavage, and photolysis, those most frequently encountered are hydrolysis and oxidation-reduction. Consequently, this section treats these two important degradation processes in detail and only briefly reviews the others.

Hydrolysis

Many pharamaceuticals contain ester or amide functional groups, which undergo hydrolysis in solution. Examples of drugs that tend to degrade by hydrolytic cleavage of an ester or amide linkage are anesthetics, antibiotics, vitamins, and barbiturates.

Ester Hydrolysis. The hydrolysis of an ester into a mixture of an acid and alcohol essentially involves the rupture of a covalent linkage between a carbon atom and an oxygen atom. Although some of these hydrolyses can be effected in pure water, in the majority of cases, the presence of a catalyst is needed to promote the reaction. These catalysts are invariably substances of a polar nature, such as mineral acids, alkalies, or certain enzymes, all of which are capable of supplying hydrogen or hydroxyl ions to the reaction mixture. The alkaline hydrolysis of an ester does not differ essentially from an acid-catalyzed hydrolysis, except that it is irreversible, and therefore quantitative, because the resultant acid is at once neutralized. On the other hand, the acid-catalyzed hydrolysis of esters is reversible and may be made essentially complete in either direction by an excess of water or alcohol.

Of the numerous schemes presented to represent the hydrolysis of esters by either alkali or acid, the one given by Walters is perhaps the clearest to visualize.[14]

For both the alkali- and acid-catalyzed hydrolysis, it is evident that the ester is cleaved at the acyl-oxygen linkage, that is, between the carbonyl carbon $\left(\begin{smallmatrix} O \\ \| \\ C \end{smallmatrix} \right)$ and the oxygen of $C_2H_5 (O - C_2H_5)$. This type of cleavage takes place for most ester hydrolytic reactions.

In practice, the general scheme employed to denote ester hydrolysis is as follows:

$$\underset{\text{ester}}{R^1 \overset{O}{\underset{\|}{-}C-OR}} + H^+ + OH^- \longrightarrow$$

$$\underset{\text{acid}}{R^1 \overset{O}{\underset{\|}{-}C-OH}} + \underset{\text{alcohol}}{HOR}$$

Alkali Catalyzed

rate-determining
addition of ionic
catalyst

Acid Catalyzed

Combination of ion with
water gives this unstable
intermediate, which
immediately breaks down
to acid or salt and alcohol.

This holds true for either acid- or alkaline-catalyzed reactions.

The general form of the kinetic equations to express acid- or base-catalyzed hydrolysis is as follows:

$$\frac{d\,(ester)}{dt} = -k\,(ester)(H^+)$$

$$\frac{d\,(ester)}{dt} = -k\,(ester)(OH^-)$$

These equations denote second-order reactions, but in studying degradation reactions of this type, it is possible to treat them as pseudo-first-order reactions. This is done by keeping the OH^- or H^+ at a considerably higher concentration than the ester concentration or by keeping the H^+ or OH^- concentrations essentially constant through the use of buffers. This would cause the previous equation to reduce to:

$$\frac{d\,(ester)}{dt} = -k\,(ester)$$

which represents a kinetic expression for a first-order reaction. Whenever possible, first-order

kinetic expressions have been employed in the study of the degradation of drugs by ester hydrolysis, but at times, second-order kinetic expressions have been employed.

A number of reports in the literature deal with detailed kinetic studies of the hydrolysis of pharmaceutical ingredients containing an ester group in the molecule. Probably one of the earliest and most thorough studies was performed on aspirin by Edwards.[15] He studied the degradation of aspirin in various buffer solutions and treated the overall reaction as pseudo-first-order.

The data in Table 26-2 represent a summary of the rates of degradation over a wide pH.

TABLE 26-2. *Aspirin Hydrolysis at Varying pH at 17°C*

pH	k (days⁻¹)	pH	k (days⁻¹)
0.53	0.578	6.0	0.120
1.33	0.0835	6.98	0.10
1.80	0.045	8.00	0.13
2.48	0.0267	9.48	0.321
2.99	0.0343	10.5	1.97
4.04	0.088	11.29	13.7
5.03	0.130	12.77	530

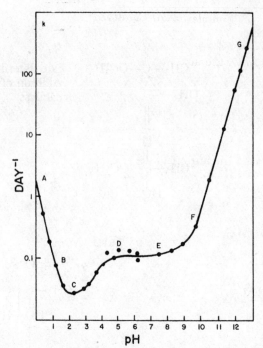

FIG. 26-19. *Overall velocity constant for aspirin hydrolysis at 17°C as a function of pH. (From Edwards, L. J.: Trans. Farad Soc., 46:723, 1950.)*

From a plot of the log k versus pH as presented in Figure 26-19, Edwards was able to postulate a reaction mechanism and determine the influence of pH on the degradation. The pH of optimum stability is at 2.4. At a pH of 5 to 7, the degradation reaction was essentially pH-independent, and at a pH above 10, the stability of aspirin was found to decrease rapidly with increase in pH. In the area in which the degradation is pH-independent, there are several reactions going on, each causing an effect of its own resulting in a cancellation of the effect of H⁺ and OH⁻, which gives a uniform rate over this pH range.

Although the use of pseudo-first-order kinetics is sufficient to define and study the degradation of aspirin, the hydrolysis of aspirin proceeds through a complex mechanism over the pH range studied, consisting of six different degradative pathways as shown below.

Other pharmaceutical materials that have been reported to degrade through ester hydrolysis are procaine, atropine, and methyl p-aminobenzoate.

These examples serve to illustrate the importance of chemical kinetic studies in evaluating the degradative pathways and overall stability of pharmaceutical compounds containing an ester group in the molecule.

As a result of the realization that a considerable number of drugs degrade through ester hydrolysis, methods to enhance the stability of pharmaceuticals undergoing this type of degradation have been under study. The following are factors to be considered:

1. *pH.* If physiologically permissible, the solution of the drug should be formulated as close as possible to its pH of optimum stability. In the event that the hydrolytic degradation of the drug is general acid and base catalyzed, that is, that the degradation is catalyzed by the acid and basic species of the buffer salt in addition to H⁺ and OH⁻, the buffer concentration should be kept at a minimum.

2. *Type of Solvent.* Partial or full replacement of water with a solvent of lower dielectric constant generally causes a considerable decrease in the velocity of ester hydrolysis.[16-26] Examples of these nonaqueous solvents are ethanol, glycols, glucose, and mannitol solutions and substituted amides.

$$CH_3COOC_6H_4COOH + H_3O^+ \xrightarrow{k_1} HOC_6H_4COOH + CH_3COOH + H^+ \qquad \text{(at low pH)}$$

$$CH_3COOC_6H_4COOH + H_2O \xrightarrow{k_2} HOC_6H_4COOH + CH_3COOH \qquad \text{(uncatalyzed)}$$

$$CH_3COOC_6H_4COOH + OH^- \xrightarrow{k_3} \left. \begin{array}{l} HOC_6H_4COOH + CH_3COO^- \\ HOC_6H_4COO^- + CH_3COOH \end{array} \right\} \qquad \text{(pH independent)}$$

$$CH_3COOC_6H_4COO^- + H_3O^+ \xrightarrow{k_4} HOC_6H_4COOH + CH_3COOH$$

$$CH_3COOC_6H_4COO^- + H_2O \xrightarrow{k_5} \left. \begin{array}{l} HOC_6H_4COOH + CH_3COO^- \\ HOC_6H_4COO^- + CH_3COOH \end{array} \right\} \qquad \text{(uncatalyzed)}$$

$$CH_3COOC_6H_4COO^- + OH^- \xrightarrow{k_6} HOC_6H_4COO^- + CH_3COO^- \qquad \text{(at high pH)}$$

3. *Complexation.* The hydrolytic rates may be influenced in two ways by complex formation, namely, by either steric or polar effects. Obviously, the attachment of a large caffeine molecule, for example, on a benzocaine molecule, can greatly affect the frequency and ease of encounter of the ester with various catalytic species (H^+, OH^-) through steric hindrance. The reaction also may be affected by the electronic influence of the complexing agent, which can alter the affinity of the ester carbonyl ion for the catalytic species. In general, the steric effect would be expected to decrease the hydrolytic rate, whereas the electronic effect may increase or decrease the reaction velocity.

Caffeine

Benzocaine

There have been several reports on the influence of complexing agents in retarding the hydrolytic deterioration of esters.[27-30] Higuchi and Lachman,[27] Lachman et al.,[28] and Lachman and Higuchi[29] have shown that caffeine complexes with local anesthetics, such as benzocaine, procaine, and tetracaine, cause a reduction of the velocity of their hydrolytic degradation. These investigators have also shown that the complexed fraction of the ester undergoes essentially no degradation.

Consequently, if it were possible to complex the total amount of drug in solution, it might be possible to stabilize it completely. Because of the limited solubility of caffeine, it has not been possible to accomplish this in the studies employing the hydrochloride salts of the local anesthetics. Guttman reported that the velocity of the base-catalyzed decomposition of riboflavin was decreased by the presence of caffeine in solution.[31] It was found that the vitamin in its complexed form with caffeine possessed negligible reactivity toward alkaline hydrolysis.

4. *Surfactants.* Using benzocaine as an example, Riegelman studied the effect of surfactants

TABLE 26-3. *Influence of Surfactant on Benzocaine Degradation at 30°C Using 0.04N NaOH*

Half-Life ($t_{1/2}$) in Minutes	Nonionic (%)	Cationic (%)	Anionic (%)
64	0	0	0
188	1.33		
324	3.3		
57		0.067	
425		1.34	
650		2.46	
420			1
1150			5

on the rate of hydrolysis of esters.[32] He found that nonionic, cationic, and anionic surfactants stabilize the drug against base catalysis, as evidenced by the data in Table 26-3.

A 5% sodium lauryl sulfate solution (anionic) caused an 18-fold increase in the half-life of benzocaine. The association of benzocaine close to the anionic head group of the surfactant made a definite barrier to the approach of the hydroxyl group into the micelle and attack on the ester linkage. When 2.46% cetyl trimethyl ammonium bromide in solution (cationic) is used, a tenfold increase in the half-life of benzocaine results. This effect is rather interesting, but can possibly be explained by the fact that although the negatively charged hydroxyl ion is attracted by the cationic group, it apparently cannot penetrate beyond this polar head into the deeper confines of the micelle wherein the benzocaine appears to be held. When a nonionic surfactant at 3.3% concentration is used, only about a four-fold to fivefold increase in half-life was obtained for benzocaine, indicating that the nonionic surfactant is a less effective stabilizer than the anionic or cationic ones. Because of the relatively high degree of hydration at the surface of the nonionic surfactant micelle, it would appear that considerable hydrolytic attack could take place within the micelle, as well as in the aqueous phase. However, this explanation of micelle protection against hydrolytic degradation of pharmaceutical compounds warrants further exploration.

5. *Modification of Chemical Structure.* A number of reports in the literature show that certain substituents added to the alkyl or acyl chain of aliphatic or aromatic esters or to the benzene ring of aromatic esters cause a decrease in the hydrolytic rate.[33-38] This may be attributed to a steric and/or polar effect of the substituent group. For example, by increasing the length of, or by branching, the acyl or alkyl chain, the rate of hydrolysis of the ester usually

Nonionic	Anionic	Cationic

Nonionic — Drug located at periphery of micelle.

Anionic — The free negative charges repel incoming OH^- ions.

Cationic — Presence of + ends attracts OH^- at low concentration. At higher concentration, the attached OH^- shields the drug from OH^-.

decreases, owing to steric hindrance. However, if an electrophilic or nucleophilic group is introduced into the acyl or alkyl side chain of aliphatic or aromatic esters, or on the benzene ring of aromatic esters, the rate of hydrolysis can be increased or decreased by the electronic effect of these groups.[39,40] For example, alkaline hydrolysis of aromatic esters is promoted by the presence of electrophilic groups on the benzene ring (halogen or NO_2), which attract electrons away from the reaction site (ester groups). The hydrolysis is retarded, on the other hand, by nucleophilic groups (CH_3, OCH_3, and NH_2), which cause electrons to move toward the point of reaction.[32] The reverse effect would be found in the case of hydrogen-ion-catalyzed hydrolysis of aromatic esters.

In general, base-catalyzed hydrolytic reactions are more affected by polar effects of substituents than is acid-catalyzed hydrolysis. On the other hand, the steric retardation of acid-catalyzed hydrolysis caused by substituents is greater than for base-catalyzed hydrolysis. The total effect produced by substituents in alkaline hydrolysis, however, is considerably greater than the effect produced in acid ester hydrolysis.[41] This is probably accounted for by the fact that in alkaline ester hydrolysis, both polar and steric effects of the substituents occur, whereas in acid ester hydrolysis, the polar effect is almost negligible.

In pharmaceutical practice, it is generally not possible to employ substituents on the drug molecule for improving stability against hydrolytic cleavage of the ester group, because in most cases, these substituents also have an effect on the physiologic activity of the drug molecule. The dipivalate ester of epinephrine, however, helps to protect the catechol ring from undergoing oxidation, thus enhancing the stability of the topical ophthalmic solution of epinephrine.

6. *Salts and Esters.* Another technique that is sometimes employed to increase the stability of pharmaceuticals undergoing degradation through ester hydrolysis is to reduce their solubility by forming less soluble salts or esters of the drug.[42–44] Usually, only the fraction of the drug that is in solution undergoes hydrolytic degradation. Garrett, in his study with acyl-salicylates, found that a compound that shows rapid hydrolysis in solution may be made to exhibit better stability than a more stable analog by reducing its solubility.[44]

Transient derivatives are nontoxic additions to drug molecules, such as hydrolyzable esters, which remain intact long enough to improve the drug bioavailability and then cleave to allow the parent compound to exert its recognized biologic activity. A transient derivative is a more soluble and/or stable form of the parent compound and permits better absorption for improved and more reproducible bioavailability. In this case, the drug modification undergoes biotransformation or hydrolysis at physiologic pH to yield the active form of the drug.

Monoesters of the antibiotics lincomycin and clindamycin have been prepared to render soluble and stable compounds suitable for injection. At pH 7.4, the antibiotics undergo biomodification to yield the active undissociated forms.

Monoesters of lincomycin with faster rates of hydrolysis were found to have greater in vivo antibacterial activity.[45,46]

Lincomycin, R groups = OH

Substitution of a hexanoate group:

$$-O-\overset{\overset{\displaystyle O}{\|}}{C}-C_5H_{11}$$

in the 2 position gives rise to hydrolysis rates at pH 7.4 in intestinal fluid, which are significantly greater than hexanoate substitution in the 3, 4, or 7 positions. The difference in enzymatic hydrolysis rates is attributed to the different steric and electronic environments of the four hydroxyl groups. Steric hindrance at the 2 position was also demonstrated by the observation that (3,3-dimethyl) butyrate hydrolyzed much more slowly than the hexanoate ester.

The phosphate esters of clindamycin undergo biomodification to release the active undissociated form. The inactive compound, clindamycin phosphate, on treatment with dephosphorylating enzymes affords the active compound clindamycin.[47] Figure 26-20 shows the percentage of hydrolysis of clindamycin phosphate esters in various enzymatic systems. The 3-phosphate ester was found to hydrolyze much more slowly and much less extensively than the 2-phosphate ester. An in vivo study in rats revealed lower blood levels for the 3-phosphate, which are probably related to the rate and degree of hydrolysis.

Amide Hydrolysis. Pharmaceutical compounds containing an amide group can undergo hydrolysis in a manner similar to that of an ester type compound. Instead of the acid and alcohol that form as a result of ester hydrolysis, hydrolytic cleavage of an amide results in the formation of an acid and an amine.

$$\underset{\text{amide}}{R-\overset{\overset{\displaystyle O}{\|}}{C}-\overset{\overset{\displaystyle H}{|}}{N}-R^1} + H_2O \longrightarrow$$

$$\underset{\text{acid}}{R-\overset{\overset{\displaystyle O}{\|}}{C}-OH} + \underset{\text{amine}}{H_2N-R^1}$$

Because of the relatively greater stability of amides as compared with structurally similar esters, there is considerably less information in the literature on quantitative chemical kinetic studies pertaining to the hydrolytic stability of such compounds. Pharmaceuticals such as nia-

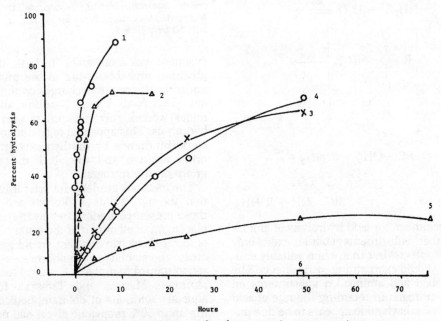

FIG. 26-20. *Percentage of hydrolysis of clindamycin phosphate esters in enzyme systems.*
1. Clindamycin—2—PO₄ in alkaline phosphatase.
2. Clindamycin—2—PO₄ in rat liver homogenate.
3. Clindamycin—2—PO₄ in human plasma.
4. Clindamycin—3—PO₄ in alkaline phosphatase.
5. Clindamycin—3—PO₄ in rat liver homogenate.
6. Clindamycin—3—PO₄ in human plasma. (From Brodasky, T. F., and Lewis, C. J.: Antibiot, 25:230, 1972.)

cinamide, phenethicillin, barbiturates, and chloramphenicol degrade by amide hydrolysis.

In a report on the stability of salicylamide and some N-substituted derivatives, Kosky postulated both basic and acid hydrolysis as mechanisms for degradation.[48] The basic hydrolysis proceeded as follows:

$$R-\overset{\overset{\displaystyle O}{\|}}{C}-NHR^1 + OH^- \underset{\text{slow}}{\rightleftharpoons}$$

$$R-\overset{\overset{\displaystyle O^-}{|}}{\underset{\underset{\displaystyle OH}{|}}{C}}-NHR^1 \xrightarrow{\text{fast}} R-\overset{\overset{\displaystyle O}{\|}}{C}-OH + R^1NH^-$$

$$RC\overset{\overset{\displaystyle O}{\|}}{}-O^- + R^1NH_2 \xleftarrow{\hspace{1cm}} \text{fast}$$

The rate-determining step in the hydroxide-ion-catalyzed reaction is the nucleophilic attack by the hydroxide ion.

The acid hydrolysis was as follows:

$$RC\overset{\overset{\displaystyle O}{\|}}{}-NHR^1 + H_3O^+ \xrightarrow{\text{fast}}$$

$$RC\overset{\overset{\displaystyle O}{\|}}{}-\overset{+}{N}H_2R^1 + H_2O \underset{\text{slow}}{\rightleftharpoons}$$

$$\left[R-\overset{\overset{\displaystyle O}{|}}{\underset{\underset{\displaystyle \overset{O}{\underset{H}{|}} \ \ H}{|}}{C}}-NH_2R \right]^+ \xrightarrow{\text{fast}}$$

$$RC\overset{\overset{\displaystyle O}{\|}}{}-OH_2^+ + R^1NH_2 \xrightarrow{\text{fast}}$$

$$RC\overset{\overset{\displaystyle O}{\|}}{}-OH + R^1NH_3^+$$

The mechanism for acid hydrolysis of amides requires that substituents should exert only weak polar effects, but that when suitably situated, they should exert strong steric effects. The effect of alkyl and aminoalkyl substituents on the amide nitrogen in retarding the rate of acid hydrolysis of salicylamide appears to be due primarily to steric hindrance.

As can be seen in Figure 26-21 in the acid medium, salicylanilide was more stable than salicylamide, which in turn was more stable than benzamide. Aminoalkyl substituents on the nitrogen increased the stability of benzamide. Sali-

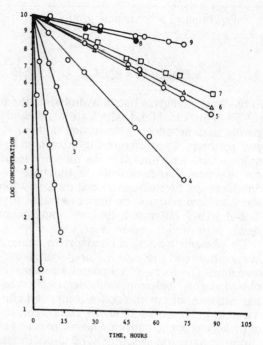

FIG 26-21. *Pseudo-first-order plot of the hydrolysis of amides in 1.0N perchloric acid at 90°. Key: 1, benzamide; 2, salicylamide; 3, N-(2-diethylaminoethyl) benzamide; 4, salicylanilide; 5, N-(2-diethylaminoethyl) salicylamide hydrochloride; 6, N-(2-dimethylaminoethyl)-salicylamide hydrochloride; 7, N-(2-diisopropylaminoethyl)-salicylamide hydrochloride; 8, N-isopentylsalicylamide; 9, N-propylsalicylamide. (From Kosky, K. T.: J. Pharmaceut. Sci., 58:560, 1969.)*

cylamide was more stable in basic than acidic medium, probably owing to the protection afforded by the negative charges on the phenolate ion. The N-alkyl and N-amino alkylsalicylamides were highly resistant to acid and base hydrolysis. This appeared to be due to combined steric hindrance by the hydroxyl group in the ortho position and the alkyl and aminoalkyl group on the nitrogen.

The methods available for retarding deterioration through amide hydrolysis are similar to those presented under ester hydrolysis. The replacement of all or part of the water with solvent of lower dielectric constant would generally increase the stability of the pharmaceutical preparation toward hydrolysis. Contrary to this generalization, Marcus and Taraszka found that aqueous solutions of chloramphenicol containing up to 50% propylene glycol had no effect on improving the stability of this antibiotic over that obtained with solutions of the antibiotic in water.[49] In fact, a slight increase in the rate of reaction was observed. Consequently, as illustrated in this study, it is unwise to make a blanket assumption that replacement of all or part of the water in a pharmaceutical preparation enhances the stability of an active ingredient. Instead, each situation must be individually evaluated with due consideration given to the mechanism of degradation. An instance in which the use of propylene glycol was found to retard amide hydrolysis is given in a report by Bodin and Taub,[50] who show that the stability of pentobarbital in solution is effectively enhanced by the use of a propylene glycol solvent system.

Ring Alteration. A hydrolytic reaction can proceed as a result of ring cleavage with subsequent attack by hydrogen or hydroxyl ion. Examples of drugs that have been reported to undergo hydrolysis by this mechanism include hydrochlorothiazide, pilocarpine, and reserpine. Quite often, equilibrium kinetics is associated with such mechanisms.

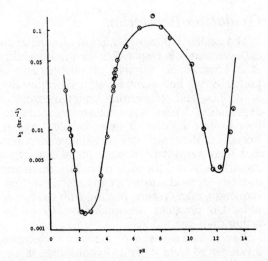

FIG. 26-22. *pH-Rate profile of the hydrolysis of hydrochlorothiazide at 60°C. (From Mollica, J. A., Rehm, C. R., and Smith, J. B.: J. Pharm. Sci., 58:635, 1969. Reproduced with permission of the copyright owner.)*

Mollica et al. reported that the hydrolysis of hydrochlorothiazide involved reversible kinetics in which the rate of forward reaction was influenced by pH, but the equilibrium constant was independent of pH.[51] The hydrolytic reaction was reported to proceed by ring opening to form an imine, which undergoes attack by water or hydroxide ion to yield a carbinolamine intermediate, which further decomposes to formaldehyde and 4-amino-6-chloro-m-benzenedisulfonamide, as shown by the following scheme:

$$I \rightleftharpoons R - N = CH_2 \rightleftharpoons$$
$$R - NH - CH_2OH \rightleftharpoons II + HCHO$$

The observed pH profile for hydrochlorothiazide, illustrated in Figure 26-22, is relatively complex and cannot be explained by ionization of reactants, but lends itself to Schiff base formation and hydrolysis.

The hydrolysis of pilocarpine in aqueous solution has been reported to involve a cyclic equilibrium process, which is catalyzed by hydrogen ion and hydroxyl ion.[52] Although uncertainty exists as to whether both the hydrogen ion and hydroxide ion catalysis are equilibrium processes, the concentration of pilocarpate and pilocarpic acid are influenced by pH. One of the schemes postulated for the cyclic mechanism is as follows:

Pilocarpine is relatively stable in solutions of acidic pH, $k_H = 1.35 \times 10^{-1}$ liters/mole/hr. As the pH increases, pilocarpine progressively becomes unstable, $k_{OH} = 7.56 \times 10^2$ liters/mole/hr. Phosphate and carbonate buffers catalyze the degradation, whereas borate does not. The addition of methylcellulose improves the stability slightly.

Oxidation-Reduction

The oxidative decomposition of pharmaceutical compounds is responsible for the instability of a considerable number of pharmaceutical preparations. For example, steroids, vitamins, antibiotics, and epinephrine undergo oxidative degradation. These reactions are mediated either by free radicals or by molecular oxygen. Because of the complexity of oxidative processes and their sensitivity to trace metal and other impurities, it is difficult to reproduce them and to establish mechanisms for the reactions. Consequently, many reports dealing with oxidation-reduction reactions are qualitative in nature rather than quantitative.

A substance is said to be oxidized if electrons are removed from it. Thus, a substance is oxidized when it gains electronegative atoms or radicals or loses electropositive atoms or radicals. Oxidation often involves the addition of oxygen or the removal of hydrogen. The simplest type of oxidation is, therefore, the elimination of an electron, as in the process:

$$Fe^{++} \longrightarrow Fe^{+++} + e^-$$

where the ferrous ion is oxidized to the ferric ion.

The most common form of oxidative decomposition occurring in pharmaceutical preparations is autoxidation, which involves a free radical chain process. In general, autoxidation may be defined as the reaction of any material with molecular oxygen. Free radicals are produced by reactions involving homolytic bond fission of a covalent bond, so that each atom or group involved retains one of the electrons of the original covalent bond. This may be depicted as follows:

$$A:B \longrightarrow A\cdot + B\cdot$$
$$CH_3:CH_3 \longrightarrow 2CH_3$$

These radicals are highly unsaturated and readily take electrons from other substances, causing oxidation. The autoxidation of an organic substance RH by a free radical chain process can be simply described as follows:

Initiation:

$$RH \xrightarrow[\text{light, heat}]{\text{activation}} R\cdot + (\dot{H})$$

Propagation:

$$R\cdot + \bar{O}_2 \longrightarrow RO_2$$
$$RO_2\cdot + RH \longrightarrow ROOH + R\cdot$$

Hydroperoxide Decomposition:

$$ROOH \longrightarrow RO\cdot + \cdot OH$$

Termination:

$$RO_2\cdot + X \longrightarrow \text{inactive products}$$
$$RO_2 + RO_2 \longrightarrow \text{inactive products}$$

The initiation of this reaction can be produced by the thermal decomposition of substances naturally present or added to the reaction mixture or possibly by light. As shown above, termination of the reaction may take place by combining two $RO_2\cdot$ radicals or by X, a free radical inhibitor. In the latter case, X generally converts the peroxy radical $RO_2\cdot$ to a hydroperoxide and becomes a resonance stabilized radical incapable of continuing the chain. Generally free radicals can best be terminated by a free radical inhibitor (e.g., sodium metabisulfite, thiourea, cysteine hydrochloride), since otherwise the product of recombination of radicals could contain sufficient energy to redissociate the molecule. In autoxidative reactions, only a small amount of oxygen is needed to initiate the reaction, and thereafter, oxygen concentration is relatively unimportant.

Heavy metals, particularly those possessing two or more valency states, with a suitable oxidation-reduction potential between them (copper, iron, cobalt, and nickel) generally catalyze oxidative deteriorations. These metals reduce the length of the induction period (the time in which no measurable oxidation occurs) and increase the maximum rate of oxidation. They can affect the rates of chain initiation, propagation, and termination, as well as the rate of hydroperoxide decomposition. In each case, their major function is to increase the rate of formation of free radicals.

Many oxidations are catalyzed by hydrogen and hydroxyl ions. This can partly be ascribed to the fact that the redox potential for many reactions depends on pH. This is particularly true for pharmaceutical compounds falling under the classification of weak acids. The system quinone/hydroquinone may be taken as a classic example to illustrate this point.

The oxidation potential may be expressed by the following simplified version of the Nernst equation:

$$E = Eo + \frac{0.06}{2} \log \frac{C_{H^+}{}^2 \cdot C_{quinone}}{C_{hydroquinone}}$$

where Eo is the so-called standard potential, E is the actual potential, 2 equals the number of electrons taking place in the change from the ox-form to the red-form, and 0.06 is a calculated approximate constant.[53] It can be seen from this equation that an increase in the concentration of hydrogen ions causes an increase in the value of E. This means that the red-form of the system is less readily oxidized when the pH is low. Since pharmaceuticals that undergo deterioration through oxidation are generally in the red-form, minimum decomposition is usually found in the pH range of 3 to 4.

Although the oxygen concentration is of importance in the autoxidation process, its significance is usually not adequately considered. When studying the rate of the reaction for an oxidation at different temperatures, it is necessary to consider both the direct effect of the temperature and the effect of temperature on the oxygen content (concentration of oxygen) of the liquid. For example, the transfer of a preparation from storage at 15 to 5°C, with a temperature coefficient of 2 for a 10°C change, causes the rate to be reduced to half its initial magnitude, owing to the direct temperature dependence of the reaction. Simultaneously, the concentration of oxygen increases by about 25%, usually resulting in an increased rate of oxidation. Examples of pharmaceuticals that degrade through oxidative pathways are shown in Table 26-4.

For the most part, oxidative degradations of pharmaceutical compounds follow first-order or second-order kinetic expressions. Guttman and Meister studied the base-catalyzed degradation of prednisolone and found that the degradation exhibited a first-order dependency on steroid concentration.[54] The rate of prednisolone disappearance from aqueous solutions increased with an increase in hydroxyl ion concentration under both aerobic and anaerobic conditions; however, the reaction mixture exposed to air showed more rapid degradation of prednisolone (Table 26-5). For example, at a hydroxide ion concentration of 0.01N, the rate constant for the overall degradation obtained under anaerobic conditions was approximately half the value of that obtained when no precautions were taken to exclude air from the system.

Trace metal impurities in buffer salts caused

TABLE 26-4. *Common Drugs That are Reported to React with Oxygen*

Amikacin	Novobiocin
Apomorphine	p-Aminobenzoic acid
Ascorbic acid	Paraldehyde
Chlorpromazine and other phenothiazines	Penicillin
	Pentazocine
Cyanocobalamin	Phenylephrine
Dexamethasone	Physostigmine
Dobutamine	Prednisolone
Epinephrine	Prednisone
Edrophonium	Procaine and related amides
Ergometrine	Reserpine
Gentamicin	Resorcinol
Heparin	Riboflavin
Hydrocortisone	Streptomycin
Isoamyl nitrite	Sulfadiazine
Isoproterenol	Thiothixene
Kanamycin	Terpenes
Methyldopate	Tetracyclines
Metaraminol	Thiamine
Metoclopramide	Tobramycin
Morphine	Turbocurarine
Neomycin	Vitamin A
Norepinephrine	Vitamin D
	Vitamin E

From Akers, M. J.: J. Parenter. Sci. Tech., 36:223, 1982.

an accelerated decomposition of prednisolone, which was first thought to be due to buffer concentration.[55] By studying the oxidative degradation with and without 0.1% disodium salt of ethylenediamine tetraacetic acid at different buffer concentrations, it was found that the solutions not containing any chelating agent degraded more rapidly as the buffer concentration increased, while the buffered solutions containing chelating agent showed that the rate of degradation was independent of the concentration of the buffer. This is clearly shown by the graphs in Figure 26-23.

These investigators also studied the influence of pH on the stability of prednisolone in borate

TABLE 26-5. *Rate Constants for the Base-Catalyzed Degradation of Prednisolone at 35°C in the Absence and Presence of Air*

Normality of NaOH	ka (Anaerobic) Hr^{-1}	ka (Aerobic) Hr^{-1}
0.01	0.0311	0.0589
0.02	0.0531	0.0839
0.03	0.071	0.110
0.04	0.103	0.097
0.05	0.120	0.110

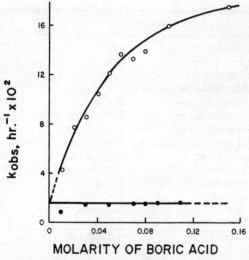

FIG. 26-23. *The effect of buffer concentration on the rate of prednisolone degradation in the presence and absence of sequestrene Na₂ at 30°, pH 10, and ionic strength 0.2. Key: ○, no EDTA; ●, 0.1% EDTA. (From Oesterling, T. O., and Guttman, D. E.: J. Pharm. Sci., 53:1189, 1964.)*

buffer with and without chelating agent. The chelating agent was found to have little effect on the degradation rate up to a pH of 8; but at higher pH, the disappearance of prednisolone occurred more rapidly from systems that were not protected by chelating agents. Using a phosphate buffer system, it was found that the solutions containing the chelating agent showed enhanced stability, beginning at pH 5 over the solutions without chelating agent. In addition, the pH dependency from 5 to 8 was very small for the system containing chelating agent, but considerable for the system without it. It is interesting to note that the influence of pH on the metal catalyzed reaction in phosphate buffer was somewhat different from the borate buffer.

Rancidity, which can affect nearly all oils and fats, is a widely known term covering many typical off-flavors formed by the autoxidation of unsaturated fatty acids present in an oil or fat. These off-flavors have a more or less distinct odor and are due to the volatile compounds that are formed upon oxidation of the oils and fats. These volatile compounds are generally short-chain monomers that are formed by cleavage of the nonvolatile hydroperoxide primary oxidation product. The free radical mechanism shown here depicts the oxidation of oils and fats that takes place in the presence of atmospheric oxygen, light, and trace amounts of catalysts.

Determination of iodine numbers can be employed as an indication of whether oxidation has taken place across the double bond.

$$R'—CH_2—CH{=}CH—R'' + O_2 \longrightarrow R'—\dot{C}H—CH{=}CH—R'' + HO_2\cdot$$

$$R'—\dot{C}H—CH{=}CH—R'' + O_2 \longrightarrow \underset{\underset{O—O\cdot}{|}}{R'—CH—CH{=}CH—R''}$$

$$\underset{\underset{O—O\cdot}{|}}{R'—CH—CH{=}CH—R''} + R'—CH_2—CH{=}CH—R'' \longrightarrow$$

$$\underset{\underset{O—OH}{|}}{R'—CH—CH{=}CH—R''} + R'—\dot{C}H—CH{=}CH—R''$$

$$2\,\underset{\underset{O—OH}{|}}{R'—CH—CH{=}CH—R''} \longrightarrow R'—CHO + R''—CH{=}CH\cdot + \cdot OH$$

hydroperoxide   nonvolatile

$$\div$$

$$R''—CH{=}CH—CHO—R' + \cdot OH$$

volatile

or

$$2\,\underset{\underset{H}{|}}{R'—\overset{\overset{O}{\|}}{C}—CH{=}CH—R''} + 2\cdot OH$$

The stability of pharmaceutical compounds undergoing oxidative degradation can be increased by several approaches.

Oxygen Content. Since, in many cases, oxidative degradation of a drug takes place in aqueous solution, it is helpful to keep the oxygen content of these solutions at a minimum. In a study to determine the oxygen content of water prepared and treated by different techniques, it was found that water in equilibrium with atmospheric oxygen contains 5.75 ml per liter of oxygen at 25°C and 9.14 ml per liter of oxygen at 4°C, and that all free oxygen is expelled from water at 100°C.[56] Freshly distilled water collected directly from the distillation apparatus and stored at 4°C in closed containers contains ¼ to ⅓ the oxygen content of water saturated with oxygen from the atmosphere. Boiling and cooling this freshly distilled water to 20°C results in almost a twofold increase in the oxygen content of the water; however, if the water is cooled in an atmosphere essentially free from atmospheric oxygen, there is no increase in oxygen content. To obtain water that contains a minimum amount of free oxygen, water after it is first boiled is purged with carbon dioxide or nitrogen gas. The oxygen content of water treated with carbon dioxide is reduced to 0.45 ml per liter at 20°C.

Since most oxidative degradations of pharmaceutical compounds are probably autoxidative in nature and involve chain reactions that require only a small amount of oxygen for initiating the reaction, reduction of oxygen concentration alone is not sufficient in many cases to prevent degradation from occurring. The traces of oxygen left may be sufficient to start a chain reaction. Consequently, it is necessary to add agents such as antioxidants and chelating agents to obtain acceptable protection against oxidative degradation.

Antioxidants. Antioxidants are added to pharmaceutical formulations as redox systems possessing higher oxidative potential than the drug that they are designed to protect, or as chain inhibitors of radical induced decomposition. In general, the effect of antioxidants is to break up the chains formed during the propagation process by providing a hydrogen atom or an electron to the free radical and receiving the excess energy possessed by the activated molecule.

Although the selection of an antioxidant can be made on sound theoretic grounds based on the difference in redox potential between the drug and antioxidant, electrometric measurements only rarely predict the efficiency of antioxidants in complex pharmaceutical systems. The effectiveness of an antioxidant or the comparative value of various antioxidants for a particular pharmaceutical preparation is best accomplished by subjecting the pharmaceutical system with the antioxidant to standard oxidative conditions and periodically assaying the formulation for both drug and antioxidant. Although this method may require maximum effort, it yields the most useful information.

It should be remembered that because of the complexity of free radical oxidative processes and their sensitivity to trace amounts of impurities, attempts to compare the effectiveness of antioxidants among different pharmaceutical systems are of limited validity.

Antioxidant materials used in pharmaceutical systems are listed in Tables 26-6 and 26-7.

Water-soluble antioxidants act by preferentially undergoing oxidation in place of the drug. Oil-soluble antioxidants serve as free radical acceptors and inhibit the free radical chain process. Sulfurous acid salts consume molecular oxygen present in solution. Structurally, other antioxidants have the property of losing a hydrogen free radical and/or an electron.

The effectiveness of these antioxidants can depend on the concentration used, whether they are used singularly or in combination, the solution pH, and the package integrity and nonreactivity.

Although sodium metabisulfite has been used extensively in the past and is still used to a considerable extent as an effective antioxidant, recent reports have indicated that the antioxidant

TABLE 26-6. *Antioxidants Commonly Used for Aqueous Systems*

Sodium sulfite	Ascorbic acid
Sodium metabisulfite	Isoascorbic acid
Sodium bisulfite	Thioglycerol
Sodium thiosulfate	Thioglycolic acid
Sodium formaldehyde	Cysteine hydrochloride
sulfoxylate	Acetylcysteine
Sulfur dioxide	

TABLE 26-7. *Antioxidants Commonly Used for Oil Systems*

Ascorbyl palmitate	Butylated hydroxy
Hydroquinone	toluene
Propyl gallate	Butylated hydroxy anisole
Nordihydroguaiaretic	α-tocopherol
acid	Lecithin

activity of this substance is inhibited by a number of compounds, that it actually undergoes degradation itself, and that it potentiates the degradation of epinephrine.[57-60]

The effectiveness of bisulfite as an antioxidant in typical pharmaceutical systems depends on the ease with which this compound is oxidized in comparison with the drug it is to protect. Substances that inhibit bisulfite oxidation may exert important effects on the overall stability of the product by decreasing the antioxidant effect of bisulfite. It has been postulated that the mechanism by which these substances inhibit sulfite activity is through the formation of coordination compounds between inhibitor and bisulfite. Typical substances that can inhibit the oxidation of bisulfite are mannitol, phenols, inorganic anions, aldehydes, ketones, and alkaloids.

It has been shown that bisulfite reacts with epinephrine to form a colorless, inactive epinephrine sulfonate, which thus indicates the need for caution in using bisulfite in formulations without performing adequate studies to determine its effect on active ingredients.[59] These investigators showed that a substantial breakdown of epinephrine takes place in the presence of bisulfite as depicted in Figure 26-24. Higuchi and Schroeter reported that the degradation of chloramphenicol induced by bisulfite appears to be considerably more complex than that found with epinephrine.[58] Loss of optical activity was found to occur at a much faster rate in the presence of bisulfite.

Riegelmen and Fisher, in their study to stabilize epinephrine against sulfite-catalyzed degradation, found that when boric acid was added to the solution, a marked stabilization of epinephrine took place.[60] They postulated that this stabilizing effect of boric acid was due to chelate formation between boric acid and the catechol grouping of epinephrine.

The epinephrine is able to form a one-to-one chelate through its dihydroxy structure, as follows:

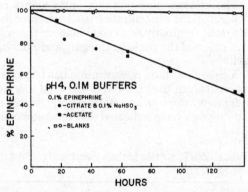

In the presence of boric acid, the rate of sulfite attack is reduced as the hydrogen ion concentration decreases. The half-life for epinephrine under the reaction conditions at pH 6.0 in the absence of boric acid was found to be 195 hours, whereas in the presence of boric acid, the half-life was found to be 267 hours. At pH 7.5, however, the half-life of epinephrine was found to be 74 hours in the absence of boric acid and 1,270 hours in its presence. It was postulated that epinephrine is increasingly chelated by the boric acid molecules as the pH is made more alkaline, and that the chelated epinephrine is far less susceptible to sulfite attack than free epinephrine.

The effectiveness of antioxidants can be enhanced through the use of synergists such as chelating agents.

Chelating Agents. Chelating agents tend to form complexes with the trace amounts of heavy metal ions inactivating their catalytic activity in the oxidation of medicaments. Examples of some chelating agents are ethylenediamine tetraacetic acid derivatives and salts, dihydroxyethyl glycine, citric acid, and tartaric acid.

pH. It is also desirable to buffer solutions containing ingredients that are readily oxidizable to a pH in the acid range. This causes an increase of the oxidation potential of the system with a concurrent increase in stability when oxidations are catalyzed by hydrogen or hydroxyl ions. The pH of optimum stability in the acid range, however, must be determined experimentally for each drug.

Solvents. Solvents other than water may have a catalyzing effect on oxidation reactions when used in combination with water or alone.

FIG. 26-24. *Percentage of epinephrine remaining in 0.1% (0.0055 molar) solutions containing 0.1% sodium bisulfite (0.0096 molar) buffered at pH 4.0 with 0.1 molar acetate or citrate. The solutions were stored in sealed, evacuated ampuls at 80°. (From Schroeter, L. C., Higuchi, T., and Schuler, E. E.: J. Am. Pharm. Assoc., Sci. Ed., 47:724, 1958.)*

Photolysis

Consideration of the decomposition of pharmaceutical compounds resulting from the absorption of radiant energy in the form of light has become more important in recent years because of the complex chemical structure of many new drugs. Degradative reactions, such as oxidation-reduction, ring rearrangement, or modification and polymerization, can be brought about by exposure to light at particular wave lengths. According to the equation $E = 2.859 \times 10^5 / \lambda$ Kcal per mole, the shorter the wave length (λ) of light, the more energy is absorbed per mole. Consequently, the radiations absorbed from the ultraviolet and violet portions of the light spectrum are more active in initiating chemical reactions than those absorbed from the other longer wave length portions of the spectrum.

In a large number of systems that are photolyzed, free radicals are products that undergo subsequent reactions. If the molecules absorbing the radiation take part themselves in the main reaction, the reaction is said to be a *photochemical* one. Where the absorbing molecules do not themselves participate directly in the reaction, but pass on their energy to other molecules that do, the absorbing substance is said to be a *photosensitizer*.

The kinetics of photochemical reactions is more complicated than the kinetics of thermal reactions because more variables are involved. The intensity and wave length of light and the size and shape of the container may greatly affect the rate of reaction. A photochemical reaction may be accompanied by a thermal reaction that is identical to the photochemical reaction opposite to it, or entirely different in character. A photochemical reaction may produce a catalyst, which then causes a thermal reaction to proceed at a measurable rate. Sometimes an induction period is necessary while a sufficient quantity of catalyst is being accumulated, to make the reaction proceed with a measurable velocity. A thermal reaction, once started, may continue after the illumination is stopped, giving an aftereffect. The energy available in a photochemical reaction is much greater than in a thermal reaction, and this fact often changes the character of the reaction.

As a result of the complexity of photolytic reactions, investigations in this area of pharmaceutical stability have been, for the most part, qualitative in nature. Only within recent years have photodegradative studies been performed on a quantitative basis. In photodegradative reactions, second-order, first-order, and zero-order reactions are possible.

Felmeister and Dischler studied the photodecomposition of chlorpromazine hydrochloride at 253.5 mμ and derived the mechanism for the free radical-mediated deterioration of chlorpromazine.[61] The ultraviolet irradiation of chlorpromazine causes the degradation to proceed through a semiquinone free radical intermediate. The semiquinone free radical disproportionates in aqueous media in both the absence and the presence of dissolved oxygen, though the loss of free radical is slightly faster in the presence of oxygen. The loss in concentration of chlorpromazine versus photons of light per liter absorbed shows that degradation follows zero-order kinetics.

Hamlin et al. studied the photolytic degradation of alcoholic solutions of hydrocortisone, prednisolone, and methylprednisolone exposed to ordinary fluorescent lighting.[62] The plots in Figure 26-25 show that the degradation follows first-order kinetics and that prednisolone and methylprednisolone show about the same rate of degradation, whereas hydrocortisone degrades about $1/7$ the rate of the other two steroids. Hence, the two double bonds present in prednisolone and methylprednisolone make these steroids more susceptible to light-catalyzed degradation than the one double bond in the A ring of hydrocortisone.

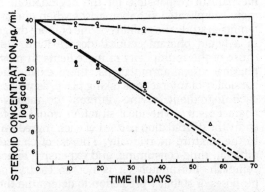

FIG. 26-25. *First-order plots of the photolytic degradation of steroids when exposed to laboratory fluorescent lighting. Hydrocortisone: X, INH assay; O, U. V. assay. Prednisolone: △, INH assay; □, U. V. assay. Methylprednisolone;* ●, *INH. (From Hamlin, W. E., Chulski, T., Johnson, R. H., and Wagner, J. G.: J. Am. Pharm. Assoc. Sci., Ed., 49:253, 1960.)*

Racemization

In such a reaction, an optically active substance loses its optical activity without changing its chemical composition. This reaction can be important to the stability of pharmaceutical formulations, since the biologic effect of the dextro form can be considerably less than that of the levo form. For example, levo-adrenaline is 15 to 20 times more active than dextro-adrenaline. Solutions of levo-adrenaline form a racemic mixture of equal parts of levo- and dextro-adrenaline with a pharmacologic activity just over half that of the pure levo compound.

The kinetics of racemization may be studied in a manner similar to hydrolytic reactions. By determining the rate constant, temperature dependency of the reaction, and dependence of the reaction on pH, it is possible to establish the optimal conditions for storage of the preparation. Racemization reactions, in general, undergo degradation in accordance with first-order kinetic principles. The racemization of a compound appears to depend on the functional group bound to the asymmetric carbon atom; aromatic groups tend to accelerate the racemization process.

Chemical and Physical Stability Testing of Pharmaceutical Dosage Forms

Chemical Stability. The information presented thus far has illustrated that it is possible, through the use of chemical kinetic principles, to study the degradation of an active drug in solution accurately, as well as determine the mechanism responsible for the degradation. A more complicated situation arises when one attempts to study the stability of one or more drugs in a liquid pharamaceutical dosage form. Because of the multiplicity of ingredients in most pharmaceutical formulations, there exists the possibility of interactions taking place, as well as each ingredient having different degradative characteristics. The ideal situation would be to study the degradation pattern of each ingredient in the mixture individually. This is, of course, difficult, time-consuming, and expensive to accomplish. Fortunately, it is not necessary for purposes of stability prediction to determine the mechanisms of degradation. In general, it is possible to evaluate the stability of any component of a pharmaceutical preparation by determining some property of the degradation as a function of time. If this function can be linearized in accordance with chemical kinetic reaction orders, the

TABLE 26-8. *Rates of Decrease of Absorbance of Prepared Extract at 500 mμ per Hour (k)*

°C	(k)
40	0.00011
50	0.00028
60	0.00082
70	0.00196

temperature dependency of the degradation can be obtained. Information of this type, obtained from exaggerated test conditions of short duration, permits the determination of the chemical stability of an active ingredient or ingredients, colorants, and antimicrobial preservatives for extended shelf storage.

The color stability of a multisulfonamide preparation was determined in this fashion. By the use of colorimetric measurements of samples subjected to thermally accelerated degradation, it was possible to predict the color stability of the preparation at room temperature, with data obtained in about 25 days.[1]

The arithmetic plots in Figure 26-2 presenting the change in absorbance at 500 mμ versus time are linear, indicating that color loss is following a zero-order reaction. The slopes of these lines were obtained, and they indicate the rate of change of color with time. These rate constants are summarized in Table 26-8.

From the data in this table, Arrhenius plots were made and are shown in Figure 26-26. The linear nature of the curve indicates its utility in predicting the rates of color loss at lower temperatures. The rate constants at the lower temperatures obtained from this plot are summarized in Table 26-9.

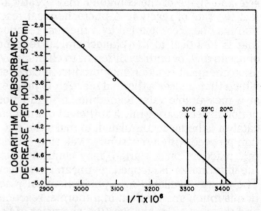

FIG. 26-26. *Plot of the logarithm of the rate of decrease in absorbance of extracted color per hour against the reciprocal of the absolute temperature (T) as obtained at 500 mμ. (From Garrett, E. R., and Carper, R. F.: J. Am. Pharm. Assoc., Sci. Ed., 44:515, 1955.)*

TABLE 26-9. *k Values Determined from Arrhenius Expression*

°C	k, Absorbance dec/hr
20	0.0000115
25	0.0000209
30	0.0000363

These rate constants can then be used to determine the time when the color has reached an undesirable level. For example, to predict the time for the absorbance to fall to 0.225 (At) from a zero time value of 0.470 (Ao), the zero-order kinetic equation At = Ao − kt is used. At 20°C, the rate constant (k) from Table 26-9 is 1.15×10^5 (absorbance decrease/hour). Rearranging the above equation to find the time, the absorbance reads 0.225 at 20°C:

$$t_{20°} = \frac{-At + Ao}{k}$$

$$= \frac{-0.225 + 0.470}{1.15 \times 10^{-5}}$$

$$= 21,304 \text{ hours}$$

$$= 887 \text{ days}$$

The predicted times for 20°, 25°, and 30°C are summarized in Table 26-10.

The thermal degradation of ascorbic acid, vitamin B_{12}, folic acid, vitamin A, d-pantothenyl alcohol, and thiamine hydrochloride in a liquid multivitamin preparation was studied by use of either zero-order or first-order treatment of the data. It was possible to predict the stability of the vitamin components maintained at room temperature from the data obtained from samples stored under accelerated test conditions.

The stability of ascorbic acid in a liquid o/w multivitamin emulsion containing sodium fluoride and vitamins A, B_6, D, and C as active ingredients was studied under accelerated storage conditions to predict its shelf-life. With zero-

TABLE 26-10. *Duration of Color (Corresponding to Estimated Point of Rejection of Absorbance of Extract, A' = 0.225)*

°Centigrade	Time
20°	887 days (ca. 2½ yr)
25°	488 days (ca. 1⅓ yr)
30°	281 days (ca. ¾ yr)

and first-order kinetic treatment of the data, it was possible to determine the pH of optimum stability, as well as the concentration of ascorbic acid to provide for a shelf-life of two years for the product. It was possible to make this estimation from 30 days of accelerated temperature study. The predicted stability was subsequently corroborated by room temperature data.[63]

Swintosky et al. used chemical kinetics to predict the shelf-life of oral penicillin G procaine suspensions from elevated temperature storage conditions.[35] The degradation of penicillin in saturated procaine penicillin solutions was found to follow a first-order reaction. Using information obtained from the Arrhenius plot of the stability data at several elevated temperatures and the solubility of penicillin at these temperatures, the authors were able to prepare aqueous suspensions of procaine penicillin of a predictable shelf-life that would be far in excess of that observed in solution, since only that fraction of the penicillin in solution undergoes degradation.

It has been shown that vitamin A acetate and palmitate encased in gelatin, acacia, and like substances, when tabletted into conventional uncoated tablets and/or chewable tablets, follow a pseudo-first-order degradation scheme.[64] An Arrhenius plot of the data obtained at several elevated temperatures for vitamin A palmitate is shown in Figure 26-27. This linear plot of the logarithm of the pseudo-first-order rate constants obtained at elevated temperatures versus absolute temperature permits an estimation of the rate constants at room temperature (25°C), and thus an estimation of the shelf-life of the vitamin in the tablet. If the rate constant is

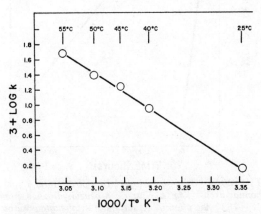

FIG. 26-27. *Rate constants (k = week⁻¹) for pseudo-first-order rate constants of vitamin A palmitate beadlets in dry-slugged, mannitol-base, multivitamin chewable tablet. Log k is plotted against reciprocal absolute temperature. (From Carstensen, J. T.: J. Pharm. Sci., 51:100, 1964.)*

placed into equation (16), the $t_{10\%}$ at 25°C is obtained. The relative stabilities of several vitamin A derivatives in the solid state are demonstrated by the zero-order plots of their degradation in Figure 26-28.[65] It was postulated that the degradation occurs almost exclusively in a liquid film at the surface of the crystal. The relative amount of material in the liquid state may be expected in these instances to determine, in some large manner, the rate of degradation. The fraction of material in the liquid state is related to the melting point of the pure crystalline solid by the following equation:

$$\ln x_1 = -\frac{Lf}{R}\left(\frac{1}{T} - \frac{1}{Tm}\right)$$

where x_1 is the mole fraction of solvent (the liquid phase), Lf is the molar heat of fusion, R, the gas constant, and Tm the melting point of the pure solid. It is evident from the plots in Figure 26-28 that in a series of vitamin A derivatives, the compound having the highest melting point is generally the most stable, all other factors being equal. Consequently, the use of chemical alteration to provide derivatives having high melting points, and hence greater stability, should prove a useful tool to the pharmaceutical formulator of solid dosage forms in instances where drug degradation poses a serious problem.

The influence of active constituents and tablet diluents on the stability of phenylephrine hydrochloride in a solid state was studied in accordance with chemical kinetic principles. For the most part, phenylephrine hydrochloride was found to degrade in accordance with zero-order kinetics. Such studies made possible the scientific development of multi-ingredient tablet formulations containing phenylephrine hydrochloride at optimal stability.

Statistical Techniques in Predicting Thermal Stability. In the last few years, it has become standard procedure to use statistics in determining the validity of the Arrhenius treatment of data.

Statistical aspects of the Arrhenius treatment of kinetic data and the prediction of stability have been covered by Carstensen and Su.[66] The authors demonstrated that when decomposition is less than 10%, which is the case for many drugs of intermediate stability and certainly those for which a New Drug Application (NDA) is being considered, zero-order and first-order degradation are practically indistinguishable, and statistical methods are greatly facilitated by the use of zero-order kinetics. Of importance is the necessity to employ at least four points to obtain reasonable accuracy in applying the Arrhenius treatment and making an extrapolation. The degree of accuracy can be calculated, and Garrett has shown there is a substantial difference between three points and more than three points.[67] In addition, the "longer" the extrapolation, the larger the scatter of points. For example, Carstensen demonstrated that if only the data shown in Table 26-11 at the three highest temperatures were used to predict stability at 25°C, using least squares for plotting, then:

$$\log k_{(25°C)} = [0.0353 - 7] \pm 1.6740$$

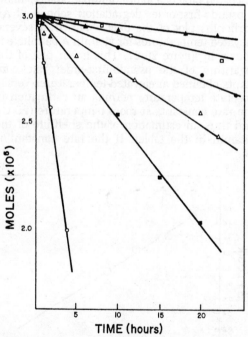

FIG. 26-28. *Solid state degradation of vitamin A compounds at 50°. Key:* ▲, *Vitamin A benzahydrazone, m.p. 181–182°;* ■, *vitamin A succinate triphenylguanidine salt, m.p. 140.0–140.5°;* ●, *vitamin A 3,4,5-trimethoxybenzoate, m.p. 85–86°;* △, *vitamin A nicotinate, m.p. 93–94°;* □, *vitamin A phthalimido-N-acetate, m.p. 111–112°;* ○, *vitamin A acetate, m.p. 57–58°. (From Guillory, J. K., and Higuchi, T. J.: J. Pharm. Sci., 51:100, 1962.)*

TABLE 26-11. *Rate Constants of Degradation of Diazepam Injection*

t°C	$1000/T$	$10^5 k_1$ (hr^{-1})	$y = 5 + \log k_1$
121	2.54	176	2.2455
110	2.61	84.3	1.9258
100	2.68	33.1	1.5198
85	2.81	10.0	1.0000
70	2.92	2.15	0.3324

which corresponds to:

$$k_{(25°C)} \text{ of } 2.30 \times 10^{-9} \text{ to } 5.12 \times 10^{-6}$$

The interval is of several orders of magnitude, and at the higher rate constant (the least stable), the drug remaining after two years would be calculated to be 81.6%.

If all the data in Table 26-11 are employed, however, then:

$$\log k_{(25°C)} = [0.2257 - 7] \pm 0.2937$$

which corresponds to:

$$k_{(25°C)} \text{ of } 8.51 \times 10^{-8} \text{ to } 3.30 \times 10^{-7}$$

The interval is much narrower, and at the higher rate constant, the drug remaining after two years would be calculated to be 98.7%.

If an Arrhenius plot of the data at the three highest temperatures listed in Table 26-11 is constructed and 95% confidence lines are included, the graph shown in Figure 26-29 results. The dotted lines represent the high and low limits around the extrapolated solid line. The further away the actual experimental points are from the extrapolation, the greater is the variation. This emphasizes the inaccuracy that results from attempts to extrapolate over too wide a temperature range.

Both Garrett and McLeod et al. used statistical procedures to determine the degree of confidence to be held in the predicted stability of a pharmaceutical preparation;[68,69] the data they used were based on accelerated storage tests. In all cases, the predicted potency was found to agree closely with the potency determined for samples stored at the temperature for as long as a year. The estimates were found to be well within the limits of error of prediction and the 95% confidence limits of a single assay.

To facilitate data processing and statistical treatment of stability information, computer programs have been developed and are commercially available.* Digital and analog computer programs have been employed to simulate drug decomposition induced during linear nonisothermal stability studies.[70,71]

Stability Data Generation and Handling. In the past few years, stability testing has been revolutionized by two highly technologic advancements—high pressure liquid chromatography (HPLC) methodology for analyzing drug product stability, and the computer for stability data acquisition, storage, analysis, and reporting. Since the FDA has become more demanding in its requirements that product expiration dates be based on stability data obtained using stability-indicating assay methods and such data analyzed by valid statistical calculations, HPLC and the computer have become essentially indispensable tools for fulfilling these requirements.

Most assay methods described in the official compendial drug monographs are not stability-indicating, that is, the assay is not capable of differentiating intact drug from one or more of its degradation products. In other words, the assay lacks specificity for the active ingredient. Nearly all new drug products being developed today use HPLC as the method of choice for analyzing the stability of the dosage form. HPLC can separate and quantitate the active ingredient from its degradation products in the dosage form. Many of the older analytic methods used as official assay methods are gradually being changed to the more specific, sensitive, and accurate HPLC method.

One disadvantage of HPLC methodology is that it is time-consuming; however, this can be overcome through automation. Thus, the role of the computer has reached new heights in managing stability testing programs. Not only can the computer control the analytic process for generating stability data, but also it has become essential in all aspects of data manipulation and reporting.

Physical Stability. Although there are a considerable number of reports in the literature

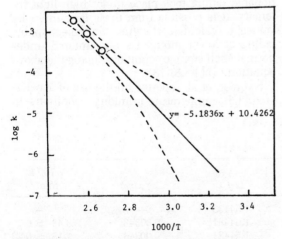

FIG. 26-29. *Arrhenius plot of degradation of diazepam in ampul solution with high and low limits. (From Carstensen, J. T., and Su, K. S. W.: Bull. Parenteral Drug Assn., 25:287, 1971.)*

*EDP Technology Inc., 1532 Third Street, Santa Monica, CA 90401 The Upjohn Company, Kalamazoo, MI.

concerned with chemical stability testing of active ingredients in pharmaceutical dosage forms, there is a conspicuous scarcity of reports dealing with physical stability testing. From both pharmaceutical and therapeutic standpoints, physical changes in the dosage form upon storage can be as serious as chemical instability of the active ingredients, sometimes more so. Examples of physical changes that can take place are crystal growth, change in crystal form, increase or decrease in dissolution rate and disintegration times, cracking of emulsions, caking of suspension, color fading, color development, and sediment or swirl development in solutions. Crystal growth in a suspension can result in a change in the rate of absorption and possibly in ineffective therapeutic levels. Crystal growth in an ointment or cream can cause skin irritation as well as poorer absorption. A change in crystal form of a steroid in suspension can result in the formation of a therapeutically inactive form of the drug.

Tablets. There have been several studies concerned with the influence of temperature and light on the color stability of tablets. In one investigation, the effect of temperature on the rate of darkening of tablet dosage forms was investigated, and it was found that the darkening was following either zero- or first-order kinetics, depending on the drug and tablet formulation.[72] For example, for tablet of drug A, which darkened in accordance with first-order kinetics, the Arrhenius plot is given in Figure 26-30, and the data in Table 26-12.

The linearity of the Arrhenius plot permits extrapolation to 25°C from the elevated temperatures. With this information, it is possible to estimate the extent of darkening at room temperature at extended storage periods. Everhard and Goodhart,[73] using certain relationships developed by Kubelka,[74] quantitated the relationship of light-catalyzed fading of colored tablets as a function of time and light intensity. Since fading is proportional to the product of time, t, and intensity of the light, I, these investigators pro-

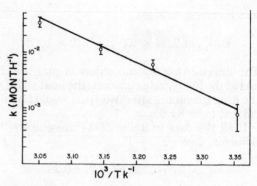

FIG. 26-30. *Logarithm of apparent rate constants k of drug A, taken from Table 26-12 and plotted as a function of reciprocal absolute temperature. (From Carstensen, J. T., Johnson, J. L., Valentine, W., and Vance, J. J.: J. Pharm. Sci., 53:1050, 1964.)*

ceeded to plot θ_t versus the product of time and intensity (Fig. 26-31). The value for θ_t was obtained from the equation $(1 - R_t)^2/2R_t$ where R_t is the measured reflectance of the tablet. The consistency of the slopes (k values) at the three different concentrations shows that the fading of the dye at the surface of the tablet is first-order. By using the product of time and intensity, each intensity condition was found to be on the same straight line for any given concentration. The general first-order equation for the straight line plots in Figure 26-31 is:

$$\ln \theta_t = -ktI + \ln \theta_t'$$

where θ_t (Kubelka-Munk function of the tablet) is the θ calculated at time, t, and θ_t' is the θ_t at $t = 0$. By determining the times at which objectionable fading took place under high light intensity, it is possible from these time-intensity values to calculate the time for objectionable fading at lower intensities encountered under normal shelf storage conditions, using the above equation (Table 26-13).

Nyquist, et al. reported on the use of accelerated light-temperature-humidity conditions in

TABLE 26-12. *Drug A*

Temp (t°C)	$10^3/T$ (°K^{-1})	Mo Stored	x-Value (%)	Log x	Log x/x_0*	100 k (Mo^{-1})
5	—	21	34.78	1.54133	—	—
55	3.05	1	35.06	1.54481	0.00348	3.48 ± 0.7
45	3.145	3	35.06	1.54481	0.00348	1.15 ± 0.23
37	3.225	6	35.07	0.54494	0.00361	0.62 ± 0.12
26	3.355	16	34.88	1.54258	0.00125	0.08 ± 0.04

*5° Value used for reference.

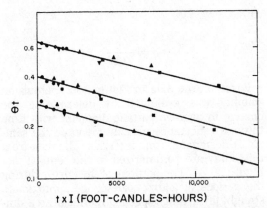

FIG. 26-31. *Plots of θ_t vs. the product of time and intensity. Key:* ●, *11 footcandles;* ▲, *50 footcandles;* ■, *80 footcandles;* ▼, *655 footcandles. Top line, 0.06% dye; middle line, 0.03%; bottom line, 0.015% dye. (From Everhard, M. E., and Goodhardt, F. W.: J. Pharm. Sci., 52:281, 1963.)*

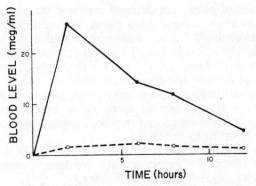

FIG. 26-32. *Decrease in blood levels when an aged tablet (------), rather than a fresh tablet (—), was administered orally to human beings.*

predicting light stability and in establishing a rapid method of evaluating light stability of white tablets.[75] Exposing tablets to a fadeometer combined with color measurement in a tristimulus colorimeter was found to be a rapid method for evaluating light stability of white tablets under various temperature and humidity conditions.

If the dissolution rate of the active ingredient from the tablet or the tablet disintegration time were to increase under extended shelf storage of the tablet formulation, the therapeutic effectiveness of the tablet medication could be seriously affected. In general, a decrease in therapeutic efficacy would take place because the active ingredient would be less readily available for absorption.

The effect of storage of phenobarbital and phenacetin tablets on the rates of dissolution has been studied for three tablet formulations.[68] Tablets prepared with gelatin or polyethylene glycol 6,000 as granulating agents changed little during storage, whereas tablets prepared with carboxymethylcellulose underwent a significant increase in dissolution rate.

It is unwise and dangerous to assume that a tablet formulation exhibiting good drug absorption will remain so throughout its shelf-life. This can be illustrated by the curves in Figure 26-32, in which the blood levels are plotted for an aged tablet and for one newly prepared. It is evident that aging of this tablet formulation results in a considerable change in drug availability.

Disperse Systems. The physical stability of an emulsion or suspension can be influenced by factors affecting the chemical stability of the emulsifier, suspending agent, antioxidant, microbiologic preservative, and active substance, as well as the physical characteristics of the disperse system.

It is an established fact that the degree of stability of an emulsion may be measured by the variation of the distribution of sizes of the dispersed droplets with time. An emulsion approaching the unstable state is characterized by the appearance of large globules as the result of coalescence and aggregation of small globules.

Lloyd has employed the relationship between reflectance of colored emulsions and the surface average diameter of their disperse phase to evaluate different emulsion stabilizers and study the kinetics of emulsion coalescence.[76] Oil-in-water emulsions containing 50% volume of the dis-

TABLE 26-13. *Time Required For Objectionable Fading at Low Light Intensities as Calculated From Accelerated Light Conditions*

Concentration of Dye (% w/w)	Hours at 540 fc	Calcd. Hours at 50 fc	Calcd. Hours at 10 fc
0.060	17	180	920
0.030	7	75	380
0.015	2	20	110

fc = footcandles

persed phase and different starches, starch derivatives, water-soluble gums, and surfactants were used. The oil phase was colored with the red dye, Scarlet B. Reflectance of the emulsions was determined at 450 mμ and the surface average particle diameters of the internal phase was determined by microscope. Upon plotting surface average particle diameter on logarithmic paper, a linear relationship becomes apparent as shown in Figure 26-33.

The relationship between percentage of reflectance (R) and surface average particle diameter (D) is expressed as follows:

$$Log\ R = -k\ log\ D + log\ c$$

or alternatively as:

$$R = \frac{c}{D^k}$$

where k and c are constants characteristic of the emulsion. Surface average particle diameter was shown to be inversely related to specific interfacial area (A) of a given emulsion as follows:

$$D = \frac{6f}{A}$$

where f is the volume fraction of the dispersed phase. Thus, the reflectance is proportional to the specific interfacial area of the emulsion raised to k power.[77]

$$R = c'A^k$$

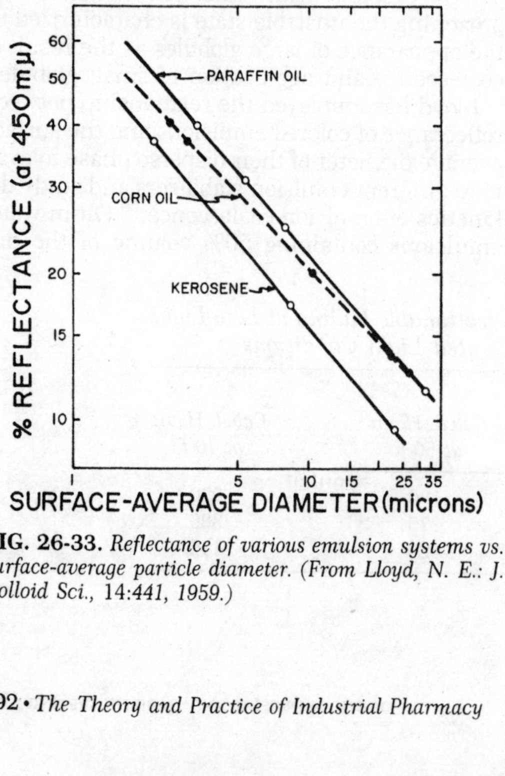

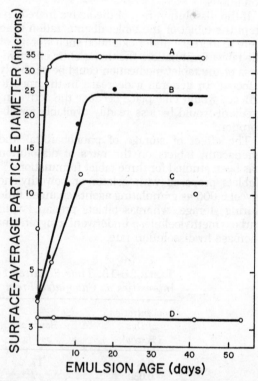

FIG. 26-33. Reflectance of various emulsion systems vs. surface-average particle diameter. (From Lloyd, N. E.: J. Colloid Sci., 14:441, 1959.)

where:

$$c' = \frac{c}{(6f)^k}$$

Based on the data in Figure 26-33, emulsion stability was evaluated by determining the change in average particle diameter with time through reflectance measurements of the sample at designated time intervals. The data from this study are summarized in the semilog plot Figure 26-34. The portions of the curves during the periods of active coalescence approximate straight lines. Since specific interfacial area simulates a concentration factor (interfacial areas per unit volume of oil), the coalescence behavior of the emulsion system in Figure 26-34 simulates a first-order reaction and can be used to estimate the physical stability of an emulsion at extended storage periods.

Van den Tempel measured the rate of coagulation of o/w emulsions according to the following simplified equation:

$$\frac{1}{n} - \frac{1}{n_0} = at$$

FIG. 26-34. Stability of paraffin oil emulsions containing various starches and starch derivatives. (From Lloyd, N. E.: J. Colloid Sci., 14:441, 1959.)

where n is the number of particles in a unit volume at time t, n_0 is the number of particles at time t_0, and a is the rate of decrease of particle concentration.[78] Plotting $\frac{1}{n}$ versus time results in a linear relationship (Fig. 26-35). The data plotted in this figure show the rate of decrease of particle concentration (coagulation) in an emulsion stabilized with dioctyl sodium sulfosuccinate.

While it is undoubtedly fundamental to study emulsion stability on the basis of size frequency analysis, the practical commercial aspect of stability is the observation of creaming and/or separation of water and oil in an emulsion. Factors involved in this observation are vibration, head space of gas, temperature, globule size, density of the phases, viscosity of the external phase, gelling, and other changes in the emulsifying agent with aging.

A scheme for expressing separation changes quantitatively is presented.[79] The separation of oil or water of quantity dV in time t depends on time and the amount of emulsion still emulsified $(1 - V)$, as well as the height at which the emulsified globule must travel to reach the separation layer and make the separated portion of the phase clear. This height is proportional to V in a cylindric vessel; however, the sedimentation velocity is not proportional to the height, but to a power of this, which can theoretically be between 0 and 1, and is usually 0.5. Errors of ±3% were reported to accompany this method of eval-

uation. The equation for sedimentation was reported as:

$$\frac{dV}{dt} = k(1 - V)V^{1/2}$$

Integration of the equation gives:

$$kt = \log \frac{1 + \sqrt{V}}{1 - \sqrt{V}}$$

By determining the half-life, the time for half the volume to separate, it is possible to readily compare a series of emulsions.

To study demulsification of oil-in-water and water-in-oil emulsions, the internal phase was colored, and the volumes of separated internal phase were measured colorimetrically at different times.[80] A graphic evaluation of the rate of internal phase separation revealed that the relationship of the percentage separated to time is exponential (Fig. 26-36). The straight lines obtained by this log-log plot indicate the following equation:

$$x = ky^a$$

$$\log x = \log k + a \log y$$

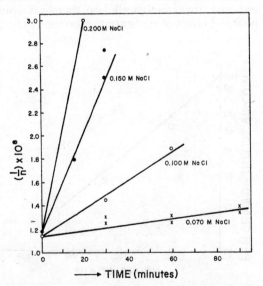

FIG. 26-35. *Decrease of particle concentration in emulsions with time. (From Van den Tempel, M.: Rec. Trav. Chim., 72:433, 1953.)*

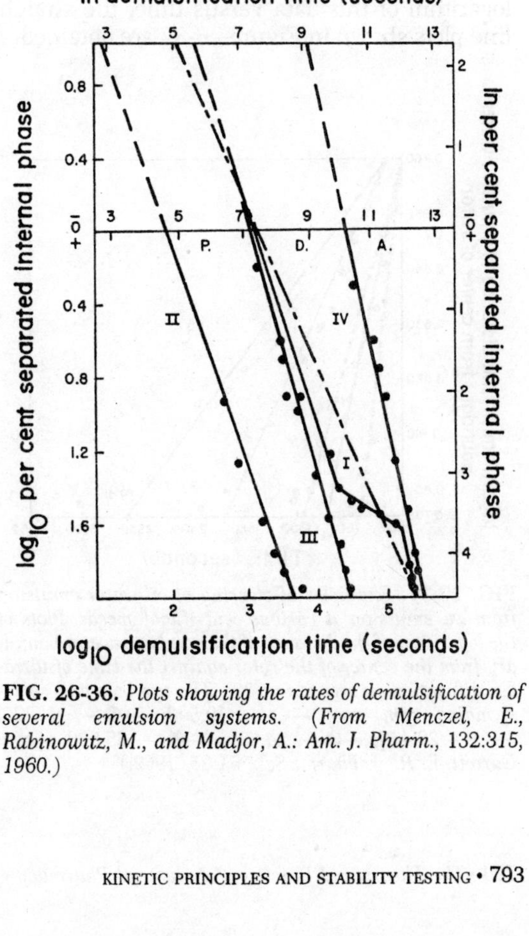

FIG. 26-36. *Plots showing the rates of demulsification of several emulsion systems. (From Menczel, E., Rabinowitz, M., and Madjor, A.: Am. J. Pharm., 132:315, 1960.)*

where y is the percentage of separated internal phase, x is time, and k and a are constants that differ from one emulsion system to another.

Whatever the rate of separation of the internal phase, the demulsification is at first nonapparent, and then it becomes apparent. It was assumed that the rate of demulsification was equal at both the nonapparent and apparent stages (negative and positive y axis of Figure 26-36) for emulsions consisting of considerable volumes of internal phase dispersion; the separation of 1% internal phase (ln = 0) renders the demulsification perceptible. A perceptible demulsification axis (PDA) was suggested, which is actually the demarcation point between apparent and nonapparent demulsification; the less the rate of demulsification, the more time is needed to reach the PDA. If the slope of the internal phase separation is drawn upward and extended into the nonapparent stage, the interception points (k) with the perceptible axis of demulsification indicate the degree of emulsion stability. When the same exponential time units are used for the x axis, as well as for the PDA, the higher the value for k, the more stable is the emulsion.

The ultracentrifuge has been suggested as a means to measure o/w emulsion stability.[81] By determining the emulsion clearing or separation at different centrifugal speeds and plotting the logarithm of this data versus time, the straight line plots shown in Figure 26-37 are obtained. A

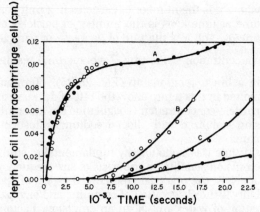

FIG. 26-38. *Increase of oil coalescence as a function of time for "bad," curve A, and "good," curves B, C, D, oil-water emulsions. The symbols and ultracentrifugal rpm at 30° are:* ⊙, *59,780;* ○, *52,640;* ●, *47,660. (From Garrett, E. R.: J. Pharm. Sci., 51:35, 1962.)*

bad emulsion was found to separate oil almost instantly following a first-order rate of separation. A good emulsion exhibited an induction period during which no detectable oil separation took place, followed by an accelerated rate of oil separation as depicted in Figure 26-38.

The viscosity aging characteristics of suspensions and suspending agents were studied by Levy.[82] The viscosity degradation curve for sodium alginate XR-C is shown in Figure 26-39, and it appears to follow a first-order degradation. For sodium alginate, the effect of concentration on stability was found to be negligible in the concentration range studied; however, in the case of sodium carboxymethylcellulose, there was a pronounced effect of concentration on the viscosity

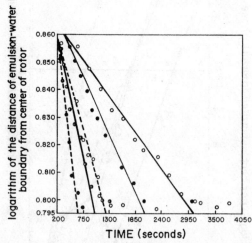

FIG. 26-37. *Examples of clearing of oil-water emulsion from i.v. emulsion at various centrifugal speeds. Plots of the logarithm of the distance of the emulsion-water boundary from the center of the rotor against the time of ultracentrifugation in seconds at 30°. The symbols and corresponding rpm are:* —○—, *12.590;* —●—, *15220;* --○-- *20,410;* —◐—, *24,630;* --●--, *35.600. (From Garrett, E. R.: J. Pharm. Sci., 51:35, 1962.)*

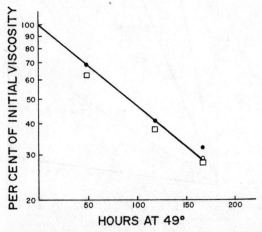

FIG. 26-39. *The viscosity stability of sodium alginate XR-C at several concentrations. (From Levy, G.: J. Pharm. Sci., 50:429, 1961.)*

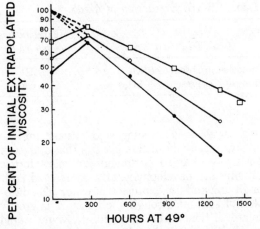

FIG. 26-40. *The decrease in the apparent viscosity of several concentrations of sodium carboxymethylcellulose (M. W. 75,000) as a function of time. (From Levy, G.: J. Pharm. Sci., 50:429, 1961.)*

stability as shown in Figure 26-40. Increase in polymer concentration results in a decrease in the rate of viscosity change.

The plots in Figure 26-41 compare the stability of sodium carboxymethylcellulose of various average molecular weights by plotting viscosity half-lives versus initial apparent viscosity. The vertical line in the figure serves to compare the viscosity half-lives of the three polymer types at a given apparent viscosity. It was indicated that if a comparison of solutions of equal concentra-

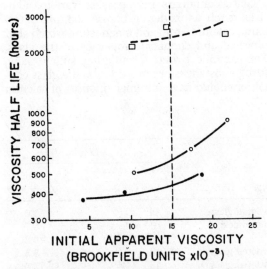

FIG. 26-41. *The viscosity half-life ($V_{1/2}$) of sodium carboxymethylcellulose solutions at 49° as a function of the initial apparent viscosity. (From Levy, G.: J. Pharm. Sci., 50:429, 1961.)*

tion rather than equal viscosity was performed, the formulator would receive a distorted picture of their relative stabilities.

None of the several methods described for evaluating the physical stability of disperse systems considered the temperature dependency of the parameters employed. For accurate utilization of the data from exaggerated temperature storage, the relationship of the change in these parameters at the different temperatures must be determined. It is realized, however, that for emulsions and suspensions, it may not be possible to exaggerate the temperatures to the extent done for solutions. In disperse systems, the physical properties at temperatures above a certain point could be completely different from those that would exist at normal temperatures of storage. For example, in formulations exhibiting thixotropic properties, a rise in temperatures above a certain value would cause a change in the properties of the preparation into a gel structure. In this physical form, the preparation would exhibit parameters that could not be extrapolated to those that would exist in the normal system. However, it is felt that through the use of elevated temperatures that are not as high as those employed for chemical reactions, valid temperature dependency data could be obtained that would be useful in the estimation of the physical stability of a product at normal storage conditions.

A significant challenge confronting pharmaceutical development and analytic scientists is the testing of new drug delivery systems for physical and chemical stability. Since most new delivery systems involve polymeric systems, protein, and genetically engineered substances, standards need to be developed for these systems, and new tests, specifications, and equipment are required to evaluate such systems.

Influence of Packaging Components on Dosage Form Stability

Faulty packaging of pharmaceutical dosage forms can invalidate the most stable formulation. Consequently, it is essential that the choice of container materials for any particular product be made only after a thorough evaluation has been made of the influence of these materials on the stability of the product and of the effectiveness of the container in protecting the product during extended storage under varying environmental conditions of temperature humidity, and light.

The materials most commonly employed as

container components for pharmaceutical preparations include glass, metal, plastic, and rubber.

Glass. Of these four materials, glass has been the container of choice for pharmaceutical dosage forms because of its resistance to decomposition by atmospheric conditions or by solid and liquid contents of different chemical composition. Furthermore, by varying the chemical composition of glass, it is possible to adjust the chemical behavior and radiation properties of the glass.

Although glass exhibits many advantages over other packaging materials, it has two principal faults, namely, the release of alkali and the release of insoluble flakes to liquids stored in the container. The USP XX acknowledges that alkali ions can be released for each of four types of glass listed in the USP compendium, as shown by the data in Table 26-14.

By decreasing the soda content in the glass or replacing the sodium oxide with other oxides, it has been possible to overcome the undesirable property of glass releasing alkali cations into solution. This is exemplified by the borosilicate glass in Table 26-14 as compared with the general purpose soda-lime glass.

Several approaches have been used to increase the resistance of glass to alkali release by surface treatment. One method consists of treating the surface of soda-lime glass to produce a fire-polished skin of silica, which is more resistant than the inner layers of glass. This surface-treated glass is represented by Type II glass in Table 26-14.

Another approach is to treat the surface of the glass with sulfur dioxide in the presence of water vapor and heat.[83] This causes the surface alkali to react with the sulfur dioxide, and the glass becomes more resistant, as shown by the data in Table 26-15, for 5-hour extractions performed with boiling water for treated and un-

TABLE 26-15. *Extraction of Alkali*

Glass Treatment	Extraction as mg Na_2O
Annealed in absence of SO_2	2.9
Annealed in presence of SO_2	0.9

treated glass. The suggested reason for the greater resistivity of this glass is that a layer of positively charged hydrogen ion glass forms, causing the development of a compacted layer on drying and the expulsion of water. The diffusion of sodium through such a layer is greatly retarded; hence, the extraction by water would be considerably reduced.

In recent years, a number of drugs have been developed that are of high potency, and consequently, of low dosage. The stability of these drugs can be readily affected by the release of soluble alkali from glass containers. As a safety factor, whenever the dosage form is a liquid, the solution should be buffered to eliminate any effect due to possible change in pH if some alkali were released from the glass.

Sometimes, insoluble flakes have been found to appear in solutions stored in glass containers. The type of glass employed plays a major role in whether flake formation takes place. For example, flake formation may occur in nonborosilicate glass immediately after autoclaving, whereas in borosilicate glass, it occurs at temperatures much higher than those normally used for autoclaving.

Glass containers may possess various additives, such as oxides of boron, sodium, potassium, calcium, iron, and magnesium which alter physical and chemical properties of the glass. For example, when formulating sulfate salts, (drug substances or antioxidants) the glass container should have minimal amounts of calcium

TABLE 26-14. *Glass Types and USP Test Limits*

Type	General Description*	Type of Test	Limits	
			Size (ml)†	ml of 0.02 N Acid
I	Highly resistant borosilicate glass	Powdered glass	All	1.0
II	Treated soda-lime glass	Water attack	100 or less	0.7
			over 100	0.2
III	Soda-lime glass	Powdered glass	All	8.5
IV	General purpose soda-lime glass	Powdered glass	All	15.0

*Description applies to containers of the type of glass usually available.

†Size indicates overflow capacity of the container source. (Data from USP XX/NF XV, United States Pharmacopeial Convention, Inc., 1982, p. 949.)

TABLE 26-16. *Parenteral Solutions Containing Barium Sulfate Crystals*

Product	Type of Glass Container	Source of Sulfate or Bisulfite Ions
Procaine hydrochloride, 2%	30-ml vial	Antioxidant
Kanamycin sulfate, 0.5 g/2 ml	2-ml vial	Drug
Meperidine hydrochloride, 100 mg/ml	1-ml vial	Antioxidant
Magnesium sulfate, 5 g/10 ml	10-ml vial (plunger) and rubber closure	Drug
Atropine sulfate, 0.5 mg/ml	1-ml ampul	Drug
Promethazine hydrochloride, 25 mg/ml	1-ml ampul	Antioxidant

From Boddapati, S., Butler, D. L., Im, S., and DeLuca, P. P., J. Pharm. Sci., 69:608, 1980. Reproduced with permission of the copyright owner, the American Pharmaceutical Association.

and barium to prevent the formation of insoluble inorganic salts.[84] Table 26-16 shows six parenteral solutions containing barium sulfate crystals, which were identified by polarizing microscopy, scanning electron microscopy with energy-dispersive x-ray analysis, micro-x-ray powder diffraction, and micro Ramon spectroscopy. Figure 26-42 shows the crystals from two solutions. On the basis that barium sulfate forms in situ,[85] the sulfate ions appear to originate from the union of the drug and/or the bisulfite ion of the antioxidant. The barium ions originate from the borosilicate glass, which can contain up to 5% BaO.[86]

Flakes are also likely to occur with phosphate, citrate, tartrate, and alkaline solutions. Pretreatment of the containers with dilute acid solution was found to delay flake formation.

Many pharmaceutical preparations exhibit physical or chemical changes due to the radiant energy of light. Light radiations can cause color development or color fading and potentiate an oxidation-reduction reaction, resulting in drug degradation, rancidity of oil formulations, and flavor and odor loss. Products exhibiting physical and chemical changes resulting from the effects of radiant energy can, in most instances, be adequately protected by the use of special glass containers. Flint glass, which is the most widely used multipurpose container material, has the disadvantage of being transparent to light rays above 300 mμ. As a result, amber glass, which has the property of shutting out certain portions of the light spectrum, has been used extensively by the pharmaceutical industry. The transmission curves for flint and amber glass shown in Figure 26-43 show that although flint glass transmits significantly from 300 mμ, amber

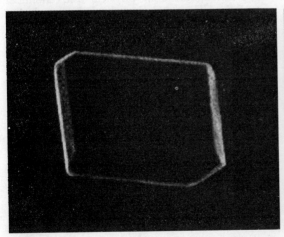 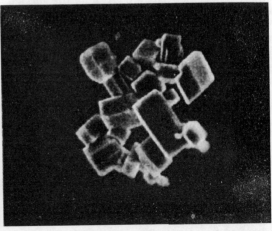

A   **B**

FIG. 26-42. *Scanning electron micrographs of barium sulfate crystals isolated from procaine hydrochloride (A) and atropine sulfate (B) (1000 × , 20 kv). (From Boddapati, S., Butler, D. L., Im, S., and DeLuca, P. P.: J. Pharm. Sci., 69:608, 1980. Reproduced with permission of the copyright owner, the American Pharmaceutical Association.)*

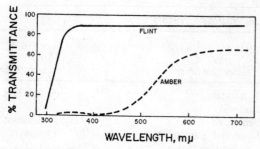

FIG. 26-43. *Transmission curves for typical flint and amber glass.*

glass does not begin to transmit to any appreciable extent until 470 mμ. Since it is known that the photochemical activity of the light radiations drops off with increasing wave length, it would be expected that the amber container would afford a product better protection against light than the flint glass. This is illustrated by the following examples.

The data in Table 26-17 show the protective effect of amber glass on the fading of dyes from the surface of tablets stored in flint and amber glass bottles.

The results in Table 26-18 summarize the stabilizing properties of amber glass on the photochemical degradation of an antihistamine injectable solution exposed to exaggerated illumination. The solutions stored in clear glass ampuls show a 36% loss of antihistamine concentration, while those in amber glass show essentially no loss in drug concentration.

The protective effect of amber glass on the darkening of sulfonamide tablets exposed to exaggerated lighting is shown in Table 26-19, where reflectance data are given for the surface of the sulfonamide tablets. It is evident that the tablets darken with storage, since the reflectance values decrease substantially when the tablets are exposed to light in an open dish. Visual observation of these tablets indicated that they had taken on a yellow-tan color; however, for the tablets stored in amber bottles, no significant change in reflectance took place, and visual observation showed no apparent darkening.

TABLE 26-17. *The Amount of Dye (%) Faded per Day When Irradiated Under Exaggerated Intensity*

Glass Sample	FD&C Blue #1	D&C Yellow #10
Flint	12.9	38.1
Amber	4.6	6.2

TABLE 26-18. *Chemical Assay for Residual Antihistamine from Solutions Stored in Clear and Amber Glass Ampuls*

Time (Weeks)	Assay (%)	
	Clear Glass	Amber Glass
0	100	100
4	83	98
8	64	98

The amber color of the glass is imparted by the addition of iron and manganese oxides, cations that are known to catalyze oxidative reactions. Studies have shown that these ions are extracted from the glass,[87] and that the decomposition rates of several drugs—thiomerosol,[88] amitriptylene,[89] and L-ascorbic acid[90]—are enhanced in amber glass containers.

The Parenteral Drug Association has published guidelines on the processing and selection of glass containers.[91] Various surface treatments are used to improve chemical resistance and decrease alkalinity. For example, exposing hot containers to sulfur dioxide reduces sodium content at the surface, and a brief treatment with ammonium bifluoride effectively cleans the surface by dissolving a portion of it.

Plastics. Although glass has many desirable properties, recent years have seen the use of more and more containers having all or part of their structure composed of plastic for the storage of pharmaceutical preparations. It should be realized that the term plastic denotes a considerable group of high-molecular-weight polymers, each having different physical and chemical properties. They include polyethylene, polypropylene, polystyrene, polyvinylchloride, and several others. Any particular plastic may be available in different densities or may be modified by certain additives that affect its chemical and

TABLE 26-19. *Influence of Light on the Photosensitivity of a Sulfonamide Tablet Formulation*

Time (Weeks)	% Reflectance at 450 mμ	
	Open Dish	Amber Bottle
0	52.6	52.6
2	41.3	52.3
4	35.6	53.6
6	31.7	53.8
8	28.9	52.9
10	25.4	—
12	23.8	51.5

physical properties. Only through studying the stability of the plastic container with the product for which it is to be used is it possible to be certain that the plastic has no effect on the preparation and that the preparation or one of its ingredients has no effect on the plastic.

A chief disadvantage of plastic containers, as compared with glass, is the problem of permeation in two directions, namely, from the solution in the container through the plastic into the ambient environment and from the ambient environment through the plastic into the preparation. In addition, materials can be leached from the plastic container into the liquid preparation, materials from the preparation can be adsorbed or absorbed onto and into the plastic container, and in certain instances, the contents of the container can chemically or physically react with the plastic components of the container, causing container deformation. The degree of permeation, leaching, sorption, diffusion, and chemical reactivity varies considerably from one plastic material to another.

The stability of a product packaged in a plastic container can be affected in several ways, owing to container permeability. The chemical, as well as the physical, stability of the tablet dosage form can be influenced considerably by penetration of water vapor from the atmosphere into the container. Penicillin tablets were found to degrade in polystyrene containers, owing to permeation of water vapor.[92] Oxygen and carbon dioxide in air can permeate through plastic containers, catalyzing the degradation of drugs that are prone to oxidation or hydrolysis. A tetracycline suspension was found to change in color and taste, owing to permeation of air through the walls of a polyethylene container.[93]

Plastic containers, when used for emulsion preparations, must be thoroughly evaluated for physical and chemical changes of the emulsion, as well as for physical changes in the container. It has been reported that certain materials in an emulsion have a tendency to migrate toward the polyethylene wall, causing either a change in the emulsion or a collapse in the container.[94] Since polyethylene has a tendency toward elastic recovery, air is continuously drawn into the plastic container, increasing the chance of oxidation and drying out of the preparation. In the case of an emulsion, the air can cause the emulsion to break down, owing to dehydration or oxidation of the oil phase. This phenomenon of package "breathing" is a major cause of product deterioration during storage in plastic containers. It can also be responsible for the loss of flavor and perfume ingredients from products packaged in plastic containers.

The property of plastics to sorb materials from solution can cause loss of drug, antibacterial agent, or other materials from solution. The curves in Figure 26-44 show the degree of binding of several commonly used antibacterial preservatives when solutions of these preservatives are in contact with the nylon barrel of a disposable syringe.[95] In nearly all instances, after one week's storage at 30°C, over 60% of the preservative is bound. When these same preservatives have been evaluated with polyethylene and polystyrene barrels, essentially no binding has been found. This clearly illustrates the importance of selecting the correct plastic material for a particular use.

Stability tests performed on Vioform Lotion packaged in plastic containers showed that the Vioform was being sorbed by the container. Lining of the container with an epoxy resin eliminated this problem. This is illustrated by the data summarized in Table 26-20, which presents reflectance data of the inside wall of the lined and unlined container. A decrease in the reflectance of the container wall is indicative of Vioform sorption by the plastic since a yellow surface reflects less light than a white surface. This is further substantiated by the increase in reflectance of the lotion with storage, indicating that the lotion is becoming lighter because of the loss in Vioform content.

Although the epoxy lining was effective in

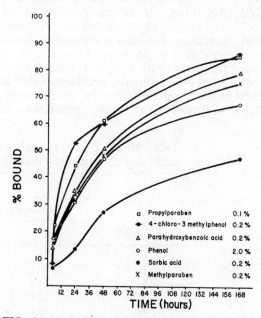

FIG. 26-44. *Binding of antibacterial preservatives by nylon as a function of time. (From Marcus, E., et al.: J. Am. Pharm. Assoc., Sci. Ed., 43:457, 1959.)*

TABLE 26-20. *Sorption of Vioform by the Plastic Container from the Lotion When Stored at 40°C.*

| | Reflectance in % | | | |
| | Unlined Container | | Lined Container | |
Time (Weeks)	Lotion	Container	Lotion	Container
0	60.0	55.0	63.0	54.5
1	60.0	48.0	61.5	53.0
2	61.0	49.5	63.0	53.0
3	65.0	50.0	61.5	54.0
4	—	49.0	63.0	53.0

eliminating the problem with Vioform lotion, it was not effective in preventing the sorption of the antibacterial agent, phenylmercuric acetate, from solution as illustrated by the data in Table 26-21.

It is evident from the results presented in Tables 26-20 and 26-21 that linings are not always effective and must be evaluated separately for each product. The ineffectiveness of the lining could be attributed to sorption of the lining itself by the preservative or to the presence of imperfections, such as pinholes in the lining, which permit penetration of the lining to the plastic.

Metals. In addition to glass and plastic, certain metals are also employed as containers for pharmaceutical products. Disperse systems, having a consistency of a soft paste, gel, cream, or ointment, can be conveniently packaged into collapsible tubes. Metals commonly used for such tubes are tin, plastic-coated tin, tin-coated lead, aluminum, and coated aluminum. Tubes constructed of a single material can readily be tested for stability with a product. Tubes having coatings present additional problems, since it must be established whether the coating material is sufficiently inert for the preparation, as

well as whether the coating completely covers the underlying material. In addition, the coating must be evaluated for ease of cracking and solvent resistance.

Tin and tin-coated tubes are usually employed because of their unreactive properties, although it has been reported that tin tubes can be corroded by chlorides or acid conditions. Vinyl and cellulose lacquers are applied to tin to increase their utility.

Coated and uncoated aluminum tubes are being used, but are not always satisfactory. It has been reported that aluminum reacts with fatty alcohol emulsions to form a white encrustation.[96] Such tubes were also found to be unstable for mercury-containing compounds. It has been stated that uncoated aluminum tubes are deleteriously affected when used for preparations outside the pH range of 6.5 to 8.0.[97] The application of an epoxy lining to the internal surfaces of aluminum tubes was found to make them more resistant to attack.

Whether the container is made of glass, plastic, or metal, it still requires a closure to contain the contents effectively. In addition to forming an effective seal on the container, the closure

TABLE 26-21. *Loss of Phenylmercuric Acetate from Solution Stored in Lined and Unlined Polyethylene Bottles*

| | % Preservative Lost | | | |
| | Unlined Container | | Epoxy-Lined Container | |
Time (Weeks)	25°C	40°C	25°C	40°C
0	0	0	0	0
1	10.0	29.3	12.4	24.6
2	11.5	38.5	—	27.0
3	20.0	35.8	15.4	37.7
4	20.0	46.2	23.9	43.9
8	33.2	57.7	27.7	58.5
12	33.7	70.0	33.2	68.8

should not react chemically or physically with the container contents to sorb material from the contents or leach material to the contents.

Rubber. Rubber of varying composition is used in pharmaceuticals and biologicals as stoppers, cap liners, and parts of dropper assemblies. A major use of the rubber stopper is that of a closure for multiple-dose vial solutions for injections. The problems that can be encountered by having rubber stoppers in contact with the liquid in the vial are the sorption of active ingredient, antibacterial preservative, or other materials into the rubber, and the extraction of one or more components of the rubber into the vial solution.

The data in Table 26-22 illustrate the influence of various rubber closures on the loss of the antimicrobial preservative chlorobutanol from vial solutions. It is evident from these data that the closures have a marked deleterious effect on preservative concentration at all temperatures. At 60°C, after 12 weeks of storage, the vials stoppered with neoprene closures and stored in an inverted position show only 8.5% residual concentration of chlorobutanol, whereas the ampuls under the same conditions of storage contain 72.4%.

The curves in Figure 26-45 show that extractives from the natural rubber closures used to stopper vials containing water for injection were leached into the water when the vials were autoclaved. It is evident from the absorption spectra of the extractives in the vial solutions that even normal autoclaving at 115°C, 10 psi for 30 min causes appreciable extractive to enter the water for injection. Subsequent storage of these vials at room temperature for the shelf-life of the pharmaceuticals, which at present is an average

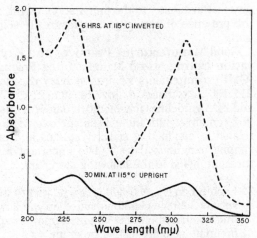

FIG. 26-45. *Leaching of extractives from rubber stoppers on multiple dose vial solutions.*

of three years, would no doubt cause further leaching of extractives in solution.

If an epoxy lining is applied to rubber stoppers, a considerable reduction results in the amount of extractive leached from the stopper by the water for injection in the vials, but there is essentially no effect on the sorption of preservative from solution. However, the use of Teflon-coated rubber stoppers essentially prevents sorption and leaching of the rubber stopper.

The presence of rubber closure extractives in the vial solutions could interfere with the chemical analysis of the active ingredient, affect the toxicity or pyrogenicity of the injectable preparation, interact with the drug or preservative to cause inactivation or loss of stability, and cause

TABLE 26-22. *Influence of Various Closures on Residual Concentration of Chlorobutanol in Vial Solutions After Storage*

			Stopper Composition					
			Natural Rubber		Neoprene Polymer		Butyl Polymer	
Temp (°C)	Storage Time (wk)	Ampul Control (%)	Upright (%)	Inverted (%)	Upright (%)	Inverted (%)	Upright (%)	Inverted (%)
25	12	100	81.00	78.7	87.3	81.0	68.1	63.8
40	2	100	76.6	63.8	61.7	59.6	68.1	61.7
—	12	97.9	74.5	57.5	53.2	46.8	66.0	66.0
50	2	97.9	59.6	57.5	57.5	46.8	66.0	61.7
—	12	91.5	57.5	42.5	46.8	38.3	59.6	57.5
60	2	95.8	57.5	53.2	51.0	46.8	51.0	48.9
—	12	72.4	57.5	42.5	29.8	8.5	46.8	46.8

physical instability to the preparation, owing to the presence of particulate matter in the solution.

Good Manufacturing Practices and Expiration Dating. Good Manufacturing Practice (GMP) requirements for drug stability (Section 211.166), expiration dating (Section 211.137), and FDA guidelines for stability studies (Section 98), contain significant and specific information related to conducting stability studies and assigning expiration dates.[98] The important features are listed in the following summary:

1. Each product's expiration date related to the specific storage condition stated on the label must be based on data obtained from an appropriate stability testing program.

2. Such a stability program would include:
   (a) numbers and sizes of containers per sample time;
   (b) testing of drug product in the marketed container-closure system at appropriate storage condition(s);
   (c) an adequate number of batches, usually at least three production batches, to be placed on long-term stability testing for a new product initially, and one production batch per year thereafter.

3. Expiration date must be derived from data obtained using reliable and specific stability-indicating assay methods for the active ingredient(s).

4. Tentative expiration dates can be assigned based upon data from accelerated stability studies as long as it can be shown that such accelerated studies are scientifically sound and that long-term studies are being conducted to confirm the predicted expiration date. It may be appropriate to utilize an increased sampling frequency toward the end of the expiration dating period. A rule of thumb for solid dosage forms allows a 2-year tentative expiration date at room temperature if the drug has retained 90% of its original potency after 90 days storage at 40°C and 75% relative humidity.

5. Long-term stability studies should attempt to determine the time at which the lower 95% confidence limit curve of the mean degradation line intersects the acceptable lower limit for drug degradation.

6. If a drug product is placed in a different packaging system, it can retain its expiration date if the repackager can assure the FDA that the repackaged container-closure system is as good as the original package and that all product specifications can be maintained throughout the dating period.

References

1. Federal Register, 43:45077, 1978.
2. The Gold Sheet, 17, Cole Palmer Werble, October 1983.
3. Garrett, E. R., and Carper, R. F.: J. Pharm. Sci., 44:515, 1955.
4. Berge, S. M., Henderson, N. L., and Frank, M. J.: J. Pharm. Sci., 72:59, 1983.
5. Woolfe, A. J., and Worthington, H. E. C.: Drug Dev. Commun., 1:185, 1974.
6. Pope, O. G.: Drug Cosmet. Ind., 127:48, 1980.
7. Free, S. M.: Considerations in Sampling for Stability. Presented before the American Drug Manufacturers Association, November 1955.
8. Blythe, R. H.: Product Formulation and Stability Prediction. Presented at the Production Section of the Canadian Pharm. Mfrg. Assoc., April 1957.
9. Kennon, L.: J. Pharm. Sci., 53:815, 1964.
10. Waltersson, J. O., and Lundgren, P.: Acta Pharm. Suec., 20:145, 1983.
11. Waltersson, J. O., and Lundgren, P.: Acta Pharm. Suec., 19:127, 1982.
12. Schlechtrull, J., et al.: Insulin II. In Handbook of Experimental Pharmacology. Vol. 32. Pt. 2. Edited by A. Hasselblatt and F. von Bruchhousen. Springer Verlag, New York, 1975, p. 760.
13. Fisher, B. V., and Porter, P. B.: J. Pharm. Pharmacol., 33:203, 1981.
14. Walters, W. A.: Physical Aspects of Organic Chemistry. 4th Ed. Van Nostrand, New York, 1959, p. 332.
15. Edwards, J. J.: Trans Farad. Soc., 46:723, 1950.
16. Blakey, W., McCombie, H., and Scarborough, H. A.: J. Chem. Soc., 129:2863, 1926.
17. Timm, E. W., and Hinshelwood, C. N.: J. Chem. Soc., 1983, p. 862.
18. Tommila, E.: Suomen Kemistilehti, 15B:9, 1942.
19. Germuth, F. G.: J. Am. Pharm. Assoc., 20:568, 1931.
20. Schultz, R. F.: J. Am. Chem. Soc., 61:1443, 1939.
21. Selvinova, A. S., and Syrkin, Y. K.: Comptes rendus Acad. Sci., 23:45, 1939.
22. Vavon, G., and Ducass, J.: J. Bull. Soc. Chim., 10:325, 1943.
23. Stinson, V. R.; J. Chem. Soc., Part III:2673, 1955.
24. Stinson, V. R.: Nature, 175:47, 1955.
25. Tommila, E., and Hella, A.: Ann. Acad. Sci., Fennicae, A2:3, 1954.
26. Bowles, W. J.: J. Pharm. Sci., 57:1057, 1968.
27. Higuchi, T., and Lachman, L.: J. Am. Pharm. Assoc., Sci. Ed., 44:532, 1955.
28. Lachman, L., Ravin, L. J., and Higuchi, T.: J. Am. Pharm. Assoc., Sci. Ed., 45:290, 1956.
29. Lachman, L., and Higuchi, T.: J. Am. Pharm. Assoc., Sci. Ed., 46:32, 1957.
30. Lachman, L., Guttman, D., and Higuchi, T.: J. Am. Pharm. Assoc., Sci. Ed., 46:36, 1957.
31. Guttman, D. E.: J. Pharm. Sci., 51:1162, 1962.
32. Riegelman, S.: J. Pharm. Sci., 49:339, 1960.
33. Smith, L., and Olsson, H.: Z. Physik. Chem., 102:26, 1922.
34. Olsson, H.: Z. Physik Chem., 125:243, 1927.

35. Paloma, M. H., and Juvala, A.: Chem. Ber., *61B*:1770, 1928.
36. Evans, D. P., and Davies, G.: J. Chem. Soc., *Part I*:339, 1940.
37. Salmi, E. J., and Lemin, R.: Suomen Kemistilehti, *20B*:43, 1947.
38. Newman, M. S.: J. Am. Chem. Soc., 72:4783, 1950.
39. Tommila, E.: Ann. Acad. Sci. Fennicae, *A57*:3, 1941.
40. Ingold, C. K.: Structure and Mechanisms in Organic Chemistry. Cornell University Press, Ithaca, 1953, p. 752.
41. Hammett, L. P.: J. Am. Chem. Soc., 74:213, 1952.
42. Swintosky, J. V., Rosen, E., Robinson, T. J., et al.: J. Am. Pharm. Assoc., Sci. Ed., 45:37, 1956.
43. Blaug, S. M., and Wesolowski, J. W.: J. Pharm. Sci., 48:691, 1959.
44. Garrett, E. R.: J. Am. Pharm. Assoc., Sci. Ed., 46:584, 1957.
45. Sinkula, A. A., Morozowich, W., Lewis, C., and Mac-Kellar, F. A.: J. Pharm. Sci., 58:1389, 1969.
46. Taraszka, M. J.: J. Pharm. Sci., 60:1414, 1971.
47. Brodasky, T. F., and Lewis, C.: J. Antibiot., 25:230, 1972.
48. Kesky, K. T.: J. Pharm. Sci., 58:560, 1969.
49. Marcus, A. D., and Taraszka, A. J.: J. Am. Pharm. Assoc., Sci. Ed., 48:77, 1959.
50. Bodin, J., and Taub, A.: J. Am. Pharm. Assoc., Sci. Ed., 44:296, 1955.
51. Mollica, J. A., Rehm, C. R., and Smith, J. B.: J. Pharm. Sci., 58:635, 1969.
52. Chung, P. H., Chin, T. F., and Lach, J. L.: J. Pharm. Sci., 59:1300, 1970.
53. Glasstone, S.: Textbook of Physical Chemistry. 2nd Ed. Van Nostrand, New York, 1954, p. 947.
54. Guttman, D. E., and Meister, P. D.: J. Am. Pharm. Assoc., Sci. Ed., 47:773, 1958.
55. Oesterling, T. O., and Guttman, D. E.: J. Pharm. Sci., 53:1189, 1964.
56. Schou, S. A., and Gredsted, A.: Dansk. Tids. Farm., 25:164, 1951.
57. Schroeter, L. C.: J. Pharm. Sci., 52:564, 1963.
58. Higuchi, T., and Schroeter, L. C.: J. Am. Pharm. Assoc., Sci. Ed., 48:535, 1959.
59. Schroeter, L. C., Higuchi, T., and Schuler, E. E.: J. Am. Pharm. Assoc., Sci. Ed., 47:724, 1958.
60. Riegelmen, S., and Fisher, E. Z.: J. Pharm. Sci., 51:206, 1962.
61. Felmeister, A., and Dischler, C. A.: J. Pharm. Sci., 53:756, 1964.
62. Hamlin, W. E., Chulski, T., Johnson, R. H., and Wagner, J. G.: J. Am. Pharm. Assoc., Sci. Ed., 49:253, 1960.
63. Tingstad, J. E., MacDonald, L. H., and Meister, P. D.: J. Pharm. Sci., 52:343, 1963.
64. Carstensen, J. T.: J. Pharm. Sci., 53:839, 1964.
65. Guillory, J. K., and Higuchi, T.: J. Pharm. Sci., 51:100, 1962.
66. Carstensen, J. T., and Su, K. S. W.: Bull. Parenteral Drug Assn., 25:287, 1971.
67. Garrett, E. R.: J. Pharm. Sci., 51:811, 1962.
68. Garrett, E. R.; J. Pharm. Assoc., Sci. Ed., 45:171, 1956.
69. McLeod, H. A., Pelletier, O., and Campbell, J. A.: Canad. Pharm. J., Sci. Ed., 55:173, 1958.
70. Zoglio, M. A., Windheuser, J. J., Vatte, R., et al.: J. Pharm. Sci., 57:2080, 1968.
71. Kay, A. I., and Simon, T. H.: J. Pharm. Sci., 60:205, 1971.
72. Carstensen, J. T., Johnson, J. B., Valentine, W., and Vance, J. J.: J. Pharm. Sci., 53:1050, 1964.
73. Everhard, M. E., and Goodhart, F. W.: J. Pharm. Sci., 52:281, 1963.
74. Kubelka, P.: J. Opt. Soc. Am., 38:448, 1948.
75. Nyquist, H., Lundgren, P., and Jansson, I., Acta Pharm. Suec., 17:148, 1980.
76. Solvang, S., and Finholt, P.: Medd. Norsk. Farm. Selsk., 31:101, 1969.
77. Lloyd, N. E.: J. Colloid Sci., 14:441, 1959.
78. Van den Tempel, M.: Rec. Trav. Chim., 72:433, 1953.
79. Lederer, E. L.: Kolloid Z., 71:61, 1935.
80. Menczel, E., Rabinovitz, M., and Madjor, A.: Am. J. Pharm., 132:315, 1960.
81. Garrett, E. R.: J. Pharm. Sci., 51:35, 1962.
82. Levy, G.: J. Pharm. Sci., 50:429, 1961.
83. Dimbley, V.: J. Pharm. and Pharmacol., 5:969, 1953.
84. Boddapati, S., and Butler, D. L., Im, S., and DeLuca, P. P.: J. Pharm. Sci., 69:608, 1980.
85. Sarrut, S., and Nezelof, C.: Presse Med., 68:375, 1960.
86. Vanga, S. V.: J. Parent. Drug. Assoc., 33:61, 1979.
87. Moretti, C.: Boll Chem. Farm. 103:69, 1964.
88. Lipper, R. A., and Nevola, M. M.: Influence of Amber Glass on the Decomposition of Thromerosol in Aqueous Solution. In press.
89. Enever, R. P., and LiWanPo, A., and Shotton, E.: J. Pharm. Sci., 66:1087, 1977.
90. Kassem, M. A., Kassem, A. A., and Ammar, H. O.: Pharm. Acta Helv., 44:611, 1969.
91. Anschel, J.: Bull Parenter. Drug Assoc., 31:47, 1977.
92. Bull, A. W.: J. Pharm. and Pharmacol., 7:806, 1955.
93. Wight, C. S., Tomlinson, J. A., and Kirmeier, S.: Drug & Cosmetic Ind., 72:766, 1953.
94. Chen, J. L., Cyr, G. N., and Langlykke, A. F.: Drug & Cosmetic Ind., 81:596, 1957.
95. Marcus, E., Kimm, H. K., and Autian, J.: J. Am. Pharm. Assoc., Sci. Ed., 48:457, 1959.
96. Boardman, L. H.: J. Pharm. and Pharmacol., 1:934, 1949.
97. Stephenson, D.: J. Pharm. and Pharmacol., 5:999, 1953.
98. Proposed Guidelines for Stability Studies for Human Drugs and Biologicals, Food and Drug Administration, Washington, DC, March 1984.

27

Quality Control and Assurance

LEON LACHMAN, SAMIR A. HANNA, *and* KARL LIN

The concept of total quality control refers to the process of striving to produce a perfect product by a series of measures requiring an organized effort by the entire company to prevent or eliminate errors at every stage in production. Although the responsibility for assuring product quality belongs principally to quality assurance personnel, it involves many departments and disciplines within a company. To be effective, it must be supported by a team effort. Quality must be built into a drug product during product and process design, and it is influenced by the physical plant design, space, ventilation, cleanliness, and sanitation during routine production. The product and process design begins in research and development, and includes preformulation and physical, chemical, therapeutic, and toxicologic considerations. It considers materials, in-process and product control, including specifications and tests for the active ingredients, the excipients, and the product itself, specific stability procedures for the product, freedom from microbial contamination and proper storage of the product, and containers, packaging, and labeling to ensure that container closure systems provide functional protection of the product against such factors as moisture, oxygen, light, volatility, and drug/package interaction. Provision for a cross referencing system to allow any batch of a product to be traced from its raw materials to its final destination in the event of unexpected difficulties is required.

Quality Assurance

The assurance of product quality depends on more than just proper sampling and adequate testing of various components and the finished dosage form. Prime responsibility of maintaining product quality during production rests with the manufacturing department. Removal of re-

sponsibility from manufacturing for producing a quality product can result in imperfect composition, such as ingredients missing, subpotent or superpotent addition of ingredients, or mixup of ingredients; mistakes in packaging or filling, such as product contamination, mislabeling, or deficient package; and lack of conformance to product registration. Quality assurance personnel must establish control or checkpoints to monitor the quality of the product as it is processed and upon completion of manufacture. These begin with raw materials and component testing and include in-process, packaging, labeling, and finished product testing as well as batch auditing and stability monitoring.

Sources of Quality Variation

Because of the increasing complexity of modern pharmaceutical manufacture arising from a variety of unique drugs and dosage forms, complex ethical, legal, and economic responsibilities have been placed on those concerned with the manufacture of modern pharmaceuticals. An awareness of these factors is the responsibility of all those involved in the development, manufacture, control, and marketing of quality products. A systematic effective quality assurance program takes into consideration potential raw material, in-process, packaging material, labeling and finished product variables.

Control of Quality Variation

Raw Materials Control

Good raw material specifications must be written in precise terminology, must be complete, must provide specific details of test methods, type of instruments, and manner of sampling, and must be properly identified. Table 27-1 lists general tests, limits, and other physical or chemical data for raw materials related to identity, purity, strength, and quality. Table 27-2 presents the quality assurance monograph for acetaminophen, USP, as an example of a specific raw material quality assurance monograph.

The FDA Current Good Manufacturing Practices (CGMP) covering raw material handling procedures are found in the Code of Federal Regulations, Title 21, Section 211.42. It simply states that "components" be received, sampled, tested, and stored in a reasonable way, that rejected material be disposed of, that samples of tested components be retained, and that appropriate records of these steps be maintained. In practice, the manufacturer physically inspects and assigns lot numbers to all raw materials re-

---

TABLE 27-1. *Raw Material Quality Assurance Monograph*

A. (Raw Material Name)
   1. Structural formula, molecular weight
   2. Chemical name(s)
   3. Item number
   4. Date of issue
   5. Date of superseded, if any, or new material
   6. Signature of writer
   7. Signature of approval

B. Samples
   1. Safety requirement
   2. Sample plan and procedure
   3. Sample size and sample container to be used
   4. Preservation sample required

C. Retest Program
   1. Retesting schedule
   2. Reanalysis to be performed to assure identity, strength, quality, and purity

D. Specifications (wherever applicable)
   1. Description
   2. Solubility
   3. Identity
      a. Specific chemical tests such as related alkaloids, organic nitrogen basis, acid moiety, or inorganic salt tests; sulfate, chloride, phosphate, sodium, and potassium tests; or other spot organic and inorganic chemical tests as needed.
      b. Infrared absorption
      c. Ultraviolet absorption
      d. Melting range
      e. Congealing point
      f. Boiling point or range
      g. Thin-layer, paper, liquid, or gas chromatography
   4. Purity and quality
      a. General completeness of solutions, pH, specific rotation, nonvolatile residue, ash, acid-insoluble ash, residue on ignition, loss on drying, water content, heavy metals, arsenic, lead, mercury, selenium, sulfate, chloride, carbonates, acid value, iodine value, saponification value.
      b. Special quality tests, particle size, crystallinity characteristics, and polymorphic forms
      c. Special purity tests, ferric in ferrous salts, peroxides and aldehydes in ether and related degradation products
   5. Assay, calculated either on anhydrous or hydrous basis
   6. Microbial limits, especially for raw materials from natural sources

E. Test Procedures
   1. Compendial, USP, or NF references
   2. Noncompendial, detailed analytical procedure, weights; dilutions; extractions; normality; reagents; instrumentation used and procedure, if any; calculations

F. Approved Suppliers
   1. List of prime suppliers and other approved alternative suppliers, if any

---

TABLE 27-2. *Acetaminophen, USP, Quality Assurance Specifications*

Item Number	Date of Issue	Superseded	Written by	Approved by
001	Jan. 1, 1984	New	J. Doe	T. Mullen

Sampling Plan		Retest Program	
Containers #	Containers to be Sampled	Schedule	Tests
1	All	2 yr	Identity IR
2–5	All		p-aminophenol
6–10	6		assay
11–18	7		
19–28	8		
29–100	9		
101	10		

$$\text{HO}\!-\!\!\left\langle\!\!\bigcirc\!\!\right\rangle\!\!-\!\text{NHCOCH}_3$$

$C_8H_9NO_2$ Mol. wt. 151.16

Chemical Formula

4′-Hydroxyacetanilide, p-hydroxyacetanilide, p-acetaminidophenol, p-acetaminophenol, p-acetylaminophenol, N-acetyl-p-aminophenol

Specifications

Description	White, odorless, crystalline powder, possessing a slightly bitter taste
Solubility	Soluble in boiling water and in sodium hydroxide TS, freely soluble in alcohol
Identity A-IR	Scan conforms to reference standard
B-UV	Scan conforms to reference standard
C-FeCl₃	Violet-blue color is produced
Melting range	168–172°C
pH (saturate solution)	5.3–6.5
Water	NMT 0.5%
Residue on ignition	NMT 0.1%
Chloride	NMT 0.014%
Sulfate	NMT 0.02%
Sulfide	No coloration or spotting of the test paper occurs
Heavy metals	NMT 0.001%
Readily carbonizable substances	No more color than Matching Fluid A
Free p-aminophenol	NMT 0.005%
p-Chloroacetanilide	NMT 0.001%
Assay	98.0–101.0% on the anhydrous basis
Completeness of solution	1 g/20 ml methanol is not less clear than an equal volume of methanol examined similarly

Test Procedures

For all tests, see USP XXI, United States Pharmacopeial Convention, Rockville, MD, 1980.

Approved Suppliers

1. S. B. Penick & Co., Lyndhurst, NJ
2. Mallinckrodt, Raleigh, NC

ceived and quarantines them until they are approved for use. Each raw material is sampled according to standard sampling procedures and is sent to the quality control laboratory for testing according to the written procedures (Table 27-2). If acceptable, it is moved to the release storage area, after being properly stickered to indicate the item number, name of material, lot number, date of release, reassay date, and signature of the quality assurance inspector. It is retested as necessary according to an established schedule to assure that it still conforms to specifications at time of use.

Quality assurance personnel should keep preservation samples of active raw materials that consist of at least twice the necessary quantity to perform all tests required, to determine whether the material meets the established specifications. These preservation samples should be retained for at least 7 years. Approved materials should be rotated so that the oldest stock is used first. Any raw material not meeting specifications must be isolated from the acceptable materials, stickered as a rejection, and returned to the supplier or disposed of promptly. To verify the supplier's conformance to specifications, further supporting assurance by means of on-site periodic inspections are pertinent to the total quality of raw materials. This procedure assures that cross-contamination does not take place because of improperly cleaned equipment or poor housekeeping practices; otherwise, contaminants could go undetected because specifications generally are not designed to control the presence of unrelated materials. In general, raw materials may be classified into two groups: (1) active or therapeutic and (2) inactive or inert.

Active or Therapeutic Materials

ANTIBIOTICS

Antibiotics are one of the few drugs for which the official analytic method appears in the Code of Federal Regulations. The USP and NF refer to the Code of Federal Regulations for specifications and analytic methods given in the individual monographs for each antibiotic. The Code of Federal Regulations, Title 21, Chapter 1, Parts 436 to 436.517 and Parts 442 and 455 contain the analytic method specifications for all antibiotics approved for human use in the United States. The number of tests required varies from one antibiotic to another. The data in Table 27-3 specify the tests required by the Code of Federal Regulations for some antibiotics.

Testing of antibiotics is usually performed either chemically, microbiologically, biologically, or by all three methods. Caution must be exercised in testing antibiotic raw material to assure that it is not altered during the sampling procedure. The sample must be taken in a relatively dry atmosphere, relatively free from dust, and free of both chemical and microbial airborne contamination, and exposure must be reduced to minimal time of sampling. Special attention should be given to the assay for potency of antibiotic raw materials. Since the potency value in terms of micrograms per milligram obtained for this material is used in calculating the number of grams or kilograms required for the working formula procedures, it is recommended that at least two separate weighings of such antibiotic raw material powder be assayed on each of three different days (six different assays using six different weighings). If all the individual results are not within the normal distribution of the group or show too much variance, additional assays should be performed until a mean potency is obtained with confidence limits of $\pm 2.5\%$ (or better) at $P = .05$.

OTHER ACTIVE MATERIALS

The current editions of the USP and NF contain monographs on most therapeutically active materials used in manufacturing. Since there is such a wide variance in the nature of the active ingredients used in manufacturing, it is impossible to summarize briefly the testing of those raw materials. One of the most important decisions to be made in raw material control is the degree of purity to be maintained for each material. It is not uncommon to find an appreciable variation in the degree of purity between samples of the same raw material purchased from different commercial sources. The selection must then result in the highest purity practical for each raw material, consistent with safety and efficacy of the final dosage form. In general, a typical raw material currently found in a compendium has a purity requirement of at least 97%. Its specifications normally include solubility, identification, melting range, loss on drying, residue on ignition, special metal testing, specific impurities that are pertinent to the method of synthesis of each individual raw material, and assay. The methods of assay are usually chemical in nature.

It should be understood that these compendial tests are intended as the minimum required from a legal point of view. For certain products, it may be necessary to require that the active ingredient specifications be far tighter than those of the comparable compendial standard. Raw materials cannot be adequately evaluated

TABLE 27-3. Tests of Some Antibiotics

	LOD	Moisture	pH	Crystallinity	Iodometric Assay*	Hydroxylamine Col. Assay*	Residue on Ignition	Heavy Metals	Melting Range or Temperature	Disintegration	Nonaqueous Titration	Special Test	Microbial Limits	ID	Specific Rotation
Ampicillin	NMT 2%		3.5–6.0	X	X	X					X		Potency† safety	X	
Cephalexin monohydrate	4–8%		3.0–5.0	X	X								Potency† safety	X	
Neomycin sulfate	NMT 8%		5.0–7.5	X									Potency† safety	X	
Tetracycline		NMT 13%	3.0–7.0	X								Absorption at 380 nm	Potency† safety	X	
Zinc bacitracin		NMT 5%	6.0–7.5							NMT 1 hr			Potency† NMT 10% Zn safety	X	
Griseofulvin	NMT 1%			X			NMT 0.2%	NMT 25 ppm	217–224°C			UV absorption specific surface area	Potency† safety	X	+348° to +364°
Erythromycin	NMT 10%		8.0–10.5	X			NMT 2%	NMT 50 ppm					Potency† safety	X	−50° to −58°
Sodium novobiocin	NMT 6%		6.5–8.5				10.5–12%						Potency†	X	

*Chemical methods of assay as alternatives to microbiologic assay are allowed for special antibiotics: iodometric and hydroxylamine colorimetric for most penicillin, cephalothin, and cephaloridine; GLC for lincomycin and clindamycin; ultraviolet spectrophotometry for chloramphenicol succinate and palmitate, and griseofulvin; colorimetric for cycloserine and troleandomycin.

†Potency is determined microbiologically using the turbidimetric assay and the diffusion plate assay.

From Code of Federal Regulations, 21 Food and Drugs, U.S. Govt. Printing Office, 1985.

and controlled without special instrumentation such as spectrophotometry; potentiometric titrimetry; column, gas (GLC), paper, thin-layer, and high-pressure liquid chromatography (HPLC); polarography; x-ray diffraction; x-ray fluorescense; spectrophotofluorimetry; calorimetry; and radioactive tracer techniques. No less demanding are the tests required for microbiologic assay, pharmacologic assay, and safety testing. For certain products, even when highly purified and well characterized raw materials are involved, specifications should include additional critical tests, such as particle size, crystal shape, and crystalline versus amorphous forms. Any of these characteristics could affect the safety or effectiveness of the final dosage form. It is a CGMP requirement that all raw materials, active or inactive, be assigned a meaningful reassay date that assures the purity and potency of the raw material at time of use. This confirms the continued stability of each raw material.

Inactive or Inert Materials

Inactive or inert materials usually make up the major portion of the final dosage form. Therefore, their physical characteristics, such as color, odor, and foreign matter, are as important as their chemical purity. Among other important specifications of inactive or inert materials are particle size, heavy metal content, arsenic, selenium, water content, microbial limit, foreign matter, residue on ignition, and pH.

Approved certified water-soluble Food, Drug and Cosmetics (FD&C) dyes, or mixtures thereof, or their corresponding lake, may be used to color oral dosage forms. The color in oral dosage forms is mainly a means of identification. The FDA determines and approves colorants for use in food and drugs with recommendation of limits, if any. Table 27-4 lists selected colors and FDA restrictions on their use. A typical analysis of a color contains identity tests and tests of total volatile matter, heavy metals, water-insoluble matter, synthesis impurities, arsenic, lead, and total color. An FD&C color lake analysis contains additional tests for chloride, sulfate, and inorganic matter.

If a flavored oral dosage form is desired, flavors or volatile oils may be used. Flavors or volatile oils are usually tested for refractive index, specific gravity, solubility, and alcohol content, if any. A GLC chromatogram can be used as a "fingerprint" for each specific flavor to help in assuring the supplier's continuous compliance to specifications. Knowledge of the presence of any synthetic FD&C dyes in a flavor formula is important for the formulator and quality control

TABLE 27-4. *Colorants*

Colorant	Restriction on Use
FD&C: Blue #1	Permanent listing for use in foods, drugs, and cosmetics
Blue #2 Green #2 Red #3 Red #40 Yellow #5 Yellow #6	Provisional listing for use in foods, drugs, and cosmetics
D&C: Blue #6 Green #5 Green #6 Orange #5 Orange #10 Orange #17	Provisional listing for use in drugs and cosmetics
Red #6 Red #7 Red #21 Red #22 Red #27 Red #28 Red #30	
Red #8 Red #12 Red #19 Red #33 Red #36	Provisional listing for use in drugs and cosmetics with restriction of NMT 0.75 mg to be ingested on a daily basis
Yellow #10	Provisional listing for use in drugs and cosmetics
Lakes of the above:	
Annatto Carotene	Permanent listing for use in foods, drugs, and cosmetics
Caramel	Permanent listing for use in foods, drugs, and cosmetics and provisional listing for use in cosmetics
Carmine	Permanent listing for use in foods, drugs, and cosmetics
Titanium dioxide	Permanent listing for use in drugs and cosmetics

Data from Food and Drug Administration, Federal Register.

personnel to assure compliance with FDA colorant regulations.

The most popular sweetening agents used are

sucrose, glucose, mannitol, lactose, crystalline and liquid sorbitol, and such artificial sweetening agents as saccharin, sodium saccharin, calcium saccharin, and aspartame.

Testing for unwanted impurities resulting from synthesis side reaction in the manufacturing procedure is essential in the analysis of sweetening agents, for example, furfuraldehyde in lactose, and reducing sugars in mannitol. Sweetening agents are usually tested for water content, heavy metals, residue on ignition, arsenic, and special tests such as specific rotation, melting range, selenium, and readily carbonizable substances.

In-Process Items Control

Conformance to compendial standards as the sole basis for judging the quality of a final dosage form can be grossly misleading. Obviously, a compendial monograph could never cover all possibilities that might adversely affect the quality of a product. The difficulty lies in part in the fact that final dosage forms are frequently produced in batches of hundreds of thousands or even millions of units. The numbers of units assayed at the end of the process is not likely to be representative of more than a small fraction of the actual production.

There is a real and significant difference between a finished product compendial standard and the quality assurance of the manufacturing process. The FDA-CGMP regulations emphasize environmental factors to minimize cross-contamination of products and errors in labeling and packaging, and the integrity of production and quality control records; however, they do little to minimize within-batch and batch-to-batch variation in the output of production. Therefore, it is an important function of the in-process quality assurance program to ensure that finished dosage forms have uniform purity and quality within a batch and between batches. This is accomplished by identifying critical steps in the manufacturing process and controlling them within defined limits.

Quality Assurance Before Start-Up

ENVIRONMENTAL AND MICROBIOLOGIC CONTROL AND SANITATION

To assure that finished dosage forms meet high standards of quality and purity, an effective sanitation program is required at all facilities where such products are manufactured. A successful extermination program must be enforced within and outside the plant to control insects and rodents. People are the mainstay of any plant housekeeping and sanitation program. Consequently, personal cleanliness and proper haircovering and clothing should be required. Floors, walls, and ceilings should be resistant to external forces, capable of being easily cleaned, and in good repair. Adequate ventilation, proper temperature, and proper humidity are other important factors. Ventilation in manufacturing departments is usually designed so that dust can be contained and removed. In such departmental operations, dust collectors, air filters, and scrubbers to clean the air are checked on a routine schedule. Air quality monitoring at the work station could indicate the adequacy of these elements.

The water supply may be potable, distilled, or deionized, and must be under adequate pressure to keep the water flowing. Deionization units should be monitored, and the resins changed or regenerated frequently, to deliver water of consistently high chemical and microbial quality as per written compendial or inhouse specifications.

Quality assurance should review and monitor the following programs, based on written procedures that specify the details of each:

Sanitation: Example is shown in Table 27-5 for one insecticide.
Cleaning: Building and equipment.
Ventilation: Filter conditions and changes; pressure gauge; humidity monitoring; temperature monitoring; microbial monitoring (Table 27-6); light intensity.
Water: Release at point of use after checking by quality control; proper flushing period and/or volume before water use.

MANUFACTURING WORKING FORMULA PROCEDURES (MWFP)

Documentation of the component materials and processing steps, together with production operation specifications and equipment to be used, make up the MWFP.

A working formula procedure should be prepared for each batch size that is produced. To attempt expansion or reduction of a batch size by manual calculations at the time of production cannot be considered good manufacturing practice.

Quality assurance personnel must review and check the working formula procedures for each production batch before, during, and after production for the following details:

TABLE 27-5. *Quality Assurance Operating Procedure*

Page	No.	
Date	Supersedes	
	NEW	Sanitation Control—Pest Control
Written by	Checked by	

Certox: Insecticide

Type of action
Kills on contact

Formula	*Approximate %*
Petroleum distillates	71.8%
Technical piperonyl butoxide*	12.0
Pyrethrine	1.2
Inert ingredients	15.0

Dilution
Dilute 1 gallon of concentrate with 4 gallons of water.

Time interval
To be used once weekly after working hours on Friday evenings.

Area designation
Floor and drains

Equipment
Spray unit for Certox
Certox concentrate
Safety equipment

Removal of waste materials
Removal of waste materials remaining in the spray units after exterminating shall be the responsibility of the exterminator.

Effectiveness inspection
It will be the responsibility of the quality assurance department to perform routine area checks to ascertain the effectiveness of the frequency of spraying.

It will be the responsibility of the area supervisor, however, to take necessary action immediately upon seeing any infestation.

Special restrictions and cautions
1. Foods should be removed or covered during treatment.
2. Do not store or use near heat or open flame.
3. Apply only as designated on area designation assignments.

Toxicity in humans
Severe allergic dermatitis and systemic allergic reactions are possible.

Toxic symptoms
Large amounts may cause nausea, vomiting, tinnitus, headache, and other CNS disturbances.

Government status
EPA Registration Number: 1748-110
Since Certox presents no significant toxicity problem, no tolerance data are available.

*equivalent to 9.6% (butylcarbityl) (6-propyl-piperonyl) ether and 2.4% related compounds.

Signature and date of issue given by a responsible production or quality assurance employee.

Proper identification by name and dosage form, item number, lot number, effective date of document, reference to a superseded version (if any), amount, lot, and code numbers of each raw material utilized.

TABLE 27-6. *Environmental Control in Manufacture of Oral Dosage Forms*

Product _____   Lot No. _____

Room _____   Date exposed _____

| Media _____ | Time of Exposure _____ | Incubation temperature ____°C Duration _____ | Date read _____ |

1—Location of Plate Exposure	Plate no.	Colony Count

2—Location of Air Sampler (m³ air/hr)	Plate no.	Colony Count

Comments

Microbiologist _____   Supervisor _____

Date Reported _____

Initialing of each step by two of the operators involved.

Calculations of both active and inactive materials, especially if there have been any corrections for 100% potencies for active ingredients used.

Starting and finishing times of each operation.

Equipment to be used and specification of its set-up.

Proper labeling of released components and equipment, indicating product name, strength, lot number, and item number.

RAW MATERIALS

Quality assurance should check the original containers of released raw materials for cleanliness before they are taken to the production department. Most raw materials, however, are weighed in an environmental control weighing area, where they are transferred to a secondary container that circulates only inside the production department. This secondary container should be properly labeled with a sticker that bears all the information on the original container label. Only released raw materials with

proper reassay dates should be allowed to enter the production department. Raw materials intended for use in specific products should be stacked and stored together in an approximate staging area with proper identification (name, dosage form, item number, lot number, weight, and signatures).

MANUFACTURING EQUIPMENT

Quality assurance personnel must ensure that manufacturing equipment is designed, located, and maintained so that it facilitates thorough cleaning, is suitable for its intended use, and minimizes potential for contamination during manufacture. Manufacturing equipment and utensils should be thoroughly cleansed and maintained in accordance with specific written directions. Whenever possible, equipment should be disassembled and thoroughly cleaned to preclude the carryover of drug residues from previous operations. Adequate records of such procedures and tests, if appropriate, should be monitored by quality assurance employees. It is good manufacturing practice to use laboratory checks whenever possible to detect trace quantities of drugs if products containing such drugs were produced on specific equipment prior to cleaning.

Prior to the start of any production operation, the quality assurance personnel should ascertain that the proper equipment and tooling for each manufacturing stage are being used. Equipment must be identified by labels bearing the name, dosage form, item number, and lot number of the product to be processed. Equipment used for special batch production should be completely separated in the production department, and all dust-producing operations should be provided with adequate exhaust systems to prevent cross-contamination and recirculation of contaminated air.

Weighing and measuring equipment used in production and quality assurance processes, such as thermometer and balances, should be calibrated and checked at suitable intervals by appropriate methods; records of such tests should be maintained by quality assurance and production personnel. Examples for such calibration methods are given in Table 27-7.

Quality Assurance At Start-Up

RAW MATERIALS PROCESSING

Only released, properly labeled raw materials are allowed in the in-processing area. Depending on the nature of the product, quality assurance personnel should check and verify that the temperature and humidity in the area are within the specified limits required for the product. If the temperature and/or humidity is beyond the specified limits, production must be informed and corrective actions taken.

TABLE 27-7. *Quality Assurance Calibration Procedure*

Page	No.
Date	Supersedes Calibration of Thermometers
Written by	Checked by

Thermometers (to be checked every 6 months)

1. Employ suitable USP melting point standards for the range of the thermometer to be tested.

2. Use USP method class I to determine the actual melting range of the standards.

3. Tag the thermometer with calibration date, next calibration date, temperature correction, if any, and signature of the person conducting the test.

The specified in-process procedure is to be checked, at each step in the process, according to written in-process quality assurance procedures.

Quality assurance personnel should verify and document the proper equipment, addition of ingredient, mixing time, drying time, filtering, and mesh size of sieves used in screening.

At certain points, samples are to be taken to the quality control laboratory for potency assay and any other testing that is necessary to ensure batch uniformity and purity.

Containers of in-process raw materials are labeled with product name, item number, lot number, and gross, tare, and net weights of the contents.

COMPOUNDING

Quality assurance personnel are responsible for ascertaining that all containers of raw materials are properly labeled and staged in the compounding staging area, that they are clean, and that manufacturing equipment is properly identified as to product, strength, item number, and lot number.

The production process begins with the set-up of the manufacturing equipment to prepare the finished dosage form within the specified limits for the particular product. At each significant step in the procedure, quality assurance personnel verify that the process is being performed in accordance with the written directions and is conforming to required standards.

A variable group of tests that are widely used for in-process controls measure characteristics including physical appearance, color, odor, thickness, diameter, friability, hardness, weight variation, disintegration time, volume check, viscosity and pH. Such in-process tests are designed to ensure control of problems that can arise during finished dosage form manufacturing.

Current Good Manufacturing Practices require that in-process quality assurance be adequately documented throughout all stages of manufacturing. Throughout the production run, in-process samples are removed and tested, and data are recorded on special forms as specified in the product's in-process monograph. The number of samples taken for testing and the type of testing obviously depend on the size of the batch and the type of product. If deviation from the specified limits occurs, the necessary corrective action is taken and recorded, and a resample is taken and tested to determine whether the quality attribute of the product is now within the limits. In some instances, as in the case of compendial weight variation or pH specifications, the deviation is such that units produced prior to the corrective action are isolated, accounted for, and rejected.

In addition to the foregoing, portions of the initial, final, and in-process samples are used for collecting average run samples for the quality control laboratory to perform final batch analysis and release.

PACKAGING MATERIALS CONTROL

The USP defines the container closure system as that device that holds the drug and is or may be in direct contact with the drug. The immediate container is that which is in direct contact with the drug at all times. The closure is a part of the container.

Packaging materials should not interact physically or chemically with the finished product to alter the strength, quality, or purity beyond specified requirements. The compendium provides specifications and test procedures for light resistance: well-closed, tightly closed, and four different types of glass containers.

Specifications and test methods are designed for containers on the basis of tests performed on the product in the container. The following features are to be considered in developing container specifications:

Properties of container tightness.

Moisture and vapor tightness regardless of container construction.

Toxicity and chemical/physical characteristics of materials needed in container construction.

Physical or chemical changes of container upon prolonged contact with product.

Compatibility between container and product.

Good Manufacturing Practices require that stability data be submitted for the finished dosage form of the drug in the container closure system in which it is to be marketed.

LABELS CONTROL

Production control issues a packaging form that carries the name of the product; item number; lot number; number of labels, inserts, and packaging materials to be used; operations to be performed, and the quantity to be packaged. A copy of this form is sent to the supervisor of label control, who in turn counts out the required number of labels. Since labels may be spoiled during the packaging operation, a definite number in excess of that actually required is usually issued; however, all labels must be accounted for at the end of the operation, and unused labels must be accounted for before their destruction.

If the lot number and expiration date of the product are not going to be printed directly on the line, the labels are run through a printing machine, which imprints the lot number and expiration date. The labels are recounted and placed in a separate container with proper identification for future transfer to the packaging department. The packaging department then requests, according to the packaging form, the product to be packaged, along with all packaging components, such as labels, inserts, bottles, vials, ampuls, stoppers, caps, seals, cartons, and shipping cases. Quality assurance personnel inspects and verifies all packaging components and equipment to be used for the packaging operation to ensure that it has the proper identification, that the line has been thoroughly cleaned, and that all materials from the previous packaging operation have been completely removed. Proper reconciliation and disposition of the unused and wasted labels should occur at the end of the packaging operation.

FINISHED PRODUCT CONTROL

Specifications. Final testing of finished product is made in the quality control laboratories. These tests are designed to determine compliance with specifications. Thus, the testing of the finished product for compliance with predetermined standards prior to release of the product for packaging and subsequent distribution is a critical factor for quality assurance. This testing, along with in-process testing, assures that each unit contains the amount of drug claimed on the label, that all of the drug in each unit is available for complete absorption, that the drug is stable in the formulation in its specific final container closure system for its expected shelf-life, and that dosage units themselves contain no toxic foreign substances.

Normally, the design of test parameters, procedures, and specifications is made during product development. It is a good manufacturing practice to base such parameters on experiences developed from several pilot and production batches. Furthermore, the results of these studies should be subjected to statistical analysis where appropriate, to appraise the precision and accuracy of each procedure correctly for each characteristic. In the long run, with additional production experience, specifications may possibly be modified to upgrade product specifications.

Bulk Product Testing. Each lot of bulk

product should be tested to ensure identity, quality, potency, and purity. Quality assurance authorizes the release for further processing based on actual physical, chemical, and/or biologic laboratory testing.

Tests required by the official compendia on the ingredients and the dosage form applies to all manufacturers of a specific compendial product. The manufacturer frequently employs alternative methods that are more accurate, specific, or economical than those in the compendia.

The manufacturer is not required to employ the official analytic procedures as long as the quality of his product complies with the compendial requirements. In the case of a legal action, however, the compendial procedures become the referee procedures for determining compliance.

Quality Assurance During Packaging Operation. If the quality control laboratory analysis confirms that the product complies with specifications, and if the quality assurance audit indicates that manufacturing operations are satisfactory, the bulk product is released to the packaging department, and production control is notified. Packaging operations should be performed with adequate physical segregation from product to product. Quality assurance personnel should periodically inspect the packaging lines and should check filled and labeled containers for compliance with written specifications. Some packaging operations, especially those using high-speed equipment, are fitted with automated testing equipment to check each container for fill and label placement. Alternatively, an operator may visually inspect all packages fed into the final cartons. Quality assurance should perform an independent inspection and select finished preservation samples at random from each lot. The preservation samples should consist of at least twice the quantity necessary to perform all tests required to determine whether the product meets its established specifications. These preservation samples should be retained for at least 1 year after the expiration date and should be stored their original package under conditions consistent with product labeling.

Quality assurance personnel should also select an appropriate size sample of the finished package product and send it to the analytic control laboratory for final testing.

Auditing. Good Manufacturing Practice requires that the manufacturing process be adequately documented throughout all stages of the operation. The history of each task, including the starting materials, equipment used, personnel involved in production and control until completed packaging is complete, should be recorded. The areas of record keeping include:

Individual components, raw materials, and packaging materials. Master formula and procedure.

Batch production.

Packaging and labeling operation.

Laboratory in-process and finished control testing.

Proper signing and dating by at least two individuals independently for each operation in the proper spaces.

Reconciliation of materials supplied with amounts of tablets produced, taking into account allowable loss limits.

Before releasing the product for distribution, quality assurance should evaluate the batch records of all in-process tests and controls and of all tests of the final product to determine whether they conform to specifications.

Concept of Statistical Quality Control

Statistical quality control (SQC) has been defined as the monitoring of quality by application of statistical methods in all stages of production. Statistical methods of investigation based on the theory of probability may be used for estimating parameters, for performing tests of significance, for determining the relationship between factors, and for making meaningful decisions on the basis of experimental evidence. The selection of an appropriate method essentially depends on the type of measurement, the sampling techniques, the design of the experiment, and the type of sample distribution (normal, binomial, or Poisson).

SQC has been used to serve (1) as a basis for improved evaluation of materials through more representative sampling techniques, and (2) as a means of achieving sharper control in certain manufacturing processes. The procedures consist of properly sampling the product, determining the quality variation of the sample, and from this data, making inferences to the entire batch under investigation. Once the characteristic data pattern of a process has been determined, the pattern can be utilized to predict the limits within which future data can be expected to fall as a matter of chance, and to determine when significant variations in the process have taken place. The objective is to determine whether the major source of observed variation is due to "chance variation," which is inevitable during the manufacturing process, or to "assignable causes," which can usually be detected and corrected by appropriate methods.

Any program of production and inspection has its own unique chance causes of variation, which cannot be controlled or eliminated and often cannot be identified. This variation represents a pool of small individual variations for which limits can be established. On the other hand, the assignable causes can usually be identified by statistical techniques, for example, the detection of an outlier or a trend or pattern. Assignable causes, by definition, are associated with something special and assignable, such as excessive variations caused by a specific machine, a specific batch of material, or a container. Therefore, the use of SQC permits the evaluation of the magnitude of "chance variation" and the detection of "assignable variation" of product quality. This may be detected by means of quality control charts.

Normal Frequency Distribution

There are many types of variation patterns in product quality. The most common pattern of data distribution is the normal curve, a symmetric, bell-shaped curve. By plotting the relative frequency of the data obtained from a large number of results along the vertical axis against the magnitude of the measured characteristic, such as tablet weight or chemical assay, on the horizontal axis, a normal frequency distribution curve is often obtained, as shown in Figure 27-1. Most statistical techniques are based on the as-

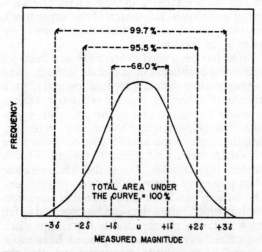

FIG. 27-1. *A normal frequency distribution curve characterized by the mean (μ) and the standard deviation (δ).*

sumption of a normal frequency distribution curve.

The normal distribution is defined completely by two parameters: the mean and the standard deviation. The observed mean ($\bar{X}$) is the arithmetic average of a series of values and is calculated by dividing the sum of such values by the number of values (N) in the series. It is expressed as:

$$\bar{X} = \frac{\Sigma X}{N} \quad (1)$$

$\bar{X}$ is the best measure of the central value of a normal distribution and is an estimate of the theoretic mean (μ). For quantitative expression of the dispersion or scatter about the central value for establishing an estimate of variation among the values, the range (R) and the standard deviation (δ) are commonly employed. The range is calculated as the arithmetic difference between the largest and the smallest value in a group of data. The standard deviation of the sample (s) is an unbiased estimate of the standard deviation of the population (δ) and is calculated from the following formula:

$$s = \sqrt{\frac{\Sigma(X - X)^2}{N - 1}} \quad (2)$$

The standard deviation is a measure of the variation expressed in the same units of measurement as the original values. Furthermore, if the distribution of measurements is normal, it permits delineation of a zone or range within which a given portion of the original observations normally lie. Thus, as seen in Figure 27-1, about 68% of all results fall within one standard deviation ($\pm 1s$) on either side of the mean, 95.5% within two standard deviations (± 2 s), and 99.7% within three standard deviations (± 3 s).

When sampling from a normal distribution, $\bar{X}$ and s are independent of each other, i.e., the dispersion or scatter as measured by s is independent of the magnitude of the $\bar{X}$. Figure 27-2 shows a series of normal probability distributions whose mean values are the same, but whose standard deviations differ. Such distributions are so constructed that the total area under each curve is unity, or 100%; thus, segments of area under the curve represent probabilities.

Both the range (R) and standard deviation (s) are measures of the variability among individuals in a group. Although R is a less efficient measure of that variability, there is a definite relationship between the two values. In fact, it is possible to obtain an estimate of s from R by di-

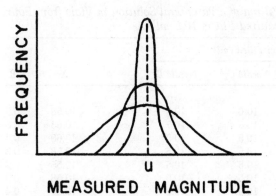

FIG. 27-2. *Frequency distributions with the same mean but different standard deviation.*

viding R by an appropriate divisor, the numerical value of which depends on the sample size (N). Divisors (D) for selected N are presented in Table 27-8. If it is known that the mean sample range calculated from a series of samples, each containing N = 4 items, has the value 6.3, then the standard deviation for the distribution of individual items can be estimated as s = 6.3/2.1 = 3.0. If s for the distribution of individual items in a certain population is 4.0, the mean sample range in samples of N = 7 could also be estimated from Table 27-8 as R = 2.7 × 4.0 = 10.8. Estimations of the standard deviation from the range are used quite extensively in industrial statistics.

Quality Control Charts

Control charts have been employed for various pharmaceutical operations and may be used as

TABLE 27-8. *Divisors for Estimating Standard Deviation from the Range*

Sample Size [N]	Divisor [D]
2	1.1
3	1.7
4	2.1
5	2.3
6	2.5
7	2.7
8	2.8
9	3.0
10	3.1
15	3.5
30	4.0
50	4.5
100	5.0
500	6.0

aids in controlling and analyzing physical, chemical, analytic, or biologic parameters of a product, such as (1) weight variation of tablets and capsules; (2) thickness of tablets; (3) volume of liquid filling in a container; (4) the number or percentage of defects in parenteral products; and (5) the number or fraction of defects in a sample of packages emanating from a packaging operation. Any measurements that could form the basis of acceptance or rejection of the product would be amenable to surveillance via the control chart.

Control charts are useful in highlighting trends for intra- and inter-batch variation by following a moving mean value of a specification, as for tablet hardness or assay. There are two basic types of quality control charts: charts based on *variable* and charts based on *attributes*. Attribute charts refer to go or no-go situations in which each sample inspected is tested to determine whether it conforms to the requirements; variable charts are based on a continuous distribution of measurements that can, in a sense, measure degrees of unacceptability. A quality control chart by variables or by attributes developed on the basis of certain quality characteristics serves as an aid in keeping the product in control.

The application of control charts to manufacturing processes can best be described by means of the following examples:

Control Charts by Variables

Example 1. During the automatic filling of a parenteral solution in vials, control of the volume filled during a production run should be established and maintained. One vial was taken at random from each of the four needles of the filling machine at designated times and the average and range of this subgroup of four was computed. The numerical data obtained for the process control record is summarized in Table 27-9 and graphically depicted in Figure 27-3. The upper curves of Figure 27-3 and $\overline{X}$ (mean) charts and the lower curves are R (range) charts. The lines connecting the points serve only to aid in visualizing the trend. The upper and lower control limits for the average (UCL_x and LCL_x) of the filled volume were calculated as shown on the lower part of Table 27-9, using the formulas:

$$UCL_x = \overline{\overline{X}} + A_2\overline{R} \qquad (3)$$
$$LCl_x = \overline{\overline{X}} - A_2\overline{R} \qquad (4)$$

where $\overline{\overline{X}}$, the grand average, is the arithmetic average of all the $\overline{X}$; $\overline{R}$, the average range, is calculated as the arithmetic average of the values of

TABLE 27-9. *Process Control Record of Automatic Filling of a Parenteral Solution in Vials from Four Filling Needles of Machine (Label Fill is 10 ml; Required Fill is 10.5 ml)*

Time the Vial is Sampled	Volume of Solution Filled (ml)				$\bar{X}$	R
	Needle A	Needle B	Needle C	Needle D		
Day 1						
8:30 a.m.	10.7	10.5	10.6	10.5	10.58	0.2
9:20	10.5	10.5	10.8	10.7	10.63	0.3
10:15	10.5	10.9	10.5	10.5	10.60	0.4
11:25	10.8	10.5	10.5	10.5	10.58	0.3
1:00 p.m.	10.5	10.7	10.5	10.5	10.55	0.2
2:00	10.5	10.8	10.5	10.5	10.58	0.3
3:10	10.6	10.5	10.9	10.6	10.65	0.4
4:00	10.5	10.5	10.7	10.7	10.60	0.2
Day 2						
8:20 a.m.	10.5	10.7	10.7	10.5	10.60	0.2
9:30	10.6	10.5	10.8	10.5	10.60	0.3
10:15	10.7	10.8	10.8	10.7	10.75	0.1
11:30	10.5	10.6	10.6	10.6	10.58	0.1
1:10 p.m.	10.4	10.5	10.5	10.8	10.55	0.4
2:20	10.5	10.6	10.4	10.9	10.60	0.5
3:30	10.6	10.6	10.5	10.8	10.63	0.3

Calculation:

$\bar{\bar{X}}$ = Grand average = 10.60
$\bar{R}$ = Average range = 0.28
$UCL_{\bar{x}} = \bar{\bar{X}} + A_2\bar{R} = 10.60 + (0.73)(0.28) = 10.80$
$LCL_{\bar{x}} = \bar{\bar{X}} - A_2\bar{R} = 10.60 - (0.73)(0.28) = 10.40$
$UCL_R = D_4\bar{R} = (2.88)(0.28) = 0.64$
$LCL_R = D_3\bar{R} = (0)(0.28) = 0$

R; and A_2, the factor for using the range to calculate three standard deviation limits for the average, is a constant that for subgroups of four has the value of 0.73. A_2 for selected sample sizes (N) are presented in the last column of Table 27-10.

TABLE 27-10. *Factors for Estimating the Three Standard Deviation Limits*

Sample Size (N)	Factors for R Chart		Factors for X Chart (A₂)
	D_3	D_4	(A_2)
2	0.00	3.27	1.88
3	0.00	2.57	1.02
4	0.00	2.28	0.73
5	0.00	2.11	0.58
6	0.00	2.00	0.48
7	0.08	1.92	0.42
8	0.14	1.86	0.37
9	0.18	1.82	0.34
10	0.22	1.78	0.31

The upper and lower control limits for the range (UCL_R and LCL_R) were calculated from the formulas:

$$UCL_R = D_4 \cdot \bar{R} \tag{5}$$
$$LCL_R = D_3 \cdot \bar{R} \tag{6}$$

where D_3 and D_4, the factors to calculate three standard deviation limits for the range, are constants, which for subgroups of four in this case have the values of 0.00 and 2.28, respectively. D_3 and D_4 for selected sample sizes (N) are tabulated in Table 27-10.

Control charts are depicted in Figure 27-3 are characterized by a vertical axis that has a scale of varying measurement, such as a mean (X), range (R), standard deviation (s), or fraction unacceptable (p), and a horizontal axis that is time-oriented. Each point in the control chart represents a value obtained from a selected number of items referred to as a subgroup. These values are plotted in sequence. The control charts as shown in Figure 27-3 consist of a solid and two horizontally parallel lines on either

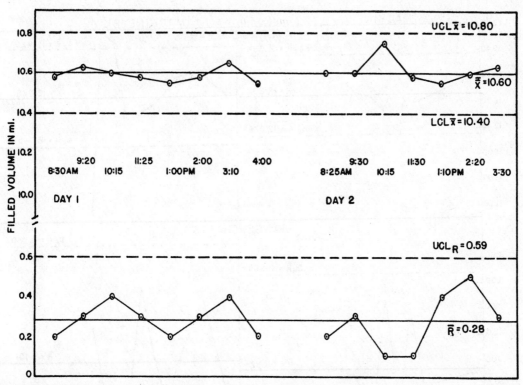

FIG. 27-3. *Control chart for automatic filling of a parenteral solution in vials. The upper curves are $\bar{x}$ (mean) charts and the lower curves are R (range) charts.*

side of the solid line. The central solid line is the target value or the historical process average and/or range. The two dotted parallel lines indicate the limits within which practically all the observed results should fall as long as the process is under normal variation (statistically controlled). The upper dotted line is the upper control limit (UCL), which is normally three standard deviations above the center line. Likewise, the lower line is the lower control limit (LCL) and is three standard deviations below the center line.

If the process is in control, the six standard deviations spread between the upper and lower control limits encompass 99.7% of the values in a normal distribution with its mean at the center line. This is the case for the example shown in Figure 27-3. The control chart of Figure 27-3 is said to show evidence of "control," since all points fall within the designated control limits.

The control chart for averages ($\bar{X}$ chart) is a measurement of the central tendency. Approximately half of the values are above the average while the other half are located below it. This would be expected if random variation is present and the process is under control. Control charts that are used for plotting sample averages are

frequently used in conjunction with a range or standard deviation chart. The control chart for ranges (R chart) indicates the variation present in a set of samples. It is advantageous to plot both the $\bar{X}$ and R charts together, because one may be in control and the other may show excessive variation.

Example 2. The performance of the filling machines for filling by weight a relatively viscous parenteral suspension in multiple dose containers can be followed with control charts.[1] Figure 27-4 shows a control chart on the performance of two machines in filling a batch of the material. Two samples were removed from the production flow and weighed approximately every 20 min, and the average and range measurements were used to construct the control chart in Figure 27-4. It can be seen that Machine A is filling vials within the predicted limits, the averages being within the control limits. Machine B shows large variation, however, as can be seen in the range chart as well as by points indicated outside the control limits on the average chart. Since the measured values fall outside the limits, causes for the process being out of control, which may be assignable, must be investigated. Some possibilities of the assignable

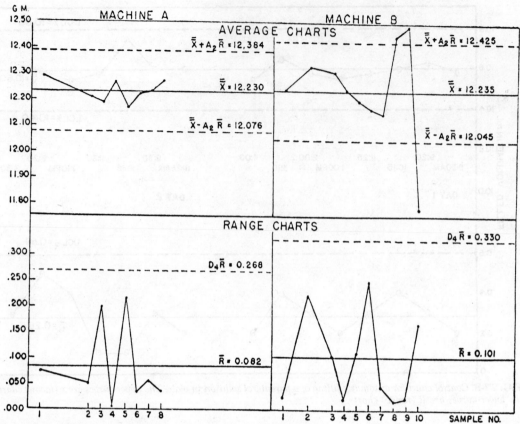

FIG. 27-4. *Control chart containing the $\bar{x}$ and R charts on comparative performance of two filling machines for a parenteral suspension.*

causes are filling machine connections, filters, filling heads, and automatic measuring equipment.

Assuming that the assignable causes for the out-of-control behavior in Machine B are found and corrected, it still may be desirable to reduce the variation as observed in the range charts of Machines A and B. This would allow the establishment of narrower control limits on the average chart, thus making it possible to reduce the overfill and still maintain the same degree of assurance of meeting the specifications. Upon intensive process investigation and improvement, it was possible to narrow the control limits on the average chart as shown in the control chart of Figure 27-5. It is worth noting here that the control limits were narrowed on both X and R charts as compared to those of Figure 27-4. Thus, the process was brought into closer statistical control, with the fill weight variation being minimized.

Control Charts by Attributes

As mentioned, when a record shows only the number of articles conforming and the number of articles failing to conform to any specified requirement (go or no-go) it is said to be a control record by attributes. It is obvious that most routine inspections of manufactured pharmaceutical products, such as the inspection of parenteral products or counting of broken tablets in a bottle, are inspections for attributes. The interest is in the number of flaws or fraction defective per batch. Thus, the weakness of attribute measurements is that gradation of quality cannot be measured. In general, variable charts are more sensitive than attribute charts, although the latter are usually easier to implement. To employ control charts for attributes, a plan with desirable properties would include the following:

1. Samples should be chosen at random.

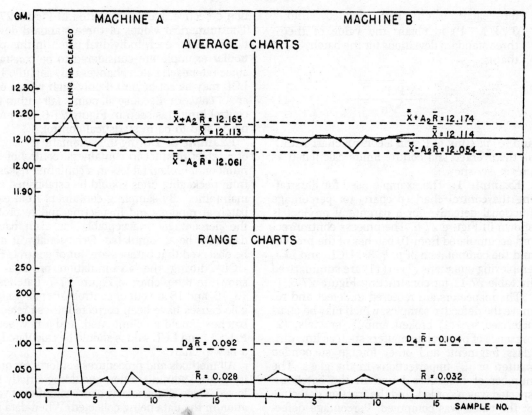

FIG. 27-5. *Control chart containing the $\bar{x}$ and R charts on performance of two filling machines after process investigation and improvement. Note that the control limits were narrowed on $\bar{x}$ and R charts as compared to that of Figure 27-4.*

2. For easier evaluation there should be a fixed number of samples (n) taken each time for inspection. Each tablet or ampul inspected is considered a sample.

3. Each sample is evaluated so that the sample is accepted or rejected, i.e., each tablet or ampul is either good or defective.

4. Each sample must be independent, i.e., each tablet or ampul, good or defective, has nothing to do with another tablet or ampul to cause it to be good or defective.

The essential steps in constructing the control charts for fraction defective are: (1) recording the number inspected, n, and the number of defectives found, d; (2) computing the fraction defective, p, which is the ratio of the number of defectives found to the total number of units actually inspected in the batch, and which is expressed as:

$$p = \frac{d}{n} \tag{7}$$

(3) computing the average fraction defective, $\bar{P}$, obtained by dividing the total number of defectives found by the total number of units inspected in a series of batches:

$$\bar{P} = \frac{\Sigma d}{\Sigma n} \tag{8}$$

(4) calculating the upper and lower control limits, UCL and LCL, through the following formulas:[2]

$$UCL = \bar{P} + \frac{3\sqrt{\bar{P}(1 - \bar{P})}}{\sqrt{n}} \tag{9}$$

$$LCL = \bar{P} - \frac{3\sqrt{\bar{P}(1 - \bar{P})}}{\sqrt{n}} \tag{10}$$

If n is different for different batches, upper and lower control limits will vary from batch to batch. To calculate the limits, first the value of $3\sqrt{\bar{P}(1 - \bar{P})}$ is computed. The value of the square root of n is calculated for each batch and divided into $3\sqrt{\overline{P}(1 - \overline{P})}$ to obtain the value of the three standard deviations for the batch, 3s, that is:

$$3s = \frac{3\sqrt{\overline{P}(1 - \overline{P})}}{\sqrt{n}} \qquad (11)$$

and (5) plotting of P's on a control chart with $\overline{P}$ as the average and control limits calculated as previously shown.

Example 1. The example used for illustrating the control chart (p chart) for percentage fractional defective for a parenteral product is shown in Figure 27-6. The process control record accumulated from 10 batches of the product and the computation of p, $\overline{P}$, 3s, UCL, and LCL employing equations (7) to (11) are summarized in Table 27-11 for constructing Figure 27-6.

The inspectors are required to detect and remove the defective samples, which may be characterized by: (1) broken ampuls or vials; (2) presence of particulate matters such as lint, dirt, glass fragment, and other foreign suspended matter; or (3) imperfections in the glass. The number of defectives found in the batch inspected was recorded, and the fraction defective of the batch was computed. Percentage defective (100 P), a more convenient value than fraction defective, has been plotted in Figure 27-6. The numerical values of three standard deviations (3s) for each individual batch in this particular example are considered to be constant, since n for each batch changes only slightly. The LCL may be set at zero if only high values of p are of concern. Because all points fall within the control limits, as seen in Figure 27-6, the product is said to be in statistical control.

Example 2. During the automatic packaging of a tablet product in containers, control of the number of broken tablets in a container released from packaging lines should be established and maintained. By sampling containers from each batch at random and inspecting and recording the percentage unacceptable for each batch, data may be accumulated. Occasionally, it may be observed that batches are out of control (P > UCL) during the accumulation of data, as shown in the p chart of Figure 27-7. Batches 6, 13, 16, and 18 are out of control. After all assignable causes have been corrected, these rejected batches should be eliminated, and a new set of P, UCL, and LCL values should be calculated for a new p chart.

All methods and procedures set forth for quality control administration should be strictly followed, since changes may cause significant variation in the data being collected. When data are being recorded, any conditions that have

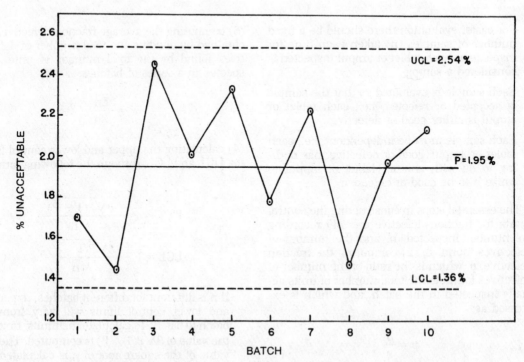

FIG. 27-6. *Control chart (p chart) for percentage of defective units inspected for a parenteral product.*

TABLE 27-11. *Process Control Record and Control Limits Calculated (for Ten Batches of a Parenteral Product)*

Batch #	Number Inspected (n)	Number Defective (d)	Fraction Defective (p)	3S	UCL	LCL
1	4956	84	0.0170	0.0059	0.0254	0.0136
2	4924	71	0.0144	0.0059	0.0254	0.0136
3	4900	120	0.0245	0.0059	0.0254	0.0136
4	4883	98	0.0201	0.0059	0.0254	0.0136
5	4891	114	0.0233	0.0059	0.0254	0.0136
6	4952	88	0.0178	0.0059	0.0254	0.0136
7	4905	109	0.0222	0.0059	0.0254	0.0136
8	4897	72	0.0147	0.0059	0.0254	0.0136
9	4868	95	0.0197	0.0059^5	0.0255	0.0135
10	4845	103	0.0213	0.0059^6	0.0255	0.0135

Calculation: $\Sigma n = 49021$

$\Sigma d = 954$

$$p = \frac{84}{4956} = 0.0170 = 1.70\%$$

$$\bar{p} = \frac{954}{49021} = 0.0195 = 1.95\%$$

$$3S = \frac{3\sqrt{0.0195[1 - 0.0195]}}{\sqrt{4956}} = 0.0059 = 0.59\%$$

$$UCL = \bar{P} + 3S = 0.0195 + 0.0059 = 0.0254 = 2.54\%$$

$$LCL = \bar{P} - 3S = 0.0195 - 0.0059 = 0.0136 = 1.36\%$$

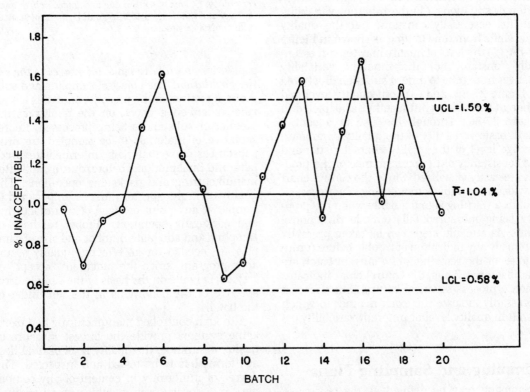

FIG. 27-7. *Control chart (p chart) for percentage of broken tablets in plastic containers.*

changed since the last sample was taken should also be recorded. These include such items as changes in machine settings and operators. In general, the control chart is plotted initially without the benefit of control limits. When sufficient historical data from at least 10 to 12 batches have been collected, the control limits computed are reasonably reliable, and the control chart can be established for future batches. As the new batches of the product are produced, the inspection data are plotted on the control chart. Close attention to control charts indicates to manufacturing personnel and control inspectors whether the product is of poor quality.

Quality Level and Inherent Variability

The ideal state of a statistically controlled process or situation is one in which both the quality level, as reflected by averages in $\bar{X}$ chart, and the inherent variability, as indicated by ranges in R chart, remain within limits predicted from ordinary variation. This is illustrated in Figure 27-8D, where the process is in the ideal state of statistical control. This situation is not always ideal in practice, however, and lack of control may be indicated in the following three different situations: (1) the inherent variability remains essentially constant, but the quality level shifts from time to time as shown in Figure 27-8A; (2) the level of quality may remain essentially constant, but the inherent variability changes from time to time, a situation illustrated in Figure 27-8B; and (3) both quality level and inherent variability shift together as depicted in Figure 27-8C. Through the use of a control chart, basic variability of the quality parameter, average level of the quality characteristic, and the consistency of the performance of the product are easily visualized. Since the control chart provides a continuous monitoring of a process, it sounds a warning signal quickly when the property being measured falls outside the control limits. As a result, steps can be taken promptly to remedy any indication of trouble before future batches or the remainder of a current batch are manufactured. Thus, the control chart indicates when a process is out of control, but does not necessarily indicate the exact manner in which a shift in quality level or inherent variability occurs.

Sampling and Sampling Plans

Sampling may be defined as *the process of removing an appropriate number of items from a*

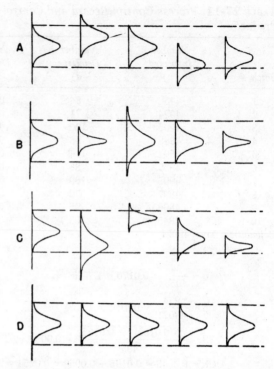

FIG. 27-8. *Examples of product quality variation during manufacturing. Key: A, lack of control due to a shifting quality level; B, lack of control due to changes in inherent variability; C, lack of control due to changes in both quality level and inherent variability; and D, an ideal statistically controlled process.*

population in order to make inferences to the entire population. The object of sampling and subsequent testing, in the present context, is to provide an effective check on the quality of the product or substances being processed. Representative of materials to be sampled are drug substances, raw materials, intermediate products, and final products before, during, and after manufacturing and packaging operations. The quality control inspector must be empowered to sample at any point or stage of manufacturing and packaging operations. Proper methods of sampling and adequate number and size of samples are needed for an effective quality assurance program, since the judgment "accept" or "reject" is made on the basis of the sample, irrespective of the conditions in the remainder of the batch.

Although controlled manufacturing and packaging systems provide the largest measure of quality assurance, the quality level of final dosage forms has to be tested and inspected. The degree of uniformity in content of any component in a dosage form is subject to an additive effect of the variabilities of the process steps. To obtain a value representative of the total population, the sample taken is most important. An improper sample may result in a value that can be biased and in error. Careful consideration of the design of the sampling plan enables these errors to be kept to a minimum. The only possible way to avoid such sampling errors is to do a 100% inspection. This normally cannot be attained practically and can also introduce errors due to personnel fatigue and other related human factors. Even if it is possible to perform 100% inspection, good sampling plans are preferred for efficient inspection.

A good statistical sampling plan should be able to pass a high percentage of acceptable batches and reject the unacceptable ones. The number of unacceptable units are controlled to rigid standards by the stringency of the sampling plan. The variety of sampling plans, procedures, and tables that can be constructed is unlimited. The advantages and disadvantages of each of several possible choices should be carefully weighed from both theoretic and practical viewpoints. Frequently, the ease of implementation weighs more heavily than the statistical procedure because overall costs and ease of application may be more important. Sometimes, trials of alternative procedures under actual operating conditions may bring to light unanticipated factors that result in the adoption of a plan that seems less efficient in theory. The choice of the most advantageous plan is determined after experiences have been accumulated.

Sampling plans based on data from measurements of attributes or variables may be constructed. As discussed previously, attribute data refer to go or no-go situations in which each piece inspected is examined or tested to determine whether it conforms to the requirements imposed by specifications; variable sampling is based on a continuous distribution of measurements, which can, in a sense, measure degrees of unacceptability covering the gray zone between accepted and rejected situations.

For practical purposes, the work involved in designing a sample plan may be greatly reduced or eliminated by use of a series of government-sponsored sampling plans such as MIL-STD-414 for variables sampling plans,[3] and MIL-STD-105D for attribute sampling plans.[4] In addition to providing a savings in time, these books have gained acceptance by industry throughout most of the United States. These publications provide sampling procedures and related reference tables for use in planning and conducting inspection. Acceptability of a batch is determined by the use of a sampling plan associated with the designated acceptable quality

level or levels. A sampling plan indicates the number of units of product from each batch to be inspected (sample size or series of sample sizes) and the criteria for determining the acceptability of the batch. The inspection level determines the relationship between the batch size and the sample size and is to be determined by the responsible authority.

The most common and distinct methods of inspection are single and double sampling methods. In single sampling, only the specified sample size is inspected before a decision is reached regarding the disposition of the batch, and the acceptance criterion is expressed as an acceptance number. In double sampling, a second sample for inspection is permitted if the first fails, and two acceptance numbers are used— the first applying to the observed number of defectives for the first sample alone, and the second applying to the observed number of defectives for the first and second samples combined. Triple and multiple samplings are merely extensions of the foregoing.

The following example illustrates the double sampling method. A sample of 50 tablets is taken. If it contains no more than two defectives, the batch is accepted. If it contains four or more defectives, it is rejected. If it contains more than two but less than four defectives, a second sample size of 50 is taken. If the two samples combined contain less than four defectives, the batch is accepted.

The construction of a statistical sampling plan normally requires that four basic quality standards be specified: (1) an acceptable quality level (AQL) (e.g., a batch of tablets is considered to be accepted if it contains 2% or less unacceptable tablets) (2) an unacceptable quality level (UQL) (e.g., the same batch of tablets is said to be rejected if it contains 4% or more unacceptable tablets); (3) the risk or error, designated as α (Producers' Risk), which is the probability of rejecting a good batch; and (4) the risk or error, designated as β (Consumers' Risk), which is the probability of accepting a bad batch. In general, the sampling scheme should be designed in such a way that the α and β errors are appropriately shared by the producer and the consumer.

The usual approach is the determination of desirable AQL, UQL, α, and β and subsequent computation of the sample size and acceptance criteria. If the AQL and UQL are close together and α and β are very small, as in the case of low-dose or potent drugs, a large sample is required for a suitable sampling plan. Conversely, the plan calls for few samples if the AQL and UQL are far apart and α and β are large. A convenient graphic method of presenting these risks, α and β, is through the operating characteristic (OC) curves, which are graphs illustrating the ability of a sampling plan to discriminate between acceptable and unacceptable batches. For every sampling plan, there is an OC curve. The OC curve is prepared by plotting the percentage of batches of a given quality that is expected to be accepted versus the quality of submitted batches expressed as percentage unacceptable.

For characteristics that may be measured on a continuous scale and for which quality may be expressed in terms of percentage unacceptable, the MIL-STD-414 may be used as a source of statistical plans if the measurements are random and independent observations follow a normal distribution. To illustrate the application of MIL-STD-414, a hypothetical example for teaching purposes is employed.[5] The tolerances of pure drug contained in the tablets in question were set at 93 to 107% of the labeled amount, and the desired quality characteristics of the tablets produced were specified at AQL = 10%, UQL = 40%, α = 10% and β = 8%. By searching through the OC curves of MIL-STD-414, Figure 27-9A was found, which most nearly corresponds to these requirements. From this OC curve, one learns that batches of AQL = 10% will be accepted 90% (α = 10%) of the time,

since the curve crosses the 10% abscissa at the 90% ordinate. By a similar operation, batches of UQL = 40% will be accepted only 8% (β) of the time. By referring to the appropriate table of MIL-STD-414, the sample size was found to be N = 10, and the acceptability criteria (or estimated percentage unacceptable) that balances the risks is 21.06%. Therefore, the final statistical plan takes the following form. Select 10 tablets at random from an inspection batch, and individually assay each tablet. From these ten determinations, estimate the percentage unacceptable in the batch. The batch will be accepted if this estimate does not exceed 21.06% unacceptable. Otherwise, the batch will be rejected.

Figure 27-9B shows an OC curve,[5] where one would pass that quality at least 95% of the time (α = 5%) if the submitted batch of material contains 10% or less unacceptable units (AQL = 10%). This same OC curve shows that a batch 20% or more unacceptable (UQL = 20%) would not pass more than 10% of the time (β = 10%). For this example, a sample size of 85 tablets is required. An ideal OC curve,[5] illustrating perfect discrimination but unrealistic stringency, is shown in Figure 27-9C. To obtain such a curve, the entire batch of products would have to be examined.

The five characteristics (AQL, UQL, α, β, and N) operating within a variable sampling plan can be seen graphically from the operating characteristic curves for sampling plans at N = 10. As shown in Figure 27-10, the horizontal scale running from 0 to 100% is the quality of submitted lots in the percentage defective, i.e., the percentage of the units in a lot that fall outside the established tolerances for the product. The vertical scale, which also runs from 0 to 100%, is the percentage of lots of a stated percentage unacceptable that are expected to be accepted under the sampling plan. For the OC curve of Figure 27-10, labeled AQL = 4%, for example, it is shown that a lot that is 4% unacceptable will be accepted 90% of the time [α = 10%] at N = 10, and a lot that is 20% unacceptable [UQL = 20%] will be accepted 20% of the time [β = 20%] at N = 10. At a given AQL, these plans are designed to greatly enlarge a probability of accepting a batch if the batch has AQL or a smaller percentage unacceptable. Figure 27-10 shows that when AQL of the product is raised, the percentage unacceptable that can be tolerated is also increased at the given α level and sample size.

The operating characteristic curves for sampling plans at AQL = 1% are illustrated in Figure 27-11. It should be noted that there are dif-

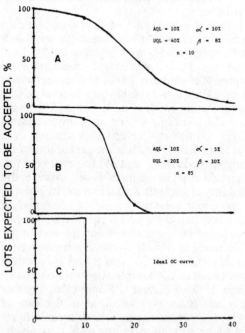

FIG. 27-9. *Examples of operating characteristic curves.*

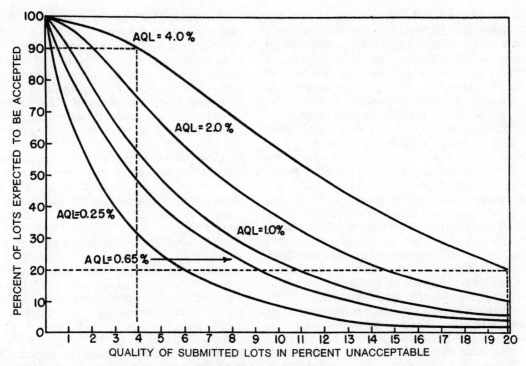

FIG. 27-10. *Operating characteristic curves for sampling plans at N = 10.*

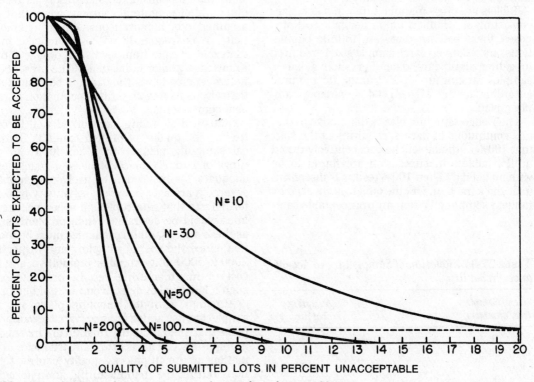

FIG. 27-11. *Operating characteristic curves for sampling plans at AQL = 1%.*

ferent curves for different sample sizes. For the OC curve labeled N = 10, it can be seen that a lot with 1% unacceptable [AQL = 1%] will be accepted 90% of the time or conversely rejected 10% of the time [α = 10%]. A lot that is 20% unacceptable [UQL = 20%] will be accepted 5% of the time [β = 5%]. As shown in Figure 27-11, at a given α level and AQL are more discriminating with larger sample sizes; for example, it will accept good lots and reject bad lots a greater percentage of the time.

When operating characteristic curves were developed for the compendial weight variation specifications, a batch of tablets containing a total of 5% underweight and overweight tablets were found to have 93% probability of being accepted when samples of 10 tablets were employed. The relations depicted in Table 27-12 show that a larger sample size increases acceptance probability. These data were obtained on the basis of a million-tablet batch.

The same curves showed that a batch with 20% unacceptable tablets had a probability of passing the weight variation test 40%, 23%, 4%, and 0% of the time as the sample size increased from 10 to 20 to 50 to 100 tablets.

Tablets are often manufactured in batch sizes consisting of a million units. For practical purposes, these batches represent infinite populations, and relatively large sample size is required to gather significant data. For such a batch, samples ranging up to 200 units are required according to the MIL-STD-414 variable sampling plan.

The Dodge sampling plan is distinctive in that it is continuous in nature, requiring at the start that 100% of the tablets be consecutively tested until p tablets in succession are found to be without defect.[6] Then 100% testing is discontinued, and a fraction, f, of the tablets is checked by random sampling. When an unacceptable sample is found, 100% testing is resumed until p tablets in succession are again found free of defect. For example, using a rotary tabletting press of 25 punches to manufacture a batch of a million tablets, let p be 50 (to contain two tablets from each punch) and f be one tablet in ten thousand. The Dodge plan then calls for testing an additional 100 tablets, thus bringing the total to 150 tablets if no operation problem is found and if the process is under control. The two advantages offered by this sampling plan are (1) it reduces the amount of testing necessary when compressing proceeds as designed and predicted, and (2) it increased the chances for detection and correction if the tablets fall out of specification.

In the application of sampling plans to pharmaceutical dosage forms, homogeneity of the samples must be emphasized. For homogeneous dosage forms such as oral or parenteral solutions, samplings are ordinarily taken with a sample size as small as one unit. If a drum of a powdered drug or excipient is known to be homogeneous, then for statistical purposes it can be thought of as a solution, and single or duplicate samples are considered sufficient to provide a reliable response. Semisolid dosage forms such as ointments, creams, and suspensions may be considered statistically as resembling oral or parenteral solutions when they are assumed to be homogeneous. To verify homogeneity, it is frequently necessary to take more than one sample from semisolid dosage forms. Knowledge and/or indication of the presence of heterogeneity allows the batch to be treated statistically as having an infinite population of variable components.

Statistical sampling has worked well in controlling the quality of printed material. Statistical sampling plans with a sensitivity in the range of 1 to 5% unacceptable were considered adequate for inspection of packaging supplies several years ago; however, sensitivity of 0.1% for defects that interrupt high-speed packaging lines would be desirable. When problems such as these arise, sampling schemes must be modified, since the cost of sampling and inspecting 3000 to 5000 units would be prohibitive, and the cost of manufacturing certain products with such a low level of defectiveness would be high.

Although attribute sampling plans are the simplest to use and to enforce, variable sampling plans that yield more information are increasing in importance. This is especially true with automation of the in-process quality control functions during the manufacturing and packaging operations.

TABLE 27-12. *Relation of Sample Size to Acceptance Probability*

Size of Samples (No. of tablets)	Acceptance Probability (%)
10	93
20	95
50	98
100	99

Control and Assurance of Manufacturing Practices

The factory inspection provision of the 1962 Amendments to the Food, Drug, and Cosmetic Act empowered the FDA to inspect drug manufacturing sites (in which drugs are processed, manufactured, packaged, and stored) for compliance with accepted standards of operations, practices, and sanitation. The regulations promulgated as a result of the 1962 Amendments require a complete and full description of the controls the manufacturer employs in the preparation of dosage forms for clinical trials as well as of the marketed products routinely produced. The law recognizes that Current Good Manufacturing Practices (CGMP) with the attendant quality control procedures, are paramount to the production of quality products. As a result, the FDA has required pharmaceutical manufacturers to commit themselves to a method of manufacturing and quality assurance for each product. The manufacturer should have performed sufficient control tests to permit an evaluation of the adequacy of the manufacturing, processing, and packaging operations.

The first CGMP regulations were issued in 1963, one year after the enactment of the 1962 Kefauver-Harris Drug Amendments. Although it took about eight years (1971) to revise them, they are in no way stagnant. In fact, the word "current," in referring to CGMP, suggests that they are dynamic, and the regulatory agency constantly updates and maintains them in relation to the current state of the art and science of drug manufacturing practices in the industry. The next revision of the CGMP took place in 1978, and these are in effect at present.

The successful application of CGMP is complex but possible if the systems governing the various phases of personnel, equipment, buildings, control records, and production procedures are at the state of proper planning and control. It should be kept in mind that CGMP is an aid and by no means a substitute for a good total quality assurance program.

Personnel. One criterion for a successful quality assurance program is the encouragement of quality consciousness in the personnel of the entire company. Proper selection, training, and motivation of production, packaging, and control personnel are vital to produce quality pharmaceuticals consistently. The degree to which the desired quality for the product is attainable is proportional to the attitudes or desires of the individuals working in production, packaging, and control. By building a sense of pride in performance and showing the importance of the contributions of these individuals in producing products that could be lifesaving, the risk of errors can be minimized. In reality, this is the basis for the so-called control of quality by the zero-defect concept, which operates through prevention rather than detection of the mistakes by properly directing and motivating personnel. Quality work and products result from this approach.

It is essential that qualified personnel be employed to supervise the formulation, processing, sampling, testing, packaging, and labeling of the drug product, and that competent staff be placed in charge of the maintenance of machinery, equipment, and sanitation. The qualified personnel are persons who by virtue of education, training, and experience have the knowledge and ability to execute the technologic assignments. The key personnel involved in the manufacture and control of the drug should assume the responsibility of assuring that the drug and the dosage form they are handling have the desired characteristics. The responsibility for keeping the manufacturing process within the CGMP regulations of the FDC Act must be delegated to the people directly involved with the various aspects of the process and their immediate supervisors. The supervisors are required to provide the necessary direction and control of the operation and be available at all times in case a question or a problem arises. The operating personnel should have the necessary authority to sign the manufacturing documents for each process for which they are responsible. The document is then countersigned by the supervisor. The signature and endorsement should appear on the proper worksheet at the completion of a production operation.

Equipment and Buildings. Equipment and buildings used in the manufacture, processing, packaging, labeling, storage, or control of drugs should be of suitable design, size, construction, and location and should be maintained in a clean and orderly manner.

The building should provide adequate space for the orderly placement of materials and equipment to minimize any risks of mixups or cross-contamination between the drugs, excipients, packaging, and labeling from the time the materials are received to the time the products are released. Adequate lighting, ventilation, dust control, temperature, and humidity should also be provided. To avoid conditions unfavorable to the integrity and safety of the product, other considerations may be required for particular operations and products, such as bacteriologic controls for preventing microbial contamination, for sanitizing work areas for parenteral preparations, and for preventing the dissemination of microorganisms from one area to another or from previous manufacturing operations.

The desired characteristics of equipment for producing quality products are numerous, and they differ from machine to machine; however, the equipment should be of suitable size, accuracy, and reproducibility. Their surfaces should be inert, nonreactive, nonabsorptive, and nonadditive so that the identity, purity, and quality of the drug substance and other components are not affected to any significant extent. The equipment should be constructed to facilitate adjustment, cleaning, and maintenance to assure the precision, reliability, and uniformity of the process and product, and to assure the exclusion of contaminants from previous and current manufacturing and packaging operations.

Control of Records. The records, such as master formula and batch production records, should be prepared and maintained in accordance with established procedures.

Master Formula Record. Master formula records for each product should be prepared, endorsed, and dated by a competent and responsible individual and should be independently checked, endorsed, and dated by another competent and responsible individual. The information contained in the records should be provided in a format and language that will not be misinterpreted by the operating personnel and the supervisor, to assure that each batch of a product can be identically reproduced.

Although the content and format may differ from product to product, the master formula record shall include the following information:

1. The name of the product, a description of the dosage form, and its strength.

2. The complete list of ingredients, designated by whole names and codes sufficiently specific to indicate any special characteristic.

3. The quantity by weight or volume of each ingredient, regardless of whether it appears in the finished product. If variations in the quantity of a particular ingredient are permitted, as is sometimes necessary in the preparation of a dosage form, an adequate statement should be provided in the record.

4. The standards or specifications of each ingredient used in the product.

5. An appropriate statement concerning any calculated excess of an ingredient.

6. Appropriate statements of theoretic yield at various stages and the termination of processing.

7. Manufacturing and control instructions, specifications, precautions, and special notations to be followed.

8. A detailed description of the closures, containers, labeling, packaging, and other finishing materials.

Batch Production Record. Batch production records should be prepared, maintained, and controlled for each batch of product. In general, they should be retained for a period of approximately five years after distribution has been completed. The batch production record shall contain an accurate reproduction of the manufacturing formula, procedure, and product specifications from the correct master formula procedure to be used in the production of a batch of product. These batch records are then sent to each of the departments involved in the production, packaging, and control of the product. The records include dates, specific code or identification numbers of each ingredient employed, weights or measures of components and products in the course of processing, results of in-process and control testing, and the endorsements of the individual performing and supervising each step of the operation.

In addition, a lot number is assigned that permits the identification of all procedures performed on the lot and their results. This lot number appears on the label of the product. This procedure facilitates a search for the details of manufacture and control history of any particular product.

Control of Production Procedures. To ensure that products have the intended characteristics of identity, strength, quality, and purity, production and the related in-process quality control (IPQC) procedures should be rigidly followed as required by the master formula record or the batch production record. To a large extent, IPQC is concerned with providing accurate, specific, and definite descriptions of procedures to be employed from the receipt of raw materials to the release of the finished dosage forms. It is a planned system to identify the materials, equipment, processes, and operators; to enforce the flow of manufacturing and packaging operations according to the established rules and practices; to minimize human error or to detect the error if and when it does occur; and to pinpoint the responsibility to the personnel involved in each unit operation of the entire process. In general, the in-process control procedures are usually rapid and simple tests or inspections that are performed when the manufacturing of a product batch is in progress. They are used to detect variations from the tolerance limits of the product so that prompt and corrective action can be taken. The in-process control procedures and tests should be openly discussed, experimentally justified, written in detail, properly explained, and in particular, rigidly enforced once they are established.

For the convenience of discussion, the actual production procedures are subdivided and discussed as manufacturing control and packaging control.

Manufacturing Control. Although the scope and structure of the manufacturing control operation differs appreciably from company to company, it is possible to highlight their common elements. The production planning department issues the formula and manufacturing worksheets bearing an identification number, title of product, and the names and quantities for all ingredients, together with a complete description of the procedures to be followed, the precautions to be taken, the equipment to be used, the lot sizes to be processed, and the suitable in-process controls to be undertaken.

Material tickets for each raw material are written and issued by the production department to the department of material stores, where the orders are filled and verified. After the materials have been sent to the production department and checked similarly, the pattern of control takes shape as production proceeds. The addition of raw materials to the batch is verified and countersigned by a qualified person. Notation is made on the manufacturing worksheet of the identifying number of each ingredient as it is used, and each unit operation is checked off as it is performed. An appropriate label is attached to each container or piece of equipment in use to identify its contents and to ensure that the in-process stage is properly designated. Any deviation from standard operating conditions, no matter how small, should be reported to both production and control personnel responsible for the product.

The in-process checking during manufacturing plays an important role in the auditing of the quality of the product at various stages of production. Duties of the auditor or the control inspector consist of checking, enforcing, and reviewing procedures and suggesting the change for upgrading the procedures when necessary.

The primary objective of an IPQC system is to monitor all the features of a product that may affect its quality and to prevent errors during processing. Only the most commonly practiced methods for parenterals, solid dosage forms (tablets and capsules), and semisolid preparations (ointments, creams, and lotions) are briefly described.

For parenteral products, the in-process quality controls are (1) checking the bulk solution, before filling, for drug content, pH, color, clarity, and completeness of solution; (2) checking the filled volume of liquids or the filled weight of sterile powders for injection in the final containers at predetermined intervals during filling; (3) testing for leakage of flame-sealed ampuls; (4) subjecting the product to physical examination (visually or mechanically) for appearance, clarity, and particulate contamination; (5) examining the sterility indicator placed in various areas of the sterilizer for each sterilization operation; (6) submitting the product for sterility testing or other predetermined biologic tests to establish the safety and other parameters of the product.

The in-process quality controls for solid dosage forms are (1) determining the drug content of the formulation; (2) checking the weight variation for tablets and capsules at predetermined intervals during manufacturing; (3) checking the disintegration and/or dissolution time, hardness, and friability of the tablets at least during the beginning, middle, and end of production or at prescribed intervals during manufacturing; (4) testing soluble tablets for compliance with solution time requirements; and (5) examining products by line inspection or other equally suitable means and removing the defective units prior to packaging.

For semisolid preparations, the following in-process controls are available: (1) checking for uniformity and homogeneity of drug content prior to the filling operations; (2) determining the particle size of the preparation when appropriate; (3) checking the appearance, viscosity, specific gravity, sediment volume, and other physical parameters at prescribed intervals; (4) testing for filling weight during the filling operation; and (5) testing for leakage on the finished jars or tubes.

At the completion of the manufacturing process as well as in-process stages, actual yields are checked against theoretic value, and the representative samples are withdrawn for laboratory testing by the control inspector according to the predetermined sampling plan. The operators actively performing the process, their supervisors, and the control inspector must all verify that the entire operation was accomplished in the prescribed manner. Occasionally, materials in bulk storage are sampled at random and are examined to determine that no detectable change has taken place, and that the batch is satisfactory for final packaging.

The batch production records and other needed documents are then delivered to the quality control office, together with the withdrawn samples of the product. These records and test results are reviewed for conformance to specifications and CGMP. The bulk finished products are held in quarantine until they are released for packaging by quality control personnel.

Packaging Control. At some time before the manufacture of a product is completed, a packaging record bearing an identification number is issued to the packaging section. This record specifies the packaging materials to be used, operations to be performed, and the quantity to be packaged. Simultaneously, requisitions are issued for the products to be packaged and for the packaging and printed materials, such as labels, containers, inserts, brochures, cartons, and shipping cases.

The packaging operation unites the product, container, and label to form a single finished unit. Not only must individual package components be correct, but they must also be assembled correctly. Prior to the start of a packaging operation, the control inspector and packaging supervisor must check and verify the line to ensure that it has been thoroughly cleaned and that all materials from the previous packaging order have been completely removed. In addition, various pieces of packaging equipment are stripped down, cleaned, and examined when an order is finished. The bulk of the product and each of the packaging components should be checked, endorsed, and dated by qualified packaging personnel with the cooperation of a control inspector. In practice, only the exact number of labels required for a batch, including a small excess, should be delivered to the labeling area after careful and meticulous inspection of each label.

In the packaging area, a large group of people work on several different products simultaneously, using high-speed packaging equipment. Therefore, the operation should be performed with adequate physical segregation of products. Dosage forms of similar color, size, and shape should not be scheduled consecutively on a line. Tablets of similar shape should not be scheduled on the neighboring packaging lines at the same time, even though the size or color may be dissimilar. Proper on-line inspection should be made during the packaging operation to ensure

absence of foreign drugs and labels, adequacy of the containers and closures, and accuracy of labeling. Proper reconciliation and disposition of the unused and wasted labels should occur at the end of the packaging operation. The yield must be justified against the theory represented by the batch size of the starting materials. Suitable and reasonable procedures should be established for action to be taken when an unexplained discrepancy exists between the number of labels issued and the number accounted for on the finished product. The common approach is for key personnel to prevent distribution of the batch in question, and of other batches of products that were packaged during the same period of time, until a satisfactory explanation can be obtained for the discrepancy.

Validation. The terms validation and qualification have, in recent years, become familiar in connection with pharmaceutical processes. Qualification is generally related to equipment and is used to determine whether the equipment operates as it was designed to in a reproducible manner. *Validation* of a process is the demonstration that controlling the critical steps of a process results in products of repeatable attributes (e.g., content uniformity) or causes a reproducible event (e.g., sterilization).

The concept of applying a systems approach to pharmaceutical manufacture and control, requiring validation of the process and qualification of equipment, facilities, personnel, and so forth, received considerable impetus when it was recognized by both the FDA and industry that sampling and testing of finished products alone cannot provide the necessary assurance of drug product quality within and between batches. The customary sample size in end product testing does not provide sufficient statistical validity for high product quality; it alone cannot verify that the various factors in the system intended to assure quality within and between batches of product are functioning as they were designed to function. Such verification can only be accomplished through identifying the critical components of the system and implementing control tests for these components, which when taken as a whole, demonstrate that their characteristics are repeatable from batch to batch of product. Consequently, a validated process is a systematic, documented program that provides a high degree of assurance that a specific process will consistently produce a product meeting its predetermined specifications and quality attributes.

The FDA, in its program guidance manual to FDA investigators, defines a validated manufacturing process as follows:

"A validated manufacturing process is one that has been proved to do what it purports or is represented to do. The proof of validation is obtained through collection and evaluation of data, preferably, beginning from the process development phase and continuing through into the production phase. Validation necessarily includes process qualification (the qualification of materials, equipment, systems, building, personnel), but it also includes the control of the entire processes for repeated batches or runs."

The FDA interprets Subpart F Section 211.100(a) and 211.110(a) of the Current Good Manufacturing Regulations for drug products to mean that pharmaceutical processes must be validated. These two sections of the regulations are presented:

Section 211.100(a)—"There shall be written procedures for production and process control designed to assure that the drug products have the identity, strength, quality and purity they purport or are represented to possess. Such procedures shall include all requirements in this subpart. These written procedures including any changes, shall be drafted, reviewed and approved by the appropriate organizational units and reviewed and approved by the quality control unit."

Section 211.110(a)—"To assure batch uniformity and integrity of drug products, written procedures shall be established and followed that describe the in-process controls, and tests or examinations to be conducted on appropriate samples of in-process materials of each batch. Such control procedures shall be established to monitor the output and to validate the performance of these manufacturing processes that may be responsible for causing variability in the characteristics of in-process material and drug product."

The documentation, including protocols, data, and results obtained from process validation and equipment qualification are important, since the validation performed should be auditable by an appropriate responsible individual who, after reviewing the records, should be able to certify the validation of the process to produce products to defined attributes consistently provided that the system validated is not altered.

Control and Assurance of Finished Products

Good manufacturing practices, well-defined specifications, sound sampling procedures, and efficient process controls do not in themselves constitute an overall quality control program. Unless the testing procedures by which the product quality is finally measured are established on an equally sound basis, the entire system may be deficient. Product failures causing rejections or recalls after market introduction are serious and can be easily detected and minimized by an effectively administered quality testing program. Therefore, the testing of the finished products for compliance with the established standards prior to release of the material for distribution is a critical factor for quality control and assurance. The testing indicates the possible deviations from perfection that occur in the batch. Product quality assurance is not complete with the release of the batch, however. The stability of the product in the marketed package should be repeatedly reconfirmed by actual physical, chemical, and biologic tests performed on several representative batches of the product over the period of its expected shelf-life. The activities associated with the control of the dosage form after manufacture are discussed briefly in this section.

Types of Specifications

The element of potential hazard to public health and the risk of violating stringent and exacting statutes render specification writing for the pharmaceutical industry quite unique. The main purpose of establishing specifications is to ensure that the characteristics of the finished dosage forms conform to appropriate standards of identity, purity, potency, quality, safety, and efficacy.

The first four types of specifications (i.e., identity, purity, potency, and quality) are distinctively analytic in nature and are embodied in specifications known as drug standards. Examples of tests for standard of identity, purity, and quality are shown in Table 27-13. These drug standards may be further delineated and illustrated by citing the typical examples in the following sections.

Standard of Identity

Identity tests are usually the distinctive qualitative chemical methods used to confirm the actual presence of the compound. For some drugs, microbiologic and pharmacologic tests also may be employed. Examples are:

1. The infrared absorption spectrum for chlorothiazide dispersed in mineral oil exhibits maxima only at the same wavelengths as that of a similar preparation of chlorothiazide reference standard.

2. Ouabain, when dissolved in sulfuric acid, produces a dark red color by transmitted light and shows a greenish fluorescence in reflected light.

TABLE 27-13. *Examples of Tests for Standards of Identity, Purity, and Quality*

Standard of Identity	Standard of Quality	Standard of Purity
Color formation	Absorbance	Color and/or odor
Precipitation	Refractive index	Clarity and/or color of solution
Decomposition	Optical rotation	Acidity or alkalinity
Derivative formation	Specific gravity	Acid of alkali
Infrared spectra	pH	Inorganic salt
Ultraviolet spectra	Viscosity	Heavy metals
Visible spectra	Melting point or range	Foreign matter
Specific reactions	Saponification value	Residue on evaporation
Cations or anions determination	Acid value	Readily carbonizable substances

3. The ultraviolet absorption spectrum of propranolol hydrochloride in methanol exhibits maxima and minima at the same wavelengths as that of a similar preparation of reference standard. The respective absorptive values at the maximum wavelength do not differ by more than 2.5%.

4. A solution of quinidine gluconate in dilute sulfuric acid exhibits a vivid blue fluorescence. On the addition of a few drops of hydrochloric acid, the fluorescence disappears.

Standards of Quality

Quality tests are usually the physical methods used to measure accurately the characteristic properties of the drug. Results are expressed as a permissible range of values for a measured property of the drug. Examples are:

1. The specific notation of propranolol hydrochloride is between $-1.0°$ and $+1.0°$ calculated on the dried basis.

2. A solution of quinidine gluconate is dextrorotary.

3. The refractive index of clofibrate is between 1500 and 1505 at 20°.

4. The specific gravity of ethanol is between 0.812 and 0.816 at 15.56°.

Standards of Purity

Purity tests are generally designed to estimate the levels of all known and significant impurities and contaminants in the drug substance under evaluation. These standards are numerically expressed as maximum tolerable limit or the absence of an impurity or contaminant based on the prescribed methods. Examples are:

1. The maximum tolerable limit of diazotizable substances of chlorothiazide is 1.0%.

2. A solution of ouabain yields no precipitate with tannic acid or with iodine to indicate the absence of alkaloids.

3. The residue on ignition of propranolol hydrochloride is not more than 0.1%.

4. After drying quinidine gluconate at 105° for 1 hour, it loses not more than 0.5% of its weight.

Based on USP XXI, standard of purity of several drug substances and their dosage forms is tabulated as illustrated in Table 27-14. Each drug substance has its specific contaminant or impurity specified at different maximum allowable limits. The limit may be as low as 0.003% of p-chlorophenol in clofibrate or as high as 5.0% of related alkaloids in ergotamine tartrate. The same contaminant or impurity present in different drug substances may not have the same maximum allowable limit. For example, m-aminophenol is a common impurity found in aminosalicylic acid, and its alkali salts at a maximum allowable limit of 0.25% and 0.20% respectively. The maximum allowable limits of levarterenol is 4.0% in epinephrine and 2.0% in epinephrine bitartrate. The limits for diazotizable substances in various diuretic thiazide compounds range from 1.0% in hydrochlorothiazide to 2.5% in trichlormethiazide. In contrast to this situation, however, the limit for 4-epianhydrotetracycline is 2.0% regardless of whether the drug substance is from tetracycline, tetracycline hydrochloride, or tetracycline phosphate complex.

The same situation exists for the maximum allowable limit of contaminant or impurity in dosage forms of the same drug substance. As shown in the last column of Table 27-14, the limits of nonaspirin salicylates in aspirin tablets, aspirin suppositories and aspirin buffered tablet are 0.3%, 1.0%, and 3.0% respectively. The maximum allowable 4-epianhydrotetracycline

Drug Substances	Contaminant or Impurity	Raw Material	Maximum Allowable Limit (%) Dosage Form
Aminosalicylic acid	m-Aminophenol	0.25	1.0 (Tablet)
Aminosalicylic sodium	m-Aminophenol	0.20	0.75 (Tablet)
Aminosalicylic potassium	m-Aminophenol	0.20	0.75 (Tablet)
Aminosalicylic calcium	m-Aminophenol	0.20	0.77 (Tablet, capsule)
Benzoylpas calcium	3'-Hydroxybenzanilide	0.1	0.2 (Tablet)
	m-Aminophenol	0.05	0.1 (Tablet)
	Aminosalicylic acid	0.2	0.4 (Tablet)
	Nonaspirin salicylates	0.1	0.3 (Tablet)
Aspirin			3.0 (Coated or buffered tablet)
			1.0 (Suppositories)
Azathioprine	Mercaptopurine	1.0	None (Tablet)
			3.0 (Injection)
Clofibrate	p-Chlorophenol	0.003	None (Capsule)
Clotrimazole	Imidazole	0.5	None (Tablet, cream, solution)
	(0-chlorophenyl) diphenylmethanol	0.5	None (Tablet, cream, solution)
Chloprocaine HCl	4-Amino-2-Chloro-benzoic acid	0.625	3.0 (Injection)
Dimercaprol	1,2,3-Trimercaptopropane and related impurities	1.5	4.5 (Injection)
Epinephrine	Levarterenol	4.0	—
Epinephrine bitrate	Levarterenol	2.0	None (Injection, inhalation, solution)
Ergotamine tartrate	Related alkaloids	5.0	None (Injection, solution)
Ergonovine maleate	Related alkaloids	2.0	None (Tablet, injection)
Estradiol valerate	Free valeric acid	0.5	2.0 (Tablet, injection)
	Free estradiol	1.0	—
Bendroflumethiazide	Diazotizable substances	1.5	3.0 (Injection)
Chlorothiazide	Diazotizable substances	1.0	None (Tablet)
Cyclothiazide	Diazotizable substances	1.0	None (Tablet, suspension)
Hydrochlorothiazide	Diazotizable substances	1.0	None (Tablet)
Hydroflumethiazide	Diazotizable substances	1.0	1.0 (Tablet)
Trichlormethiazide	Diazotizable substances	2.5	None (Tablet)
Probenecid	p-Bis (di-n-propyl) carbamylbenzene-sulfonamide	0.5	None (Tablet)
Penicillamine	Mercury	0.002	None (Capsule)
Prednisolone sodium phosphate	Free prednisolone	1.0	None (Injection, solution)
Phenacetin	p-Chloroacetanilide	0.03	None (Capsule)
Tetracycline	4-Epianhydrotetracycline	2.0	3.0 (Suspensions)
Tetracycline HCl	4-Epianhydrotetracycline	2.0	3.0 (Capsule, injection, tablet)
			None (Topical solution, ophthalmic suspension and ointment)
Tetracycline phosphate complex	4-Epianhydrotetracycline	2.0	3.0 (Capsule, injection)

Data compiled from USP XXI, United States Pharmacopeial Convention, Rockville, MD, 1980.

limit is prescribed at 3.0% for tetracycline hydrochloride capsules, injections, and tablets; however, none is described for ophthalmic suspensions, topical solutions, and ophthalmic ointments. A similar situation is found for azathioprine, with the maximum limit of mercaptopurine set at 3.0% for azathioprine injection, but no limit described for the tablet dosage form. Even more striking is the fact that the maximum limit for some contaminant or impurity is set for drug substance but is not required for its dosage forms. Examples are mercaptopurine in azathioprine, p-chlorophenol in clofibrate, p-chloroacetanilide in phenacetin, levarterenol in epinephrine, and diazotizable substances in most of the diuretic thiazides.

Standards of Potency

Potency tests are assays that estimate the quantity of active ingredient in the drug. Employing physical, chemical, biologic, pharmacologic, or microbiologic means, these quantitative tests yield the strength or potency of the drug substance. Examples are:

1. Chlorothiazide contains not less than 98.0% and not more than 100.5% of $C_7H_6ClN_3O_4S_2$, calculated on the dried basis.

2. Ouabain contains not less than 95.0% and not more than 100.5% of $C_{29}H_{44}O_{12}.8H_2O$.

3. Propranolol hydrochloride contains not less than 98.0% and not more than 101.5% of $C_{16}H_{21}NO_2.HCl$ calculated on the dried basis.

4. Quinidine gluconate contains not less than 99.0% and not more than 100.5% of total alkaloid salt, calculated on the dried basis as:

$$C_{20}H_{24}N_2O_2.C_6H_{12}O_7$$

Its content of dihyroquinidine gluconate is not more than 20.0% by weight of its content of total alkaloid salt, calculated as:

$$C_{20}H_{24}N_2O_2.C_6H_{12}O_7.$$

Examples of standards of potency for several drug substances and their dosage forms are listed in USP XXI and are demonstrated in Table 27-15. For drug substance, most of the chemically synthesized raw materials have a lower specification limit of at least 97% potency with the exception of antibiotics such as chloramphenicol, ampicillin, and tetracycline hydrochloride, which in general have a lower potency limit of 90% or more. As shown in Table 27-15, different dosage forms of the same drug substance are assigned the same specification limits, such as 90.0 to 130.0% for chloramphenicol capsules, ophthalmic solutions, and ophthalmic ointments, and 95.0 to 110.0% for all dosage forms containing promazine hydrochloride. As shown in Table 27-15, however, different dosage forms of the same drug substance may be assigned different specification limits as well. Using ephedrine sulfate as an example, limits are 90.0 to 110.0% for syrups, 92.0 to 108.0% for capsules, 95.0 to 105.0% for injections, and 93.0 to 107.0% for tablets and nasal solutions. It should be noted that the positive and negative specification limits are generally symmetric around the potency for most of the dosage forms. Therefore, in many cases, the potency range is expressed in the form of 100 ±10% or 100 ±7% than 90 to 110% or 93 to 107%.

A drug substance is suitable for use if the totality of data derived from these four attributes shows that it meets all of the specifications.

In general, specifications should provide for the maintenance of reasonable standards, while allowing a sensible degree of latitude for manu-

TABLE 27-15. *Standard of Potency of Different Dosage Forms Having Same Limits*

	Standard of Potency Expressed as Percentage of Claim	
Drug Substance	*Raw Material*	*Dosage Forms*
Amitriptyline HCl	99.9–100.5	90.0–110.0 (Injection, tablet)
Chloramphenicol	≥90.0	90.0–130.0 (Capsule, ophthalmic solution, ointment)
Chlorpromazine HCl	98.0–101.5	95.0–105.0 (Injection, syrup, tablet)
Digoxin	97.0–103.0	95.0–110.0 (Injection, elixir, tablet)
Fluphenazine HCl	97.0–103.0	95.0–110.0 (Injection, oral solution, elixir, tablet)
Griseofulvin	90.0–105.0	90.0–115.0 (Oral suspension, tablet, capsule)
Meperidine HCl	98.0–101.0	95.0–105.0 (Injection, syrup, tablet)
Reserpine	97.0–101.0	90.0–110.0 (Injection, elixir, tablet)
Promazine HCl	97.0–101.5	95.0–110.0 (Injection, oral solution, syrup, tablet)

Data compiled from USP XXI, United States Pharmacopeial Convention, Rockville, MD, 1980.

TABLE 27-16. *Utilization of Historical Batch Data to Guide the Specification for Standard of Purity*

Drug substance:	An experimental antihypertensive
Proposed limit of purity:	1% of an impurity
Method:	High-pressure liquid chromatography for an impurity
Detection limit:	0.1%
Batch record:	0.2 0.2 0.3 0.1 <0.1 0.3 <0.1 0.1 0.1 0.3
Acceptable limit:	0.6%
"House" limit:	0.5%

facturing variations or tolerances, and acceptable latitude for analytic errors, particularly in control techniques. To guide in the appropriate development of specifications, historical data accumulated from batch analyses of the drug substance or the drug product are usually the best source. The relevance of historical batch records to establish meaningful specifications is illustrated in Table 27-16 for standard of purity, and in Table 27-17 for standard of potency, respectively. Proposed limits usually become acceptable limits, which must be realistic and relevant to the actual historical batch analysis record and to the sensitivity or reproducibility of method.

Specifications and procedures that are designed to test the product quality consist of a series of statements and methods of evaluating the physical, chemical, and biologic characteristics of the dosage form. The in vivo clinical testing of lot to lot of product is replaced, out of necessity, with a series of in vitro laboratory tests, which are correlated to reflect the clinical performance of the drug substance formulated in the product.

Specifications are also used in the procure-

TABLE 27-17. *Utilization of Historical Batch Data to Guide the Specification for Standard of Potency.*

Drug substance:	Antihypertension
Proposed potency limits:	93.0–107.0%
Method:	Chloroform extraction followed by UV spectrophotometry
Reproducibility:	±2%
Batch record:	99.3 98.4 103.4 97.9 101.3 98.9 101.8 99.7 98.6 100.4
Acceptable limits:	95.0–105%
"House" limits:	96.0–104%

ment of drug substance, excipients, reagents, packaging, and printed materials. The incoming materials and the finished products are checked against the specifications to an extent sufficient to determine the compliance and the acceptability of the materials and products. Therefore, the specifications set forth as the standard should be discriminating enough to differentiate good or acceptable material from inferior or rejectable material. The specifications should be practical and realistic, however, and they should reflect those parameters necessary to define the product as well as to permit manufacture of the product to a defined quality level. In developing specifications for purchased material, the vendor's capability to supply the material should also be considered.

In the development of specifications, the following objectives should be carefully considered: (1) to ascertain which physical, chemical, and biologic characteristics of dosage form are critical, which are important, which are helpful, and which are not particularly important but are useful; (2) to decide which dosage form characteristics shall be established as the criteria for evaluating routine production batches; (3) to establish the appropriate test methods for evaluating the selected criteria; and (4) to determine the acceptable tolerances and limits for each of the dosage form characteristics.

In deciding the elements that will contribute to the making of a satisfactory specification for a drug, the first question to be asked must always be "For what purpose is the specification needed?" No single set of requirements meets all possible situations.

Specifications for New Products

During the development of any new drug, there must be a rigorous investigation of both the chemical and physical properties of the material. A knowledge of the synthetic and appropriate testing by nuclear magnetic resonance, infrared spectroscopy, and mass spectrometry route usually provides strong evidence of structure, together with hints as to the identity of possible by-products that might be present. Specific chemical reactions may give further confirmation of structure. As frequently happens, possible contaminants bear a close structural relationship to the drug substance. Two percent or 3% of such substances may produce no readily detectable effect even by infrared spectroscopy. It is necessary to recognize the presence of impurities present at such low levels, however, because the contaminant might have an undesirable or even harmful effect. Thus, it is reasonable that its presence should be defined and controlled.

Although, ideally, a drug should be absolutely pure, this is generally not feasible in practice. A more practical approach is to require that the material to be subjected to pharmacologic and clinical trial is prepared to be as pure as is economically reasonable and then characterized as fully as possible with respect to its impurity content. If the trials prove satisfactory and acceptable, then the aim should be to ensure that subsequent batches of material should be at least as "clean" as the trial material. It is essential that the total identity of the material being used, including both its major and minor constituents, be known. Only in this way can the results of clinical trials be meaningful for a new drug.

Specifications for Well-Established Products

It is important to bear in mind that material synthesized on a pilot scale for clinical trial work may not be the same as material synthesized in a full-scale manufacturing process, especially in respect to its pattern of minor constituents.

What is a tolerable level of impurity in a drug? This question, of course, has no answer. Every impurity in each drug must be considered as a separate and individual case. If the impurity has been shown to have, or is suspected to have, undesirable properties, it should be limited as rigorously as possible.

Official Specifications

The manufacturer's specifications are designed to be applied to the drug at the time of manufacture or quite shortly thereafter. An official specification, on the other hand, should be designed to apply to the material at any time during its period of possible use. An official specification is likely to be somewhat less stringent, especially with regard to changes due to slight decomposition. As an obvious example, a manufacturer's release specification for content of free salicylic acid in aspirin would need to be considerably more stringent than that of a pharmacopoeia, which applies to the shelf-life of the drug.

There is another complicating factor arising when the specification is intended to apply to the drug independent of its source. A specification developed for the drug using a particular manufacturing process that is designed to limit certain known impurities may fail to control other impurities that might arise by use of a different route of synthesis.

Specifications for a product are developed not only to assure product quality but also to detect and identify impurities. There are two major kinds of impurities: product-nonspecific impurities, which are introduced externally into the product during processing, and product-specific impurities, which appear as by-products or degraded products of the drug substances as well as excipients used in the product. Therefore, the test parameters should be designed, and the testing procedures for the specifications should be established, so that the tests are capable of detecting product-specific as well as product-nonspecific impurities.

Today, many countries require the establishment of interim specifications when the product is registered for clinical trials. Therefore, the analytic methodology for the drug in a dosage form must be developed at the initial stages of product development. The early provisional specifications may be less rigorous than subsequently provided since they are often based on experiences from only a few small batches. Seldom does a drug manufacturer base his specifications on observations made on a single development batch. The stability, potency, and other critical characteristics of the product should be finalized only after several pilot and production batches have been produced. The results of these studies should be subjected to statistical analysis to appraise correctly the magnitude of the variation involved for each characteristic, thereby establishing firm specifications for each characteristic. A specific method of analysis must be developed early in the program to perform stability studies adequately. Even at this stage, the experience with the product is usually still limited.

A description of the tests and reagents for various official drugs and their dosage forms are available from the official compendia. From content uniformity to dissolution tests, and from identity tests to assay procedures, each section outlines specific procedures that are mandatory for the proper control of the product.

All drug specifications listed in pharmacopeias have been verified in collaborating laboratories of pharmaceutical companies and academic institutions. The pharmacopoeia issued for a country is the legal standard of that nation. The specifications in a pharmacopoeia are so designed that the tests and the requirements for acceptance are applicable to all manufacturers' products. This means that anyone who manufactures a product of that type should conform with those specifications. It should be recognized that the specifications set in the compendium are minimum standards to which the product is expected to conform at any time during its expiry date period. A partial list of official

TABLE 27-18. *Partial List of Pharmacopeias and Other Books of Standards*

Country	Pharmacopeia or Other Standards
Federal Republic of Germany	Deutsches Arzneibuch and supplements
France	Pharmacopee Francaise
Japan	The Pharmacopeia of Japan
Sweden	Pharmacopeia Nordica
Switzerland	Pharmacopeia Helvetica and its supplements
Union of Soviet Socialist Republics	State Pharmacopeia of the Union of Soviet Socialist Republics
United Kingdom	British Pharmacopeia; The Pharmaceutical Codex
United States of America	The United States Pharmacopeia/National Formulary; Code of Federal Regulations, 21 Foods & Drugs
World Health Organization	Pharmacopeia Internationales

compendia from several countries and WHO is presented in Table 27-18. A compendium is a collection of monographs of drug substances and drug products. "Official" as used in "official compendium" signifies governmental authorization. As defined in the FD&C Act of 1938, the phrase "official compendium" means the Official United States Pharmacopeia, Official Homeopathic Pharmacopeia of the United States, Official National Formulary, or any of their supplements.

The complexity of quality control testing can be more clearly understood from the quality control profiles of a hypothetical parenteral dosage form containing sulfadimethoxide as an active ingredient (Table 27-19), and a hypothetical tablet dosage form containing glutethimide as the active ingredient (Table 27-20). For manufacturing the parenteral sulfadimethoxide injection, there are seven items or raw materials to be tested and cleared by quality control laboratory according to the specifications designed for each item. There are approximately 70 tests required prior to the release of these seven items for compounding. Similarly, a large number of tests are required to accept eight items for fabricating glutethimide tablets. There are approximately 80 tests that need to be performed to determine the acceptability of these eight ingredients. Based on the examples shown in Tables 27-19 and 27-20, the average number of quality control tests required to accept or reject a raw material is approximately ten. It is evident that the total number of tests required by the official compendia on the ingredients in the dosage form are numerous. In addition to these tests are added the quality control tests on the finished dosage

TABLE 27-19. *Quality Control Profile of Various Raw Materials Used in a Proposed Parenteral Sulfonamide Injection*

Item	Function	Tests Required
Sulfadimethoxine, NF XVI	Antibacterial	Appearance; solubility; identity; melting range; ultraviolet absorption; loss on drying; residue on ignition; content of heavy metals; assay.
Glycerine, USP XXI	Cosolvent	Appearance; solubility; identity; color; specific gravity; residue on ignition; contents of chloride, sulfate, arsenic, and heavy metals; limit of chlorinated compound; readily carbonizable substances; limit of fatty acids and esters.
Benzyl alcohol, NF XVI	Preservative	Appearance; solubility; identity; specific gravity; distilling range; refractive index; residue on ignition; limits for aldehyde and chlorinated compounds.
Sodium bisulfite, NF XVI	Antioxidant	Appearance; solubility; identity; contents of arsenic, iron, and heavy metals; assay.
Disodium edetate, USP XXI	Chelator	Appearance; solubility; identity; pH; loss on drying; contents of calcium and heavy metals; assay.
Sodium hydroxide, NF XVI	pH adjuster	Appearance; solubility; identity; insoluble substances and organic matters; contents of potassium and heavy metals; assay.
Water for injection, USP XXI	Solvent	Appearance; reaction; chloride, sulfate, ammonia, calcium, carbon dioxide and heavy metals; total solids and oxidizable substances; pyrogen test.

Data compiled from USP XXI/NF XVI, United States Pharmacopeial Convention, Rockville, MD, 1980.

TABLE 27-20. *Quality Control Profile of Various Raw Materials Used in a Proposed Glutethimide Tablet*

Item	Function	Tests Required
Glutethimide, USP XXI	Depressant	Appearance; solubility; identity; melting range; ultraviolet absorption; loss on drying; residue on ignition; assay.
Tragacanth, NF XVI	Binder	Appearance; identity; karaya gum; microbial limits, arsenic, lead, heavy metals.
Lactose, USP XXI	Diluent	Appearance; solubility; identity; specific rotation; residue on ignition; heavy metals; clarity and color of solution, microbial limits, pH, water, alcohol soluble residue.
Talc, USP XXI	Glidant	Appearance; identity; loss on ignition; acid-soluble substances; water-soluble iron; reaction and soluble substances.
Magnesium stearate, NF XVI	Lubricant	Appearance; solubility; identity; loss on drying; lead content; assay.
Polyethyleneglycol 4000, NF XVI	Binder and lubricant	Appearance; solubility; viscosity; completeness and color of solution; pH, acidity; average molecular weight; residue on ignition; arsenic; heavy metals, limit of ethylene glycol and diethylene glycol, ethylene oxide average molecular weight.
Alcohol, USP XXI	Solvent	Appearance; solubility; specific gravity; nonvolatile residue; water-insoluble substance; aldehydes and other foreign organic substances; methyl ketones, methanol and other alcohol content; fusel oil constituents, amyl alcohol and nonvolatile, carbonizable substances.
Purified water, USP XXI	Solvent	Appearance; reaction; heavy metals content, total solids; bacteriologic purity, oxidizable substance, carbon dioxide, calcium ammonia, sulfate, chloride, pH.

forms of sulfadimethoxide injection and glutethimide tablets according to the product specifications.

Procedures in the compendium apply to all manufacturers of a particular product, whereas the quality control procedures of the manufacturer are intended to apply specifically to his own product. The pharmaceutical industry frequently employs alternative methods, which may be more accurate, specific, sensitive, and economical than those in the compendium. The manufacturer is not required to employ procedures in the official compendium as long as the quality of his product ultimately meets the requirements in the compendium for identity, quality, potency, and purity. In the case of a legal action, the test methods in the compendium are the basis for determining compliance.

Container components should not interact physically or chemically with the product to alter its identity, purity, quality, or potency beyond the official allowances. Usually, the major component of the container is glass or plastic. The official compendium provides for several types of glass and several classes of plastic to be used with various pharmaceutical products. Examples of quality control profiles of three major packaging materials are shown in Table 27-21. Specifications designed for containers are meaningful only if they have been selected on the basis of tests performed on the product in the container. The following features are to be considered before container specifications are set: (1) physical changes of container upon prolonged contact with the product; (2) moisture and gaseous permeability of the container; (3) compatibility between the container and the product; and (4) toxicity and safety.

Testing Program and Method

Total quality assurance certifies that each received lot of raw material or each manufactured batch of product meets the established quality

TABLE 27-21. *Quality Control Profile of Various Packaging Materials USP XXI/NF XVI*

Item	Function	Test Required
1. High-density poly-ethylene containers	Containers for capsules and tablets	Multiple internal reflectance, thermal analysis, light transmission, water vapor permeation, extractable substances, nonvolatile residue, heavy metals.
2. Glass		
Highly resistant, borosilicate glass (Type II)	Parenteral use	Light transmission, chemical resistance—powdered glass test.
Treated soda-lime glass (Type II)	Acidic and neutral parenteral preparation	Light transmission, chemical resistance—water attack at 121° test.
Soda-lime glass (Type III)	Parenteral and nonparenteral preparation	Light transmission, chemical resistance—powdered glass test.
General purpose soda-lime glass	Nonparenteral articles, i.e., oral or topical use	Light transmission, chemical resistance—powdered glass test.
3. Elastomeric closure for injection	Parenteral use	Biologic test—acute systemic toxicity, intracutaneous reactivity; physicochemical test—turbidity, reducing agents, heavy metals, pH change, total extractables.

Data compiled from USP XXI/NF XVI, United States Pharmacopeial Convention, Rockville, MD, 1980.

standards. It provides for the authorization of the release of the approved raw materials for manufacturing, and the release of the manufactured product to the market, based on actual laboratory testing—physical, chemical, microbiologic, and at times, biologic.

Outlines of various quality control tests for different properties of the product are presented here to illustrate the scope of various laboratory testing.

1. *Physical and chemical tests*—Tests for appearance, color, odor, identity, optical rotation, specific gravity, pH, solubility, viscosity, disintegration time hardness, friability, average weight or volume per unit, weight or volume variation, content uniformity, dissolution profile, polymorphic form, particle size, moisture content, and assay for active ingredient(s), impurities, contaminants, or degradation products.

2. *Biologic and microbiologic tests*—Macrobiologic or microbiologic assays, and tests for potency, safety, toxicity, pyrogenicity, sterility, histamine, phenol coefficient, antiseptic activity, and antimicrobial preservative effectiveness tests.

Most therapeutic agents are substances of known chemical structure or composition and can be assayed by quantitative physicochemical

means. The standard purity statement for the active ingredient in the dosage form usually permits a wider variation than that for the active ingredient itself. Through purity and identity tests, the quality of the drug alone is established, and its level of impurities restricted, as in the limiting tests for chloride, sulfate, and heavy metals. The assay measures the concentration of this previously accepted drug in the dosage form.

When a physicochemical assay method is not possible, a macrobiologic or microbiologic procedure is employed. Biologic testing of drugs may be quantitative or qualitative in nature; it utilizes intact animals, animal preparations, isolated living tissues, or microorganisms. Biologic methods are employed in the following situations: (1) when adequate chemical assay has not been devised for the drug substances, although its chemical structure has been established (e.g., insulin); (2) when chemical structure of the drug substance has not been fully elucidated (e.g., parathyroid hormone); (3) when the drug is composed of a complex mixture of substances of varying structure and activity (e.g., digitalis and posterior pituitary); (4) when it is impossible or impractical to isolate the drug from its interfering substances, although the drug itself can be analyzed chemically (e.g., isolation of vitamin D from certain irradiated oils); (5) when the biologic activity of the drug substance is not defined by the chemical assay (as when active and inactive isomers of methylphenidate cannot be differentiated by the chemical method); and (6) when specificity, sensitivity, or practicality dictates the use of biologic rather than chemical assay procedures.

The accuracy of biologic tests does not approach that which is expected with good chemical methods. Accuracy within ±20% of the true value is good, and within ±10% is excellent, for most bioassays. Consequently, it is useful and advisable to supplement the biologic tests with select physicochemical tests when possible. Some official quantitative and qualitative biologic tests are summarized in Tables 27-22 and 27-23 respectively. Some biologic tests require as long as a month for completion; others may take only a few hours. Therefore, bioassays are often expensive and inconvenient.

To minimize the source of error resulting from animal variation during biologic tests, reference standards or pure drug substances and standard reference preparations are used, where possible, for comparison of their potency with the potency of unknown preparations to be tested. A reference standard is the specific active principle of the drug in its purest obtainable form. The principle of using tests in which reference materials are employed is based upon successive testing of the unknown and standard preparations on two groups of similar animals, as in the case of digitalis and tubocurarine, or on the same animal or organ, as in the case of posterior pituitary and epinephrine. The potency of the unknown can therefore be expressed as a percentage of the standard, although other methods of computation have been devised to improve the reliability of the results.

Increasing emphasis on microbiologic attributes of nonsterile products has generated additional responsibility in the quality control of raw materials, especially those derived from animal or botanical origin. In recognition of this increased concern regarding the possible contamination of nonsterile products with pathogenic or otherwise objectionable microorganisms, the USP XXI has included microbiologic quality control test procedures. These are designed to monitor nonsterile drug products for possible adulteration with microorganisms such as Salmonella species, Escherichia coli, certain species of Pseudomonas, and Staphylococcus aureus. Medicinal substances of natural and mineral origin are likely to be contaminated with bacteria, while synthetic medicinal substances tend to be bacteriologically clean in comparison. Nevertheless, solutions, suspensions, and semisolid dosage forms of these synthetic medicines tend to acquire bacterial contamination from excipients, manufacturing processes and environment, and containers. At the present time, there are many monographs in the USP XXI requiring freedom from one or more of the aforementioned organisms. Typical examples are given in Table 27-24.

The microbial flora associated with various raw materials can vary considerably. Standard plate-counting procedures are familiar and popular methods. In addition, broth enrichment

TABLE 27-22. *Partial List of Official Quantitative Biologic and Microbiologic Tests*

Biologic Tests	
Drug and Dosage Form	*Test Animal(s)*
Insulin	Rabbit
Digitalis and the related cardiac glycosides	Pigeon
Parathyroid	Dog
Posterior pituitary	Rat
Tubocurarine chloride	Rabbit
Microbiologic Tests	
Drug and Dosage Form	*Test Organism(s)*
	Microbiologic assay
Calcium pantothenate	Lactobacillus plantarum
Cyanocobalamin	Lactobacillus leichmannii
Penicillin	Staphylococcus aureus
Other antibiotics	(Varied according to the antibiotics)
Antimicrobial preservatives	Antimicrobial preservations—effectiveness
	Candida albicans, Aspergillus niger, Escherichia coli, Pseudomonas aeruginosa, Staphylococcus aureus

TABLE 27-23. *Partial List of Official Qualitative Biologic Tests*

Products to be Tested	Test
Preparations of liver or stomach	Antianemia tests
Antiseptics, disinfectants, fungicides, germicides	Antibacterial tests
Preparations containing toxoids	Antigenic test
Water, USP	Bacteriologic purity tests
Gelatin	Bacterial content
Protein hydrolysate injection	Biologic adequacy test
Protein hydrolysate injection	Nonantigenicity test
Diagnostic diphtheria toxin, influenza virus vaccine, and smallpox vaccine	Potency tests
Parenteral products, radioactive pharmaceutical, transfusion and infusion assemblies	Pyrogen test/bacterial endotoxin test
Most antibiotics, transfusion and infusion assemblies	Safety tests
Parenteral and ophthalmic products, antibiotics, sutures, all surgical dressings, transfusion and infusion assemblies	Sterility tests
Chloramphenicol, streptomycin, chlorotetracycline, tetracycline, liver injection	Test for depressor substances
Adrenal cortex injection	Test for pressor substances
Suramin sodium and preparations containing toxoids	Toxicity tests
Pharmaceutical articles, from raw materials to finished products	Microbial limit tests

TABLE 27-24. *Typical Pharmaceutical Materials Required by Official Compendia to Ensure Freedom from Specific Objectionable Microorganisms*

USP XXI			
Absence of Escherichia Coli	Absence of Salmonella	Absence of Escherichia Coli and Salmonella	Absence of Salmonella and Pseudomonas
Alumina and magnesia oral suspension	Dehydrocholic acid	Gelatin	Chymotrypsin
Aluminum hydroxide gel	Digitalis capsules		
	Pectin	Pancrelipase	
Milk of magnesia	Thyroid	Activated charcoal	
	Trypsin (crystallized)		
	Pancreatin		

NF XVI			
—	Absence of Salmonella	Absence of Escherichia Coli and Salmonella	Absence of Salmonella, Escherichia Coli, Staphylococcus Aureus, and Pseudomonas Aeruginosa
—	Acacia	Starch	
	Agar	Alginic acid	Caramel

Data compiled from USP XXI/NF XVI, United States Pharmacopeial Convention, Rockville, MD, 1980.

procedures are used to detect low levels of microorganisms. The following categories of raw materials are often contaminated with various microbial flora and should be thoroughly investigated: processed water, colors, dyes, pigments, talcs, starches, clays, fillers, natural gums, and thickening agents. It is important to consider the pharmaceutical process when a limit is established for the number of microorganisms per gram of raw material. Samples should be taken throughout the production cycle on a random basis to evaluate the microbiologic spectrum of the process. This serves as an indicator of sanitation and good manufacturing practices.

The final dosage form is often statistically sampled and tested for microbiologic attributes. Here again, the absence of pathogens is important, and the total count gives a measure of microbiologic normality. The hazard of microbial contamination is related to the intended area of use for the product. For parenteral products, the dictum is that any viable microorganism is a health hazard. Even for orally administered products, the presence of E. coli and Salmonella species are always objectionable, and the presence of Pseudomonas species, C. albicans, Enterobacter species and mycotoxin-producing fungi are usually objectionable since these organisms have been implicated as agents of diseases in foods. Further examples of objectionable microorganism contamination are tabulated in Table 27-25.

Microbiologic testing of sterile products (injection and ophthalmic) for the antimicrobial efficacy of added antimicrobial agents, for sterility, and for pyrogenicity are discussed in detail in Chapters 21, "Sterilization," and 22, "Sterile Products."

Traditionally, pyrogen testing is performed on rabbits, and observations are made for febrile response. A recent innovation in pyrogen testing is the use of an in vivo limulus amebocyte lysate (LAL) test, which is capable of detecting the more potent endotoxin pyrogens. Manufacturers of nonantibiotic injectable products may substitute the LAL test for the official rabbit pyrogen assay as an end product endotoxin test immediately upon a supplemental submission to the FDA, provided that the firm has validated the test for the particular drug product. On the other hand, antibiotic drug makers and manufacturers of biologicals who change manufacturing controls are required to submit to the agency for advance approval a full statement describing the

TABLE 27-25. *Partial List of Objectionable Organisms in Pharmaceuticals*

Intended Area of Product Application	Examples of Objectionable Organisms	
	Always Objectionable	*Usually Objectionable*
Oral products	Escherichia coli Salmonella sp.	Pseudomonas sp. Enterobacter sp. Enterotoxigenic Staphylococcus aureus Myocotoxin-producing fungi Candida albicans
Parenteral products	Any viable microorganism	
Ophthalmic preparations	Pseudomonas aeruginosa	Other Pseudomonas sp. Staphylococcus aureus
Genitourinary tract products	Escherichia coli Proteus mirabilis Serratia marcescens Pseudomonas aeruginosa Pseudomonas multivorans	Klebsiella sp. Acinetobacter anitratus
Products for surface wounds and damaged epithelium	Pseudomonas aeruginosa Staphylococcus aureus Klebsiella sp. Serratia marcescens Pseudomonas multivorans Pseudomonas putida Clostridia perfringens	
Topical products	Pseudomonas aeruginosa Staphylococcus aureus Klebsiella sp. Serratia marcescens	Pseudomonas multivorans Pseudomonas putida Clostridia perfringens Clostridia tetani Clostridia novyi

proposed change supported by the validated data.

An important aspect of dosage form control is the safety or toxicity test that is performed on the finished dosage form to guard against adventitious adulterations of pharmaceuticals. Analytic assays of drugs may not detect impurities or errors unforeseen in formulation, whereas in vivo testing may qualitatively show a change in a predetermined response to a specific drug dosage.

The use of reference standards has been extended beyond biologic assays, so that today they are required for many pharmacopeial assays and tests. This reflects the extensive use of modern chromatography and spectrophotometry, which require measurements relative to a reference standard to attain accurate and reproducible results. For example, a set of standards is provided for checking the reliability of apparatus used for melting point determinations. There are also pure specimens of steroids suitably diluted with an inert diluent for use in the chromatographic identification of steroids.

Reference standards are prepared and distributed by the USP. A similar program providing international standards is maintained by the World Health Organization, which is concerned mainly with standards for serums, vaccines, toxins, vitamins, and endocrine extracts. In general, the critical characteristics of the specimens selected as standards are determined independently in three or more laboratories.

The traditional and conventional gravimetric and volumetric assay methods are being supplemented by newer instrumental methods. Pharmaceutical analysis now includes such techniques as partition or absorption chromatography, gas-liquid chromatography, high pressure liquid chromatography, ultraviolet and infrared spectrophotometry, complexometry, chelatometry, nonaqueous titrimetry, fluorometry, polarography, differential scanning calorimetry, x-ray spectroscopy, nuclear magnetic resonance, autoradiography, thermogravimetric analysis, and mass spectroscopy. Thus, the analytic work required may range from the standardized elemental analysis of the compound to the highly specialized and sophisticated chemical or instrumental functional group determination.

Just as there are differences between samples and between replicate determinations on the same sample, there are also variations between technicians, instruments, and laboratories. These variations for the most part can be measured, and their significance determined. Such knowledge provides for the most accurate appraisal of the data and optimal confidence in the results. If the error in the analytic methods employed for product testing is not understood, the possibility of rejecting a finished product may be due to the test methods and not to inferior products.

Occasionally, outside laboratories may be used to augment the testing capacity and capability of the manufacturer. It is advisable that the facilities and personnel of the outside laboratories be evaluated before they are engaged. The quality control personnel of the manufacturer should evaluate and endorse the results submitted by the outside laboratories.

Quality of Analytic Methodologies

The quality of a method has to be characterized, monitored, measured, and validated. The nature of the analytic methods may be physical, chemical, microbiologic, biologic, or a combination of these types.[7,8] The quality of analysis is built in during its design stage, validated in its development stage, and confirmed in its utilization stage.

Parameters of Quality Analysis. The selection of an analytic method may be based on one or more of the following quality criteria or parameters, which serve as the foundations of a quality analysis:

1. Specificity
2. Sensitivity (limit of detection)
3. Linearity
4. Precision
5. Accuracy
6. Ruggedness
7. System Suitability

These important quality parameters of an analytic method are briefly described in this section.

Specificity is an important quality criterion. Analysis of a component of a mixture may interfere with other components of the mixture. If this occurs, the analytic method is nonspecific for the component under investigation. With a specific method, the concentration of the component can be completely measured regardless of what other compounds are present in the sample. Ideally, for chromatographic analysis, a specific method should be capable of resolving from the peak of interest all other components, including impurities, contaminants, excipients, and degradation products. In general, baseline resolution from other peaks or spots is accepted as adequate resolution for good specificity. It is not necessary, however, to have clean baseline separation among components that are not to be quantified. Furthermore, the integrity of the peak should be verified by collecting the peak fraction and chromatographing it by another solvent system or chromatographic method. It can also be further verified by wavelength-ratio techniques for direct comparisons to a standard.

Sensitivity pertains to the ease of detection. Analysts usually try to develop methods in which sensitivity has a constant value in a range as large as possible. Limit of detection gives the minimum concentration of a component that can be detected by the analytic method. As a rule, whenever a sample contains a compound in a very low concentration, the signal from the instrument will be small. Therefore, uncertainty exists as to whether the signal comes from noise produced by the instrument, from the method, or from the actual component to be measured. This gives rise to the term limit of detection. The analyst should determine the lowest detectable quantity of major component of interest at the most sensitive instrument settings. This detection limit is usually taken to be twice the signal-to-noise ratio. For determining the detection limit of minor components, the analyst must determine the smallest amount of contaminants, impurities, precursors, or degradation products quantifiable as weight percent of major component in the presence of this major component. This limit of detection is usually taken as ten times the signal-to-noise ratio; however, the minimum quantifiable levels of these substances should be no more than 50% of the limit set in the specifications for these substances.

Linearity of method gives the characteristic trend of such parameters as absorbance, peak height, peak area, or response ratio as a function of concentration of component to be measured. At least five different concentrations of a standard solution should be employed and spanned 80 to 120% or even 50 to 150% of the expected working concentration range. By plotting the concentration versus response, the linearity of the observed data points can be visualized. The test of linearity can be accomplished by fitting the data points to a curve of the form:

$$y = mx^n + b$$

For perfect linearity, $n = 1$. Once the concentration-response equation is known, one can calculate the maximum error to be expected from deviations in linearity and the possible error to be anticipated from use of a single point standard within the acceptable assay range of the method.

Precision is a quality criterion referred to the reproducibility of measurement within a set number of independent replicate measurements of the same property. Thus, it refers to the dispersion of a set about its central value and is generally expressed as the standard deviation of a series of measurements obtained from one sample. Usually, the precision of a method is established during the development stage by the multiple analyses of samples judged to be typical of the material that is to be analyzed. These analyses usually do not account for any additional sources of variation such as day-to-day fluctuation, laboratory-to-laboratory variation, small modification in technique, varying skill of analysts, undetected operational or instrumental factors, and other unexpected systematic errors.

Methods used to estimate the precision within a batch suffer from certain drawbacks. The most straightforward consists in the replicate analysis of a few selected samples and the subsequent calculation of the standard deviation. Unless random sampling is used, the samples selected may not be representative of the batch. In any analytic system, the precision of determination varies over the concentration range of the samples. This fact must be taken into account if the concentration range is wide. In a system in which the substance determined occurs in the same matrix in all the samples, the standard deviation of measurement increases with concentration, usually as a linear function. If all the duplicate determinations were made within a batch of analyses, the method would give an estimate only of the within-batch precision rather than of the overall characteristics of the analytic system. If the same procedure were used on many successive batches, a valid estimate of the overall variance would be obtained, consisting of the sum of the within-batch variances and the variance due to any systematic differences between batches.

Table 27-26 illustrates the precision data for the three sulfonamide assays in trisulfapyramidine suspensions by a stability-indicating high pressure liquid chromatographic (HPLC) method of analysis.[9] Analyses were performed by two analysts over a 2-day period, and results were calculated as percentage of theory on a weight basis. Each sample represents a freshly prepared suspension, and as shown in Table 27-26, the relative standard deviations ranged from ±2.1 to ±3.1%.

An example of a precision study during a method transfer from research laboratory to rou-

TABLE 27-26. *Precision Data for Trisulfapyrimidines in a Suspension Containing 200 mg of Each Drug per 5 ml by a Stability-Indicating HPLC Method.*

Sample	Theoretic Percentage		
	Sulfadiazine	Sulfamethazine	Sulfamerazine
1	105.0	103.5	103.8
2	105.6	104.0	103.5
3	106.6	104.1	103.8
4	100.6	99.6	102.1
5	107.6	109.6	112.2
6	106.7	103.4	107.3
7	104.7	105.3	106.4
8	106.6	105.7	108.0
Mean	105.4	104.4	105.9
SD	±2.2	±2.8	±3.3
RSD, %	±2.1	±2.7	±3.1

From Elrod, L., Cos, R. D., and Plasz, A. C.: J. Pharm. Sci., *161*:71, 1982. Reproduced with permission of the copyright owner, the American Pharmaceutical Association.

tine microbiologic laboratory for an erythromycin dosage form is illustrated in Table 27-27.

In general, the quality control laboratory determines the precision of the method on six rep-

licates of a representative composite sample containing 18 to 24 times the amount of drug needed for one assay. A separate determination of the precision of the system is made, considering only the error attributable to the operating system and not the error attributable to sample handling and preparation. The measure of system precision is performed by repeatedly analyzing aliquots of a single standard solution, recording responses, and calculating the relative standard deviation of the response.

Accuracy is defined as the closeness of a measured value to its true value. It normally refers to the difference between the mean of the set of results and the value accepted as the true or correct value for the quantity measured. As a rule, results of analysis of the unknown are compared with the results obtained from the analysis of standards or reference materials. The analyst should prepare six samples of drug in matrix spanning 80 to 120% or even 50 to 150% of the expected content, assaying each of those synthetic samples. The acceptance criterion in the accuracy test is expressed in terms of the standard deviation of the method as determined in the precision test, since the deviation from theory depends on the error inherent in the method itself. As acceptance criteria, recovery of drug expressed as percentage of theory must be ± 4s

TABLE 27-27. *Comparison of Microbiologic Assay of Erythromycin Dosage Form at Two Different Laboratories.*

Claimed Level Erythromycin Conc. (%)	Sample Designation	Concentration of Erythromycin Potency Found			
		Routine Laboratory		Research Laboratory	
		Day 1	Day 2	Day 1	Day 2
80	a	77	79	79	84
	b	85	77	85	86
	c	80	86	70	86
	d	78	80	80	80
	e	83	84	78	84
	f	81	79	79	87
100	a	102	108	94	120
	b	105	103	108	92
	c	97	110	108	102
	d	101	107	115	102
	e	104	102	97	106
	f	98	108	105	115
120	a	130	135	115	147
	b	132	118	110	140
	c	133	130	124	120
	d	128	127	111	140
	e	131	133	117	133
	f	130	130	122	126

of the theoretic value at all levels where s is the relative standard deviation obtained in the precision test. The range of 4s units is intended, and preferred, to cover the additional error possibly introduced in preparing the synthetic samples for accuracy testing.

Ruggedness tests describes the influence of small but reasonable alterations in the procedures of the quality of analysis.[10]

Examples of these minor variations are source and age of reagents, concentration and stability of solutions and reagents, heating rate, thermometer errors, column temperature, humidity, voltage, fluctuation, variations of column to column, plate to plate, analyst to analyst and instrument to instrument, and many others. Eight measurements suffice to investigate seven variables when the appropriate experimental design is employed. The various types of interlaboratory checks should be carried out to ensure that the analyst who developed the method is not the only one who can obtain satisfactory results from the procedure, and that all details are written into the testing directions and are not inadvertently omitted. With the widespread use of automatic injectors for HPLC systems, it is necessary to check and validate the length of time for which prepared solutions or reagents are stable. The stability of these solutions should be checked over a period of 12 to 24 hours if an automated method of running samples overnight is practiced in the laboratory.

System-suitability tests help to answer the question, "How good and reliable is the performance of a given analytic system on a given day?" FDA and the compendia have recommended system suitability tests for inclusion in all HPLC procedures.[11,12] System, in this context, means all components of the analysts, hardware, solvents, and electronics considered together. System-suitability tests are composed of a system's precision measurement and a system's powers of resolution measurement to check the performance of the analytic system on a given day. System-suitability testing differs from method validation testing. Validation of analytic method is generally initiated at the method development stage and is finalized by demonstrating that the method is scientifically sound and technically adequate for a particular drug. Therefore, validation is often done only once. System-suitability testing should be on a continuing basis, however.

The measurement of system precision is most easily made by employing replicate aliquots of the same solution. Signal responses such as peak height, peak area, and response ration derived from these aliquots are determined, and

the relative standard deviation is calculated to indicate the system's precision as compared with the historical data. The second part of each system-suitability test is the system's powers of resolution. The most useful measurement of such power is the calculation of the resolution between two closely eluting chromatographic peaks for which the resolution is considered critical. Normally, the separation between the peak of interest and a second peak eluting close to it is chosen as the resolution factor to be calculated.

Although system-suitability tests are recommended for all HPLC methods, it is suggested that they can be used in some manner for all analytic methods adopted for drug products.

With the background knowledge of specificity, sensitivity, linearity, precision, accuracy, and ruggedness of an analytic method, it is relatively easy to derive the confidence and reliability of the analytic data obtained with the method. With the use of a formal validation procedure and a system-suitability test, each new method is sure to meet the same performance standards, minimizing the problems encountered in daily routine analysis and in interlaboratory method transfer or method change.

To select an appropriate method, the analyst should have a thorough knowledge of the physicochemical properties of a drug, degradation products, degradation mechanisms, and degradation reaction rates. One can then develop a specific method suitable for monitoring the stability of an active ingredient or formulation. The methodology used for kinetic studies (solid state or solution) can generally be considered scientifically suitable for monitoring decomposition.

For the purpose of this brief presentation, stability-indicating methods are classified as electrometric methods, solvent extraction methods, spectrophotometric methods, and chromatographic methods.

Electrometric Methods. Titrimetric methods (aqueous or nonaqueous) that can be used for the precise analysis of the active ingredient most often do not offer the desired specificity for the analysis of pharmaceutical products. If the decomposition products do not interfere with the titration, however, e.g., formation of nonbasic degradation products of an organic amine or amine hydrochloride, then one may be able to utilize titrimetry. Alternatively, by employing suitable extraction procedures for eliminating possible interferences from excipients and/or decomposition products, one can use titrimetry for monitoring the stability of products.

Solvent Extraction Methods. It is possible to extract acidic, neutral, or basic compounds selectively from organic solvents on the basis of the partition behavior of their ionized and unionized species. The USP/NF compendia utilize a double-extraction procedure as the preferred method of analysis for organic nitrogeneous bases. This procedure provides some degree of specificity, because it may possibly remove compounds that are neutral or acidic or that have more polar substituents that could arise upon degradation. It does not, however, eliminate isomers or other closely related basic substances. Therefore, the validity of this approach for monitoring stability should be demonstrated prior to its utilization.

Spectrophotometric Methods. Direct spectrophotometric determination such as colorimetric analysis or ultraviolet determination is widely used in pharmaceutical analysis but usually lacks selectivity. The selectivity or specificity can be improved through separation or by reaction of an appropriate functional group. For example, the reactions that produce a colored product are generally measured in the visible region of the spectrum. As examples of colorimetric analysis, carboxylic acid derivatives such as lactams, amides, lactones, and esters are converted to the corresponding hydroxamic acids by reacting with hydroxylamine hydrochloride in an alkaline medium. The hydroxamic acid is then allowed to react with ferric chloride in the presence of dilute acid to produce red-violet ferric hydroxamate for colorimetric determination. Owing to its limited sensitivity, IR analysis is primarily used for identification of decomposition products and has found few quantitative applications in stability evaluation. An increasing number of applications are being found for nuclear magnetic resonance (NMR) spectroscopy, since it offers specificity along with simplicity of operation, but it, too, lacks sensitivity and precision.

Chromatographic Methods. Many stability-indicating methods entail some form of chromatography: paper, thin-layer (TLC), column, gas (GLC), and liquid (HPLC). The latter two techniques not only offer sharp separation but also provide precise methods of quantitation. Less than a decade ago, paper chromatography was used extensively in pharmaceutical analysis. This technique has rapidly given way to TLC, GLC, and HPLC. Of these three techniques, HPLC has the most widespread application. Several applications of recent interest are summarized in Table 27-28. With this technique, a compound can be chromatographed in several ways, and most important, the volatility required for GLC is not a limitation. The problems due to thermal instability are not encountered because most separations are carried out at

ambient or low temperatures. Of various chromatographic techniques employed in stability evaluations, GLC and HPLC provide the most useful quantitative information.

Stability-Indicating Methods. One of the major characteristics for a quality analytic method for pharmaceuticals is its ability to determine distinctively the parent compound from the degradation products. The current trend in stability-indicating methods is based on direct chromatography or derivatization chromatography. These approaches are used extensively in stability evaluation of pharmaceutical products. When it is not possible to determine the intact drug directly because of interfering substances, it is desirable to precede the final analysis with a separation procedure. This step can be solvent extraction or chromatographic separation.

The USP and NF provide yet another approach to evaluating stability. This approach entails monitoring the content of a decomposition product, e.g., salicylic acid in aspirin and disulfonamide in hydrochlorothiazide, while utilizing an assay for the drug itself that may not be totally stability-indicating. In some ways, this approach provides a more rigorous control of product stability. In the examples cited, the presence of 1 to 4% of a decomposition product render the item unsuitable; thus, much tighter limits are being applied to these products as compared with those that must meet the rubric limits for potency. These examples also illustrate that different standards are used to define product stability.

TABLE 27-28. *Some Applications of HPLC to Pharmaceutical Products*

Mode of HPLC	Drug Substance or Type of Product
Anion exchange	Ampicillin, barbiturates, prostaglandins A_2 and B_2
Cation exchange	Imidazolines, tetracyclines, trisulfapyrimidines, xanthines
Anion and cation exchange	Water-soluble vitamins, analgesics such as aspirin and acetaminophen
Absorption	Benzodiazepines, carbamazepine, phenytoin, phenobarbital, riboflavin
Partition	Corticosteroids
Reversed phase partition	Ergotamine, nortriptyline, procaine, synthetic estrogens
Ion exchange and reversed phase partition	Androsterone and dehydroepiandrosterone

Automated Continuous System for Assay Procedures

Automation usually enhances the quality, quantity, and efficiency of an operation. Its introduction into the analytic laboratory has dramatically changed the traditional look, capability, precision, and acceptability of most of our conventional analytic disciplines. The use of automated instrumentation of pharmaceutical analysis, data handling, and data storage is certainly on the rise. Within the last decade, and especially during the last few years, great strides have been made in a diversity of instrumental approaches to automated chemical, microbiologic, enzymatic, and other assays. Since automated continuous testing has great potential use for routine testing, it is not surprising that some pharmaceutical manufacturers are initiating automated control methods that are capable of sampling, analyzing, and accepting or rejecting. The use of these methods permits the analysts to cope with the increasing number of samples required to ensure product quality. Automated continuous assay procedures enhance the reliability of data and provide immediate feedback on process control with tremendous savings in time.

In the quality control laboratory, where a sufficiently large number of similar dosage forms or dosage units must be subjected routinely to the same type of examination, automated methods of analysis provide for far more efficient and precise testing than manual methods. Such automated methods have been found especially useful in testing the content uniformity of tablets and capsules and in facilitating methods requiring precisely controlled experimental conditions. Many manufacturing establishments, as well as the laboratories of regulatory agencies, have found it convenient to utilize automated methods as alternatives to pharmacopeial methods.

As a general practice, before an automated method for testing an article is adopted as an alternative, it is advisable to ascertain that the results obtained by the automated method are equivalent in accuracy and precision to those obtained by the prescribed pharmacopeial method. It is necessary to monitor the performance of the automated analytic system continually, by assaying standard preparations of known composition that have been frequently interspersed among the test preparations.

Many of the manual methods given in the pharmacopeia can be adapted for use in semi-automated or fully automated equipment, incorporating either discrete analyzers or continuous flow systems and operating under a variety of conditions. On the other hand, an analytic scheme devised for a particular automated system may not be readily transposable for use either with a manual procedure or with other types of automated equipment.

Compendial methods for testing drugs are based largely on ultraviolet absorption measurements. After extraction of dilution, the sample must exhibit maxima and minima at the same wavelengths as those of a similar solution of the reference standard, and the respective wavelength of maximum absorption should not differ significantly. Based on this principle, the Autoanalyzer, an automated continuous system for repetitive spectral scanning, was developed. This equipment is capable of accepting tablet, capsule, powder, solution, and suspension samples for analysis as required. The Autoanalyzer is, in fact, a mechanical chemist that can automatically perform designated tests at a much greater speed than a trained analyst. It has been utilized to perform many chemical microbiologic, biologic, and clinical tests, as well as to implement production in-process control.

Besides the Autoanalyzer produced by Technicon Company, there are other automated systems for drug analysis, such as Titralyzer from Fischer Scientific Company. Recent advances in automation and computerization have improved the efficiency and economics of laboratory performance. For example, numerous companies have developed dedicated gas-liquid or high efficiency liquid chromatographic systems that permit on-line sample analysis and data handling. One such system utilizes an automatic sample injector, which is time-sequenced and connected to a gas-liquid chromatograph that has been preset for a specific analysis. The signal from the gas-liquid chromatographic detector is digitized, and the computer automatically prints out such parameters as retention time, area under the curve, and concentration of the drug. Such automated data processing provides multiple analysis with minimum supervision and with a savings in time. Dedicated gas-liquid chromatographic systems are offered by such companies as Hewlett-Packard and Waters Associates, Inc. These and other suitable automated procedures have been developed for the analysis of phenothiazine derivatives, erythromycin, tolbutamide, vitamins A and B_6, amitriptyline hydrochloride, and various steroid dosage forms.

As previously discussed, HPLC is one of the most important analytic techniques to be given various degrees of automation in recent years. Its proven versatility and fast-growing ability to supply fundamental information and quality control data have stimulated the development of a completely automated HPLC system. In addition, the great advances in minicomputer science and microprocessor technology, such as Technicon Solid Prep Sample II and Peristaltic Pump III, have provided the extra dimension needed to automate fully most of the hardware components and flow-of-operation and data-management processes. The system has proved to be successful for the routine analyses of fat-soluble vitamins in more than nine different multivitamin formulations. The productivity has been at least three times greater than the conventional manual procedures. The continuous flow analyses with automated HPLC systems are especially useful in content uniformity analyses, which require large volumes of samples. When the microprocessor is properly programmed, the system can be easily adapted for reliable, around-the-clock, unattended operation in each specific application.

Microbiologic assays have always been time-consuming and tedious. Following the successful assay in fermentation media of streptomycin and penicillin (the first two antibiotics whose assay was automated), a variety of automated systems have been devised and applied successfully in turbidimetric and respirometric assays. For example, plates used in the microbiologic assay of several antibiotics are being prepared and read automatically, with the data recorded magnetically and the results analyzed and recorded by computer.

Among the requirements in the current USP/NF is a content uniformity test for tablets and capsules containing 50 mg or less of active ingredient. In the event that general strength dosage forms of the active ingredient are available below and above 50 mg per tablet or capsule, then all strengths require a content uniformity test. It is only through the use of automated procedures that the analytic burden is manageable.

One may expound any number of good reasons to automate laboratory procedures. Automated systems may enable a laboratory to provide new services more quickly, with increased reliability, in greater abundance, or at lower cost. Any of these benefits may justify consideration of an automated instrument. In any case, the total economic effect must be considered.

Associated Activities

Stability Studies. There are legal, moral, economic, and competitive reasons, as well as reasons of safety and efficacy, to monitor, predict, and evaluate drug product stability. The aim of quality control stability testing is to en-sure that batches of the released product are maintained within specification limits throughout their stated period of shelf storage. Stability testing of the product during development and scale-up stages is employed to define the recommended expiration date and storage conditions for inclusion on the label and to establish a product stability profile. Therefore, quality control stability testing after product is released to the market is for the verification and confirmation of this profile.

The stresses and hazards to which products are exposed during their passage from the manufacturing plant to the distribution chain and to the consumer can be environmental, mechanical, or contaminant in nature. Environmental stresses such as extreme temperatures, high moisture, intense light, and radiation are common, and mechanical hazards such as vibration, sudden drop, inversion, shock, and deformation are not unusual. Elevated temperature, especially if coupled with high relative humidity, is known to cause and accelerate physical deterioration and chemical degradation. Mechanical stresses have shown to cause such problems as liquid spillage, tablet chipping, and package deformation and breakage. Therefore, quality control of the marketed product does not stop at the final release of the product from the manufacturing site. A reserve sample of at least two times the quantity of product required to conduct all the quality control tests performed on the batch of product should be retained for at least one year after the expiration date.

Section 505-(b) of the CFR law as stated on the New Drug Application Form specifically describes the requirements for stability information as:

"A complete description of, and data derived from studies of the stability of, the drug, including information showing the suitability of the analytical methods used. Describe any additional stability studies under way or contemplated. Stability data should be submitted for any new drug substance, for the finished dosage form of the drug in the container in which it is to be marketed, and if it is to be put in solution at the time of dispensing, for the solution to be prepared as directed. State the expiration date(s) that will be used on the label to preserve the identity, strength, quality, and purity of the drug until it is used. If no expiration date is proposed, the applicant must justify its absence."

Under the regulations for antibiotic drugs, an expiration date is required for the product label of any antibiotic drug. These regulations are detailed in the Antibiotic Application, FD Form 1675 (1/71), as follows:

"A completed description of, and data derived from stability studies of the potency and physical characteristics of the drug, including information showing the suitability of the analytical methods used. Describe any additional stability studies underway or contemplated. Stability data should be submitted for any new antibiotic, for the finished dosage form of the drug in the container including a multiple-dose container in which it is to be marketed, and if it is to be put into solution at the time of dispensing, for the solution prepared as directed. The expiration date needed to preserve the identity, strength, quality, and purity of the drug until it is used."

The most desirable stability data are from actual shelf-life studies using products in the container-closure systems stored under labeled conditions. For introducing new products to the market, however, or for making material changes in the process, formula, or container-closure system of existing products, one cannot wait until all the needed stability data at room temperature are generated. Therefore, appropriately designed and executed short-term (e.g., 3-month) accelerated stability studies have been accepted by the FDA as data bases for use in extrapolating longer room-temperature expiration dates. Use of accelerated data is obviously not a substitute for actual shelf-life study. It is a means of predicting shelf-life of a product based on scientific principles and guided by experience. This method of shelf-life prediction based on short-term accelerated stability data is currently well-utilized by pharmaceutical scientists. An example is demonstrated in Table 27-29.

The manufacturer is asked to confirm the shelf-life stability of the product on production batches by taking the first several batches of the product or by taking batches at certain intervals of time during the first year of manufacture, and in subsequent years at least one additional production batch, and subjecting them to extended shelf-life testing at ambient storage conditions. At each sampling, which is generally performed on a yearly or semiannual basis, the samples are tested for physical, chemical, and biologic properties according to the standards set forth in the monographs of the official compendia or to the specifications established by the manufacturer.

The stability of the product should be evaluated in the container in which it is marketed. The expiration date and storage conditions should appear on the label of the product. Experience in the pharmaceutical industry has shown that there can be a considerable delay between the manufacture of a product and its eventual utilization by the consumer. To avoid deterioration of drugs and finished products during storage, the adequacy of warehouse and other storage facilities requires proper attention. To assist in assuring the stability of the dosage forms during transportation and storage, indication of the proper storage condition should appear on the label.

Since 1979, expiration dates have been required on prescription and over-the-counter drug products with limited exceptions. The FDA considers a product misbranded when it is labeled with an expiration date not supported by suitable stability data. The expiration date of a drug product must appear on the immediate

TABLE 27-29. *Comparison of Shelf-life Predicted from Short-Term Accelerated Stability Study and Shelf-Life Obtained by Long-Term Room Temperature Study*

Parenteral Formulation	Apparent Heat of Activation (kcal/mole)	Shelf-Life Prediction, t (in Years) 10% Extrapolated from Short-Term Accelerated Stability Testing Data	Calculated from Long-Term Room Temperature Stability Data
Steroid A	22.1	3.4	3.4
Antihypertensive A	18.6	9.0	9.4
Antihypertensive B	17.4	11.5	18.5
Local anesthetic hydrochloride	30.4	14.6	14.6
Diagnostic agent	26.3	20.0	28.2
Antidepressant	17.3	1.5	1.5
Antibiotic S (bio. assay)	28.5	1.3	1.3
Antibiotic V (chem. assay)	25.1	2.9	3.0
Sulfonamide G (suspension)	20.4	9.0	10.0

container and also on the outer package. When single dose containers are packaged in individual cartons, however, the expiration date may properly appear on the individual carton instead of on the immediate product container.

Furthermore, the current GMP regulations provide specific information as to the stability characteristics of pharmaceutical products and their expiration dating. These GMP regulations indicate that the Commissioner of the FDA concludes, "The interests of the consumers must be served by the establishment of valid expiration dates for all products, and Sections 211.166 of the GMP regulations set forth basic guidelines for stability studies for all drugs, which studies will be used to establish expiration dates."

Product Identification Systems. To ensure the quality of a product, the unit doses are (1) individually packaged and labeled and (2) imprinted with an assigned code for the purpose of identification. The first procedure is usually termed the unit dose packaging concept. Single unit doses for medication—tablets, capsules, or parenterals—are individually sealed in packages that have been imprinted with complete identifying data. Thus, the danger of error is substantially reduced.

The second procedure in identifying the products is called the unit code system. Various techniques have been employed for this method. The codes vary in complexity, for example, a system adopts alphabetical and numerical combinations. A drug product code composed of nine characters to be used by pharmaceutical manufacturers for inclusion in the National Drug Code Directory has been developed and has been used by the FDA to establish a uniform code system for dosage forms. The nine-character code would identify the labeler, the dosage form, the strength of the product, and the number of product units in the package. In the case of tablets or capsules, those parts of the code identifying the drug and its strength would be used on each unit of the dosage form. Interestingly, any product not identified would be termed misbranded unless compliance were impractical and the FDA granted an exemption.

Adulteration, Misbranding, and Counterfeiting. An adulterated, misbranded, or counterfeited drug is a fraud to the public. Such products can seriously endanger the health and safety of the person taking the medication, since there is no guarantee that the ingredients are safe, of highest quality, or of labeled potency. A situation of this nature may mislead the physician because his patient's response may differ from the response expected.

A drug product may be deemed adulterated because of various defects or shortcomings, as discussed in Section 501 of the Federal FDC Act. According to the law, a drug is considered adulterated if it does not meet the quality and purity characteristics it is represented to possess.

According to Section 502 of the Federal FDC Act, the major reason for considering a drug to be misbranded is the mislabeling of the product. To safeguard the manufacturer from marketing adulterated or misbranded products, the establishment of a total quality control system concerned with the dosage form, package, and labeling prior to release for distribution is essential.

Maintenance, Storage, and Retrieval of Records. The proper control of records (master formula, batch production, and packaging records) in manufacturing operations has been discussed in a previous section of this chapter. Suitable maintenance storage and retrieval of records for dosage form control are mandatory in assuring product quality.

Product distribution records should be organized systematically for each manufactured product. Complete records of the distribution of each batch of product must be maintained in a manner that would facilitate its recall if necessary. Such records should include the batch or control numbers identifying the batch of product distributed, the date and quantity shipped, and the name and address of the consignee. Such records should be retained for at least two years after the batch of product has been distributed or at least one year after the drug's expiration date, whichever is longer.

For the vast amounts of records maintained in a quality assurance program, the storage and retrieval of these records when needed can be time-consuming if done manually. The application of computer systems in the storage and retrieval of data in this area is inescapable.

In general, records of data converted to digitized form are stored on computer tapes, cards, or discs, or in case storage. The choice of storage medium depends on the volume, pattern of use, type of data, and cost factors. Case memory is the fastest, most expensive and most accessible type of memory. Disc storage is available for large volumes of data, and its almost random access features are particularly useful. Magnetic tape is compact and provides relatively cheap storage. The main disadvantage of tape is that if the data to be retrieved does not occur in the same sequence as that in which it is stored on the tape, the whole tape must be searched for the requested information.

The importance of batch or control numbers must be re-emphasized. The establishment of these identification numbers for the products manufactured is the direct key by which the entire quality assurance program in production, control, storage, and distribution can be readily unlocked. As an indirect assurance of the product quality to the consumer, this identification number not only opens the correct file without delay should the need arise, but also facilitates recall of that particular product from the market should it become necessary.

Complaints. Suitable systems should be provided to investigate and follow up the complaints regarding deteriorated, adulterated, misbranded, or counterfeited products. Often, useful information can be generated from detailed investigation of the reason for complaint; the investigation may be physical, chemical, or biologic in nature. Complaints should be recorded and carefully evaluated by competent and responsible personnel, and the complaint files should indicate the action taken.

Return of Goods. Inevitably, a certain fraction of distributed product is returned for one reason or another. Returned products should be properly handled by capable individuals and correctly recorded in a manner that prevents confusion and the possibility of errors. On receipt, each should be listed on an appropriate form, giving the name and address of the sender, the batch or control numbers of the returned product, the reason for returning the product, and the estimated condition of the product. The product should then be analyzed by physical, chemical, or biologic methods whenever possible and stored in an orderly manner pending issuance of credit and a decision for disposal.

Recall Procedures. The need to establish an effective drug recall system by the pharmaceutical manufacturers is evident inasmuch as hundreds of recalls are made annually. In general, product recalls may be initiated by the manufacturer, by the regulatory agency, by government seizure through the courts, or by the manufacturer at the request of the regulatory agency. The last category applies to the majority of recalls. If the products to be recalled have been distributed only to the warehouses of the manufacturer or the distributor, the hazard to the public health may not be serious. The recall can be effected rapidly and easily. When recall involves the local pharmacist, the physician, or the public, however, the problem becomes complicated, and complete recall may be hampered. It then becomes necessary to enlist the aid of public communication systems to reach the consumer. An effective system for product recall requires, in addition to the efforts of pharmaceutical manufacturers, a careful system of record-keeping at all levels of product distribution, from manufacturer to ultimate consumer.

Adverse Effects. Quality of marketed products can be further ensured if competent personnel are assigned to evaluate the significance and severity of each side reaction or adverse effect reported by the physician who prescribes the medicinals, the drug surveillance group of the hospital, published scientific results, and even the regulatory agency. An effective product information system should be established to evaluate and accumulate these reports on the safety, potency, adverse reactions, clinical side effects, and drug abuse problems of the marketed product and to prepare appropriate replies and reports in this area.

Summary

The professional, social, and legal responsibilities that rest with the pharmaceutical manufacturers for the assurance of product quality are tremendous. It is only through well-organized, adequately staffed, and accurately performed process and dosage form control before, during, and after production that adequate quality assurance of the product can be achieved. It should be realized that no amount of dosage form testing and control can maintain and assure product quality unless good manufacturing practices are implemented systematically and process control is practiced vigorously. Product quality must be built into, and not merely tested in, the product.

The pharmaceutical manufacturer assumes the major responsibility for the quality of his products. The manufacturer is in a position (1) to control the sources of product quality variation, namely materials, methods, machines, and men, (2) to ensure the correct and most appropriate manufacturing and packaging practices, (3) to assure that the testing results are in compliance with the standards or specifications, and (4) to assure product stability and to perform other activities related to product quality through a well-organized total quality assurance system.

For the total quality assurance system to function effectively, certain basic operational rules should be established and should always prevail. First, control decisions must be based solely on considerations of product quality. Second, the operation must adhere rigidly to the established standards or specifications as determined by systematic inspection, sampling, and testing, and should constantly strive for improving the levels of the current standards or specifications. Third, the facilities, funds for personnel, and environment necessary for personnel to perform their responsibilities effectively should be adequately provided. Last but not least, the control decisions should be independent administratively, and they must not yield to, or be overruled by, production or marketing personnel under any circumstances. Because the control decision can involve the health of the consumer and the reputation of the manufacturer, the climate necessary for making judicious decisions is essential. In times of major disagreement, the control decisions should be subjected to review only at the highest level of management.

References

1. Noel, R. H.: Indus. Quality Control, 7:14, 1950.
2. Grant, E. L: Statistical Quality Control. 3rd Ed. McGraw-Hill, New York, 1964.
3. Military Standard Sampling Procedures and Tables for Inspection by Variables for Percent Defective (MIL-STD-414). Superintendent of Documents, U.S. Government Printing Office, Washington, DC, June 1957, and Notice 1 of May 1968.
4. Military Standard Sampling Procedures and Tables for Inspection by Attributes (MIL-STD-105-D). Superintendent of Documents, U.S. Government Printing Office, Washington, DC, April 1963, Notice 1 of November 1963, and Notice 2 of March 1964.
5. Breunig, H. E. and King, H. P.: J. Pharm. Sci., 51:1187, 1962.
6. Dodge, H. L.: Ann. Math. Statistics, 14:264, 1962.
7. Zarembo, J. E., J. Assoc. Off. Anal. Chem., 65:542, 1982.
8. Kateman, G., and Pijpers, F. W.: Quality Control in Analytical Chemistry. Wiley-Interscience, New York, 1981.
9. Elrod, L., Cox, R. D., and Plasz, A. C.: J. Pharm. Sci., 71:161, 1982.
10. Youden, W. J.: Statistical Techniques for Collaborative Tests. Association of Official Analytical Chemists, Washington, DC, 1972.
11. Roman, R.: Pharmacopeial Forum, 8:2237, 1982.
12. Guidelines for the Analytical Validation of HPLC Method. Pharmacopeial Forum, 9:2789, 1983.

28

Drug Regulatory Affairs

WILLIAM R. PENDERGAST *and* RAYMOND D. McMURRAY*

The laws and regulations governing the pharmaceutical industry were adopted to protect the consuming public by attempting to provide drugs of consistent quality, purity, and efficacy. The Federal Food, Drug and Cosmetic Act (the Act) is a living document in that it is amended frequently and interpreted constantly.[1] The Act may be imperfect, but careful attention to its provisions plus an effort of good faith by all persons concerned with drug manufacturing can produce the type of product for which the Act and its regulations strive.

Even though the applicable laws and regulations may change with regard to specifics, there are, nonetheless, many constants applicable generally. This chapter serves as an overview of some of the more important laws and regulations.

The text describes the Federal Food, Drug and Cosmetic Act, treats briefly other Federal acts and regulations bearing on pharmaceutical manufacturing, looks at the structure, powers, and duties of the Food and Drug Administration (FDA), describes state and local laws and regulations, and finally, covers the protection of industrial property and product liability.

Definitions

The terms most commonly used in this chapter are defined as they are in the Act:

Drug. Sec. 201(g)(1):[2] The term "drug" means (A) articles recognized in the official United States Pharmacopoeia, official Homeopathic Pharmacopoeia of the United States, or official National Formulary, or any supplement to any of them; and (B) articles intended for use in the diagnosis, cure, mitigation, treatment, or prevention of disease in man or other ani-

mals; and (C) articles (other than food) intended to affect the structure or any function of the body of man or other animals; and (D) articles intended for use as a component of any article specified in clause (A), (B), or (C); but does not include devices or their components, parts, or accessories.

Label. Sec. 201(k):[3] The term "label" means a display of written, printed, or graphic matter upon the immediate container of any article; and a requirement made by or under authority of this Act that any word, statement, or other information appearing on the label shall not be considered to be complied with unless such word, statement, or other information also appear[s] on the outside container or wrapper, if any there be, of the retail package of such article, or is easily legible through the outside container or wrapper.

Labeling. Sec. 201(m):[4] The term "labeling" means all labels and other written, printed, or graphic matter (1) upon any article or any of its containers or wrappers, or (2) accompanying such article.

New Drug. Sec. 201(p):[5] The term "new drug" means—(1) any drug (except a new animal drug or an animal feed bearing or containing a new animal drug) the composition of which is such among experts qualified by scientific training and experience to evaluate the safety and effectiveness of drugs, as safe and effective for use under the conditions prescribed, recommended, or suggested in the labeling thereof, except that such a drug not so recognized shall not be deemed to be a "new drug" if at any time prior to the enactment of this Act it was subject to the Food and Drugs Act of June 30, 1906, as amended, and if at such time its labeling contained the same representations concerning the conditions of its use; or (2) any drug (except a new animal drug or an animal feed bearing or containing a new animal drug) the composition of which is such that such drug, as a result of investigations to determine its safety and effectiveness for use under such conditions, has become so recognized, but which has not, otherwise than in such investigations, been used to a material extent or for a material time under such conditions.

New Animal Drug. Sec. 201(w):[6] The term "new animal drug" means any drug intended for use for ani-

*Deceased.

mals other than man, including any drug intended for use in animal feed but not including such animal feed—(1) the composition of which is such that such drug is not generally recognized, among experts qualified by scientific training and experience to evaluate the safety and effectiveness of animal drugs, as safe and effective for use under the conditions prescribed, recommended, or suggested in the labeling thereof; except that such a drug not so recognized shall not be deemed to be a "new animal drug" if at any time prior to June 25, 1938, it was subject to the Food and Drug Act of June 30, 1906, as amended, and if at such time its labeling contained the same representations concerning the conditions of its use; or (2) the composition of which is such that such drug, as a result of investigations to determine its safety and effectiveness for use under such conditions, has become so recognized but which has not, otherwise than in such investigations, been used to a material extent or for a material time under such conditions; or (3) which drug is composed wholly or partly of any kind of penicillin, streptomycin, chlortetracycline, chloramphenicol, or bacitracin, or any derivation thereof, except when there is in effect a published order of the Secretary declaring such drug not to be a new animal drug on the grounds that (A) the requirement of certification of batches of such drug, as provided for in section 512(n), is not necessary to insure that the objectives specified in paragraph (3) thereof are achieved and (B) that neither subparagraph (1) nor (2) of this paragraph (w) applies to such drug.

Animal Feed. Sec. 201(x):[7] The term "animal feed," as used in paragraph (w) of this section, in section 512, and in provisions of this Act referring to such paragraph or section, means an article which is intended for use for food for animals other than man and which is intended for use as a substantial source of nutrients in the diet of the animal, and is not limited to a mixture intended to be the sole ration of the animal.

Brief History of the Federal Food, Drug, and Cosmetic Act

Approximately 100 years after its founding, during the later phases of Reconstruction following the Civil War, the Congress of the United States came to realize that all matters of public health and safety could not be lodged solely in the states, and that certain measures had to be taken to protect the population in these vital areas. On August 30, 1890, there was enacted a law prohibiting the importation into the United States of adulterated or unwholesome food, drugs, or liquors. Thus began the federal interest in regulating unwholesome consumer products.

In 1906, realizing the limitations of a statute concerned only with the importation of unfit foods, drugs, and liquors, Congress passed the Wiley Act to prevent "the manufacture, sale, or transportation of adulterated or misbranded or poisonous or deleterious foods, drugs, medicines, and liquors and for regulating traffic therein." This was the first concept of regulating the *introduction* into interstate commerce of unfit foods and drugs and was based on the Commerce Clause of the Constitution of the United States granting power to Congress "to regulate commerce with foreign nations, and among the several states."[8] The concept of misbranding as well as adulteration thus was introduced into the law, and violation again was subject to seizure and confiscation.

Even though the 1906 Act was a great step forward, it soon became apparent that prohibitions in the law were not sufficiently stringent. The ever-expanding industrial economy, including the practice of pharmacy on an industrial scale, made it apparent that even though amendments could be passed to fill specific gaps, there were areas requiring further controls. Although the law prohibited crude adulteration and misbranding of drugs, its less than precise language did not provide a suitable vehicle for policing medical claims. For instance, an attempt was made in 1912 to plug this loophole by an amendment prohibiting any false statement of curative or therapeutic effect on the labeling of drugs. This effort was thwarted when it was held that that language required a showing that there was fraudulent intent in making the claim. Simply proving a medical claim to be false was insufficient.

Another important defect of the 1906 Act was that it did not require testing of new drug products to show their safety prior to marketing. Spurred on by several unfortunate instances, some involving deaths, due at least in part to the lack of pretesting, the current law was enacted on June 27, 1938: the Federal Food, Drug and Cosmetic Act. This is the basic federal law under which foods, drugs, medical devices, diagnostic products, and cosmetics are regulated today. Now, more than 45 years later, that Act begins to look like a patchwork quilt after many amendments through the years, which have affected both substance and procedure.[9] Incidentally, the 1938 Act dropped its concern with liquor.

The 1938 Act contained the first "new drug" provisions, which required that drugs not generally recognized as safe, by experts qualified to make that judgment, under the conditions of use stated on the label, had to be marketed under a procedure by which a "New Drug Application" (NDA) was filed. The NDA had to contain convincing evidence to show that the drug was safe for its intended purpose. The Act also provided the following:

1. The label of each drug had to state the name of each active ingredient, and the amount of certain specific substances, whether active or not, enumerated in the Act.

2. Therapeutic claims that were false or misleading were not actionable without a showing of fraudulent intent.

3. The manufacture and sale of devices were brought under the law.

4. The Government was given limited authority to make factory inspection to ensure compliance with the law.

5. Cosmetics were brought under the law and were required to be nondangerous, and properly labeled and packaged.

Since 1938, the Act has carried a provision that the label of a drug must bear adequate directions for use. It became apparent in practice, however, that certain drugs and drug products of necessity had to be administered by or under the direction of a licensed practitioner, because of the inability of a layman to diagnose his condition, choose an effective treatment, and recognize a cure or mitigation. Many products were so restricted, but it was not until the Durham-Humphrey Amendment of 1951 that the concept of a "prescription drug" was introduced into the Act. The Amendment was, in fact, an exception to the provision that all drugs must bear adequate directions for use on their labels. A label bearing the so-called prescription legend, CAUTION, FEDERAL LAW PROHIBITS DISPENSING WITHOUT PRESCRIPTION, by dint of this exception, was deemed to bear adequate directions for use. The sale of these had to be restricted to an order by a licensed practitioner, and the labeling on or within the package had to have adequate information for use from which such practitioner might safely prescribe the drug.

In the years immediately following World War II, pharmaceutical research expanded rapidly, and in ever-increasing numbers, more drugs aimed at specific disease, primarily prescription products, became available. With the great strides in research, production, and marketing in the pharmaceutical industry, there grew an increasing concern among the federal lawmakers with the problem of the adequacy of procedures employed in the testing and distribution of these new drug products. In particular, there was concern for proof of effectiveness and for the need to ensure a clear disclosure of possible side effects along with a need to require advertising and promotion not only to be positive, but also to point out the possible harmful side effects of these new drugs.

Kefauver-Harris Amendments

The Drug Amendments of 1962 amended the basic 1938 Act in an attempt to establish stronger controls over research manufacturing, advertising, promotion, sale, and use of drugs, and to ensure their quality, safety, and effectiveness.[10]

New Drugs

Probably the most significant provisions of the 1962 Drug Amendments relate to "new drugs." The definition of a "new drug" was expanded beyond that of the original 1938 definition, for which lack of general recognition by qualified experts as to a drug's *safety* for its intended purpose was the sole criterion. Now the test was that unless it was generally recognized by such experts to be both safe and *effective* for its intended purpose, the product must seek approval under the New Drug Application procedure set forth in the Act at Section 505. There was also introduced into the law the concept of "substantial evidence of effectiveness," which was defined to mean:

. . . adequate and well-controlled investigations, including clinical investigations, by experts qualified by scientific training and experience to evaluate the effectiveness of the drug involved, on the basis of which it could fairly and responsibly be concluded by such experts that the drug will have the effect it purports or is represented to have under the conditions of use prescribed, recommended, or suggested in the labeling or proposed labeling thereof.[11]

The Federal Food, Drug and Cosmetic Act, as now written, prohibits the interstate shipment of a new drug that is not covered by an approved new drug application, unless such shipment is made for investigational purposes and is in accordance with the regulations governing the use of investigational drugs, which are designed to obtain evidence demonstrative of the safety and effectiveness of an investigational new drug for the purposes for which it is intended to be used.[12]

A drug may be considered "new" because of its composition, its use, its dosage, or its dosage form. It can readily be understood that a drug that contains as its active ingredient a new chemical entity would be considered to be a new drug; however, a drug may be new owing to the composition of inactive ingredients, the proportion of ingredients, active or inactive, or the combination of ingredients, active or inactive.

A drug's recommended new use or change in recommended dosage, dosage form, or route of administration also can cause it to be considered a new drug. The basis for a drug's "newness" determines what steps must be taken to obtain an approved new drug application.[13]

Investigational New Drugs. The factor of "newness" that requires the greatest amount of work is the presence of a new chemical entity. The activities involved in obtaining new drug approval in such instances are briefly set forth in the following paragraphs. (Forms FD-1571, FD-1572, and FD-1573, which are required for sponsorship of new drug clinical testing and statements of the investigations are available from the Food and Drug Administration, 5600 Fishers Lane, Rockville, MD 20852.)

After its synthesis, a new chemical entity is normally subjected to a "screening" process, which involves initial testing of the drug in a small number of animals of different species (usually three) plus microbiologic tests to detect any beneficial effects of the chemical. Although serendipity does play a certain part in this effort, the approach is generally quite controlled, based on the known structure of the compound. Today, in addition to the usual LD_{50} and acute and chronic toxicity studies, tests involving teratogenicity, mutagenicity, and carcinogenicity are often conducted.

If the initial screening proves the new chemical to be worthy of further investigation, more extensive animal tests for its suspected properties are conducted. If the properties are similar to those of a drug already on the market, the two compounds may be tested against each other to determine their relative merits.

Animal tests are designed to determine:

1. The relative toxicity of the new chemical. These tests would include acute toxicity and LD_{50} tests to determine toxic dosage, as well as median and long-term toxicity tests for harmful effects on the animal and on various specific organs, such as the eyes, liver, and brain.

2. The probable or possible effect of the chemical in human drug use, including areas of interest for study, dosage, and probable side effects.

Animal tests or "preclinical investigations," as they are also termed, are designed with particular regard to possible future testing of the drug in humans, or "clinical investigation."

Preclinical tests, therefore, are designed with the following considerations: (1) the expected duration of administration of the drug to human beings; (2) the age groups and physical status of the intended human subjects with special consideration for infants, pregnant women, or the aged; and (3) the expected effects of the drug in humans.

Prior to the institution of clinical testing in humans, a Notice of Claimed Investigational Exemption for a New Drug (Form FD-1571) must be filed with the Food and Drug Administration by the sponsor. This form is also referred to as an IND, or investigational new drug application.

This notice is required to set forth:

1. The best available descriptive name of the drug, including, to the extent known, the chemical name and structure of any new drug substance (a new chemical entity).

2. A complete list of components of the drug.

3. The quantitative composition of the drug.

4. The name and address of the supplier of any new drug substance if other than the sponsor (the person or firm submitting the IND) and a description of the preparation (chemical synthesis or other method of manufacture) of any new drug substance.

5. A statement of the methods, facilities, and controls used for the manufacture, processing, and packaging of the new drug.

6. A statement covering all information available to the sponsor derived from preclinical investigations and any clinical studies and experience with the drug.

7. Copies of labels for the drugs and informational material that will be supplied to investigators. This material must describe the preclinical studies with the drug and describe all relevant hazards, side effects, contraindications, and other information pertinent to use of the drug by the investigator.

8. A description of the scientific training and experience considered appropriate by the sponsor to qualify an investigator as a suitable expert to investigate the drug.

9. The names and curriculum vitae of all investigators.

10. An outline of the planned investigations of the drug in humans. These investigations are divided into three phases. The first two phases are termed "clinical pharmacology" studies.

Phase 1 is the initial introduction of the drug into humans for the purpose of determining toxicity, metabolism absorption, elimination, safe dosage range, and other pharmacologic action.

Phase 2 covers the initial trials for specific therapeutic effect and is conducted on a limited number of patients.

Phase 1 and 2 studies are limited in nature and should be very closely controlled by the sponsor.

Phase 3 is termed the "clinical trial" of the new drug and is intended to assess its safety and effectiveness in one or more particular indications.

The regulations provide for a 30-day waiting period, after which, if the FDA has not responded negatively, the clinical trials may commence.

Specific information on the planned studies for all phases of the investigation must be submitted to the Food and Drug Administration in the IND before work is begun. These may be submitted sequentially and not necessarily concurrently. To avoid any delays at this point, most sponsors discuss the planned tests and the test substance with the FDA beforehand. In this way, false starts and wasted efforts are minimized.

The sponsor of an investigational new drug is required to:

1. Keep records of shipment of the drug to each investigator.

2. Monitor the progress of the investigations of the drug and report on these investigations to the FDA at intervals not exceeding one year.

3. Promptly investigate and report to the FDA and to investigators findings associated with use of the drug that may suggest significant hazards, contraindications, side effects, or precautions pertinent to the safety of the drug.

4. Refrain from promoting the drug as being "safe" or "effective."

5. Obtain from clinical investigators a signed Statement of Investigator form (Form FD-1572 for investigations in Phase 1 or 2 clinical pharmacology and Form FD-1573 for Phase 3 clinical trails), setting forth the investigator's curriculum vitae and his commitments, some of which are:

   A. The investigator will maintain required records of the study.

   B. The drug will only be given to patients under his supervision or under the supervision of named investigators responsible to him.

   C. The investigator will:
      (1) inform patients that they are involved in an investigational drug study, and
      (2) obtain their consent for this involvement except when this is not feasible or not in the best interests of the patient.

An important facet of any clinical testing under an IND is its supervision by Institutional Review Boards (IRBs). To assure, so far as possible, that all humans subjected to the investiga-tional testing are protected from unnecessary risk, the FDA requires that the sponsor of any such test have it reviewed and approved by a board of nongovernment employees. This Board is directed to assure the protection of the rights and welfare of any humans subject to such a test.

The FDA has detailed regulations describing the makeup of those Boards, how they are to function, the records they are to keep, and their role in the drug approval process.[14] In brief, there must be five members who cumulatively possess the requisite expertise to evaluate the drug, the proposed tests, and the local community attitudes toward such studies. Both sexes must be represented, there must be at least one member whose primary concerns are nonscientific (such as a member of the clergy), and no member of the IRB can have a conflicting interest. The sponsor has the responsibility of selecting this Board, but if it fails to meet FDA standards or fails to function according to FDA regulations, the agency can refuse to approve any NDA incorporating a study done under the supervision of such an IRB.[15] Today, most major institutions engaged in clinical research have at least one IRB established.

New Drug Application. In 1985, the FDA revised its regulations governing NDAs in a number of ways designed to speed up the review process. These new regulations and the Agency's discussion of them appear in the Federal Register of February 22, 1985, beginning on page 7452. The sponsor, upon completion of a sufficient amount of clinical work to demonstrate the safety and effectiveness of the new drug for the use or uses for which it is intended, may then submit a new drug application (NDA) to the FDA (FD Form 356). This application must include (1) detailed reports of the preclinical (animal) studies; (2) reports of all clinical (human) studies; (3) information on the composition and manufacture of the drug and on the controls and facilities used in its manufacture; and (4) samples of the drug and its labeling. Under the new rules, summaries of the data must be provided, and the full case reports of each person who received the drug are needed only in limited circumstances.

Material previously submitted to the FDA in the IND or in periodic reports must be included by reference in the NDA.

NDAs for new chemical entities are usually very involved submissions running into thousands of pages in total. The information contained therein must be sufficient to justify the claims made in the proposed labeling for the drug as to effectiveness, dosage, and safety, and foreign data can be used. The exact wording that may be used in the labeling of a drug usually is decided by an exchange between the sponsor and the FDA.

Once a new drug application is approved, any significant change in the manufacturing, control, packaging, or other physical properties of the drug, or any change in its labeling that may have an effect on safety and effectiveness relative to either the drug itself or the manner in which it is used must be covered by a supplemental new drug application.

The requirements of an NDA for prescription and over-the-counter drugs are similar. It is extremely rare, however, that any new chemical entity would be approved by the FDA for over-the-counter sale for reasons of lack of sufficient data to support the safety in use of a totally "new" drug. Since the basic test is the ability to provide on the label adequate direction for use, most applications specifically for over-the-counter drugs would tend to be supplemental applications, mainly on the particular showing that the drug might be safely used without direct medical supervision.

Once approved, several conditions must be met in connection with an NDA. First, advertising must be submitted to FDA on a routine basis. It is especially important that introductory advertising be submitted with some promptness. Second, reports of human clinical experience are required on the following basis. The first reports are due at intervals of three months, beginning with the date of approval of the application, during the first three years, and annually thereafter.

Records reflecting clinical experience with the drug must be retained, and they must be available for inspection. The reports required at the aforementioned intervals must include unpublished reports of clinical experience, studies, investigations, and tests conducted by the applicant or reported to him, unpublished reports of animal experience, experience involving the chemical, or physical properties of the drug, and any information that might affect the safety or efficacy of the product. These may be submitted on Forms FD-1639, FD-2253, or FD-2252.

The FDA requires immediate reporting of information concerning any mixup in a drug or its labeling with another article; information concerning any bacteriologic or any significant chemical, physical, or other changes, or deterioration in the drug; or any failure of one or more distributed batches of the drug to meet the specifications established for it in the New Drug Application. This information could, of course, form the basis for a recall.

Certain other information must be transmitted as soon as possible—in any event, within 15 working days of receipt. This information would pertain to serious and unsuspected side effects, injury, toxicity, sensitivity reaction, or incidents associated with clinical use, studies, investigations, or tests, whether or not they are determined to be attributable to the drug, or information concerning any unusual failure of the drug to exhibit its expected pharmacologic activity.

Supplements to NDA. The 1985 rules also change the requirements for supplements. Supplements are required if there is a proposed change in the drug or its labeling (with exceptions), and the changes cannot be put into place until FDA approves them. Any number of these changes may be made, but a separate submission must be made for each.

The regulation provides for certain changes that can be made without the approval of a supplemental application, if such change is fully described in the next periodic report. These changes are:

1. Any change made to comply with an official compendium.

2. A different container size or closure system for solid oral dosage forms.

3. Change in a description of a drug that does not involve a change in a dosage strength or form.

4. An editorial or minor change in labeling.

5. Deletion of a color ingredient.

6. Inclusion of additional specifications and methods without deletion of those described in the approved application.

7. Addition of reasonable expiration data based on FDA approved protocol.

It is a good general rule, when considering to make any material changes, to anticipate that a supplement to the approved NDA will be needed unless specifically covered by the language of the aforementioned enumerated exceptions.

Abbreviated New Drug Applications. By regulation published in final form on April 24, 1970, the Food and Drug Administration amended Section 130.4 of the New Drug Regulations,[16] to provide for the filing of a short form NDA, where it is found that it is not necessary to provide the FDA with all the information called for in Section 505 of the Act. Findings may be directed to specific drugs individually, or as in the case of the Drug Efficacy Study Implementation (DESI) reviews, the DESI announcement may state that only the submission of an abbreviated NDA may need to be made. Information submitted in an abbreviated NDA may be limited to a table of contents, label and labeling copy, a statement as to the prescription or OTC nature of the drug, and the components of the new drug. In lieu of the broader NDA statements concerning the full composition of the drug and a detailed description of the methods used in—and the facilities and controls used for—the manufacture, processing, and packaging of the drug required under items 7 and 8 of the NDA form, the following items are necessary:

1. Include the composition of the drug, stating the name and amount of each ingredient, whether active or not, contained in a stated quantity of the drug in the form in which it is to be distributed.

2. Identify the place where the drug will be manufactured, processed, packaged, and labeled and the name of the supplier of the active ingredient(s).

3. Identify any person other than the applicant who performs a part of those operations and designate the part.

4. Include certifications from the applicant and from any person identified in subdivision (3) of this subparagraph that the methods used in, and the facilities and controls used for, the manufacture, processing, packing, and holding of the drug are in conformity with current good manufacturing practice in accord with Part 133 of this chapter (21CFR Section 133).

5. Assure that the drug dosage form and components will comply with the specifications and tests described in an official compendium, if such article is recognized therein, or, if not listed or if the article differs from the compendium drug, that the specifications and tests applied to the drug and its components are adequate to assure their identity, strength, quality, and purity.

6. Outline the methods used in, and the facilities, and controls used for, the manufacture, processing, and packing of the drug.

If the finding that the drug requires only an abbreviated new drug application also specifies that there must be included adequate data to assure the biologic availability of the drug, and for preparations claiming sustained action, such data should show that the drug is available at a rate of release that will be safe and effective.

Recent Legislation. In 1984, Congress passed the Drug Price Competition and Patent Term Restoration Act of 1984. This bill promises to have far-reaching effects on the pharmaceutical industry. In brief, it provides the following.

For the first time, there is now in place a statutory mechanism for obtaining FDA approval of generic equivalents of previously approved pharmaceuticals. Thus, the ANDA mechanism put into place for pre-1962 products during the course of the DESI review has now been extended by statute to post-1962 drugs, subject to certain conditions.

If the FDA agrees that a particular pharmaceutical is appropriate for an abbreviated new drug application, companies wishing to market it can submit ANDAs, which usually contain bioequivalency data and certain other detailed information, to obtain agency approval. Full clinical studies are not needed. The processing of abbreviated applications should proceed rapidly. As President Reagan has said, "[This] legislation will speed up the process of federal approval of inexpensive generic versions of many brand name drugs, [and] make the generic versions more widely available to consumers . . . ." He estimated that the American consumer would save more than $1 billion over the ten-year period following 1984.

The second section of the new law provides a mechanism to grant drug companies up to 5 years additional patent protection for new drugs to compensate for some of the years of patent life lost as a result of the time-consuming testing required by the FDA. Under this provision, the Patent Office, working in collaboration with FDA, can grant up to 5 years additional time of patent protection to certain new pharmaceutical entities depending on the length of time for which these entities were required to go through the regulatory review process. The FDA, which is charged with the responsibility for computing the regulatory review time period, will not grant any additional time for delays caused by the neglect or mistakes of the pharmaceutical company.

At the time of this writing, the FDA is only beginning to implement the many provisions of this complex law, and no new regulations have yet been promulgated specifying all of the details that must be met. Many generic equivalents have already been approved for post-1962 drugs, however, and undoubtedly, this new legislation will encompass a large part of the efforts of many pharmaceutical companies for years to come.

New Animal Drugs and Animal Feed. Effective August 1, 1969, the Act was amended to include definitions of "new animal drug" and "animal feed."[17] The same amendment, the Animal Drug Amendment of 1968, also added a new section 512 to the Act, which requires applications for new animal drug to be filed with reference to new animal drugs and provides for certain registrations of animal feeds containing new animal drugs. Regulations quite similar to those involving drugs for human use have been adopted by the Bureau of Veterinary Medicine, and forms for an Animal New Drug Application and a Medicated Feed Application are Forms FD-356V and 1800 respectively.

Certification of Drugs. Insulin and antibiotics are the two classes of drugs requiring certification, although certain antibiotics may be exempt from certification. The FDA, acting under the mandate of the Act, has adopted regulations to ensure that each batch has the characteristics of identity, strength, quality, and purity prescribed in such regulations.

Application for certification must be made to the Commissioner. For insulin, the information that must be contained in a request for certification is set forth in 21 CFR Section 164.2.

In 1982, the FDA published a regulation that exempts virtually all antibiotics from the requirement of obtaining batch certification.[18] For 20 years, companies marketing approved antibiotics had been required to submit assay results and samples of each manufacturing batch for FDA testing and evaluation. The purpose of this exercise was to assure batch-to-batch integrity and uniformity, and this testing was paid for by the companies involved and was both costly and time-consuming (a batch could not be released for sale until FDA passed it). Apparently finding the exercise no longer justified, the FDA dropped it. Batch confirmation continued to be required for insulin products.[19]

Recalls

While the FDA has no statutory authority to require the recall of a pharmaceutical, the agency nevertheless has published, in the interest of public safety, extensive regulations concerning recalls and has set up a detailed mechanism for the recall of drugs from the marketplace. Recalling a drug is one of the most difficult decisions facing a manufacturer or distributor, for such an act has important ramifications, ranging from a company's relationships with the FDA to potential product liability litigation. Therefore, recalls should be entered into only after the most careful evaluation of the problem, and once begun, they must be completed as rapidly and efficiently as possible. FDA regulations provide extensive guidelines to determine (1) what products should be recalled (and to what level) and (2) the precise mechanism for recall that would most likely achieve the desired goal. In addition to these regulations, the FDA has also made available its own regula-

tory procedures manual, which defines in even greater detail the recall mechanism and FDA's involvement in it. All companies manufacturing or distributing pharmaceutical products should have officials and employees that are fully informed as to these regulations and FDA procedures, so that accurate and appropriate decisions can be made.

The FDA classifies all recalls into one of three categories. Category I recall represents an emergency situation in which the drug poses a hazard that is immediate, long-range, and life-threatening. Such recalls require special mechanisms and a close relationship with the FDA, since a public warning must be issued, and the product must be recalled to the consumer level.

The second type of recall is Category II, a priority situation in which the consequences of the offending drug remaining on the market may be immediate, long-range, or potentially life-threatening. In general, such recalls must be made to the retail or dispensing level, and occasionally, the FDA issues press releases to inform the public. The final recall classification is Category III. This is a routine situation in which the threat of life is remote or nonexistent. Such recalls include products that are technically illegal because they are adulterated or misbranded in some respect or another, for example, labeling violations not involving a health hazard. Such recalls are required only to the wholesale level, and press releases are usually not issued.

In addition to such formal recall mechanisms, there are occasions that require companies to remove products from the market when there are no violations of the law involved. This is often done for reasons totally unrelated to the FDA or to the integrity of the product. It is important for companies to appreciate that such market withdrawals are not recalls and are not subject to FDA regulations.

Removal of a product that is still entirely under the direct control of the manufacturer, even though it may have been shipped interstate to one or more branch warehouses, also is not classified as a recall, provided no stock has been distributed to the trade. These removals are termed "stock recoveries" and do not appear on the public recall list. Usually, however, checks are made on the adequacy of these retrievals to cover ultimate disposition of the merchandise.

Drug Efficacy Study Implementation (DESI) Review

A particularly controversial provision of the 1962 Amendments concerns drugs already on the market that had effective NDAs under the old law, i.e., during the period from 1938 to 1962. A two-year period of grace was provided for the manufacturer to supply substantial evidence of effectiveness to support the claims on the previously cleared labeling, since the 1938 Act required proof of safety only.

To cope with the overwhelming burden of such a review, FDA enlisted the services of the National Academy of Sciences, National Research Council (NAS/NRC) to help. The NAS/NRC set up a series of panels to which drugs were assigned on the basis of the medical disciplines in which they were used, e.g., Ophthalmic Panel, Dermatology Panel, and Cardiology Panel. Manufacturers of drugs affected were invited to submit data to these panels in addition to the data already contained in their NDAs. Upon an evaluation of these data, the panels rated the drugs on effectiveness for their labeled indications as follows:

1. Effective

1a. Effective, but . . . [20]

2. Possibly effective

3. Probably effective

4. Ineffective

The panels worked independently, and frequently, a drug would be judged effective for one of its uses by one panel and less than effective, i.e., ratings 1a through 4, for another of its uses by another panel. These apparent differences were not resolved by joint panel meetings, but were treated as independent judgments having equal weight.

The extent of the problem can be seen in the fact that the NAS/NRC Panels returned 2824 reports covering approximately 3700 drugs manufactured by 237 companies. The Panels began submitting reports on October 11, 1967, and the last report was submitted on April 15, 1969. The FDA attempted to implement these reports by publishing findings in the Federal Register, and in the case of drugs that were probably or possibly effective, the drug would be allowed to remain on the market for periods of 12 months and 6 months respectively, to allow for further clinical trials to support efficacy. After these periods, if no work had been done, a notice of withdrawal was prepared and published in the Federal Register. This gave rise to requests for hearings under the appropriate sections of the Act. In all cases, hearings were denied based on a finding by the Secretary that no issue of fact

had been presented on the face of the petitioning papers to require a hearing.

The apparent slowness with which the Food and Drug Administration was implementing the NAS/NRC Reports gave rise to litigation, wherein the American Public Health Association and the National Council of Senior Citizens brought an action against the then acting Secretary of the Department of Health, Education and Welfare and the Commissioner of the Food and Drug Administration to make public all the reports theretofore not public, and in addition, to speed up the process.[21] This resulted in a memorandum by Judge Bryant of the United States District Court for the District of Columbia, wherein the court concluded that there is no compelling reason why the NAS/NRC Reports not then public should not be immediately released, and that it would be an abuse of agency discretion to refuse to make such reports public. In addition, the court would set a deadline for the FDA to complete its evaluation of all drugs with regard to efficacy, and in October 1972, Judge Bryant threw open to public inspection all of the remaining reports. He set certain timetables (1) for implementing either a removal of less than effective classifications or a withdrawal of the NDAs, (2) for allowing certain drugs to remain on the market if good reason was shown by the FDA, pending a longer-term implementation, and (3) for requiring reports to the Court of the progress of the DESI review implementation program. Therefore, with the exception of less than effective drugs, which may be continued past the cutoff date because of public health considerations, all implementation would be finished by final order of FDA at least by October 10, 1976. The FDA did not appeal Judge Bryant's ruling.

The FDA once again failed to perform under court order, and the plaintiffs went before Judge Bryant for a further order, which resulted in a settlement stipulation calling for the final regulatory action in all cases to be taken by June 1984. The stipulation set certain priorities within which the classes of drugs to be dealt with were specified. Periodic reports of progress were to be made by the FDA to Judge Bryant.

In its own attempt to give some notice to practitioners that the drug they were planning to prescribe had received a rating of less than effective by the NAS/NRC Panels, the FDA promulgated a regulation that became final on February 12, 1972. It required that the less than effective evaluation be called to the practitioner's attention by including a statement prominently in the labeling, and surrounding it with an appropriate border. Since most package insert labeling is printed black on white, this regulation promptly became known as the "Black Box" regulation. Thus, during the period of implementation ordered by Judge Bryant, all products rated less than effective must be so designated, in the "Indications" section of the package insert or on the label within an appropriate border, as follows:

Based on a review of this drug by the National Academy of Sciences/National Research Council and/or information, FDA has classified the indication(s) as follows:
(a statement of the probably or possibly effective status in paragraph form appears here)
Final classification of the less than effective indications requires further investigation.

From the beginning, enforcement of the NAS/NRC findings was not without its problems; resolving these problems ultimately required recourse to the Supreme Court of the United States. First, there was the spectre of the so-called "grandfather clause" of the Kefauver-Harris Bill, which it was claimed, protected certain drugs within its definition from ever having to be proven effective.[22] Second, it was claimed that certain drugs that were identical or similar to NDA drugs reviewed by NAS/NRC were unaffected by the findings of such review because they had been marketed in imitation of such drugs, but had not themselves had an NDA ("me-too" drugs). This claim was made in the face of FDA's proposed notice in February and final notice in October of 1972 that DESI notices of findings were equally applicable to identical, related, or similar drug products even though such products had never had an NDA.

Third, there was a controversy regarding which body, the FDA or the courts, had jurisdiction to decide whether a drug was a "new drug"—that is, that it was not generally recognized as safe and effective. Finally, there was the question whether a manufacturer had an absolute right to a hearing before FDA prior to withdrawal of his NDA or whether FDA could administratively decide that no hearing was warranted because, on the face of the documents offered in support of the drug, there was not "substantial evidence" of safety and/or efficacy.

These cases were fought vigorously through the lower courts, and the importance of their outcomes was deemed to be so great that the Supreme Court granted writs of certiorari, that is, it agreed to hear argument on the issues. They were resolved in June 1973.

The first case is the so-called Bentex case.[23] In this case, a group of drug companies marketing pentylenetetrazol had filed suit against the FDA, alleging that their products were generally recognized as safe and effective and therefore were not new drugs. They asked to be exempt from the regulatory results of an NAS/NRC panel report, which had found that other companies' pentylenetetrazols, which were the subject of new drug applications, lacked substantial evidence of efficacy. This meant that the question before the court was whether a so-called "me-too" drug could be subject to the NAS/NRC results, even if it had never held an NDA and even if it might meet the literal requirements of the grandfather clause. The Supreme Court held that such products are subject to the NAS/NRC results.

Thus, "me-too" products must meet the standards announced by the FDA for NDA drugs, notwithstanding any other legal arguments that the "me-too" manufacturers might make. The court held that the FDA has jurisdiction to decide, with administrative finality, the new drug status of individual drugs or classes of drugs. The FDA, according to the Supreme Court, should not be required to litigate on a case-by-case basis the new drug status of each drug on the market. All of this means that henceforth FDA may say with great finality whether a product is a new drug and, in particular, can say that "me-too" products are new drugs and must come off the market if the NDA drug they are imitating is required to come off the market.

The second case before the Supreme Court involved a bioflavonoid product.[24] In this instance, a lower court had held that the courts had jurisdiction to determine whether a product was protected by the grandfather clause, and that the FDA did not have authority to decide this question conclusively. The lower court also had held that the manufacturer's own "me-too" versions of its NDA drug were subject to the NDA procedures. The Supreme Court held that the phrase "any drug," as used in the grandfather clause, is used in a generic sense, which means that the "me-toos," whether products of the same or of different manufacturers, covered by an effective NDA, are not exempt from the efficacy requirements of the 1962 Amendments. Thus, the grandfather clause has been further narrowed so that it applies *only* to those drugs that meet the definition in the grandfather clause *and* are not "me-toos" of other drugs that did have NDAs.

The third decision involves the important question of a drug company's rights to administrative hearings before the FDA. This is the Hynson, Westcott, & Dunning decision.[25] In this case, a lower court had ruled that the company had presented enough evidence, in its request for a hearing to revoke a new drug application, to entitle that company to a hearing. In this decision, the Supreme Court sustained the summary judgment mechanism instituted by FDA to determine whether administrative hearings must be held. Under this mechanism, a drug company must present, in its hearing request, substantial evidence that the drug is effective, and if the FDA concludes that such evidence has not been presented, no hearing is granted, and the drug is removed from the market without hearing. The Supreme Court has sustained this mechanism. In the event that the FDA denies a hearing, the Supreme Court has ruled that a court of appeals, in reviewing this administrative action, "must determine whether the Commissioner's findings accurately reflect the study in question, and, if they do, whether the deficiencies he finds *conclusively* render the study inadequate or uncontrolled . . . "

Perhaps the most important statement in the Hynson, Westcott & Dunning decision regards a problem other than hearing requests. It had long been accepted that a drug could be an "old drug" if there was sufficient expert medical opinion declaring it to be generally recognized as safe and effective. It was further thought that this opinion could be just that—opinion—and need not be based on any particular type of scientific data. The Supreme Court has now severely narrowed this thinking and has ruled that a drug can be an old drug, based on a consensus of expert opinion, "only when that expert consensus is founded upon 'substantial evidence' as defined in Section 505(d)." This means that a drug can be an old drug only if there is substantial evidence of efficacy by well-controlled studies that demonstrate that the product is in fact effective. Lower federal courts have followed this discussion, and there now remains no question as to the validity of this doctrine.

The final case before the Supreme Court involved CIBA.[26] Here, a lower court had ruled that the FDA had the authority, in an administrative hearing, to determine whether a product was a new or old drug. CIBA had appealed this decision. The Supreme Court held, in a manner consistent with the previous three decisions, that the agency does have such jurisdiction, and that, therefore, when a company has had one

opportunity to litigate the new drug issue before FDA, it may not later try to litigate it in another forum, such as a federal court.

A final chapter in this controversy, the status of "me-too" or generic equivalent drugs, was finally decided in 1983. All through the late fifties and sixties, and well into the seventies, companies continued to market their unapproved versions of drugs that had gone through the NDA process, relying on various legal arguments and an FDA policy of allowing such marketing—a policy that seemingly conceded that NDAs were unnecessary for generic drugs. As the DESI Review moved on and the ANDA policy was put into effect, however, a more definitive resolution of this problem was needed.

Following a series of lawsuits involving the generic drug industry, one finally reached the Supreme Court.[27] There the Court ruled that generic versions of drugs that had gone through an NDA process (be it NDA or ANDA) also had to go through a similar procedure. The main reason for this decision was the Court's reliance on the fact that changes in inactive ingredients such as colors, stabilizers, binders, or the like could affect the safety or efficacy of an active ingredient. Thus, each should be separately approved by the FDA. With that ruling, the last issue of the DESI Review was resolved, so that the question of whether there are any drugs that do not require FDA approval is largely academic.

OTC Review

Another practice of FDA, similar to the NAS/NRC reviews, is the appointment of panels of experts to review the safety and efficacy of all over-the-counter drugs (OTC drugs). As with the NAS/NRC, these OTC panels have been assigned products on a category basis, e.g., analgesics, antacids, and anesthetics. Each OTC panel is to review products in each category, as well as published literature and data supplied, on call, from manufacturers. After the review, a "monograph" is to be published in the Federal Register setting forth the panel's evaluation of all the data and its decision regarding the ingredients that may be included in products for the indications related to the panel's investigation. The monograph will also set forth allowable claims, permissible combinations, contents, and dosage ranges, as well as permissible dosage forms and routes of administration. Manufacturers may request a hearing to add substances or change any of the recommendations of the monograph, after which it will be published in the Federal Register in final form and will become law. OTC preparations falling outside the monograph in any particular will be deemed to be new drugs and will require approved NDAs.

This process is still underway, and while several final monographs have been published,[30] most remain in the administrative process—which some believe will not be finished before the end of this century.

Further 1962 Drug Amendments

Other provisions of the 1962 Amendments relate to:

1. Immediate registration with the FDA upon first engaging in the manufacture, repacking, or relabeling of drugs, and then registration annually thereafter, with inspections to be made at least once every two years.

2. Strengthened factory inspections with respect to establishments concerned with prescription drugs.

3. A requirement that procedures employed by manufacturers must conform to "current good manufacturing practice." This permits the Government to be in a better position to oversee operations without the necessity of interstate shipment of a product, which would be in violation of the law.

4. The "established name" or nonproprietary name must be designated on the label.

5. Prescription drug advertising must provide a "brief summary relating to side effects, contraindications, and effectiveness" so as to give the physician a balanced picture of the desirability of its use.

6. All antibiotics are subject to certification procedures.

Labeling Requirements

The following serve to summarize the principal requirements for the labeling of both OTC products and prescription drugs subsequent to the passage of the 1962 Drug Amendments.

Over-The-Counter Drugs. The labeling for OTC products is governed by Section 502(f) of the Federal Food, Drug and Cosmetic Act, which states:

Section 502. A drug . . . shall be deemed to be misbranded—Unless its labeling bears (1) adequate directions for use; and (2) such adequate warnings against use in those pathological conditions or by children where its use may be dangerous to health, or against unsafe dosage or methods or duration of ad-

ministration or application, in such manner and form, as are necessary for the protection of users.

"Adequate directions of use" has been defined in the Regulations as meaning directions under which the layman can use a drug safely and for the purposes for which it is intended.[29]

The label of an over-the-counter drug must name, but need not state the quantity of proportion of, the active ingredients, except for any habit-forming ingredient covered by Section 502(d). The latter also requires that the statement "Warning—May be habit forming" appear on the label "in juxtaposition" with the name of such ingredient, or any of the substances specified in Section 502(e) of the Act.

Warning Notices. A drug may be deemed to be misbranded if it does not contain, in addition to adequate directions for use, adequate warnings against use in certain pathologic conditions (or by children) in which its use may be dangerous to health, or warnings against unsafe dosage or methods or duration of administration or application, in such manner and form as are necessary for the protection of users. Thus, a manufacturer, packager, or distributor must warn against all known hazards. To aid in making these uniform, suggested warning statements for most known hazards are set forth in Sections 369 and 310.201 of the Regulations.[30] These warning statements must contain the full meaning of those suggested, but need not use the identical wording.

Prescription Drugs. The specific requirements for the labeling of a prescription drug are set forth in Part 201.50, Subpart B of the Regulations. It need not bear "adequate directions for use" if it complies with the requirements set forth in that Section, namely, speaking to the practitioner, it must bear "labeling," on or within the package from which the drug is to be dispensed, that sets forth adequate information for its use. This information includes indications, effects, dosages, routes, methods, frequency and duration of administration, relevant hazards, contraindications, side effects, and precautions " . . . under which practitioners licensed by law to administer the drug can use the drug safely and for the purposes for which it is intended, including all purposes for which it is advertised or represented . . . "

With respect to all drugs, Section 502(b) of the act requires the label to provide an accurate statement of the quantity of the contents in terms of weight, measure, or numerical count, as well as the name and place of business of the manufacturer, packer, or distributor.

The label of a prescription drug intended for

oral administration must contain the quantity or proportion of each active ingredient.

If the drug is intended for parenteral administration, the quantity or proportion of all inactive ingredients must also be stated on the label, except that ingredients added to adjust the pH or to make the drug isotonic may be declared by name and a statement of their effect. If the vehicle is water for injection, however, it need not be specifically named.

If the drug is for other than oral use, but is not for parenteral use, e.g., ointment or suppository, the names of all inactive ingredients must be set forth except that flavorings and perfumes may be designated as such without naming their specific components.

Color additives may be designated as coloring without being specifically named, unless this is required in a separate section of the color additive regulations, and trace amounts of harmless substances added solely for individual product identification need not be named.

Warning Notices. The only specific warning required on a prescription label or on the outer container of the package, if the label is too small to accommodate this statement, is: "Caution: Federal law prohibits dispensing without prescription."

Package Inserts. A package insert is not specifically required with any drug; however, since all drugs, whether prescription or over-the-counter, must bear labeling with adequate directions for use if the label of the drug does not permit sufficient space to set forth all the required information, a package insert must be included to contain this required information. Package inserts and labels containing directions for use must include the date of the latest revision of the piece.

In order to satisfy the requirements of Section 201.100 of the regulations, package inserts that are generally included in prescription drug packages must bear "adequate information for its use, including indications, effects, dosages, routes, methods, and frequency and duration of administrations, and any relevant hazards, contraindications, side effects, and precautions under which practitioners licensed by law to administer the drug can use the drug safely and for the purposes for which it is intended, including all purposes for which it is advertised or represented." In order to present the information in a uniform manner, FDA has issued labeling policies,[31] setting forth the format, order, and section headings for package inserts as follows:

Description
Actions

Indications
Contraindications
Warnings
Precautions
Adverse Reactions
Dosage and Administration
Overdosage (Where Applicable)
How Supplied

Optionally, the package insert may contain the following:

Animal Pharmacology and Toxicology
Clinical Studies
References

and other special warnings or precautions peculiar to that particular drug product, which must appear conspicuously in the beginning of the package insert for special attention by physicians and by patients for purposes of safety.

"Contraindications" warn against those conditions in which the drug must not be used because it may actually cause harm to the patient, as through aggravation of an existing condition such as high blood pressure or glaucoma. "Warnings" are utilized in connection with those situations in which the use of the drug might cause a serious problem, such as causing abortion in a pregnant patient. "Precautions" describe instances in which the use of the drug should be closely supervised to avoid undesired side effects that are annoying but not of a serious nature. "Adverse Reactions" warn the physician to look for drug-related conditions that have been known to occur even when the drug is used at the recommended dosage level. These must be taken into account by the physician when he judges the benefit-to-risk ratio of the drug. Adverse reactions warned against need not appear in all patients at all times, but the physician must be made aware of the possibility in order to make a considered judgment in prescribing the drug.

Drug Listing Act of 1972

By the terms of the Kefauver-Harris Amendment of 1962, all producers of drugs and drug products were required to register their establishments with FDA.[32] The effect of registration was twofold: (1) it gave the Food and Drug Administration an updated list of all legitimate manufacturers, and (2) by the operation of the amendment, it required inspection of these producers at least once every two years. It did not, however, provide the Food and Drug Administration with a list of the types of drugs produced at each of these establishments, or with formulas for the many thousands of such drugs. Since the 1962 Amendment required that drugs, whether prescription or over-the-counter, which were deemed to be less than effective come off the market, FDA was faced with the almost insurmountable job of locating all such drugs and taking appropriate action. Regulations have been promulgated, however, under Section 2 of the Drug Listing Act to ensure that sufficient data be sent to the FDA and be computerized for easy handling.

Once the data are fully computerized and classes of drugs can be identified, the FDA intends to use the broad new powers, which it gained in June of 1973 by dint of the four landmark Supreme Court decisions already cited, to move against drug entities deemed to be less than effective. With the DESI and OTC Reviews affecting virtually every drug currently on the market, and with the Supreme Court mandate, FDA feels it need not proceed on a case-by-case basis, but merely needs to locate violative drugs and notify the producer that it intends to take action. If the producer persists in marketing the violative drug, not only will seizure and injunction follow, but use of the criminal penalties of the Act will increase.

Current Good Manufacturing Practice (GMP)

Perhaps the most significant addition to the law is the concept of "current good manufacturing practice" (GMP). This is a requirement that drugs, and the methods used in, or the facilities or controls used in their manufacture, processing, packing, or holding conform with those practices that will assure that such drugs meet the requirements of the Act as to safety, and have the identity, strength, quality, and purity characteristics that they purport or are represented to possess. If they do not, they are adulterated.[33]

What does this mean to a manufacturing pharmacist? The requirement is so broadly stated that it casts a tremendous burden of proof on the Food and Drug Administration, especially in cases where there are arguable variables in methodology, procedure, or equipment. It also casts a heavy burden on the industrial pharmacist, however, because it requires him to produce drug products by using manufacturing practices that are both *current* and *good*. In other words, he must keep up with advances and adopt those that will increase assurance of drug integrity according to the requirements of the Act.

"Current good manufacturing practice" is nowhere defined in the Act or in the regulations. The regulations concern themselves with specific criteria for buildings, equipment, personnel, components, master formula and batch production records, production and control procedures, product containers, packaging and labeling, laboratory controls, distribution records, stability, and complaint files.[34]

These regulations had been promulgated under the general regulatory powers granted in Section 701(a) of the Act. Before the Supreme Court decisions of 1973, these regulations were thought to be interpretive only—not having the force and effect of law. Now, however, it has been held that Section 701(a) regulations *do* have such an effect, and therefore all regulations adopted in final form by FDA must be considered as being a pronouncement of the law, unless and until they are successfully challenged in court.

It would be well, therefore, for the industrial pharmacist to know just what an FDA inspector looks for,[35] both in a sanitary inspection and in a good manufacturing practice inspection. (These may take place separately, but are usually simultaneous.) The generally accepted sanitary inspection checklist is as follows:

1. Human behavior
   (a) Personal hygienic practices of the employees
   (b) Supervision to which employees are subjected

2. Infestation
   (a) Rats, mice, and other vermin
   (b) Flies, roaches, water bugs, and other insects

3. Conditions of equipment and utensils
   (a) Provisions for cleaning these articles

4. Conditions of raw materials
   (a) Sanitary conditions of water and ice supplies

5. Toilets, washing facilities, and their accessibility

6. The plant
   (a) Surroundings, structure in relation to rodent and insect exclusion, cleanliness, and "cleanability"

7. Waste disposal, including methods of sewage disposal of the plant and of other buildings in immediate surroundings, when this information may be of significance

8. Conditions of storage and handling of products, particularly those subject to insect and rodent infestation after the finished product is produced

Under GMP, the inspector will concern himself with other aspects of pharmaceutical manufacturing.

1. Buildings shall be maintained in a clean and orderly manner and shall be of suitable size, construction, and location to facilitate adequate cleaning and maintenance and proper operation in the manufacturing, processing, packing, labeling, or holding of a drug.

2. Equipment used for the manufacture, processing, packing, labeling, holding, testing, or control of drugs shall be maintained in a clean and orderly manner and shall be of suitable design, size, construction, and location to facilitate cleaning, maintenance, and operation.

3. Personnel must be adequate in number and background of education, training, and experience or combination thereof to ensure that the drug has the safety, identity, strength, quality, and purity that it purports to possess, and they must also be in good health.

4. Components and other materials used in the manufacture, processing, and packaging of drug products and materials necessary for building and equipment maintenance must be stored and handled in a safe, sanitary, and orderly manner, with adequate measures taken to prevent mixups and cross-contamination affecting drugs and drug products. They must be withheld from use until they have been identified, sampled, and tested for conformance with established specifications and are released by a materials approval unit.

5. Master production and control records for each drug product and each batch size of drug product shall be prepared, dated, and signed or initialed by a competent and responsible individual, and shall be independently checked, reconciled, dated, signed, or initialed by a second competent and responsible individual to assume uniformity from batch to batch.

6. Production and control procedures shall include all reasonable precautions to assure that the drugs produced have the safety, identity, strength, quality, and purity they are purported to possess, including but not limited to double checking of selection; weighing and measuring of components; the addition of ingredients during the process; proper identification of all containers, lines, and equipment; adequate cleaning facilities to prevent contamination and mixups; appropriate precautions to minimize microbiological and other contamination of the drug or the cross-contamination of any other drugs; adequate in-process checking of weights, measures, and counts at appropriate intervals, and the taking and maintaining of representative samples in process.

7. Product containers and their components must be tested and found to be suitable for their intended use and should not be reactive, additive, or absorptive so as to affect the safety, identity, strength, quality, or purity of the drug or its components.

8. Packaging and labeling operations shall be adequately controlled to assure that only those drug products that have met the standards and specifications established in their master production and control records shall be distributed; to prevent mixups between drugs during filling, packaging, and labeling operations; to assure that correct labels and labeling are employed for the drug; and to identify the finished product with a lot or control number that permits determination of the history of the manufacture and control of the batch.

9. Laboratory controls must include the establishment of scientifically sound and appropriate specifications, standards and test procedures to assure that components, in-process drugs, and finished products conform to appropriate standards of identity, strength, quality, and purity.

10. Distribution records must be kept so that the distribution of each lot of drug can be readily determined to facilitate its recall if necessary, and so that a first-in, first-out warehouse system can be used.

11. Stability of finished drug products must be assured by appropriate means.

12. Suitable expiration dating of drug products must be instituted, especially for those liable to deterioration, so that the drug meets appropriate standards of identity, strength, quality, and purity at the time of use.

13. Complaint files must be maintained, carrying records of all written and oral complaints regarding each product, and an investigation of each complaint must be made and recorded in writing.

Food and Drug Administration (FDA)

The enforcement of the Federal Food, Drug and Cosmetic Act is the responsibility of the Food and Drug Administration, which is a part of the Department of Health and Human Services. The agency is administered by a Commissioner, a Deputy Commissioner, and six Associate Commissioners. It is broken down, at the headquarters level, into five Centers, namely, Foods (which includes cosmetics), Drugs, Devices, Radiological Health, and Veterinary Drugs (which includes veterinary devices).

FDA maintains a headquarters building in the District of Columbia, but its main headquarters activities are at 5600 Fishers Lane, Rockville, MD 20852. There are ten regions and 17 district offices located throughout the United States. These local offices have the prime responsibility for the day-to-day monitoring of manufacturers of products falling within their jurisdiction. New drug applications, food additive petitions, product and plant registration, and the like are handled centrally. Inspectors generally work out of the various district offices, and they, together with their own local laboratory facilities and under the direction of a director, are the prime contact with manufacturers to ensure that products meet regulatory standards.

Inspections may be made without warning during reasonable business hours and may encompass the buildings in which drugs are manufactured or in which raw materials or bulk drugs are held, including vehicles in which such drugs are held or are being transported. Section 704 of the Act gives wide latitude to the scope of inquiry, which may be made into all areas of plant administration, from housecleaning to the qualifications of those responsible for production and quality control, as well as production records, formulas, assays, and all quality-control documents kept in the regular course of business.

Following the adoption of the 1962 Amendments, all plants manufacturing pharmaceutical products were required to be registered. The requirement also included a mandate that FDA inspect each such establishment at least once every two years. Such inspections cannot be refused if made at a reasonable hour and if the inspector shows proper credentials and presents a formal "Notice of Inspection." At the conclusion of an inspection, an inspector may take samples, for which he is required to give a receipt,[36] and if requested, to provide for payment for the articles taken. In addition, if the inspection warrants it, a report of deficiencies noted by the inspector is written out and delivered to the person in charge of the establishment. These reports can form the basis for regulatory action should they be serious enough or if, on a subsequent inspection, the deficiencies have not been satisfactorily corrected.

FDA Enforcement Powers

Inasmuch as the Federal Food, Drug and Cosmetic Act is a criminal statute, FDA activities are discussed in terms of enforcement. If necessary, legal action can be taken against any party violating the Act. Such action can take one of the following forms.

1. Seizure.[37] Whenever FDA believes that a drug product that has traveled in interstate commerce, or is being held for shipment into interstate commerce, is in some way violative of the Act, a so-called monition or complaint against the articles themselves is drawn up and presented to the United States Attorney in the District where the goods are located. He then proceeds to make this case *ex parte* (without an adversary present) before a Federal Judge sitting

in that district. The monition is an *in rem* proceeding, that is, it is a proceeding against the articles to be seized for condemnation. Since the articles themselves are the defendant in the case, the owner, usually the manufacturer, if he wishes to resist the seizure, becomes an "intervenor," that is, alleging ownership, he files a claim for the goods and thus becomes the litigant. Under the law, seizure can be made in only one district of one quantity of the product unless: (1) the Commissioner of Food and Drugs finds that the goods represent a significant hazard to health, or (2) he finds that the drug is claimed to be a new drug, in which case multiple seizures may take place. Drugs seized can be destroyed if there is no intervenor or if intervention is not successful. After intervention, the drugs can, under proper safeguards, be released back to the intervenor for relabeling to bring them in compliance with the Act, or they can be returned to the manufacturer under bond for reworking if that will cure the misfeasance.

2. Injunction.[38] An injunction is a legal term describing a court-directed prohibition against a person, firm, or corporation doing a particular act. Generally, in the case of industrial pharmacy, it can be against the production of a drug not in compliance with GMP or the selling or shipping of such drug in interstate commerce, or against certain advertising or promotion found to be violative of the Act. The issuance of an injunction is not a function of the FDA. FDA must go to court and prove to a Federal District Judge that there is a violation of the law sufficient to cause him to invoke the extraordinary remedy of injunction. The burden of proof is on FDA, and because of the extraordinary nature of the remedy, it is a heavy burden. Injunction is a regulatory tool rarely used.

3. Criminal Prosecution.[39] Criminal action may be taken against persons, corporations, or responsible officers. A penalty of $1,000 or one year in jail for an unintentional first offense may be exacted, or $10,000 and three years if the offense was committed with intent to defraud or mislead, or by a previous offender. The latter form of action is relatively rare, and would normally involve a wanton disregard of the law.

Prior to the institution of criminal proceedings, however, Section 305 of the Act provides for an informal hearing procedure whereby the manufacturer may present to an FDA hearing officer explanations for and circumstances behind the activities cited.[40] The hearing officer may receive documentary as well as oral evidence, after which he prepares a report, uniformly dictated in the presence of the respondent. He asks the respondent to agree that the facts so stated are those presented by him, and in addition, gives the respondent a chance to add explanatory matter to the report. The hearing report, with the hearing officer's recommendation, is then forwarded to the compliance branch in Washington for final disposition. This informal hearing procedure is important, both for the manufacturer and for the FDA. It affords the manufacturer a hearing at a level higher than that of the inspector, and it gives the FDA a chance to reevaluate its regulatory thinking in the light of such explanation. Thus, the procedure avoids unnecessary litigation and acts as a buffer against precipitous action, either by the regulating authority or by the regulated industry.

Other Federal Laws Affecting the Industry

There are other laws with which the industrial pharmacist should be familiar. Perhaps the most important is the Fair Packaging and Labeling Act, which is administered by both the Food and Drug Administration and the Federal Trade Commission (FTC). The Fair Packaging and Labeling Act is designed primarily to protect the consumer by requiring a prominent display of statements of net contents and ingredients on the principal display panel of consumer packaging. The law has certain specific requirements concerning the placement and size of this information. Violation of the provisions of this Act might lead to seizure by FDA or to a cease and desist order from the FTC.

Often the product development chemist is involved in helping to create advertising claims and copy. To do this, he should understand the regulatory agency concerned with these matters. The FTC (Federal Trade Commission), operating under the Federal Trade Commission Act, has jurisdiction over the advertising and promotion of all consumer products including drugs and cosmetics. This authority extends to all advertising media and is concerned with deceptive advertising practices and with promotion that is deemed to be false and misleading. Since there is some overlap between the jurisdictions of the FTC and the FDA, there has been an agreement between these agencies to the effect that, in general, the FTC would monitor advertising of OTC drugs and cosmetic products insofar as false and misleading claims might be concerned, whereas the FDA would have responsibility for drug labeling and all advertising relating to prescription drugs. The reason for this agreement, of course, is to avoid unnecessary duplication of enforcement procedures. The agencies have a close working relationship, with the FTC relying in large measure on FDA for its scientific expertise.

Since the industrial pharmacist is generally involved with FDA inspections, it might be interesting to note in passing that the federal statutes relating to crimes and criminal procedure make it a crime to forcibly assault, resist, oppose, impede, intimidate, or interfere with an FDA inspector during the performance of his official duties. Any such offense carries with it a fine of not more than $5,000 or imprisonment for not more than 3 years, or both. If any of the aforementioned acts entails the use of a dangerous weapon, the fine may be as high as $10,000 and the imprisonment up to 10 years, or both.

The Color Additives Amendments of 1960, which are a part of the Federal Food, Drug and Cosmetic Act, specify that no product is to contain any unsafe color additive. An unsafe color additive is defined in Section 706(a) 21 USC 376 of the Act as a drug ingredient that has been added for purposes of color only, but not in conformity with a regulation issued under the Act, or not from a batch certified in accordance with proper regulation, or not otherwise exempt from regulation by FDA.

The Post Office Department prohibits shipments of poisons, explosives, or injurious or fraudulent materials through the mails and has jurisdiction over drugs falling within this definition. Violations are subject to seizure and fine.

The Alcohol Tax Division of the Internal Revenue Service has jurisdiction over the use of alcohol in the formulation of drugs. Specially denatured alcohol may be purchased for industrial use at a fully taxed price. After manufacture of the drug, using such denatured alcohol, the manufacturer may file a claim showing that it has been used in the manufacture of a product unfit for beverage purposes. This qualifies the manufacturer for a recovery of most of the tax, known as a tax "drawback."

Should the industrial pharmacist be involved in the manufacture of narcotics or other controlled substances, such manufacture is within the ambit of the Controlled Substances Act and regulations thereunder. The Drug Enforcement Agency (DEA) maintains a quota system for the manufacture of controlled substances and generally monitors this production by the use of established yield ratios. Periodic inspection by agents of the DEA are made for the purposes of verifying accountability and security against loss. Regulations are not only concerned with manufacture of controlled substances, but also with provisions against the diversion of these drugs.

If a hearing becomes necessary under any provision of the Federal Food, Drug and Cosmetic Act or the Controlled Substances Act, it is conducted under the provisions of the Administrative Procedure Act, unless a specific hearing procedure is set forth in the principal Act.[41] Records, letters, memoranda, and other documents pertaining to particular drugs and/or to matters pertinent to a hearing may be requested under the provisions of the Freedom of Information Act. The FDA generally allows inspection of all such documents except (1) internal memoranda relating to the regulatory aspects of the administration; (2) INDs or NDAs and the material contained therein withdrawn or otherwise expired NDAs or INDs lie in a gray area, with the FDA leaning toward disclosure, but with the overwhelming sentiment of the industry being that these should remain confidential; and (3) materials marked confidential upon submission on request of the FDA by a regulated company. Such material will remain confidential unless called for by a third party, at which time the party claiming confidentiality must prove to the satisfaction of the FDA that the material is indeed confidential; the test is generally whether or not the release of such material will place the person, firm, or corporation submitting it at a competitive disadvantage.

Finally, there are several other acts that are too specialized for discussion here, but that may also be of interest to the industrial pharmacist. Their titles are fairly indicative of the subject matter of the contents:

Animal Welfare Act
Caustic Poison Act
Controlled Substances Act
Controlled Substances Import and Export Act
Drug Abuse Office and Treatment Act
Hazardous Substances Act
Insecticide, Fungicide and Rodenticide Act (Economic Poisons Act)
Poison Prevention Packaging Act of 1970
Virus Serum and Toxin Act of 1944

State and Local Regulations

The right of any governmental authority to pass laws for the protection of its citizens is an inherent one. This right is called the "police power," and it is the basis upon which laws regulating drugs and drug products, and their manufacture, distribution, and sale are predicated. It is not unusual for such laws to exist in large municipalities as well as at the state and federal levels. These laws generally deal with misbranding and adulteration, false advertising, and the maintenance of sanitary conditions. In order to sort out the proper jurisdiction under which a particular manufacturing operation is conducted, a body of law known as "preemption" has evolved.

The doctrine of preemption means that when a greater and a lesser authority (i.e., a state and municipality or the federal government and the state) both regulate a particular activity such as the production of pharmaceutical products, and find they are in conflict, the highest authority is most often deemed to have preempted the regulatory field, and the law of the higher authority prevails.

As with all general rules, the doctrine of preemption has subrules. For example, if an operation is strictly an intrastate one, and there is no interstate commerce involved, the federal law cannot attach. Similarly, if there is an overriding "local" concern, as for example a more stringent control of the holding or transportation of narcotics for legitimate local reasons, then the more stringent local rule would apply.

Lest it be thought that a strictly intrastate business, if it embraces the practice of industrial pharmacy, might be conducted only under state law, the courts have increasingly taken the view that the federal law is applicable on a very broad scale. For example, it has been held that if any component used in the manufacture of a drug has at any time been shipped in interstate commerce, federal jurisdiction attaches. Since most components in a drug have been purchased and shipped from an out-of-state supplier, one can readily understand that an almost universal federal jurisdiction applies to the regulation of drug products.

There is a uniform state Food, Drug and Cosmetic Bill, which is patterned largely after the federal statute, and which has been endorsed by the Executive Committee of the Association of Food and Drug Officials of the United States. It has been adopted in many states, and with certain modifications, those states dealing with the manufacture of drugs, even if they themselves do not use the uniform statute, lean heavily on federal law and definitions. The District of Columbia is, of course, regulated by the federal Act.

Most states provide purity, labeling, and packaging requirements that are applicable to a "drug," and these are defined most frequently in language identical or similar to that of the federal Act. All but 17 states prohibit the marketing of a new drug (which is defined in federal terms) until a new drug application has been filed with FDA and has been approved. The drug labeling requirements of each of the states, as governed by their local laws, appear in Table 28-1.

Intellectual and Industrial Property

The term "intellectual and industrial property" generally is understood to refer to patents, trademarks, and copyrights. There is often uncertainty, however, regarding the rights each of these embraces and the manner in which each is obtained. There is also that nebulous something called "know-how" and that further something called "trade secrets." Perhaps most important for the industrial pharmacist is the ability to recognize the rights, duties, and obligations inherent in each of these concepts—as applied to others as well as to himself.

Briefly, a *patent* is a statutory grant of monopoly for a period of years during which an inventor can exclude others from making, using, or selling his invention. The right is absolute as long as the validity of the patent is upheld. A *trademark,* on the other hand, does not derive its value or indeed its validity from a statutory grant. The right to the exclusive use of a trademark is derived primarily from the common law in that it must be properly used by the person claiming ownership, and such use may be challenged by another even though there is a federal or state registration. *Registration* is merely a procedural tool in that it serves as notice of use and claim of ownership. A *copyright* (often confused with a trademark) is a statutory grant given to creators of artistic or literary works, so that they might enjoy the fruits of their intellectual labors for a period of years without fearing plagiarism or other copying.

Know-how is a term widely used to describe the accumulated knowledge of a person, a group of persons, or, in some instances, a corporate entity. It describes the general intelligence concerning either the manufacturing, or particular steps in the manufacturing, of a product or products and embraces the experience of years, largely empiric, that is generally claimed to impart particular qualities of elegance or superiority to the product manufactured in that manner. "Know-how," if not patentable, is carefully husbanded by the owner and usually passed on only to those who need to know in order to continue the production of the product. In general, it is knowledge that is common, but that involves a particular application within the production procedure to accomplish its beneficial results.

Trade secrets, on the other hand, are generally those bits of knowledge or ingenuity that may well be patentable, but for reasons best known to the keeper of the secrets, are not imparted to the general public. One explanation for the keeping of a trade secret is that if it is exposed in a patent, it can only be monopolized for a short period of years, generally 17, after which it can be used by others with impunity. As long as the secret is kept a secret, its use can be exclusive for an indefinite period. The law recognizes and protects genuine trade secrets. Each of these subjects are discussed subsequently, with emphasis being placed on patents because they represent the most likely area of industrial property and intellectual protection for the industrial pharmacist.

Patents

Nature of the Grant. In the United States, the protection of industrial property by patent has its genesis in the Constitution, Article I, Section 8, which states:

The Congress shall have Power . . . to promote the Progress of Science in useful Arts, by securing, for limited Times to Authors and Inventors the exclusive Right to their respective Writings and Discoveries.

This recognition, by those farsighted founders of this country, of the essential means of promoting industrial advance has been the backbone of technologic and economic growth in the United States since its inception. By rewarding the inventive mind with a monopoly, others are prompted to absorb the teaching and improve on it. A patent is a right granted by the United States Government to an inventor to exclude others from making, using, and selling his invention for a period of years (usually 17) in exchange for the benefits to be gained by disclosing the invention to others and to have the knowledge in the public domain following the period of exclusive use.

Most countries of the world have patent laws. They vary so widely in their requirements that it would be impossible to enumerate the differences in this chapter. It is useful to know, however, that since the general rule in foreign countries is to grant a patent to the first party filing for it, such filing should be done as rapidly as possible after the issuance of the United States Patent. Some measure of protection is afforded to the United States patent owner by an international Convention to which the United States belongs. The convention provides that a patent application filed in a foreign country within one year of its first filing in a Convention country is given the earlier filing date. The following discussion relates only to United States Patent law.

Requirements. To be patentable, an invention must be new, useful, and not obvious to one skilled in the art to which the invention pertains. To be new, the article must be novel, that is, of a novelty requiring more than the use of journeymen skills in the field to which the invention applies. And newness alone does not support patentability.

The requirement that the development not be obvious is the main criterion for patentability. An invention or development may not be obvious for several reasons. The results obtained from the use of the development are unexpected, that is, they are outside the general theory pertaining to the combination of the various ingredients. This concept is also related to lack of obviousness that might come about by way of synthesization, with unexpected results arising from the utilization of two or more known features in a combination resulting in something greater than a mere sum of known effects. The invention may relate to new compositions of matter as in the synthesis of a new chemical entity, which must not be an obvious variation of the prior art compounds or compositions. The invention might also be a new approach to solving technical problems or even for the production of a new plant strain.

To be useful, the invention must be able to be reduced to practice, and must perform in a predictable manner in accordance with the claims made for such performance in the Patent application. For other than pharmaceutical inventions, utility is rarely a problem. The United States Patent Office has taken an increasingly stringent position with respect to utility data for pharmaceuticals, particularly those intended for the treatment of serious illness. The claims for utility should be written clearly and concisely with as much detail as possible to prove that the product will perform in a uniform manner with a predictable result. Patent coverage can be obtained on compositions of matter, apparatuses, new processes of manufacture, new article of manufacture, and asexually reproduced plants.

For the sake of completeness, it should be mentioned that design patents may be issued. These are generally for nonfunctional elements of an article of manufacture. The period of design patent exclusivity is much shorter, running usually for a period of 7 years.

Finally, in addition to being new, useful, and not obvious, the invention must not be barred by having been previously known, used, or sold publicly in the United States, or patented or described in a publication anywhere in the world before the invention by the applicant, or more than one year prior to the filing of the application obtaining a patent.

Since strong proof of the date of conception is the inventor's best insurance for obtaining his patent, he should keep careful notes, preferably in a bound notebook, giving a brief description of the invention and the manner in which it is expected to work. This record should be dated by the inventor, and should be witnessed by at least one other person who is able to understand the invention. Often, in an interference or a litigation involving two or more claimants, this early record can be controlling.

An *interference* is a procedural device used by the Patent Office and is declared when different inventors have applied for the same invention. Since uncorroborated testimony of the inventor as to the date of invention is not admissible, a failure to make early disclosure records as noted above can lead to the loss of valuable rights. The attesting witness might have to give testimony at a later date, and therefore the fullest explanation of the invention and the manner in which it operates should be given to the witness, since he will later have to describe in detail that which was explained to him.

Although it is not necessary to reduce an invention to practice, there must be in the application enough detail to enable one skilled in the art to practice it. Patent applications for pharmaceuticals generally are not filed until the utility of the pharmaceutical has been determined, and this, in a sense, is "reduction to practice."

When an invention is made and sufficient data gathered to prove it useful, the next step should be a disclosure to a patent attorney, who will then follow several prescribed steps to obtain the patent. He will usually want to do a search of the prior art in an effort to determine novelty. Such a search is not required by the rules of the Patent Office, but a careful patent attorney will want the information so as not to waste the time and money of his client or the time of the patent examiner.

Once satisfied that the invention has all the elements of patentability, the patent attorney draws up the application, the principal portions of which are the specification and the claims. The specification is a detailed description of the invention, including general and preferred versions, with necessary supporting data when ap-

Table 28-1. *Drug Labeling Requirements Chart*[*]

State	Name and Place of Business	Quantity of Contents	Name of Drug	Names of Ingredients	Quantity or Proportion of Certain Ingredients	Directions for Use	"Habit-Forming" Warning	Precaution Against Deterioration	Warnings Where Use May Be Dangerous	Special Labeling Requirements for Official Drugs
AL	X	X			X		X			
AK	X	X	X	X	X	X	X	X	X	X
AZ	X	X	X	X	X	X	X	X	X	X
AR	X	X	X	X	X	X	X	X	X	X
CA	X	X	X	X	X	X	X	X	X	X
CO	X	X	X	X	X	X	X	X	X	X
CT	X	X	X	X	X	X	X	X		X
DE					X					X
DC[†]										
FL	X	X	X	X	X	X	X	X	X	X
GA	X	X	X	X	X	X	X	X	X	X
HI	X	X	X	X	X	X	X	X	X	X
ID	X	X	X	X	X	X	X	X	X	X
IL	X	X	X	X	X	X	X	X	X	X
IN	X	X	X	X	X	X	X	X	X	X
IA	X	X	X	X	X	X	X	X	X	X
KS	X	X	X	X	X	X	X	X	X	X
KY	X	X	X		X	X	X	X	X	X
LA	X	X	X	X	X	X	X	X		X
ME	X	X	X	X	X					
MD	X	X	X	X	X	X	X	X	X	X
MA	X		X	X	X	X	X	X	X	X
MI	X									

MN	X	X	X	X	X	X	X	X
MS								X
MO	X	X	X	X	X	X	X	X
MT	X	X	X	X	X	X	X	X
NE	X				X			X
NV	X	X	X	X	X	X	X	X
NH	X	X	X	X	X	X	X	X
NJ	X	X	X	X	X		X	X
NM	X	X	X	X	X	X	X	X
NY	X	X	X	X	X	X	X	X
NC	X	X	X	X	X	X	X	X
ND	X	X	X	X	X	X	X	X
OH	X	X	X	X	X	X	X	X
OK	X	X	X	X	X		X	X
OR	X	X	X	X	X	X	X	X
PA	X	X	X	X	X	X	X	X
RI	X	X	X	X	X	X	X	X
SC					X			
SD					X			
TN	X	X	X	X	X	X	X	X
TX	X	X	X	X	X	X	X	X
UT	X	X	X	X	X	X	X	X
VT	X	X	X	X	X	X	X	X
VA	X	X	X	X	X	X	X	X
WA	X	X	X	X	X	X	X	X
WV								
WI								
WY	X	X		X	X			X

*Any specific provision of any state law as applied to a particular manufacturing plant or operation should, of course, be checked by a person qualified to make a judgment as to the applicability of the statute and its provisions.

†The provisions of the Federal Act are applicable to commerce within the District of Columbia.

plicable. A specification also may include drawings, graphs, or any other aids to the understanding of the invention. If the prior art search has uncovered references, these may also be included in the specification, and distinguishing features of the invention for which patent is sought should be set forth. All of this is designed to enable one skilled in the art to understand the invention and to employ it.

Perhaps the most critical part of the application is the section containing claims, which appear as a series of numbered paragraphs setting forth the scope of the patent protection sought. These claims are important because, when a patent is granted, the claims form the basis of exclusivity and determine whether another has infringed on the issued patent. Beginning with the first of the numbered paragraphs, claims are presented in the order of the broadest protection sought to the narrowest embodiment of the invention. Since the claims determine infringement, they should include all of the elements of the invention, because no patent protection is accorded subject matter disclosed in the specification, only subject matter specifically claimed in the claims section.

Once all specifications and claims are written, the necessary formal documents, including an oath by the inventor, are completed, an attorney is appointed, and the application is filed with the Patent Office and receives an application number and a filing date. It is thereafter examined by a patent examiner, who is generally a person trained or skilled in the art relating to the invention. Should questions arise in the mind of the examiner, he asks in writing for clarification or limitation or other remedial steps. These are called Office Actions, to which responses by the inventor are invited—indeed, are mandatory if the patent is to be issued. Following these actions, the application is allowed in all of its parts, in some of its parts, or in a restricted way, or it is finally rejected. There is an appeal procedure from final rejection, but if it is not successful, the application either becomes abandoned or may be further appealed to the Patent Office Board of Appeals, which is the final agency review. The Board is a tribunal of three highly qualified Patent Office experts who pass on the merits of the examiner's and the applicant's positions. The decision of the Board may be appealed to the Court of Customs and Patent Appeals or to any United States District Court having jurisdiction. Elapsed time from application to allowance without an appeal is generally considered to be more than two years but less than four. Appeals, of course, may make the time span longer.

General Comments. Since the benefits derived from a patent are manifold, certain restrictions must be kept in mind both by the inventor and by those who would use the invention. A patent grants the right to exclude others from making, using, and selling the invention, but this right may be restricted if the patent is subordinate to another. For instance, a new chemical entity that has been granted a patent may be taken by a second inventor and combined with another compound to form a new and useful compound, the properties of which were not obvious to those skilled in the art. Thus, to practice the teaching of the second invention, one would of necessity have to reward the original inventor.

Licensing is a system of rewarding the original inventor and to otherwise authorize the practice of the invention by persons other than the inventor. The license grants the right to make, to use, or to sell the invention, or any appropriate combination of these rights. A licensor is usually given periodic payments, called royalties, for the term of the patent. Of course, it is also possible, after negotiation, to purchase the rights to a patent from the inventory by an outright lump sum payment.

Patent licensing is a delicate endeavor today, since there have been decisions in the antitrust area which tend to restrict the types of license that might be granted. For instance, it has been held in certain cases to be a violation of the antitrust laws to license an invention in only one area of the marketplace and not in another—for example, to license the use of the invention in oral dosage forms to one licensee and in parenteral dosage forms to another licensee. Inattention to these important interdictions (which at this writing tend to become more and more restrictive) could lead to the imposition of fines, both on the licensor and the licensee, or in more aggravated cases, the loss of patent protection entirely.

Applications for patents in the United States are submitted in the name of the inventor, and he personally receives the grant of patent. In the larger industrial centers, including pharmaceutical manufacturers, it is common practice for the inventor to assign the patent application to his employer in consideration of his continued employment, that is, inasmuch as he was hired to do the research and was given the facilities to do it by the employer, he is expected to make the proper assignment. Usually, a contract covers this right of the employer to receive and benefit from the inventions of his employee. When no such contract exists and the inventor balks at an assignment, a legal doctrine of "shop right" becomes operative. This is a right that belongs to the employer, who has implicitly been given the right to use the invention because he supplied the necessary support for the inventor, and allows him to use the patent even though title remains in the name of the inventor.

If there is more than one inventor, that is, if two or more individuals have contributed to the conception and/or the reduction to practice of the invention, each contributor is separately named and becomes a "co-inventor." The important thing to remember about co-inventors is that each may separately exploit the patent, unless there is a contractual agreement among them to act in concert. Therefore, one having an interest as a licensee in a patent for which there are co-inventors, especially if that interest is exclusive, should either obtain a license from all or have the noncontracting inventors agree on the licensing document to the exclusivity of the license granted.

An inventor can stop an infringement by applying to a Federal court for relief, which is generally available in two forms. One is *injunction,* that is, a judicially imposed restriction against the infringer from continuing to make, use, or sell the invention; the other involves an award of damages to the inventor for past infringement.

Since there can be no infringement prior to the issuing of the patent, the inventor who wishes to exclude others even during the pendancy of his application can mark his product with the phrases "Patent Pending" or "Patent Applied For." These phrases serve as warnings to putative infringers that they make, use, or sell the invention at their peril. Notices on goods that bear patent numbers, of course, refer to already issued patents, and infringement after issue can result in damages generally based on the measure of sales lost by the patent holder.

Finally, it should not be overlooked that issued patents in any particular field are a rich source of research data. Further, because countries foreign to the United States may issue patents earlier than the U.S. Patent Office, foreign inventions should be monitored, as they are often the first indication of new technologic developments in the United States.

Trademarks

A trademark, unlike a patent, is not a statutory grant of monopoly. A trademark is any word, name, symbol, or device that a manufacturer or trader places on his goods to distinguish them from goods manufactured or sold by others. The validity of a trademark is tested by its proper use,

not by the fact of registration. The registration of a trademark may be accomplished either in a state having a trademark registration statute or at the Federal level. To be registered in the United States Patent Office, the trademark must be used on goods that have actually travelled in interstate commerce.

Thus, the application for a trademark must await the first use of that mark in interstate commerce, the date of which, along with the date of its first use anywhere, must appear on the application. The trademark must not be descriptive of the goods or any of its properties (although it may be "suggestive"); it must not be so similar to prior registrations as to cause confusion as to the source of origin of the goods; it must not be immoral or deceptive; and it must not utilize the flag or insignia of the United States or the portrait or likeness of any living individual without that individual's consent. Trademark protection extends over a period of 20 years, and is renewable indefinitely as long as the trademark continues to be used by its owner. Ownership of a trademark is transferable by assignment, and the use thereof is able to be licensed.

A trademark represents good will. The considerable value of such good will often cannot be determined in units of absolute dollars. For instance, if by some quirk of massive misfortune, all the Coca-Cola bottling plants in the United States should burn down today, there would be no question that because of the extensive good will in that trademark alone, the necessary financing could be had to begin to rebuild the plants tomorrow.

A registered trademark may be infringed by others who use the same mark or a similar mark on the same or similar goods or on goods that travel in the same channels of trade. The legal determination for an infringement is whether the second user of the mark confuses the buying public regarding the originator of the goods on which the mark appears.

Since the axiom is that trademark rights are gained only by proper use, it is possible to have an infringement of an unregistered mark. An action for such infringement is generally couched in terms of the law of unfair competition, of which the trademark laws have uniformly been held to be a subdivision.

A word trademark is a name; it is a special part of the language having unusual characteristics. It should always be used in conjunction with a generic or descriptive term, for instance, Librium, brand of chlordiazepoxide. The use of a descriptive or generic term preserves the function of the trademark as a symbol pointing to the source of origin and not as a descriptive term for the article itself. The trademark might be rendered invalid if it is not used at all or if it is used improperly, that is, if it falls into the common language to describe the article. Prime examples of trademarks that have been lost by such improper use are aspirin, cellophane, and escalator. Trademark owners jealously guard their rights, and more popular trademarks become the subject of letters to publishers or printers to remind them that the trademark should always be printed either in all-caps or at least in initial caps, generally with quotation marks and *never* in the possessive.

A claim to trademark rights is generally printed by the claimant on the goods and in advertisements relating to the goods. Prior to Federal registration, the symbol "TM" is generally used in conjunction with the mark. After registration, the symbol ® or the phrases "Trademark Registered," "Trademark Registered in the United States Patent Office," or "TM Reg. U.S. Pat. Off." are used. These notices serve, as with patent notices, to tell would-be infringers that they adopt this mark at their peril. Infringement and unfair competition actions may be brought in United States District Courts in the case of Federally registered trademarks or in state courts on counts of unfair competition. Damages are awarded against infringers based on an assessment of the damage that the infringement has caused to the goodwill of the trademark owner.

A trade name, for which registration also is permitted, is distinguishable from a trademark in that the trade name identifies the manufacturer or trader rather than the goods themselves. For instance, Schering-Plough Inc. is a trade name identifying a manufacturer; Coricidin is that manufacturer's well-known brand name for a product for the relief of the symptoms of colds.

Unfair Competition

The law of unfair competition is almost as old as the common law itself. Essentially, it is the effort of the law to referee in the marketplace and to maintain fair and open competition among traders. It covers a vast array of commercial wrongs, some of which, e.g., the Patent and Trademark laws, have been codified. Complaints in the area of unfair competition generally seek relief under the principles of both equity and law. That is, they seek specific performance or specific nonperformance (injunction), which is an outgrowth of the ancient laws of equity, or they seek money damages (law), or both. In all of

the jurisdictions in the United States today, both law and equity relief can be sought in one court rather than in separate courts, which our common law adopted from the ancient English practice, but which has now been uniformly replaced by the single jurisdiction system.

One possible grievance in an unfair competition action is interference with a contractual relationship. Such interference could take the form of commercial disparagement, that is, disparagement of the name of a company or of its product; the hiring of an employee to gain insight into the prior employer's business practices or customers; or some other inducement of a breach of contract by one party to the detriment of another.

The law of unfair competition also provides for protection of know-how and trade secrets, which are as much a property right as a patent or a trademark. Although the theft or disclosure of these is actionable, anyone innocently receiving knowledge of a trade secret or know-how in the usual course of his business may practice such knowledge with impunity. This points up the peril of attempting to keep commercial secrets, since their only protection lies in their freedom from theft. For this reason, when secret information is received or given, it is usually done on the basis of a "confidential disclosure." It should be given in writing, with the receiver acknowledging and promising to maintain its confidentiality.

Finally, the law of unfair competition prevents the palming-off of the goods of one trader as being those of another, as in false advertising and in misleading statements made by sales personnel. Recent decisions have narrowed the scope of this type of protection in that elements of an article not protected by United States patents or trademark registrations may be copied with impunity. Thus, nonfunctional features, even though they are unique with the original user and might serve to indicate origin, cannot be held exclusively unless the originator can show that these nonfunctional features have gained "secondary meaning," and are attributed in the minds of purchasers with the originator only and with no one else. In other words, it serves to identify the goods as coming from a particular manufacturer or trader.

Copyrights

A copyright is a statutory grant of monopoly for a period of years. Generally, it is for 27 years renewable for another 27 years by the copyright owner or his heirs or assigns. After that, the copyrighted material falls into the public domain and can be used by anyone.

Copyright protection may be granted for works of art and literature, and a copyright carries with it, as does a patent, the right to exclude others from reproducing the work of art or literature without compensation to the copyright owner. A copyright is obtained by the filing of an application on which is stated the nature of the work; in the case of published literature or music, a copy is filed with the Library of Congress. For works of art, such as painting and sculpture, generally a picture will suffice. The danger inherent in the publication of a copyrightable work lies in the fact that rights gained through copyright might be lost if a proper copyright notice is not placed on the article *before* it is published or otherwise made public. Thus, a musical composition performed before an audience or a book disseminated widely without a printed claim of copyright almost invariably causes that work of art to fall immediately into the public domain. Since it is so easy to lose copyright rights, competent advice should be sought whenever a new work of art or literature is to be made available for public sale or use. The Copyright Office in the Library of Congress supplies the forms necessary for copyright application, but since application is an after-the-fact event, advice concerning proper notice should be sought at an early stage in the development of the work of art or literature.

Copyright rights are commonly claimed by the use of the phrase: Copyright, year, name of the copyright claimant. The symbol © might also be used as: © year, name of claimant.

Product Liability

The manufacture of a product that is to be purchased for use or consumption carries with it the responsibility to make that product as free from hazard as possible. The law of product liability is a common law concept. Broadly stated, it gives redress to a purchaser based on the concept of breach of contract or of negligence, or some combination of the two. The breach of contract, a legal fiction, holds that there is an implied warranty of merchantability of the goods for their intended use, that is, if used in the manner prescribed by the manufacturer or seller, there will be no hazard inuring to the purchaser or user. Increasingly, state laws are being so broadened as to remove the need for a direct relationship (as at the old common law) between the purchaser and the seller. The anomalous situation, for instance, wherein a child hurt by a product bought by a parent could not recover because the purchase was not made by the person injured (the privity doctrine), has largely been abandoned. The implication of liability has been so broadened that virtually anyone using the product and being hurt can, upon a showing that the product was properly used (or at least not abused), be compensated for the injury.

The other concept is that of negligence, that is, the product or food was manufactured in such a way that it contained a defect that should have been eliminated or discovered by the manufacturer. Thus, the article, when placed in the hands of the consumer, carries with it an inherent danger even if properly used. The burden on pharmaceutical manufacturers is especially heavy, their product by its very nature being potentially dangerous; however, strict adherence to current good manufacturing practices and stringent quality control are the pharmaceutical manufacturer's best protection.

References

1. 21 United States Code (USC) 301 et seq.
2. 21 USC 321 (g) (1).
3. 21 USC 321 (k).
4. 21 USC 321 (m).
5. 21 USC 321 (p).
6. 21 USC 321 (w), which was added by Section 102(e) of the Animal Drug Amendments of 1968, PL 90-399, 90th Congress, effective August 1, 1969.
7. 21 USC 321 (x), which was added by Section 102(e) of the Animal Drug Amendments of 1968, ibid.
8. Constitution of the United States, Section 8, "The Congress shall have Power . . . To regulate Commerce with foreign Nations, and among the several states, and with the Indian tribes . . . "
9. Insulin Amendment of 1941.
   Antibiotic Amendments of 1945, 1947, 1949, and 1962.
   Prescription Drug (Durham-Humphrey) Amendment of 1951.
   Pesticides (Miller) Amendments of 1954.
   Procedural (Hale) Amendments of 1954 and 1956.
   Food Additives Amendment of 1958.
   Color Additives Amendment of 1960.
   Drug (Kefauver-Harris) Amendments of 1962.
   Drug Abuse Control Amendments of 1965.
   Animal Drug Amendments of 1968.
   Controlled Substances Act of 1970.
   Drug Listing Act of 1972.
   Vitamins and Minerals Amendment of 1976.
   Medical Device Amendment of 1976. (This "amendment" is itself longer than the basic act.)
10. Kefauver-Harris Amendments, Public Law (PL) 87-781, 87th Congress, October 10, 1962.
11. Section 102(c) of the Drug Amendments of 1962, amending Section 505(d) (21 USC 355 (d)) of the 1938 Act.
12. 21 Code of Federal Regulations (CFR) Part 312.
13. 21 CFR 310(h).
14. 21 CFR 56.101–56.124 (1983 ed.).
15. IRBs must keep detailed records of their proceedings,

and if they refuse to make those records available to the FDA, the agency may refuse to evaluate any IND data involving such an IRB. 21 CFR 56.115(c) (1983 ed.).

16. 21 CFR 314.1(f).
17. Section 201(w) (21 USC 321(w)) and Section 201(x) (21 USC 321(x)) respectively.
18. 21 CFR 433.1 (1983 ed.). This proposal was made on May 4, 1982 (47 FR 19954), and published in final form on September 7, 1982 (47 FR 39155).
19. 21 CFR 429.40 (1983 ed.).
20. This classification, which no longer exists, was meant to provide for the situation in which a particular drug entity might be considered to be effective, but its use must be restricted to certain dosage ranges or must not be in combination with other drugs, or must be administered in some special way. Since the "but" was not a uniform consideration, however, these classifications were returned to the panels for their determination of the effectiveness of the drug, and if there were conditions on such effectiveness, these were to be stated in proposed labeling.
21. American Public Health Association and National Council of Senior Citizens v. John G. Veneman, Acting Secretary of HEW, and Charles Edwards, Commissioner of FDA, 349 F. Supp. 1311, DC, 1972.
22. Section of 107(c)(4) of Public Law 87-781, provided: In the case of any drug which, on the day immediately preceding the enactment date, [October 10, 1962] (A) was commercially used or sold in the United States, (B) was not a new drug as defined by Section 201(p) of the Basic Act as then in force and (C) was not covered by an effective application under Section 505 of that Act, the amendments to Section 201(p) made by this Act under conditions prescribed, recommended, or suggested in labeling with respect to such drug on that day.
23. Casper W. Weinberger, Secretary of Health, Education & Welfare et al. v. Bentex Pharmaceuticals, Inc., et al., 412 U.S. 645, 1973.
24. USV Pharmaceutical Corporation v. Weinberger, 412 U.S. 655, 1973.
25. Casper W. Weinberger, Secretary of Health, Education & Welfare, et al. v. Hynson, Westcott & Dunning, Incorporated, 412 U.S. 609, 1973.
26. CIBA Corporation v. Weinberger, 412 U.S. 640, 1973.
27. United States v. Generix Drug Co., 103 S. Ct. 1298 (1983).
28. For example, for antacids, 21 CFR 331.1 et seq. (1983 ed.), and for antiflatulent products, 21 CFR 332.1 et seq. (1983 ed.).
29. " . . . alpha eucaine, barbituric acid, beta eucaine, bromal, cannabis, carbromal, chloral, coca, cocaine, codeine, heroin, marijuana, morphine, opium, paraldehyde, peyote, or sulfonmethane; or any chemical derivative of such substance, which derivative of such substance has been by the Secretary, after investigation, found to be, and by regulations designated as, habit forming . . . "
30. 21 CFR 131 and 130.102; recodified as 369 and 310.201 respectively.
31. 21 CFR 201.56.
32. Section 510 of the Act (21 USC 360).
33. Section 501(a)(2) of the Act, 21 USC 351(a)(2).
34. Current Good Manufacturing Practice Regulations appear at 21 CFR Parts 210 (general), 211 (finished pharmaceuticals), 229 (blood and allergenic products). Section 211.1 states:
(a) The criteria in §211.20–211.115, inclusive, shall apply in determining whether the methods used in, or the facilities or controls used for, the manufacture, processing, packing, or holding of a drug conform to or are operated or administered in conformity with current good manufacturing practice to assure that a drug meets the requirements of the act as to safety, and has the identity and strength, and meets the quality and purity characteristics, which it purports or is represented to possess, as required by Section 501(a)(2)(B) of the act.
(b) The regulations in this part permit the use of precision automatic mechanical or electronic equipment in the production and control of drugs when adequate inspection and checking procedures are used to assure proper performance.
35. Section 704 21 USC 374 of the Act gives FDA the right for purposes of enforcing the Act, upon the presentation by the Inspector of appropriate credentials and a written notice to the owner, operator or agent in charge, the authority to enter at reasonable time, and to inspect at reasonable times and within reasonable limits and in a reasonable manner, any factory warehouse or establishment in which drugs are manufactured, processed, packed, or held for introduction into interstate commerce, or after such introduction, or to enter any vehicle being used to transport or haul such drug in interstate commerce. This Section does not apply to pharmacies which operate under applicable local laws and practitioners licensed by law to prescribe or administer drugs.
36. 21 CFR 1.106(b)(3).
37. Section 304 of the Act, 21 USC §334.
38. Section 302 of the Act, 21 USC §332.
39. Section 303 of the Act, 21 USC §333.
40. 21 USC 335.
41. Section 701(c) of the Act (21 USC 371 (c)) and regulations promulgated thereunder 21 CFR Part 12.

Index

Page numbers in *italics* refer to illustrations; page numbers followed by a t refer to tables; page numbers followed by an n refer to notes.

structure factors affecting suspension formulation, 486–487
Crystal bridging, in suspensions, 484
Crystallinity, consolidation of powders and, 73–74
  preformulation research on, 176–180, *177, 178,* 178t, *179, 180*
Curve stripping, 202
Cutting mill(s), *37,* 37t, 41–42
Cyclone product, 61

D value, 620–621, *620*
  in preservative efficacy testing, 553–554
Dalton's law, 591
Deaeration, in soft capsule manufacture, 406
  See also *Aeration*
Debye length, 111
Decompression, in tabletting, 83–85, *84*
Deficit plot, 199, *199*
Defoamer(s), in emulsion formation, 512
Deformation of solids, 71, *71, 72*
  elastic, *72, 72*
  plastic, 72–73, *72*
Degradation, general acid-base catalysis of, 768–769, *769*
  ionic strength and, 769–770, *769, 770*
  order of reaction and, 761–764
  pathways of, 772–786
  pH and, 764, *764, 765*
  temperature and, 765–768, *766, 767,* 767t, *768*
Degree(s) of freedom, 247
Demulsification, 529, 793–794, *793*
Density, of aerosols, measurement of, 616
  of powders, 70–71
  of tablet granules, 315–316
  preformulation measurements of, 183, *183*
Dental cone(s), 333–334
Depot formulation(s), 654
Dermis, *535, 536*
Desensitizing agent(s), in flavoring liquid pharmaceuticals, 470
Desorption, 120–121
Device(s), for sterile products, 651
Dew point, 49
Dextrose, as tablet diluent, 327
Diametric compression test of tablet strength, 297
Diatomite, as filter aid, 150, 151t
Dielectric constant, solubility and, 461–462
Differential scanning calorimetry, solid characterization by, 179–180, *179, 180*
Differential thermal analysis, solid characterization by, 179–180
Diffuse double-layer theory, 111, *111,* 112t, 506–507, *506*
Diffusion, Fick's law and, 5, 221
  molecular, in fluid mixing, 5
  solids mixing by, 15–16
Diffusion testing, 158–159
Dilatant behavior, 125, *125, 127,* 128
Diluent(s), for capsule formulations, 389–392
  for tablets, 321t, 325–327
Dimensionless group(s), 12
Dimethylacetamide (DMA), as accelerant in semisolids, 539
  as cosolvent in liquid pharmaceuticals, 461
Dimethylformamide (DMF), as accelerant in semisolids, 539
Dimethylsulfoxide (DMSO), as accelerant in semisolids, 539

Dioctyl-phthalate test method, 738, *738*
Diosna mixer/granulator, 322–323, *323*
Dip coating, 372
Dip tube(s), for aerosols, 595
  quality control for, 613–614
Disc mill(s), 42
Disinfection, surface, 636, 659–660
Disintegrant(s), in tablets, 321t, 328
Disintegration, tablet excipients and, 329, *330*
Disintegration test, for enteric coated tablets, 331–332, 367
  for tablets, 301, *301*
Disperse system(s). See *Emulsion(s); Suspension(s)*
Dispersion method(s), of emulsification, heat and, 508–509
  of suspension formation, 488
Disposition, 197–204
  multicompartment model of, 204
  one-compartment model of, 198, *198*
  two-compartment model of, 202–204, *202*
Dissociation constant (pKa), determination of, in preformulation research, 185–186, *185*
  drug absorption and, 222
Dissolution, of soft capsules, 410
  preformulation research on, 189, *189, 190,* 190t
Dissolution testing, of suppositories, 587
  of tablets, 301–303, *303*
Distribution, 202–204, *202, 204*
Dixon Criteria for Testing an Extreme Mean, 257, 257t
Dosage form(s), design of, 169–289
  evaluation of, in product development, 234–239, *236,* 237t, 238t, *238,* 239t, 240t
  See also particular dosage forms
Dosage regimen(s), biopharmaceutic considerations in development of, 232–233, *232*
  for sustained release formulations, 439–440, *440*
Dosage replacement factor, in suppository formulation, 585
Dosator(s), on hard-shell capsule filling machines, instrumentation of, 95–97, *96, 97*
Dose dependence, in dosage form evaluation, 235, 236–237, *236,* 237t, *238*
Dowicil 200, as preservative in semisolids, 553
Driacoater system, *347, 348–349, 351*
Drop-weight method, 109
Drug(s), animal, new, 856–857, 862–863
  certification of, 863
  defined, 856
  generic, approval of, 862, 866
  "me-too," regulatory requirements for, 865–866
  new, 858–863
    applications, 860–862
    defined, 856
    investigational, 859–860
    1938 provisions on, 857
  over-the-counter, approval of, 861
    labeling requirements for, 867
    review of safety and efficacy of, 866–867
  prescription, 858
    labeling requirements for, 867–868
Drug complex(es). See *Complexation*
Drug Efficacy Study Implementation Review, 863–866
Drug Enforcement Agency, 872–873
Drug Listing Act (1972), 868–869
Drug Price Competition and Patent Term Restoration Act (1984), 862
Drug release test(s), in vivo response prediction from in vitro data, 449

Drug standard(s), 833–837, 834t, 835t, 836t, 837t
Dry-bulb temperature, 49
Dry-bulb thermometer, 50, 50
Dryer(s), classification of, 55, 56
  conveyor, 57
  flash, 62, 62
  fluidized-bed. See Fluidized-bed dryer(s)
  freeze, 63–64
  horizontal vibrating conveyor, 59–60, 60
  microwave, 64
  moving-bed, 55, 57–58
  pan, 58
  pneumatic, 55, 60–62
  spray. See Spray dryer(s)
  static-bed, 55–57
  tray, 55–57, 57
  truck, 55–57
  tunnel, 57
  turbo-tray, 57–58, 58
Drying, 47–65
  behavior of solids during, 52–55, 53
  definition of, 47
  flash, 62
  freeze. See Freeze drying
  in pilot plant operation, 690–692
  loss on, 52
  microwave, 64
  purpose of, 47
  rate of, method of determining, 52n
  specialized methods of, 62–64
  spray. See Spray drying
  theory of, 50–52
  unsaturated surface, 53
Durham-Humphrey Amendment (1951), 858
Dust collection, 736–739, 738. See also Ventilation
DVLO theory, 112–113
Dye(s). See Colorant(s)

Eccrine gland(s), 535, 536
Economic order quantity, 751–753, 752
Ejection force(s), in tabletting, 81
Electrolyte(s), particle aggregation and, 481–482, 482
Electrometric method(s), 848
Electron accelerator(s), sterilization by, 629–630, 629
Electrophoretic method, for emulsion shelf life
      assessment, 531
  for suspension stability evaluation, 494
Electrostatic charge. See Surface charge
Electrostatic coating, 372
Elimination, 198–202
  capacity limitations on, 216–218
  defined, 197
  effects of disease on, 218–220
  factors affecting, 208–220
  presystemic, 223–225
Elimination rate constant, 198
Embedded matrix concept, sustained release
      formulations using, 442–444, 443, 445, 452
Emulsifiable concentrate(s), 512
Emulsification, 508–510
  descriptive theory of, 504–508, 505, 506
  low-energy, 510, 559–560, 562
  mechanical equipment for, 510–512, 511
  spontaneous, 511–512
Emulsifier(s), auxiliary, 518–519
  choice of, in emulsion formulation, 513
  defined, 502
  in cocoa butter suppositories, 576
  in semisolids, 541–543

mixed, 505, 505
  HLB value determination for, 516
  in semisolids, 542
Emulsion(s), 502–533
  aerosols using, 604–605
  applications and utility of, 503–504
  basic chemical principles related to, 100–122
  clear. See Microemulsion(s)
  defined, 502
  external (continuous) phase of, 502
  filling equipment for, 668
  formulation of, 512–526
    phase ratio in, 513
    practical examples, 523–526
  internal (disperse, discontinuous) phase of, 502
  inversion of, 502, 509
  lipid phase ingredients for, 513, 513t
  micellar, 503
  multiple, 502–503
    formation of, 519
  parenteral, 523, 655
  production aspects of, 512
  safety of, 512
  scale-up considerations with, 704–705
  semisolid, manufacture of, 555–560, 560, 561, 562
  shelf life assessment for, 527–532, 530
  sources of microbial contamination in, 520
  stability of, 526–527
    chemical, 512, 529
    kinetic vs. thermodynamic, 100–101, 526
    physical, 529–531, 791–794, 792, 793, 794, 795
  symptoms of instability in, 526–527
  types of, 507, 508t
  viscosity of, 519
    shelf life and, 529–531, 530
Encapsulation. See Capsule(s); Microencapsulation
End-folded wrapper(s), 724–725, 725
Enteric coating(s), 331–332, 366–368
Epidermis, 535–536, 535
Epinephrine, degradation of, 784, 784
Epoxy resin, for aerosol container coating, 607
Equilibrium moisture content, 54, 54
Equilibrium relative humidity, 54–55
Equilibrium solubility, crystal growth and, 116–117, 117t
Equipment, calibration of, 813, 813t
  for sterile products processing, cleaning of, 664, 666
  quality control procedures for, 812–813, 813t, 829–830
  selection of, in pilot plant operation, 684
  See also particular types of equipment and under
      particular dosage forms and processes
Error sum of squares, 273
Erweka KEA dedusting and polishing machine, 394–395, 395
Erweka tester, 298
Ester hydrolysis, 772–777
  prevention of, 774–777
Estradiol, preparation of suspension of, 488
Ethanol, in aerosols, reactions with aluminum
      containers, 607
  in water-based aerosols, 600
Ethylcellulose, as granulating agent, 328
  in film coating, 365
Ethylene oxide, sterilization with, 551, 551t, 634–635, 634t
Eutectic point, 64
Excipient(s), for capsule formulations, 389–392
  for sterile products, 642–644, 642t–643t

Fluidity, 124
Fluidized-bed coater(s), 350–351, 352, 360–361
Fluidized-bed dryer(s), 55, 58–60, 59, 60
  scale-up considerations with, 691–692
Fluidized-bed granulator-dryer, 59, 59
Fluidized-bed spray granulator(s), 339–340, 339
Fluorocarbon(s), as aerosol propellants, 589–590, 590t, 592
  limitations on use of, 606, 607
Foam(s), aerosols dispensed as, 604–605
  actuators for, 596, 598, 599
  testing for stability, 616–617
Foam depressant(s), in emulsion formation, 512
Foaming, in emulsion formation, 512
Food and Drug Administration (FDA), 870–874
  enforcement powers of, 871–872
  packaging regulations of, 731–732
  stability testing requirements of, 760, 802
Food, Drug and Cosmetic Act (1938), history of, 857–858
Food, Drug and Cosmetic Bill, state, 873
Force-displacement curve(s), 86, 86
Form/fill/seal system, 728–729, 729
Forward flow test, 159
Fragrance(s). See Perfume(s)
Freedom of Information Act, 873
Freeze drying, 62–64, 63, 672–673
  formulations for, 653
Freeze-thaw cycling technique, for suspension stability evaluation, 494
Freundlich equation, 120
Friabilator, 88, 299, 299
Friability, of granules, 316
  of tablets, 88, 299
Friction, effects of, in powder compaction, 79
Friedman's two-way analysis, 287–288
Froude number, 12
Fusion bonding, 73
Fusion process, for anhydrous ointment manufacture, 555
Fusion welding, 73

Gamma ray(s), sterilization by, 629–630
Gas(es), inert, in sterile solutions, 653
Gaseous filtration flow rate formula, 153
Gastrointestinal tract, presystemic metabolism in, 223–224
Gel(s), 534, 548
  scale-up considerations with, 705–706
Gel strength of gelatin, 400
Gelatin, as granulating agent, 327
  for hard capsules, 374–375
    manufacture of, 375
  for soft capsules, 400–401, 400t, 401t
    manufacture of, 406
  glycerinated, as suppository base, 577, 583
Gelsiccation. See Freeze drying
Germall II, in semisolids, 552–553
Gibbs equation, 103–104
Glass, 645–649, 646t–647t, 648t, 711–712. See also under Container(s)
  advantages of, 711
  alkali release by 796, 796t
  amber, 649, 712
    light protection by, 797–798, 798, 798t
  borosilicate, 646t–647t, 712
  chemical resistance of, 648, 712
  colored, 712
  composition of, 711

"flint," 491
  light transmission by, 797–798, 798, 798t
  insoluble flake formation and, 796–797, 797t, 797
  manufacture of, 711–712
  soda-lime, 646t–647t, 712
  stability and, 796–798
  types and test limits for, 648t, 796t
Glatt coater, 349, 351
Glidant(s), 79
  in tablets, 321t, 328
Glomerular filtration, 209
Glomerular filtration rate, 209
Glomerulus, 209
Glucose, liquid, as granulating agent, 327
  in liquid pharmaceuticals, 469
Glycerin, as suppository base, 577
Glycerinated gelatin, as suppository base, 577, 583
Glycerine, in semisolids, 544
Good Manufacturing Practices (GMP), 733, 869–870
  in pilot plant operation, 686
  quality control and, 829–833
Gral mixer/granulator, 323–324, 325
Granulation, 76–78, 317–324. See also Tablet granulation(s)
  compression, 318–320, 319
    scale-up considerations with, 698, 698
  dry, 317–320, 318t
    common tablet ingredients in formulas for, 344
    scale-up considerations with, 697–698, 698
  dust collection specifications for, 739
  facilities for, 741, 741
  scale-up considerations with, 687–690, 688, 689, 690, 691, 692, 693
  stability during, preformulation research on, 194
  wet, 76–77, 76, 77, 320–324
    common tablet ingredients in formulas for, 343
    scale-up considerations with, 687–688
    state-of-the-art processing, 338
Granulator(s), 322–324, 323, 324, 325, 341–342, 341, 342
  fluid bed spray, 339–340, 339
  oscillating, 693, 694
Granulator-dryer, fluidized-bed, 59, 59
Granule(s), density of, 315–316
  encapsulated slow release, 451–452
  properties of, affecting tabletting, 77, 87–88, 87
  strength of, 77–78, 316
Gravimetric filling, 476
Gravimetric method for measuring humidity, 50
Gravity filler, for liquids, 668
Gravity nutzch, 159–160
Griffith theory of cracks and flaws, 30
Grinding. See Milling
Grossing syrup(s), 356
Gum(s), as auxiliary emulsifiers, 518, 518t, 523

Hair follicle(s), 535, 536
Hammer mill(s), 37t, 37, 38–40, 38, 39, 693–694, 695
Hard butter, manufacture of, 576
Hardness of tablets, 297–299
  variation in, 314
Hartnett capsule imprinting machine, 395, 397
Heat, in emulsion formation, 508–509
Heat of activation, 192, 765
Heat of solution, 187–188, 188
Heckel plot(s), 82–83, 83
Helical flight mixer(s), 17
Helipath, in emulsion shelf life assessment, 530, 531
Helium pycnometer, 69–70, 70

Hepatic clearance, 200, 212–214, *213*
Hepatic dysfunction, drug elimination and, 220, 220t
Hepatic extraction ratio, 212–213, *213*
Hi-Coater system, 347, 348, *351*
Hildebrand's solubility parameter, 461
Histogram, data display using, 250, *250*
HLB temperature. See *Phase inversion temperature*
HLB value, 514–517, 515t, 516t
Höfliger and Karg capsule filling equipment, 380, *381, 382, 383*
Hofmeister series, 113, 482
Hole theory, 152
Homogenizer(s), for emulsion formation, 510–511, *511, 512*
  for semisolid manufacture, 560–561
  rotor-stator. See *Colloid mill(s)*
Honey, in liquid pharmaceuticals, 469
Hopper flow rate(s), 317
Humectant(s), in semisolids, 544
Humidity, 48–50
  absolute, 49
  encapsulation and, 703
  measurement of, 50
  relative, 49
    equilibrium, 54–55
  saturation, 49
Humidity chart, 48–50, *48*
Hydrate(s), 177–178, *177*
Hydrocarbon(s), as aerosol propellants, 589, 590, 590t, *593*, 606–607
  standards for glass containers, 599–600
  in semisolids, 540, 544
Hydrocarbon wax(es), in semisolids, 540
Hydrochlorothiazide, stability studies on, 779, *779*
Hydrocolloid(s), as emulsifiers, 518–519, 518t
Hydrocortisone, degradation of, 785, *785*
Hydrogenation, in suppository base manufacture, 576
Hydrolysis, drug degradation by, 772–779
Hydrophilic material(s), 480, 481
  increasing wettability by use of, 480
Hydrophilic-Lipophilic Balance, 514–517, 515t, 516t
Hydrophobic material(s), 480, 481
Hydrotrophy, solubility and, 466
Hydroxyl value, of suppository bases, 569
Hydroxymethylcellulose, in sustained release matrix tablets, 454
Hydroxypropyl cellulose, as granulating agent, 327–328
  in film coating, 365
Hydroxypropyl methylcellulose, as granulating agent, 327
  in film coating, 365
  in formulation of dispersed suspensions, 490
Hydroxypropyl methylcellulose phthalate, in film coating, 368
Hygrometer(s), 50
Hygroscopicity, of suppositories, 583
  preformulation research on, 181–182
Hynson, Westcott, & Dunning decision, 866
Hypothesis, null, 251
Hypothesis testing, 251–255
  of binomial data, 260–261

Identification marking(s), on hard capsules, 395, *397*
  on tablets, 296–297
Identification system(s), 853
Identity, standards of, 833–834, 834t
Immersion-sword system, 348, *350*
Immersion-tube system, 348, *350*
Impeller(s), for fluid mixing, 6–7, *7*

Incomplete block design, 278
Independence, in statistics, 245
Indomethacin, biliary clearance of, 214–215, 215t
Inhaler(s), metered-dose, 596–597
Injunction, 871
Inspection(s), FDA, 869–871
  penalties for interfering with, 872
Inspissation, 626–627
Institutional Review Board(s), 860
Instrumentation, of hard-shell capsule filling machines, 95–97, *96, 97*
  of tablet machines, 89–95, *94*
Insulin, certification of, 863
  preparation of suspension of, 488
Integrity testing, of filtration systems, 157–159, 633
Interesterification, in suppository base manufacture, 576
Interface(s), in emulsions and suspensions, 100, *101*
  of powder with air, 66–67, *66*
  solid-liquid, adsorption at, 119–121, *119*
Interfacial film(s), 107–108, *107, 108*, 504–506, *505, 506*
Interfacial tension, in emulsions, 504
  See also *Surface tension*
Interference, in patent law, 875
Interparticle force(s), between surfaces, 111–113, *112, 113, 114*, 507
Intestinal flora, drug absorption and, 223
Intrinsic reaction velocity, 212
Inventory(-ies), 747
  ABC classification of, 748, *748*
  conversion of, to months of supply, 749, 749t
  management of, 747–748
    systems for, 753–755
  reporting and analysis of, 749, 749t
Inversion, of emulsions, 502, 509
Iodine value, of suppository bases, 569, 575
Ion(s), potential determining, 110
Ion-exchange resin(s), for purified water system, 473
Ion-exchange resin complex(es), sustained release formulations using, 450–451
Ionic strength, drug degradation and, 769–770, *769, 770*
Ionizing radiation(s), sterilization by, 629–630, *629*
Iron, in soft gelatin capsules, 400
Irrigating solution(s), standards for, 639
Isoelectric point, 110
Isotonicity, in parenteral preparations, 644, 655

Jelly(-ies), as bases for semisolids, 548

Kaolin, in suspensions, preservative interaction with, 491
Kefauver-Harris Amendments (1962), 858–870
Kelvin element, 139, *139*
Kelvin equation, 103
Kick's equation, 31
Kidney(s), physiology of, 209–211
Kneading mixer(s), 11, *11*
Know-how, 874, 880

Labeling, defined, 856
  equipment for, 745–746
  of sterile products, 676
  quality control of, 814
  requirements for, 867–868
    state laws, 876t–877t
Labor, costs of, 758–759, 758t
Lactose, as tablet diluent, 326

coating materials for, 415–416, *415*, 416t
core materials for, 414, 414t
equipment and processing for, 419
fundamental considerations in, 414–419
methodology of, 419–428, 419t
problems of, 413
release properties and, 417–419, *418*
stability enhancement by, 416–417, *417*
sustained-release formulations using, 417–419, *418*
Microfiltration, 166
Microindentation test(s), 88
Micromelting range test, for suppository bases, 586
Micronizer(s), 37, 37t, 41
Microscopy, fine particle characterization using, 182–183
   particle size distribution measurement by, 26–27
   solid characterization by, 178–179
Microsquashing, 72
Microwave drying, 64
Mill(s), attrition, 37t
ball, 40–41
colloid. See *Colloid mill(s)*
cutting, 37, 37t, 41–42
disc, 42
fluid-energy, 37, 37t, 41
hammer, 37t, *37*, 38–40, *38*, *39*, 693–694, *695*
pebble, 40
revolving, 37t
rod, 40
roller, 11, *11*, 37, 37t, 42
selection of, 43, 44t, 45t
tube, 40
types of, 37–42, *37*, 37t
Milling, 21–46
closed-circuit, 38
dry, 45
energy use in, 30, 31
equipment for. See *Mill(s)*
factors influencing, 42–43
open-circuit, 38
pharmaceutical applications of, 21–22
rate of, 36–37
scale-up considerations with, 692–695
techniques of, 43–45
wet, 45
See also *Comminution*
Mineral oil, as lubricant, 328
   in semisolids, 540
Minim per gram factor, 404, 405t
Minimum threshold level, 471
Misbranding, 853
Mixer(s), granulating, 321–324, *322*, *323*, *324*, *325*
   scale-up considerations with, 687–688, *688*, *689*, *690*, *691*, *692*
helical flight, 17
kneading, 11, *11*
mathematical analysis of operation of, 11–13
mulling, 11
planetary, *689*
rheologic measurements and, 144
ribbon blender, 17, *18*
selection of, for fluid mixing, 10–13
   for solids mixing, 18–19
sigma blade, *688*
tumbling, for solids, 17–18, *17*
twin shell, *17*, *690*
Mixer-dryer processer, double-cone, 340, *340*
Mixer-granulator(s), See *Mixer(s), granulating*

Mixing, 3–20
batch, of fluids, 6–8
   of solids, 17–18
continuous, of fluids, 8–9, *8*, *9*
   of solids, 18
convective, of solids, 15
diffusive, of solids, 15–16
equipment for. See *Mixer(s)*
inadequate, tablet weight variation from, 314
measures of degree of, 18–19
of fluids, 3–13
   equipment for, 6–13
   fundamentals of, 3–6
   time dependence of mechanisms in, 5–6, *6*
of solids, 13–19
   equipment for, 17–19
   fundamentals of, 13–17
   power requirements for, 19
   scale-up considerations with, 687, 695–696, 697
   segregation mechanisms in, 16–17, 19
   surface charges in, 16
polyphase, equipment for, 10–11
shear, of solids, 15
Moisture content, 52
critical, 53
equilibrium, 54, *54*
in powder compaction, 75–76, *75*
Molasses, in liquid pharmaceuticals, 469
Mold release agent(s), in suppository manufacture, 584–585
Molding of suppositories, in-package, 582
methods of, 580–581, *581*
scale-up considerations with, 708–709
Monadic test(s), 265–267, *266*
Monosodium glutamate, in flavoring liquid pharmaceuticals, 470
Monsanto hardness tester, 297
Mottling. See *Color, variation in*
Moving-bed dryer(s), 55, 57–58
Mulling mixer(s), 11
Multiorifice-centrifugal process, microencapsulation by, 419t, 425–426, *425*

Narcotics, regulations on, 872–873
Nauta mixer-processor, 340–341, *341*
Negligence, product liability and, 881
Nephelometer, filtration effectiveness assessment with, 154, *154*
Nephron(s), 209
Nernst equation, 780–781
New drug(s). See under *Drug(s)*
New Drug Application(s), 860–862
Nitrile polymer(s), 715, 718t–719t
Nonisothermal kinetic method, 768
Normal curve, standard, 248, 248t
Normal distribution, 246–250, *246*, *247*, *248*, 248t, *249*, *250*, 816–817, *816*, *817*, 817t
Noyes-Whitney equation, 189, 221
Null hypothesis, 251
Nutzch, gravity, 159–160
Nylon, 714, 720–721t

Ointment(s), 534
anhydrous, fusion process for manufacture of, 555
greaseless, bases for, 548
ophthalmic, bases for, 548
scale-up considerations with, 705–706
white, as semisolid base, 544

for emulsions, 704–705
for liquid dosage forms, 703
for semisolids, 705–706
for solid dosage forms, 687–703
for suppositories, 706–709
for suspensions, 703–704
personnel requirements for, 682
preparation of master manufacturing procedures in, 685–686
process evaluation in, 684–685
quality assurance in, 686
reporting responsibilities in, 681–682
space requirements for, 682–683
Pipet method, for particle size distribution measurement, 28–29, 28, 29t
pKa. See Dissociation constant
Planetary mixer(s), 689
Plasma clearance, 200–201
Plasma half-life, 198, 198
approach to steady state and, 206, 206
biliary recycling and, 215–216
Plasma renal clearance rate. See Renal clearance
Plastic(s), 645, 646t–647t, 712–716, 718t–719t, 720t–721t. See also under Container(s)
additives in, 645, 646t–647t, 712–713
advantages of, 645, 712
collapsible tubes of, 717
tamper-resistant seals for, 730
drug-plastic considerations, 715–716, 798–800, 799, 800t
thermoplastic, 645, 646t–647t
for closures, 723
thermosetting, for closures, 723
types of, 645, 646t–647t, 713–715, 718t–719t, 720t–721t
Plastic closure(s), 723
Plastic component(s), for sterile products, cleaning of, 665–666
Plasticizer(s), in film coating, 368–369
in gelatin soft capsules, 400
Plastoelasticity, 83
Plate process for soft capsule manufacture, 398
Plug flow, 127, 143, 143
Plug strength tester, 75
Pneumatic dryer(s), 55, 60–62
Pohlman liquid whistle, 511, 511
Point of zero charge, 110, 110
Poiseuille's equation, 131
Poisson ratio, 80, 84
Polishing, of coated tablets, 356, 356, 358
facilities for, 743, 744
of solutions, 667
Polyacrylic acid, in formulation of dispersed suspensions, 490
Polyamide. See Nylon
Polycarbonate, 714–715, 720t–721t
Polyethylene, 713, 718t–719t, 720t–721t
collapsible tubes of, 717
Polyethylene glycol(s), as lubricant, 328
as suppository base, 577–578, 578t, 583–584
in film coating, 366
in semisolids, 544, 547–548
Polyethylene terephthalate (PET), 715
Polyethylene-polypropylene, 645
Polymer(s), acrylate, in film coating, 366, 368
carboxyl vinyl, as auxiliary emulsifiers, 518
in sustained release matrix tablets, 453–454, 453t
nitrile, 715, 718t–719t

Polymerization, microencapsulation by, 427–428
sustained release capsules using, 452
Polymorphism, preformulation studies of, 178, 178, 180–181, 181, 230–231
suspension stability and, 487
Polyol(s), in semisolids, 544
Polyolefin(s), 645
Polypropylene, 645, 713, 718t–719t, 720t–721t
for film wrapping, 724
Polystyrene, 714, 718t–719t, 720t–721t
Polyvinyl acetate phthalate, in film coating, 368
Polyvinyl chloride (PVC), 713–714, 718t–719t, 720t–721t
blister packs of, 727
Polyvinylpyrrolidone, as granulating agent, 328
Porcelain candle(s), sterile filtration with, 155–156
Porosity, 69
applied force and, in tabletting, 81–83, 82, 83
Potency, standards of, 836–837, 836t, 837t
Pouch(es), 728–729, 729
Povidone, in film coating, 365–366
Powder(s), angle of repose of, 67, 68, 317
compression and consolidation of. See Compaction of powders
effect of applied forces on, 71–76, 71
electrostatic forces in, 16, 67
flow properties of, preformulation research on, 183–184, 184t
flow rates of, 67, 69, 183–184
free surface energy of, 66, 66
granulation of. See Granulation
insoluble, in semisolids, 544
interface of, with air, 66–67, 66
mass-volume relationships of, 68–71
volume of, measurement of, 69–70, 70
wetting of, 117–119, 117, 118, 118t, 480–481
See also Particle(s); Solid(s)
Powdered glass test, 648, 712
Power, of statistical tests, 265
Power Law Equation, 125–126
Power number, 12
Powr Flo system, 607
Precautions, on package inserts, 868
Precipitation method(s), of suspension formation, 487–488
Precision, 846–847, 847t
Precoating technique, 151
Prednisolone, degradation of, 781–782, 781t, 782, 785, 785
precipitation of, 487
Preemption, 873
Prefilter(s), 153–154, 153, 154, 154t
Preformulation, 171–196, 172, 173, 176
biopharmaceutics in, 229–231
bulk characterization in, 176–184
molecular optimization in, 171–176
reporting of findings, 194–195
Prescription drug(s). See under Drug(s)
Preservative(s), for emulsions, 520–522, 521t, 522t
for liquids, 466–468, 467t
for semisolids, 549–554
testing of, 550, 550t, 553–554, 554
for suspensions, 491
inactivation of, 491. See also under Paraben(s)
solubilities of, 552, 553t
Press(es), See Tablet press(es)
Pressure filling of aerosols, 610, 610, 612–613
Pressure pump filler, for liquids, 668

Preval system, 608, *609*
Privity doctrine, 881
Probability distributions, 246–250, 246t, *246, 247, 248,*
    248t, *249, 250*
Probenecid, antibiotics with, 234
    renal transport and, 210
Procainamide, sustained release formulation design,
    433–437, 435t, *436*
Prodrug(s), 172–175, *173, 176,* 223
    in sustained release formulations, *441,* 442
Product development, biopharmaceutics and
        pharmacokinetics in, 226–239
    design variables in, 231–234
    See also particular dosage forms
Product liability, 881
Production management, 733–759
Promulgen(s), 543
Propellant(s), for aerosols, 589–591, 590t, *592, 593*
        identification of, in product testing, 616
        quality control for, 613
        selection of, 606–607
        stability testing of, 609
Propeller(s), for fluid mixing, 6–7
    side-entering, 8
Propiolactone, sterilization by, 635–636
Propylene glycol, in semisolids, 544
Pseudoplastic behavior, 125, *125,* 127, *127*
Psychrometer, sling, 50, *50*
Psychrometric chart, 48–50, *48*
Psychrometry, 47–50
Pump(s), positive displacement, for semisolid product
        transfer, 706, *707*
Purchase price variance report, 756, 757t
Purger, for aerosols, 611–612
Purity, standards of, 834–836, 834t, 835t, 837t
Pycnometer, helium, 69–70, *70*
Pyrogen(s), source and elimination of contamination
        with, 641
Pyrogen testing, 674–675, *675,* 844–845

Qualification, 832
Quality, standards of, 834, 834t
Quality control, 804–855. See also particular dosage
        forms and processes
    charts for, 817–824, *819, 820, 821, 822, 823*
    costs of, 759
    in pilot plant operation, 686
    in-process, 810–814, 830–832
    of finished products, 814–815, 833–854
    of raw materials, 804–810, 805t, 806t, 812, 839,
        839t, 840t
    statistical, 815–824
    testing program and method for, 840–845

R value, 80
Rabbit pyrogen assay, 674, 675, 844
Racemization, drug degradation by, 786
Radiation(s), ionizing, sterilization by, 629–630, *629*
    ultraviolet. See *Ultraviolet light*
Rancidity, 782
    of suppositories, 585
Random model, 272, 274–275
Randomized block(s), 273–274
Range, 250, 816–817
Raoult's law, 591
"Rat-holding," 314, *314*
Reaction(s), complex, 770–772
    consecutive, 771

first-order, 762–763, *762, 763*
opposing (reversible), 770–771
order of, drug degradation and, 761–764
pseudo-first-order, 763–764, *764*
pseudo-zero-order, 761–762
second-order, 771
side, 771–772
zero-order, 761–762, *761, 762*
Reaction velocity constant, 763
Recall(s), 854, 863
Reciprocating die process for soft capsule manufacture,
    399
Reconciliation, of liquid product yield, 745
    of tablet yield, 742, *743*
Reconstitution, 62
Record(s), maintenance, storage and retrieval of, 853–
        854
    product distribution, 853
    quality control of, 830
Redispersibility, evaluation of, in suspension stability
        tests, 493
Re-esterification, in suppository base manufacture, 576–
        577
Reference standard(s), for quality control tests, 842,
        845
Registration of trademarks, 874, 879
Regression, in data analysis, 278–283
    simple linear, 278–279
    weighting in, 282
Regulation(s), 856–882. See also *Food and Drug
        Administration*
    definitions relating to, 856–857
    state and local, 873–874
Renal clearance, 199–200, *199, 200,* 201
    calculation of, 210–211
    experimental techniques using, 211
Renal excretion, experimental techniques for study of,
        211
    mechanisms of, 209–211
Renal impairment, drug elimination and, 219–220,
        219, 219t
Renal tubule(s), 209
    carrier-mediated transport across, 210–211
    passive transport across, 209–210
Replacement factor, for suppositories, 585
Repose angle, 67, *68,* 317
Reservoir aerosol-type delivery system, 597
Return of goods, 854
Reverse osmosis system, for preparing Water for
        Injection, 664
Revolving mill(s), 37t
Reynolds number, 12
Rheology, 123–145
    aging effects in, 130–131, *130*
    artifactual observations in, from plug flow or slippage
        planes, 143
    definitions and fundamental concepts in, 123–126
    graphic presentation of data in, 128–131
    properties influencing behavior in, 126–128
    specialized pharmaceutical applications of, 140–144
    types of instruments used in, 131–139
Rheometer(s), extrusion, 133–134, *133*
Rheopexy, *127,* 128
Ribbon blender, 17, *18*
Ring alteration, hydrolysis by, 779
Ring-detachment method, 109–110
Rinser(s), for new containers, 665, *665, 666*
Rittinger's equation, 31–32

Solid(s), amorphous (*Continued*)
    microscopic appearance of, 178
    analytic methods for characterization of, 178–180,
        178t
    classification of, based on drying behavior, 53–54
    drying of, 52–55, 53
    effect of applied forces on, 71, 71
    finely divided, as emulsifiers, 518
    in soft capsules, 403–406, 405t
    mixing of, 13–19
        batch, 17–18
        continuous, 18
        equipment for, 17–19
        fundamentals of, 13–17
    sterile, filling equipment for, 668–669, 669, 670
    stress-strain curve for, 29–30, 29
    See also *Particle(s); Powder(s)*
Solid-fat index, 569, 569
Solidification point, of suppository bases, 569
Solubility, drug absorption and, 221
    equilibrium, crystal growth and, 116–117, 117t
    in liquid pharmaceutical formulation, 457–466
    of hard capsules, treatments affecting, 395–396
    pH and, 186–187, 187, 458–460, 459, 460
    preformulation studies of, 184–189, 229–230
Solubility analysis technique, 464–465, 465
Solubilization, in liquid pharmaceutical formulation,
        462–464, 464
    preformulation research on, 188, 188
Solubilizing agent(s), 463t
Solution(s), aerosol systems using, 597–600
    "regular," 461
    reverse micellar, 508
    sterile. See *Sterile product(s)*
    See also *Liquid(s)*
Solvate(s), 177–178, 177
Solvent(s), in film coating, 368
        safety considerations with, 354
    in granulation, safety considerations with, 689–690
Solvent evaporation, microencapsulation by, 419t, 427
Solvent extraction method(s), 848–849
Sorbitol, as tablet diluent, 327
    in semisolids, 544
    paraben binding and, 465, 466
Sorption, by plastic containers, 716, 799–800, 800t
Soudronic system, for welding aerosol containers, 592
Specific reaction rate, 763
Specific surface, 21
Specifications, 833–840
    for new products, 837–838
    for well-established products, 838
    official, 838–840, 839t
Specificity, 845–846
Spectrophotometric method(s), 849
Spore(s), resistance of, to sterilization processes, 619,
        620t
Spray congealing, 62
    microencapsulation by, 419t, 426, 427
Spray dryer(s), 60–61, 61
    wet granulation using, 338–339
Spray drying, 61–62
    microencapsulation by, 419t, 426–427
Spread, measures of. See *Range; Standard deviation*
Stability, drug absorption and, 223
    enhancement of, by microencapsulation, 416–417,
        417
    of aerosols, 608–610
    of coated tablets, 370–371

of emulsions, 526–527
    chemical, 512
    kinetic, 526
of hard capsules, 392
of liquid pharmaceuticals, 471–473
of soft gelatin capsules, 404–406, 408–410, 408
of suppositories, testing of, 583
    typical problems of, 587–588
of suspension aerosols, 603–604
of suspensions, 794–795, 794, 795
    crystal factors in, 486–487
    evaluation of, 492–495
    kinetic vs. thermodynamic, 100–101
    yield value and, 142–143, 142
of sustained release formulations, 448
of tablets, 790–791, 790t, 790, 791t, 791
of toxicology formulations, 190–191
    packaging components and, 795–802
    physical, 798–795
    preformulation analysis of, 190–194, 191t, 192, 193t
    testing, 760–803, 851–853, 852t
        analytic methods for, 848–849
        chemical, 786–788, 786t, 786, 787t
        FDA requirements for, 760, 802
        fitting lines to data from, 279–282, 279t, 280
        high pressure liquid chromatography in, 789, 849,
            849t
        theoretic considerations in, 761–772
    thermal, statistical techniques in prediction of, 788–
        789, 788t, 789
Stability-indicating method(s), 849
Stainless steel, 703
    aerosol containers of, 594, 600t
Standard deviation, 247, 816–817, 817t
Starch, as disintegrant, 328
    as granulating agent, 327
    as tablet diluent, 326–327
Static-bed dryer(s), 55–57
Statistical inventory control, 753–754, 754t, 755
Statistical significance. See *Significance*
Statistics, 243–289
    descriptive, 244
    in quality control, 815–824
    inference and estimation using, 250–263
    introductory concepts in, 244–250
    nonparametric, 285–288
Steady state, 206–208, 206, 207, 208
Stearic acid, as lubricant, 328
    in semisolids, 541
Stearyl alcohol, in semisolids, 541
Sterile product(s), 639–677
    additives in, 652–653
    compounding, 667
    development of, 639–656
    devices for, 651
    filling procedures for, 667–669, 668, 669, 670
    filtration of, 667
    formulation of, 652–656
        route of administration and, 639–640, 655–656
    packaging of, 675–676
    production of, 656–673, 657
        automated, 669, 670, 671–672
        environmental control in, 658–661, 662t–663t
        facilities for, 657–663, 659
        personnel for, 661–663
        processing, 663–673
    quality control for, 656, 673–675, 675, 831
    sealing, 668, 670, 671

Suspension(s), formulation of (*Continued*)
    crystal structure factors in, 486–487
    illustrative examples, 495–500
    parenteral, 654–655
  in soft capsules, 403–404, 405t
  parenteral, bioavailability of, 500
    formulation of, 654–655
  particle interactions and behavior in, 481–484, *482, 483*
  preparative techniques for, 491–492
  scale-up considerations with, 703–704
  sedimentation rates of, 484–486
  stability of, 794–795, *794, 795*
    crystal factors in, 486–487
    evaluation of, 492–495
    kinetic vs. thermodynamic, 100–101
    yield value and, 142–143, *142*
  theoretic considerations with, 479–487
  wetting and, 480–481
  with high solids content, 497, 497t
  with low solids content, examples of formulations, 496–497, 496t
  with wetting and aggregating agents, examples of formulations, 495–496
Sustained release formulation(s), 430–456
  advantages of, 430–431
  controlled release technology for, 455–456, *455*
  design of, 233, 431–433, *433, 434*
    implementation of, 440–446
  disadvantages of, 431
  dosage form modification approaches to, 442–446
  drug availability measurement, in vitro, 446–448, *447*
    in vivo, 448–450, *449*
  drug modification approaches to, 440–442, *441*
  drugs unsuitable for, 431, 431t
  microencapsulation for, 417–419, *418*
  multiple dosing with, 439–440, *440*
  practical formulation of, 450–455
  product evaluation and testing of, 446–450
  theory of, 431–440
  with first-order release approximation, 437–439, 437t, 438t, *438*
  with zero-order release approximation, 433–437, 434t
Sweat gland(s), *535, 536*
Sweetening agent(s), in liquids, 468–469, *469*, 470t
  in tablets, 321t, 329
  testing of, 809–810
Synchrowax(es), 540
System-suitability test(s), 848

t distribution, 250–251, *251*
t test, 251–253, 252t
  independent two-sample, 254
  one-sided, 255
  one-sided vs. two-sided, 252, 259
  with paired samples, 254–255
Tablet(s), 293–345
  advantages of, 293–294
  buccal, 333
  capping of, 88–89, *88*, 311–312, 701
  challenges in design, formulation and manufacture of, 295
  chewable, 333
  chocolate-coated, 332
  coated, evaluation of, 363–364
    manufacture of. See *Tablet coating*
  compressed, 329–330

  multiple, 330–331
  compression of. See *Tabletting*
  delayed-action, 331–332
  depot (implantation), 334
  disadvantages of, 294
  disintegration of, 301, *301*
  dispensing, 335
  dissolution of, 301–303, *303*
  double impression on, 314
  drug content and release from, 299–303
  effervescent, 334–335
  enteric coated, 331–332, 366–368
  evaluation of, 296–303
  excipients for, 321t, 324–329, *330*
    future trends in, 336
  film-coated, 332–333. See also *Film coating*
  for oral ingestion, 329–333
  for preparing solutions, 334–336
  for use in oral cavity, 333–334
  future trends in, 336–342
  gastric retention, 337
  general appearance of, 296–299
  hardness and friability of, 297–299
    devices for testing, 297–298, *298, 299, 299*
  hypodermic, 335
  identification markings on, 296–297
  in-process quality control for, 831
  international considerations in formulation of, 329
  lamination of, 88–89, *88*, 311–312
  manufacture of, computer control of, 342
    improvements, 337–342, 338t
    See also particular processes
  matrix, for sustained release, 453–455, 453t
  mottling of, 297, 313
  of slow release granulations, 452
  organoleptic properties of, 297
  physical stability of, 790–791, 790t, *790*, 791t, *791*
  picking and sticking of, 312–313
  potency uniformity of, 300–301
  properties of, 295–296
    affecting coating, 347–348
  purity of, 301
  repeat-action, 331
  role of, in therapy, 293
  scale-up considerations with, 687–702
  size and shape of, 296
  strength of, 86–89
  sublingual, 333
  sugar-coated, 332. See also *Sugar coating*
  sustained release, 336–337, 442, 453–455, 453t
  types and classes of, 329–336, 331t
  vaginal, 334
  weight variation in, 300, 300t, 309–311, *311*, 313–314
Tablet coating, 346–373
  automation of, 354, *355*
  dust collection specifications for, 739
  equipment for, 348–352, *349, 350, 351, 352, 354*
  facilities for, 354, 742–743, *744*
  future trends in, 336, 372
  history of, 346
  parameters of, 352–354
  principles of, 346–354
  processes of, 354–362
  quality control in, 370
  scale-up considerations with, 701–702
  specialized, 372
  stability testing in, 370–371

tablet properties affecting, 347–348
  See also *Film coating; Sugar coating*
Tablet crushing strength. See *Hardness of tablets*
Tablet granulation(s), 314–317
  basic characteristics of, 314–315
  flow properties of, 316–317
    tablet weight variation from problems with, 313–314, *314*
  manufacture of. See *Granulation*
  properties of, 315–317
  slow release, 452
Tablet press(es), 303–306
  capabilities of, 700t
  counters for, 742, *743*
  eccentric, 79
  facilities for, 741–742, *742*
  instrumentation of, 89–95
    signal processing with, 94, *94*
  mechanized feeders for, 309, *310*
  multi-station rotary, 303–304, *305*, 306t, *307*
    instrumentation of, 92–93, *92, 93, 94*
  single-punch, 303, *304*
    instrumentation of, 90–92, *90, 91, 92*
  tooling for, 306–309, *308*
    problems related to, 312, 314
Tablet triturate(s), 335–336
Tabletting, 303–314
  decompression in, 83–85, *84*
  dust collection specifications for, 739
  ejection forces in, 81
  energy involved in, 85–86, 85t, *85*, 86t, *86*
  equipment for, auxiliary, 309–311
    See also *Tablet press(es)*
  facilities for, 741–742, *742*
  force-volume relationships in, 81–83, *82, 83*
  in-process quality control of, 311
  processing problems in, 311–314
  rheologic measurements and, 144
  scale-up considerations with, 699–701
Tackiness, measurement of, 143
Talc, as lubricant, 328
Tank(s), for liquid pharmaceutical manufacture, 474
Tape seal(s), 730
Taub's rule, 119, *119*
Technicon Autoanalyzer, 850
Temperature, adiabatic saturation, 50
  crystal growth and, 117
  drug degradation and, 765–768, *766, 767*, 767t, *768*
  dry-bulb, 49
  emulsion shelf life assessment and, 528
  filtration efficiency and, 152
  in semisolid production, scale-up considerations, 706
  in suppository manufacture, 708–709
  solubility and, in preformulation research, 187–188, *188*
  viscosity and, 152, 152t
  wet-bulb, 49–50
Test(s), biologic, 841–842, 842t, 843t
  in quality control, 840–845
    automated continuous system for, 850–851
    quality of analytic methods, 845–849
  microbiologic, 842–844, 842t, 843t, 844t
    automated, 851
  of bulk product, 814–815
  See also under *Stability;* particular test methods and parameters
Theobroma oil. See *Cocoa butter*
Theo-Dur (sustained-release theophylline), 336–337

Theophylline, blood levels from different dosage forms, 568, *568*
  sustained-release, 336–337
Thermal analysis, differential, solid characterization by, 179–180
Thermogravimetric analysis, solid characterization by, 179–180, *179*
Thermometer(s), dry-bulb, 50, *50*
  wet-bulb, 50, *50*
Thiamine hydrochloride tablet(s), ingredients for, 344
Thief, sampling using, 245
Thixotropy, 127–128, *127*, 480
Tin, collapsible tubes of, 717
  drug stability and, 800
Tinplate, aerosol containers of, 592, 600t, 607
Titralyzer, 850
Titrimetric method(s), 848
Tolbutamide, disposition of, in hepatic disease, 220, 220t
Tonicity, of parenteral preparations, 644, 655
Topo granulator, 341–342, *341*
Torque, 472–473, 722
Toxicity test(s), 845
Toxicology studies, preclinical, biopharmaceutic considerations in, 227
  stability in formulations for, 190–191
Trade name, 879
Trade secret(s), 874, 880
Trademark(s), 874, 879–880
Tragacanth, as granulating agent, 327
Transformation(s), in statistics, 278
Transient derivative(s), 776
Tray dryer(s), 55–57, *57*
Triangle test(s), of consumer acceptance, 267–268
Troche(s), 333
Truck dryer(s), 55–57
Tube(s), collapsible, 716–720
  metal, drug stability and, 800
  tamper-resistant seals for, 730–731
Tube mill(s), 40
Tukey's multiple range method, 272–273
Tumbling mixer(s), 17–18, *17*
Tunnel dryer(s), 57
Turbine(s), for fluid mixing, 7, *7*
Turbo-tray dryer(s), 57–58, *58*
Turbulent flow, in fluid mixing, 4
Turnover, 749
Twin shell mixer(s), *17, 690*
Tyler Standard Scale, 27, 27t
Tyndallization, 626–627

Ultrafiltration, membrane, 166–167, *167*
  membrane filters for, 149, 166–167
Ultrasonifier(s), in emulsion formation, 511, *511*
Ultraviolet light, sterilization using, 628–629, 628t
  surface disinfection using, 659–660
Unfair competition, 879
United States Standard Scale, 27, 27t
Urea, closures of, 723
Urinary excretion, 198–199, *199*
Urine, pH of, renal clearance of drugs and, 210

Vacuum crimper, for aerosols, 611–612
Vacuum filling, 476–477, *477*
  for sterile liquids, 668
Vacuum film coating, 372
Validation, 832–833